Encyclopedia of Medical Immunology

Ian R. MacKay • Noel R. Rose
Editors-in-Chief

Jordan Scott Orange • Javier Chinen
Editors

Encyclopedia of Medical Immunology

Immunodeficiency Diseases

With 73 Figures and 69 Tables

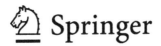 Springer

Editors-in-Chief

Ian R. MacKay
Department of Biochemistry
and Molecular Biology
Monash University
Clayton, Victoria, Australia

Noel R. Rose
Center for Autoimmune Disease Research
Department of Molecular Microbiology
and Immunology
Department of Pathology
Johns Hopkins University
Baltimore, MA, USA

Editors

Jordan Scott Orange
Department of Pediatrics
Columbia University Vagelos
College of Physicians and Surgeons
NewYork-Presbyterian Morgan
Stanley Children's Hospital
New York, NY, USA

Javier Chinen
Division of Allergy and Immunology
Department of Pediatrics
Baylor College of Medicine
Texas Children's Hospital
The Woodlands, TX, USA

ISBN 978-1-4614-8677-0   ISBN 978-1-4614-8678-7 (eBook)
ISBN 978-1-4614-8679-4 (print and electronic bundle)
https://doi.org/10.1007/978-1-4614-8678-7

This Springer imprint is published by the registered company Springer Science+Business Media, LLC, part of Springer Nature.
The registered company address is: 233 Spring Street, New York, NY 10013, U.S.A.

Introduction

The concept of an encyclopedia derives from the Greek words for gathering together or "encircling" knowledge and learning. Indeed, Diderot and the French encyclopedists of the mid eighteenth century aimed to bring together all of the world's knowledge in one giant publication. Our ambitions today are more modest but "encapsulating" existing knowledge of a defined topic is still a reasonable basis for decision making in the present and planning for the future. The Encyclopedia of Medical Immunology follows in the encyclopedist tradition. At the present time, however, progress is proceeding at such a rapid pace that a static volume, no matter how extensive, could never do justice to this dynamic subject. Thus our present encyclopedia is based on the concept that articles will be linked to current research and updated on a regular basis. The reader needs to gain an understanding of medical immunology not only at the date of publication, but on a continuing basis.

The immune system, as a vital component of normal physiology, participates in establishing and maintaining the well-being of the host. Its core responsibility is to prevent or control infection and malignancy. Immune functions can be divided into constituative and adaptive. Inherited innate immunity takes its origins from most primitive cellular functions of recognition and nutrition. In animals, it evolved through invertebrates as a group of formed barriers and a system of cells and cell products for promptly dealing with harmful invaders or preventing clonal amplification of malignant cells. In vertebrates, in addition to innate immunity, an adaptive immune system provides a more focused and potent response, but one that requires more time to mobilize. It utilizes a novel system of hypermutation and recombination to provide a sufficiently broad repertory of receptors to recognize and eliminate, in principle, any potential microbial invader. In establishing and maintaining such a wide repertory of recognition structures, the adaptive immune system inevitably recognizes many epitopes on molecules within the body of the host. Thus, the same protective effector mechanisms of the healthy immune system, if out of control, can produce harm in the form of the immune mediated disorders described in these Volumes.

The most frequent disorders of the immune system are deficiencies. If the immune system fails to perform its core function of protection, infectious or malignant disease can follow. Most of these immune failures result from germ line inheritance of mutations in genes regulating the innate or adaptive immune systems. The most frequent sign of an immune deficiency disease is infection due to one or more of the myriad microorganisms that inhabit the human environment.

A second group of immune-related illnesses results from loss of normal immunologic homeostasis. The regulatory devices that normally limit immune responses are inadequate. The failure may result from deficiencies, either inherited or acquired, of the overall regulatory machinery. Rather than a decrease in homeostatic regulation, immune disease can result from augmented immune responses. Powerful adjuvants, providing the non-antigenspecific signals, may overcome even normally functioning immune regulation.

Both types of immune-mediated disease are considered in our encapsulated knowledge. Allergies result from exposures to foreign substances that are harmless in the majority of individuals. As a group, allergic diseases affect at least 10% of the population and appear to be increasing over time in many populations. In contrast to an exaggerated response to foreign antigens, auto-immunity is the consequence of the "forbidden" recognition of some antigens in the host's body. Like allergic disease, autoimmune disease represents an uncontrolled immune response. Because allergic and autoimmune diseases can occur in different organ systems in the body, they can differ greatly in their clinical presentation, even though they share many genetic and regulatory features.

The goal in all medical immunology is to alleviate or prevent illness. If a disease is related to an inadequate immune response or to an overwhelming challenge, an intervention in the form of vaccination is a historically proven approach. Preventive vaccinations may be the most successful public health measure of the twentieth century. New vaccines directed to oncoming newly emerging infectants or subtypes remains a major goal of current immunologic research. Potential adverse effects of vaccines also require constant attention. These days vaccines are being tested as a way of limiting or reducing malignant tumors.

Immunotherapy is a more modern success story as biological agents such as monoclonal antibodies and receptor-blocking ligands are increasingly available for control of diseases due to immunological derangement. The need for an Encyclopedia of Medical immunology is compelling. Our encyclopedia is divided for convenience into the four subject areas discussed above: Immune deficiency diseases, allergic diseases, autoimmune diseases and vaccines. Each of these areas has significant and immediate relevance to medical practice and public health. Each is a growing area of research.

By bringing together these different areas in one comprehensive publication, the encyclopedia illustrates and emphasizes the fundamentals of the immune response. For immunity to play its part in good health, it must maintain homeostasis within itself and with all other physiologic systems. The challenges to maintaining immunologic good health are both internal and external. In the face of changes in the environment, including climate, infectious agents and industrial exposures, human survival places a need for constant recalibration of the immune system. Internally, the effects of aging, hormonal changes, the microbiome and life cycle events (e.g. puberty, pregnancy) also require readjustment of immunologic homeostasis. Interventions are designed to restore immunologic balance, to repair innate or induced deficiencies and to strengthen immune responses.

As Editors-in-Chief, we trust that the users will find this "encirclement" of a body of knowledge will prove helpful for decision making in promoting immunologic health and reducing immunologic disorders.

Clayton, Victoria, Australia   Ian R. Mackay
Boston, MA, USA   Noel R. Rose
October 2020   Editors-in-Chief

Preface

The field of primary immunodeficiency (PID) has changed drastically over the decades since the first diseases were phenotypically defined in the 1930s through 1950s. In fact, the name of the field has even changed and it now can also be referred to as the inborn defects of immunity (IEI). PID – now IEI – emerged from a small series of conditions that were identified owing to a characteristic set of clinical and immunological features that most notably included susceptibility to microbial infections. Specifically, patients with the original described IEIs presented with infections – either recurrently, severely, or unusually. As we now appreciate, particular IEIs lead to very specific infectious susceptibility – some even limited to a single organism within a limited age range. IEIs result from inherent defects, mostly genetic, that interrupt the way the immune system functions. That said, we now appreciate that it is not solely increased susceptibility to infections by external environment agents that defines this family of diseases where immunity breaks down, but also dysregulation of the immune tolerance to elements of the internal environment. In particular, patients with IEI can characteristically experience increased autoinflammation, autoimmunity, and cancer. In the case of autoinflammation, the initiation of a response is either pathologically amplified or cannot be curtailed. In autoimmunity, the immune response becomes confused and attacks the self as opposed to foreign materials. With cancer, the immune system fails to detect and eradicate abnormal growth or loss of growth control.

In all cases of IEI, defects in immunity result in an abnormal immune homeostasis relative to the internal and external environments. As the field of IEI entered the genetic era, it became clear that rare clinical presentations were teaching us as to what the specific value of individual genes were with regards to true immunological purpose. Key examples emerged including the relevance of the *IL2RG* gene to lymphocyte development and the cytoskeletal regulator *WASP* with regards to accessing immune cell function. Just over 20 years ago the number of diseases identified as PIDs crossed 50 in number and many of these had genetic and resulting immunological mechanisms identified. In recent years, and into the genomic era, we have experienced explosive growth in the number of IEIs, largely owing to unbiased genetic approaches. The international union of immunological societies (IUIS) has met every other year to catalogue and classify IEIs and has most recently (in 2019) listed over 400 individual conditions. While our initiative for this volume began in 2015 and is already behind the current classification document, we aspired to have an encyclopedic and alphabetic listing of the individual IEIs complementary to the largely tabular IUIS classification and listing of the diseases. Readers are able to find a brief description of each the IEIs, searched by alphabetical order and by immunological classification. We do hope that it will serve as a reference to those trying to learn more about these conditions and advance the well-being and understanding of patients in the midst of their diagnostic journeys.

Tremendous appreciation and gratitude must be directed to the numerous authors who contributed individual chapters in this volume. Each represents a critical passion of the author and undoubtedly defines fundamental lessons learned from patients through both discovery, suffering, and healing. Specific recognition must also be provided to the section editors, Drs. Antonio Condino-Neto, Raphaela Golbach-Mansky, Joris van Montfrans, Maite de la Morena, Robert Nelson, Jolan Walter, Elena Perez, Kathleen Sullivan, Stuart Turvey, and Klaus Warnatz who have curated a tremendous collection of chapters and authors to bring forward meaningful perspectives. They represent an international group of top experts in IEIs. Their reach throughout the field, efforts, and tenacity have made this volume a reality. We would also like to specifically acknowledge the efforts of Francisco (Tony) A. Bonilla, M.D., Ph. D., who served as an editor of this volume through some of the initial phases of this project and whose efforts were essential to its completion. Most importantly we would like to recognize the patients and their families who have taught us all as investigative physicians as to the meaning of both science and healing and have undoubtedly inspired our collective devotion to this collection.

The Woodlands, TX, USA   Jordan Scott Orange
New York, NY, USA   Javier Chinen
October 2020   Editors

List of Topics

About the Editors-in-Chief

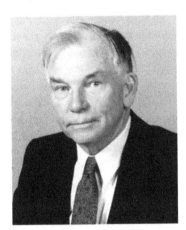

Ian R. Mackay's research career, mostly directed to autoimmunity, began in 1956 in the Clinical Research Unit (CRU) of the Walter & Eliza Hall Institute and Royal Melbourne Hospital (RMH), Melbourne, Australia. It comprehended associations between disorders of immunological function and clinical expressions in diseases of obscure causation. Research laboratories in the Hall Institute and supervision of a 27-bed general medical ward in the adjacent RMH encouraged one to think of autoimmunity holistically rather than via any single disease. A particular interest in autoimmunity and liver and a collaboration with D Carleton Gajdusek pointed to autoimmune responses in causation of two major entities, chronic active hepatitis and primary biliary cirrhosis (PBC). The detection of autoimmune reactivity of a monoclonal plasma paraprotein was a key element in Burnet's formulation of the Clonal Selection Theory of Acquired Immunity. Mackay's later return to PBC in the molecular era (1980s) in research with M Eric Gershwin resulted in cloning and identification of the gene for the disease-associated "mitochondrial" autoantigen of PBC, the E2 subunit of pyruvate dehydrogenase complex (PDC-E2). In autoimmune hepatitis, levels in serum of transaminase enzymes were found to reflect ongoing hepatocellular damage, so providing a monitor of efficacy of immunosuppressive drugs prednisolone and azathioprine, and, in the 1960s, the first long-term treatment trial established their benefit. This drug combination remains today as the standard therapy for autoimmune hepatitis.

In the early 1960s, Mackay became sufficiently convinced of the reality of autoimmunity to compile with F MacFarlane Burnet the first authoritative text (1963). Thereafter, he made research contributions on numerous autoimmune diseases, thyroiditis, multiple sclerosis, myasthenia gravis, pemphigus, and gastritis. With "Reg" Strickland, gastritis was separated into Type A (autoimmune) and Type B (later, bacterial) gastritis, foreshadowing bacterial infection in peptic ulcer disease. Mackay became a major protagonist for the early development of the specialty of Clinical Immunology and with Senga Whittingham laid out specifications for the practice of this specialty. In the 1980s, the RMH drew on the CRU to establish an AIDS service, and observations made on human papillomavirus (HPV) infection in rectal swabs of homosexual men led to Ian Frazer's development in Brisbane of an HPV vaccine for prevention of virus-induced cervical cancer.

In 1987, Mackay relocated to the Department of Biochemistry, Monash University, where with Merrill Rowley an autoimmunity laboratory was established for further investigation of PBC, Type 1 (autoimmune) diabetes, and rheumatoid arthritis. The laboratory sought to identify in various autoimmune diseases molecular epitopes (autoepitopes) using contemporary techniques including antibody screening of phage-displayed random peptide libraries. A notable achievement arising from collaborations at Monash with James Whisstock, Gus Fenalti, and others was the crystallization of both isoforms of glutamic acid decarboxylase (GAD) 65 and 67, revealing the 3D structure and "molecular positioning" of the reactive antibody epitopes of the autoantigenic 65kD isoform and differences from the non-autoantigenic 67 kD isoform. This work is ongoing.

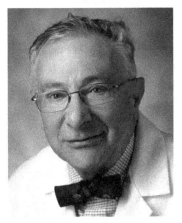

Noel R. Rose received his basic training in microbiology at Yale University followed by Ph.D. and M.D. degrees at the University of Pennsylvania and State University of New York at Buffalo. He was appointed to the faculty at Buffalo in 1951, where he began his research career. His early studies under the tutelage of Professor Ernest Witebsky searched properties of the organ-specific antigens that characterize the unique functions of normal and malignant cells. In the course of these investigations, he discovered that he could produce an autoimmune disease in the thyroid gland by immunization with the major thyroid protein, thyroglobulin. Until that time, it was generally accepted that in only a few "privileged sites" in the body were such pathogenic autoimmune responses possible. These studies opened the modern era of research on the autoimmune diseases and set the direction of Rose's career since then. In the 1960s, he investigated the requisite conditions for inducing autoimmune disease and the delineation of the basic immunologic and pathological processes. He included studies on other organs, such as the pancreas, as well as allergic diseases. In 1971, he and his colleagues discovered the first major gene that is responsible for susceptibility to autoimmune diseases and proved that it was a member of the major histocompatibility complex. At that time, he moved his laboratory to Wayne State University in Detroit, where he and his colleagues carried out detailed studies on the genes responsible for autoimmune disease of the thyroid gland. He also performed early experiments of the regulatory role of the thymus-derived lymphocytes and other studies related to unique enzymes of specialized cells, especially prostatic cancer. In 1981, Rose moved to Johns Hopkins University, where he created a department devoted to studies of immunity and infection. He directed much of his research to infectious agents and chemicals that induce autoimmune disease. A major effort was devoted to developing an experimental model of autoimmune heart disease produced in genetically prepared mice by infection with a virus that led work to the first identification of a well-defined antigen responsible for cardiac inflammation. Investigations on this model revealed a stepwise process that leads from infection to initial harmless autoimmunity to later life-threatening autoimmune disease.

In addition to his research, Rose has been deeply involved in the clinical practice of immunology. He directs a diagnostic immunology laboratory; he serves as expert consultant to the World Health Organization and as Director of the WHO Collaborating Center for Autoimmune Disorders. He chaired the first committee on clinical immunology of the American Association of Immunologists and was Co-founder of the Clinical Immunology Society. He was Editor-in-Chief of the first six volumes of the *Manual of Clinical Immunology* co-sponsored by the American Association of Immunologists and the American Society for Microbiology.

Throughout his career, Rose has had the opportunity of working with a number of leading investigators including Pierre Grabar at the Pasteur Institute, Paris, Henry Isliker at the Swiss Institute for Cancer Research, Sir James Gowans at Oxford University, and Sir Gustav Nossal and Ian Mackay at the Walter and Eliza Hall Institute in Australia. While at the Hall Institute, Rose was invited to prepare a book describing the broad area of autoimmune disorders. He joined with Mackay in producing the first volume of the book *The Autoimmune Diseases*, which is now in its sixth edition.

At Johns Hopkins, he taught students, continues to teach in medicine and public health, and directed an active research laboratory. He also headed the Center for Autoimmune Disease Research, which facilitated communication and collaboration among specialists in the different facets of autoimmune disease research.

In 2015, Rose was appointed Emeritus Professor in Medicine and Public Health and moved to Boston. There he is Senior Lecturer in Pathology (part time). He continues to teach and mentor graduate students and fellows, organize periodic conferences on new developments in autoimmune disease, and consult with the U.-S. Department of Health and Human Services on vaccine safety.

About the Editors

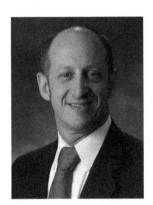

Jordan Scott Orange, M.D., Ph.D., is the Reuben S. Carpentier Professor and Chairman of the Department of Pediatrics at Columbia University and the Pediatrician-in-Chief at NewYork-Presbyterian Morgan Stanley Children's Hospital. Previously, he was Professor, Vice Chair for Research, and Chief of Immunology/Allergy/Rheumatology at Baylor College of Medicine and Director of the Center for Human Immunobiology at Texas Children's Hospital. Prior to that he was the Jeffrey Modell Endowed Chair of Immunology Research at the Children's Hospital of Philadelphia (CHOP). Dr. Orange completed baccalaureate and M.D./Ph.D. degrees at Brown University, Pediatric Residency at CHOP, and Allergy/Immunology/Rheumatology Fellowship at Boston Children's Hospital. He is an elected member of the National Academy of Medicine and the American Society for Clinical Investigation and was the recipient of the 2017 E. Mead Johnson Award from the Society for Pediatric Research and the 2018 O'Donnell Prize in Medicine from the Texas Academy of Medicine, Engineering and Science. Dr. Orange's research focuses on the cell biology of intercellular immune interactions, the immunological synapse, novel causes of primary immunodeficiency, and mechanistic insights gained from inborn defects of immunity. While being credited with the discovery of several diseases, his specific focus has been upon those that impair the defenses of natural killer (NK) cells and has led him to focus on the defects that impair NK cell development or function as a major contribution to clinical immunodeficiency. Dr. Orange's work has been continuously funded by the NIH, and he has over 300 publications.

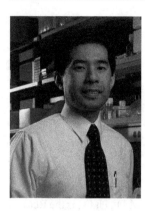

Javier Chinen, M.D., Ph.D., is an Associate Professor of Allergy and Immunology in the Department of Pediatrics at Baylor College of Medicine and Chief of Service of the David Clinic for Allergy and Immunology at Texas Children's Hospital The Woodlands. He received his medical degree from the University Cayetano Heredia in Lima, Peru, and his Ph.D. Immunology degree from Baylor College of Medicine.

Dr. Chinen currently practices as a clinical immunologist, and is a teacher and a researcher. He has a focused interest in the diagnosis and management of patients with inborn errors of immunity, particularly children with severe combined immunodeficiencies. Among his contributions in this area, Dr. Chinen's research efforts have included the early exploration of gene therapy for X-linked SCID at the National Institutes of Health and the description of the natural history of patients with partial DiGeorge Syndrome. He is actively involved in the outcome evaluation of the newborn screening program for SCID in Texas. Dr. Chinen is an Associate Editor for the *Journal of Allergy and Clinical Immunology* and an author of chapters on aspects of immunodeficiencies for *Rudolph's Textbook of Pediatrics*, *Feigin and Cherry Textbook of Pediatrics Infectious Diseases*, and Rich's *Clinical Immunology Principles and Practice*.

Section Editors

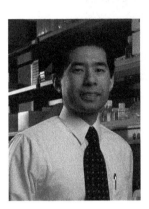

Javier Chinen
Division of Allergy and Immunology
Department of Pediatrics
Baylor College of Medicine
Texas Children's Hospital
The Woodlands, TX, USA

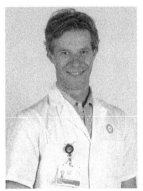

Joris M. van Montfrans
Department of Pediatric Immunology and Infectious Diseases
Wilhelmina Children's Hospital
University Medical Center Utrecht (UMCU)
Utrecht, The Netherlands

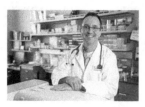

Stuart E. Turvey
Division of Allergy and Clinical Immunology
Department of Pediatrics and Experimental Medicine Program
British Columbia Children's Hospital
The University of British Columbia
Vancouver, BC, Canada

Willem-Alexander Children's Hospital
Leiden University Medical Center
Leiden, The Netherlands

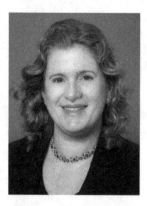

Jolan Walter
University of South Florida
St. Petersburg, FL, USA

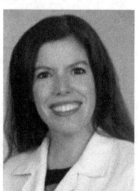

Elena E. Perez
Allergy Associates of the Palm Beaches
North Palm Beach, FL, USA

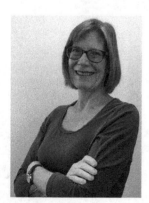

Kathleen Sullivan
Wallace Chair of Pediatrics
Division of Allergy Immunology
The Children's Hospital of Philadelphia
Philadelphia, USA

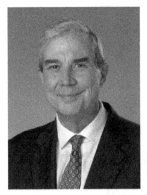

Robert P. Nelson
Divisions of Hematology and Oncology
Stem Cell Transplant Program
Indiana University (IU) School of Medicine and
the IU Bren and Simon Cancer Center
Indianapolis, IN, USA

Pediatric Immunodeficiency Clinic
Riley Hospital for Children at Indiana University
Health
Indianapolis, IN, USA

Medicine and Pediatrics Indiana University
School of Medicine
Immunohematology and Transplantation
Indianapolis, IN, USA

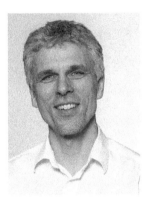

Klaus Warnatz
Department of Rheumatology and Clinical
Immunology and Center for Chronic
Immunodeficiency
University Medical Center and
Unversity of Freiburg
Freiburg, Germany

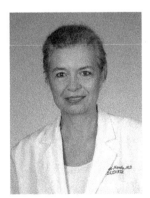

Raphaela Goldbach-Mansky
Translational Autoinflammatory Diseases Section
(TADS)
National Institute of Allergy and Infectious Dis-
eases (NIAID)
National Institutes of Health (NIH)
Bethesda, MD, USA

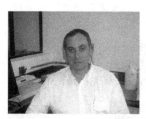

Antonio Condino-Neto
Department of Immunology
Institute of Biomedical Sciences – University of
São Paulo
São Paulo, SP, Brazil

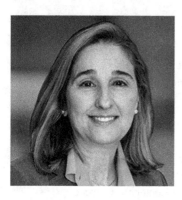

M. Teresa de la Morena
Department of Pediatrics and
Division of Immunology
Seattle Children's Hospital and
University of Washington
Seattle, WA, USA

Contributors

Ivona Aksentijevich Inflammatory Disease Section, National Human Genome Research Institute (NHGRI), Bethesda, MD, USA

Mary Armanios Johns Hopkins University School of Medicine, Baltimore, MD, USA

John P. Atkinson Division of Rheumatology, Department of Medicine, Washington University School of Medicine, St. Louis, MO, USA

Sara Barmettler Division of Rheumatology, Allergy and Immunology, Massachusetts General Hospital, Boston, MA, USA

Jenna R. E. Bergerson Laboratory of Clinical Immunology and Microbiology, National Institutes of Allergy and Infectious Diseases (NIAID), National Institutes of Health (NIH), Bethesda, MD, USA

Catherine M. Biggs Department of Pediatrics, BC Children's Hospital, University of British Columbia, Vancouver, BC, Canada

Donald B. Bloch Division of Rheumatology, Allergy and Immunology, Department of Medicine and the Anesthesia Center for Critical Care Research of the Department of Anesthesia, Critical Care, and Pain Medicine, Harvard Medical School and Massachusetts General Hospital, Boston, MA, USA

Bruna Bombassaro Division of Clinical Immunology and Allergy, Department of Clinical Medicine, State University of Campinas (UNICAMP), Campinas, Brazil

Arturo Borzutzky Department of Pediatric Infectious Diseases and Immunology, School of Medicine, Pontificia Universidad Católica de Chile, Santiago, Chile

Anne M. Bowcock Icahn School of Medicine at Mount Sinai, New York, NY, USA

Adeeb A. Bulkhi Department of Internal Medicine, College of Medicine, Umm Al Qura University, Makkah, Saudi Arabia

Division of Allergy and Immunology, Department of Internal Medicine, Morsani College of Medicine, University of South Florida, Tampa, FL, USA

Sonia Caccia "Luigi Sacco" Department of Biomedical and Clinical Sciences, University of Milan, Milan, Italy

Scott W. Canna University of Pittsburgh and UPMC Children's Hospital of Pittsburgh, Pittsburgh, PA, USA

Javier Chinen Division of Allergy and Immunology, Department of Pediatrics, Baylor College of Medicine, Texas Children's Hospital, The Woodlands, TX, USA

Ivan K. Chinn Section of Immunology, Allergy, and Retrovirology, Texas Children's Hospital, Houston, TX, USA

William T. Shearer Center for Human Immunobiology, Texas Children's Hospital, Houston, TX, USA

Department of Pediatrics, Baylor College of Medicine, Houston, TX, USA

Herberto Jose Chong-Neto Division of Allergy and Immunology, Department of Pediatrics, Federal University of Parana Medical School, Curitiba, Brazil

Debora Carla Chong-Silva Division of Allergy and Immunology, Department of Pediatrics, Federal University of Paraná, Curitiba, Brazil

Marco Cicardi Department of Biomedical and Clinical Sciences Luigi Sacco, University of Milan, Milan, Italy

ASST Fatebenefratelli Sacco, Milan, Italy

Antonio Condino-Neto Department of Immunology, Institute of Biomedical Sciences – University of São Paulo, São Paulo, SP, Brazil

Edward W. Cowen Dermatology Branch, National Institute of Arthritis and Musculoskeletal and Skin Diseases, National Institutes of Health, Bethesda, MD, USA

Melissa L. Crenshaw Division of Genetics, Johns Hopkins All Children's Hospital, St. Petersburg, FL, USA

Virgil A. S. H. Dalm Internal Medicine, Clinical Immunology, Erasmus MC, Rotterdam, The Netherlands

Adriana A. de Jesus Translational Autoinflammatory Diseases Section (TADS), National Institute of Allergy and Infectious Diseases (NIAID), National Institutes of Health (NIH), Bethesda, MD, USA

M. Teresa de la Morena Department of Pediatrics and Division of Immunology, Seattle Children's Hospital and University of Washington, Seattle, WA, USA

Esther de Vries Tranzo, TSB, Tilburg University, Tilburg, the Netherlands

Laboratory for Medical Microbiology and Immunology, Elisabeth-Tweesteden Hospital, Tilburg, the Netherlands

Beata Derfalvi Department of Pediatrics, IWK Health Centre, Dalhousie University, Halifax, NS, Canada

Christian Drouet GREPI EA7408, University Grenoble Alpes, Grenoble, France

Ilona DuBuske Division of Allergy and Immunology, University of Cincinnati, Cincinnati, OH, USA

A. Durandy INSERM UMR 1163, Human Lymphohematopoiesis Laboratory, Paris, France

Imagine Institute, Université Paris Descartes, Sorbonne Paris Cité, Paris, France

Zoya Eskandarian Institute for Immunodeficiency, Center for Chronic Immunodeficiency, Medical Center, Faculty of Medicine, Albert-Ludwigs-University of Freiburg, Freiburg, Germany

Faculty of Biology, Albert-Ludwigs-University of Freiburg, Freiburg, Germany

Amos Etzioni Ruth Children Hospital, Faculty of Medicine, Technion, Haifa, Israel

Jack Farah Institute of Molecular Biology, Armenian National Academy of Sciences, Yerevan, Republic of Armenia

Anders Fasth Department of Pediatrics, Institute of Clinical Sciences, Sahlgrenska Academy at University of Gothenburg, Gothenburg, Sweden

Polly J. Ferguson Rheumatology, Allergy and Immunology, Department of Pediatrics, University of Iowa Carver College of Medicine, Iowa City, IA, USA

Thomas G. Fox Department of Pediatrics, Section of Pediatric Infectious Diseases, Indiana University School of Medicine, Riley Hospital for Children, Indianapolis, IN, USA

Department of Pediatrics, Division of Pediatric Infectious Disease, Emory University School of Medicine, Atlanta, GA, USA

Alexandra F. Freeman Laboratory of Clinical Immunology and Microbiology, National Institutes of Allergy and Infectious Diseases (NIAID), National Institutes of Health (NIH), Bethesda, MD, USA

Joost Frenkel Department of Pediatrics, University Medical Center Utrecht, Utrecht, The Netherlands

Shan Yu Fung BC Children's Hospital Research Institute, University of British Columbia, Vancouver, BC, Canada

María Isabel García-Laorden Department of Immunology, Gran Canaria Dr. Negrín University Hospital, Las Palmas de Gran Canaria, Spain

CIBER de Enfermedades Respiratorias (CIBERES), Instituto de Salud Carlos III, Madrid, Spain

Megha Garg Translational Autoinflammatory Diseases Section (TADS), National Institute of Allergy and Infectious Diseases (NIAID), National Institutes of Health (NIH), Bethesda, MD, USA

Peter Garred Laboratory of Molecular Medicine, Department of Clinical Immunology, Section 7631 Rigshospitalet, Faculty of Health and Medical Sciences, University of Copenhagen, Copenhagen, Denmark

Christina Gavino Research Institute-MUHC (RI-MUHC), Montréal, QC, Canada

Ninette Genster Laboratory of Molecular Medicine, Department of Clinical Immunology, Section 7631 Rigshospitalet, Faculty of Health and Medical Sciences, University of Copenhagen, Copenhagen, Denmark

Arije Ghannam GREPI EA7408, University Grenoble Alpes, Grenoble, France

KininX SAS, Grenoble, France

Berhane Ghebrehiwet The Department of Medicine, Stony Brook University, New York, NY, USA

Health Sciences Center, Stony Brook University School of Medicine, New York, NY, USA

Silvia Giliani Department of Molecular and Translational Medicine, University of Brescia, Brescia, Italy

Vera Goda Pediatric Hematology and Stem Cell Transplantation Department, South-Pest Central Hospital, United Szent Istvan and Szent Laszlo Hospital Budapest, Budapest, Hungary

Raphaela Goldbach-Mansky Translational Autoinflammatory Diseases Section (TADS), National Institute of Allergy and Infectious Diseases (NIAID), National Institutes of Health (NIH), Bethesda, MD, USA

Bodo Grimbacher Institute for Immunodeficiency, Center for Chronic Immunodeficiency, Medical Center, Faculty of Medicine, Albert-Ludwigs-University of Freiburg, Freiburg, Germany

DZIF – German Center for Infection Research, Satellite Center Freiburg, Freiburg, Germany

CIBSS – Centre for Integrative Biological Signalling Studies, Albert-Ludwigs University, Freiburg, Germany

RESIST – Cluster of Excellence 2155 to Hanover Medical School, Satellite Center Freiburg, Freiburg, Germany

Institute of Immunity and Transplantation, Royal Free Hospital, University College London, London, UK

Anete Sevciovic Grumach Faculdade de Medicina ABC, Santo Andre, SP, Brazil

David Hagin Allergy and Clinical Immunology Unit, Department of Medicine, Tel-Aviv Sourasky Medical Center, Tel Aviv, Israel

Sackler Faculty of Medicine, University of Tel Aviv, Tel Aviv, Israel

Lennart Hammarström Karolinska Institute, Stockholm, Sweden

Eric P. Hanson Division Chief, Pediatric Rheumatology Department of Pediatrics, Medical and Molecular Genetics, Riley Hospital for Children and Indiana University School of Medicine Herman B. Wells Center for Pediatric Research, Indianapolis, IN, USA

Merja Helminen Tampere Center for Child Health Research, Tampere University Hospital, Tampere, Finland

Kyla Jade Hildebrand Division of Allergy & Immunology, Department of Pediatrics, Faculty of Medicine, University of British Columbia, Vancouver, BC, Canada
British Columbia Children's Hospital Research Institute, Vancouver, BC, Canada

Hal M. Hoffman Division of Pediatric Allergy, Immunology, and Rheumatology, University of California, San Diego and Rady Children's Hospital, San Diego, CA, USA

Rodrigo Hoyos-Bachiloglu Department of Pediatric Infectious Diseases and Immunology, School of Medicine, Pontificia Universidad Católica de Chile, Santiago, Chile

Armenuhi A. Hyusyan Institute of Molecular Biology, Armenian National Academy of Sciences, Yerevan, Republic of Armenia

Anuja Java Division of Nephrology, Department of Medicine, Washington University School of Medicine, St. Louis, MO, USA

Jerold Jeyaratnam Department of Pediatrics, University Medical Center Utrecht, Utrecht, The Netherlands

Jay J. Jin Division of Pediatric Pulmonology, Allergy, and Sleep Medicine, Indiana University School of Medicine, Riley Hospital for Children at Indiana University Health, Indianapolis, IN, USA

Sonia Joychan Division of Allergy and Immunology, University of South Florida/Johns Hopkins All Children's Hospital, Tampa, FL, USA

Soma Jyonouchi Division of Allergy and Immunology, Department of Pediatrics, The Children's Hospital of Philadelphia, Philadelphia, PA, USA

Daniel L. Kastner National Human Genome Research Institute, National Institutes of Health, Bethesda, MD, USA

Stefan H. E. Kaufmann Max Planck Institute for Infection Biology, Berlin, Germany
Hagler Institute for Advanced Study at Texas A&M University, College Station, TX, USA

Lisa J. Kobrynski Children's Healthcare of Atlanta, Department of Pediatrics, Emory University School of Medicine, Atlanta, GA, USA

Larysa V. Kostyuchenko Department of Clinical Immunology and Allergology, Danylo Halytsky Lviv National Medical University, West-Ukrainian Specialized Children's Medical Center, Lviv, Ukraine

Sven Kracker INSERM UMR 1163, Human Lymphohematopoiesis Laboratory, Paris, France

Imagine Institute, Université Paris Descartes, Sorbonne Paris Cité, Paris, France

Anne Sophie Kubasch Department of Pediatrics, Medizinische Fakultät Carl Gustav Carus, Technische Universität Dresden, Dresden, Germany

Taco W. Kuijpers Department of Pediatric Immunology, Rheumatology and Infectious Diseases, Emma Children's Hospital, Amsterdam University Medical Center (Amsterdam UMC), Amsterdam, The Netherlands

Attila Kumánovics Department of Pathology, University of Utah, Salt Lake City, UT, USA

Caroline Y. Kuo Allergy and Immunology, David Geffen School of Medicine at the University of California, Los Angeles, Los Angeles, CA, USA

Marija Landekic Research Institute-MUHC (RI-MUHC), Montréal, QC, Canada

Gaetana Lanzi Department of Molecular and Translational Medicine Organisation; University of Brescia, Angelo Nocivelli Institute for Molecular Medicine, Brescia, Italy

Min Ae Lee-Kirsch Department of Pediatrics, Medizinische Fakultät Carl Gustav Carus, Technische Universität Dresden, Dresden, Germany

Jennifer W. Leiding Department of Pediatrics, Division of Allergy and Immunology, University of South Florida at Johns Hopkins – All Children's Hospital, St. Petersburg, FL, USA

Denise Leite-Caldeira Division of Clinical Immunology and Allergy, Department of Clinical Medicine, State University of Campinas (UNICAMP), Campinas, Brazil

M. Kathryn Liszewski Division of Rheumatology, Department of Medicine, Washington University School of Medicine, St. Louis, MO, USA

Vassilios Lougaris Pediatrics Clinic and Institute for Molecular Medicine A. Nocivelli, Department of Clinical and Experimental Sciences, University of Brescia and ASST-Spedali Civili of Brescia, Brescia, Italy

Michelle A. Lowes The Rockefeller University, New York, NY, USA

Henry Y. Lu Department of Pediatrics and Experimental Medicine Program, British Columbia Children's Hospital, The University of British Columbia, Vancouver, BC, Canada

Aniko Malik Department of Pediatrics, Semmelweis University, Budapest, Hungary
Pediatric Immunology, IWK Health Centre, Halifax, NS, Canada

Eli Mansour Division of Clinical Immunology and Allergy, Department of Clinical Medicine, State University of Campinas (UNICAMP), Campinas, Brazil

Michel J. Massaad Department of Experimental Pathology, Immunology, and Microbiology, and Department of Pediatrics and Adolescent Medicine, American University of Beirut, Beirut, Lebanon
Department of Pediatrics, Division of Immunology, Boston Children's Hospital, Harvard Medical School, Boston, MA, USA

Yoshinori Matsumoto Princess Margaret Cancer Center, University Health Network, University of Toronto, Toronto, ON, Canada
Department of Nephrology, Rheumatology, Endocrinology and Metabolism, Okayama University Graduate School of Medicine, Dentistry and Pharmaceutical Sciences, Okayama, Japan

Karine R. Mayilyan Institute of Molecular Biology, Armenian National Academy of Sciences, Yerevan, Republic of Armenia

Michael F. McDermott Leeds Institute of Rheumatic and Musculoskeletal Medicine (LIRMM), St James's University Hospital, Leeds, UK

Lauren Metterle Department of Dermatology and Cutaneous Surgery, University of South Florida Health Morsani College of Medicine, Tampa, FL, USA

Dror Mevorach Rheumatology Research Center, Department of Medicine, Hadassah-Hebrew University, Jerusalem, Israel

Joshua D. Milner Laboratory of Allergic Diseases, NIAID, NIH, Bethesda, MD, USA
Department of Pediatrics, Columbia University Irving Medical Center, New York, NY, USA

Isabela Mina Division of Immunology and Allergy, Department of Pediatrics, Ribeirão Preto Medical School, University of São Paulo, Ribeirão Preto, Brazil

Gina A. Montealegre Sanchez Translational Autoinflammatory Diseases Section (TADS), National Institute of Allergy and Infectious Diseases (NIAID), National Institutes of Health (NIH), Bethesda, MD, USA

Luis Murguia-Favela Pediatric Immunology and Allergy, Alberta Children's Hospital, Calgary, AB, Canada

The University of Calgary, Calgary, AB, Canada

Robert P. Nelson Divisions of Hematology and Oncology, Stem Cell Transplant Program, Indiana University (IU) School of Medicine and the IU Bren and Simon Cancer Center, Indianapolis, IN, USA

Pediatric Immunodeficiency Clinic, Riley Hospital for Children at Indiana University Health, Indianapolis, IN, USA

Medicine and Pediatrics, Indiana University School of Medicine, Immunohematology and Transplantation, Indianapolis, IN, USA

Peter E. Newburger Department of Pediatrics, Division of Hematology/Oncology, University of Massachusetts Medical School, Worcester, MA, USA

Eric Oksenhendler Department of Clinical Immunology, Hôpital Saint-Louis, Paris, France

Amanda K. Ombrello National Human Genome Research Institute, National Institutes of Health, Bethesda, MD, USA

Jordan Scott Orange Department of Pediatrics, Columbia University Vagelos College of Physicians and Surgeons, NewYork-Presbyterian Morgan Stanley Children's Hospital, New York, NY, USA

Seza Ozen Department of Pediatric Rheumatology, Faculty of Medicine, Hacettepe University, Ankara, Turkey

Bhumika Patel Asthma, Allergy and Immunology of Tampa Bay, Tampa, FL, USA

Elena E. Perez Allergy Associates of the Palm Beaches, North Palm Beach, FL, USA

Alessandro Plebani Pediatrics Clinic and Institute for Molecular Medicine A. Nocivelli, Department of Clinical and Experimental Sciences, University of Brescia and ASST-Spedali Civili of Brescia, Brescia, Italy

Robert J. Ragotte Nuffield Department of Medicine, University of Oxford, Oxford, UK

Nikita Raje Department of Pediatrics, Children's Mercy Hospital, Kansas City, MO, USA

University of Missouri–Kansas City School of Medicine, Kansas City, MO, USA

Pediatric Allergy, Asthma and Immunology Clinic, Children's Mercy Hospital, Kansas City, MO, USA

Mike Recher Immunodeficiency laboratory and Immunodeficiency Clinic, Medical Outpatient Unit and Department Biomedicine, University Basel Hospital, Basel, Switzerland

Ismail Reisli Meram Medical Faculty, Division of Pediatric Allergy and Immunology, Department of Pediatrics, Necmettin Erbakan University, Konya, Turkey

Nicholas L. Rider Section of Immunology, Allergy and Retrovirology, Department of Pediatrics, Baylor College of Medicine, Texas Children's Hospital, Houston, TX, USA

Hannah Roberts Division of Allergy and Clinical Immunology, Department of Pediatrics, BC Children's Hospital, University of British Columbia, Vancouver, BC, Canada

Carlos Rodríguez-Gallego Department of Immunology, Gran Canaria Dr. Negrín University Hospital, Las Palmas de Gran Canaria, Spain

Cristine Secco Rosario Department of Pediatrics, Federal University of Paraná, Curitiba, Brazil

Nelson Augusto Rosario Federal University of Paraná, Curitiba, Brazil

Carlos D. Rose duPont Children's Hospital, Thomas Jefferson University, Philadelphia, USA

Robert Rottapel Princess Margaret Cancer Center, University Health Network, University of Toronto, Toronto, ON, Canada

Department of Medicine, Department of Medical Biophysics and Department of Immunology, University of Toronto, Toronto, ON, Canada

Division of Rheumatology, St. Michael's Hospital, Toronto, ON, Canada

Persio Roxo-Junior Division of Immunology and Allergy, Department of Pediatrics, Ribeirão Preto Medical School, University of São Paulo, Ribeirão Preto, Brazil

Jacob Rozmus Department of Pediatrics, BC Children's Hospital and The University of British Columbia, Vancouver, BC, Canada

Hafize Emine Sönmez Department of Pediatric Rheumatology, Faculty of Medicine, Hacettepe University, Ankara, Turkey

Nicole P. Safina Department of Pediatrics, Children's Mercy Hospital, Kansas City, MO, USA

University of Missouri–Kansas City School of Medicine, Kansas City, MO, USA

Division of Clinical Genetics, Children's Mercy Hospital, Kansas City, MO, USA

Carol Saunders Center for Pediatric Genomic Medicine, Children's Mercy Hospital, Kansas City, MO, USA

Department of Pathology and Laboratory Medicine, Children's Mercy Hospital, Kansas City, MO, USA

University of Missouri–Kansas City School of Medicine, Kansas City, MO, USA

Elizabeth C. Schramm Sevion Inc, Anthro Bio Inc, St. Louis, MO, USA

Catharina Schuetz Pediatric Immunology, Technical University Dresden, Dresden, Germany

Gesmar Rodrigues Silva Segundo Pediatrics Allergy and Immunology, Universidade Federal de Uberlandia, Uberlandia, Brazil

Lucia Seminario-Vidal Department of Dermatology and Cutaneous Surgery, University of South Florida Health Morsani College of Medicine, Tampa, FL, USA

Svetlana O. Sharapova Research Department, Belarusian Research Center for Pediatric Oncology, Hematology and Immunology, Minsk, Belarus

Raz Somech Pediatric Department, Allergy and the Immunology Services, "Edmond and Lily Safra" Children's Hospital, Sackler School of Medicine, Tel Aviv University, Tel Aviv, Israel

Jeffrey Modell Foundation Center, Sackler School of Medicine, Tel Aviv University, Tel Aviv, Israel

Sheba Medical Center, Tel Hashomer, Sackler School of Medicine, Tel Aviv University, Tel Aviv, Israel

Ana Flavia Bernardes Sousa Division of Clinical Immunology and Allergy, Department of Clinical Medicine, State University of Campinas (UNICAMP), Campinas, Brazil

Panida Sriaroon Department of Pediatrics, Division of Allergy and Immunology, University of South Florida/Johns Hopkins All Children's Hospital, Tampa, FL, USA

Tali Stauber Pediatric Department, Allergy and the Immunology Services, "Edmond and Lily Safra" Children's Hospital, Sackler School of Medicine, Tel Aviv University, Tel Aviv, Israel

Jeffrey Modell Foundation Center, Sackler School of Medicine, Tel Aviv University, Tel Aviv, Israel

Sheba Medical Center, Tel Hashomer, Sackler School of Medicine, Tel Aviv University, Tel Aviv, Israel

Deborah L. Stone National Human Genome Research Institute, National Institutes of Health, Bethesda, MD, USA

Gunnar Sturfelt Department of Rheumatology, University Hospital of Skåne, Lund, Sweden

Chiara Suffritti Department of Biomedical and Clinical Sciences Luigi Sacco, University of Milan, Milan, Italy

ASST Fatebenefratelli Sacco, Milan, Italy

Victoria Tüngler Department of Pediatrics, Medizinische Fakultät Carl Gustav Carus, Technische Universität Dresden, Dresden, Germany

Isabelle Thiffault Center for Pediatric Genomic Medicine, Children's Mercy Hospital, Kansas City, MO, USA

Department of Pathology and Laboratory Medicine, Children's Mercy Hospital, Kansas City, MO, USA

University of Missouri–Kansas City School of Medicine, Kansas City, MO, USA

Lennart Truedsson Dept. of Laboratory Medicine, Section of Microbiology, Immunology and Glycobiology, Lund University, Lund, Sweden

Stuart E. Turvey Division of Allergy and Clinical Immunology, Department of Pediatrics and Experimental Medicine Program, British Columbia Children's Hospital, The University of British Columbia, Vancouver, BC, Canada

Willem-Alexander Children's Hospital, Leiden University Medical Center, Leiden, the Netherlands

Mirjam van der Burg Department of Pediatrics, Willem-Alexander Children's Hospital, Leiden University Medical Center, Leiden, The Netherlands

Joris M. van Montfrans Department of Pediatric Immunology and Infectious Diseases, Wilhelmina Children's Hospital, University Medical Center Utrecht (UMCU), Utrecht, The Netherlands

Menno C. van Zelm Department of Immunology and Pathology, Central Clinical School, Monash University, Melbourne, VIC, Australia

Department of Respiratory Medicine, The Alfred Hospital, Melbourne, VIC, Australia

The Jeffrey Modell Diagnostic and Research Centre for Primary Immunodeficiencies, Melbourne, VIC, Australia

Lilly M. Verhagen Department of Pediatric Immunoloy and Infectious Diseases, Wilhelmina Children's Hospital, Utrecht, The Netherlands

Donald C. Vinh Infectious Disease Susceptibility Program, McGill University Health Centre (MUHC) and Research Institute-MUHC (RI-MUHC), Montréal, QC, Canada

Department of Medicine, Division of Infectious Diseases & Medical Microbiology, McGill University Health Centre, Montréal, QC, Canada

Department of Human Genetics, McGill University, Montréal, QC, Canada

Luke A. Wall Section of Allergy Immunology, New Orleans, LA, USA

Department of Pediatrics, Louisiana State University Health Sciences Center and Children's Hospital, New Orleans, LA, USA

Jolan Walter University of South Florida, St. Petersburg, FL, USA

Suzanne C. Ward Dermatology Branch, National Institute of Arthritis and Musculoskeletal and Skin Diseases, National Institutes of Health, Bethesda, MD, USA

Klaus Warnatz Department of Rheumatology and Clinical Immunology and Center for Chronic Immunodeficiency, University Medical Center and University of Freiburg, Freiburg, Germany

Levi B. Watkin Department of Pediatrics, Baylor College of Medicine, Center for Human Immunobiology, Division of Allergy, Immunology, and Rheumatology, Texas Children's Hospital, Houston, TX, USA

Carine H. Wouters Department of Microbiology and Immunology, KU Leuven – University of Leuven, Leuven, Belgium

Pediatric Rheumatology, University Hospitals Leuven, Leuven, Belgium

Maddalena Wu Department of Biomedical and Clinical Sciences Luigi Sacco, University of Milan, Milan, Italy

ASST Fatebenefratelli Sacco, Milan, Italy

Christina Yee Division of Immunology, Boston Children's Hospital & Harvard Medical School, Boston, MA, USA

Regina M. Zambrano Section of Clinical Genetics, New Orleans, LA, USA

Department of Pediatrics, Louisiana State University Health Sciences Center and Children's Hospital, New Orleans, LA, USA

Andrea Zanichelli Department of Biomedical and Clinical Sciences Luigi Sacco, University of Milan, Milan, Italy

ASST Fatebenefratelli Sacco, Milan, Italy

Julia Zinngrebe Department of Pediatrics and Adolescent Medicine, Ulm University Medical Center, Ulm, Germany

A

Activated PI3-Kinase Delta Syndrome (APDS)/p110d-Activating Mutations Causing Senescent T Cells, Lymphadenopathy, and Immunodeficiency (PASLI)

Sven Kracker
INSERM UMR 1163, Human
Lymphohematopoiesis Laboratory, Paris, France
Imagine Institute, Université Paris Descartes,
Sorbonne Paris Cité, Paris, France

Synonyms

p110δ-Activating mutations causing Senescent T cells, Lymphadenopathy, and Immunodeficiency (PASLI) (Lucas et al. 2014a) and PASLI-R1 in patients with mutations in *PIK3R1* (Lucas et al. 2014b).

Definition

An immunodeficiency defined by *PIK3CD* gain-of-function mutations encoding for the p110δ catalytic subunit of the phosphatidylinositol3-kinase delta (PI3K δ) (activated PI3K delta syndrome (APDS) 1) (Angulo et al. 2013) or by autosomal dominant mutations in *PIK3R1* encoding the regulatory subunit p85α (APDS2) (Deau et al. 2014).

Prevalence

So far (2018), over 100 patients with mutations in *PIK3CD* and over 50 patients with mutations in *PIK3R1* have been identified (Lougaris et al. 2015; Coulter et al. 2016; Elkaim et al. 2016; Crank et al. 2014; Kracker et al. 2014; Wentink et al. 2017; Petrovski et al. 2016; Tsujita et al. 2016; Takeda et al. 2017; Dulau Florea et al. 2017; Heurtier et al. 2017).

Clinical Presentation

Most APDS patients present with recurrent bacterial respiratory tract infections and lymphoproliferation. Pneumonia (85%), bronchiectasis (60%), and lymphadenopathies/splenomegaly (75%) were frequently observed in APDS1 patients, often with childhood onset (Coulter et al. 2016). Other complications reported include herpes virus (especially EBV and CMV) infections and reactivations (49%), autoimmune-induced cytopenia (17%), and occurrence of B lymphomas (diffuse large B cell, marginal zone, non-Hodgkin lymphomas) that affected 13% of APDS patients (Coulter et al. 2016; Kracker et al. 2014). Neurodevelopmental delay was reported for APDS patients (19%) indicating a function of p110δ in cells from the central nervous system (Coulter et al. 2016).

APDS2 is a combined immunodeficiency with a variable clinical phenotype and complications

© Springer Science+Business Media LLC, part of Springer Nature 2020
I. R. Mackay et al. (eds.), *Encyclopedia of Medical Immunology*,
https://doi.org/10.1007/978-1-4614-8678-7

such as severe bacterial and viral infections, lymphoproliferation, and lymphoma similar to APDS1 (Elkaim et al. 2016). Growth retardation (45%) and mild neurodevelopmental delay (31%) were frequently noticed for APDS2 patients (Elkaim et al. 2016). These clinical complications together with microcephaly, joint extensibility, and increased glucose levels in the blood, although rarely reported for APDS2 patients, suggest disturbed PI3K signaling also in non-lymphoid lineage cells (Elkaim et al. 2016; Petrovski et al. 2016).

Genetics

Several different GoF mutations of p110δ responsible for APDS1 (E81K (Takeda et al. 2017; Heurtier et al. 2017), G124D (Takeda et al. 2017; Heurtier et al. 2017), N334 K (Lucas et al. 2014a), R405C (Rae et al. 2017), C416R (Crank et al. 2014), E525K (Lucas et al. 2014a), E525A (Tsujita et al. 2016), R929C (Wentink et al. 2017), E1021K (Angulo et al. 2013), and E1025G (Dulau Florea et al. 2017)) have been reported so far; the most frequent of them being E1021K located in the kinase domain. The GoF *PIK3CD* mutations are next to the kinase domain located in the adapter-binding domain and the linker between the adapter-binding domain, the protein kinase C homology-2 (C2) domain, and the helical domain of p100δ. The GoF *PIK3CD* mutations in those domains are located in parts involved in the interaction with the regulatory PI3K subunit (Takeda et al. 2017; Heurtier et al. 2017).

Heterozygous mutations in *PIK3R1* affecting the splice donor or splice acceptor site of exon 11 (coding exon 10) result in alternative splicing and deletion of exon 11 which encodes a part of the PI3Kδ−interacting domain of p85α are responsible for APDS2 (Deau et al. 2014; Elkaim et al. 2016). A missense mutation N546 K in p85α located in the inter-SH2 domain of p85α (Wentink et al. 2017) also increases PI3Kδ activity.

Of note, SHORT syndrome, which is a rare autosomal dominant multisystem disease due to loss-of-PI3K activity, is also caused by heterozygous mutations in the *PIK3R1* gene. Mutations causing SHORT syndrome (e.g., p.R649W, p.N636Tfs*, and p.Y657*) are affecting especially the C-terminal part of p85α (Chudasama et al. 2013; Dyment et al. 2013; Thauvin-Robinet et al. 2013).

Immunological Phenotype

Class IA PI3Ks are composed of a p110 catalytic subunit (p110α, p110β, or p110δ) and a regulatory subunit (p85α, p55α, p50α, p85β, or p55γ) that regulates the stability, cellular localization, and function of p110. Class IA PI3Ks convert phosphatidylinositol 4,5-bisphosphate into phosphatidylinositol 3,4,5-trisphosphate, an important phospholipid secondary messenger (Okkenhaug 2013). Expression of the p110δ catalytic subunit is restricted mainly to leukocytes, whereas p110α and p110β are ubiquitously expressed. The widely expressed p85α regulatory subunit is the predominant regulatory subunit in lymphocytes.

PI3Kδ is expressed in both T and B lymphocytes, and patients suffer from a very variable immunodeficiency, which can present as a partial humoral or combined defect; patients can evolve into a profound combined immunodeficiency. A large proportion of patients was previously diagnosed as CSR-Ds because of increased IgM and reduced IgG (essentially IgG2 and IgG4) and IgA levels in serum, impaired antibody responses (especially to polysaccharide antigens), and a strongly decreased number of switched B cells contrasting to a strikingly increased number of transitional B cells. Somatic hypermutation frequency was found normal in the decreased CD27+ B cell subset (Angulo et al. 2013). Besides the B cell defect, patients suffer from T lymphopenia, decreased numbers of naïve CD4+ and CD8+ T cells, increased number of CD8 senescent CD57+ T cells, defective proliferation to antigens, and increased activation-induced cell death indicating an intrinsic T cell defect (Angulo et al. 2013; Deau et al. 2014; Lucas et al. 2014a).

Diagnosis

Diagnosis is made by genetic analysis of *PIK3CD* and *PIK3R1*, respectively. Suspicion should be raised in patients with respiratory tract infections, lymphoproliferative disease, dysgammaglobulinemia especially with elevated serum IgM, and expansion of transitional B cells. Functional analysis includes the evaluation of ribosomal protein S6 phosphorylation (Ser235/236) in B lymphocytes and AKT phosphorylation (Ser473) in IL2 propagated T cell blasts of patients (Lucas et al. 2014a; Heurtier et al. 2017).

Management

Treatment of APDS1 and APDS2 patients is very much dependent on the clinical presentation: successful hematopoietic stem cell transplantation was reported (Nademi et al. 2016; Kuhlen et al. 2016) and should be considered for severe forms. Ig replacement therapy is indicated for the patients with a predominant humoral defect. Inhibition of the mTOR pathway by rapamycin has shown its efficacy especially for patients presenting with lymphoproliferation (Lucas et al. 2014a; Coulter et al. 2016). Interesting perspectives for the future may be represented by specific inhibitors of PI3Kδ, currently on trial (Rao et al. 2017).

References

Angulo I, Vadas O, Garcon F, Banham-Hall E, Plagnol V, Leahy TR, et al. Phosphoinositide 3-kinase delta gene mutation predisposes to respiratory infection and airway damage. Science. 2013;342(6160):866–71. Epub 2013/10/19.

Chudasama KK, Winnay J, Johansson S, Claudi T, Konig R, Haldorsen I, et al. SHORT syndrome with partial lipodystrophy due to impaired phosphatidylinositol 3 kinase signaling. Am J Hum Genet. 2013;93(1):150–7.

Coulter TI, Chandra A, Bacon CM, Babar J, Curtis J, Screaton N, et al. Clinical spectrum and features of activated phosphoinositide 3-kinase delta syndrome: a large patient cohort study. J Allergy Clin Immunol. 2016;139:597.

Crank MC, Grossman JK, Moir S, Pittaluga S, Buckner CM, Kardava L, et al. Mutations in PIK3CD can cause hyper IgM syndrome (HIGM) associated with increased cancer susceptibility. J Clin Immunol. 2014;34(3):272–6. Epub 2014 Mar 8.

Deau MC, Heurtier L, Frange P, Suarez F, Bole-Feysot C, Nitschke P, et al. A human immunodeficiency caused by mutations in the PIK3R1 gene. J Clin Invest. 2014;124(9):3923–8.

Dulau Florea AE, Braylan RC, Schafernak KT, Williams KW, Daub J, Goyal RK, et al. Abnormal B-cell maturation in the bone marrow of patients with germline mutations in PIK3CD. J Allergy Clin Immunol. 2017;139(3):1032–5.e6. Epub 2016/10/05.

Dyment DA, Smith AC, Alcantara D, Schwartzentruber JA, Basel-Vanagaite L, Curry CJ, et al. Mutations in PIK3R1 cause SHORT syndrome. Am J Hum Genet. 2013;93(1):158–66.

Elkaim E, Neven B, Bruneau J, Mitsui-Sekinaka K, Stanislas A, Heurtier L, et al. Clinical and immunologic phenotype associated with activated phosphoinositide 3-kinase delta syndrome 2: a cohort study. J Allergy Clin Immunol. 2016;138(1):210–8.e9.

Heurtier L, Lamrini H, Chentout L, Deau MC, Bouafia A, Rosain J, et al. Mutations in the adaptor-binding domain and associated linker region of p110delta cause activated PI3K-delta syndrome 1 (APDS1). Haematologica. 2017;102:e278. Epub 2017/04/22.

Kracker S, Curtis J, Ibrahim MA, Sediva A, Salisbury J, Campr V, et al. Occurrence of B-cell lymphomas in patients with activated phosphoinositide 3-kinase delta syndrome. J Allergy Clin Immunol. 2014;134:233. Epub Epub ahead of print.

Kuhlen M, Honscheid A, Loizou L, Nabhani S, Fischer U, Stepensky P, et al. De novo PIK3R1 gain-of-function with recurrent sinopulmonary infections, long-lasting chronic CMV-lymphadenitis and microcephaly. Clin Immunol. 2016;162:27–30. Epub 2015 Oct 31.

Lougaris V, Faletra F, Lanzi G, Vozzi D, Marcuzzi A, Valencic E, et al. Altered germinal center reaction and abnormal B cell peripheral maturation in PI3KR1-mutated patients presenting with HIGM-like phenotype. Clin Immunol. 2015;159(1):33–6.

Lucas CL, Kuehn HS, Zhao F, Niemela JE, Deenick EK, Palendira U, et al. Dominant-activating germline mutations in the gene encoding the PI(3)K catalytic subunit p110delta result in T cell senescence and human immunodeficiency. Nat Immunol. 2014a;15(1):88–97. Epub 2013 Oct 28.

Lucas CL, Zhang Y, Venida A, Wang Y, Hughes J, McElwee J, et al. Heterozygous splice mutation in PIK3R1 causes human immunodeficiency with lymphoproliferation due to dominant activation of PI3K. J Exp Med. 2014b;211(13):2537–47.

Nademi Z, Slatter MA, Dvorak CC, Neven B, Fischer A, Suarez F, et al. Hematopoietic stem cell transplant in patients with activated PI3K delta syndrome. J Allergy Clin Immunol. 2016;139:1046. Epub 2016/11/17.

Okkenhaug K. Signaling by the phosphoinositide 3-kinase family in immune cells. Annu Rev Immunol. 2013;31:675–704.

Petrovski S, Parrott RE, Roberts JL, Huang H, Yang J, Gorentla B, et al. Dominant splice site mutations in PIK3R1 cause hyper IgM syndrome, lymphadenopathy and short stature. J Clin Immunol. 2016;36(5):462–71. Epub 2016/04/15.

Rae W, Gao Y, Ward D, Mattocks CJ, Eren E, Williams AP. A novel germline gain-of-function variant in PIK3CD. Clin Immunol. 2017;181:29–31. Epub 2017/06/05.

Rao VK, Webster S, Dalm V, Sediva A, van Hagen PM, Holland S, et al. Effective "activated PI3Kdelta syndrome"-targeted therapy with the PI3Kdelta inhibitor leniolisib. Blood. 2017;130(21):2307–16. Epub 2017/10/04.

Takeda AJ, Zhang Y, Dornan GL, Siempelkamp BD, Jenkins ML, Matthews HF, et al. Novel PIK3CD mutations affecting N-terminal residues of p110delta cause activated PI3Kdelta syndrome (APDS) in humans. J Allergy Clin Immunol. 2017;140(4):1152–6.e10. Epub 2017/04/18.

Thauvin-Robinet C, Auclair M, Duplomb L, Caron-Debarle M, Avila M, St-Onge J, et al. PIK3R1 mutations cause syndromic insulin resistance with lipoatrophy. Am J Hum Genet. 2013;93(1):141–9.

Tsujita Y, Mitsui-Sekinaka K, Imai K, Yeh TW, Mitsuiki N, Asano T, et al. Phosphatase and tensin homolog (PTEN) mutation can cause activated phosphatidylinositol 3-kinase delta syndrome-like immunodeficiency. J Allergy Clin Immunol. 2016;138:1672.

Wentink M, Dalm V, Lankester AC, van Schouwenburg PA, Scholvinck L, Kalina T, et al. Genetic defects in PI3Kdelta affect B-cell differentiation and maturation leading to hypogammaglobulineamia and recurrent infections. Clin Immunol. 2017;176:77–86. Epub 2017/01/21.

ADA and PNP Deficiency

Beata Derfalvi

Department of Pediatrics, IWK Health Centre, Dalhousie University, Halifax, NS, Canada

Introduction/Background

Adenosine deaminase (ADA) deficiency (OMIM# 608958) and purine nucleoside phosphorylase (PNP) deficiency (OMIM# 164050) are two genetic deficiencies of purine metabolism. The ADA gene on chromosome 20q13.12 encodes adenosine deaminase, an enzyme that catalyzes the irreversible deamination of adenosine and deoxyadenosine in the purine catabolic pathway. The PNP gene localized on chromosome 14q11.2 encodes purine nucleoside phosphorylase, an enzyme that catalyzes the reversible phosphorolysis of the purine nucleosides and deoxynucleosides (inosine, guanosine, deoxyinosine, and deoxyguanosine) (Fig. 1).

Both enzymes are ubiquitous, and defective ADA or PNP proteins are unable to effectively detoxify several naturally occurring methylated adenosine compounds of the purine salvage pathway; this results in "metabolic poisoning" that manifests its most deleterious effects in dividing cells such as lymphocytes. Although these defects primarily affect lymphocyte development, viability, and function, they also impact multiple organ systems and are considered systemic metabolic disorders (Whitmore and Gaspar 2016). The primary immunodeficiency called ADA deficiency is a consequence of ADA1 enzyme deficiency. ADA has two isoenzymes, ADA1 and ADA2, of which ADA1 is largely intracellular and widely distributed in various tissues, with the highest amounts found in the thymus, brain, and gastrointestinal tract. As a result, the major source of ADA replacement therapy was bovine intestine until 2018 when recombinant bovine ADA was first introduced.

ADA2 is more abundant in serum and is secreted by the monocyte-macrophage system. The deficiency of ADA2 (DADA2) is a completely different disease entity, a new autoinflammatory disorder characterized by an early-onset vasculopathy with livedoid skin rash associated with systemic manifestations, CNS involvement, and variable severity of CVID-like immunodeficiency. This condition is secondary to autosomal-recessive mutations of the CECR1 (Cat Eye Syndrome Chromosome Region 1) gene on chromosome 22q11.1, which encodes for the enzymatic protein ADA2.

Prior to the introduction of newborn screening (NBS) for SCID, ADA deficiency was diagnosed in approximately 40% of autosomal-recessive forms and 20% of all cases of severe combined immunodeficiency (SCID); since then, the relative frequency of SCID-ADA deficiency has decreased to 10% among all variants (Fischer et al. 2015). PNP deficiency, also inherited in an autosomal-recessive fashion, is less frequent, with

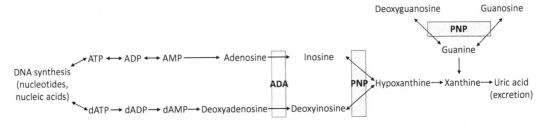

ADA and PNP Deficiency, Fig. 1 Schematic presentation of ADA and PNP metabolic pathways

fewer than 100 patients identified worldwide; hence, literature is limited.

Clinical Presentation

ADA deficiency presents with clinical and immunological manifestations typical of SCID or in a less severe form as "delayed/late"-onset combined immunodeficiency (CID). PNP-deficient patients exhibit T cell dysfunction with normal B-cell function and a variable degree and extent of immunodeficiency.

Age-Related Clinical Presentations of ADA Deficiency

ADA deficiency presents with a broad clinical spectrum in terms of onset and severity of immunodeficiency-related infections and impact on non-immunological organ systems. There are three major clinical phenotypes in ADA deficiency:

Neonatal/Infantile Onset
Clinically indistinguishable from SCID, except for bony abnormality in half of the patients. Affected patients suffer from disseminated viral (mainly herpes and respiratory tract viruses), fungal (thrush caused by *Candida albicans*), and opportunistic (*Pneumocystis jiroveci*) infections, but bacterial infections, especially sepsis, are not uncommon. All these infections are the consequences of a marked and progressive depletion of T, B, and NK lymphocytes and an absence of both humoral and cellular immune function. ADA-deficient infants exhibit failure to thrive,

and maternal T cell engraftment can cause graft-versus-host disease (GVHD).

Delayed or Late Onset
Diagnosed from 3 years of age until early adulthood and presents as a combined immunodeficiency with recurrent bacterial otitis and sinopulmonary infections, often resulting in chronic pulmonary insufficiency. Septicemia, especially caused by *Streptococcus pneumoniae*, is not uncommon. Persistent viral warts, recurrent herpes zoster and *Candida* infections, asthma, allergies, and immune abnormalities such as elevated serum concentration of IgE, as well as eosinophilia and lymphopenia, are the characteristics. Autoimmunity is frequently observed. Late-onset patients may retain 2–5% of normal ADA1 activity.

Partial ADA Deficiency
A benign condition without immunodeficiency, identified upon analysis of blood relatives of affected individuals. ADA activity is very low or absent in erythrocytes but 5–80% in nucleated cells. *ADA* genotype has a major effect on clinical phenotype, to the extent that it determines the level of exposure to ADA substrates.

Clinical Presentation of PNP Deficiency
The most common infectious complications are recurrent bacterial and viral, upper and lower respiratory tract infections. PNP-deficient patients often suffer from opportunistic infections caused by *Aspergillus fumigatus*, mycobacteria, JC virus, and *P. jiroveci*. Disseminated varicella and persistent herpes simplex virus infections were also observed.

Noninfectious Manifestations of ADA and PNP Deficiencies

Immune dysregulation is common in delayed or late-onset phenotype. The clinical spectrum of immune dysregulation includes multiple forms of autoimmunity, such as autoimmune cytopenia (hemolytic anemia, immune thrombocytopenia), type 1 diabetes mellitus, hypothyroidism, hepatitis, and glomerulonephritis in both ADA and PNP deficiencies. Lupus and central nervous system vasculitis were only described in PNP deficiency (Sauer et al. 2012). Malignancy, especially EBV-related lymphoma, was also observed. Patients with ADA deficiency have susceptibility to a rare mesenchymal tumor of the skin known as dermatofibrosarcoma protuberans.

Syndromic Features in ADA Deficiency

Neurological abnormalities include neurosensorial deafness, cognitive and behavioral impairments, developmental delay, hypotonia, nystagmus, and seizures. Many of these impairments are both a consequence of the metabolic disturbance in ADA deficiency and dependent on the degree of deficiency. Skeletal abnormality may occur in costochondral junctions, detectable by lateral view of chest radiograph or by physical exam (similar to "rachitic rosary"). Kidney abnormalities result in impaired renal function secondary to mesangial sclerosis. Additional abnormalities such as pyloric stenosis and adrenal cortical fibrosis might reflect the effects of infectious agents rather than primary effects due to ADA deficiency (Hirschhorn and Candotti 2006; Grunebaum et al. 2013; Flinn and Gennery 2018).

Syndromic Features in PNP Deficiency

Neurological abnormalities develop in over 50% of PNP-deficient patients. Neurodevelopmental delay often precedes the onset of immunodeficiency. Spastic paresis such as spastic diplegia or tetraparesis (may be confused with cerebral palsy), tremor, hyper- or hypotonia, ataxia, retarded motor development, behavioral difficulties, and mental retardation are observed (Hirschhorn and Candotti 2006).

Diagnosis/Laboratory Testing

ADA Deficiency

Immunological abnormalities include progressive lymphopenia affecting all compartments (T, B, and natural killer (NK) cells). Since the generation of T cells and thymic function is normal, TREC assay will only decrease after the accumulation of toxic purine pathway metabolites and death of naïve lymphocytes. In this case, patients may be identified by newborn SCID screening. ADA deficiency is, however, the only form of SCID that might be missed by newborn screening if the progression of loss of lymphocytes is slower.

In the neonatal-onset form, T cells do not proliferate in response to mitogen and antigen stimulation, and immunoglobulins are undetectable or very low around 4–6 months of age, after loss of transplacental maternal immunoglobulin G (IgG).

In milder forms with some residual ADA activity, there is only mild lymphopenia, but markedly reduced lymphocyte proliferation to mitogens such as phytohemagglutinin (PHA) is observed. Antibody deficiency is usually IgG2 subclass deficiency and poor vaccine response to antigens such as *S. pneumoniae* polysaccharides. IgE is elevated, and eosinophilia is often present (Grunebaum et al. 2013) (Table 1).

The diagnosis of ADA deficiency is established in an individual with <1% of normal ADA catalytic activity in erythrocyte lysates or – if transfused – in extracts of other cells (e.g., blood mononuclear cells, fibroblasts). Increased levels of dATP and deoxyadenosine in urine can also aid the diagnosis (Hershfield 2017). In the United States, the reference laboratory for ADA functional assays including enzyme activity and measurements of toxic metabolites is at Dr. Michael Hershfield's laboratory at Duke University School of Medicine.

The diagnosis can be supported by identification of biallelic pathogenic variants (homozygous or compound heterozygous) in the ADA gene by next-generation sequencing (NGS). In case of variants of unknown significance, functional assays for ADA catalytic

ADA and PNP Deficiency, Table 1 Immune abnormalities in ADA and PNP deficiencies (Grunebaum et al. 2013; Flinn and Gennery 2018)

ADA deficiency	PNP deficiency
Thymus: severe thymus atrophy, maturation defect in thymic epithelial cells including the absence of medullary thymic epithelial cells with autoimmune regulator (AIRE) expression	Marked depletion of lymphoid tissues (thymus, tonsils, lymph nodes, and spleen) Only plasma cells can be identified in the spleen, lymph nodes, and intestines
Absent or markedly diminished CD3+ T lymphocytes, CD4/CD8 ratio often reversed, absent T cell receptor excision circles in severe neonatal forms, reduced CD4 + CD25 + FoxP3+ Treg cells	Marked T cell lymphopenia, absence of T cell receptor excision circles
Abnormal T cell function: absent to markedly reduced proliferation to mitogens (PHA), absent to trace proliferation to antigens, abnormal CD4+ T cell TCR/CD28-driven activation	Abnormal T cell function: lack of lymphocyte response to mitogenic stimulation
Absent or markedly diminished B-cell count Abnormal B-cell function: absent or low IgG (in late onset especially IgG2), absent or very low specific antibody titers, excess autoreactive transitional and mature naïve B-cell clones, reduced B-cell receptor and Toll-like receptor functions	Variable B-cell deficiency; immunoglobulin levels might be normal, but absent vaccine-specific antibodies

activity, measurement of protein expression, and toxic metabolites are needed to confirm the association. This is especially important in the era of gene therapy when the immunodeficiency can be corrected by transduction with the normal ADA gene.

PNP Deficiency

Immunological abnormalities include progressive decline in the number of T cells, while B and NK cells are often spared. T cell function, measured by stimulation of lymphocyte proliferation with antigen and mitogen, is abnormal. PNP deficiency is not frequently associated with profound B-cell defects. Immunoglobulin levels might be within normal range, but specific antibody responses are poor (Table 1). Radiochemical or spectrophotometric assays that reveal the absence of PNP activity in erythrocyte lysates can confirm the diagnosis. Low serum and urinary levels of uric acid support the diagnosis. Rarely, serum uric acid is within the pediatric normal range; therefore, PNP deficiency should not be ruled out in the absence of hypouricemia. Urine levels of inosine, deoxyinosine, guanosine, and deoxyguanosine are characteristically high. Homozygous mutation of the PNP gene by NSG can confirm the diagnosis.

Genotype-Phenotype Correlation

Correlations between specific mutations, residual ADA activity, metabolite concentration, age at onset, and severity of disease appear to be present in ADA deficiency; however, other genetic and nongenetic factors (e.g., infections) can modify the phenotype in patients with identical pathogenic gene variants. Somatic mosaicism, due to de novo mutations during embryogenesis and resulting in only a proportion of cells that carry the inherited disease-causing gene variant, can significantly modify the clinical phenotype (Hershfield 2003). Because of the low numbers of PNP-deficient patients described in the literature, there is no genotype-phenotype correlation established for this disease.

Treatment/Prognosis

ADA Deficiency

If immune function is not restored, children with ADA-deficient SCID rarely survive beyond 1 to 2 years of age.

Infections are treated with specific antibiotic, antiviral, and antifungal agents. *P. jiroveci* prophylaxis is recommended with trimethoprim-sulfamethoxazole.

Antibody deficiency requires immunoglobulin replacement therapy (IgRT) via either intravenous or subcutaneous route.

Enzyme replacement therapy (ERT) with polyethylene glycol-modified ADA (PEG-ADA) administered weekly (30 U/kg) by intramuscular injection is recommended to stabilize the metabolic status of patients until autologous or allogenic hematopoietic stem cell transplantation (HSCT) is available. This is a lifesaving but not curative treatment for patients lacking a donor or awaiting gene therapy. Dosage regimen may be individualized, based on monitoring of PEG-ADA levels in plasma and toxic metabolite levels (dATP or total dAdo nucleotides: the sum of dAMP, dADP, and dATP) in erythrocytes. Periodic testing for anti-ADA antibodies is also recommended, since in approximately 10% of cases, neutralizing antibodies impair the effect of ERT. ERT has resulted in the development of protective, although not normal, T cell immunity in 80% of treated patients, and approximately half of PEG-ADA-treated patients have been able to discontinue IgRT. No toxic or hypersensitivity reactions to PEG-ADA have been reported, but there have been examples of several manifestations of immune dysregulation, including autoimmunity, malignancies, and progression of chronic pulmonary insufficiency (Sauer et al. 2012). The need for prolonged use of PEG-ADA for several years has been reported among patients who received and failed HSCT therapy. The expenses of few years prolonged PEG-ADA replacement therapy near the cost of HSCT. Therefore, it is still recommended medically and financially that patients be offered HSCT, if needed, even repeatedly.

Restoration of a functional immune system is essential for long-term survival. The preferred treatment is HSCT from an HLA-identical relative (usually a sibling) since this has a superior outcome in terms of overall survival as well as immune recovery in comparison to transplant from matched unrelated or haploidentical donors (Hirschhorn and Candotti 2006; Flinn and Gennery 2018).

Gene therapy with retroviral vectors has been pursued on over 200 ADA-deficient patients in clinical trials. Specifically, ex vivo autologous hematopoietic stem cells (CD34+ enriched cell fraction) are transduced with retrovirus containing the ADA cDNA sequence. Although the insertion site in the genome is not directed, ADA retroviral vectors are not associated with increased risk of malignancy, unlike first-generation IL2RG gene therapy trials. The patients require reduced intensity conditioning before the transfusion of modified stem cells. The ex vivo stem cell retroviral vector ADA gene therapy (Strimvelis™) is the first genetic treatment for SCID that received approval by the European Medicines Agency in 2016. Currently, lentiviral studies are ongoing that show great promise with high transduction rate. In summary, a high level (50–90%) of gene correction in T, B, and NK cells has been detected in all variants of gene therapy, leading to an efficient systemic detoxification and immune recovery, but there is significant risk of autoimmunity post gene therapy. No leukemic or oncogenic events have been reported, indicating that ADA-SCID gene therapy has a favorable risk/benefit profile; however, long-term safety needs to be monitored.

Genetic counseling is recommended, to reduce morbidity and mortality through early diagnosis and treatment. If the pathogenic variants in the proband have been identified by molecular genetic testing, carrier testing for at-risk family members and prenatal testing for pregnancies are recommended. Alternatively, relatives at risk can be evaluated by assaying ADA catalytic activity in red blood cells (Hirschhorn and Candotti 2006).

PNP Deficiency

HSCT is the treatment of choice in PNP deficiency, but overall prognosis is poor. Even when engraftment is successful, the neurological deficit does not improve (Grunebaum et al. 2013).

Cross-References

- ▶ Evaluation of Suspected Immunodeficiency, Genetic Testing
- ▶ Management of Immunodeficiency, Antibiotic Therapy
- ▶ Management of Immunodeficiency, Bone Marrow Transplantation
- ▶ Management of Immunodeficiency: Gene Therapy
- ▶ Management of Immunodeficiency, IgG Replacement (IV)
- ▶ Management of Immunodeficiency, IgG Replacement (SC)

References

Fischer A, Notarangelo LD, Neven B, Cavazzana M, Puck JM. Severe combined immunodeficiencies and related disorders. Nat Rev Dis Prim. 2015;1:15061.

Flinn AM, Gennery AR. Adenosine deaminase deficiency: a review. Orphanet J Rare Dis. 2018;13(1):65.

Grunebaum E, Cohen A, Roifman CM. Recent advances in understanding and managing adenosine deaminase and purine nucleoside phosphorylase deficiencies. Curr Opin Allergy Clin Immunol. 2013;13(6): 630–8.

Hershfield MS. Genotype is an important determinant of phenotype in adenosine deaminase deficiency. Curr Opin Immunol. 2003;15(5):571–7.

Hershfield M. Adenosine deaminase deficiency. 2006 Oct 3 [Updated 2017 Mar 16]. In: Adam MP, Ardinger HH, Pagon RA, Wallace SE, Bean LJH, Stephens K, editors. GeneReviews® [Internet]. Seattle: University of Washington, Seattle; 1993–2018. Available from: https://www.ncbi.nlm.nih.gov/books/NBK1483/

Hirschhorn R, Candotti F. Immunodeficiency due to defects of purine metabolism. In: Ochs HD, Smith CIE, Puck JM, editors. Primary immunodeficiency diseases. 2nd ed. New York: Oxford University Press; 2006. p. 169–96.

Sauer AV, Brigida I, Carriglio N, Aiuti A. Autoimmune dysregulation and purine metabolism in adenosine deaminase deficiency. Front Immunol. 2012;3:265.

Whitmore KV, Gaspar HB. Adenosine deaminase deficiency – more than just an immunodeficiency. Front Immunol. 2016;7:314.

AD-HIES

- ▶ Autosomal Dominant Hyper IgE Syndrome

Aicardi-Goutières Syndrome (AGS1–AGS7)

Victoria Tüngler, Anne Sophie Kubasch and Min Ae Lee-Kirsch
Department of Pediatrics, Medizinische Fakultät Carl Gustav Carus, Technische Universität Dresden, Dresden, Germany

Synonyms

Familial infantile, with intracranial calcification and chronic cerebrospinal fluid lymphocytosis; Pseudotoxoplasmosis syndrome

Definition

Aicardi-Goutières syndrome (AGS) is a genetically defined inflammatory encephalopathy with onset in infancy with clinical features reminiscent of an in utero acquired viral infection including basal ganglia calcification, microcephaly, leukodystrophy, and cerebrospinal fluid (CSF) lymphocytosis. It is caused by predominantly recessive loss-of-function mutations in the deoxyribonuclease *TREX1* (AGS1, MIM#225750); the three subunits of ribonuclease H (RNase H2) encoded by *RNASEH2B* (AGS2, MIM#610181), *RNASEH2C* (AGS3, MIM#610329), and *RNASEH2A* (AGS4, MIM#610333); the triphosphohydrolase and ribonuclease *SAMHD1* (AGS5, MIM#612952); and the RNA-editing enzyme *ADAR* (AGS6, MIM#615010). AGS subtype 7 is caused by autosomal dominant or de novo gain-of-function mutations in *IFIH1* (AGS7, MIM#615846) encoding the dsRNA sensor MDA5.

Introduction and Background

First described by Aicardi and Goutières in 1984, AGS is a rare immune-mediated inflammatory disorder mainly affecting the brain (Aicardi and Goutieres 1984). The cardinal features comprise a subacute encephalopathy with cerebrospinal

Aicardi-Goutières Syndrome (AGS1–AGS7), Table 1 Clinical findings in Aicardi-Goutières syndrome

Symptoms	Laboratory	Neuroimaging
Common Irritability, dystonia Truncal hypotonia Spastic tetraplegia Progressive microcephaly Seizures Profound developmental delay	**Common** CSF lymphocytosis Increased IFN-α in CSF Interferon signature in blood	**Common** Bilateral intracerebral calcifications, especially in the basal ganglia Progressive cerebral atrophy Leukodystrophy
Less common Sterile pyrexia Chilblain lesions Hepatosplenomegaly Arthritis	**Less common** Increased neopterin in CSF Elevated liver enzymes Thrombocytopenia Autoantibodies	**Less common** Intracerebral vasculopathy Bilateral striatal necrosis

CSF cerebrospinal fluid, *IFN* interferon

fluid (CSF) pleocytosis and raised levels of CSF interferon (IFN)-α along with radiologic evidence of intracranial calcifications, cerebral white matter abnormalities, and brain atrophy (Table 1). The clinical picture mimics congenital viral infection despite the absence of evidence for an infectious cause. AGS is a genetically defined disease and in most cases inherited as an autosomal recessive trait. All seven genes that have been implicated in AGS thus far encode proteins involved in the metabolism or the immune recognition of endogenous nucleic acids including both DNA and RNA (Lee-Kirsch 2017). Thus, a loss of function of the nucleic acid-degrading enzymes, TREX1 and RNase H2, or the RNA-editing enzyme ADAR results in the intracellular accumulation of nucleic acid species that activate nucleic acid sensors, which subsequently initiate a type I IFN-mediated innate immune response. Type I IFN plays a central role in the immune defense against viral infections. Normally, type I IFN signaling is activated by pattern recognition receptors upon sensing of viral nucleic acids which initiates antiviral programs through the modulation of innate and adaptive immune responses. An inappropriate chronic activation of type I IFN causes autoinflammation and may also induce a loss of immune tolerance leading to autoimmunity. AGS belongs to a group of immunological disorders characterized by a constitutive type I IFN activation that are referred to as type I interferonopathies (Lee-Kirsch 2017).

Genetics

AGS is a genetically heterogeneous disorder and caused by mutations in seven nonallelic genes, including *TREX1* (AGS1), *RNASEH2B* (AGS2), *RNASEH2C* (AGS3), *RNASEH2A* (AGS4), *SAMHD1* (AGS5), *ADAR* (AGS6), and *IFIH1* (AGS7) (Table 2) (Lee-Kirsch 2017). The AGS subtypes 1 to 5 are inherited in an autosomal recessive manner and caused by biallelic loss-of-function mutations, although rare de novo dominant-negative mutations in *TREX1* have been described. Similarly, AGS subtype 6 is caused by loss-of-function mutations in *ADAR* that may be inherited as autosomal recessive trait or occur as heterozygous de novo mutation, while AGS subtype 7 is caused by autosomal dominant or de novo dominant gain-of-function mutations (Table 2).

Pathogenesis

AGS causing gene mutations lead to disturbances in the intracellular metabolism or the sensing of nucleic acids. TREX1 functions as a cytosolic deoxyribonuclease with high specificity for single-stranded DNA (ssDNA). TREX1 deficiency results in intracellular accrual of ssDNA metabolites, which activate DNA sensing pathways leading to type I IFN induction (Lee-Kirsch 2017). *RNASEH2A*, *RNASEH2B*, and *RNASEH2C* encode the three subunits of the

Aicardi-Goutières Syndrome (AGS1–AGS7), Table 2 Aicardi-Goutières syndrome subtypes

Subtype	Gene	Inheritance	Protein function
AGS1	*TREX1*	Autosomal recessive, de novo dominant	3′ Repair exonuclease; cytosolic deoxyribonuclease
AGS2	*RNASEH2B*	Autosomal recessive	Ribonuclease H2, subunits A, B, C; ribonucleotide excision repair
AGS3	*RNASEH2C*		
AGS4	*RNASEH2A*		
AGS5	*SAMHD1*	Autosomal recessive	SAM domain and HD domain-containing protein 1; dNTP degrading triphosphohydrolase, ribonuclease
AGS6	*ADAR*	Autosomal recessive, de novo dominant	Adenosine deaminase, RNA-specific; editing of dsRNA
AGS7	*IFIH1*	Autosomal dominant, de novo dominant	IFN-induced helicase C domain-containing protein 1; pattern recognition receptor for dsRNA

dNTP deoxynucleoside triphosphate, *dsRNA* double-stranded ribonucleic acid, *IFN* interferon

RNase H2 complex that removes ribonucleotides misincorporated into genomic DNA (Reijns et al. 2012). A lack of RNase H2 promotes DNA damage and leads to enhanced formation of DNA repair metabolites, which also activate DNA sensing pathways (Gunther et al. 2015). The deoxynucleoside triphosphate (dNTP) triphosphohydrolase SAMHD1 degrades dNTPs required for DNA synthesis during replication and has also ribonuclease activity. Loss of SAMHD1 causes cell cycle arrest and DNA damage due to imbalances in dNTP pools (Kretschmer et al. 2015). Type I IFN activation may be caused by DNA damage repair metabolites. ADAR catalyzes the deamination of adenosine to inosine in dsRNA. This chemical modification prevents the sensing of endogenous dsRNA as nonself (Liddicoat et al. 2015). Gain-of-function mutations in *IFIH1* encoding MDA5, a pattern recognition receptor for long dsRNA, increase receptor affinity resulting in enhanced type I IFN signaling (Lee-Kirsch 2017).

Clinical Manifestation

In its classical form, AGS presents during the first year of life as a subacute encephalopathy after a period of apparently normal development.

Neurological Manifestations
Neurologic symptoms are the most prominent. Patients usually present with severe irritability,

feeding difficulties, dystonic movements, leading to progressive microcephaly, truncal hypotonia, and spastic tetraplegia (Table 1). Typically, the encephalopathic period lasts a few months and may be accompanied by intermittent sterile pyrexia and seizures. AGS usually causes permanent neurological damage and results in loss of skills with severe developmental delay. During the early phase of the disease, examination of CSF often reveals lymphocytosis and increased levels of IFN-α (Lebon et al. 1988). Neuroimaging findings include bilateral symmetric calcifications, particularly within the basal ganglia or the periventricular area extending into the white matter, leukodystrophy, as well as cerebral atrophy (Fig. 1a, b). Owing to its clinical and neuroimaging findings, AGS is often misdiagnosed as congenital viral infection, although serologic tests for the typical infectious causes such as cytomegaly, rubella, herpes simplex, as well as toxoplasmosis remain negative. At later stages, the clinical course of AGS remains static and is characterized by severe neurological impairment, although few patients show further episodes of disease progression. The intrafamilial variability can be high with one sibling presenting with classic AGS and the other with only mild spasticity and normal intellectual abilities (Lee-Kirsch 2017).

Other Manifestations
Concomitant extraneurologic symptoms include cold-induced inflammatory cutaneous lesions at

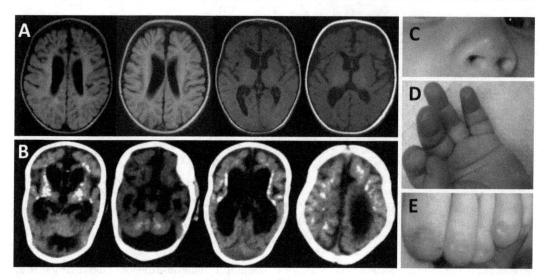

Aicardi-Goutières Syndrome (AGS1–AGS7), Fig. 1
Neuroimaging findings and cutaneous signs in Aicardi-Goutières syndrome. (**a**) Magnetic resonance imaging of a patient with AGS3 showing extensive white matter abnormalities with an anteroposterior gradient in addition to cortical atrophy. (**b**) Computed tomography imaging of a patient with AGS4 demonstrating marked brain atrophy with prominent cerebellar atrophy as well as symmetrical calcifications of the basal ganglia and periventricular region extending throughout the cerebrum. (**c–e**) Typical chilblain lesions on nose, finger tips, and toes presenting as erythematosus painful swellings in a patient with AGS1. (Adapted from (Ramantani et al. 2010) with permission from John Wiley & Sons, Inc.)

acral location referred to as chilblain lesions (Fig. 1c–e). In addition, some patients develop signs of autoimmunity such as arthritis, oral ulcers, antinuclear antibodies or other autoantibodies, reduced complement, or lymphopenia (Ramantani et al. 2010; Cuadrado et al. 2014). A small group of patients already presents either prenatally with intracranial calcification and intrauterine growth retardation or at birth with hepatosplenomegaly, elevated liver enzymes, and thrombocytopenia along with neurologic findings.

In addition, there is also phenotypic variability depending on the genetic cause. Thus, patients with *RNASEH2B* mutations tend to show a milder course of the disease with a later onset, while patients with *SAMHD1* mutations may present with intracerebral large artery disease (du Moulin et al. 2011). On contrast, patients with *ADAR* mutations may present with bilateral striatal necrosis without any signs of leukodystrophy. Mutations in *ADAR*, *IFIH1*, and *RNASEH2B* may also present as nonsyndromic spastic paraplegia (Crow et al. 2014).

Laboratory Findings

Patients with AGS typically show lymphocytosis and increased IFN-α in the CSF. In addition, increased levels of neopterin in CSF as a nonspecific sign of inflammation have also been described. While IFN-α in the CSF tends to gradually decrease over the course of the disease, AGS patients consistently exhibit an increased expression of IFN-stimulated genes in peripheral blood cells, which is also referred to as interferon signature (Rice et al. 2013). Less specific laboratory findings include thrombocytopenia, autoantibodies, or raised liver function tests.

Diagnosis

AGS should be taken into consideration in an individual with symptoms, neuroimaging, and laboratory findings listed in Table 1 after exclusion of congenital infection and other metabolic or neurodegenerative disorders. Although the finding of a chronic interferon signature in blood in an infant with typical neurological symptoms is highly suggestive of AGS, the definitive diagnosis of AGS can only be established by molecular genetic analysis.

Treatment

Currently, there is no causal therapy for AGS available. Treatment strategies are based on symptomatic and supportive therapies. However, based on the knowledge gained recently on disease pathology more targeted treatment concepts are emerging. Given the central role of a constitutive activation of the type I IFN axis in AGS pathogenesis, immunomodulation by inhibition of uncontrolled type I IFN signaling using for example Janus kinase (JAK) inhibitors may represent a promising therapeutic approach. However, further clinical studies are required to test the potential therapeutic benefit of such intervention.

References

Aicardi J, Goutieres F. A progressive familial encephalopathy in infancy with calcifications of the basal ganglia and chronic cerebrospinal fluid lymphocytosis. Ann Neurol. 1984;15(0364–5134 (Print)):49–54.

Crow YJ, Zaki MS, Abdel-Hamid MS, Abdel-Salam G, Boespflug-Tanguy O, Cordeiro NJV, Gleeson JG, Gowrinathan NR, Laugel V, Renaldo F, Rodriguez D, Livingston JH, Rice GI. Mutations in ADAR1, IFIH1, and RNASEH2B presenting as spastic paraplegia. Neuropediatrics. 2014;45(6):386–93.

Cuadrado E, Vanderver A, Brown KJ, Sandza A, Takanohashi A, Jansen MH, Anink J, Herron B, Orcesi S, Olivieri I, Rice GI, Aronica E, Lebon P, Crow YJ, Hol EM, Kuijpers TW. Aicardi–Goutières syndrome harbours abundant systemic and brain-reactive autoantibodies. Ann Rheum Dis. 2014; https://doi.org/10.1136/annrheumdis-2014-205396.

du Moulin M, Nürnberg P, Crow YJ, Rutsch F. Cerebral vasculopathy is a common feature in Aicardi–Goutières syndrome associated with SAMHD1 mutations. Proc Natl Acad Sci. 2011;108(26):E232.

Gunther C, Kind B, Reijns MA, Berndt N, Martinez-Bueno M, Wolf C, Tungler V, Chara O, Lee YA, Hubner N, Bicknell L, Blum S, Krug C, Schmidt F, Kretschmer S, Koss S, Astell KR, Ramantani G, Bauerfeind A, Morris DL, Cunninghame Graham DS, Bubeck D, Leitch A, Ralston SH, Blackburn EA, Gahr M, Witte T, Vyse TJ, Melchers I, Mangold E, Nothen MM, Aringer M, Kuhn A, Luthke K,

Unger L, Bley A, Lorenzi A, Isaacs JD, Alexopoulou D, Conrad K, Dahl A, Roers A, Arcon-Riquelme ME, Jackson AP, Lee-Kirsch MA. Defective removal of ribonucleotides from DNA promotes systemic autoimmunity. J Clin Invest. 2015;125(1558–8238 (Electronic)):413–24.

Kretschmer S, Wolf C, Konig N, Staroske W, Guck J, Hausler M, Luksch H, Nguyen LA, Kim B, Alexopoulou D, Dahl A, Rapp A, Cardoso MC, Shevchenko A, Lee-Kirsch MA. SAMHD1 prevents autoimmunity by maintaining genome stability. Ann Rheum Dis. 2015;74(3):e17. https://doi.org/10.1136/annrheumdis-2013-204845. Epub 2014 Jan 20.

Lebon P, Badoual J, Ponsot G, Goutieres F, Hemeury-Cukier F, Aicardi J. Intrathecal synthesis of interferon-alpha in infants with progressive familial encephalopathy. J Neurol Sci. 1988;84(0022–510X (Print)):201–8.

Lee-Kirsch MA. The type I Interferonopathies. Annu Rev Med. 2017;68:297–315.

Liddicoat BJ, Piskol R, Chalk AM, Ramaswami G, Higuchi M, Hartner JC, Li JB, Seeburg PH, Walkley CR. RNA editing by ADAR1 prevents MDA5 sensing of endogenous dsRNA as nonself. Science. 2015;349(6252):1115–20.

Ramantani G, Kohlhase J, Hertzberg C, Innes AM, Engel K, Hunger S, Borozdin W, Mah JK, Ungerath K, Walkenhorst H, Richardt HH, Buckard J, Bevot A, Siegel C, von SC, Ikonomidou C, Thomas K, Proud V, Niemann F, Wieczorek D, Hausler M, Niggemann P, Baltaci V, Conrad K, Lebon P, Lee-Kirsch MA. Expanding the phenotypic spectrum of lupus erythematosus in Aicardi-Goutieres syndrome. Arthritis Rheum. 2010;62(1529–0131 (Electronic)):1469–77.

Reijns MA, Rabe B, Rigby RE, Mill P, Astell KR, Lettice LA, Boyle S, Leitch A, Keighren M, Kilanowski F, Devenney PS, Sexton D, Grimes G, Holt IJ, Hill RE, Taylor MS, Lawson KA, Dorin JR, Jackson AP. Enzymatic removal of ribonucleotides from DNA is essential for mammalian genome integrity and development. Cell. 2012;149(1097–4172 (Electronic)):1008–22.

Rice GI, Forte GM, Szynkiewicz M, Chase DS, Aeby A, Abdel-Hamid MS, Ackroyd S, Allcock R, Bailey KM, Balottin U, Barnerias C, Bernard G, Bodemer C, Botella MP, Cereda C, Chandler KE, Dabydeen L, Dale RC, De Laet C, De Goede CG, Del TM, Effat L, Enamorado NN, Fazzi E, Gener B, Haldre M, Lin JP, Livingston JH, Lourenco CM, Marques W Jr, Oades P, Peterson P, Rasmussen M, Roubertie A, Schmidt JL, Shalev SA, Simon R, Spiegel R, Swoboda KJ, Temtamy SA, Vassallo G, Vilain CN, Vogt J, Wermenbol V, Whitehouse WP, Soler D, Olivieri I, Orcesi S, Aglan MS, Zaki MS, Abdel-Salam GM, Vanderver A, Kisand K, Rozenberg F, Lebon P, Crow YJ. Assessment of interferon-related biomarkers in Aicardi-Goutieres syndrome associated with mutations in TREX1, RNASEH2A, RNASEH2B, RNASEH2C, SAMHD1, and ADAR: a case-control study. Lancet Neurol. 2013;12(1474–4465 (Electronic)):1159–69.

AIFEC

▶ NLRC4-Associated Autoinflammatory Diseases

AILJK – Autoimmune Interstitial Lung, Joint, and Kidney Disease

▶ COPA Syndrome

AIPDS Autoinflammation, Panniculitis, and Dermatosis Syndrome

▶ OTULIN Deficiency-Associated Disease Spectrum

Alpha Polypeptide

▶ CD8 Alpha (CD8A) Deficiency

Alymphoid Cystic Thymic Dysgenesis

▶ Winged Helix Deficiency (FOXN1)

Amylopectinosis

▶ LUBAC Deficiencies

Anhidrotic Ectodermal Dysplasia with Immunodeficiency (EDA-ID), Autosomal-Dominant

Jacob Rozmus
Department of Pediatrics, BC Children's Hospital and The University of British Columbia, Vancouver, BC, Canada

Synonyms

Human IkB-alpha gain of function

Definition

Autosomal-dominant EDA-ID (OMIM # 612132) is an immune deficiency with ectodermal dysplasia caused by germline heterozygous gain-of-function mutations in *NFKBIA* which encodes IkB-alpha.

Introduction

The NF-kB signaling cascade is comprised of transcription factors that are normally sequestered in an inactive state in the cytoplasm through an association with inhibitory proteins such as IkB-alpha. Signaling through a variety of cell surface receptors involved in innate (TLRs, IL-1Rs, TNFRs) and adaptive (TCR and BCR) immunity triggers the phosphorylation of two key serine residues (S32 and S36) leading to its dissociation and subsequent proteasomal degradation. Once free from inhibition, NF-kB transcription factors are free to translocate to the nucleus and initiate cell-specific gene expression programs. Autosomal-dominant EDA-ID is associated with gain of function mutations in *NFKBIA* that reduce the degradation of IkB-alpha, thus impairing NF-kB signaling.

Genetics

Autosomal-dominant EDA-ID was first described in 2003 (Courtois et al. 2003). To date only 14 patients with 11 mutations have been described in the literature (Boisson et al. 2017). All mutations associated with autosomal-dominant EDA-ID enhance the inhibitory capacity of IkB-alpha to block NF-kB activation by preventing its phosphorylation on S32 and S36 and subsequent degradation. Mutations belong to one of two groups: (1) missense mutations (point mutations) affecting S32, S36, or neighboring amino acids and (2) nonsense mutations (truncation mutations) that lead to the production of a mutant protein that skips S32 or S36 limiting its ability to be degraded (Petersheim et al. 2017). IkB-alpha point mutations were shown to accumulate at higher levels compared with truncation mutations in transfected cells and are associated with more severe disease and greater impairment of NF-kB signaling in patient cells.

Disease Manifestations

Leukocytes from patients with autosomal-dominant EDA-ID have impaired Toll/interleukin-1 receptor (TIR), tumor necrosis factor receptor (TNFR1), and CD40 responses to stimuli. T-cell function mediated through TCR engagement is impaired. Most patients also had abnormally large total B-cell numbers but with a reduction or absence of memory B cells. Dysgammaglobulinemia was often detected, and patients had only low levels or no antibodies to vaccine antigens. Impaired NF-kB-mediated responses in innate and adaptive immune cells lead to a clinical phenotype consisting of multiple, severe infections caused by bacteria, fungi, and viruses beginning in early infancy.[2] Bacterial infections include upper respiratory infections and pneumonia due to *Klebsiella*, *Pseudomonas aeruginosa*, or *Haemophilus influenza* and sepsis or meningitis due to *Streptococcus* or *Staphylococcus aureus*. Three patients developed mycobacterial infection caused by the BCG vaccine.

Multiple patients suffered chronic mucocutaneous candidiasis and severe viral infections caused by rotavirus, norovirus, parainfluenza virus, RSV, and CMV. The majority of patients also presented with recurrent diarrhea and/or colitis without a clear inflammatory or infectious cause. Lastly, 13 of the 14 patients had varying presentations of anhidrotic ectodermal dysplasia including sparse hair, abnormal or missing teeth, and inability to sweat.

Diagnosis

Laboratory evaluation should include quantitative immunoglobulins, measurement of vaccine antibody titers, flow cytometry for B-cell subpopulations, T-cell proliferation to specific antigens, and Toll-like receptor assays. Sequencing of the gene for *NFKBIA* will confirm the diagnosis.

Treatment

The outcome and treatment of all 14 patients has been reported.[2] One patient died prior to 1 year of age. The 11 remaining patients underwent allogeneic hematopoietic stem cell transplantation (HSCT) to correct the underlying hematological abnormalities of which 6 died after HSCT from bacterial sepsis ($n = 3$), progressive neurodegenerative disease ($n = 1$), acute respiratory distress ($n = 1$), or cerebellar hemorrhage ($n = 1$). Of the five cases who underwent successful HSCT, all still have the EDA phenotype and four still have persistent partial immunodeficiency and are on intravenous immunoglobulin (IVIG) replacement therapy due to engraftment difficulties. For the two remaining patients without HSCT, both patients are on IVIG therapy and one has been receiving anti-tuberculosis treatment, recombinant IFN-gamma therapy as long-term antimycobacterial treatment, and antibiotic prophylaxis. The published cases suggest that HSCT is a high-risk undertaking that requires further investigation.

Cross-References

▶ Anhidrotic Ectodermal Dysplasia with Immunodeficiency (EDA-ID), X-linked

References

Boisson B, Puel A, Picard C, Casanova JL. Human IkBalpha gain of function: a severe and syndromic immunodeficiency. J Clin Immunol. 2017;37(5):397–412.

Courtois G, Smahi A, Reichenbach J, et al. A hypermorphic IkappaBalpha mutation is associated with autosomal dominant anhidrotic ectodermal dysplasia and T cell immunodeficiency. J Clin Invest. 2003;112(7):1108–15.

Petersheim D, Massaad MJ, Lee S, et al. Mechanisms of genotype-phenotype correlation in autosomal dominant anhidrotic ectodermal dysplasia with immune deficiency. J Allergy Clin Immunol. 2017;143:1060. e3. Pii: S0091-6749(17)30984-3

Anhidrotic Ectodermal Dysplasia with Immunodeficiency (EDA-ID), X-linked

Jacob Rozmus
Department of Pediatrics, BC Children's Hospital and The University of British Columbia, Vancouver, BC, Canada

Synonyms

IKK-gamma deficiency; NF-kappa-B essential modulator (NEMO) deficiency

Definition

X-linked recessive EDA-ID (OMIM # 300291) is an immune deficiency with hypohidrotic ectodermal dysplasia caused by hypomorphic hemizygous mutations in *IKBKG* which encodes IKK-gamma/NF-kappa-B essential modulator (NEMO).

Introduction

The NF-B signaling cascade is comprised of transcription factors that are normally sequestered in an inactive state in the cytoplasm. They are held in an inactive state through their interaction with IkB inhibitors. In response to a variety of immune and inflammatory stimuli, the IkB molecules become phosphorylated by an IkB kinase (IKK) core complex on two critical serine residues. This is a prerequisite to recognition by UBE2D3 leading to polyubiquitination and subsequent proteasomal degradation. This releases the NF-kB transcription factors and allows them to translocate into the nucleus where they initiate distinct profiles of gene expression depending on the cell type. NEMO/IKK-gamma is the regulatory subunit of the IKK core complex which also includes two kinases, IKK-alpha and IKK-beta, that is, responsible for phosphorylating the IkB inhibitors and releasing the transcription factors. The clinical manifestations of X-linked EDA-ID are characterized by hypomorphic mutations in the NEMO gene that impair NF-kB signaling in a wide variety of cell types.

Genetics

The 23-kb human *IKBKG* gene is composed of ten exons with four alternative noncoding first exons on the human X-chromosome (Xq28). It is located in a region with a sequential duplication comprising a partial nonfunctional truncated pseudogene copy. Human IKK-gamma is a 419-amino acid protein with a predicted molecular weight of 48 kDa composed of two coiled-coil regions (CC1 – aa 100–194, CC2 – aa 260–292), a UBAN (ubiquitin binding in ABIN and NEMO proteins) domain, a leucine zipper (LZ) domain (aa 322–343), a proline-rich region, and a zinc finger (ZF) domain (aa 389–419) (Maubach and Naumann 2017). The activity of NEMO depends on its dimerization and its ability to interact with linear or K63-linked polyubiquitin chains. NEMO is normally recruited to polyubiquitin scaffolds assembled by upstream signaling events which in turn facilitates the recruitment, phosphorylation, and activation of the catalytic IKK subunits,

IKK-alpha and IKK-beta, by TAK1 (TGF-beta activated kinase 1), which is also recruited concomitantly to the ubiquitin scaffolds (Israël 2010). This allows the kinase subunits to phosphorylate IkB inhibitors leading to their proteasomal degradation and inducing nuclear translocation of NF-kB transcription factors.

XR-EDA-ID caused by hypomorphic NEMO mutations was first described in 2000 (Zonana et al. 2000). Up to 100 male patients have been reported with more than 40 different mutations leading to impaired NEMO function. All known X-linked EDA-ID causing hypomorphic mutations either impair (1) protein expression, or (2) protein folding, or (3) polyubiquitin binding of NEMO, all essential for NEMO activation (Hubeau et al. 2011). Mutations span the entire NEMO gene and the variety and severity of clinical manifestations including infectious susceptibilities, auto-inflammatory diseases, and ectodermal dysplasia is strongly related to which specific NEMO protein domains are affected (Fusco et al. 2015). For example, mutations in the NEMO ZF domain causes a severe impairment in humoral immunity and dendritic cell function due to a specific impairment in c-Rel activation in response to CD40 (Temmerman et al. 2016). Mutations in the CC2 domain have no effect on protein expression but lead to a loss in the oligomer stability thereby altering IKK complex assembly which reduces TNF-alpha and LPS-induced NF-kB activation in B and T cells (Vinolo et al. 2006).

Disease Manifestations

NF-kB activation is down-stream of numerous cell surface receptor families involved in innate and adaptive immunity including B cell receptor (BCR), T cell receptor (TCR), tumor necrosis factor (TNFR), Toll (TLR), and interleukin-1 receptor superfamilies. The development of ectodermal tissues is associated with the ectodysplasin receptor which is homologous to members of the TNF receptor superfamily. The various clinical manifestations of XR-EDA-ID result from impaired NF-kB signaling via these signaling pathways.

Common immune defects include variable defects in T cell proliferation, antibody deficiency, impaired antibody response to polysaccharide, and impaired NK cell cytotoxicity (Kawai et al. 2012; Nishikomori et al. 2004).

Affected patients suffer from bacterial sinopulmonary and invasive infections, mostly caused by pyogenic bacteria such as *S. pneumoniae, S. aureus,* and *H. influenza* and mycobacteria (Döffinger et al. 2001; Carrol et al. 2003; Picard et al. 2011). This is due to impaired functioning of innate immunity receptors such as TLRs and IL-1Rs and poor serum-antibody response to polysaccharide antigens (Ku et al. 2005). Pneumocystis jiroveci pneumonia has also been reported. Severe herpes virus infections have been reported may be due to the deficient natural killer cell cytotoxicity (Orange et al. 2002). Some patients present with a hyper IgM phenotype due to impaired co-stimulation by CD40 (Jain et al. 2004). Autoimmune and inflammatory diseases including hemolytic anemia, arthritis, and inflammatory bowel disease-like colitis have also been described (Mizukami et al. 2012). Osteopetrosis and lymphedema occurs in a severe subset of patients (Dupuis-Girod et al. 2002). In addition to immune defects, there are varying degrees of ectodermal dysplasia including conical teeth, fine sparse hair, and absence of sweat glands due to impaired NF-kB activation via the ectodysplasin/EDAR signaling pathway (Courtois and Israël 2011).

Diagnosis

Laboratory evaluation should include quantitative immunoglobulins, measurement of vaccine antibody titers, functional analysis of NK cells, and Toll-like receptor assays. Patients can have low IgG but elevated IgM and IgA. Vaccine antibodies should be checked as antibody responses to polysaccharide antigens are often reduced. There is usually a deficiency of NK cell cytotoxicity. There is decreased inflammatory cytokine production from peripheral blood mononuclear cells after stimulation with TLR ligands. Sequencing of the gene for *IKBKG* will confirm the diagnosis. The presence of a NEMO pseudogene makes it difficult to perform genetic analysis using genomic DNA; the mutation should be identified by sequencing analysis of NEMO cDNA.

Treatment

Patients should receive immunoglobulin replacement therapy (Perez et al. 2017). Prophylactic antibiotics should be considered for patients who continue to have infections despite immunoglobulin replacement. Vaccination with BCG should be avoided (Karaca et al. 2016). Hematopoietic stem cell transplantation should be considered in patients with a severe clinical immunodeficiency phenotype. A recent review of HSCT in 29 patients with hypomorphic IKBKG/NEMO mutations reported a global survival rate of 74% at a median follow-up after HSCT of 57 months (Miot et al. 2017). Preexisting mycobacterial infection and colitis were associated with poorer HSCT outcome. Critical genetic and immune studies aimed at identifying patients with NEMO deficiency at risk of mycobacterial infection are needed (Chandrakasan et al. 2017). HSCT will not correct the ectodermal dysplasia seen in patients.

References

Carrol ED, Gennery AR, Flood TJ, et al. Anhidrotic ectodermal dysplasia and immunodeficiency: the role of NEMO. Arch Dis Child. 2003;88(4):340–1.

Chandrakasan S, Marsh RA, Uzel G, et al. Outcome of patients with NEMO deficiency following allogeneic hematopoietic cell transplant. J Allergy Clin Immunol. 2017;139(3):1040–3.

Courtois G, Israël A. IKK regulation and human genetics. Curr Top Microbiol Immunol. 2011;349:73–95.

Döffinger R, Smahi A, Bessia C, et al. X-linked anhidrotic ectodermal dysplasia with immunodeficiency is caused by impaired NF-kappaB signaling. Nat Genet. 2001;27(3):277–85.

Dupuis-Girod S, Corradini N, Hadj-Rabia S, et al. Osteopetrosis, lymphedema, anhidrotic ectodermal dysplasia, and immunodeficiency in a boy and incontinentia pigmenti in his mother. Pediatrics. 2002;109(6):e97.

Fusco F, Pescatore A, Conte MI, et al. EDA-ID and IP, two faces of the same coin: how the same IKBKG/NEMO mutation affecting the NF-kB pathway can cause immunodeficiency and/or inflammation. Int Rev Immunol. 2015;34(6):445–59.

Hubeau M, Ngadjeua F, Puel A, et al. New mechanism of X-linked anhidrotic ectodermal dysplasia with immunodeficiency: impairment of ubiquitin binding despite normal folding of NEMO protein. Blood. 2011;118(4):926–35.

Israël A. The IKK complex, a central regulator of NF-kappaB activation. Cold Spring Harb Perspect Biol. 2010;2(3):a000158.

Jain A, Ma CA, Lopez-Granados E, et al. Specific NEMO mutations impair CD40-mediated c-Rel activation and B cell terminal differentiation. J Clin Invest. 2004;114(11):1593–602.

Karaca NE, Aksu G, Ulusoy E, et al. Disseminated BCG infectious disease and hyperferritinemia in a patient with a novel NEMO mutation. J Investig Allergol Clin Immunol. 2016;26(4):268–71.

Kawai T, Nishikomori R, Heike T. Diagnosis and treatment in anhidrotic ectodermal dysplasia with immunodeficiency. Allergol Int. 2012;61(2):207–17.

Ku CL, Yang K, Bustamante J, et al. Inherited disorders of human toll-like receptor signaling: immunological implications. Immunol Rev. 2005;203:10–20.

Maubach G, Naumann M. NEMO links nuclear factor-kB to human diseases. Trends Mol Med. 2017;23(12): 1138–55.

Miot C, Imai K, Imai C, et al. Hematopoietic stem cell transplantation in 29 patients hemizygous for hypomorphic IKBKG/NEMO mutations. Blood. 2017;130(12):1456–67.

Mizukami T, Obara M, Nishikomori R, et al. Successful treatment with infliximab for inflammatory colitis in a patient with X-lined anhidrotic ectodermal dysplasia with immunodeficiency. J Clin Immunol. 2012; 32(1):39–49.

Nishikomori R, Akutagawa H, Maruyama K, et al. X-linked ectodermal dysplasia and immunodeficiency caused by reversion mosaicism of NEMO reveals a critical role for NEMO in human T-cell development and/or survival. Blood. 2004;103(12):4565–72.

Orange JS, Brodeur SR, Jain A, et al. Deficient natural killer cell cytotoxicity in patients with IKK-gamma/ NEMO mutations. J Clin Invest. 2002;109(11):1501–9.

Perez EE, Orange JS, Bonilla F, et al. Update on the use of immunoglobulin in human disease: a review of evidence. J Allergy Clin Immunol. 2017;139(3S):S1–S46.

Picard C, Casanova JL, Puel A. Infectious diseases in patients with IRAK-4, MyD88, NEMO, or IkBalpa deficiency. Clin Microbiol Rev. 2011;24(3):490–7.

Temmerman ST, Ma CA, Borges L, et al. Impaired dendritic-cell function in ectodermal dysplasia with immune deficiency is linked to defective NEMO ubiquitination. Blood. 2016;108(7):2324–31.

Vinolo E, Sebban H, Chaffotte A, et al. A point mutation in NEMO associated with anhidrotic ectodermal dysplasia with immunodeficiency pathology results in destabilization of the oligomer and reduces lipopolysaccharide and tumor necrosis factor-mediated NF-kappa B activation. J Biol Chem. 2006;281(10): 6334–48.

Zonana J, Elder ME, Schneider LC, et al. A novel X-linked disorder of immune deficiency and hypohidrotic ectodermal dysplasia is allelic to incontinentia pigmenti and due to mutations in IKK-gamma (NEMO). Am J Hum Genet. 2000;67(6):1555–62.

Antibody Replacement Therapy

▶ Management of Immunodeficiency, IgG Replacement (IV)

APLAID – Autoinflammatory PLCG2-Associated Antibody Deficiency and Immune Dysregulation

▶ PLAID and APLAID

APOL1

▶ APOL-1 Variants, Susceptibility and Resistance to Trypanosomiasis

APOL-1 Variants, Susceptibility and Resistance to Trypanosomiasis

Luis Murguia-Favela
Pediatric Immunology and Allergy, Alberta Children's Hospital, Calgary, AB, Canada
The University of Calgary, Calgary, AB, Canada

Synonyms

APOL-1: Apolipoprotein L1; APOL1; Human serum's trypanosome-killing component; Sleeping sickness; Trypanosomiasis: African trypanosomiasis

Definition

African trypanosomes are flagellate protozoans that are transmitted to mammals after inoculation by flies of the genus *Glossina*, also known as tsetse flies. Chronic infection with these parasites is fatal if untreated. In humans, the disease is also called "sleeping sickness" and affects thousands of people per year in sub-Saharan Africa (Pays et al. 2014).

Apolipoprotein L1 (APOL-1), an ionic channel-forming protein, is the lytic component of the innate immune system that protects humans against infection from the majority of the African trypanosomes, except for *Trypanosoma brucei rhodesiense* in East Africa and *Trypanosoma brucei gambiense* in West Africa. These two species have evolved mechanisms to become resistant to lysis mediated by APOL-1 (Cooper et al. 2016).

In recent years, variants of APOL-1 have been identified that either knock down the trypanolytic activity of the protein and thus predispose the carrier to infections by atypical trypanosomes (Cuypers et al. 2016), or are able to lyse and kill the East African *Trypanosoma brucei rhodesiense* by hindering the resistance mechanism of the parasite. The latter variants were found in a subset of Old World monkeys (Cooper et al. 2016) but now also in some humans with African ancestry (Genovese et al. 2010). Part of the importance of knowing about these variants is the potential for developing alternative therapeutic options for infected patients, who currently receive medications that are mostly unsatisfactory (Cooper et al. 2016).

Trypanosomiasis

Trypanosomes are protozoan parasites that are able to infect a wide variety of mammals and cause major public health and agricultural development problems in Africa. Only two of the subspecies are able to infect humans: *Trypanosoma brucei gambiense* in West Africa and *Trypanosoma brucei rhodesiense* in East and Southern Africa. These cause a debilitating and

A

many times fatal human disease that is often referred to as sleeping sickness. The western parasite (>97% of all cases of trypanosomiasis) typically causes a chronic disease, whereas the eastern one results in an acute and rapidly progressing disease (Cooper et al. 2016).

Trypanosomiasis caused by *T.b. gambiense* is characterized by an early hemolymphatic phase associated with nonspecific symptoms such as intermittent fever and headache, followed by a meningoencephalitic phase where the parasite invades the central nervous system leading to the characteristic neurological disorder and death if left untreated. In *T.b. rhodesiense* infection, the symptoms are very similar, yet the progression is more rapid. Also, an inoculation "chancre" is often observed at the site of the bite by the tsetse fly, in contrast with *T. b. gambiense* infection in which the occurrence of the chancre is rare (Bucheton et al. 2011).

Hundreds of thousands of trypanosomiasis cases occurred in the first part of the twentieth century due to exploitation of tsetse-infested areas. Systematic screening and treatment of millions of people lead to almost a halt in transmission by the 1960s. However, the disease progressively flared up again since the 1970s and reached almost half a million cases at the end of the last century (Bucheton et al. 2011).

Despite efforts to improve diagnosis and treatment, trypanosomiasis continues to be an important public health issue in Africa. Current antitrypanosomal drugs are mostly unsatisfactory due to toxicity, difficulty to follow regimens, and the emergence of resistance (Cooper et al. 2016).

Human Immunity Against Trypanosomes

The ability to control parasitemia in trypanosomiasis in humans involves at least four mechanisms: (1) antibody/complement lysis, (2) antibody-mediated phagocytosis, (3) innate immunity in terms of trypanolytic complexes in human serum (i.e. APOL-1), and (4) release of trypanotoxic molecules such as reactive nitrogen intermediates or reactive oxygen radicals by macrophages, cells

that provide the first line of defense (Bucheton et al. 2011).

With regards to the innate immunity mechanism against trypanosomes, it is now known that these parasites are lysed by APOL-1, a component of human high-density lipoprotein (HDL) particles that are also characterized by the presence of haptoglobin-related protein (Vanhollebeke et al. 2008).

APOL-1 is one of the six members of the APOL gene family. The function of these proteins is mainly unknown and only humans, gorillas, and baboons express the APOL1 gene. APOL-1 was first discovered within the high-density lipoprotein 3 (HDL-3) particle (Limou et al. 2015).

APOL-1 is the trypanolytic protein that provides resistance against *Trypanosoma brucei* infection (Vanhamme et al. 2003). The parasite internalizes the protein through endocytosis and is then transported to the lysosomes. APOL-1 is bound to an HDL particle but is released after progressive acidification of the environment within the lysosome. APOL-1 then forms an ionic channel in the lysosomal membrane that causes an influx of ions, which provokes osmotic swelling, and death of the parasite (Pérez-Morga et al. 2005; Limou et al. 2015). Haptoglobin-related protein (HPR), another primate-specific protein, is involved in targeting the complex that contains APOL-1 to the parasite after association with hemoglobin (Pays et al. 2014). Thus, in humans, the presence of haptoglobin-related protein has diverted the function of the trypanosome haptoglobin-hemoglobin receptor to elicit innate host immunity against the parasite (Vanhollebeke et al. 2008).

The APOL-1 protein has a pore-forming domain, a pH-sensitive membrane-addressing domain, and an SRA-interacting domain (Vanhollebeke and Pays 2006) and shares some structural and functional similarities with bacterial colicins (from different strains of *E. coli*), diphtheria toxin, and mammalian Bcl-2 family members, which suggest a similar activity for all these proteins. Interestingly, the diphtheria pathway through the infected cell is highly comparable to APOL-1's pathway in the trypanosome (Limou et al. 2015).

Furthermore, other studies suggest that APOL-1 may have other protective roles in innate immunity in general and not just for protection against trypanosomal infection. It is known that APOL genes are upregulated by pro-inflammatory cytokines such as IFNγ and TNF, and also that APOL-1 can ameliorate other parasitic infections such as leishmaniasis (Limou et al. 2015; Samanovic et al. 2009) and even restrict in vitro replication of HIV-1 in macrophages (Taylor et al. 2014).

Evasion of Human Immune Responses by Trypanosomes

Being extracellular parasites that are continually exposed to the host's immune system, African Trypanosomes have evolved sophisticated evasion mechanisms to survive in the chronically infected host (Bucheton et al. 2011).

One of the first mechanisms that prevents the immediate elimination of trypanosomes is the parasite's ability to limit early on the production of tumor necrosis factor by myeloid cells. This is caused by the stress-induced activation of adenylyl cyclases of the trypanosome plasma membrane when the parasite is phagocytosed, leading to the release of cyclic AMP by the parasite into the myeloid cells, the consecutive activation of protein kinase A, and inhibition of TNF synthesis (Salmon 2012).

After that, the main strategy is by antigenic variation in which the variant surface glycoproteins (VSG), the main surface antigens of the parasite, change continuously to avoid antibody-mediated clearance (Hall et al. 2013).

Most importantly, and as part of an arms race against human immunity, trypanosomes have evolved different mechanisms to resist the killing by APOL-1. T.b. rhodesiense evolved a serum resistance associated (SRA) glycoprotein that binds to APOL-1 within the lysosome to prevent its toxicity (Vanhamme et al. 2003), whereas T.b. gambiense has a specific glycoprotein (TgsGP) that forms hydrophobic β-sheets that stiffen the endolysosomal membrane to prevent the insertion and thus toxicity of APOL-1. Also, the uptake of

this protein by the parasite is limited and the degradation is enhanced (Uzureau et al. 2013).

SRA in T.b. rhodesiense is derived from a mutated VSG. Instead of being targeted to the plasma membrane, as would normally occur for other VSGs, SRA is targeted to the endolysosomal system where it encounters APOL-1 and binds strongly to it (Pays et al. 2014).

The mechanism of resistance is different for T. b. gambiense as TgsGP does not interact directly with APOL-1 but rather inhibits its toxicity by inducing endosomal membrane stiffening. This process prevents or slows down insertion of APOL-1 into the membrane and results in its degradation by endosomal proteases (Pays et al. 2014). The lysosomal cathepsin I is known to be the main cysteine protease involved in APOL-1 degradation, and it seems that, in *Trypanosoma brucei*, APOL-1 is prone to efficient degradation by cathepsin I, unless it is inserted into endosomal membranes, where it will generate ionic pores.

As mentioned above, there are two additional processes which are necessary for full resistance of T.b. gambiense to human serum, both responsible for reducing the intracellular levels of APOL-1: the limitation of its uptake and increased degradation. The reduced uptake results from the inactivation by a single point mutation of the receptor that allows entry of the APOL-1-containing complex into the parasite, known as T. brucei surface receptor for haptoglobin-hemoglobin or TbHpHbR (Kieft et al. 2010). The increased degradation comes from lowering endosomal pH, causing earlier acidification of endosomes which enables faster cysteine protease-mediated digestion of APOL-1 (Uzureau et al. 2013).

APOL-1 Variants and Their Consequences

APOL-1 variants that confer either susceptibility or resistance to African trypanosomiasis have been found in humans and other primates.

Recently, a patient in Ghana infected with an atypical T.b. gambiense lacking the TgsGP defense mechanism against APOL-1 was found to have homozygous missense substitution in the membrane-addressing domain of APOL-1, which knocked down the trypanolytic activity, allowing the trypanosome to avoid APOL-1 mediated immunity. It is thought that populations with this variant may be at increased risk of contracting trypanosomiasis (Cuypers et al. 2016).

On the other hand, APOL-1 variants that confer resistance to trypanosomiasis have been found in African-American and western African populations. The two genotypes known as G1 and G2 have been found to confer resistance to *T.b. rhodesiense* but, unfortunately, they do so at the expense of high probability of developing end-stage kidney disease in homozygotes. The resistance is owed to reduced interaction of these APOL-1 variants with SRA (Genovese et al. 2010).

The pathophysiology behind the development of kidney disease in those expressing these variants is an area of active research. APOL proteins share structural and functional similarities with proteins of the BCL2 family, as mentioned above, which control apoptosis and autophagy. APOL-1 could then be contributing to glomerulosclerosis by apoptosis, autophagy and/or endocytosis and lysosomal stimulation (Limou et al. 2015). Autophagy is a recognized major pathway in kidney function and disease, and some propose that APOL-1 may be interfering with autophagy in podocytes, leading to progressive kidney sclerosis (Pays et al. 2014). Furthermore, the fact that APOL-1 circulates with HDL particles is suggestive of a role in lipid transport and metabolism, which could be very important to maintain the plasma membranes of podocytes (Limou et al. 2015).

There is currently no evidence for natural APOL-1 variants that confer resistance to *T.b. gambiense* in humans. However, an APOL-1 variant was recently found in a West African baboon species that is able to kill both *T.b. rhodesiense* and *T.b. gambiense*. This variant could be a potential candidate for anti-trypanosomal therapies targeted at all pathogenic trypanosome species. Indeed, this knowledge has led to the experimental design of APOL-1 variants that are able to kill

these parasites and could eventually be used as therapeutic tools (Cooper et al. 2016).

Conclusions

Trypanosomiasis is a potentially fatal parasitosis that affects thousands of people in sub-Saharan Africa. The two species that cause the disease in humans are *T.b. rhodesiense* and *T.b. gambiense*. An evolutionary arms race between these protozoa and humans has led to the development of mechanisms of resistance to each other's killing. One such important factor in humans is APOL-1, a protein that ultimately lyses the lysosomal membrane of the parasite, leading to its death. Thus, APOL-1 should be considered as part of the innate immunity's armament in humans.

As it would be expected, genetic variations of the APOL-1 protein can lead to either increased susceptibility or resistance to infection by these and other *Trypanosoma* species. Finding and understanding these variants could lead to therapeutic alternatives against this public health concern.

Cross-References

▶ Evaluation of Suspected Immunodeficiency, Overview
▶ Innate Immune Defects, Clinical Presentation

References

Bucheton B, MacLeod A, Jamonneau V. Human host determinants influencing the outcome of *Trypanosoma brucei gambiense* infections. Parasite Immunol. 2011;33:438–47.

Cooper A, Capewell P, Clucas C, Veitch N, Weir W, Thomson R, Raper J, MacLeod A. A primate APOL1 variant that kills *Trypanosoma brucei gambiense*. PLoS Negl Trop Dis. 2016;10(8):1–20.

Cuypers B, Lecordier L, Meehan CJ, Van den Broeck F, Imamura H, Büscher P, Dujardin JC, Laukens K, Schnaufer A, Dewar C, Lewis M, Balmer O, Azurago T, Kyei-Faried S, Ohene SA, Duah B, Homiah P, Mensah EK, Anleah F, Franco JR, Pays E, Deborggraeve S. Apolipoprotein L1 variant associated with increased susceptibility to trypanosome infection. MBio. 2016;7(2):e02198–15.

Genovese G, Friedman DJ, Ross MD, Lecordier L, Uzureau P, Freedman BI, Bowden DW, Langefeld CD, Oleksyk TK, Uscinski Knob AL, Bernhardy AJ, Hicks PJ, Nelson GW, Vanhollebeke B, Winkler CA, Kopp JB, Pays E, Pollak MR. Association of trypanolitic APOL1 variants with kidney disease in African Americans. Science. 2010;329:841–5.

Hall JP, Wang H, Barry JD. Mosaic VSGs and the scale of *Trypanosoma brucei* antigenic variation. PLoS Pathog. 2013;9:e1003502.

Kieft R, Capewell P, Turner CMR, Veitch NJ, MacLeod A, Hadjuk S. Mechanism of Trypanosoma brucei gambiense (group 1) resistance to human trypanosome lytic factor. PNAS. 2010;107(37):16137–41.

Limou S, Dummer P, Nelson GW, Kopp JB, Winkler CA. APOL1 toxin, innate immunity and kidney injury. Kidney Int. 2015;88(1):28–34.

Pays E, Vanhollebeke B, Uzureau P, Lecodier L, Pérez-Morga D. The molecular arms race between African trypanosomiasis and humans. Nat Rev Microbiol. 2014;12:575–84.

Pérez-Morga D, Vanhollebeke B, Paturiaux-Hanocq F, Nolan DP, Lins L, Homblé F, Vanhamme L, Tebabi P, Pays A, Poelvoorde P, Jacquet A, Brasseur R, Pays E. Apolipoprotein L-1 promotes trypanosome lysis by forming pores in lysosomal membranes. Science. 2005;309:469–72.

Salmon D. Adenylate cyclases of Trypanosoma brucei inhibit the innate immune response of the host. Science. 2012;337:463–6.

Samanovic M, Molina-Portela MP, Chessler AD, Burleigh BA, Raper J. Trypanosome lytic factor, an antimicrobial high-density lipoprotein, ameliorates *Leishmania* infection. PLoS Pathog. 2009;5(1):e1000276.

Taylor HE, Khatua AK, Popik W. The innate immune factor apolipoprotein L1 restricts HIV-1 infection. J Virol. 2014;88(1):592–603.

Uzureau P, Uzureau S, Lecordier L, Fontaine F, Tebabi P, Homblé F, Grélard A, Zhendre V, Nolan DP, Lins L, Crowet JM, Pays A, Felu C, Poelvoorde P, Vanhollebeke B, Moestrup SK, Lyngsø J, Pedersen JS, Mottram JC, Dufourc EJ, Pérez-Morga D, Pays E. Mechanism of *Trypanosoma brucei gambiense* resistance to human serum. Nature. 2013;501:430–4.

Vanhamme L, Paturiaux-Hanocq F, Poelvoorde P, Nolan DP, Laurence L, Van Den Abbeele J, Pays A, Tebabi P, Van Xong H, Jacquet A, Moguilevsky N, Dieu M, Kane JP, De Baetselier P, Brasseur R, Pays E. Apolipoprotein L-1 is the trypanosome lytic factor of human serum. Nature. 2003;422:83–7.

Vanhollebeke B, Pays E. The function of apolipoproteins L. Cell Mol Life Sci. 2006;63(17):1937–44.

Vanhollebeke B, De Muylder G, Nielsen MJ, Pays A, Tebabi P, Dieu M, Raes M, Moestrup SK, Pays E. A haptoglobin-hemoglobin receptor conveys innate immunity to *Trypanosoma brucei* in humans. Science. 2008;320:677–81.

APOL-1: Apolipoprotein L1

▶ APOL-1 Variants, Susceptibility and Resistance to Trypanosomiasis

Arp Actin-Related Protein

▶ Wiskott-Aldrich Syndrome Deficiency

AT

▶ Ataxia-Telangiectasia (ATM)

Ataxia-Telangiectasia (ATM)

Sara Barmettler
Division of Rheumatology, Allergy and Immunology, Massachusetts General Hospital, Boston, MA, USA

Synonyms

AT; ATM

Introduction/Background

Ataxia-telangiectasia (AT) is an autosomal recessive genetic disorder due to mutations in the ATM gene, characterized by progressive cerebellar ataxia, oculocutaneous telangiectasias, abnormal eye movements, neurologic abnormalities, and immune deficiency.

Pathogenesis

Ataxia-telangiectasia is caused by homozygous mutations in the ATM (AT mutated) gene, located on chromosome 11q22.3 (Gatti and Perlman

1993). ATM is involved in the detection of DNA damage and is expressed in all tissues of the body. ATM is important in cell cycle progression (Ambrose and Gatti 2013) and stalls the progression of the cell cycle in the presence of DNA damage to allow the cell to repair the damage. ATM kinase phosphorylates the tumor suppressor protein p53, which serves as a transcriptional activator of genes that cause cell cycle arrest/apoptosis. In the absence of ATM kinase, p53 does not become phosphorylated and cannot prevent the cell from moving into the next phase of the cell cycle (Khanna et al. 1998).

Clinical Presentation

The estimated incidence for AT is 1:40,000–100,000 live births (Gatti and Perlman 1993). AT is an autosomal recessive disorder. There are a number of clinical manifestations including progressive cerebellar ataxia, oculocutaneous telangiectasias, abnormal eye movements, neurologic abnormalities, and immune deficiency.

Ataxia is the earliest clinical manifestation and can be variable in onset. Manifestations of progressive cerebellar dysfunction include gait and truncal ataxia, head tilting, slurred speech, oculomotor apraxia, and abnormal ocular saccades. Many children initially appear healthy in the first year of life; however, these patients can be slow to develop gait fluidity. Some patients have delayed walking and ataxia in infancy. Gross and fine motor skills deteriorate over time, and patients develop dysarthria and complex movement disorders. Many AT patients are wheelchair dependent by the second decade of life.

Telangiectasias of the blood vessels are seen on the bulbar conjunctivae and nose, face, pinnae, and neck. These often appear around 3–5 years of age. Eye movements are often normal initially, and patients later develop voluntary and involuntary saccades. Patients may have oculomotor apraxia, which is the inability to coordinate head and eye movements with shifting the gaze rapidly. Visual performance progressively deteriorates over time.

Cognitive impairment can be mild to moderate and presents early in patients with AT. This may become more severe over time. Initiation of speech is often delayed, and speech is slowed with inappropriate emphasis on words or syllables. Aspiration is common, due to progressive difficulty with chewing and swallowing. Other motor difficulties are extrapyramidal and include dystonia, myoclonus, tremor, chorea, delayed reaction time, facial hypomimia, and peripheral axonal neuropathy.

Immune deficiency affects up to 70% of AT patients (Gatti and Perlman 1993), with variability in presentation, and can include cellular and humoral immune deficiency. Decreased survival has been associated with patients with a high IgM phenotype with hypogammaglobulinemia, as well as patients with low IgG2 subclasses (van Os et al. 2017). Patients often have increased sinopulmonary infections, which may also be due to aspiration.

Pulmonary complications in AT include recurrent sinopulmonary infections, bronchiectasis, interstitial lung disease, pulmonary fibrosis, and neuromuscular abnormalities including dysphasia, aspiration, and respiratory muscle weakness. Progressive pulmonary disease is a major cause of morbidity and mortality in patients with AT.

Patients with AT have an increased risk for malignancy, particularly leukemia and lymphoma. Patients are susceptible to damage caused by ionizing radiation and chemotherapeutic agents.

Laboratory Findings/Diagnostic Testing

The diagnosis of AT is established by characteristic clinical findings (in particular, progressive cerebellar ataxia) and the presence of biallelic mutations in the ATM gene. In patients with the characteristic clinical findings, a serum alpha fetoprotein (AFP) at least two standard deviations above normal age can help to confirm the diagnosis. Of note, the AFP level does not correlate with disease severity, and AFP levels can be difficult to interpret in the first year of life.

Proposed diagnostic criteria for AT include (Conley et al. 1999):

• Definitive diagnosis: Patient with either increased radiation-induced chromosomal breakage in cultured cells or progressive cerebellar ataxia with disabling mutations on both alleles of ATM

- Probable diagnosis: Patient with progressive cerebellar ataxia and three of the following four findings:
  1. Ocular or facial telangiectasia
  2. Serum IgA at least 2 standard deviations (SD) below normal for age
  3. AFP at least 2 SD above normal for age
  4. Increased radiation-induced chromosomal breakage in cultured cells
- Possible diagnosis: Patient with progressive cerebellar ataxia and at least one of the four following findings:
  1. Ocular or facial telangiectasia
  2. Serum IgA at least 2 SD below normal for age
  3. AFP at least 2 SD above normal for age
  4. Increased radiation-induced chromosomal breakage in cultured cells

Humoral and cell-mediated immune deficiency can manifest as immunoglobulin deficiency, poor response to polysaccharide vaccines, oligoclonal gammopathy, lymphopenia, and T-cell lymphopenias. This T-cell lymphopenia has led to some AT patients being identified on the newborn screen for severe combined immunodeficiency (SCID) using quantification of T-cell receptor excision circles (TRECs). Of note, this only identifies patients who have profoundly decreased circulating naïve T cells, so TRECs alone will not identify all patients with AT. Several functional and molecular assays have been utilized to assist in the identification of ATM cases (Cousin et al. 2018). Rapid immunoblotting assay for ATM protein can be performed, which shows depleted protein in most patients with ATM (Chun et al. 2003). Other lab findings include serum immunoglobulin A (IgA) at least 2 standard deviations below normal for age and increased spontaneous and radiation-induced chromosome fragility in cultured cells.

Management

Management is focused on treating disease manifestations as well as increased surveillance and prevention of morbidity in AT. These disease manifestations include infections, immune deficiency, dysphagia, pulmonary disease, and malignancy (Gatti and Perlman 1993).

Acute infections should be treated promptly. AT patients are susceptible to sinopulmonary infections, and prophylactic antibiotics should be considered in patients with recurrent infections. In patients with hypogammaglobulinemia (low IgG) and/or impaired specific antibody production with recurrent infections, immunoglobulin replacement should be considered. Patients who are able to mount an appropriate immune response to vaccines should receive the pneumococcal and influenza vaccines.

Given that many patients with AT struggle with aspiration due to difficulties with coordinating swallowing, swallow evaluation is important. Gastrostomy tubes are considered in some patients to reduce the risk of aspiration and maintain nutrition in symptomatic children. Nutritional status should be monitored carefully.

Physical and occupational therapies are critical to minimize contractures, scoliosis, and deconditioning.

Pulmonary function should be monitored over time with yearly spirometry, as well as MRI monitoring for bronchiectasis and consolidation. Chest clearance techniques and cough assist devices should be considered in patients with respiratory muscle weakness, and noninvasive ventilation is necessary for some patients who suffer from chronic respiratory failure. Glucocorticoids have been used in patients with interstitial lung disease or ataxia; however, data is limited regarding benefit, optimal dosing, and duration of therapy.

Given the increased susceptibility of AT patients to ionizing radiation and radiomimetic chemicals due to the DNA repair defect, unnecessary diagnostic testing involving radiographs/ionization radiation should be avoided when possible and used with caution.

Patients with AT and female family members with heterozygous mutations in ATM should have earlier breast cancer screening. The age of screening is dependent on the type of mutation in the ATM gene.

Prognosis

AT has a poor prognosis due to its multisystem involvement. There is currently no disease-modifying treatment that exists for the ataxia or progressive cerebellar neurodegeneration. Research is ongoing regarding potential therapies for patients with AT.

Consideration has been given to preemptive allogeneic hematopoietic stem cell transplantation (alloHSCT) with a reduced intensity conditioning regimen to restore immune competence and prevent malignancy. This has been described in a case report with 6-year follow-up, with good outcomes (Bakhtiar et al. 2018). Given that conventional treatment protocols of malignant disease using radio- and/or chemotherapy have high morbidity and mortality in AT patients, the preemptive treatment strategy may benefit these patients.

The average life expectancy was historically ~25 years of age (van Os et al. 2017), with many patients suffering from progressive pulmonary disease or malignancy; however, survival has been improving over time.

Cross-References

► Ataxia-Telangiectasia-Like Disorder (ATLD)

References

Ambrose M, Gatti RA. Pathogenesis of ataxia-telangiectasia: the next generation of ATM functions. Blood. 2013;121(20):4036–45.

Bakhtiar S, Woelke S, Huenecke S, Kieslich M, Taylor AM, Schubert R, et al. Pre-emptive allogeneic hematopoietic stem cell transplantation in Ataxia telangiectasia. Front Immunol. 2018;9:2495.

Chun HH, Sun X, Nahas SA, Teraoka S, Lai CH, Concannon P, et al. Improved diagnostic testing for ataxia-telangiectasia by immunoblotting of nuclear lysates for ATM protein expression. Mol Genet Metab. 2003;80(4):437–43.

Conley ME, Notarangelo LD, Etzioni A. Diagnostic criteria for primary immunodeficiencies. Representing PAGID (Pan-American Group for Immunodeficiency) and ESID (European Society for Immunodeficiencies). Clin Immunol Orlando Fla. 1999;93(3):190–7.

Cousin MA, Smith MJ, Sigafoos AN, Jin JJ, Murphree MI, Boczek NJ, et al. Utility of DNA, RNA, protein, and functional approaches to solve cryptic immunodeficiencies. J Clin Immunol. 2018;38(3):307–19.

Gatti R, Perlman S. Ataxia-telangiectasia. In: Adam MP, Ardinger HH, Pagon RA, Wallace SE, Bean LJ, Stephens K, et al., editors. GeneReviews® [Internet]. Seattle: University of Washington; 1993. [cited 2019 Jan 21]. Available from: http://www.ncbi.nlm.nih.gov/books/NBK26468/.

Khanna KK, Keating KE, Kozlov S, Scott S, Gatei M, Hobson K, et al. ATM associates with and phosphorylates p53: mapping the region of interaction. Nat Genet. 1998;20(4):398–400.

van Os NJH, Jansen AFM, van Deuren M, Haraldsson A, van Driel NTM, Etzioni A, et al. Ataxia-telangiectasia: immunodeficiency and survival. Clin Immunol. 2017;178:45–55.

Ataxia-Telangiectasia Variant 1 (AT-V1)

► Nijmegen Breakage Syndrome (NBS1)

Ataxia-Telangiectasia-Like Disorder (ATLD)

Sara Barmettler
Division of Rheumatology, Allergy and Immunology, Massachusetts General Hospital, Boston, MA, USA

Synonyms

ATLD

Introduction/Background

Ataxia-telangiectasia-like disorder (ATLD) is a rare, autosomal recessive disorder characterized by ataxia and oculomotor apraxia that is caused by mutations in the MRE11 gene. ATLD shares many features with ataxia-telangiectasia (AT), thus giving rise to the name.

Pathogenesis

ATLD is caused by mutations in the MRE11A gene. MRE11A encodes a protein that is involved in double-strand DNA break recognition and repair (Stewart et al. 1999). Cells from patients with MRE11A mutations were found to have chromosomal instability, increased sensitivity to ionizing radiation, and defective induction of stress-activated signal transduction pathways (Stewart et al. 1999).

Clinical Presentation

Patients with ATLD have progressive ataxia without telangiectasias. The patients share many clinical features with AT; however, the reported cases have been notable for slower progression of the disease with longer survival (Delia et al. 2004).

In contrast to AT, extra-neurological features such as telangiectasias, elevated alpha-fetoprotein (AFP), and reduced immunoglobulin levels have not been described in ATLD (Fernet et al. 2005). Tumor development has also not been described in ATLD, unlike AT (Fernet et al. 2005).

There has been one report of two siblings with cerebellar vermis hypoplasia as a central feature of nephronophthisis-related ciliopathies (NPHP-RC) who were found to have a homozygous truncation mutation of MRE11 (Chaki et al. 2012).

There is some evidence to suggest that the phenotypic variations in ATLD may correspond to genotypic differences (Miyamoto et al. 2014).

Laboratory Findings/Diagnostic Testing

Cells of patients with ATLD have been shown to have increased susceptibility to radiation, consistent with a DNA repair defect (Stewart et al. 1999).

The diagnosis of ATLD is made when biallelic mutations in MRE11A are found by sequencing. Unlike AT, patients with ATLD have normal ATM protein levels (Stewart et al. 1999). Additionally,

patients have been described to have normal immunoglobulins, α-fetoprotein, lysosomal enzymes, lipoproteins, and vitamin E levels (Delia et al. 2004).

Management

The management of ATLD is similar to ataxia-telangiectasia. Given the rarity of cases, there are no guidelines or recommendations for management that have been published to date. Please see the section on "Management" in AT for further details.

Prognosis

There have only been a few reported cases of ATLD, and thus, the prognosis is unclear. There is a slower reported rate of neurodegeneration in ATLD than for patients with AT, with most ATLD patients reported to be ambulatory into their teenage years.

Cross-References

▶ Ataxia-Telangiectasia (ATM)

References

Chaki M, Airik R, Ghosh AK, et al. Exome capture reveals ZNF423 and CEP164 mutations, linking renal ciliopathies to DNA damage response signaling. Cell. 2012;150(3):533–48. https://doi.org/10.1016/j.cell.2012.06.028.

Delia D, Piane M, Buscemi G, et al. MRE11 mutations and impaired ATM-dependent responses in an Italian family with ataxia-telangiectasia-like disorder. Hum Mol Genet. 2004;13(18):2155–63. https://doi.org/10.1093/hmg/ddh221.

Fernet M, Gribaa M, Salih MAM, Seidahmed MZ, Hall J, Koenig M. Identification and functional consequences of a novel MRE11 mutation affecting 10 Saudi Arabian patients with the ataxia telangiectasia-like disorder. Hum Mol Genet. 2005;14(2):307–18. https://doi.org/10.1093/hmg/ddi027.

Miyamoto R, Morino H, Yoshizawa A, et al. Exome sequencing reveals a novel MRE11 mutation in a patient with progressive myoclonic ataxia. J Neurol

Sci. 2014;337(1–2):219–23. https://doi.org/10.1016/j.jns.2013.11.032.

Stewart GS, Maser RS, Stankovic T, et al. The DNA double-strand break repair gene hMRE11 is mutated in individuals with an ataxia-telangiectasia-like disorder. Cell. 1999;99(6):577–87.

ATLD

▶ Ataxia-Telangiectasia-Like Disorder (ATLD)

ATM

▶ Ataxia-Telangiectasia (ATM)

Autoinflammation with Infantile Enterocolitis

▶ NLRC4-Associated Autoinflammatory Diseases

Autosomal Dominant Anhidrotic Ectodermal Dysplasia with Immunodeficiency (AD-EDA-ID)

Adeeb A. Bulkhi
Department of Internal Medicine, College of Medicine, Umm Al Qura University, Makkah, Saudi Arabia
Division of Allergy and Immunology, Department of Internal Medicine, Morsani College of Medicine, University of South Florida, Tampa, FL, USA

Synonyms

EDA-ID; HED-ID; Hypohidrotic ectodermal dysplasia with immunodeficiency; IkB-alpha gain of function

Introduction

Anhidrotic ectodermal dysplasia with immunodeficiency (EDA-ID) is a group of disorders characterized by ectodermal tissue (ED)-related abnormalities including conical teeth, decrease/absent sweat glands, fine sparse hair, and increase susceptibility to severe infections. The disorder is linked to abnormalities of activation of nuclear factor kappa-light-chain-enhancer of activated B cells (NF-κB) pathways (Fig. 1). Normally, in the canonical pathway, NF-κB activation occurs once external stimuli activate IκB kinase (IKK) complex that constitutes of a heterodimer of the catalytic IKKα and IKKβ units and a regulatory IKKγ unit also called NF-κB essential modulator (NEMO). Activated IKK complex phosphorylates NF-κB inhibitor α (IκBα) at serine 32 and 36 residues and therefore promotes its ubiquitination and degradation. Subsequently, NF-κB transcription factor dimer (p50/RelA) is released from an inhibited state and translocated to the nucleus to activate target genes linked to inflammation. This pathway is triggered by several receptors (e.g., CD40, Toll-like receptor (TLR), T- and B-cell antigen receptor (TCR/BCR), and tumor necrosis factor α (TNF-α) receptor). In contrast, non-canonical activation of NF-κB pathway may occur with B-cell activating factor receptor (BAFFR), LTβR, and CD40 and will promote lymphorganogenesis by nuclear translocation of a second variant of NF-κB transcription factor dimer (p52/RelB). Interaction between these two pathways has been discovered through immune evaluation of patients with mutations in *NFKBIA* that result in deficiency IκBα.

There are two forms of EDA-ID, X-linked (XL)(OMIM #300291) and autosomal dominant (AD) (OMIM #164008) EDA-ID. Mutations in *IKBKG* encoding NEMO are hemizygous, whereas gain-of-function (GOF) mutations in *NFKBIA* gene encoding IκBα are heterozygous. A mutation to *NFKBIA* gene leads to continued inhibition of NF-κB activation when the pathway is triggered.

Autosomal Dominant Anhidrotic Ectodermal Dysplasia with Immunodeficiency (AD-EDA-ID), Fig. 1 After stimulation of NF-κB classical pathway receptors (CD40, TNF−α, TCR/BCR, TRLs) with appropriate stimuli, the IκB kinase (IKK) is activated. IKK constitutes of a heterodimer of the catalytic IKKα, IKKβ, and regulatory IKKg subunits also coined as NF-κB essential modulator (NEMO). Normally, IKK phosphorylates NF-κB inhibitor α (IκBα) that results in its ubiquitination, protein degradation, and in turn release of NF-κB (p50/RelA) to translocate to the nucleus and stimulate genes expression. However, in IκBα gain of function (GOF) mutations, IκBα is not accessible for phosphorylation and consequently unable to liberate NF-κB to apply its effect. Furthermore, in point mutation (missense), sequestration of IκBα with p50/RelA also inhibits activation of NF-κB (p52/RelB) via non-canonical pathway. Abbreviations: *CD40* Cluster of Differentiation 40, *TNF-a* Tumor Necrosis Factor-alpha, *TCR/BCR* T cell receptor/B cell receptor, *TLRs* Toll-like Receptors, *RANK* Receptor Activator of Nuclear Factor κ B, *CD30* Cluster of Differentiation 30

Clinical Presentation

Characteristic Clinical Features of Ectodermal Dysplasia (EDA) and Beyond

The first case of AD-EDA-ID with heterozygous *NFKBIA* mutation was discovered in 2003 (Courtois et al. 2003). Unlike XL-EDA-ID, almost all patients reported with AD-EDA-ID mutations presented with EDA early in life. Abnormalities of embryonic ectodermal tissues are evident during the physical examination (hair, teeth, nail, sweat glands) as NF-κB activation is an essential step in their development via ectodysplasin/ectodysplasin signaling pathway. The most apparent signs of EDA are anhidrosis or hypohidrosis due to lack of functional sweats glands followed by teeth abnormalities (i.e., conical shaped), sparse hair, and mental retardation, respectively. Other developmental features like neurological deficits, osteopetrosis, and lymphedema have not reported. Lymph nodes are usually small or absent, mainly in patients with missense mutations. Autoimmunity is not uncommon which can present as lupus, juvenile idiopathic arthritis, autoimmune thyroiditis, or autoinflammation. Patients can present with recurrent diarrhea and/or colitis.

Infectious Features

Patients present with broad-spectrum severe infections (viruses, bacteria, and fungi) at an early age. Patients commonly present with recurrent upper respiratory tract infections including pneumonia; however, severe sepsis and meningitis also occur. Mycobacterial infections have been reported in a few cases. Fungal infections in the form of chronic mucocutaneous candidiasis (CMC) and pulmonary pneumocystosis have been described. While they still occur, viral infections caused by rotavirus, respiratory syncytial virus (RSV), cytomegalovirus (CMV), parainfluenza virus, norovirus, and sapovirus are less frequent. Patients are usually unable to mount fever due to impaired of the IL-1R and TLR signaling.

Immunological Features

The defect in innate immunity is variable and not well characterized. Monocytes and neutrophils appear normal in count and function. Unlike XL-EDA-ID, NK cell counts and function are also generally within normal range except in three reported cases; however, functional studies were reported only in one case (Boisson et al. 2017). There are no reports of innate lymphoid cell counts or proportions. The defect in adaptive immunity is less variable compared to innate immunity. The most observed defect is T lymphocytosis with an abundance of naïve CD4 and CD8 T cells and decreases memory T-cell fraction. The proportion of γ/δ T cells is low or absent. Limited evidence shows impaired polarization of naïve CD4 T cells to Th1 and Th17. T-cell proliferation with mitogens phytohemagglutinin A (PHA) or concanavalin A (ConA) is generally intact. T-cell proliferation to antigen stimulation was variable from intact to absent in a couple patients. T-cell proliferation with α-CD3 alone was impaired in almost all the cases; however, adding α-CD28 restored the proliferation of these T cells. The B-cell compartment is significantly affected. Total B cells are typically high but can be normal. Nonetheless, switched memory B cells are either low or absent. Immunoglobulin

levels are almost always abnormal and vary between high IgM with or without low IgG/IgA and low IgM with or without high IgG/IgA. Dysgammaglobulinemia is common with impaired antibodies response to vaccine antigens.

Diagnosis and Laboratory Testing

Anhidrotic ectodermal dysplasia features are a helpful indicator for early diagnosis of AD-EDA-ID. It is almost observed in all cases of AD-EDA-ID. To clinically diagnose EDA, at least two of the following seven features need to be seen: (1) lessened skin pigmentation; (2) sparse or absent scalp and body hair; (3) reduced, absent, or malfunctioned sweat glands; (4) dark and wrinkled periorbital skin; (5) hypodontia, anodontia, or conically shaped front teeth; (6) low nasal bridge and small nose with underdeveloped alae nasi; and (7) frontal bossing with prominent supraorbital ridges.

Broad-spectrum infections, the absence of tonsils and lymph nodes, and autoimmune manifestations can be important clues for diagnosis.

Laboratory studies may include complete blood count (typically normal), lymphocyte enumeration (naïve lymphocytosis in T- and B-cell compartments with low to absent memory cells), immunoglobulin levels and vaccine titers (antibodies' response postimmunization is always poor), and functional assay for T-cell proliferation (stimulated by mitogen, antigen, and interleukins). The definitive diagnostic tool for AD-EDA-ID is genetic testing for *NFKBIA* gene mutations (Ohnishi et al. 2012). In case of variant of unknown significance, molecular studies are recommended to evaluate IκBα expression and NFKB nuclear translocation (signaling of canonical and noncanonical NKFB pathways).

Genotype–Phenotype Correlation

By 2018, 13 more cases have been described, and a scoring system with excellent genotype-phenotype correlation was proposed based on infections, ED-related abnormalities, antibody responses, lymphocyte counts, and memory subsets (Petersheim et al. 2018). The majority of patients had de novo nonsense (truncation mutation) or missense (point mutation) at or close to serine 32 and 36 residues. IκBα missense point mutations result in higher level of mutant protein with increased cytoplasmic sequestration and higher level of impairment of NF-κB (p50/RelA) than truncating mutations. Furthermore, missense mutations also affected the noncanonical NF-κB pathway supported by the molecular studies and absence of tonsils and lymph nodes in this cohort. Overall, patients with missense *NFKBIA* mutations had more severe disease.

Treatment/Prognosis

It is recommended that AD-EDA-ID patients get immunized with conjugated and non-conjugated bacterial vaccines (e.g., *Streptococcus pneumoniae*, *H. influenzae*, and *Neisseria meningitidis*). Live vaccines including BCG should be avoided. If no response is mounted to vaccines, initiation of immunoglobulin replacement therapy (IgRT) is indicated. As patients are usually unable to mount fever, if an infection is suspected, early empirical intravenous antibiotics should be administered. It is highly recommended to initiate prophylaxis antibiotics against *Pneumocystis jirovecii* and *Candida albicans* with cotrimoxazole and an antifungal drug (e.g., fluconazole) (Kawai et al. 2012). In the event of mycobacterial infection, antimycobacterial treatment along with recombinant interferon γ (rIFN-γ) should be started. Hematopoietic stem cell transplantation (HSCT) has been attempted for patients with both missense (n = 6) and truncating mutations (n = 2) (Petersheim et al. 2018). In this small study, HSCT was partially successful. Half of the patients are alive after HSCT, and all patients with missense *NFKBIA* mutations continue to remain on IgRT for recurrent infection. The outcome of HSCT in one patient with truncating *NFKBIA* is excellent with no infections and off IgRT. However, another patient with truncating *NFKBIA* is doing well on IgRT without the need for HSCT. Therefore, the indication for HSCT in this complex group of AD-EDA-ID is unclear.

Cross-References

▶ Anhidrotic Ectodermal Dysplasia with Immunodeficiency (EDA-ID), Autosomal-Dominant
▶ Anhidrotic Ectodermal Dysplasia with Immunodeficiency (EDA-ID), X-linked

References

Boisson B, Puel A, Picard C, Casanova JL. Human IkappaBalpha gain of function: a severe and syndromic immunodeficiency. J Clin Immunol. 2017;37(5):397–412.

Courtois G, Smahi A, Reichenbach J, Doffinger R, Cancrini C, Bonnet M, et al. A hypermorphic IkappaBalpha mutation is associated with autosomal dominant anhidrotic ectodermal dysplasia and T cell immunodeficiency. J Clin Invest. 2003;112(7):1108–15.

Kawai T, Nishikomori R, Heike T. Diagnosis and treatment in anhidrotic ectodermal dysplasia with immunodeficiency. Allergol Int. 2012;61(2):207–17.

Ohnishi H, Miyata R, Suzuki T, Nose T, Kubota K, Kato Z, et al. A rapid screening method to detect autosomal-dominant ectodermal dysplasia with immune deficiency syndrome. J Allergy Clin Immunol. 2012;129(2):578–80.

Petersheim D, Massaad MJ, Lee S, Scarselli A, Cancrini C, Moriya K, et al. Mechanisms of genotype-phenotype correlation in autosomal dominant anhidrotic ectodermal dysplasia with immune deficiency. J Allergy Clin Immunol. 2018;141(3):1060–73. e3

Autosomal Dominant Hyper IgE Syndrome

Jenna R. E. Bergerson and Alexandra F. Freeman
Laboratory of Clinical Immunology and Microbiology, National Institutes of Allergy and Infectious Diseases (NIAID), National Institutes of Health (NIH), Bethesda, MD, USA

Synonyms

AD-HIES; Job's syndrome; STAT3 loss of function

Introduction

Autosomal dominant hyperimmunoglobulin E syndrome (AD-HIES)(OMIM#147060), also known as Job's syndrome, is a primary immunodeficiency characterized by elevated immunoglobulin E (IgE), eczema, infections, and multiple connective tissue, skeletal, and vascular abnormalities. First described in 1966 by Davis et al., it was initially characterized by the triad of eosinophilia, eczema, and recurrent skin and pulmonary infections (Davis et al. 1966). Shortly thereafter, in 1972, Buckley et al. recognized that an elevated IgE levels was a part of this clinical spectrum, giving rise to the name hyperimmunoglobulin E syndrome. Dominant-negative heterozygous mutations in signal transducer and activator of transcription 3 (STAT3) were identified in 2007 as the link between recurrent infections and connective tissue abnormalities (Holland et al. 2007; Minegishi et al. 2007). Many cases are sporadic, but when familial, all individuals who carry the mutations express disease manifestations. Gender preference is not seen, and disease-causing mutations have been found in all ethnic groups.

STAT3 has been shown to be essential for embryogenesis, as homozygous STAT3 knockout mice do not survive. The majority of disease-causing mutations occur in the SH2 or the DNA-binding domains and are either short in-frame deletions or missense mutations that result in normal STAT3 protein expression but decreased function. While there are no clear genotype-phenotype correlations, there is a modest increase in some of the non-immunologic features, like high palate, wide nose, and scoliosis, in those with mutations in the SH2 domain (Sowerwine et al. 2012).

STAT3 is expressed widely and mediates various pathways involved in wound healing, host defense, and vascular remodeling, consistent with its multi-system clinical phenotype. Multiple cytokines transduce signal using STAT3, including interleukin (IL)-6, IL-10, IL-11, IL-17, IL-21, IL-22, IL-23, leukemia inhibitory factor, oncostatin M, cardiotrophin-1, cardiotrophin-like cytokine, and ciliary neurotrophic factor (Fig. 1).

One of the defining immunologic abnormalities in this disease is failure of Th17 cells to differentiate, leading to impaired upregulation of antimicrobial peptides at epithelial surfaces, which results in Candida and *Staphylococcus aureus* infections. Interestingly, impaired IL-11 signaling has been shown to cause craniosynostosis, delayed tooth eruption, and supernumerary teeth in three consanguineous families in Pakistan with IL-11R alpha mutations due to lack of STAT3 transduction.

STAT3 also plays an important role in the regulation of matrix metalloproteinases (MMPs), and as expected those with STAT3 deficiency have abnormal levels of MMP (Sowerwine et al. 2012). Such a defect in tissue remodeling likely explains the vascular aneurysms, poor lung healing after infection, and characteristic facial features with porous skin seen in this population.

Earlier diagnosis of AD-HIES through greater recognition of clinical phenotype and advanced genetic testing is allowing for implementation of preventative antimicrobial therapies prior to development of significant comorbidities and is significantly improving the quality of life and life span of those affected.

Clinical Presentation

Immunologic and Infectious Complications

AD-HIES is characterized by eczematous rashes, skin abscesses, recurrent sinopulmonary infections, and mucocutaneous candidiasis. Pustular or eczematoid eruptions on the face and scalp typically begin in the first few weeks of life and persist frequently through the teenage years. Biopsies of such lesions are often characterized by eosinophilia. This eczematoid rash is often exacerbated by *Staphylococcus aureus*, and as such, control of eczema is typically most successful with topical or systemic anti-staphylococcal therapy. Recurrent skin infections starting in early childhood, usually *S.aureus* abscesses, can also be a common skin manifestation in this disease. While drainage from these lesions is purulent, other signs of inflammation are often absent. Whereas typical skin infections are

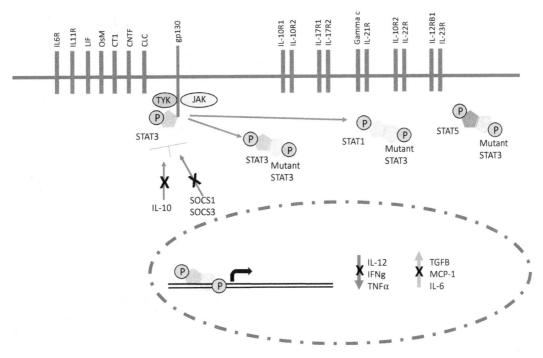

Autosomal Dominant Hyper IgE Syndrome, Fig. 1 The signaling and inhibitions of STAT3 are shown, with areas of special emphasis for the dominant-negative mutants shown. Green STAT3 depicts the AD mutant form of the molecule; each heterodimer it is part of results in inhibited function. STAT3 is directly involved in signaling of hematological and extra-hematological receptors; classes of receptors known to activate STAT3 include the common beta chain gp130, type I and II interferons, IL-12, IL-23, receptor tyrosine kinases, and the IL-10 family of cytokines. After stimulation of the cell, JAKs phosphorylate a key tyrosine residue of STAT3 and the resulting phosphorylated STAT3 forms homo- and heterodimers that are translocated to the nucleus, where they activate a complex array of genes, depending on the stimulus and cell type. The "X" indicates where a normal function is inhibited. STAT3 is involved in IL-10 signaling and expression, both of which are affected in AD-HIES. IL, interleukin; LIF, leukemia inhibitory factor; OsM, oncostatin M; CT1, cardiotrophin-1; CNTF, ciliary neurotrophic factor; CLC, cytokine-like factor 1; R, receptor

characterized by warmth and erythema, these abscesses lack those features and are considered "cold" abscesses.

Recurrent pulmonary infections begin in the first several years of life and are predominantly caused by *S. aureus*, *Streptococcus pneumoniae*, and *Haemophilus* species. Much like the absence of typical inflammatory signs with abscess formation, the systemic signs that classically accompany lung infections are often diminished leading to delayed diagnosis. There may be absence of fever, a normal white blood cell count, and fairly normal inflammatory markers despite radiographic signs that demonstrate new lung infiltrate. However, despite a lack of systemic inflammation, local airway inflammation is present, and copious airway secretions are seen. Such pyogenic pneumonias typically respond well to antibiotic therapy; however, frequent delay in diagnosis often leads to infectious complications like empyema, pneumatocele formation, and bronchiectasis. Aberrant healing following lung infection likely explains the increased frequency of pneumatoceles and bronchiectasis.

Once such pulmonary parenchymal damage has occurred, the spectrum of pathogenic organisms more closely mimics those seen in cystic fibrosis. Pulmonary nontuberculous mycobacteria infection occurs at a rate similar to that seen in cystic fibrosis, as does infection with gram-negative organisms like *Pseudomonas aeruginosa*. Bronchiectasis and pneumatoceles also lead to chronic infection with filamentous

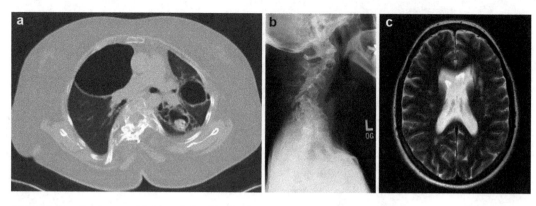

Autosomal Dominant Hyper IgE Syndrome, Fig. 2 Clinical imaging from patients with AD-HIES. (**a**). 46-year-old female with pneumatoceles and an Aspergilloma. (**b**). 56-year-old woman with severe cervical spine degenerative disease. (**c**). T2-weighted images of a brain MRI of a 45-year-old woman demonstrating multiple hyperintensities

molds such as *Aspergillus* and *Scedosporium*, and fungal balls within pneumatoceles can form (Fig. 2a). These chronic infections are the cause of significant morbidity and mortality as they may cause hemoptysis and can become increasingly resistant to antimicrobial agents over time.

While resection of pneumatocele is appealing, the abnormal healing that presumably led to the pneumatoceles can also cause complications post-surgery, and there is a high rate of complication such as bronchopleural fistulae (Freeman and Olivier 2016). Avoidance of surgery stems from the concern of impaired healing as well as the anesthetic risks due to impaired lung function in the late stages of the disease.

While the majority of pulmonary mold infections are seen in areas of pre-existing parenchymal damage, occasionally features of allergic bronchopulmonary aspergillosis (ABPA) are seen. Making this diagnosis in a syndrome defined by high IgE levels is complicated, as not surprisingly antigen-specific serologies may be falsely positive to many allergens. Diagnosis, therefore, must be made using typical radiographic findings in addition to clinical response to corticosteroids, antifungal therapy, and omalizumab treatment.

Mucocutaneous candidiasis can present as disease of the nails, oropharynx, esophagus, and vaginal mucosa. Opportunistic infections can also be seen in AD-HIES. *Pneumocystis jiroveci*

pneumonia has been reported in infants as their first pneumonia. Endemic fungi can disseminate, and lead to gastrointestinal disease, such as with histoplasmosis and *Cryptococcus*, or meningitis, with *Coccidioides* and *Cryptococcus*.

Reactivation of viral infections, specifically VZV, has been observed in this population at significantly increased rates. Work by Siegel et al. found that nearly one third of AD-HIES patients had a history of herpes zoster, starting as early as the second decade of life. Rates of VZV reactivation were 6–20-fold higher than the rate of herpes zoster in the general population over the same decades of life. Similarly, rates of herpes zoster recurrence in AD-HIES were significantly higher than those of the general population. This impaired control of chronic viral infections is proposed to be due to the observed defect in central memory T cells seen in AD-HIES patients (Siegel et al. 2011).

Interestingly, despite the elevated total and antigen-specific IgE, those with loss of function STAT3 mutations are less susceptible to clinical food allergy and anaphylaxis compared to other highly atopic patients. Work by Hox et al. demonstrated STAT3 signaling is essential for mast cell mediator-induced vascular permeability and that this is impaired in patients with AD-HIES (Hox et al. 2016).

Similar to many other primary immunodeficiencies, there is an increased incidence of both

Hodgkin's and non-Hodgkin's lymphoma. There does not seem to be any relationship with EBV infection and malignancy in this population (Yong et al. 2012). As STAT3 is an oncogene, the development of lymphoma is paradoxical, and further investigation is necessary to understand the mechanism of tumorigenesis in patients with loss of function STAT3 mutations.

Non-Immunologic Manifestations

What makes AD-HIES unique among many primary immunodeficiency disorders is the multi-system involvement with vascular, GI, and musculoskeletal manifestations. Characteristic facial features usually manifest during adolescence and are characterized by a prominent forehead and chin, deep-set eyes, a broad nose, and porous skin. Failure to shed primary teeth is common, and if not surgically removed prior to the emergence of secondary teeth, then dental crowding is seen. Other abnormalities of the oral cavity can be seen, including a high-arched palate, hard palate midline sagittal fibrotic thickening, deep grooves on the tongue, and buccal mucosa with multiple mucosal fissures (Sowerwine et al. 2012). An increased frequency of aphthous stomatitis is also seen during the teenage/early adolescent years (unpublished observations). Additionally, some degree of craniosynostosis is typically seen in the skull but does not usually require surgical correction.

Other musculoskeletal abnormalities include hyperextensible joints, scoliosis, minor trauma fractures, and osteopenia. Scoliosis is present in many patients and may be severe enough to warrant surgical correction. Interestingly, wound healing following orthopedic surgeries is not usually complicated, as it is for pulmonary surgery. Approximately half of all AD-HIES individuals have minimal trauma fractures, and many have osteopenia. However, there is no direct correlation between bone mineral density and propensity to fracture. The joints are typically hyperextensible, and this may be responsible for the significant arthritis seen at younger ages than in the general population. Degenerative cervical spine disease in the fourth and fifth decade of life can cause neurological deficits and may require surgical stabilization (Fig. 2b).

Vascular abnormalities have more recently been recognized and include aneurysms, dilation and tortuosity of middle-sized arteries, and lacunar infarcts. Reported arterial abnormalities in AD-HIES include coronary artery aneurysms, bilateral berry aneurysms of the carotids, and a middle cerebral artery mycotic aneurysm. Further investigation of vascular abnormalities in a large AD-HIES cohort using cardiac CT and MRI found that coronary artery aneurysms and tortuosity are a common feature of the disease. These radiologic findings occurred in 70% of AD-HIES patients compared to 21% of the control group, and 37% of AD-HIES patients had aneurysms versus 3% in the non-HIES group (Sowerwine et al. 2012; Yong et al. 2012). The coronary artery aneurysms have resulted in myocardial infarction in several individuals, and therefore screening in adults is warranted as antiplatelet therapies such as aspirin may be indicated to minimize the risk of clot forming within the aneurysm. An increased incidence of hypertension was also seen in the AD-HIES group. A subsequent investigation demonstrated that coronary vessel walls are significantly thicker in AD-HIES than in healthy subjects, indicative of atherosclerosis being present but not leading to narrowing. The enlarged coronary lumen in AD-HIES, compared to CAD patients, is suggestive that disordered tissue remodeling associated with STAT3 mutations is responsible for these findings (Abd-Elmoniem et al. 2017).

Central nervous system abnormalities are found on imaging of AD-HIES patients at an incidence much higher than the general population. Focal hyperintensities are seen on brain MRI in the majority of individuals with AD-HIES. These lesions are predominantly white matter hyperintensities (Fig. 2c). The incidence of these lesions does seem to increase in number with age, although patients with AD-HIES are found to have these focal hyperintensities at a much younger age than would be expected in the general population. Similar brain lesions are also frequently found as incidental findings in the elderly. In the elderly, the focal hyperintense lesions are indistinguishable from those found in AD-HIES patients, and they have been associated with increased blood pressure, smoking, previous silent strokes, and other vascular risk factors. However, the clinical significance of these lesions in AD-HIES patients remains unknown as they are usually not associated with neurologic abnormalities. They may represent focal areas of demyelination, and whether they are due to ischemia, infection, or poor astrocyte activity is still unknown (Sowerwine et al. 2012). Overall, cognitive functioning in AD-HIES patients who develop early onset of these white matter hyperintensities is intact. In fact, these patients in one study scored in the average to high average range. However, the development of focal brain lesions may be a risk factor for relative weakness in specific areas like visual-spatial skills and working memory. Additionally, Chiari 1 malformations have also been found in a higher incidence in AD-HIES patients, but generally have not required surgical correction.

The gastrointestinal manifestations in STAT3 deficiency are consistent with both the immune abnormalities and the connective tissue findings seen in this disorder. This includes infections of the GI tract with Candida and other endemic fungal organisms related to the impaired epithelial host immunity presumably. There is also overlap between patients with STAT3 deficiency and those with connective tissue disorders like Marfan's and Ehlers-Danlos syndromes; specific to the GI tract, those findings include diagnoses like diverticula and perforation. One large cohort of patients with STAT3 deficiency were analyzed for type and frequency of GI disorders. Interestingly, 60% of these patients reported one or more GI symptoms with the most prevalent being gastroesophageal reflux disease (GERD) and dysphagia. Another predominant patient report was of food impaction, which is likely related to the increased incidence of chronic eosinophilic esophagitis (EoE) found in this cohort. Chronic EoE also likely contributed to the esophageal rings, linear furrows, diverticula, and upper esophageal strictures seen on endoscopy. Evidence of underlying GI dysmotility and colonic perforation was also reported, which is likely related to issues of abnormal connective tissue repair and impaired mucosal healing, as discussed above. It should be mentioned that this cohort of patients did not have an increased incidence of inflammatory bowel disease (IBD) as is seen with many other disorders of immune dysregulation (Arora et al. 2017). This is perhaps related to the absence of Th17 cells in STAT3-deficient patients, as increased IL-17 signaling has been observed in IBD.

Laboratory Findings/Diagnostic Testing

As indicated by the name of the syndrome, the most consistent laboratory finding is an elevated serum IgE level. The peak is typically greater than 2000 IU/mL, but the level tends to decrease or even normalize with increased age. The IgE level does not correlate with disease activity or severity. The complete blood count is typically normal, but aberrations in the white blood cells can be seen with a relative neutropenia. As previously mentioned, the white blood cell count often fails to increase in response to infection. Eosinophilia is also common. Serum IgG and IgM are usually normal, and serum IgA is normal or low. However, specific antibody responses can be impaired. Lymphocyte phenotyping often reveals diminished memory T and B cells and very low IL-17-producing T cells.

Treatments/Prognosis

The main target of therapy for AD-HIES involves the prevention and treatment of infections. Since AD-HIES patients can lack the classic signs of infection, like fevers, chills, or rigors, a careful history, physical exam, and relevant imaging are important to initiate timely therapies.

Prophylactic antibiotics targeting *S. aureus* (e.g., trimethoprim/sulfamethoxazole) are useful to decrease the frequency of pyogenic pneumonia, with the goal of preventing the development of pneumatoceles and bronchiectasis. Control of skin disease, exacerbated by *S. aureus*, also is benefited by oral anti-staphylococcal therapy, along with topical antiseptics like dilute bleach baths or chlorhexidine washes. Recurrent abscesses are usually controlled with good skin care and anti-staphylococcal maintenance therapy. Oftentimes, however, despite even aggressive skin care and decolonization of bacteria on the skin, infections in the axilla and groin can persist.

Antifungal prophylaxis may be of help in AD-HIES patients with chronic or recurrent *Candida* infections like onychomycosis. Those who have evidence of mold colonization or infection of the lung should be treated with antifungal agents with activity against molds, such as posaconazole. Anti-*Aspergillus* prophylaxis should also be considered for any AD-HIES patient with pneumatoceles, as they are at higher risk for development of *Aspergillus* infections in these areas of parenchymal lung damage. In areas with endemic mycoses, antifungal prophylaxis such as fluconazole for *Coccidioides* or itraconazole for *Histoplasma* should be strongly considered.

The management of lung disease in the setting of chronic infection with parenchymal lung injury is difficult. Airway clearance techniques such as secretion clearance devices and nebulized hypertonic saline should be utilized as in other patients with bronchiectasis. However, the benefits that aggressive airway management can offer must be balanced by the increased risk of hemoptysis that some with AD-HIES face. Those most at risk for acute episodes of hemoptysis include those with extensive bronchiectasis, infected pneumatoceles, or mycetomas, likely from abnormal vasculature associated with chronic infection. In such cases, antimicrobial therapy should be optimized, and inhaled airway irritants should be withheld during acute episodes of hemoptysis. Patients should be counseled for when to seek emergent evaluation should hemoptysis occur. Also complicating the manner in which airway clearance is delivered is the increased risk for minimal trauma fractures, thus limiting

the use of devices like the percussive vest (Freeman and Olivier 2016).

Immunoglobulin replacement, administered by either intravenous or subcutaneous routes, has also been shown to significantly decrease the incidence of sinopulmonary infections. Furthermore, many AD-HIES patients likely benefit from such treatment as this population has diminished memory B cells and specific antibody production with age. Prophylaxis combining oral antimicrobials and immunoglobulin replacement should be strongly considered in patients with recurrent pulmonary infections or parenchymal lung damage (Yong et al. 2012; Sowerwine et al. 2012).

Routine vaccination according to an age-appropriate schedule is recommended. The majority of patients are able to make antibodies in response to protein and polysaccharide-based vaccines. These vaccines are usually tolerated well, with the exception of the 23-valent pneumococcal vaccine in which fever and large areas of edema and erythema develop around the injection site, oftentimes requiring systemic steroids (unpublished observations). For this reason, avoidance of the 23-valent pneumococcal vaccine should be considered in this population.

Optimal therapy for GI disorders remains to be determined. Experience with the use of oral or topical corticosteroid therapy for EoE is limited in this population, and it is reasonable to be concerned about using such a therapy in these patients who are already prone to both infections and osteoporosis. The use of long-term acid suppression for GERD, with either proton-pump inhibitors (PPI) or H2 blockers, raises similar concerns.

The role of hematopoietic stem cell transplantation (HSCT) in AD-HIES is unclear, particularly as some of the disease manifestations are of non-hematopoietic origin. The first two reports of HSCT in AD-HIES patient were deemed failures; the first suffered from lymphoma and died in the posttransplant period, and the second reported recurrence of AD-HIES features 4 years posttransplant despite full donor engraftment (Sowerwine et al. 2012; Yong et al. 2012).

However, more recent reports of transplantation in this patient population indicate that HSCT may be an important therapeutic option in patients with severe disease manifestations. Two children transplanted with high-grade non-Hodgkin's lymphoma, subsequently found to have STAT3 mutations, were successfully transplanted with improvement in immunologic and non-immunologic features of their underlying disease. One would not expect resolution of non-immunologic features, but improvement in osteoporosis and resolution of characteristic facial features were noted (Goussetis et al. 2010). A recent report of two Japanese patients followed for more than 8 years posttransplant showed normalization of IL-17 and IgE levels, even in the one patient with persistently mixed chimerism studies. While overall frequency of infections and hospitalizations decreased substantially, both patients still suffered from pulmonary complications following HSCT (Yanagimachi et al. 2016). Such reports suggest that HSCT to correct immunological defects before severe complications arise may be of benefit for AD-HIES patients with frequent and severe infections.

In summary, AD-HIES is characterized by mutations in STAT3 which result in both immunologic defects leading to infection susceptibility, as well as somatic features involving connective and vascular tissues, the brain, the gastrointestinal tract, and the skeleton. Knowledge of the genetic basis for the disease and improving understanding of the pathogenesis are allowing for earlier diagnosis and initiation of antimicrobial therapies, particularly anti-staphylococcal, prior to developing troublesome skin infections or parenchymal lung damage. As recognition and control of infections are improving, these patients are living longer, and our focus must turn to better understanding somatic aliments like scoliosis, atherosclerosis, aneurysms, and osteoporosis.

References

Abd-Elmoniem KZ, Ramos N, Yazdani SK, Ghanem AM, Holland SM, Freeman AF, et al. Coronary atherosclerosis and dilation in hyper IgE syndrome patients: depiction by magnetic resonance vessel wall imaging and pathological correlation. Atherosclerosis. 2017;258:20–5. https://doi.org/10.1016/j.atherosclerosis.2017.01.022.

Arora M, Bagi P, Strongin A, Heimall J, Zhao X, Lawrence MG, et al. Gastrointestinal manifestations of STAT3-deficient hyper IgE syndrome. J Clin Immunol. 2017;37(7):695–700. https://doi.org/10.1007/s10875-017-0429-z.

Davis SD, Schaller J, Wedgwood RJ. Job's syndrome. Recurrent, "cold," staphylococcal abscesses. Lancet. 1966;1(7445):1013–5.

Freeman AF, Olivier KN. Hyper IgE syndromes and the lung. Clin Chest Med. 2016;37(3):557–67. https://doi.org/10.1016/j.ccm.2016.4.016.

Goussetis E, Peristeri I, Kitra V, Traeger-Synodinos J, Theodosaki M, Osarra K, et al. Successful long-term immunologic reconstitution by allogenic hematopoietic stem cell transplantation cures patients with autosomal dominant hyper-IgE syndrome. J Allergy Clin Immunol. 2010;126(2):392–4. https://doi.org/10.1016/j.jaci.2010.05.005.

Holland SM, DeLeo FR, Elloumi HZ, Hsu AP, Uzel G, Brodsky N, et al. STAT3 mutations in the hyper IgE syndrome. N Engl J Med. 2007;357(16):1608–19. https://doi.org/10.1056/NEJMoa073687.

Hox V, O'Connell MP, Lyons J, Sackstein P, Dimaggio T, Jones N, et al. Diminution of signal transducer and activator of transcription 3 signaling inhibits vascular permeability and anaphylaxis. J Allergy Clin Immunol. 2016;138(1):187–99. https://doi.org/10.1016/j.jaci.2015.11.024.

Minegishi Y, Saito M, Tsuchiya S, Tsuge I, Takada H, Hara T, et al. Dominant-negative mutations in the DNA-binding domain of STAT3 cause hyper-IgE syndrome. Nature. 2007;448(7157):1058–62. https://doi.org/10.1038/nature06096.

Siegel AM, Heimall J, Freeman AF, Hsu AP, Brittain E, Brenchley JM, et al. A critical role for STAT3 transcription factor signaling in the development and maintenance of human T cell memory. Immunity. 2011;35(5):806–18. https://doi.org/10.1016/j.immuni.2011.09.016.

Sowerwine KJ, Holland SM, Freeman AF. Hyper-IgE syndrome update. Ann N Y Acad Sci. 2012;1250:25–32. https://doi.org/10.1111/j.1749-6632.2011.06387.x.

Yanagimachi M, Ohya T, Yokosuka T, Kajiwara R, Tanaka F, Goto H, et al. The potential and limits of hematopoietic stem cell transplantation for the treatment of autosomal dominant hyper-IgE syndrome. J Clin Immunol. 2016;36(5):511–6. https://doi.org/10.1007/s10875-016-0278-1.

Yong PF, Freeman AF, Engelhardt KR, Holland SM, Puck JM, Grimbacher B. An update on the hyper-IgE syndromes. Arthritis Res Ther. 2012;14(6):228. https://doi.org/10.1186/ar4069.

Autosomal Recessive CGD (NCF-1, NCF-2, CYBA, NCF4)

Antonio Condino-Neto[1] and Peter E. Newburger[2]
[1]Department of Immunology, Institute of Biomedical Sciences – University of São Paulo, São Paulo, SP, Brazil
[2]Department of Pediatrics, Division of Hematology/Oncology, University of Massachusetts Medical School, Worcester, MA, USA

Chronic Granulomatous Disease (CGD) is a primary immunodeficiency which was originally characterized in the 1950s as a clinical entity affecting male infants and termed "fatal granulomatous disease of childhood". CGD is characterized by early onset of severe recurrent infections affecting mainly the natural barriers of the organism such as the respiratory tract and lymph nodes, and eventually internal structures such as liver, spleen, bones, and brain. The estimated incidence of this disease is approximately 1/250,000 live births per year. CGD can also present with abnormal inflammatory responses, which often result in the dysregulated granuloma formation in inflamed tissues (Arnold and Heimall 2017).

Phagocytes, such as monocytes/macrophages, contain a membrane-associated nicotinamide adenine dinucleotide phosphate – reduced form (NADPH)-oxidase that produces superoxide and other reactive oxygen intermediates involved in microbicidal, tumoricidal, and inflammatory activities. Defects in NADPH oxidase activity lead to defective superoxide production and predisposes the patient to severe, life-threatening infections, generally by catalase positive pathogens, which demonstrate the importance of the oxygen-dependent microbicidal system in host defense (Arnold and Heimall 2017). Phagocyte NADPH oxidase activation results in conversion of molecular oxygen to superoxide anion. Superoxide dismutase converts superoxide anion to hydrogen peroxide. In neutrophils, myeloperoxidase (MPO) catalyzes the production of hypochlorous acid from hydrogen peroxide

and chloride ions (Arnold and Heimall 2017). The terminal electron donor to oxygen is a unique low-midpoint-potential flavocytochrome b, cytochrome b_{558}, a heterodimer composed of a 91 kDa glycoprotein (termed gp91-$phox$, for *glycoprotein 91* kDa of *phagocyte oxidase*), and a 22 kDa nonglycosylated polypeptide (p22-$phox$). Upon activation, the cytoplasmic subunits p47$phox$, p67$phox$, p40$phox$, and rac protein translocate to the membrane-bound cytochrome b_{558}.

Biallelic pathogenic variants in *CYBA*, *NCF1*, *NCF2*, and *NCF4* (Matute et al. 2009) cause autosomal recessive CGD (AR-CGD) (Roos et al. 2017). Mutations in *CYBB* cause X-linked CGD. In the Western world, AR-CGD corresponds to approximately 30% of all CGD cases. In populations with high consanguinity, AR-CGD may be the predominant form of the disease (Arnold and Heimall 2017).

NCF2 (GenBank accession number M32011) encodes p67-phox, one of the cytoplasmic components of the NADPH oxidase. Located at chromosome 1q25, the gene has 11 exons and spans 15 kb of genomic DNA. It is responsible for approximately 5% of CGD cases (Roesler et al. 2000).

The clinical presentation of AR-CGD is similar to X-linked CGD and influenced by residual NADPH oxidase function. However, because AR-CGD generally features more available residual function, survival is superior to that in X-linked CGD.

Clinical Presentation

CGD should be suspected in children with failure to thrive, early onset of recurrent pneumonias, lymphadenitis, liver abscess, osteomyelitis, and skin infections (pyoderma, abscesses or cellulitis). Other clinical manifestations include granuloma formation, especially genitourinary and gastrointestinal (often initially pyloric, and later esophageal, jejunal, ileal, cecal, rectal, and perirectal), colitis, presenting as frequent stooling and fistulae or fissures. This may be the sole finding in some individuals. Abnormal wound healing caused by excessive granulation may also occur.

A single infection by a characteristic organism – e.g., BCG, *Serratia* spp., *Burkholderia cepatia,* or *Chromobacterium violaceum* – should raise immediate suspicion of CGD.

Clinicians should be familiar with local epidemiology and be aware of unusual microorganisms as causative pathogens when evaluating CGD patients with infections. Special attention to these pathogens should be given to CGD patients after returning from endemic regions. Microbiological confirmation must be pursued, and appropriate anti-microbial regimen should be given. BCG vaccine is contraindicated in CGD and should be withheld for neonates who have a family history of CGD or suspected primary immunodeficiency disease until excluded by appropriate investigations.

Treatment/Prognosis

Prophylaxis in CGD
Standard infection prophylaxis for CGD includes an antibacterial agent, a mold-active antifungal agent, and recombinant interferon-γ.

Antibacterial Prophylaxis
Trimethoprim-sulfamethoxazole has been used for decades in CGD. This agent has been proven to be safe and effective in reducing bacterial infections. Trimethoprim-sulfamethoxazole is active against most of bacterial pathogens that cause infection in CGD, including *S. aureus*, *Burkholderia* spp., and *Nocardia* spp. In CGD patients who are allergic or intolerant of trimethoprim-sulfamethoxazole, alternative agents (e.g., cephalexin or doxycycline) with anti-staphylococcal activity should be used as prophylaxis.

Antifungal Prophylaxis
Prevention of invasive aspergillosis and other filamentous fungal diseases relies on avoiding environments where high levels of fungal spores are expected (e.g., playing on mulch or wood chips, gardening, and building renovations) and mold-active antifungal prophylaxis. Itraconazole prophylaxis has been shown to be safe and

effective in patients with CGD. Other mold-active azoles are voriconazole and posaconazole.

Recombinant Interferon-γ
Recombinant interferon-γ has been widely used as prophylaxis in patients with CGD for approximately 25 years. In a randomized trial, recombinant interferon-γ reduced in 70% the incidence of serious infections and was beneficial regardless of age, the use of prophylactic antibiotics, or the type of CGD (X-linked or autosomal recessive). The benefit of prophylactic recombinant interferon-γ may result from augmentation of oxidant-independent pathways, as well as an increase in oxidase activity in variant CGD cases with residual NADPH oxidase function. Long-term recombinant interferon- γ has been generally well tolerated in CGD, with fever being the most frequent side effect.

Treatment of Infections in CGD
Invasive bacterial infections (e.g., pneumonia, osteomyelitis, and deep soft tissue infections) require prolonged antibiotic therapy. Bacterial infections involving bone or viscera frequently require surgery. Decisions about surgical intervention must be individualized based on the pathogen, location and extent of disease, and likelihood of response to antibacterial treatment alone.

Voriconazole was shown to be superior to conventional amphotericin B as primary therapy for aspergillosis. Lipid formulations of amphotericin B, posaconazole, isavuconazole, and echinocandins are additional options for therapy of invasive aspergillosis in patients who are intolerant to voriconazole or who have refractory disease. In addition to antifungal therapy, debridement or resection of infected tissue may be required. This is particularly the case for refractory aspergillosis or extension of fungal disease to vertebrae or chest wall.

Granulocyte Transfusions
Adjunctive granulocyte transfusions have been used for severe or refractory infections in CGD patients, based on the likelihood that a proportion of normal neutrophils can augment host defense in CGD neutrophils by providing a source of

diffusible ROS. Hydrogen peroxide generated by normal neutrophils can diffuse into CGD neutrophils and provide the necessary substrate to generate hypochlorous acid and hydroxyl anion in vitro. Alloimmunization is a potential complication when performing granulocyte transfusion, as this can be a major stumbling block to allogeneic stem cell transplantation.

Hematopoietic Stem Cell Transplantation
Allogeneic hematopoietic stem cell transplantation is usually curative in CGD and is becoming accepted as a standard of care. AR-CGD patients with low or no residual function of the NADPH oxidase should be considered for bone marrow transplant.

Prognosis
Since the advent of prophylactic antibiotics, antifungals, and recombinant interferon-γ, the prognosis for patients with CGD has improved. Patients living to their 30s and 40s are now common. The production of residual ROS is a predictor of survival in patients with CGD.

Survival rates are variable but improving; approximately 50% of patients survive to age 30–40 years. Infections are less common in adults than in children, but the propensity for severe life-threatening bacterial infections persists throughout life. Fungal infections remain a major determinant of survival in CGD. Currently, the annual mortality rate is 1.5% per year for persons with autosomal recessive CGD. Morbidity secondary to infection or granulomatous complications remains significant for many patients.

Cross-References

▶ CYBB X-linked Chronic Granulomatous Disease (CGD)

References

Arnold DE, Heimall JR. A review of chronic granulomatous disease. Adv Ther. 2017;34(12):2543–57. https://doi.org/10.1007/s12325-017-0636-2.

Matute JD, Arias AA, Wright NA, Wrobel I, Waterhouse CC, Li XJ, Marchal CC, Stull ND, Lewis DB, Steele M, Kellner JD, Yu W, Meroueh SO, Nauseef WM, Dinauer MC. A new genetic subgroup of chronic granulomatous disease with autosomal recessive mutations in p40 phox and selective defects in neutrophil NADPH oxidase activity. Blood. 2009;114(15):3309–15. https://doi.org/10.1182/blood-2009-07-231498.

Roesler J, Curnutte JT, Rae J, Barrett D, Patino P, Chanock SJ, Goerlach A. Recombination events between the p47-phox gene and its highly homologous pseudogenes are the main cause of autosomal recessive chronic granulomatous disease. Blood. 2000;95(6):2150–6.

Roos D, Tool ATJ, van Leeuwen K, de Boer M. Biochemical and genetic diagnosis of chronic granulomatous disease. In: Seger RA, Roos D, Segal BH, Kuijpers TW, editors. Immunology and immune system disorders. Chronic granulomatous disease genetics, biology and clinical management. New York: Nova Science Publishers; 2017. p. 231–300.

B

B Cell Lymphoma/Leukemia 10 Deficiency

Robert P. Nelson
Divisions of Hematology and Oncology, Stem Cell Transplant Program, Indiana University (IU) School of Medicine and the IU Bren and Simon Cancer Center, Indianapolis, IN, USA
Pediatric Immunodeficiency Clinic, Riley Hospital for Children at Indiana University Health, Indianapolis, IN, USA
Medicine and Pediatrics, Indiana University School of Medicine, Immunohematology and Transplantation, Indianapolis, IN, USA

Synonyms

CARMEN; c-E10; CARD containing molecule enhancing NF-kB

Definition

Immune signaling adaptor

Introduction/Background

B Cell Lymphoma/Leukemia 10 (BCL10) is an important member of a family of molecules that transduce signals from MHC-peptide-immunoreceptors on naïve T and B-lymphocyte cell membranes to the nucleus. BCL10 was discovered as a target of the translocations of t(1; 14) (p22; q32) that cause mucosa-associated lymphoid tissue (MALT) lymphoma and is one of the three components of the caspace recruitment domain (CARD)–BCL10–MALT1 (CBM) complex that links the triggering of antigen receptors to activation of nuclear factor kappa-light-chain-enhancer of activated B cells (NF-κB) (Spencer 1999; Thome and Weil 2007). Murine homozygous BCL10 mutations lead to either embryological demise or severe immunodeficiency characterized by impaired antigen receptor, phorbol myristate acetate (PMA), or ionomycin-induced activation and lymphoid cell proliferation. The mouse knockout fails to connect antigen receptor signaling in B and T cells to NF-kB activation (Ruland et al. 2001).

Torres, working with the JL Casanova et al., characterized the genotype and phenotype of a human autosomal-recessive BCL10 deficiency in a child with combined immunodeficiency and impaired innate host defense. This particular description of a human monogenic disorder of immunity represents a model for the comprehensive, detailed, incisive characterization of a patient by the collaborative application of genetic, molecular biological, and functional immunological techniques that illuminate the fundamental connectivity between systems of human host defense, hematopoiesis and aberrancies of inflammation, autoimmunity, and cancer. Although the child died at 3 years of age, the effects of BCL10 deficiency appeared signal pathway- and cell type-dependent. Clinical findings were somewhat similar to BCL10 adaptive immune deficiency observed in mice, features specific to the patient within various cell populations were also described (Torres et al. 2014).

Function

The BCL10 protein resides in breast, thymus, and lymphoid tissues and its expression is abundant in germinal centers, moderate in the marginal zone, and weak in the mantle zone B cells. BCL10 promotes activation of NF-κB transcription factors by modulating ubiquitination of NEMO (Zhou et al. 2004). BCL10 is also a binding partner with tumor necrosis factor receptor-associated factor 2 (TRAF2), whereby low levels of BCL10 expression promote the binding of TRAF2, while overexpression induces NFKB downstream of TRAF2 to impair apoptosis (Yoneda et al. 2000).

Innate Defense
BCL10 transduces activation signals emanating from antigen-presenting cells and augments natural killer (NK) cytokine expression. The enzyme Interleukin-1 receptor-associated kinase 1 (IRAK-1) recruits BCL10 to the lipopolysaccharide (LPS)/Toll-like receptor 4 (TLR4), which propagates signal to activate NFKB. Lack of Bcl10 impairs receptor-mediated generation of GM-CSF and chemokines and reduces the generation of IFN-gamma in NK cells (Liu et al. 2004).

Adaptive Immunity
Stimulation of TCR or BCR induces signal transduction cascades through CARD11, which recruits Bcl10 and MALT1 to lipid rafts important to lymphocyte activation and development (Lin and Wang 2004). BCL110−/− mice that survive gestation are defective in antigen receptor, PMA, or Ionomycin-induced activation. Early tyrosine phosphorylation, mitogen-activated protein kinase (MAPK), and activated protein 1 (AP-1) activation and Ca2+ signaling appear normal, but antigen receptor-induced NF-kB activation is absent. Bcl10 is essential for the development of all mature B cells and its absence impedes

conversion from transitional type 2 to mature follicular B cells, decreasing marginal zone and B1 B cells. Bcl10-deficient follicular and marginal zone B cells fail to proliferate normally and Bcl10-deficient marginal zone B cells fail to activate NF-kB efficiently after stimulation with lipopolysaccharide (Lin and Wang 2004). Furthermore, Bcl10-deficient marginal zone B cells appear not to capture antigens and Bcl10-deficient mice fail to initiate humoral responses, which leads to an inability to clear blood-borne bacteria.

Cancer
Translocations of t(1; 14) (p22; q32) result in frameshift mutations within the carboxyl terminal domain that truncates BCL 10 and causes MALT lymphoma, which is the most common subset of extranodal Hodgkin lymphomas with predilection for the gastrointestinal tract. Mutant BCL-10 overexpression inhibits pro-apoptosis activity, conferring a survival advantage for MALT B-cells, while constitutive NFKB activation propagates antiapoptotic and proliferative signals mediated via its transcriptional targets (Willis et al. 1999).

Clinical Presentation

History
Beginning at 6 months, the patient recurrent otitis, encephalitis of unknown etiology, oral candidiasis, diaper dermatitis with *Candida albicans* superinfection, and respiratory infections. He experienced active chronic colitis and prolonged diarrhea due to *Campylobacter jejuni* infection, acute gastroenteritis secondary to adenovirus, and diarrhea caused by *Clostridium difficile* (Ruland et al. 2001).

Combined T and B cell immunodeficiencies, in general, are likely to be children below 18 years of age with recurrent infections and a birth history with normal or low T cell excision circles (TRECs) at newborn screening. A positive family history is helpful but de novo defects also occur, so that a negative family history does not rule out the condition. Given the broad functionality of BCL10, infectious pathogens might be those with high-grade encapsulated bacterial pathogens and/or opportunists. There may be autoimmune manifestations, enteritis, persistent or recurrent dermatological manifestations, cognitive impairment, and developmental delay or failure to thrive due to illness or consequences of infection or inflammatory disease. One would not expect cardiovascular structural defects or radiographic evidence of an absent thymus.

Physical

Signs of failure to thrive, atypical distribution or severe atopic dermatitis, oral candidiasis, and small stature are potentially present; however, there are no specific, unusual or unique pathognomonic physical features that distinguish this particular defect from other combined immunodeficiencies or primary immunodeficiencies affecting other pathways.

Laboratory Findings

Total serum immunoglobulins were low. A hallmark finding may be an immuno-phenotype characterized by a profound deficit in memory T and B cells. Over 95% of the patient's B cells were naïve (Torres et al. 2014). A distinguishing feature that points to BCL10 as the defect causing the combined immunodeficiency is the finding of intact myeloid cell response to pathogen-associated molecular pattern molecules (PAMPs) but deficient NF-kappa B-mediated fibroblast function. The effects of BCL10 deficiency were dependent on the signaling pathway and cell type affected. A defective adaptive immune response was consistent with the murine knockout; however, the BCL10 deficiency in the child resulted in normal myeloid cell responses to pathogen-associated molecular pattern molecules (PAMPs) but deficient NF-kB-mediated responses in fibroblasts.

Treatment/Prognosis

The first clinical decision to make is whether to take care of the patent locally or consider referral to a center that has a multidisciplinary center for the management of these conditions, as exist for several of the classical immunodeficiency diseases. The patient and family may need input from social services regarding health care options and avenues to care that are either available or not.

General treatment considerations of immunocompromised patients apply. Inactivated immunizations are recommended but live vaccines are not. Extreme isolation or avoidance of normal schooling may not be necessary or recommended. Prompt medical evaluation for early unusual consequences of infection is important to the care of patients with combined immunodeficiencies. There may be extension to the usual course of treatment for individual infectious episodes. Particular attention is given to address inflammatory conditions that may require iatrogenic immunosuppression and anti-inflammatory therapy that exacerbate or synergistically add to the immunodeficiency's "potency" overall. Other measures include the use of prophylactic antibiotics as indicated with guidance informed by serial assessments of clinical and laboratory findings, including antibody production capacity, the latter to alert the clinician to the need for immunoglobulin replacement therapy (Ballow et al. 2018). Early high-complexity care requires consideration, ideally before morbid complications ensue that may prohibit eligibility for curative immuno-reconstitution efforts such as hematopoietic cell transplantation.

Cross-References

▶ Caspase Recruitment Domain 11, CARD11
▶ Evaluation of Suspected Immunodeficiency, Overview
▶ MALT1 Deficiency

References

Ballow M, Paris K, de la Morena M. Should antibiotic prophylaxis be routinely used in patients with antibody-mediated primary immunodeficiency? J Allergy Clin Immunol Pract. 2018;6:421–6.

Lin X, Wang D. The roles of CARMA1, Bcl10, and MALT1 in antigen receptor signaling. Semin Immunol. 2004;16:429–35.

Liu Y, Dong W, Chen L, et al. BCL10 mediates lipopolysaccharide/toll-like receptor-4 signaling through interaction with Pellino2. J Biol Chem. 2004;279:37436–44.

Ruland J, Duncan GS, Elia A, et al. Bcl10 is a positive regulator of antigen receptor-induced activation of

NF-kappaB and neural tube closure. Cell. 2001;104:33–42.

Spencer J. Aggressive mucosa associated lymphoid tissue lymphomas are associated with mutations in Bcl10. Gut. 1999;44:778–9.

Thome M, Weil R. Post-translational modifications regulate distinct functions of CARMA1 and BCL10. Trends Immunol. 2007;28:281–8.

Torres JM, Martinez-Barricarte R, Garcia-Gomez S, et al. Inherited BCL10 deficiency impairs hematopoietic and nonhematopoietic immunity. J Clin Invest. 2014;124:5239–48.

Willis TG, Jadayel DM, Du MQ, et al. Bcl10 is involved in t(1;14)(p22;q32) of MALT B cell lymphoma and mutated in multiple tumor types. Cell. 1999;96:35–45.

Yoneda T, Imaizumi K, Maeda M, et al. Regulatory mechanisms of TRAF2-mediated signal transduction by Bcl10, a MALT lymphoma-associated protein. J Biol Chem. 2000;275:11114–20.

Zhou H, Wertz I, O'Rourke K, et al. Bcl10 activates the NF-kappaB pathway through ubiquitination of NEMO. Nature. 2004;427:167–71.

B-Actin Deficiency

Raz Somech and Tali Stauber
Pediatric Department, Allergy and the Immunology Services, "Edmond and Lily Safra" Children's Hospital, Sackler School of Medicine, Tel Aviv University, Tel Aviv, Israel
Jeffrey Modell Foundation Center, Sackler School of Medicine, Tel Aviv University, Tel Aviv, Israel
Sheba Medical Center, Tel Hashomer, Sackler School of Medicine, Tel Aviv University, Tel Aviv, Israel

Synonyms

Baraitser-Winter Syndrome 1; Chromosome 7p22 deletion

Definition

Beta-actin (ACTB), one of the actin isoforms, is an important cytoskeletal protein. Mutations in the ACTB gene were found in Baraitser-Winter cerebrofrontofacial syndrome. In one patient, immunodeficiency of neutrophils was identified.

Introduction

Actins are a family of highly conserved cytoskeletal proteins that play fundamental roles in nearly all aspects of eukaryotic cell biology. The ability of a cell to divide, move, endocytose, generate contractile force, and maintain shape is reliant upon functional actin-based structures. The importance of the cytoskeleton in mounting a successful immune response is evident from the wide range of defects that occur in actin-related primary immunodeficiencies (PIDs). Actin isoforms are grouped according to expression patterns: muscle actins predominate in striated and smooth muscle (ACTA1 and ACTA2, respectively), whereas the two cytoplasmic non-muscle actins, gamma-actin (ACTG1) and beta-actin (ACTB), are found in all cells and differ by only four amino acids at their conserved N-terminal ends. Beta-actin protein is encoded by ACTB located at 7p22.1 and has five known splice variants (Moulding et al. 2013).

Compared with myopathy and angiopathy-associated defects of muscle isoactins, mutations of beta-actin and gamma-actin isoforms lead to a wider spectrum of diseases that include deafness, cancer, and skeletal and developmental disorders.

Several different nonlethal mutations of ACTB were identified in Baraitser-Winter cerebrofrontofacial syndrome (Verloes et al. 2015). This is an autosomal dominant trait with craniofacial, visceral, and muscular involvement due to gain-of-function mutations in ACTB or ACTG1. Major features include hypertelorism, bilateral ptosis, ocular colobomata, metopic ridging, and trigonocephaly. The nose is wide, short, and upturned. Skeletal defects comprise short stature, dorsal kyphosis, anteverted shoulders, and limited joint movements with slightly flexed elbows and knees. Neurological anomalies occur in the form of motor delay, intellectual deficiency, and agyria or pachygyria. Other ACTB mutations were found to be associated with juvenile-onset dystonia (Procaccio et al. 2006), which is a severe autosomal dominant disorder of movement with involuntary muscle contractions, associated with neurosensory hearing loss, pronounced facial defects with bilateral ptosis and hypertelorism, intellectual deficiency, and structural brain defects. Perhaps, however, juvenile-onset dystonia should merely be taken as a variant within the spectrum of Baraitser-Winter cerebrofrontofacial syndrome (Rivière et al. 2012).

Clinical Presentation

To date there has been only one case report of immunodeficiency secondary to ACTB mutation (Nunoi et al. 1999). A 12-year-old female patient presented with recurrent infections, photosensitivity, and mental retardation. She also had abnormalities in neutrophil chemotaxis, superoxide production, and membrane potential response. Laboratory investigation of peripheral blood cells identified an abnormal actin protein. Sequencing of the actin gene revealed a heterozygous G-1174 to A substitution, predicting a glutamic acid 364 to lysine substitution in beta-actin. Though no defect in cell-free polymerization of actin was detected, this defect lies in a domain important for binding to profilin and other actin-regulatory molecules, and the mutant actin bound to profilin less efficiently than normal actin did. By 15 years of age, she had developed cardiomegaly, hepatomegaly, and hypothyroidism. At that time, she presented with persistent fevers, and, despite intensive therapy, she died from septicemia (Hundt et al. 2014).

References

Hundt N, Preller M, Swolski O, Ang AM, Mannherz HG, Manstein DJ, Müller M. Molecular mechanisms of disease-related human β-actin mutations p.R183W and p.E364K. FEBS J. 2014;281(23):5279–91.

Moulding DA, Record J, Malinova D, Thrasher AJ. Actin cytoskeletal defects in immunodeficiency. Immunol Rev. 2013;256(1):282–99. Erratum in: Immunol Rev. 2016;271(1):293

Nunoi H, Yamazaki T, Tsuchiya H, Kato S, Malech HL, Matsuda I, Kanegasaki S. A heterozygous mutation of beta-actin associated with neutrophil dysfunction and recurrent infection. Proc Natl Acad Sci U S A. 1999;96(15):8693–8.

Procaccio V, Salazar G, Ono S, Styers ML, Gearing M, Davila A, Jimenez R, Juncos J, Gutekunst CA, Meroni G, Fontanella B, Sontag E, Sontag JM,

Faundez V, Wainer BH. A mutation of beta -actin that alters depolymerization dynamics is associated with autosomal dominant developmental malformations, deafness, and dystonia. Am J Hum Genet. 2006;78(6):947–60.

Rivière JB, van Bon BW, Hoischen A, Kholmanskikh SS, O'Roak BJ, Gilissen C, Gijsen S, Sullivan CT, Christian SL, Abdul-Rahman OA, Atkin JF, Chassaing N, Drouin-Garraud V, Fry AE, Fryns JP, Gripp KW, Kempers M, Kleefstra T, Mancini GM, Nowaczyk MJ, van Ravenswaaij-Arts CM, Roscioli T, Marble M, Rosenfeld JA, Siu VM, de Vries BB, Shendure J, Verloes A, Veltman JA, Brunner HG, Ross ME, Pilz DT, Dobyns WB. Nat Genet. 2012;44(4):440–4, S1–2.

Verloes A, Di Donato N, Masliah-Planchon J, Jongmans M, Abdul-Raman OA, Albrecht B, Allanson J, Brunner H, Bertola D, Chassaing N, David A, Devriendt K, Eftekhari P, Drouin-Garraud V, Faravelli F, Faivre L, Giuliano F, Guion Almeida L, Juncos J, Kempers M, Eker HK, Lacombe D, Lin A, Mancini G, Melis D, Lourenço CM, Siu VM, Morin G, Nezarati M, Nowaczyk MJ, Ramer JC, Osimani S, Philip N, Pierpont ME, Procaccio V, Roseli ZS, Rossi M, Rusu C, Sznajer Y, Templin L, Uliana V, Klaus M, Van Bon B, Van Ravenswaaij C, Wainer B, Fry AE, Rump A, Hoischen A, Drunat S, Rivière JB, Dobyns WB, Pilz DT. Eur J Hum Genet. 2015;23(3):292–301.

Baff-Receptor Deficiency

Klaus Warnatz
Department of Rheumatology and Clinical Immunology and Center for Chronic Immunodeficiency, University Medical Center and University of Freiburg, Freiburg, Germany

Definition

The immunodeficiency is defined by deleterious mutations in TNFRSF13C encoding for B cell-activating factor receptor (Baff-R).

Prevalence

So far only two patients with deleterious mutations in TNFRSF13C have been published encoding for Baff-R (Warnatz et al. 2009). However, several patients have been identified carrying point mutations which may contribute to the manifestation of antibody deficiency, but the evidence is less strict, since these variants are also found in healthy people and the immunological presentation doesn't reflect the expected phenotype of an absent BAFF-R function.

Clinical Presentation

Deleterious mutations. The index patient had upper airway infections since childhood, the first pneumonia at age 37 and was diagnosed at age 57 after his third pneumonia. His older sister never presented with a remarkable susceptibility to infections until old age. Neither BAFF-R deficient person developed autoimmunity, abnormal lymphoproliferation, nor other signs of immune dysregulation (Warnatz et al. 2009). Additional patients with P21R+/−H159Y genetic variants have a highly variable presentation from asymptomatic to infection – only or complex presentation of CVID, selective IgA deficiency, or IgM deficiency (Lougaris et al. 2016; Pieper et al. 2014; Losi et al. 2005).

Genetics

A homozygous 24-bp in-frame deletion (del89–96) mutation led to absent protein expression. Several point mutations which may contribute to immunodeficiency have been reported in *TNFRSF13C*. The most prominent ones are P21R and H159Y (Lougaris et al. 2016; Pieper et al. 2014; Losi et al. 2005).

Immunological Phenotype

BAFF-R belongs to the TNF-receptor family. It is a transmembrane molecule which is expressed on B cell subpopulations. Its single known ligand is BAFF (synonym, Blys). During B cell differentiation, BAFF-R is first expressed on transitional B cells. Its expression is partly depending on B cell receptor signals. After engagement with its ligands, it forms trimers which can bind

BAFF triggering PI3K and especially alternative NF-kB signals.

Its signal is essential for sufficient B cells survival especially at the transitional stage which will subsequently allow for further maturation into the naïve B cell stage. Thus, complete BAFF-R deficiency in mice and men is characterized by severely reduced B cell counts, and the analysis of the subpopulations reveals a relative expansion of transitional B cells (Warnatz et al. 2009; Yan et al. 2001). Serum IgG and IgM were reduced in both siblings, while IgA was normal or even elevated reflecting the preserved IgA production in the gastrointestinal mucosa.

The reduction in BAFF binding by the described point mutations is not sufficient to cause the typical phenotype, but it has been shown that the P21R mutation interferes with the multimerization of the complex (Pieper et al. 2014) and might contribute to the immunodeficiency.

Diagnosis

Diagnosis is made by genetic analysis of *TNFRSF13C*. The diagnosis of complete BAFF-R deficiency is suggested by a hypogammaglobulinemia sparing IgA, a severe reduction of B cells with a block at the transitional B cell stage and the lack of BAFF-R surface expression.

Therapy

No specific therapy is available. Patients who suffer from infection should be placed on immunoglobulin replacement therapy. There is no experience with stem cell transplantation. While this disease should be in general transplantable, the mild phenotype did not require this therapy in the reported patients.

References

Losi CG, Silini A, Fiorini C, Soresina A, Meini A, Ferrari S, et al. Mutational analysis of human BAFF receptor TNFRSF13C (BAFF-R) in patients with common variable immunodeficiency. J Clin Immunol. 2005;25(5):496–502.

Lougaris V, Baronio M, Moratto D, Cardinale F, Plebani A. Monoallelic BAFFR P21R/H159Y mutations and familiar primary antibody deficiencies. J Clin Immunol. 2016;36(1):1–3.

Pieper K, Rizzi M, Speletas M, Smulski CR, Sic H, Kraus H, et al. A common single nucleotide polymorphism impairs B-cell activating factor receptor's multimerization, contributing to common variable immunodeficiency. J Allergy Clin Immunol. 2014;133(4):1222–5.

Warnatz K, Salzer U, Rizzi M, Fischer B, Gutenberger S, Bohm J, et al. B-cell activating factor receptor deficiency is associated with an adult-onset antibody deficiency syndrome in humans. Proc Natl Acad Sci U S A. 2009;106(33):13945–50.

Yan M, Brady JR, Chan B, Lee WP, Hsu B, Harless S, et al. Identification of a novel receptor for B lymphocyte stimulator that is mutated in a mouse strain with severe B cell deficiency. Curr Biol. 2001;11(19):1547–52.

"Bamboo Hair"

▶ Comel-Netherton Syndrome (*SPINK5*)

Baraitser-Winter Syndrome 1

▶ B-Actin Deficiency

Barth Syndrome

Persio Roxo-Junior and Isabela Mina
Division of Immunology and Allergy, Department of Pediatrics, Ribeirão Preto Medical School, University of São Paulo, Ribeirão Preto, Brazil

Definition

Barth syndrome (synonyms: X-linked cardioskeletal myopathy, neutropenia and abnormal mitochondria, 3-methylglutaconic aciduria type II, endocardial fibroelastosis type 2), is a mitochondrial disease (Rezaei et al. 2009; Imai-Okazaki et al. 2018) that presents phenotypic and allelic heterogeneity (Imai-Okazaki et al. 2018). This syndrome is characterized by neutropenia, dilated cardiomyopathy, hypocholesterolemia, aciduria, skeletal myopathy, growth retardation, and cognitive impairment (Rezaei et al. 2009; Imai-Okazaki et al. 2018; Jefferies 2013).

The syndrome was firstly described by Barth et al. in a large Dutch family.

Introduction

Barth syndrome is an X-linked recessive disease generally caused by mutations in the *TAZ* gene (Rezaei et al. 2009; Imai-Okazaki et al. 2018; Jefferies 2013), which encodes the tafazzin protein. Tafazzin is a phospholipid acyltransferase that is involved in remodeling cardiolipin, which is necessary to maintain mitochondrial structure.

The mutations in *TAZ* gene lead to modifications in cardiolipin composition and to the decline in its total concentration in many tissues and organs, such as granulocytes, fibroblasts, and heart and skeletal muscle (Rezaei et al. 2009).

As cardiolipin is a specific mitochondrial phospholipid, abnormal characteristics of this protein may cause a decrease in mitochondrial respiratory chain complex activity and an oxidative phosphorylation deficiency (Rezaei et al. 2009; Imai-Okazaki et al. 2018).

Clinical Presentation

Patients with Barth syndrome present clinical disorders associated with the decrease or changes in composition of cardiolipin in many tissues and organs.

The disease is characterized by dilated cardiomyopathy or isolated left ventricular abnormalities, proximal skeletal myopathy, short stature, neutropenia, hypocholesterolemia, cognitive dysfunction, and organic aciduria (Imai-Okazaki et al. 2018; Kang et al. 2016; Steward et al. 2010).

However, this syndrome presents a phenotypic heterogeneity. So clinical manifestations may differ greatly among patients, and they may present variation even in cardiac phenotypes (Imai-Okazaki et al. 2018).

Various degrees of neutropenia are observed in different patients with Barth syndrome (Rezaei et al. 2009), and it can be associated with bacterial infections and consequently sepsis (Jefferies 2013). The neutropenia may be persistent or intermittent and leads to respiratory and dermatologic infections (Jefferies 2013), besides chronic aphthous stomatitis generally caused by fungus like *Candida* infections (Rezaei et al. 2009).

Laboratory Findings and Diagnostic Testing

Elevated urinary organic acid excretion in addition to neutropenia and hypocholesterolemia, especially when associated with dilated cardiomyopathy, should lead to suspicion to Barth syndrome (Rezaei et al. 2009; Imai-Okazaki et al. 2018).

Despite Barth syndrome is characterized to present various degrees of neutropenia, the neutrophils seem to have normal function (Rezaei et al. 2009).

Another biochemical abnormality detected in patients with the disease is an elevated monolysocardiolipin/cardiolipin (MLCL/CL) ratio in blood sample. This is a noninvasive test and has been described that the accumulation of MLCL is specific for Barth syndrome and that the MLCL/CL ratio is a better diagnostic marker than the CL (Imai-Okazaki et al. 2018).

Furthermore, the definitive diagnosis may be obtained by genetic analysis. However, because of the allelic heterogeneity, besides direct screening of the *TAZ* gene on the X chromosome, another genetic analysis, such as whole exome sequencing, may be necessary if the *TAZ* gene screening is negative and the patient is clinically suspect. Various mutations have been previously detected in patients with the disease, including frameshift, nonsense, missense, and splice site mutations (Imai-Okazaki et al. 2018).

Treatment and Prognosis

It is greatly recommended a multidisciplinary approach in the management of patients with Barth syndrome (Reynolds 2015).

Previously, Barth syndrome was considered an early and lethal childhood disease. Even though mortality is still highest in the first 4 years of life, there are patients living until adulthood because of the improvements in the management of neutropenia and infections, skeletal myopathy, and cardiac disease. So, early diagnosis and prompt treatment can improve the prognosis of patients with Barth syndrome (Imai-Okazaki et al. 2018).

Granulocyte colony-stimulating factor (GCSF) may be used in periods of neutropenia to elevate absolute neutrophil numbers, associated with prophylactic antibiotics if clinically necessary (Reynolds 2015).

For short stature, growth hormone (GH) supplementation is not routinely indicated, unless documented central GH deficiency. Despite the decreased levels of GH have been reported in patients less than 15 years old, its levels generally are normal or higher than normal controls at the end of adolescence. As it has been evidenced that arginine depletion may be associated with low growth rates in patients with Barth syndrome, arginine supplementation is a possible treatment in these cases (Reynolds 2015).

The treatment of myocardial dysfunction is essential to prolong life, alleviate symptoms, and provide a better quality of life. The dilated cardiomyopathy can be treated by medical and surgical options, and the treatment must be specific to each cardiac phenotype (Jefferies 2013).

Patients with Barth syndrome also should be benefited by specific dietary interventions (Wintergerst et al. 2017).

References

Imai-Okazaki A, Kishita Y, Kohda M, Yatsuka Y, Hirata T, Mizuno Y, et al. Barth syndrome: different approaches to diagnosis. J Pediatr. 2018;193:256–260

Jefferies JL. Barth syndrome. Am J Med Genet C Semin Med Genet. 2013;163C(3):198–205.

Kang SL, Forsey J, Dudley D, Steward CG, Tsai-Goodman B. Clinical characteristics and outcomes of cardiomyopathy in Barth syndrome: the UK experience. Pediatr Cardiol. 2016;37(1):167–76.

Reynolds S. Successful management of Barth syndrome: a systematic review highlighting the importance of a flexible and multidisciplinary approach. J Multidisc Healthc. 2015;8:345–58.

Rezaei N, Moazzami K, Aghamohammadi A, Klein C. Neutropenia and primary immunodeficiency diseases. Int Rev Immunol. 2009;28(5):335–66.

Steward CG, Newbury-Ecob RA, Hastings R, Smithson SF, Tsai-Goodman B, Quarrell OW, et al. Barth syndrome: an X-linked cause of fetal cardiomyopathy and stillbirth. Prenat Diagn. 2010;30(10):970–6.

Wintergerst U, Kuijpers TW, Rosenzweig SD, Holland SM, Abinun M, Malech HL, Rezaei N. Phagocytes defects. In: Rezaei N, Aghamohammadi A, Notarangelo LD, editors. Primary immunodeficiency diseases: definition, diagnosis, and management. 2nd ed. Springer; Verlag, Berlin, Heidelberg. 2018. p. 279–80.

BCG and Novel Tuberculosis Vaccine Candidates in the Context of Immunodeficiencies

Stefan H. E. Kaufmann
Max Planck Institute for Infection Biology, Berlin, Germany
Hagler Institute for Advanced Study at Texas A&M University, College Station, TX, USA

Definitions

Tuberculosis: a chronic infectious disease caused by a bacterial pathogen which is a global health threat.

Vaccination: introduction of foreign material to induce a protective immune response against a pathogen or the disease it causes.

Subunit vaccine: a material composed of selected antigens to protect against the pathogen or the disease it causes. Generally given together with an adjuvant or expressed by a viral vector.

Antigen: material that is recognized by the immune response.

Adjuvant: material that improves the immune response against antigen.

Viral vector: a virus which expresses antigens.

Killed bacterial vaccine: a killed bacterial pathogen used as vaccine.

Live bacterial vaccine: an attenuated bacterium used as vaccine.

Attenuation: process by which a pathogen loses its capacity to cause disease, but maintains its capacity to stimulate immunity.

Immunity: host response against invading microbes or antigens introduced into the host.

Preventive vaccine: a vaccine given before disease develops to prevent the disease.

Therapeutic vaccine: a vaccine given after the disease has emerged to ameliorate or cure disease.

Preexposure vaccine: a vaccine given before the etiologic pathogen has infected the host.

Postexposure vaccination: a vaccine given after the etiologic pathogen has infected the host.

Overview

Tuberculosis (TB) is a chronic infectious disease that has been around for millennia. It was the major cause of death in densely populated urban areas around the turn of the nineteenth to the twentieth century, was considered under control by the end of the twentieth century, and then reemerged to become the most deadly infectious disease caused by a single agent (Kaufmann and Winau 2005; Global Tuberculosis Report 2018). In 2017, 10 million new cases of active TB and 1.6 million TB deaths were recorded (Global Tuberculosis Report 2018). At first sight this might be surprising because efficient drug therapy became available in the second half of the twentieth century, and a vaccine, bacille Calmette–Guérin (BCG), was introduced into clinical practice in 1924 (Calmette et al. 1927; Zumla et al. 2014). Yet, treatment is complex, requiring several drugs given over a period of 6 or more months (Pai et al. 2016). Incomplete compliance with drug treatment has led to an ever-increasing global incidence of multidrug-resistant (MDR) TB, which is difficult to cure with a success rate of only 50%. The vaccine BCG shows good, though sometimes unsatisfactory, protection against severe extrapulmonary disease in infants and is largely ineffective against pulmonary TB, notably in adolescents and adults (Colditz et al. 1994, 1995; Roy et al. 2014). As further complication, BCG is a live vaccine which is contraindicated in infants with any type of immunodeficiency (Duncan and Hambleton 2014; Ewa Anna et al. 2007; Norouzi et al. 2012; Nunes-Santos and Rosenzweig 2018; Poyhonen et al. 2019; Talbot et al. 1997). Hence, prospects about the future of TB range from highly pessimistic estimates (All-Party Parliamentary Group on Global Tuberculosis 2015) to highly optimistic proclamation of the World Health Organization (WHO) to eliminate TB by 2050 (Stop TB Partnership 2015; The End TB Strategy 2015). The latter claim was modified by the WHO to a more modest proposal to reduce morbidity and mortality due to TB by 90% or 95%, respectively, between 2015 and 2035 (Stop TB Partnership 2015; The End TB Strategy 2015). In any case, the future of TB depends on the development of better intervention measures, i.e., better drugs, better diagnostics, and better vaccines (Abu-Raddad et al. 2009; Kaufmann 2010; Pai et al. 2016). While each of these individual intervention measures will contribute to reduced global TB burden, a concerted action is needed: drugs are indispensable for short-term reduction while vaccines are essential for long-term control of the disease (Abu-Raddad et al. 2009; Kaufmann 2010; Ottenhoff and Kaufmann 2012; Pai et al. 2016; Zumla et al. 2014).

Pathogen/Disease

TB is manifested primarily in the lung, although other organs can be affected, as well (Ottenhoff and Kaufmann 2012). It is characterized by the formation of granulomatous lesions, which are the focus of both protection and pathology (Barry et al. 2009; Gengenbacher and Kaufmann 2012; Ulrichs and Kaufmann 2006). Worldwide, some 1.7 billion individuals are considered infected with the causative agent *Mycobacterium*

tuberculosis (Mtb) without clinical disease (Kaufmann 2010; Global Tuberculosis Report 2018). This chronic stage has been termed latent TB infection (LTBI). It is characterized by containment of Mtb by the immune response, which contains the pathogen in a dormant stage but fails to eradicate it (Gengenbacher and Kaufmann 2012). Although sterile eradication occurs in few cases, the majority of individuals live with LTBI lifelong. Dormant Mtb are in a mode of low replicative and metabolic activity in which they cause little harm to the host, but largely resist drug treatment and immune control. Dormant Mtb persist in well-structured solid granulomas, which are primarily composed of macrophages, T lymphocytes, dendritic cells, B lymphocytes, and neutrophils (Barry et al. 2009; Gengenbacher and Kaufmann 2012; Ulrichs and Kaufmann 2006).

Solid granulomas prevail in LTBI. Dysregulation of acquired immunity leads to necrosis, and ultimately to liquefaction of the lesion, providing fertile conditions for Mtb, which now assumes high metabolic and replicative activity (Barry et al. 2009; Gengenbacher and Kaufmann 2012; Ulrichs and Kaufmann 2006). Granuloma caseation causes severe damage of the lung, dissemination of Mtb to other tissue sites, and spread to the environment. Active TB disease has developed and patients are highly contagious. Progression to active TB disease is characterized by a continuum of granuloma alterations from solid to necrotic to caseous lesions (Barry et al. 2009; Gengenbacher and Kaufmann 2012; Ulrichs and Kaufmann 2006). The more severe the disease, the more prevalent caseation and liquefaction become. Yet, the different granuloma stages coexist in a single patient (Lin et al. 2014). During active disease, Mtb is in a metabolically active mode and is spread to contacts. During the active and dormant stages, Mtb expresses different antigens with consequences for vaccine design (Andersen and Kaufmann 2014; Andersen and Scriba 2019).

In short, the vast majority of infections with Mtb lead to LTBI characterized by solid granulomas which contain Mtb without clinical consequences for the host. Less than 10% of individuals with LTBI progress to active TB characterized by increasing transition from solid to caseous lesions accompanied by loss of control of Mtb. A major cause for loss of protective immunity is coinfection with the human immunodeficiency virus (HIV) (Ronacher et al. 2015; Global Tuberculosis Report 2018). Indeed, individuals with LTBI who become coinfected with HIV are at tenfold higher risk of developing active TB disease within the following 12–24 months.

Immune Protection

Both T lymphocytes and B lymphocytes are stimulated during TB (Jacobs et al. 2016; Li and Javid 2018; Lu et al. 2016; O'Garra et al. 2013; Ottenhoff and Kaufmann 2012). General agreement, however, exists that T cells are the major mediators of protective immunity (O'Garra et al. 2013; Ottenhoff and Kaufmann 2012). This is because Mtb persists in the intracellular compartment of professional and nonprofessional phagocytes with macrophages in granulomas being a major site of residence. Thus, macrophage activation by cytokines from T lymphocytes is considered critical for protection. However, antibodies could be involved in prevention of infection (PoI) with Mtb (Jacobs et al. 2016; Li and Javid 2018; Lu et al. 2016, 2019). This mechanism needs to be studied in more depth to determine whether it can be harnessed for future vaccination strategies aimed at PoI. Virtually all current TB vaccination strategies are focused on stimulation of T lymphocytes to contain Mtb and thereby preventing reactivation of active TB (prevention of disease (PoD)) (Kaufmann 2010, 2013). Hence, vaccination strategies focus on arrest of solid granulomas to prevent transition into necrotic caseous granulomas which serve as fertile soil for Mtb growth and are the cause of damage of the affected organ, typically the lung. CD4 T lymphocytes with T helper 1 (TH1) functions, i.e., potent interferon-γ (IFN-γ) production likely combined with secretion of interleukin-2 (IL-2) and tumor necrosis factor-α (TNF-α) are considered major mediators of protection (O'Garra et al. 2013; Ottenhoff and Kaufmann 2012). It is likely

that they are transiently supported by CD4 T cells of TH17 type which produce IL-17 which attracts neutrophils to the site of action (O'Garra et al. 2013; Ottenhoff and Kaufmann 2012). In addition, CD8 T lymphocytes are considered to significantly contribute to protection against TB by expressing cytolytic activity and secreting IFNγ and TNF-α (Ottenhoff and Kaufmann 2012). By lysing infected host cells, these cells can release Mtb from cellular sanctuaries facilitating uptake by monocytes with high antibacterial capacities (Ottenhoff and Kaufmann 2012). Of note, protection in TB is partial and not complete as underlined by the failure of most individuals with LTBI to achieve sterile eradication. The critical role of cell-mediated immunity in general and of CD4 T cells in particular is best illustrated by the fact that TB is the most frequent cause of death in HIV-infected individuals (Ronacher et al. 2015).

Even after successful drug treatment of TB patients, ca. 10% will undergo recurrence within 12 months after completion of treatment (Mirsaeidi and Sadikot 2018; Pai et al. 2016; Rosser et al. 2018). This is either due to relapse of bacteria that were hiding away from drug action or due to reinfection. Current TB vaccination strategies therefore also consider vaccines for prevention of recurrence (PoR). Moreover, neither Mtb infection nor any vaccine candidate has succeeded in reliable sterile Mtb eradication in animal models, thus far (Ottenhoff and Kaufmann 2012).

Because of the critical role of T lymphocytes in immunity and the failure to achieve complete protection, correlates of TB risk and surrogates of protection remain ill-defined (Ottenhoff et al. 2012; Sadoff and Wittes 2007). It is hoped that immune markers based on (i) antigen-specific T cell responses, (ii) cytokine levels in serum, and (iii) specific antibody responses may lead to better immune correlates and surrogates (Ottenhoff et al. 2012; Sadoff and Wittes 2007). But this goal is far from being accomplished. Most biomarker studies on TB have focused on transcriptomics and metabolomics (Kaufmann et al. 2015; Suliman et al. 2018; Weiner and Kaufmann 2014; Weiner et al. 2018; Zak et al. 2016). Diagnostic signatures which discriminate active TB from LTBI with high specificity and sensitivity have been developed (Weiner and Kaufmann 2014), and a biosignature which diagnoses incipient TB is currently being developed (Suliman et al. 2018; Weiner et al. 2018; Zak et al. 2016). This signature allows prognosis of active TB prior to its clinical diagnosis because of the high sensitivity of transcriptomics and metabolomics (Suliman et al. 2018; Weiner et al. 2018; Zak et al. 2016). Ultimately, these approaches can lead to:

- Prognostic biosignature for stratification of study participants at high risk to develop TB during the duration of the vaccine trial.
- Predictive biomarkers of clinical endpoints, prior to clinical diagnosis of active TB disease in vaccine trials (Kaufmann et al. 2015; Sadoff and Wittes 2007; Townsend and Arron 2016).

BCG: Its Benefits and Drawbacks

The TB vaccine, BCG, was developed in the first decades of the twentieth century and is still the only licensed TB vaccine (Calmette et al. 1927). After introduction of BCG into TB-control programs, there was a standstill in TB vaccine research and development until the end of the twentieth century (Andersen and Kaufmann 2014). In the meantime, it became clear that BCG only protects against severe extrapulmonary disease primarily in infants (Colditz et al. 1994, 1995; Pai et al. 2016; Roy et al. 2014). The failure of BCG to protect against pulmonary TB, which is the most prevalent disease form and the main source of transmission, has fueled attempts to develop novel vaccination strategies (Kaufmann 2013). BCG was generated by attenuation of *Mycobacterium bovis*. Although it is a live vaccine, it is considered safe for immunocompetent individuals, but principally immunodeficiencies are contraindications for BCG immunization (Eibl and Wolf 2015; Principi and Esposito 2014). This not only includes patients with severe combined immune deficiency (SCID), but also patients with impaired innate immunity, notably type I cytokine signaling (e.g., IL-12, IFN-γ)

pathways, chronic granulomatous disease (CGD), and deficiencies in toll-like receptors (TLR) (Duncan and Hambleton 2014; Ewa Anna et al. 2007; Norouzi et al. 2012; Nunes-Santos and Rosenzweig 2018; Poyhonen et al. 2019; Talbot et al. 1997). Although the role of antibodies in control of TB remains controversial, generally BCG immunization is not recommended in patients with minor antibody deficiencies (Eibl and Wolf 2015). Moreover, exposure to HIV during pregnancy which causes risk of potential HIV transmission from mother to baby is contraindicated (Ronacher et al. 2015). Therefore, care needs to be taken to determine the immune status of infants before immunization.

As a corollary, WHO has recommended that novel TB vaccines must be safer **or** more efficacious than BCG. Obviously, both criteria, namely, better safety and efficacy, would be most desirable. Subunit vaccines and killed bacterial vaccines are likely to be safer than BCG and may be considered for certain immunodeficient patients following recommendations for current licensed vaccines for these patients (Eibl and Wolf 2015; Principi and Esposito 2014). Also, viable TB vaccines may be considered, provided they show a markedly better safety profile.

Novel TB Vaccine Candidates Under Clinical Development

Because of the high proportion of Mtb-infected individuals, preventive vaccination strategies against TB can not only be restricted to immunization of naïve individuals, i.e., pre-exposure with Mtb, but also need to consider post-exposure immunization of individuals with LTBI. The current BCG vaccine is given once immediately after birth and hence pre-exposure with Mtb. Although neonates have been the prime target population for BCG since its introduction (Calmette et al. 1927), in the past, BCG has been administered to adults and adolescents to booster the immune response, including vaccines with LTBI. Certain adverse events have been recorded after repeated BCG vaccination, yet a single BCG booster during LTBI generally did not cause adverse events

(Dantas et al. 2006; Karonga Prevention Trial Group 1996; Kaufmann 2013). Notably, several lines of evidence suggest that BCG immunization partially protects against infection with Mtb (Michelsen et al. 2014; Nemes et al. 2018; Soysal et al. 2005; Verrall et al. 2019a, b). This issue has been tested recently in a formal clinical trial (Nemes et al. 2018). Participants were Mtb and HIV uninfected and had received BCG as infants. The study revealed no protection against initial infection as measured by early IFN-γ release assay (IGRA) conversion. IGRA is an indicator of Mtb infection by measuring an antigen-specific immune response mostly of CD4 T cells (Diel et al. 2011). Notably, sustained IGRA conversion was reduced in study participants immunized with BCG compared to controls (Nemes et al. 2018). These findings provide strong evidence for the capacity of BCG to prevent stable infection, most likely due to rapid elimination of initial but transient Mtb infection (Ginsberg 2019).

Both pre- and post-exposure vaccination aim to achieve PoD. Pre-exposure vaccines encounter active Mtb whereas post-exposure vaccines are confronted mostly with dormant Mtb (Andersen and Scriba 2019; Gengenbacher and Kaufmann 2012). Hence, the two types of vaccines should be equipped with different antigens. More desirably they should comprise both types of antigens to act as multistage vaccines (Andersen and Kaufmann 2014; Andersen and Scriba 2019).

A few vaccine candidates are being developed with the objective to treat high-risk individuals, including TB patients with HIV coinfection, patients with MDR-TB, or both (Groschel et al. 2014). These therapeutic vaccines are given in adjunct to chemotherapy.

Yet, most efforts of TB vaccine development are in the area of preventive vaccination. Current candidates of this type have the objective to achieve PoD leaving LTBI unaffected. Although it is generally accepted that sterile eradication of Mtb would be the preferred goal of TB vaccination, the more humble approach of PoD leaving LTBI unaffected appears more realistic. The possibility for PoI by vaccination is currently being considered as an alternative to PoD. Obviously, vaccines for PoI must be given pre-exposure with

Mtb. Evidence has been presented that infant vaccination with BCG can reduce the risk of Mtb infection later in life (Michelsen et al. 2014; Soysal et al. 2005; Verrall et al. 2019a, b).

Ongoing Clinical Vaccine Trials

Vaccine candidates undergoing clinical assessment can be grouped as: (i) viral-vectored, (ii) adjuvanted antigen formulations, (iii) killed whole cell vaccines, or (iv) recombinant viable vaccines (Table 1).

Viral-vectored and adjuvanted antigen formulations are subunit vaccines, which comprise a limited number of Mtb protein antigens (Table 1). They are generally considered for booster vaccination subsequent to BCG prime.

Viral vectors for TB antigens include human and chimpanzee adenovirus (Ad) as well as modified vaccinia virus Ankara (MVA). The most widely used antigen expressed by viral vectors is the mycolyl transferase antigen (Ag)85 expressed by both BCG and Mtb in three homologous forms (Ag85A, Ag85B, and Ag85C). MVA85A expressing Ag85A was clinically the most advanced TB vaccine but failed to show efficacy in infants and in adults (Ndiaye et al. 2015; Tameris et al. 2013). It remains in the clinical trial pipeline as part of novel prime-boost combinations (see below) and different routes of immunization (Manjaly Thomas et al. 2019; Satti et al. 2014; Stylianou et al. 2015). Ag85A has also been tested with a replication-deficient Ad5 vector (Ad5Ag85A) (Smaill et al. 2013). It has been complemented with Ag85B and the virulence factor TB10.4 in an Ad35-vectored vaccine, which completed phase IIa but apparently is not being continued (Abel et al. 2010; Churchyard et al. 2015; Tameris et al. 2015). All these vaccines have been found to be safe and immunogenic. A recent addition is the TB/FLU-04L vaccine candidate based on a replication-deficient H1N1 influenza strain expressing Ag85A and the virulence factor ESAT-6 (Sergeeva et al. 2017). Although detailed information on this candidate could not be found in the public domain, it has been registered under

BCG and Novel Tuberculosis Vaccine Candidates in the Context of Immunodeficiencies, Table 1 Promising preventive tuberculosis vaccine candidates in clinical trials

Agent	Strategy	Type	ClinicalTrials.gov Identifier of representative trial (phase; P)
Viral-vectored			
MVA85A (aerosol/ intradermal)	Boost	Viral vector (Modified Vaccinia Ankara)	NCT 01954563 (PI, completed)
Ad5Ag85A	Boost	Viral vector (Replication deficient Adeno Virus)	NCT 02337270 (PI)
ChAdOx1.85A + MVA85A	Prime-boost	Viral vector (Chimpanzee Adeno Virus)	NCT 03681860 (PII)
TB-FLU-04L	Boost	Viral vector (Replication deficient Influenza Virus)	NCT 02501421 (PI, completed)
Protein-adjuvant formulations			
Hybrid 56:IC31	Boost	Protein/adjuvant	NCT 03512249 (PII)
ID93:GLA-SE	Boost	Protein/adjuvant	NCT 03806686 (PII)
M72:AS01	Boost	Protein/adjuvant	NCT 01755598 (PIIb, completed)
Viable vaccines			
MTBVAC	Prime	Genetically attenuated *M. tuberculosis*	NCT 02933281 (PII)
VPM1002	Prime (Boost)	Recombinant bacille Calmette-Guérin (rBCG)	NCT 03152903 (PIII)
Killed vaccines			
Dar-901	Boost	Killed whole-cell *M. obuense*	NCT 02712424 (PII)
Vaccae	Boost	Killed whole-cell *M. vaccae*	NCT 01979900 (PIII)
M. indicus pranii (M w)	Boost	Killed whole-cell *M. indicus pranii*	NCT 00265226 (PIII)

clinical trial.gov website (Table 1). Moreover, novel prime-boost vaccinations (on top of BCG prime) with different viral vectors are under development. These include Ad35-expressing Ag85A, Ag85B, and TB10.4 followed by booster with MVA85A-expressing Ag85A only (Hokey et al. 2014; Walsh et al. 2016) and a prime with chimpanzee Ad (ChAdx1.85A) followed by MVA boost with both vectors exclusively expressing Ag85A (Stylianou et al. 2015). The antigens used in all these constructs are primarily produced by active Mtb although they may also be found in dormant Mtb (Andersen and Kaufmann 2014; Andersen and Scriba 2019; Gengenbacher and Kaufmann 2012).

Protein adjuvant vaccines generally comprise fusion proteins from Mtb formulated in T cell-stimulating adjuvants (Table 1). These include vaccines of the so-called hybrid (H) antigen family, which all contain Ag85B (Andersen and Kaufmann 2014). H1 expresses a fusion protein

of Ag85B and ESAT-6 (Van Dissel et al. 2010). In the H4 vaccine, ESAT-6 had been exchanged by TB10.4 (Geldenhuys et al. 2015) and the H56 vaccine contains Rv2660c in addition to Ag85B and ESAT-6 (Luabeya et al. 2015; Suliman et al. 2019). The exchange of ESAT-6 with TB10.4 in the H4 and H56 vaccines has been done to avoid cross-reactivity in IGRA tests, which contain ESAT-6 protein as test antigen. IGRAs are being widely used for diagnosis of Mtb infection, but do not discriminate between LTBI and active TB disease (Diel et al. 2011). A recent PoI trial revealed no protection by the H4 vaccine and hence the vaccine will probably not be further developed (Ginsberg 2019; Nemes et al. 2018). H56 had been designed as a multistage (pre- and post-exposure) vaccine (Andersen and Kaufmann 2014; Andersen and Scriba 2019): Ag85B and ESAT-6 are primarily expressed by active Mtb during the early stage of infection, whereas Rv2660c is a characteristic dormancy antigen expressed during LTBI although its expression as protein by Mtb has been questioned (Houghton et al. 2013). The H series of TB vaccines is generally adjuvanted with IC31, a formulation of cationic peptides and a synthetic TLR-9 agonist. More recently, H1 has also entered clinical testing with the CAF01 adjuvant comprising a cationic liposome vehicle combined with an immunomodulatory glycolipid (Van Dissel et al. 2014). Two other adjuvanted TB vaccines are currently undergoing clinical testing. The vaccine M72:AS01E is currently the most advanced TB subunit vaccine (Kumarasamy et al. 2016; Penn-Nicholson et al. 2015; Van Der Meeren et al. 2018). Recent data from a phase IIb trial in HIV uninfected individuals with LTBI revealed ca. 50% PoD afforded by M72:AS01E over unvaccinated controls after a mean of 2.3 years of follow-up (Van Der Meeren et al. 2018). A BCG control was not included in this trial. This study is still ongoing (Ginsberg 2019; Van Der Meeren et al. 2018). The vaccine M72:AS01E comprises the antigens Rv1196, a member of the PPE family and Rv0125, a peptidase. The PPE genes are highly polymorphic and hence may facilitate immune evasion of Mtb through antigenic variation (Deng and Xie 2012). The adjuvant AS01E used for this construct is composed of liposomes into which a TLR4 agonist had been incorporated. The vaccine ID93 comprises a fusion protein of four different antigens, namely, the PPE family protein Rv2608, the virulence factors Rv3619 and Rv3620, and the dormancy-associated protein Rv1813 (Bertholet et al. 2010; Penn-Nicholson et al. 2018). The adjuvant GLA-SE is composed of a synthetic TLR4 agonist in an oil-in-water emulsion. The H56, M72, and ID93 vaccines are considered as multistage vaccines for pre- and post-exposure application.

Two viable TB vaccines are currently progressing through the clinical pipeline (Table 1). MTBVAC has been attenuated by independent deletions in two genes: *phoP*, a transcription factor for Mtb virulence factors, and *fadD26*, involved in synthesis of phthiocerol dimycocerosates, a non-proteinaceous virulence factor of Mtb (Aguilo et al. 2017; Spertini et al. 2015). Thus, this vaccine fulfils the requirement of the WHO of two

independent deletions for Mtb-derived vaccines (Walker et al. 2010). This vaccine has successfully completed a phase I trial in adults (Spertini et al. 2015). The recombinant (r)BCG vaccine VPM1002 has been endowed with the pore-forming listeriolysin in a urease-deficient background (Grode et al. 2005; Nieuwenhuizen et al. 2017). Urease deficiency allows for acidification of the intraphagosomal milieu so that listeriolysin secreted by VPM1002 in phagosomes of macrophages or dendritic cells witnesses an optimal pH. This allows perturbation of the phagosomal membrane resulting in higher vaccine efficacy and safety. VPM1002 has already successfully completed two phase I trials in adults as well as a phase IIa trial in infants demonstrating its safety and immunogenicity. It has completed a phase II trial which will be succeeded by a phase III trial in HIV exposed and unexposed infants (Grode et al. 2013; Loxton et al. 2017; Nieuwenhuizen et al. 2017). These viable TB vaccines have the primary objective to replace BCG in infant vaccination and they are also considered as post-exposure vaccines for adults. In fact, in 2018 VPM1002 has already started a phase III trial for PoR in India. In high endemic areas, 10% of successfully drug-treated TB patients undergo recurrence due to reinfection or relapse within 12 months after completion of drug therapy (Mirsaeidi and Sadikot 2018; Pai et al. 2016; Rosser et al. 2018).

Three killed whole cell vaccines have been developed for therapy, namely, the fragmented Mtb vaccine RUTI (Nell et al. 2014; Vilaplana et al. 2010), and the whole bacterial vaccines based on *M. vaccae* (Butov et al. 2013; De Bruyn and Garner 2003; Efremenko et al. 2013; Groschel et al. 2014; Weng et al. 2016; Yang et al. 2011) (one of these retyped as *M. obuense*, see below) or *M. indicus pranii* (Mayosi et al. 2014). Preparations of *M. vaccae* have passed phase III therapy trials, however with controversial outcome of therapeutic efficacy (De Bruyn and Garner 2003; Groschel et al. 2014; Weng et al. 2016). Yet, one preparation has been approved for adjunct therapy in China (Efremenko et al. 2013; Weng et al. 2016). Killed *M. indicus pranii* (M. w) failed to show a therapeutic effect against tuberculous pericarditis (Mayosi et al. 2014), but has been licensed in India for specific TB indications (Groschel et al. 2014; Sharma et al. 2017). Three killed whole cell vaccines are currently in the preventive TB vaccine pipeline (Table 1). A vaccine based on killed *M. obuense* (previously *M. vaccae*, see above) had shown signs of efficacy in a phase III trial with HIV-infected participants with prior BCG vaccination (Von Reyn et al. 2010). It has been reformulated and is currently tested as a preventive vaccine under the name DAR901 (Von Reyn et al. 2017).

Conclusion and Future Outlook

The landscape of TB vaccine development has changed remarkably over the last two decades. It would be unreasonable to expect an outcome of 100% protection, i.e., complete PoD in all study participants (Kaufmann et al. 2015). Rather, we should consider it a first success when a vaccine shows PoD over the duration of a clinical trial of 2–4 years in >50% of vaccinated study participants, compared to controls (mostly BCG vaccination). Hence, the results of the clinical trial with M72:AS01E vaccine revealing ca. 50% protection over unvaccinated controls represents an important step forward (Ginsberg 2019; Van Der Meeren et al. 2018). Obviously, a vaccine which shows better protective efficacy and safety than BCG would be most valuable. Yet, because of the high rate of coinfections with Mtb and HIV, a vaccine that is safer than BCG even if its efficacy is only non-inferior to BCG would be a major step forward, notably for immunization of neonates. Although focus on safety is generally laid on subunit vaccines and killed vaccines, viable vaccines can be constructed which are safer than BCG. Thus, the recombinant BCG vaccine VPM1002 has completed a phase II trial and will soon start a phase III trial in HIV exposed and unexposed neonates to assess whether it is safer and more efficacious than BCG. Preclinical data in immunocompromised experimental animals strongly support this notion (Nieuwenhuizen et al. 2017).

With a growing number of TB vaccine candidates passing through the clinical trial pipeline

(Kaufmann et al. 2015), financial issues gain increasing relevance. With a steady ascent from phase I trials at cost of half a million USD to phase II trials at cost of 2.5–10 million USD to phase III trials at cost of 25–50 million USD, cost reduction becomes mandatory (Kaufmann et al. 2015). To achieve this goal, rational candidate selection must be implemented as early as possible based on solid criteria. More preclinical studies in relevant animal models, notably nonhuman primates (Flynn et al. 2015), and small-scale experimental medicine trials have been proposed (Kaufmann et al. 2015). Moreover, trials on PoI, rather than PoD would be less costly. Also, PoR trials will be less costly since they comprise a smaller number of study participants and shorter trial duration. Finally, controlled human challenge experiments have strongly promoted vaccine development for malaria (Sauerwein et al. 2011; Spring et al. 2014) and other infectious diseases, and the feasibility of developing a relevant and safe human challenge model for TB is currently under discussion (Minassian et al. 2012).

Complementing this selection strategy, biosignatures predicting risk of progression to active TB in individuals with LTBI allow stratifying high-risk study participants for clinical trials (Ottenhoff et al. 2012; Weiner and Kaufmann 2014). Biosignatures for progression to active TB have been described recently and more studies in this direction are on their way (Suliman et al. 2018; Weiner et al. 2018; Zak et al. 2016). Stratification could reduce numbers of study participants and shorten trial duration.

Phase II b/III trials should be monitored as extensively as possible for biomarkers indicative for vaccine efficacy and failure (Kaufmann et al. 2015; Ottenhoff et al. 2012; Weiner and Kaufmann 2014). Ultimately, this will allow definition of signatures of vaccine efficacy and safety, of value not only for the ongoing trial but also for future development of next-generation vaccine candidates. After all, we have to view TB vaccine development as an iterative process without a one-fits-all solution. Although there is still a long way to go, it is a worthwhile endeavor, which will help meet the WHO's target to reduce

TB morbidity and mortality to <1 million and <100,000, respectively, by 2035 (Stop TB Partnership 2015; Global Tuberculosis Report 2018; The End TB Strategy 2015).

TB is most prevalent in low to middle income countries with more than one million cases each in China, India, and the African continent and the situation is getting worse due to heightened incidences of drug-resistant TB (Global Tuberculosis Report 2018). Hence, it is generally accepted that a better vaccine than BCG is urgently needed to ultimately control this devastating threat. The development of TB vaccines that are at least as safe as and more efficacious than BCG remains a high priority despite the risk of vaccine-related adverse events in immunodeficient individuals. Yet, the portfolio of novel vaccines is sufficiently broad (Table 1) to hope for a vaccine that is not only more efficacious but also safer than BCG and therefore appropriate for individuals with immunodeficiency disorders.

Cross-References

▶ CYBB X-Linked Chronic Granulomatous Disease (CGD)
▶ Innate Immune Defects, Clinical Presentation
▶ Unclassified Primary Antibody Deficiency (unPAD)

Conflict of Interest SHEK is coinventor of a vaccine against tuberculosis (VPM1002) currently undergoing clinical trial testing.

References

Abel B, Tameris M, Mansoor N, et al. The novel tuberculosis vaccine, AERAS-402, induces robust and polyfunctional CD4+ and CD8+ T cells in adults. Am J Respir Crit Care Med. 2010;181:1407–17.

Abu-Raddad LJ, Sabatelli L, Achterberg JT, et al. Epidemiological benefits of more-effective tuberculosis vaccines, drugs, and diagnostics. Proc Natl Acad Sci U S A. 2009;106:13980–5.

Aguilo N, Gonzalo-Asensio J, Alvarez-Arguedas S, et al. Reactogenicity to major tuberculosis antigens absent in BCG is linked to improved protection against *Mycobacterium tuberculosis*. Nat Commun. 2017;8:16085.

All-Party Parliamentary Group on Global Tuberculosis. The price of a pandemic: counting the cost of MDR-TB. London. 2015. http://www.appg-tb.org.uk/#!publications/cghg

Andersen P, Kaufmann SH. Novel vaccination strategies against tuberculosis. Cold Spring Harb Perspect Med. 2014;4:pii: a018523.

Andersen P, Scriba TJ. Moving tuberculosis vaccines from theory to practice. Nat Rev Immunol. 2019; https://doi.org/10.1038/s41577-41019-40174-z.

Barry CE 3rd, Boshoff HI, Dartois V, et al. The spectrum of latent tuberculosis: rethinking the biology and intervention strategies. Nat Rev Microbiol. 2009;7:845–55.

Bertholet S, Ireton GC, Ordway DJ, et al. A defined tuberculosis vaccine candidate boosts BCG and protects against multidrug-resistant *Mycobacterium tuberculosis*. Sci Transl Med. 2010;2:53ra74.

Butov DA, Efremenko YV, Prihoda ND, et al. Randomized, placebo-controlled phase II trial of heat-killed *Mycobacterium vaccae* (Immodulon batch) formulated as an oral pill (V7). Immunotherapy. 2013;5:1047–54.

Calmette A, Guérin C, Boquet A, et al. La vaccination préventive contre la tuberculose par le "BCG". Paris: Masson et Cie; 1927. p. 1–250.

Churchyard GJ, Snowden MA, Hokey D, et al. The safety and immunogenicity of an adenovirus type 35-vectored TB vaccine in HIV-infected, BCG-vaccinated adults with CD4(+) T cell counts >350 cells/mm(3). Vaccine. 2015;33:1890–6.

Colditz GA, Brewer TF, Berkey CS, et al. Efficacy of BCG vaccine in the prevention of tuberculosis. Meta-analysis of the published literature. JAMA. 1994;271:698–702.

Colditz GA, Berkey CS, Mosteller F, et al. The efficacy of bacillus Calmette-Guerin vaccination of newborns and infants in the prevention of tuberculosis: meta-analyses of the published literature. Pediatrics. 1995;96:29–35.

Dantas OM, Ximenes RA, De Albuquerque MF, et al. A case-control study of protection against tuberculosis by BCG revaccination in Recife, Brazil. Int J Tuberc Lung Dis. 2006;10:536–41.

De Bruyn G, Garner P. *Mycobacterium vaccae* immunotherapy for treating tuberculosis. Cochrane Database Syst Rev. 2003;1:CD001166.

Deng W, Xie J. Ins and outs of *Mycobacterium tuberculosis* PPE family in pathogenesis and implications for novel measures against tuberculosis. J Cell Biochem. 2012;113:1087–95.

Diel R, Goletti D, Ferrara G, et al. Interferon-gamma release assays for the diagnosis of latent *Mycobacterium tuberculosis* infection: a systematic review and meta-analysis. Eur Respir J. 2011;37:88–99.

Duncan CJ, Hambleton S. Host genetic factors in susceptibility to mycobacterial disease. Clin Med. 2014;14(Suppl 6):s17–21.

Efremenko YV, Butov DA, Prihoda ND, et al. Randomized, placebo-controlled phase II trial of heat-killed

Mycobacterium vaccae (Longcom batch) formulated as an oral pill (V7). Hum Vaccin Immunother. 2013;9:1852–6.

Eibl MM, Wolf HM. Vaccination in patients with primary immune deficiency, secondary immune deficiency and autoimmunity with immune regulatory abnormalities. Immunotherapy. 2015;7:1273–92.

Ewa Anna B, Beata W-K, Malgorzata P, et al. Disseminated bacillus Calmette-Guérin infection and immunodeficiency. Emerg Infect Dis. 2007;13:799–801.

Flynn JL, Gideon HP, Mattila JT, et al. Immunology studies in non-human primate models of tuberculosis. Immunol Rev. 2015;264:60–73.

Geldenhuys H, Mearns H, Miles DJ, et al. The tuberculosis vaccine H4:IC31 is safe and induces a persistent polyfunctional CD4 T cell response in South African adults: a randomized controlled trial. Vaccine. 2015;33: 3592–9.

Gengenbacher M, Kaufmann SHE. *Mycobacterium tuberculosis*: success through dormancy. FEMS Microbiol Rev. 2012;36:514–32.

Ginsberg AM. Designing tuberculosis vaccine efficacy trials – lessons from recent studies. Expert Rev Vaccines. 2019;18:423–32.

Global Tuberculosis Report. World Health Organization. 2018. www.who.int/tb/publications/global_report/en/

Grode L, Seiler P, Baumann S, et al. Increased vaccine efficacy against tuberculosis of recombinant *Mycobacterium bovis* bacille Calmette-Guérin mutants that secrete listeriolysin. J Clin Invest. 2005;115: 2472–9.

Grode L, Ganoza CA, Brohm C, et al. Safety and immunogenicity of the recombinant BCG vaccine VPM1002 in a phase 1 open-label randomized clinical trial. Vaccine. 2013;31:1340–8.

Groschel MI, Prabowo SA, Cardona PJ, et al. Therapeutic vaccines for tuberculosis – a systematic review. Vaccine. 2014;32:3162–8.

Hokey D, O'dee DM, Graves A, et al. Heterologous primeboost with Ad35/AERAS-402 and MVA85A elicits potent CD8+ T cell immune responses in a phase I clinical trial (VAC7P.969). J Immunol. 2014;192:141.114.

Houghton J, Cortes T, Schubert O, et al. A small RNA encoded in the Rv2660c locus of *Mycobacterium tuberculosis* is induced during starvation and infection. PLoS One. 2013;8:e80047.

Jacobs AJ, Mongkolsapaya J, Screaton GR, et al. Antibodies and tuberculosis. Tuberculosis. 2016;101: 102–13.

Karonga Prevention Trial Group. Randomised controlled trial of single BCG, repeated BCG, or combined BCG and killed *Mycobacterium leprae* vaccine for prevention of leprosy and tuberculosis in Malawi. Lancet. 1996;348:17–24.

Kaufmann SH. Future vaccination strategies against tuberculosis: thinking outside the box. Immunity. 2010;33:567–77.

Kaufmann SHE. Tuberculosis vaccines: time to think about the next generation. Semin Immunol. 2013;25:172–81.

Kaufmann SHE, Winau F. From bacteriology to immunology: the dualism of specificity. Nat Immunol. 2005;6:1063–6.

Kaufmann SH, Evans TG, Hanekom WA. Tuberculosis vaccines: time for a global strategy. Sci Transl Med. 2015;7:276fs278.

Kumarasamy N, Poongulali S, Bollaerts A, et al. A randomized, controlled safety, and immunogenicity trial of the M72/AS01 candidate tuberculosis vaccine in HIV-positive Indian adults. Medicine. 2016;95:1–10.

Li H, Javid B. Antibodies and tuberculosis: finally coming of age? Nat Rev Immunol. 2018;18:591–6.

Lin PL, Ford CB, Coleman MT, et al. Sterilization of granulomas is common in active and latent tuberculosis despite within-host variability in bacterial killing. Nat Med. 2014;20:75–9.

Loxton AG, Knaul JK, Grode L et al. Safety and immunogenicity of the recombinant mycobacterium bovis BCG vaccine VPM1002 in HIV-unexposed newborn infants in South Africa. Clin Vaccine Immunol. 2017;24: e00439–16.

Lu LL, Chung AW, Rosebrock TR, et al. A functional role for antibodies in tuberculosis. Cell. 2016;167:433. e414–43.e414.

Lu LL, Smith MT, Yu KKQ, et al. IFN-gamma-independent immune markers of *Mycobacterium tuberculosis* exposure. Nat Med. 2019;25:977–87.

Luabeya AK, Kagina BM, Tameris MD, et al. First-in-human trial of the post-exposure tuberculosis vaccine H56:IC31 in *Mycobacterium tuberculosis* infected and non-infected healthy adults. Vaccine. 2015;33: 4130–40.

Manjaly Thomas Z-R, Satti I, Marshall JL, et al. Alternate aerosol and systemic immunisation with a recombinant viral vector for tuberculosis, MVA85A: a phase I randomised controlled trial. PLoS Med. 2019;16: e1002790.

Mayosi BM, Ntsekhe M, Bosch J, et al. Prednisolone and *Mycobacterium indicus pranii* in tuberculous pericarditis. N Engl J Med. 2014;371:1121–30.

Michelsen SW, Soborg B, Koch A, et al. The effectiveness of BCG vaccination in preventing *Mycobacterium tuberculosis* infection and disease in Greenland. Thorax. 2014;69:851–6.

Minassian AM, Satti I, Poulton ID, et al. A human challenge model for *Mycobacterium tuberculosis* using *Mycobacterium bovis* bacille Calmette-Guerin. J Infect Dis. 2012;205:1035–42.

Mirsaeidi M, Sadikot RT. Patients at high risk of tuberculosis recurrence. Int J Mycobacteriol. 2018;7:1–6.

Ndiaye BP, Thienemann F, Ota M, et al. Safety, immunogenicity, and efficacy of the candidate tuberculosis vaccine MVA85A in healthy adults infected with HIV-1: a randomised, placebo-controlled, phase 2 trial. Lancet Respir Med. 2015;3:190–200.

Nell AS, D'lom E, Bouic P, et al. Safety, tolerability, and immunogenicity of the novel antituberculous vaccine RUTI: randomized, placebo-controlled phase II clinical trial in patients with latent tuberculosis infection. PLoS One. 2014;9:e89612.

Nemes E, Geldenhuys H, Rozot V, et al. Prevention of *M. tuberculosis* infection with H4:IC31 vaccine or BCG revaccination. N Engl J Med. 2018;379:138–49.

Nieuwenhuizen NE, Kulkarni PS, Shaligram U, et al. The recombinant bacille Calmette-Guerin vaccine VPM1002: ready for clinical efficacy testing. Front Immunol. 2017;8:1147.

Norouzi S, Aghamohammadi A, Mamishi S, et al. Bacillus Calmette-Guerin (BCG) complications associated with primary immunodeficiency diseases. J Inf Secur. 2012;64:543–54.

Nunes-Santos CJ, Rosenzweig SD. Bacille Calmette-Guerin complications in newly described primary immunodeficiency diseases: 2010–2017. Front Immunol. 2018;9:1423.

O'Garra A, Redford PS, Mcnab FW, et al. The immune response in tuberculosis. Annu Rev Immunol. 2013;31:475–527.

Ottenhoff TH, Kaufmann SH. Vaccines against tuberculosis: where are we and where do we need to go? PLoS Pathog. 2012;8:e1002607.

Ottenhoff TH, Ellner JJ, Kaufmann SH. Ten challenges for TB biomarkers. Tuberculosis. 2012;92(Suppl 1): S17–20.

Pai M, Behr MA, Dowdy D, et al. Tuberculosis. Nat Rev Dis Primers. 2016;2:16076.

Penn-Nicholson A, Geldenhuys H, Burny W, et al. Safety and immunogenicity of candidate vaccine M72/AS01E in adolescents in a TB endemic setting. Vaccine. 2015;33:4025–34.

Penn-Nicholson A, Tameris M, Smit E, et al. Safety and immunogenicity of the novel tuberculosis vaccine ID93 + GLA-SE in BCG-vaccinated healthy adults in South Africa: a randomised, double-blind, placebo-controlled phase 1 trial. Lancet Respir Med. 2018;6:287–98.

Poyhonen L, Bustamante J, Casanova JL, et al. Life-threatening infections due to live-attenuated vaccines: early manifestations of inborn errors of immunity. J Clin Immunol. 2019;39:376–90.

Principi N, Esposito S. Vaccine use in primary immunodeficiency disorders. Vaccine. 2014;32:3725–31.

Ronacher K, Joosten SA, Van Crevel R, et al. Acquired immunodeficiencies and tuberculosis: focus on HIV/AIDS and diabetes mellitus. Immunol Rev. 2015;264:121–37.

Rosser A, Marx FM, Pareek M. Recurrent tuberculosis in the pre-elimination era. Int J Tuberc Lung Dis. 2018;22:139–50.

Roy A, Eisenhut M, Harris RJ, et al. Effect of BCG vaccination against *Mycobacterium tuberculosis* infection in children: systematic review and meta-analysis. BMJ. 2014;349:g4643.

Sadoff JC, Wittes J. Correlates, surrogates, and vaccines. J Infect Dis. 2007;196:1279–81.

Satti I, Meyer J, Harris SA, et al. Safety and immunogenicity of a candidate tuberculosis vaccine MVA85A delivered by aerosol in BCG-vaccinated healthy adults: a phase 1, double-blind, randomised controlled trial. Lancet Infect Dis. 2014;14:939–46.

Sauerwein RW, Roestenberg M, Moorthy VS. Experimental human challenge infections can accelerate clinical malaria vaccine development. Nat Rev Immunol. 2011;11:57–64.

Sergeeva MV, Pulkina AA, Vasiliev KA, et al. Safety and immunogenicity of cold-adapted recombinant influenza vector expressing ESAT-6 and Ag85A antigens of *M. tuberculosis*. Vopr Virusol. 2017;62:266–72.

Sharma SK, Katoch K, Sarin R, et al. Efficacy and safety of *Mycobacterium indicus* pranii as an adjunct therapy in Category II pulmonary tuberculosis in a randomized trial. Sci Rep. 2017;7:3354.

Smaill F, Jeyanathan M, Smieja M, et al. A human type 5 adenovirus-based tuberculosis vaccine induces robust T cell responses in humans despite preexisting anti-adenovirus immunity. Sci Transl Med. 2013;5: 205ra134.

Soysal A, Millington KA, Bakir M, et al. Effect of BCG vaccination on risk of *Mycobacterium tuberculosis* infection in children with household tuberculosis contact: a prospective community-based study. Lancet. 2005;366:1443–51.

Spertini F, Audran R, Chakour R, et al. Safety of human immunisation with a live-attenuated *Mycobacterium tuberculosis* vaccine: a randomised, double-blind, controlled phase I trial. Lancet Respir Med. 2015;3:953–62.

Spring M, Polhemus M, Ockenhouse C. Controlled human malaria infection. J Infect Dis. 2014;209(Suppl 2): S40–5.

Stop TB Partnership. The global plan to stop TB 2016–2020. WHO. 2015. www.stoptb.org/assets/documents/global/plan/GlobalPlanToEndTB_TheParadigmShift_2016-2020_StopTBPartnership.pdf

Stylianou E, Griffiths KL, Poyntz HC, et al. Improvement of BCG protective efficacy with a novel chimpanzee adenovirus and a modified vaccinia Ankara virus both expressing Ag85A. Vaccine. 2015;33:6800–8.

Suliman S, Thompson E, Sutherland J, et al. Four-gene pan-African blood signature predicts progression to tuberculosis. Am J Respir Crit Care Med. 2018;197:1198–208.

Suliman S, Luabeya AKK, Geldenhuys H, et al. Dose optimization of H56:IC31 vaccine for tuberculosis-endemic populations. A double-blind, placebo-controlled, dose-selection trial. Am J Respir Crit Care Med. 2019;199:220–31.

Talbot EA, Perkins MD, Silva SF, et al. Disseminated bacille Calmette-Guerin disease after vaccination: case report and review. Clin Infect Dis. 1997;24: 1139–46.

Tameris MD, Hatherill M, Landry BS, et al. Safety and efficacy of MVA85A, a new tuberculosis vaccine, in infants previously vaccinated with BCG: a randomised, placebo-controlled phase 2b trial. Lancet. 2013;381:1021–8.

Tameris M, Hokey DA, Nduba V, et al. A double-blind, randomised, placebo-controlled, dose-finding trial of the novel tuberculosis vaccine AERAS-402, an adenovirus-vectored fusion protein, in healthy, BCG-vaccinated infants. Vaccine. 2015;33:2944–54.

The End TB Strategy. World Health Organization. 2015. http://www.who.int/tb/strateg/end-tb/en/

Townsend MJ, Arron JR. Reducing the risk of failure: biomarker-guided trial design. Nat Rev Drug Discov. 2016;15:517–8.

Ulrichs T, Kaufmann SHE. New insights into the function of granulomas in human tuberculosis. J Pathol. 2006;208:261–9.

Van Der Meeren O, Hatherill M, Nduba V, et al. Phase 2b controlled trial of M72/AS01E vaccine to prevent tuberculosis. N Engl J Med. 2018;379:1621–34.

Van Dissel JT, Arend SM, Prins C, et al. Ag85B-ESAT-6 adjuvanted with IC31 promotes strong and long-lived *Mycobacterium tuberculosis* specific T cell responses in naive human volunteers. Vaccine. 2010;28:3571–81.

Van Dissel JT, Joosten SA, Hoff ST, et al. A novel liposomal adjuvant system, CAF01, promotes long-lived *Mycobacterium tuberculosis*-specific T-cell responses in human. Vaccine. 2014;32:7098–107.

Verrall AJ, Alisjahbana B, Apriani L, et al. Early clearance of *Mycobacterium tuberculosis*: the INFECT case contact cohort study in Indonesia. J Infect Dis. 2019a; https://doi.org/10.1093/infdis/jiz168.

Verrall AJ, Schneider M, Alisjahbana B, et al. Early clearance of *Mycobacterium tuberculosis* is associated with increased innate immune responses. J Infect Dis. 2019b; https://doi.org/10.1093/infdis/jiz147.

Vilaplana C, Montane E, Pinto S, et al. Double-blind, randomized, placebo-controlled phase I clinical trial of the therapeutical antituberculous vaccine RUTI. Vaccine. 2010;28:1106–16.

Von Reyn CF, Mtei L, Arbeit RD, et al. Prevention of tuberculosis in bacille Calmette-Guerin-primed, HIV-infected adults boosted with an inactivated whole-cell mycobacterial vaccine. AIDS. 2010;24:675–85.

Von Reyn CF, Lahey T, Arbeit RD, et al. Safety and immunogenicity of an inactivated whole cell tuberculosis vaccine booster in adults primed with BCG: a randomized, controlled trial of DAR-901. PLoS One. 2017;12:e0175215.

Walker KB, Brennan MJ, Ho MM, et al. The second Geneva consensus: recommendations for novel live TB vaccines. Vaccine. 2010;28:2259–70.

Walsh DS, Owira V, Polhemus M, et al. Adenovirus type 35-vectored tuberculosis vaccine has an acceptable safety and tolerability profile in healthy, BCG-vaccinated, QuantiFERON (R)-TB Gold (+) Kenyan adults without evidence of tuberculosis. Vaccine. 2016;34:2430–6.

Weiner J 3rd, Kaufmann SH. Recent advances towards tuberculosis control: vaccines and biomarkers. J Intern Med. 2014;275:467–80.

Weiner J 3rd, Maertzdorf J, Sutherland JS, et al. Metabolite changes in blood predict the onset of tuberculosis. Nat Commun. 2018;9:5208.

Weng H, Huang J-Y, Meng X-Y, et al. Adjunctive therapy of *Mycobacterium vaccae* vaccine in the treatment of multidrug-resistant tuberculosis: a systematic review and meta-analysis. Biomed Rep. 2016;4:595–600.

Yang XY, Chen QF, Li YP, et al. *Mycobacterium vaccae* as adjuvant therapy to anti-tuberculosis chemotherapy in never-treated tuberculosis patients: a meta-analysis. PLoS One. 2011;6:e23826.

Zak DE, Penn-Nicholson A, Scriba TJ, et al. A blood RNA signature for tuberculosis disease risk: a prospective cohort study. Lancet. 2016;387:2312–22.

Zumla AI, Gillespie SH, Hoelscher M, et al. New anti-tuberculosis drugs, regimens, and adjunct therapies: needs, advances, and future prospects. Lancet Infect Dis. 2014;14:327–40.

Berlin Breakage Syndrome

▶ Nijmegen Breakage Syndrome (*NBS1*)

Bimp2

▶ CARD14-Mediated Psoriasis and Pityriasis Rubra Piliaris (PRP)

Blau Syndrome

Carine H. Wouters[1,2] and Carlos D. Rose[3]
[1]Department of Microbiology and Immunology, KU Leuven – University of Leuven, Leuven, Belgium
[2]Pediatric Rheumatology, University Hospitals Leuven, Leuven, Belgium
[3]duPont Children's Hospital, Thomas Jefferson University, Philadelphia, USA

Synonyms

Early onset sarcoidosis; Pediatric granulomatous arthritis

Definition

Blau syndrome is a monogenic granulomatous autoinflammatory disease presenting with poly-arthritis, rash, panuveitis and systemic manifestations resulting from gain-of-function point mutations at or near the NOD domain of the *NOD2* gene.

Introduction

Blau syndrome (BS) is an inflammatory disorder considered part of the spectrum of pediatric sarcoidosis and as such primarily characterized by the presence of non-caseating epithelioid giant cell granulomas in a variety of tissues and organ systems. The clinical phenotype associated with an autosomal dominant inheritance pattern was described in 1985 (Blau 1985). In 2001 a mutation in the nucleotide-binding oligomerization domain 2/caspase activation recruitment domain 15 *(NOD2/CARD15)* was found in four patients with Blau syndrome and with this discovery the first monogenic autoinflammatory granulomatous disease was described (Miceli-Richard et al. 2001). Blau syndrome (BS) and Early Onset Sarcoidosis (EOS) constitute the familial and sporadic forms of this pediatric disease characterized by a triad of polyarthritis, uveitis and rash. Visceral and vascular manifestations beyond the classic triad have since been documented in 29–48% of patients with BS ratifying its true systemic nature (Rose et al. 2009, 2015).

BS is a rare disease and epidemiologic studies focusing specifically on its prevalence do not exist. An approximation can be gathered by looking at sarcoidosis registries. The Danish National Registry included 48 children within a cohort of 5536 patients with sarcoidosis, resulting in a calculated overall incidence for childhood sarcoidosis of 0.29/100,000/year. The incidence ranged from 0.06/100,000/year for children below 5 years old to 1.02/100.000/year for children 14–15 years old (Byg et al. 2003). It is in the younger age group where most cases with BS are found.

Genetics

Blau syndrome shows an autosomal dominant inheritance which matches the postulated gain-of-function mutation in *NOD2*. Over the years, a growing number of genetic mutations of *NOD2* have been published and reported in the Infevers Registry (Infevers: an online database for auto-inflammatory mutations 2017). Substitutions R334W (Arginine to Glutamine in position 334) and R334Q (Arginine to Tryptophan) are by far the most common. More recently, using targeted deep *NOD2* sequencing, germline mosaicism or gonosomal somaticism were found in patients who were negative for NOD2 mutations by Sanger sequencing (De Inocencio et al. 2015). *NOD2* mutations can be seen in patients with the complete clinical triad but also in both incomplete and expanded phenotypes. Incomplete penetrance in asymptomatic carrier status has rarely been reported (Saulsbury et al. 2009).

Pathogenesis

The *NOD2* gene encodes a 1,040 amino-acid protein composed of three main functional domains namely two amino-terminal Caspase Recruitment Domains (CARDs), a central Nucleotide Binding Oligomerization Domain (NOD/NACHT), and carboxyterminal Leucine-Rich repeats [LRRs]. The NOD2 protein is a member of the family of NOD-like receptor cytosolic proteins [NLRs] involved in pathways of inflammation, apoptosis and phagocytosis. The two amino-terminal CARD domains of NOD2 have an important role in the mediation of nuclear factor NFκB activation and secretion of pro-inflammatory cytokines, resulting from CARD-CARD interactions between NOD2 and a pivotal downstream kinase protein receptor-interacting protein kinase 2 [RIP2]. The centrally located NOD domain mediates self-oligomerization of NOD2 followed by downstream activation of effector molecules. The LRR region is structurally related to the LRR regions of the Toll-like receptors which are pattern recognition molecules of the innate immune system, sensing and binding molecular motifs specific to pathogens. NOD2 like other NLR proteins occurs in two states: a tense comma shaped auto-inhibited state, and a relaxed NOD domain exposure state after ligand engagement. NOD domain exposure is a pre-requisite for NOD2 oligomerization and downstream pathway activation (Boyle et al. 2014). Hydrophobic forces and salt bond interactions within the four subdomains of the NOD domain as well as ADP binding maintain the "tight" inactive state (Maekawa et al. 2016). NOD2 oligomerization renders a CARD domain scaffold allowing for interaction with a CARD-containing RIP2 kinase and downstream pathway activation.

The downstream effects of *NOD2* auto-activating mutations associated with BS, and their relationship with both granuloma formation and clinical phenotype are not yet understood. Consistent with the autosomal-dominant inheritance pattern and according to early experimental work, NOD2 mutations associated with BS are gain-of-function variants. Transient transfection assays performed in vitro using plasmids with powerful promoters that over-express *NOD2* have found that mutations associated with Blau syndrome cause excessive NF-κB and MAPK activation compared to the wild-type form of *NOD2* (Kanazawa et al. 2005). Yet, experiments using patients' circulating mononuclear and asymptomatic R314Q-knock-in mice show attenuated cytokine production in response to MDP (Dugan et al. 2015). These apparently contradictory data, one could conceive that the gain-of-function effect is not demonstrable in human PBMCs due to a phenomenon of attenuation and/or unknown modulating factors. Although RIP2 activation following NOD2 oligomerization in BS is well-documented, one should bear in mind that there are more than 30 proteins binding NOD2 with different degrees of affinity. Several of the NOD2 binding partners directly influence autophagy. The role of NOD2 in autophagy is of great interest since many of the interacting proteins bind NOD2 at the cytoskeleton and cell membrane where the cell fusion machinery involved in multinucleation and granuloma formation.

Clinical Manifestations

Blau syndrome features a clinical phenotype of polyarthritis, dermatitis and uveitis. In recent years, because of the availability of genetic testing, a more protean clinical picture than initially conceived is being unveiled.

The initial manifestations include the typical exanthema followed within months by a symmetrical polyarthritis. Ocular involvement tends to occur later in the disease course.

Cutaneous Involvement
The rash varies in color from pale pink with varied degrees of tan to intense erythema. The lesions appear on the trunk mainly dorsally and later extend to the face and limbs with accentuation of the tan color on extensor surfaces, where it may become scaly brownish over time. The lesions are tiny (5–7 mm), round, and barely palpable. At onset, the rash often shows a very fine desquamation, which may lead to confusion with atopic dermatitis. Over the course of the years the rash waxes and wanes. With time, the desquamation predominates, and, in adolescence, it may mimic ichthyosis vulgaris.

Subcutaneous nodules, often located in the lower limbs, are the second most common dermatological manifestation and may be clinically indistinguishable from erythema nodosum. The nodules are mildly tender and resolve without atrophy or pigmentation, even in patients with recurrent episodes. Erysipelas-like lesions have been observed as well, and in one case an urticarial rash showed typical histological features of leukocytoclastic vasculitis (Rose et al. 2006).

Articular Disease
The majority of patients present with a polyarticular symmetrical or additive arthritis, affecting large and small peripheral joints and tendon sheaths. The most frequently joints involved comprise wrists, knees, ankles and PIP joints. A characteristic feature of both synovitis and tenosynovitis is the exuberance of the swelling. The distal flexor tendons of the digits, the extensor and peroneal compartments, and the flexor groups of the carpus can reach significant size. The synovial

outpouching can acquire a cystic appearance in the dorsum of carpus and tarsus. Despite the prominent "boggy" synovitis, pain and morning stiffness appear to be moderate and are overall well tolerated. Except for the proximal interphalangeal joints, where a characteristic flexion contracture described as "camptodactyly" can be seen, the range of motion is relatively well preserved, at least in childhood. The course of the arthritis is variable, and erosive changes are mostly rare and modest. However, limited joint mobility and joint contractures may develop with time; ulnar deviations, wrist subluxations, and joint space narrowing have been described (Rose et al. 2006).

Ocular Disease

An insidious granulomatous iridocyclitis and posterior uveitis can evolve into a severe destructive panuveitis. Of the clinical triad components, the ocular disease exhibits the most somber functional prognosis. It tends to start within the first 2 years of disease as an asymptomatic uveitis. Over time characteristic iris nodules, focal synechiae and clumpy keratic precipitates at the limbus appear, and cataract and increased intraocular pressure ensue. Nodules may also occur in the conjunctivae and, in this location, offer an early biopsy site and diagnostic clue.

Visceral and Systemic Involvement

It has become apparent that the clinical phenotype of BS is not restricted to the classic triad. According to an ongoing prospective cohort study, systemic and visceral involvement affects 48% of patients with BS (Rose et al. 2015). A myriad of clinical manifestations including granulomatous and interstitial nephritis, chronic renal insufficiency, small vessel vasculitis, interstitial pneumonitis, peripheral and mediastinal (excluding hilar) lymphadenitis, pericarditis, cranial neuropathy (VII cranial nerve), and parotitis have been documented in recent studies (Rose et al. 2009).

Systemic symptoms including prolonged fever can be a presenting manifestation and may recur during first few years of the disease (Rose et al. 2009; Arostegui et al. 2007).

Takayasu-like arteritis was recently reported in a girl with BS (Khubchandani et al. 2012). Arterial hypertension with normal digital vascular imaging was observed in 25% of patients from an international registry (Rose et al. 2009).

Laboratory Testing

Peripheral blood cell counts are usually within normal limits, although mild anemia, leucopenia, or lymphopenia can be seen. Levels of C-Reactive Protein were only mildly elevated compared to healthy volunteers, and did not correlate with articular disease activity in a BS cohort study (Rose et al. 2015). Elevation of angiotensin converting enzyme (ACE) is not consistent, and the value of serum ACE levels in diagnosing and managing BS remains unclear. Hypercalciuria and hypercalcemia result from overproduction of 25-hydroxyvitamin D-1 α-hydroxylase by macrophages in granulomas. Hypercalciuria can lead to nephrocalcinosis and nephrolithiasis, both complications being documented in the international prospective BS cohort (Rose et al. 2015).

Diagnosis

The diagnosis of BS rests on genetic confirmation of a *NOD2* mutation in the context of either a typical clinical phenotype and/or the demonstration of characteristic non-caseating granulomatous inflammation.

Pathology

Typical non-caseating epithelioid and multinucleated giant cell granulomas can be documented in biopsies of skin, synovium, lymph node, kidney or liver. The skin biopsy has shown the best yield among patients with the classical granulomatous dermatitis. A synovial membrane biopsy can offer a good alternative particularly in patients whose rash has resolved or appears inactive. Blau granulomas display a distinct morphology characterized by large polycyclic granulomas with dense lymphocytic coronas. They reflect an exuberant inflammatory response, which is in line with a gain-of-function mutation in *NOD2*. Using immunohistochemistry, a predominance of CD68+ macrophages and CD4+T lymphocytes and an abundant inflammatory cytokine expression in situ is typically observed (Janssen et al. 2012).

Genetic Testing

NOD2 mutations were found in 98% of the patients of the International Pediatric Granulomatous Arthritis Registry exhibiting the classic triad phenotype with either a sporadic or a familial form (Rose et al. 2006).

Imaging

Hand X-Rays show a symmetrical non-erosive arthropathy with a number of characteristic dysplasia-like bone changes. Some of the most frequently observed deformities including a biconcave radius, carpal crowding, a short plump distal ulna and a thin second metacarpal diaphysis are characteristic and may allow recognition of BS on a single wrist X-Ray view. The radiographic picture which we dubbed the "Blau hand" is very different from the "rheumatoid hand" (Rose et al. 2015).

Differential Diagnosis

The diagnosis of BS in a child with granulomatous inflammation requires a concerted effort to exclude chronic infections, notably mycobacterial and fungal, by appropriate staining and cultures.

In geographic areas endemic for tuberculosis, granulomatous arthritis should raise the suspicion of TB. Monoarticular granulomatous synovitis can be seen in patients with foreign body arthritis. Penetration of thorns from Yucca plants, sea urchin spines and other inert foreign bodies are not that unusual in exposed children and should be suspected in the appropriate clinical scenario.

A challenging differential diagnosis for BS polyarthritis with uveitis is polyarticular juvenile idiopathic arthritis (JIA). In addition, adults with BS may be incorrectly diagnosed as rheumatoid arthritis or spondyloarthropathy.

BS needs to be differentiated from other systemic inflammatory disorders associated with granulomatous inflammation in children, such as Crohn's disease. Although BS does not affect the gastrointestinal tract some extra-intestinal manifestations could be confusing including arthritis, uveitis, hepatitis, cutaneous vasculitis and erythema nodosum. Patients with granulomatosis with polyangiitis (Wegener's) often have granulomatous inflammation of the upper respiratory tract, a biopsy will reveal signs of small-vessel vasculitis.

Large vessel vasculitis can be a presentation of Blau syndrome therefore among patients with abdominal aortitis, renal artery stenosis, Takayasu's like syndrome and aortic root disease, Blau syndrome needs to be considered (Khubchandani et al. 2012).

Various primary immunodeficiency disorders can present with granulomatous inflammation without an identifiable infectious cause, and should be excluded by evaluation of neutrophil function, analysis of circulating lymphocyte subsets and serum levels of immunoglobulins (Rose et al. 2014).

Treatment

Evidence-based data on the optimal treatment for Blau are nonexistent. Moderate- to low-dose daily corticosteroid therapy is effective to control uveitis and joint disease, but the side effects of prolonged use may become unacceptable. In a prospective Blau cohort study, more than two-thirds of Blau patients received medical therapy for several years, often combining systemic steroids, immunosuppressive and/or biologic drugs to control both uveitis and arthritis (Rose et al. 2015). Methotrexate at a dosage of 10–15 mg/m^2 once weekly reportedly was effective in suppressing articular disease activity and may be steroid sparing. TNF antagonists were the most commonly used biological therapy. Infliximab and Adalimumab were found to control chronic arthritis and visceral manifestations in a number of patients; however, the effect on uveitis activity is less convincing (Rose et al. 2015). A good response to IL-1 inhibition with Anakinra was reported in a single case (Arostegui et al. 2007) and clinical benefit on refractory uveitis in a

4-year old boy with Canakinumab for 6 months has also been reported (Simonini et al. 2013). Tocilizumab has been used in isolated cases, yet at present its efficacy remains unknown.

Antihypertensive medication may be required in patients who developed arterial hypertension with or without obvious renal involvement. ACE inhibitors have been effective in the few documented cases (Rose et al. 2015).

Prognosis

In the prospective BS cohort study, articular and ocular disease were still active after more than 10 years of systemic therapy. At the baseline evaluation, active ocular inflammation was seen in more than one third of patients and was associated have with moderate to severe visual impairment in 27% and 15% of patients respectively. There was no decrease in inflammatory activity and a progressive loss of visual acuity during 3 years of follow-up (Rose et al. 2015). Arthritis seems nondestructive, especially during the first years, but as the disease progresses, flexion deformities, camptodactyly, and less frequently erosions can be observed. Persistent joint swelling is common, with active arthritis in 70% of patients and a median joint count of 15 in patients with more than 10 years of evolution. Twenty eight percent of patients graded their functional disability as moderate or severe (Rose et al. 2015). Severe hypertension in four patients and visceral involvement, including glomerulonephritis with renal failure (one patient) and interstitial pneumonitis (one patient) was seen among 45 participants in our international retrospective registry (Rose et al. 2009). These findings underline the need for careful surveillance throughout the disease course. Anti-TNF therapy was effective in controlling one case of Blau glomerulonephritis (Rose et al. 2009) and increase in the dose of corticosteroids was effective in controlling interstitial pneumonitis in another patient (Rose et al. 2009). Conversely, pulmonary arterial hypertension was the cause of death in one patient at the age of 23 years (CDR, personal observation).

References

Arostegui JI, Arnal C, Merino R, Modesto C, Antonia CM, Moreno P, et al. NOD2 gene-associated pediatric granulomatous arthritis: clinical diversity, novel and recurrent mutations, and evidence of clinical improvement with interleukin-1 blockade in a Spanish cohort. Arthritis Rheum. 2007;56:3805–13.

Blau EB. Familial granulomatous arthritis, iritis, and rash. J Pediatr. 1985;107:689–93.

Boyle JP, Parkhouse R, Monie TP. Insights into the molecular basis of the NOD2 signaling pathway. Open Biol. 2014. https://doi.org/10.1098/rsob.140178.

Byg KE, Milman N, Hansen S. Sarcoidosis in Denmark 1980–1994. A registry-based incidence study comprising 5536 patients. Sarcoidosis Vasc Diffuse Lung Dis. 2003;20:46–52.

De Inocencio J, Mensa-Vilaro A, Tejada-Palacios P, et al. Somatic NOD2 mosaicism in Blau syndrome. J Allergy Clin Immunol. 2015;136:484.

Dugan J, Griffiths E, Snow P, Rosenzweig H, Lee E, Brown B, Carr DW, Rose CD, Rosenbaum J, Davey MP. Blau syndrome-associated Nod2 mutation alters expression of full-length NOD2 and limits responses to muramyl dipeptide in knock-in mice. J Immunol. 2015;194:349–57.

Infevers: an online database for autoinflammatory mutations. http://fmf.igh.cnrs.fr/ISSAID/infevers/ lastupdated 10/29/2014. Accessed 8 July 2017.

Janssen CE, Rose CD, DeHertogh G, Martin T, Badeer-Meunier B, Cimaz R, Harjacek M, Quartier P, Cate RT, Tomee C, Desmet VJ, Fischer A, Roskams T, Morphological WCH. Immunohistochemical characteristics of granulomas in the NOD-2-related Pediatric granulomatous disorders Blau syndrome and Crohn's disease. J Allergy Clin Immunol. 2012;129: 1076–84.

Kanazawa N, Okafuji I, Kambe N, Nishikomori R, Nakata-Hizume M, Nagai S, et al. Early-onset sarcoidosis and CARD15 mutations with constitutive nuclear factor-kappaB activation: common genetic etiology with Blau syndrome. Blood. 2005;105:1195–7.

Khubchandani RP, Hasija R, Touitou I, Khemani C, Wouters CH, Rose CD. Blau arteritis resembling Takayasu disease with a novel NOD2 mutation. J Rheumatol. 2012;39:1888–92.

Maekawa S, Ohto U, Shibata T, Miyake KShimizu T. Crystal structure of NOD2 and its implications in human disease. Nature Comm. 2016. https://doi.org/10.1038/ncomms11813.

Miceli-Richard C, Lesage S, Rybojad M, Prieur AM, Manouvrier-Hanu S, Hafner R, et al. CARD15 mutations in Blau syndrome. Nat Genet. 2001;29:19–20.

Rose CD, Wouters CH, Meiorin S, et al. Pediatric granulomatous arthritis: an international registry. Arthritis Rheum. 2006;54:3337–44.

Rose CD, Arostegui JI, Martin TM, Espada G, Scalzi L, Yague J, et al. NOD2-associated pediatric granulomatous arthritis, an expanding phenotype: study of an international registry and a national cohort in Spain. Arthritis Rheum. 2009;60:1797–803.

Rose CD, Neven B, Wouters CH. Granulomatous inflammation: the overlap of Immunodeficiencies and inflammation. Best Pract Res Clin Rheumatol. 2014;28:191–212.

Rose CD, Pans S, Casteels I, Anton J, Bader-Meunier B, Brissaud P, et al. Blau syndrome: baseline data from a prospective multicenter cohort study of clinical, radiological and functional outcomes. Rheum (Oxford) 2015; 54:1008–16.

Saulsbury FT, Wouters CH, Martin TM, Austin CR, Doyle TM, Goodwin KA, et al. Incomplete penetrance of the NOD2 E383K substitution among members of a pediatric granulomatous arthritis pedigree. Arthritis Rheum. 2009;60:1804–6.

Simonini G, Xu Z, Caputo R, De LC, Pagnini I, Pascual V, et al. Clinical and transcriptional response to the long-acting interleukin-1 blocker canakinumab in Blau syndrome-related uveitis. Arthritis Rheum. 2013;65:513–8.

BLNK Deficiency

Vassilios Lougaris and Alessandro Plebani
Pediatrics Clinic and Institute for Molecular Medicine A. Nocivelli, Department of Clinical and Experimental Sciences, University of Brescia and ASST-Spedali Civili of Brescia, Brescia, Italy

Definition

B-cell linker protein (BLNK) deficiency (OMIM #613502) is a rare primary immunodeficiency characterized by reduced serum levels of all immunoglobulin classes in the absence of peripheral B cells (peripheral B cells <2%). To date, a small number of patients have been described. BLNK deficiency is caused by biallelic deleterious mutations in the gene encoding for BLNK.

Pathogenesis

Early B cell development takes place in the bone marrow. An important maturational step is the progression form the pro-B to the pre-B stage (Espeli et al. 2006; Rudin and Thompson 1998; Bartholdy and Matthias 2004). This passage depends on the expression of a functional B cell receptor composed of the μ heavy chain (*IGHM*; OMIM*147020), Igα (*CD79A*; OMIM*112205), Igβ (*CD79B*; OMIM*147245), VpreB, and λ5 (*IGLL1*; OMIM*146770) that initiates downstream signalling necessary for early B cell differentiation through kinases such as BTK and BLNK (OMIM*604615). Over the years, animal models and in vitro studies have underlined the importance of each of the pre-BCR components and associated transcription factors for the transition from pro-B to pre-B stage of maturation, suggesting that deficiency of these proteins may be responsible for agammaglobulinemia in humans (Conley and Cooper 1998).

BLNK (also called SLP-65) is activated after BCR cross-linking and initiates the downstream signaling cascade. Since mutations in pre-BCR components have been found to cause agammaglobulinemia and BLNK acts downstream of this complex, *BLNK* was evaluated as a candidate gene. In 1999, Minegishi et al. reported on the first male patient with mutations in *BLNK* resulting in agammaglobulinemia. Bone marrow analysis showed a specific block at the pro-B to pre-B stage, and additional experiment concluded that BLNK is essential for B cell development once the pre-BCR is expressed. In 2014, the second case of BLNK deficiency was reported by Lagresle-Peyrou et al.: a male patient carrying a homozygous mutation in the BLNK gene leading to a premature stop codon with a B cell differentiation block at the bone marrow at the pre-BI stage. In 2015, Naser Eddin et al. described two siblings with a homozygous frameshift mutation in BLNK resulting in a developmental arrest at the pre-BI to pre-BII stage at the bone marrow.

Clinical Presentation

The first patient with BLNK deficiency described by Minegishi et al. in 1999 presented a clinical history of pneumonia and recurrent otitis media in the first year of life. The first immunological workup evidenced undetectable serum IgG, IgA, and IgM levels in the absence of peripheral B cells. Once on regular IVIG therapy and during an 18-year period of follow-up, his clinical history was complicated with chronic otitis and sinusitis, hepatitis C acquired from immunoglobulin product, and a protein-losing enteropathy episode during adolescence. The patient described by Lagresle-Peyrou et al. presented a clinical history of recurrent otitis and lung infections. Diagnosis of agammaglobulinemia was made at the age of 6 years, Immunoglobulin serum levels were undetectable and peripheral B cells were absent. He was put on IVIG with good clinical response. The male patient described by Naser Eddin et al. was diagnosed with agammaglobulinemia at the age of 6 months. His clinical history included recurrent otitis media, diarrhea, and positive family history. During follow-up, and under IVIG regular treatment, he developed worsening of the intestinal symptoms with associated arthritis, and progessive skin manifestations including hypercheratosis and edema. Peripheral blood PCR resulted positive for enterovirus. His older sister was diagnosed with agammaglobulinemia at the age of 12 months. Her clinical history included recurrent otitis media and sinopulmonary infections. Although IVIG was initiated, lung infections persisted over time leading to the development of bronchiectasis. She is currently on antibiotic prophylaxis and IVIG. Of note, her PCR resulted negative for enterovirus.

Diagnosis

Immunological work-up in BLNK deficient patients shows low levels of serum immunoglobulins in the complete absence of peripheral B cells. Once BTK mutations are excluded for male patients, genetic screening for mutations in components of the pre-BCR and downstream signaling molecules such as BLNK should be performed.

Management

As in other forms of primary humoral immunodeficiencies, immunoglobulin replacement treatment should be undertaken once the immunological diagnosis of agammaglobulinemia is established. Currently two options for administration are available: intravenous or subcutaneous. Commonly, a dose of 400 mg/kg/dose every three to 4 weeks is sufficient to maintain pre-infusion IgG levels >500 mg/dl that should be able to reduce the number of infectious episodes, especially that of invasive infections.

Antibiotic usage should be undertaken for every infectious episode, and in some case, prophylactic regimen may also be prescribed.

Considering the limited number of affected patients, long-term follow-up is not well known. Nonetheless, in case of lung involvement (bronchiectasis, chronic lung disease), lung physiotherapy should be taken into consideration.

References

Bartholdy B, Matthias P. Transcriptional control of B cell development and function. Gene. 2004;327:1–23.

Conley ME, Cooper MD. Genetic basis of abnormal B cell development. Curr Opin Immunol. 1998;10(4):339–406.

Espeli M, Rossi B, Mancini SJ, Roche P, Gauthier L, Schiff C. Initiation of pre-B cell receptor signaling: common and distinctive features in human and mouse. Semin Immunol. 2006;18:56–66.

Lagresle-Peyrou C, Millili M, Luce S, Boned A, Sadek H, Rouiller J, Frange P, Cros G, Cavazzana M, André-Schmutz I, Schiff C. The BLNK adaptor protein has a nonredundant role in human B-cell difefrentiation. J Allergy Clin Immunol. 2014;134(1):145–54.

Minegishi Y, Rohrer J, Coustan-Smith E, Lederman HM, Pappu R, Campana D, Chan AC, Conley ME. An essential role for BLNK in human B cell development. Science. 1999;286:1954–7.

Naser Eddin A, Shamriz O, Keller B, Alzyoud RM, Unger S, Fisch P, Prus E, Berkun Y, Averbuch D, Shaag A, Wahadneh AM, Conley ME, Warnatz K, Elpeleg O, Stepensky P. Enteroviral infection in a patient with BLNK adaptor protein deficiency. J Clin Immunol. 2015;35(4):356–60.

Rudin CM, Thompson CB. B-cell development and maturation. Semin Oncol. 1998;25:435–46.

Bloom Syndrome

Svetlana O. Sharapova
Research Department, Belarusian Research
Center for Pediatric Oncology, Hematology and
Immunology, Minsk, Belarus

Synonyms

Bloom-Torre-Machacek syndrome; Congenital telangiectatic erythema

Definition

Bloom syndrome (BS) is a rare autosomal recessive disorder, which is caused by homozygous or compound heterozygous mutations in the RecQ DNA helicase gene *BLM*. The most prominent features include severe pre- and postnatal growth retardation, variable immune deficiencies, increased risk for malignancies, a recognizable facial appearance usually with distinctive sun-sensitive erythematous skin lesions, feeding difficulties in infants and young children, and, later in life, male infertility and an increased risk to develop diabetes mellitus (Kaneko and Kondo 2004; Arora et al. 2014).

Introduction/Background

Dr. David Bloom, a practicing dermatologist in New York City, discovered this disorder in 1954 (Bloom 1954) and asked Dr. German in 1963 to study metaphase chromosomes from cultured cells of his three patients with the syndrome (Passarge 2016). From 1965 on over the next 30 years, James L. German and his coworkers systematically studied Bloom's syndrome in depth, culminating in the identification in 1995 of the *BLM* gene (*RECQL3* helicase gene) as encoding a DNA helicase at chromosome 15q26.1 (Passarge 2016). The gene contains 4437 base pairs and encodes 1417 amino acids

to create the BLM protein, which is found in the nuclear matrix of growing cells (de Renty and Ellis 2017). BLM protein expression peaks in the S and G2/M phases of the cell cycle consistent with its role in DNA replication and recombination (de Renty and Ellis 2017).

Cells from individuals with BS are characterized by increases in chromosomal aberrations, including chromatid gaps and breaks, telomere associations, and quadriradial (Qr) chromosomes, which result from unresolved recombination between homologous chromosomes. Other common abnormalities at metaphase include chromosome fragmentation, lagging chromosomes at anaphase, and anaphase bridges. There is an excess of telophase cells with a chromatid strand stretched between them and increased micronuclei formation. BS cells exhibit increased mutation rates. In molecular genetic analysis, the genomic instability in BS includes elevated mitotic homologous recombination and unequal sister-chromatid exchange (de Renty and Ellis 2017).

BS occurs in all national and ethnic groups rarely but is more frequently diagnosed in Ashkenazi Jews due to a founder effect (German et al. 2007). About 300 cases have been reported in the worldwide BS registry (de Renty and Ellis 2017; German et al. 2007; Bouman et al. 2018), one-third of whom are of Central and Eastern European (Ashkenazi) Jewish background. Males are fourfold more affected by Bloom syndrome than females.

Clinical Presentation

Facial dysmorphism and physical examinations. a narrow face, a high anterior hairline, malar flattening, small ears with attached ear lobes, increased posterior angulation of the ears, a prominent nose, a retrognathia, and small jaw. Patients with BS have a characteristically high-pitched voice, short stature, and reduced subcutaneous fat content with normal muscle development. Patients with BS often have long limbs and oversized ears, hands, and feet (Arora et al. 2014).

The typical facial erythema mainly presents during the first or second year of life and tends to worsen after sun exposure. It varies from a minimal involvement (e.g., faint blush of the cheeks) to a bright red erythematous lesion resembling lupus erythematosus. It mainly affects the face although the neck, the forearms, and dorsa of the hands can be involved as well. However, it has been described that in a small percentage of individuals with Bloom syndrome, this erythematous rash is not present at all (Kaneko and Kondo 2004; Arora et al. 2014; Bouman et al. 2018). Other dermatological conditions found in BS include poikiloderma, telangiectatic erythema of the face in a butterfly distribution, and photosensitivity that may lead to cheilitis, crusting, bleeding, blistering, or erythema on any part of the body exposed to UV radiation (Arora et al. 2014).

Growth retardation. The most striking clinical feature of BS is small but proportional body size. Birth weight for persons with BS ranges from 0.7 to 3.2 kg with mean term weights of 1.89 kg ± 0.35 kg for boys and 1.87 kg ± 0.35 kg for girls. Mean birth lengths are similarly reduced with 43.4 cm ± 4.4 cm for BS boys and 43.8 cm ± 2.8 cm for BS girls (de Renty and Ellis 2017).

Recurrent infections. Patients with BS may also present with gastrointestinal infections. Gastroesophageal reflux is common and likely the most important risk factor for infections of the upper respiratory tract, the middle ear, and the lung that occur repeatedly in BS (Arora et al. 2014). Chronic obstructive pulmonary disease also appears at unusually early ages (Kaneko and Kondo 2004).

Fertility. Men with BS appropriately examined have had azoospermia or severe oligospermia. Women with BS, although often fertile, enter menopause prematurely. Eleven women with BS followed in the BS Registry have become pregnant at least once; seven of them have delivered a total of eleven healthy babies of normal size.

Intelligence. Intellectual abilities of affected persons vary, being clearly limited in some and normal in others. Some persons with BS are reported to have a lack of interest in learning and do poorly in school in courses requiring abstract thought. However, others have excelled in school, with some earning graduate degrees.

Malignancies. Cancer is the most frequent medical complication in BS and the most common cause of death. Although the wide distribution of cell types and anatomic sites of cancer resemble that in the general population, it occurs more frequently and at much earlier ages in BS. Development of multiple cancers in a single individual is also much more common than in non-BS individuals. In persons younger than age 20 years, leukemia is the most diagnosed type of cancer. In adult patients, colon cancer is the most common solid tumor (Arora et al. 2014; de Renty and Ellis 2017).

Laboratory Findings/Diagnostic Testing

Bloom syndrome is diagnosed primarily by bromodeoxyuridine chromosomal analysis, which allows for the visualization of chromosomes during cell reproduction. The cells are analyzed for increased sister chromatid exchanges, gaps, breaks, and an increased number of quadriradial chromatid configurations (four-armed chromosomes that result from recombination between two homologous chromosomes, which remain unresolved during the process), typical of BS (Arora et al. 2014).

Immunoblot and immunohistochemical analysis for the detection the BLM protein may be used in case of normal cytogenetic study (de Renty and Ellis 2017).

Among immunologic abnormalities many patients have reduced immunoglobulins (IgM and IgA more often), which leads to increased susceptibility for pneumonia, bronchiectasis, and chronic lung disease.

Molecular analysis of the *BLM* gene is used for detecting mutations. More than 60 different

BS-causing mutations of *BLM* have been reported (Kaneko and Kondo 2004; German et al. 2007).

Treatment

A multidisciplinary approach is required to manage patients with Bloom syndrome. Supplemental feeding does not improve linear growth. Growth hormone administration to children with BS seems ineffective to increase growth rate or adult height. Furthermore, it may increase the risk to develop tumors. Antibiotic prophylaxis and therapy are helpful to control infections. Diabetes mellitus is managed according to standard guidelines. Dermatologic recommendations include frequent skin screenings and avoidance of sun exposure to reduce risk of skin cancer.

Individuals with Bloom syndrome have an enhanced sensitivity to DNA damaging agents such as chemical mutagens and ionizing radiation due to the underlying defect in DNA repair. Serious side-effects and complications during chemoradiation treatment have been described in literature. Modifications of standard chemoradiation therapy might be proposed for individuals with Bloom syndrome (Bouman et al. 2018).

Prognosis

The prognosis of BS patient is generally poor, with mortality in the second or third decade of life, due to increased frequency of malignancy (Arora et al. 2014). The population of persons with BS is relatively young. The oldest person in the Bloom Syndrome Registry is 53 years old, and the average age at death is below 30 years of age (de Renty and Ellis 2017).

References

Arora H, Chacon AH, Choudhary S, et al. Bloom syndrome. Int J Dermatol. 2014;53(7):798–802.

Bloom D. Congenital telangiectatic erythema resembling lupus erythematosus in dwarfs; probably a syndrome entity. AMA Am J Dis Child. 1954;88:754–8.

Bouman A, van Koningsbruggen S, Karakullukcu MB, et al. Bloom syndrome does not always present with sun-sensitive facial erythema. Eur J Med Genet. 2018;61:94–97. pii: S1769-7212(17)30478-0.

de Renty C, Ellis NA. Bloom's syndrome: why not premature aging?: A comparison of the BLM and WRN helicases. Ageing Res Rev. 2017;33:36–51.

German J, Sanz MM, Ciocci S, et al. Syndrome-causing mutations of the BLM gene in persons in the Bloom's syndrome registry. Hum Mutat. 2007;28(8):743–53.

Kaneko H, Kondo N. Clinical features of Bloom syndrome and function of the causative gene, BLM helicase. Expert Rev Mol Diagn. 2004;4(3):393–401.

Passarge E. James L. German, a pioneer in early human genetic research turned 90. Am J Med Genet A. 2016. 170A:1564–5.

Bloom-Torre-Machacek Syndrome

► Bloom Syndrome

C1 Deficiency and Associated Disorders

Berhane Ghebrehiwet
The Department of Medicine, Stony Brook
University, New York, NY, USA
Health Sciences Center, Stony Brook University
School of Medicine, New York, NY, USA

Abbreviations

cC1q	The collagen domain of C1q
cC1qR	Receptor for cC1q
CCP	Complement control protein
CR	Calreticulin (another name for cC1qR)
CUB C1r/ C1s	Uegf and bone morphogenetic protein-1 type protein
EGF	Epidermal growth factor
gC1q	The globular heads of C1q
gC1qR	Receptor for gC1q

Introduction

The complement system is a strictly regulated and highly complex effector system whose major function is to recognize and eliminate pathogens as well as altered self-antigens. Therefore, it constitutes a very powerful arm of the innate and adaptive immune systems with unique ability to discriminate self from nonself and eliminate "danger" through a wide array of processes that include phagocytosis and cytolytic mechanisms. Although there are three interdependent pathways of complement activation – classical, alternative, and lectin – only the role of the classical pathway and the consequences of deficiency in any of the components that initially trigger its activation are discussed here. The first component of complement (Table 1) is a multimolecular complex comprising of one molecule of C1q and the Ca^{2+}-dependent tetramer – C1r-C1s-C1s-C1r – which give rise to the pentameric complex: $C1q.C1r_2.C1s_2$ found in plasma. Each molecule within this complex plays a sequential and highly specific role. The role of C1q is to serve as a recognition unit of immune complexes as well as pathogen-associated molecular patterns (bacterial, viral, or parasitic ligands) and modified-self "danger" signals (Cooper 1985; Arlaud et al. 2001). Recognition of any of these signals is then readily translated into a highly specific and orderly intramolecular rearrangement culminating in C1 activation that sequentially sets in motion the classical pathway of complement – the primary mediator of adaptive humoral immunity. Therefore, deficiency in any of the components of C1 results in susceptibility to infections due to failure to activate the classical pathway and eliminate pathogens (Cooper 1985; Arlaud et al. 2001). Not surprisingly therefore, numerous pathogenic microorganisms have evolved an evasive mechanism to avoid destruction by complement using a number of strategies that include molecular mimicry, enzymatic degradation, as well as expression

© Springer Science+Business Media LLC, part of Springer Nature 2020
I. R. Mackay et al. (eds.), *Encyclopedia of Medical Immunology*,
https://doi.org/10.1007/978-1-4614-8678-7

C1 Deficiency and Associated Disorders, Table 1 Components of the C1 complex

Proteins	Mr (kDa)	Chain structure	Mr (kDa) each chain	Plasma concentration (µg/ml)	Chromosomal location
C1q	460	18 (6A,6B,6C)	A = 28 B = 26 C = 24	80–100	1p34–1p36.3
C1r[a]	86–90	1	86–90	50	12p13
C1s[a]	80–83	1	80–83	50	12p13

[a]C1r and C1s circulate in plasma either as a pentamolecular complex with C1q (C1q. C1s-C1r-C1r-C1s) or as a Ca^{2+} dependent tetramolecular complex – C1s-C1r-C1r-C1s – in the absence of C1q

of regulatory proteins that interfere at various steps of complement activation.

C1q Structure and Function

Human C1q (460 kDa) is a collagen-like and structurally complex hexameric glycoprotein, which displays a unique "bouquet-of-flowers-like" structure (Fig. 1) when viewed under the electron microscope (Calcott and Muller-Eberhard 1972; Shelton et al. 1972). It is comprised of six globular "heads" or "domains" that are linked via six collagen-like "stalks" to a fibril-like central region resulting in two unique structural and functional domains: the collagen-like region (cC1q) and the globular "head" or domain (gC1q). The C1q molecule (Fig. 1a, b) is made up of three incredibly similar but distinct polypeptide chains – A, B, and C – that are arranged to form six triple helical strands with three peptide chains – A, B, and C – forming one strand (Reid 1985). Within each strand, the A and B chains are linked to each other by a disulfide bond, whereas the C chain – which is associated with the AB chains of a strand through strong non-covalent forces – is disulfide linked to the C chain of an adjacent strand to form a doublet, with three doublets forming an intact C1q molecule (Fig. 1a). Therefore, when analyzed by SDS-PAGE, the typical AB and CC dimers are visualized at approximately 58 and 48 kDa, respectively, and upon reduction, the individual A, B, and C chains fall apart and migrate with an apparent molecular weights of 28, 25, and 24 kDa, respectively (Fig. 1c). The three chains are the product of three distinct genes, which are highly clustered and aligned $5' \Rightarrow 3'$, in the same orientation, in the order A-C-B on a 24 kb stretch of DNA on chromosome 1p (Table 1) (Sellar et al. 1991). The assembly of C1q in a 1:1:1 from its three chains therefore requires precisely synchronized transcription of the three C1q genes.

The crystal structure of the trimeric gC1q signature domain reveals a compact jellyroll β-sandwich fold similar to that of the multi-functional tumor necrosis factor (TNF) ligand family (Shapiro and Scherer 1998; Gaboriaud et al. 2007) suggesting that C1q arose by divergence from a primordial recognition molecule of the innate immune system. The evolutionary connection between C1q-like proteins and TNFs, which control many aspects of inflammation, adaptive immunity, apoptosis, and energy homeostasis, not only illuminates the shared diverse functions of these two important groups of molecules but also explains why C1q has retained some of its ancestral "cytokine-like" activities (Shapiro and Scherer 1998).

Although C1q is capable of binding to a plethora of membrane proteins to induce various cellular functions, there are nonetheless two distinct, well-characterized cell surface proteins with affinity for either the collagen domain (cC1qR) or the globular head region (gC1qR/p33) (Ghebrehiwet et al. 2001). However, because subsequent studies have shown that cC1qR shares sequence identity with calreticulin (CR), it is also referred to as cC1qR/CR.

As a classical pattern recognition molecule with unique ability to sense a wide variety of targets, C1q can engage a broad range of repeating molecular patterns via its heterotrimeric gC1q domain including pathogen surfaces and altered self-structures including nascent ligands expressed on apoptotic cells (Gaboriaud et al.

The structure of C1q

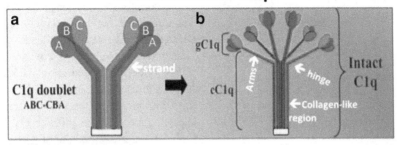

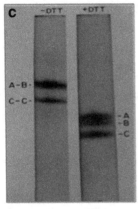

C1 Deficiency and Associated Disorders, Fig. 1 The intact C1q molecule (**b**) is assembled from 18 individual chains (6A, 6B, and 6C). The chains are organized to form six individual strands (**a**), and each strand is comprised of single A, B, and C chains. In each strand, the A chain is disulfide linked to the B chain, whereas the C chain is disulfide linked to the C chain of a neighboring strand to form a doublet (**a**). The figure in (**c**) depicts the SDS-PAGE migration profile of C1q purified from serum. The left lane (−DTT) shows the AB (~58 kDa) and CC (~48 kDa) dimers under nonreducing conditions, and the right lane (+DTT) shows individual A (~28 kDa), B (~25 kDa) and C (~24 kDa) chains under reducing conditions

2007; Païdassi et al. 2008). This in turn leads to enhanced phagocytosis, to target cell lysis as well as, to generation of inflammatory signals. Although C1q is able to bind to diverse self and nonself structures with either its cC1q or gC1q domains, it is the multivalence gC1q domains that characterize its unique versatility and diversity (Gaboriaud et al. 2007).

Pathological Disorders Associated with C1q Deficiency

In addition to its traditional role in the classical pathway of complement activation, C1q has also has emerged as a critical catalyst in an expanding list of pathological disorders that includes sepsis, meningitis, pneumonia, as well as autoimmune diseases such as rheumatoid arthritis and systemic lupus erythematosus (SLE). SLE is a prototype of a systemic autoimmune disease, which affects close to 750,000 individuals in the USA and a much higher number worldwide with a frequency that varies by race and ethnicity with higher rates reported among Black and Hispanic people (Lahita 1999). Although it is a rare multifactorial disease characterized by chronic or episodic inflammation in several organ systems, there is convincing clinical evidence, which shows that homozygous deficiency in any of the classical pathway proteins – C1q, C1r, C1s, as well as C4 and C2 – is a predictor for SLE (Pickering et al. 2000). Among these proteins however, C1q takes center stage in relevance as homozygous deficiency or hereditary deficiency due to mutation in the C1q gene has been shown

C1 Deficiency and Associated Disorders, Table 2 Genetic C1 deficiency and disease association

Protein	Inherited deficiency	Frequently found mutation	Disease association
C1q	Autosomal recessive	g2687C to T→ stop codon	SLE, recurrent bacterial infections, pneumonia, sepsis, and cancer
C1r	Autosomal recessive	Not known	SLE, bacterial infections, rhinobronchitis, impaired immune adherence
C1s	Autosomal recessive	Mutation in exon 6 at position 938	SLE, bacterial infection, impaired immune adherence

to be a powerful susceptibility factor for the development of SLE. The most frequent mutation (Table 2) is in the A chain of C1q in which a substitution in the messenger RNA of C at position 2687 by T results in a stop codon (Skattum et al. 2011). In another patient, a loss of Taq I restriction site within the B chain at the position coding for residue 150 also resulted in the termination codon (McAdam et al. 1988). Therefore, on the basis of data accumulated to date, the most probable cause of genetic deficiency in C1q appears to be point mutations in the A, B, or C genes thereby preventing a normal assembly of the C1q molecule. Regardless, the vast majority of the known individuals ($\leq$100 reported to date) with C1q deficiency are known to have developed clinical syndromes closely related to SLE. Although individuals with congenital complement deficiency constitute only a small cohort of all human SLE, this strong association implicates an important role for C1q in the regulation of SLE.

Recent studies also reveal that C1q can enhance chemotaxis, modulate angiogenesis, and regulate trophoblast migration (Ghebrehiwet et al. 2012). Deficiency in C1q therefore would result in pathological disorders in which these functions are relevant. These include preeclampsia (Hong et al. 2009), Alzheimer's disease (Stephan et al. 2013) and cancer (Singh et al. 2011). For example, pregnant C1q-/-mice have been shown to reproduce the key features of human preeclampsia that correlate with increased fetal death. Treatment of the C1q-/- mice with the cholesterol-lowering drug, pravastatin, prevented the onset of preeclampsia by apparently restoring trophoblast invasiveness, placental blood flow, and angiogenic balance (Hong et al. 2009). Another disease in which the role of C1q has been slowly taking center stage is Alzheimer's disease. Age-related cognitive decline is caused by an impacted neuronal circuitry. Recent studies, which show that C1q levels increase by as much as 300-fold in the normal aging mouse and human brain, would suggest that C1q is involved in triggering an immune attack against the synapses (Stephan et al. 2013). Most significantly, the concentration of C1q was predominantly localized in close proximity to synapses in regions of the brain such as the hippocampus, substantia nigra, and piriform cortex, which have been identified to be vulnerable in neurodegenerative diseases. In contrast, aged C1q-deficient mice exhibited significantly less cognitive and memory decline as evidenced by certain hippocampus-dependent behavior tests compared with their wild-type littermates (Stephan et al. 2013).

Previous experimental data have also suggested that C1q plays a role in suppression of tumor cell proliferation (Ghebrehiwet et al. 2012). The mechanistic underpinning of this function was intimated by recent observations, which showed that C1q induces apoptosis of prostate cancer cells by activating the tumor suppressor molecule WW domain containing oxidoreductase (WWOX or WOX1) and destabilizing cell adhesion. Conversely, downregulation of C1q enhanced prostate hyperplasia and cancer formation due to failure of WOX1 activation (Hong et al. 2009). These are only few examples of a long list of disorders in which C1q is directly or indirectly involved in triggering or contributing to the pathology.

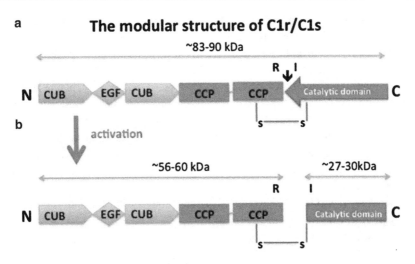

C1 Deficiency and Associated Disorders, Fig. 2 The structure of C1r and C1s is almost identical and consists of two **CUB** (C1r/C1s, Uegf and bone morphogenetic protein-1 type protein), **EGF** (epidermal growth factor), and **CCP** (complement control protein) modules, in the order depicted (**a**). In both cases, enzymatic activation involves cleavage of a single Arg-Ile bond (**b**) with the catalytic domain located in the C-terminal fragment of the disulfide-linked single chain (Adapted from Arlaud et al. 2001)

Structure and Pathological Disorders Associated with C1r and C1s Deficiency

As described above, C1r and C1s are the first proteases responsible for setting in motion the downstream events that occur during activation of the classical pathway. The two proteins, which are modular serine proteases located on human chromosome 12p13 (Tables 1 and 2), form a calcium-dependent tetramer, C1s-C1r-C1r-C1s, and circulate in plasma either as a pentameric complex in association with C1q or as an independent tetramer in the absence of C1q. Both C1r and C1s display remarkably similar structural organization in that both are single-chain zymogens (Fig. 2) of approximately 83–90 kDa and upon activation – which involves cleavage of a single Arg-Ile bond – each is converted to a single chain comprised of a non-catalytic A chain of approximately 56–60 kDa single-chain protease disulfide-bonded to a catalytic B chain of approximately 27–30 kDa. Starting from the N-terminus, the structural organization of the two proteases is identical and comprises of several distinct modules that include CUB, EGF, and CCP modules (Fig. 2). Within macromolecular C1, the C1s-C1r-C1r-C1s tetramer is located between the collagen-like arms of C1q and adopts a "figure 8"-type

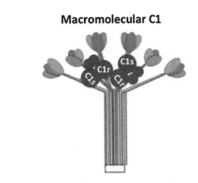

C1 Deficiency and Associated Disorders, Fig. 3 The C1 complex is made up of C1q and the C1s-C1r-C1r-C1s tetramer positioned between the arms of the C1q molecule in a manner that allows contact of the catalytic domains of C1r and C1s to each other. This positioning is presumed to facilitate cleavage of C1s by C1r

configuration in a manner that allows contact of the catalytic domains of C1r and C1s (Fig. 3). Such configuration facilitates cleavage of C1s by C1r (Arlaud et al. 2001). The conversion of C1r to an active protease is the first step in the initiation of the classical pathway. Although the mechanism is not well known, it is believed that recognition of an activator by C1q induces a conformational change within the pentameric C1 that allows autocatalytic activation of C1r, and activated C1r then cleaves proenzyme C1s into a disulfide-linked single-chain enzyme (Fig. 2). The natural substrates of C1s are C4 and C2, which are sequentially cleaved into C4a and C4b and C2a and C2b, respectively, with the larger fragments forming the major C3-converting enzyme – C4b-C2a – that sets in motion the classical pathway of complement.

Although the primary site of synthesis for both C1r and C1s is the liver, both are also synthesized by a vast array of tissues and cell types (Ghebrehiwet et al. 2012). Deficiency in either C1r (Day et al. 1971) or C1s (Amano et al. 2008) is relatively rare with fewer than 20 cases reported to date, and because of their shared chromosomal localization, deficiency of C1r will almost certainly result in deficiency in C1s. A mutation at position 938 in exon 6 of the C1s cDNA has been shown to create a premature stop codon generating splice variants of C1s mRNA transcripts in normal human cells (Amano et al. 2008). The splice variants are derived from the skipping of exon 3 and from the use of an alternative $3'$ splice site within intron 1 which increases the size of exon 2 by 87 nucleotides (Amano et al. 2008). Because of their close association and interdependent function within the C1 complex, deficiency in C1q or in either of the proteases will result in susceptibility to infections including sepsis, meningitis pneumonia, defective immune responsiveness, and increased risk of autoimmune disorders including SLE.

Diagnosis and Treatment of Diseases Associated with C1 Deficiency

Routine screening for complement deficiency by measurement of CH50 – which measures functional activity of complement – should provide an initial indication of whether an individual has normal, low, or absent CH50. While low levels of CH50 may indicate ongoing consumption due to infection, the absence of CH50 would almost invariably indicate complete deficiency in any of the components shared by all the pathways, i.e., classical, alternative, or lectin. Therefore, further screening should be tailored on the basis of the disease that the patient is suspected of having. For example, a patient while suspected SLE or rheumatoid arthritis could be screened for C1 deficiency, meningitis or sepsis could be due to deficiency in C3 or C9.

Because deficiency in the early complement components would almost invariably predispose one to upper respiratory infections or autoimmune diseases, and there is no treatment for C1 deficiency to date, prophylactic treatment with antibiotics or vaccinations against associated infections (e.g., meningococcal or *H. influenza*) is recommended for C1 deficient individuals.

References

Amano MT, Ferriani VP, Florido MP, Resis ES, Delcolli MI, Azzolini AE, et al. Genetic analysis of complement C1s deficiency associated with systemic lupus erythematosus highlights alternative splicing of normal C1s gene. Mol Immunol. 2008;45:1693–702.

Arlaud GJ, Gaboriaud C, Thielens NM, Rossi V, Bersch B, Hernandez J-F, et al. Structural biology of C1: dissection of a complex molecular machinery. Immunol Rev. 2001;180:136–45.

Calcott MA, Muller-Eberhard HJ. C1q protein of human complement. Biochemistry. 1972;11:3443–50.

Cooper NR. The classical complement pathway: activation and regulation of the first complement component. Adv Immunol. 1985;37:151–216.

Day NK, Geiger H, Stroud R, de Bracco M, Mancado B, Windhorst D, Good RA. C1r deficiency: an inborn error associated with cutaneous and renal disease. J Clin Investig. 1971;51:1102–8.

Gaboriaud C, Païdassi H, Frachet P, Tacnet-Delorme P, Thielens NM, Arlaud GJ. C1q: a versatile pattern recognition molecule and sensor of altered self. In: Kilpatrick D, editor. Collagen-related lectins in innate immunity (Research Signpost), vol. 81; 2007. p. 1–15.

Ghebrehiwet B, Lim BL, Kumar R, Feng X, Peerschke EI. gC1q-R/p33, a member of a new class of multifunctional and multicompartmental cellular proteins, is involved in inflammation and infection. Immunol Rev. 2001;180:65–77.

Ghebrehiwet B, Hosszu K, Valentino A, Peerschke EIB. The C1q family of proteins: insights into the emerging non-traditional functions. Front Immunol. 2012;3. pii:52.3:1–9.

Hong Q, Sze C-I, Lin S-R, Lee M-H, He R-Y, Schultz L, Chang J-Y, Chen S-J, Boackle RJ, Hsu L-J, Chang N-S. Complement C1q activates tumor suppressor WWOX to induce apoptosis in prostate cancer cells. PLoS One. 2009;4(6):e5755.

Lahita RG. Systemic lupus erythematosus. Third ed. NY: Academic Press, New York; 1999.

McAdam RA, Goundis D, Reid KBM. A homozygous point mutation results in a stop codon in the C1q B-chain of a C1q deficient individual. Immunogenetics. 1988;27:259–64.

Païdassi H, Tacnet P, Garlatti V, Darnault C, Ghebrehiwet B, Gaboriaud C, Arlaud GJ, Frachet P. C1q binds phosphatidylserine and likely acts as a multiligand bridging molecule in apoptotic cell recognition. J Immunol. 2008;180:2329–38.

Pickering MC, Botto M, Taylor PR, Lachmann PJ, Walport MJ. Systemic lupus erythematosus, complement deficiency, and apoptosis. Adv Immunol. 2000;76:227–34.

Reid KBM. Molecular cloning and characterization of the complementary DNA and gene coding for the B chain subcomponent C1q of the human complement system. Biochem J. 1985;231:729–35.

Sellar GC, Blake DJ, Reid KBM. Characterization and organization of the genes encoding the A-, B-, and C-chains of human complement subcomponent C1q. Biochem J. 1991;274:481–91.

Shapiro L, Scherer PE. The crystal structure of a complement-1q family of protein suggests an evolutionary link to tumor necrosis factor. Curr Biol. 1998;8:335–8.

Shelton E, Yonemasu K, Stroud RM. Ultrastructure of the human complement component C1q. Proc Natl Acad Sci U S A. 1972;69:65–8.

Singh J, Ahmed A, Girardi G. Role of complement component C1q in the onset of preeclampsia in mice. Hypertension. 2011;58:716–24.

Skattum L, van Deuren M, van der Poll T, Truedson L. Complement deficiency states and associated infections. Mol Immunol. 2011;48:1643–55.

Stephan AH, Madison DV, Mateos JM, Fraser DA, Lovelett EA, Coutellier L, Kim L, Tsai H-H, Huang EJ, Rowitch DH, Berns DS, Tenner AJ, Shamloo M, Barres BA. A dramatic increase of C1q protein in the CNS during normal aging. J Neurosci. 2013;33:13460–74.

C5b-C9 Deficiency

Anete Sevciovic Grumach
Faculdade de Medicina ABC, Santo Andre, SP, Brazil

Synonyms

LCCD: Late component complement deficiency
TCC: Terminal complement complex
Complement System, C5, C6, C7, C8, C9, component

Definition

C5b-C9 represents the terminal pathway of complement system. Complete genetic deficiency of any of those components can lead to increased risk of meningococcal disease, often recurrent infections caused by unusual serogroups.

C5b-9

Three major activation pathways, the classical, the alternative, and the lectin pathway, lead to a common pathway, the terminal complement system that consists of components five to nine. All pathways lead to cleavage of C3, and when additional C3b molecules are bound to the C3 convertases, this results in formation of C5 convertases (C4b2a3b) and subsequently cleavage of C5. This splits C5 into the small C5a molecule, and the larger C5b molecule, which is the initial component of the membrane attack complex (MAC). C5a is a strong chemotactic factor and an anaphylatoxin; it has an immunostimulatory role which also participates in the pathological process including the response to sepsis (Grimnes et al. 2011). The C5b fragment can then form a complex with C6, C7, C8, and a number of C9 molecules creating the MAC (C5b-C9). On cell membranes, MAC is capable of forming transmembrane channels through which ions migrate, leading to cell lysis and cell death.

Components six to nine are related plasma proteins, which differ in size and complexity. Components C6, C7, and C9 are single-chain serum proteins which interact with each other to become a functional unit and are also biochemically and structurally very similar (Würzner et al. 1998). Furthermore, they are coded by closely linked genes in proximity on chromosome 5p13. All genes are also strongly structurally related and likely derived from one common ancestor (Würzner et al. 1998). Both the C6 and C7 genes are polymorphic and are close homologues of the C8α, C8β, and C9 genes (Hobart et al. 1995). C8A, C8B, and C8G genes encode the α-, β-, and γ-subunits of C8, respectively. Genetic linkage and chromosomal localization studies have established that C8A and C8B are linked closely on chromosome 1p32. Significant protein sequence similarity exists between C8α and C8β and also the other terminal components, C6, C7, and C9, whereas C8γ is a member of the lipocalin family and is not related to any other complement component. The C8G gene is located on 9q22.3–q32 close to a cluster of other lipocalin genes (Lovelace et al. 2011).

C5b-9 Deficiency/Late Component Complement Deficiency (LCCD)

Genetically determined human deficiencies of any of the terminal complement components are associated with increased susceptibility to *Neisseria meningitidis* and *N. gonorrhoeae* infections indicating that the serum bactericidal function of MAC is important for the defense against neisserial infections (Ross and Densen 1984; Figueroa and Densen 1991; Sjoholm et al. 2006; Würzner et al. 1992). These organisms either possess a capsular polysaccharide, which precludes successful phagocytosis, or can invade cells and propagate intracellularly. *Neisseriae* are capable of intracellular survival. The association between the inabilities to form the lytic plug of the complement system with infection by these organisms implies that extracellular lysis is of major physiological importance as a mechanism of killing these organisms (Walport 1993). In either case, phagocytosis is ineffective. Fortunately, these organisms are susceptible to the serum bactericidal effect of MAC.

Meningococci colonize the nasopharynx of 5–15% of individuals in areas of non-endemicity, and a larger proportion of individuals may be colonized during epidemics of invasive disease (Ross and Densen 1984). At the time of birth, individuals have bactericidal antibodies (transplacental transfer of maternal antibodies) against meningococci. These maternal antibodies however disappear after a few months. After maturation of their own immune system and after contact with pathogenic as well as nonpathogenic *Neisseria* and cross-reacting gram-negative bacteria, individuals develop meningococcal antibodies (Bols et al. 1993).

Terminal complement pathway and properdin deficiencies expose the patients to a higher risk of invasive meningococcal infections, reaching up to 5000–7000 times in comparison with general population (Figueroa and Densen 1991; Mayilyan 2012; Platonov et al. 1992). In European countries, 61% of *Neisseria meningitidis* infections occurred in patients with terminal pathway defects (Turley et al. 2015). Unusual meningococcal serogroups (particularly Y, W-135, and X) usually infect patients with complement deficiencies (Figueroa and Densen 1991; Ross and Densen 1984), and the frequency of these among patients with meningococcal disease caused by these serogroups is also increased (Fijen et al. 1989).

While the average age at the onset of the first meningococcal infection is 3 years in the general population, and 56% occurs before 5 years, the average age for complement deficiency patients is 17 years, and only 10% of the cases occur before 5 years of age. Previous infection with meningococcus in this group of immunodeficient patients does not reduce the risk of new episodes; relapses occur in 7.6% of those with deficiency of C5-C9, and recurrent disease (new infection more than 1 month after a previous episode) occurs in 45% (Ross and Densen 1984; Andreoni et al. 1993; Rosa et al. 2004). This could be explained in part by the fact that antibodies against subcapsular antigens, although bactericidal and protective, are poor opsonins; they offer little protection in patients with complement deficiency, as these patients do not have the proteins needed for the expression of bactericidal activity (Andreoni et al. 1993; Rosa et al. 2004). On the other side, in individuals with terminal complement deficiency, opsonization involving C3 and immunoglobulin prevents many other invasive infections by other bacterial species (Figueroa and Densen 1991; Pallares et al. 1996).

Multiple reports of autoimmune findings have been recorded (C5 deficiency with SLE-like symptoms, C6 deficiency with SLE-like symptoms and MPGN, C7 deficiency with scleroderma, rheumatoid arthritis, and with SLE-like syndrome, C9 deficiency, and IgA nephropathy), but no firm associations have been established (Frank 2000;

Pickering et al. 2000; Barilla-La Barca and Atkinson 2003; O'Neil 2000; Yoshioka et al. 1992).

Prevalence

In a study of 7732 patients from Netherlands with meningococcal disease, the prevalence of complement deficiency was 3% (Fijen et al. 1999). When patients with unusual serotypes were examined, the prevalence of any complement deficiency was 33%, and the prevalence of C8 deficiency was 23% (Le Bastard et al. 1989). Platonov et al. (1993) evaluated 262 patients with meningococcal infection admitted to a hospital in Moscow for LCCD and four of them had their first episode of meningococcal infection (1.5%). Among patients with recurrent meningitis or meningococcemia in previous Soviet Union (USSR), 30% had LCCD. The median age of the individuals with LCCD at the time of this study was 27 years (range, 9–62), and the median age at the time of the first episode of meningococcal disease was 15 years (range, 1–46) (Platonov et al. 1993). According to the epidemic occurrence of meningococcal disease in previous USSR, prevalence of functional LCCD in the general population could be estimated as approximately 12 persons per 100,000. In Japan, a frequency of 11 per 100,000 was observed after evaluating 145,640 blood donors, similar to USSR observation (Inai et al. 1989). In countries where meningococcal disease is less common, the proportion of individuals with LCCD is higher.

Inheritance

Generally most inherited disorders of the complement system leading to deficiency are autosomal recessive except for deficiency of C1-INH (autosomal dominant), deficiency of properdin (X-linked) and MBL, and Factor I deficiencies (autosomal codominant) (Pettigrew et al. 2009). Complement deficiencies are usually caused by null alleles. These are alleles that do not produce functional protein. In most cases, heterozygotes produce one half of the normal plasma level of a specific complement protein, and homozygotes of null alleles usually produce undetectable levels. Interestingly, individuals who are heterozygotes for a null allele usually have normal total complement activity in a total hemolytic assay (CH50) (Pettigrew et al. 2009).

Ethnicity

Both the frequency of different types of complement deficiency and the frequency of diseases associated with these deficiencies depend on the ethnic composition of the population and the incidence of the diseases in the population (Figueroa and Densen 1991). Complete C6 deficiencies have been reported in Japan and Afro-Americans living in the USA. The same defects had also been reported in the Western Cape, South Africa, as well as occurring in a patient from Afro-Caribbean origin. It has been reported in Netherlands too. Family studies have revealed some C6D (C6-deficient) siblings of index cases who have suffered no infections at all (Orren and Potter 2004; Zhu et al. 2000). C7 deficiency can occur with a relatively high frequency in certain populations as Jews of Moroccan Sephardic descent living in Israel or Irish individuals (Würzner et al. 1998; Halle et al. 2001). C8 is composed of three different subcomponents termed α, β, and γ. C8 α–γ deficiency has been predominantly reported amongst Afro-Caribbeans, Hispanics, and Japanese, whereas C8β deficiency is by far the most frequent in Caucasians (Ross and Densen 1984; Tedesco 1986; Inai et al. 1989; Ram et al. 2010; Mayilyan 2012). In contrast to the situation in Japan, where C9 deficiency has a very high incidence (0.045–0.104%) (Fukumori and Horiuchi 1998), it is a rare finding in Europe (Table 1).

C5 Deficiency

C5 deficiency (C5D) has been diagnosed worldwide (Schejbel et al. 2013). It has been found in approximately 7% of Black African meningococcal disease cases in the Western Cape (Owen et al. 2015). The

C5b-C9 Deficiency, Table 1 Components of terminal pathway of complement system, alleles, and chromosomal localization

Component	Alleles	Chromosome	Ethnicity
C5	C5	9q33-q34	Black Africans
C6	C6	5p13	Japanese, Africans, Afro-Americans, Afro-Caribbeans, Hispanics
C7	C7	5p13	Moroccan Sephardic Jews, Irish
C8 α-chain	C8A	1p32	Afro-Caribbeans, Hispanics, Japanese
C8 β-chain	C8B	1p32	Caucasians
C8 γ-chain	C8G	9q34.3	Afro-Caribbeans, Hispanics, Japanese
C9	C9	5p14-p12	Japanese

system in patients with C5 deficiency is normal up to factor C3. It contains normal opsonic activity which is mainly due to normal C3 levels but fails to generate adequate chemotactic activity and, even more important, lacks serum bactericidal activity of "serum-sensitive" bacteria such as *Neisseria* (Bols et al. 1993). C5 deficiency differs from deficiency of other terminal components in that C5a is not formed during activation. Since C5a is both a strong chemotactic factor and an anaphylatoxin, it could be expected that this deficiency would have other consequences regarding infection susceptibility. In the case of a meningococcal infection, opsonophagocytosis and intracellular killing could achieve elimination of meningococci by phagocytes, but this mechanism is hampered by defective chemotaxis (Figueroa and Densen 1991; Bols et al. 1993). However, the bacterial etiology in systemic infections does not differ (Figueroa and Densen 1991).

Nowadays, patients treated with a monoclonal antibody against C5 behave as genetically C5-deficient patients. That drug links specifically to C5 fraction of complement with high affinity, preventing the formation of C5-9 and leading to meningococcal susceptibility. According to French health system, meningococcal vaccination is recommended and prophylactic antibiotics with penicillin (Haut conseil de la santé publique 2012)

C6 Deficiency

Some individuals with inherited C6 deficiency who appeared to lack C6 by conventional hemolytic complement assays were unequivocally shown by a sensitive ELISA to have C6 at a

concentration of 1–2% of normal mean (Würzner et al. 1991). Their C6 was able to integrate itself into the terminal complement complex (TCC) upon complement activation (Würzner et al. 1991). It was, furthermore, hemolytically active but structurally abnormal, as it was 14% smaller than normal C6. This condition has been designated subtotal C6 deficiency (C6SD). In contrast, the majority of C6-deficient individuals investigated by sensitive hemolytic assays and ELISA were found to completely lack C6 functional and antigenic activity and have been designated "quantitatively zero C6 deficient" (C6Q0) (Orren et al. 1992; Würzner et al. 1995). C6SD subjects do not appear to be more susceptible to neisserial infection than the population at large (Würzner et al. 1995). Some individuals come from families in which family members who are totally C6 deficient were ascertained by their history of meningococcal infection. Thus, we may assume that the C6SD subjects in these families were exposed to meningococci but did not become ill, perhaps because their very small amount of C6 protected them. If this assumption is true, C6SD subjects will be less likely to be identified than C6Q0 patients, who were ascertained because of meningococcal disease either in themselves or in a sibling (Ross and Densen 1984). C6 deficiency can be associated with subtotal C7 deficiency (Würzner et al. 1998).

C7 Deficiency

It is not always possible to distinguish genotypic total C7 deficiency from subtotal deficiency. A study of a patient with virtually no C7 in his circulation showed that he carried the same C6/C7D defects as the other C6/C7SD subjects, as well as another C7 defect. The presence of C5b6 in the circulation led to a consumption of the low amounts of secreted C7. In contrast, patients with the combined deficiency apparently do not have sufficient C6 to allow the production of C5b6, and these subjects have detectable levels of C7 in the circulation (Würzner et al. 1998; Fernie et al. 1996).

C8 Deficiency

C8 is an oligomeric protein composed of three nonidentical subunits (α, 64 kDa; β, 64 kDa; γ, 22 kDa). These subunits are arranged asymmetrically as a covalently linked α–γ heterodimer with a non-covalently associated β-chain. The α-subunit has a domain that interacts with the β-subunit, and it provides the binding site for C9 on C5b-8. The β-subunit has a domain that specifically allows recognition and binding of C8 to C5b-7. The γ-subunit, the function of which remains uncertain, is linked to the α-subunit by a disulfide bond. C8 deficiency may result from lack of the α–γ-chain or the β-chain (Arnold et al. 2009; Ross and Densen 1984).

C9 Deficiency

C9 deficiency leads to incomplete membrane attack complex formation and may therefore predispose to recurrent neisserial infections (Figueroa and Densen 1991). C9-deficient individuals have still some bactericidal activity (Nagata et al. 1989). The formation of the C5b-8 complex in absence of C9 has some protective effect, and it has been shown that sera from C9-deficient individuals can support lysis of antibody-coated sheep erythrocytes although the reaction is 100-fold slower than with normal serum (Lint et al. 1980).

Diagnosis

Recurrent infections caused by *N. meningitidis* (or *N. gonorrhoeae*) should raise suspicion of a complement deficiency (Grumach and Kirschfink

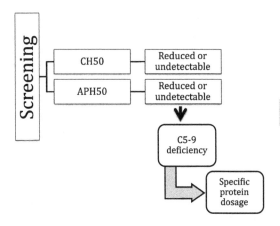

C5b-C9 Deficiency, Fig. 1 Laboratorial diagnosis of C5-9 deficiency

2014). In the case of deficiency of a factor of the classical or terminal pathway, the total hemolytic complement level (CH50) will be undetectable or very low. Hemolytic assay evaluation alternative pathway (AP50) is also undetectable in the case of terminal components of complement system.

After this screening test, the determination of individual complement factors is mandatory. Low levels of multiple factors point to an acquired deficiencies. Many individuals may not be diagnosed because individuals with only one episode of meningococcal infection are seldom investigated (Orren and Potter 2004; de Marcellu et al. 2015) (Fig. 1).

Treatment

Prevention of disease in patients with known terminal component complement deficiency relies on antibiotic prophylaxis, vaccination, and hygienic measures (Skattum et al. 2011).

Antibodies against meningococcal polysaccharide capsule confer protection by the induction of complement-mediated bacteriolysis and by stimulation of Fc-mediated or C3b-mediated opsonophagocytosis (Schlesinger et al. 1994; Platonov et al. 2003). Vaccination can enhance opsonophagocytosis (Gomez-Lus et al. 2003), and vaccination with the tetravalent polysaccharide capsule vaccines A, C, Y, and W135 is recommended for terminal complement-deficient individuals (Centers for Disease Control and Prevention 2013; Platonov et al. 1995). Although in Europe and the USA, infections in complement-deficient individuals are frequently with the rare serogroup W135 or Y strains (Orren et al. 1994), serogroup B strains were nevertheless found responsible for about 20% of all infections in deficient patients (Ross and Densen 1984); moreover, in South Africa, serogroup B infections represented almost 50% of infections in complement-deficient individuals (Orren and Potter 2004). In the last years, vaccination against invasive meningococcal capsular group B disease is available and effective (Ladhani et al. 2014).

Antibiotic prophylaxis was used to protect the more vulnerable patients. And previous studies showed that antibiotics did lessen the risk of recurrent infections but frequently have poor patient acceptance and carry the risk of generating antibiotic-resistant strains (Potter et al. 1990; Schwartz 1991; Morgan and Orren 1998; Kuruvilla and de la Morena 2013).

The use of antibiotics as well as booster vaccination is in keeping with previous studies, which have shown that meningococcal vaccination reduces but does not eliminate the risk of meningococcal disease (Platonov et al. 2003).

Prognosis

Lower mortality from meningococcal disease had been reported in the deficient individual as compared with complement-sufficient persons (Platonov et al. 1993). However, there is no convincing evidence that primary meningococcal infection is milder in complement-deficient individuals (Orren and Potter 2004). It has been suggested that the generation of membrane attack complexes during excessive complement activation in meningococcal disease in complement-sufficient individuals may contribute to the activation and injury of circulating blood leukocytes and endothelial cells during meningococcal disease and that the absence of this effect may contribute to the lower mortality in individuals with LCCD (Brandtzaeg et al. 1989; Ross and Densen 1984; Platonov et al. 1993) (Table 2).

C5b-C9 Deficiency, Table 2 Clinical characteristics of meningococcal meningitis in patients with C5b-C9 deficiency

	LCCD	General population
Neisseria infection	42%	0.0072%
Male/female	3.3:1	1.3:1
Age of first episode	17 years	3 years
Recurrence	45%	0
Therapeutic failure	6.3%	0.6%
Serogroups	Y = 44%	Y = 11%
Mortality	2.9%	19%

Modified from Ross and Densen (1984)

References

Andreoni J, Käyhty H, Densen P. Vaccination and the role of capsular polysaccharide antibody in prevention of recurrent meningococcal disease in late complement component-deficient individuals. J Infect Dis. 1993;168:227–31.

Arnold DF, Roberts AG, Thomas A, Ferry B, Morgan BP, Chapel HA. Novel mutation in a patient with a deficiency of the eighth component of complement associated with recurrent meningococcal meningitis. J Clin Immunol. 2009;29:691–5.

Barilla-LaBarca ML, Atkinson JP. Rheumatic syndromes associated with complement deficiency. Curr Opin Rheumatol. 2003;15:55–60.

Bols A, Janssens J, Petermans W, Stevens E, Bobbaers H. Recurrent meningococcal infections in a patient with congenital C5 deficiency. Acta Clin Belg. 1993;48(10):42–7.

Brandtzaeg P, Mollnes TE, Kierulf P. Complement activation and endotoxin levels in systemic meningococcal disease. J Infect Dis. 1989;160:58–65.

Centers for Disease Control and Prevention. Prevention and control of meningococcal disease. Recommendations of the advisory committee on immunization practices. Morbidity and mortality weekly report. 2013;62:2.

de Marcellus C, Taha MK, Gaudelus J, Fremeaux-Bacchi-V, de Pontual L, Guiddir T. Complement terminal fraction deficiency revealed at first invasive meningococcal infection. Arch Pediatr. 2015;22(3):296–9.

Fernie BA, Würzner R, Orren A, Morgan BP, Potter PC, Platonov AE, Vershinina IV, Shipulin GA, Lachmann PJ, Hobart MJ. Molecular bases of combined subtotal deficiencies of C6 and C7; and theis effects in combination with other C6 and C7 deficiencies. J Immunol. 1996;157:3648–57.

Figueroa JE, Densen P. Infectious diseases associated with complemente deficiencies. Clin Microbiol Rev. 1991;4:359–95.

Fijen CA, Kuijper EJ, Hannema AJ, Sjöholm AG, van Putten JP. Complement deficiencies in patients over ten years old with meningococcal disease due to uncommon serogroups. Lancet. 1989;2:585–8.

Fijen CA, Kuijper MT, Bulte MT, Daha MR, Dankert J. Assessment of complement deficiency in patients with meningococcal disease in the Netherlands. Clin Infect Dis. 1999;28:98–105.

Frank MM. Complement deficiencies. Pediatr Clin N Am. 2000;47:1339–54.

Fukumori Y, Horiuch T. Terminal complemente componente deficiencies in Japan. Exp Clin Immunogenet. 1998;15:244–8.

Gomez-Lus ML, Giménez MJ, Vázquez JA, Aguilar L, Anta L, Berrón S, Laguna B, Prieto J. Opsonophagocytosis versus complemente bactericidal killing as effectors following Neisseria meningitidis group C vaccination. Infection. 2003;31:51–4.

Grimnes G, Beckman H, Lappegård KT, Mollnes TE, Skogen V. Recurrent meningococcal sepsis in a presumptive immunocompetent host shown to be complement C5 deficient-a case report. APMIS. 2011;119(7):479–84.

Grumach AS, Kirschfink M. Are complement deficiencies really rare? Overview on prevalence, clinical importance and modern diagnostic approach. Mol Immunol. 2014;61(2):110–7.

Halle D, Elsten D, Geudalia D, Sasson A, Shinar E, Schlesinger M, Zimran A. High prevalence of complement C7 deficiency among healthy blood donors of Moroccan Jewish ancestry. Am J Med Genet. 2001;99:325–7.

Haut conseil de la santé publique. Avis relatif à l'antibioprophylaxie et la caccination méningococcique des personnes traitées par eculizumab (Soliris 300 mg solution à diluer pour perfusion), séance du 8 novembre 2012.

Hobart MJ, Fernie BA, DiScipio RG. Structure of the human C7 gene and comparison with the C6, C8A, C8B and C9 genes. J Immunol. 1995;154:5188–94.

Inai S, Akagaki Y, Moriyama T, Fukumori Y, Yoshimura K, Ohnoki S, Yamaguchi H. Inherited deficiencies of the late-acting complement components other than C9 found among healthy blood donors. Int Arch Allergy Appl Immunol. 1989;90:274–9.

Kuruvilla M, de la Morena MT. Antibiotic prophylaxis in primary immune deficiency disorders. J Allergy Clin Immunol Pract. 2013;1:573–82.

Ladhani SN, Cordery R, Mandal S, Christensen H, Campbell H, Boirrow R, Ramsay ME, PHE VaPIBI Forum Members. Preventing secondary cases of invasive meningococcal capsular group B (Men B) disease using a recently-licensed, multi-component, protein-based vaccine (Bexsero®). J Infect. 2014;69:470–80.

Le Bastard D, Riou JY, Konczaty H, Bourrillon A, Guibourdenche M. Neisseria meningitidis: Sérogroupe Y A propos de trente-huit observations. Pathol Biol. 1989;37(78):901–7.

Lint TF, Zeitz HJ, Gewurz H. Inherited deficiency of the ninth component of complement in man. J Immunol. 1980;125:2252–7.

Lovelace LL, Cooper CL, Sodetz JM, Lebioda L. Structure of human C8 protein provides mechanistic insight into membrane pore formation by complement. J Biol Chem. 2011;286(20):17585–92.

Mayilyan KR. Complement genetics, deficiencies, and disease associations. Protein Cell. 2012;3:487–96.

Morgan BP, Orren A. Vaccination against meningococcus in complement-deficient individuals. Clin Exp Immunol. 1998;114:327–9.

Nagata M, Hara T, Aoki T, Mizuno Y, Akeda H, Inaba S, Tsumoto K, Ueda K. Inherited deficiency of ninth component of complement: an increased risk of meningococcal meningitis. J Pediatr. 1989;11:260–4.

O'Neil KM. Complement deficiency. Clin Rev Allergy Immunol. 2000;19:83–108.

Orren A, Potter PC. Complement component C6 deficiency and susceptibility to Neisseria meningitidis infections. SAMJ. 2004;94(5):345–6.

Orren A, Würzner R, Potter PC, Fernie BA, Coetzee S, Morgan BP, Lachmann PJ. Properties of a low molecular weight complement component C6 found in human subjects with subtotal C6 deficiency. Immunology. 1992;75:10–6.

Orren A, Caugant DA, Fijen CAP, Dankert J, van Schalkwyk EJ, Poolman JT, Coetzee GJ. Characterization of strains of Neisseria meningitides recovered from complement -normal and complement-deficient patients in the Cape, South Africa. J Clin Microbiol. 1994;32:2185–91.

Owen EP, Würzner R, Leisegang F, Rizkallah P, Whitelaw A, Simpson J, Thomas AD, Harris CL, Giles JL, Hellerud BC, Mollnes TE, Morgan BP, Potter PC, Orren A. A complement C5 gene mutation, c.754G>A:p.A252T, is common in the Western Cape, South Africa and found to be homozygous in seven percent of Black African meningococcal disease cases. Mol Immunol. 2015;64(1):170–6.

Pallares DE, Figueroa JE, Densen P, Giclas PC, Marschall GS. Invasive Haemophilus influenza type b infection in a child with familial deficiency of the beta subunit of the eigth component of complement. J Pediatr. 1996;128:102–3.

Pettigrew HD, Teuber SS, Gershwin E. Clinical significance of complement deficiencies. Ann N Y Acad Sci. 2009;1173:108–23.

Pickering MC, Botto M, Taylor P. Systemic lupus erythematosus, complement deficiency, and apoptosis. Adv Immunol. 2000;76:227–324.

Platonov AE, Beloborodor VB, Gabrilovitch DI, Khabarova VV, Serebrovskaya LV. Immunological evaluation of late complement component-deficient individuals. Clin Immunol Immunopathol. 1992;64(2):98–105.

Platonov AE, Beloborodov VB, Pavlova LI, Vershinina IV, Kayhty H. Vaccination of patients deficient in a late complement component with tetravalent meningococcal capsular polysaccharide vaccine. Clin Exp Immunol. 1995;100:32–9.

Platonov AE, Beloborodov VB, Vershinina IV. Meningococcal disease in patients with late complement component deficiency: studies in the U.S.S.R. Medicine. 1993;72(6):374–92.

Platonov AE, Vershinina IV, Kuijper EJ, Borrow R, Käyhty H. Long term effects of vaccination of patients deficienct in a late complemente componente with a tetravalente meningococcal polysaccharide vaccine. Vaccine. 2003;11:4437–47.

Potter PC, Frasch CE, van der Sande WJM, Cooper RC, Patel Y, Orren A. Prophylaxis against *Neisseria meningitidis* infections and antibody responses in patients with deficiency of the sixth component of complement. J Infect Dis. 1990;161:932–7.

Ram S, Lewis LA, Rice PA. Infections of people with complement deficiencies and patients who have undergone splenectomy. Clin Microbiol Rev. 2010;23:740–80.

Rosa DD, Pasqualotto AC, de Quadros M, Prezzi SH. Deficiency of the eighth component of complement associated with recurrent meningococcal meningitis – case report and literature review. Braz J Infect Dis. 2004;8(4):328–30.

Ross SC, Densen P. Complement deficiency states and infection: epidemiology, pathogenesis and consequences of neisserial and other infections in an immune deficiency. Medicine (Baltimore). 1984;63(5):243–73.

Schejbel L, Fadnes D, Permin H, Lappegård KT, Garred P, Mollnes TE. Primary complement C5 deficiencies – molecular characterization and clinical review of two families. Immunobiology. 2013;218(10):1304–10.

Schlesinger M, Grienberg R, Levy J, Kayhty H, Levy R. Killing of meningococci by neutrophils: effect of vaccination on patients with complement deficiency. J Infect Dis. 1994;170:449–53.

Schwartz B. Chemoprophylaxis for bacterial infections: principles and application to meningococcal infections. Rev Infect Dis. 1991;13(Suppl. 2):S170–3.

Sjöholm AG, Jönsson G, Braconier JH, Sturfelt G, Truedsson L. Complement deficiency and disease: an update. Mol Immunol. 2006;43(1–2):78–85.

Skattum L, van Deuren M, van der Poll T, Truedsson L. Complement deficiency states and associated infections. Mol Immunol. 2011;48:1643–55.

Tedesco F. Component deficiencies. The eighth component. Prog Allergy. 1986;39:295–306.

Turley AJ, Gathmann B, Bangs C, Bradbury M, Seneviratne S, Gonzalez-Granado LI, et al. Spectrum and management of complement immunodeficiencies (excluding hereditary angioedema) across Europe. J Clin Immunol. 2015; https://doi.org/10.1007/s10875-015-0137-5.

Walport MJ. Inherited complemente deficiency – clues to the physiological activity of complemente in vivo. Q J Med. 1993;86:355–8.

Würzner R, Orren A, Potter P, Morgan BP, Ponard D, Späth P, Brai M, Schulze M, Happe L, Götze O. Functionally active complement proteins C6 and C7 detected in C6- or C7-deficient individuals. Clin Exp Immunol. 1991;83:430–7.

Würzner R, Orren A, Lachmann PJ. Inherited deficiencies of the terminal components of human complement. Immunodefic Rev. 1992;3:123–47.

Würzner R, Hobart MJ, Fernie BA, Mewar D, Potter PC, Orren A, Lachmann PJ. Molecular basis of subtotal complement C6 deficiency a carboxy-terminally truncated but functionally active C6. J Clin Invest. 1995;95:1877–83.

Würzner R, Witzel-Schlömp K, Tokunaga K, Fernie BA, Hobart MJ, Orren A. Reference typing report for complement componentes C6, C7 and C9 including mutations leading to deficiencies. Exp Clin Immunogenet. 1998;15:268–85.

Yoshioka K, Takemura T, Akano N, Okada M, Yagi K, Maki S, Inai S, Akita H, Koitabashi Y, Takekoshi Y. IgA nephropathy in patients with congenital C9 deficiency. Kidney Int. 1992;42(5):1253–8.

Zhu Z, Atkinson TP, Hovanky KJ, Boppana SB, Dai YL, Densen P, Go RC, Jablecki JS, Volanakis JE. High prevalence of complement component C6 deficiency among African-Americans in the South-Eastern USA. Clin Exp Immunol. 2000;119:305–10.

Calcium Channel Defects (STIM1 and ORAI1)

Christina Yee
Division of Immunology, Boston Children's Hospital & Harvard Medical School, Boston, MA, USA

Synonyms

CRAC channelopathy; ORAI1 deficiency; STIM1 deficiency

Introduction/Background

Calcium channel defects are rare syndromic immune deficiencies in which defective store-operated calcium release leads to severely impaired activation of T lymphocytes and natural killer (NK) cells. This syndrome, also known as CRAC channelopathy, results from inherited mutations in ORAI1 (ORAI Calcium

Release-Activated Calcium Modulator 1) or STIM1 (Stromal Interaction Molecule 1) and is characterized by combined immune deficiency, autoimmunity, myopathy, and ectodermal dysplasia. While affected patients may have preserved T cell numbers and proliferation studies, T cell activation and function of cytolytic effectors and regulatory T cells are severely impaired. The immune phenotype includes combined immune deficiency with recurrent bacterial and viral infections, as well as autoimmune cytopenias and viral-associated lymphoproliferation. Relatively more severe immune impairment is associated with ORAI1 deficiency, and immune dysregulation is more commonly associated with STIM1 deficiency. Other clinical features of calcium channel defects include hypohidrosis, muscular weakness, and dental enamel defects. Hematopoetic stem cell replacement is the definitive therapy for combined immune deficiency due to ORAI1 and STIM1 deficiency.

Store-Operated Calcium Entry and CRAC Channels

The transmembrane calcium channel proteins ORAI1 and STIM1 are part of the family of CRACs (Ca^{2+} release activated channels) required for lymphocyte activation and immune defense (reviewed in Lacruz and Feske (2015)). Activation of lymphocytes and natural killer cells (NK) through cell surface receptors such as the T cell receptor (TCR), NK receptors, or G-coupled protein receptors results in tyrosine kinase and G-protein activation in the receptor complexes, which then triggers a complex system of second messenger signaling (Fig. 1). Phospholipase C (PLC) produces inositol 1,4,5-triphosphase (IP3), which in turn binds its receptor on the ER (endoplasmic reticulum) membrane. IP3 binding triggers the process of Store-Operated Calcium Release (SOCE). Intracellular Ca^{2+} stores are released from the ER, causing depletion of Ca^{2+} from the ER. STIM1 and other sensors recognize the drop in ER calcium, and in turn, signal for the entry of extracellular calcium across the plasma membrane via store-mediated CRAC channels such as ORAI1, ORAI2, and ORAI3. Ca^{2+} influx

into the cell activates calcineurin to dephosphorylate NFAT-family transcription factors. Dephosphorylated NFAT proteins are then imported from the cytoplasm to the nucleus, where the activated NFAT proteins bind to transcription complexes at NFAT-specific promoters, resulting in cytokine secretion and proliferative responses key to lymphocyte and NK cell activation.

ORAI1

ORAI1 (also known as CRACM2 or TMEM142a) is a transmembrane protein required for CRAC-mediated entry of Ca^{2+} ions across the plasma membrane (Feske et al. 2006). Under resting conditions, ORAI1 exists predominantly as a dimer in the plasma membrane. During store-operated calcium entry, in response to release of calcium from the ER, ORAI1 organizes into tetramers and acts as the pore-forming subunit of the CRACs, through which extracellular calcium ions enter the cell to activate NFAT translocation to the nucleus, and thereby trigger lymphocyte activation. ORAI1 is widely expressed in many cell types but has nonredundant activation function in T lymphocytes, natural killer cells, skeletal muscle, and ectodermal cells.

STIM1

Like ORAI1, STIM1 is a transmembrane protein required for store-operated calcium channel function. The role of STIM1 differs from that of ORAI1. STIM1 acts as a sensor of calcium release from the endoplasmic reticulum and as an activator of CRAC channel function in the plasma membrane, through its binding to ORAI1. STIM1 is expressed primarily in the ER membrane rather than the plasma membrane. After cell surface receptor signaling activates Ca^{2+} release from the ER, the drop in Ca^{2+} levels inside the ER triggers a conformational change in STIM1. The activated STIM1 forms multimers which migrate to the ER-plasma membrane junctions. Accumulated STIM1 collects in complexes (puncta) at these junctions, which then recruit ORAI1 to the complexes to activate CRAC function and Ca^{2+} entry across the plasma membrane.

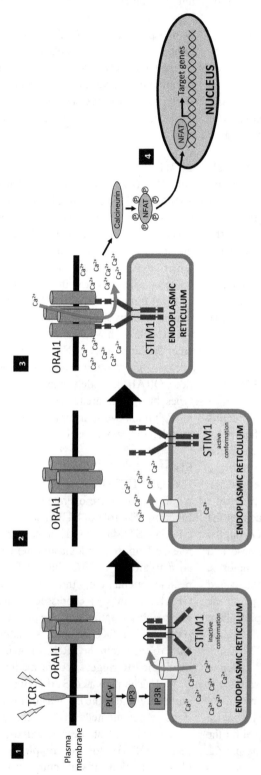

Calcium Channel Defects (STIM1 and ORAI1), Fig. 1 Lymphocyte activation through the T-cell receptor requires ORAI1 and STIM1 for store-operated calcium entry. (1) ORAI1 is located in the plasma membrane and STIM1 is found in the endoplasmic reticulum (ER) membrane. Stimulation of the T-cell receptor (TCR) triggers tyrosine kinase activation at the TCR complex, which produces an activation cascade in which activated phospholipase C (PLC) produces inositol 1,4,5-triphosphase (IP3), which in turn binds its receptor (IP3R) on the ER membrane. IP3 binding triggers the process of store-operated calcium release (SOCE) of intracellular Ca^{2+} store from the ER. (2) Depletion of Ca^{2+} from the ER results in a conformational change of STIM1 into the active form. (3) Activated STIM1 translocates to the ER-plasma membrane junctions, where active oligomers of STIM1 interact with cytoplasmic domain of ORAI1 and activate its CRAC function. Extracellular calcium crosses the plasma membrane through the activated calcium channel. (4) The influx of Ca^{2+} ions into the cell activates calmodulin and calcineurin to dephosphorylate transcription factors from the NFAT (nuclear factor of activated T cells) family. Dephosphorylated NFAT proteins then translocate from the cytoplasm into the nucleus, where activated NFAT proteins bind to transcription complexes at NFAT-specific promoters. The resulting transcriptional activation leads to cytokine secretion and proliferative responses, which are key to T lymphocyte activation

ORAI1 and STIM1 Deficiency

Combined immune deficiency with features of autoimmunity has been described in several kindreds due to homozygous or compound heterozygous mutations in ORAI1 and STIM1 (reviewed in Lacruz and Feske (2015)). Influx of Ca^{2+} into cells through CRAC channels is severely impaired due to frameshift, splice site, or missense mutations which result in loss of protein expression, or function of either ORAI1 or STIM1, or from impaired ORAI1-STIM1 interaction. Loss of NFAT-dependent transcriptional activation downstream of store-operated calcium entry leads to severely impaired T lymphocyte activation, with decreased cytokine production and proliferation. The defect of CRAC calcium channel function also results in decreased cytotoxic T cell effector activity and NK cell cytotoxicity. Decreased numbers and function of regulatory T cells (Treg) may also lead to immune dysregulation and autoimmunity (Lian et al. 2017). Variable platelet dysfunction has also been reported.

Clinical Presentation

Human patients with deficiency of ORAI1 or STIM1 present with a syndrome of combined immune deficiency, myopathy, and ectodermal dysplasia (reviewed in Lacruz and Feske (2015)). Inheritance of CRAC channelopathy is autosomal recessive. Affected patients typically present early in life with severe, recurrent bacterial, viral, and fungal infections. Autoimmune cytopenias, lymphoproliferation, and chronic diarrhea or colitis are also common. Affected patients typically have failure to thrive, developmental delay, and hypotonia. Ectodermal dysplasia is commonly associated and may manifests as impaired sweating (anhydrosis), dental enamel maturation defects (dentogenesis imperfecta), nail dysplasia, and (in STIM1 deficiency) iris hypoplasia. Due to the combination of congenital muscular weakness and impaired immune responses, pneumonia and interstitial lung disease are frequent, and sepsis with bacterial pathogens may occur. Inability to control viral infections may lead to persistent viremia or viral-driven lymphoproliferative disease.

ORAI1 Deficiency

Patients with autosomal recessive mutations in ORAI1 have all presented with severe combined immune deficiency (as first detailed in Feske et al. (2006) and reviewed in Lacruz and Feske (2015)). Recurrent sinopulmonary infections are common in ORAI1-deficient patients, with *Chlamydia pneumoniae* and *Streptococus pneumoniae* pneumonia reported as well as persistent cytomegalovirus (CMV) pneumonitis. Patients with ORAI1 deficiency frequently have difficulty controlling viral infections including *Pneumocystis jiroveci*, respiratory syncytial virus, parainfluenza virus type-3, and adenovirus, as well as chronic CMV. Bacterial and viral sepsis, urinary tract infections including pyelonephritis, and neurologic infections (meningitis and encephalitis) have also been reported, as well as chronic diarrhea due to persistent rotavirus infection and mucocutaneous candidiasis. Patients may fail to develop effective primary response to vaccine-strain *mycobacterium tuberculosis* (BCG), with absent PPD testing after vaccination and BCG-itis. Some patients have also been vulnerable to opportunistic pathogens such as Toxoplasma and scabies.

ORAI1-deficient patients may also have autoimmunity and immune dysregulation, though usually not to the degree seen in STIM1-deficient patients. Autoimmune hemolytic anemia (Coombs' positive), neutropenia, and thrombocytopenia with GI bleeding have been reported as well as antiphospholipid syndrome. Lymphadenopathy, hepatosplenomegaly, and posttransplant EBV-associated lymphoproliferative disease may occur, though not as universally as in STIM1 deficiency. Hemophagocytic lymphohistiocytosis in the setting of persistent CMV viremia has been described in a patient with ORAI1 deficiency (Klemann et al. 2017).

Loss of ORAI1 calcium channel function in other cell types also results in extra-immune manifestations. Muscular hypotonia (weakness) and anhydrosis (diminished sweating) have been noted or suspected in all ORAI1-deficient patients reported to date, with atrophy of type II fibers documented in one patient. Facial dysmorphism and small thymus has also been reported.

STIM1 Deficiency

Patients with autosomal recessive STIM1 defects share a similar phenotype of severe viral, bacterial, and fungal infections, as well as autoimmunity due to impaired immune regulation and extra-immune features of myopathy and ectodermal defects (as first described in Picard et al. (2009) and reviewed in Lacruz and Feske (2015)). Frameshift, splice site mutations and missense mutations have been reported to result in decreased STIM1 protein expression and/or loss of function. Generally, STIM1-deficient patients have presented with less severe combined immune deficiency and more prevalent autoimmunity, in comparison to ORAI1-deficient patients.

Recurrent sepsis, otitis, pneumonia, and dental infections have been reported with *Chlamydiae pneumoniae*, *Streptococcus pneumoniae*, and *Escherichia coli* observed as frequent bacterial pathogens. STIM1-deficient patients have also susceptibility to viral infections including enterovirus and herpesviruses including CMV, EBV, VZV, HSV, and HHV8. Inability to control CMV may lead to persistent CMV viremia or pneumonitis.

STIM1-deficient patients commonly have impaired immune regulation. Most STIM1-deficiency patients described have been reported to have had some form of autoimmune cytopenia such as AIHA or ITP which may result in splenomegaly, hepatomegaly, or lymphadenopathy. Patients may also present with eczema, chronic diarrhea, arthritis, or colitis. EBV-associated lymphoproliferation and HHV6-associated Karposi's sarcoma have been reported in STIM1-deficient patients, which may result from a combination of impaired inability to control viral infections with abnormal immune regulation.

Extra-immune features of STIM1 mutation are similar to those found in ORAI1 deficiency, including myopathy, anhidrosis, and dental enamel defects. Iris hypoplasia has been specifically found in STIM1 deficiency, though mydriasis (dilation of the pupil of the eye) was also reported in at least patient with an ORAI1 mutation (Lian et al. 2017). Clinical presentation may be variable; a subset of patients with decreased STIM1 protein and abnormal SOCE have been reported to have hypohidrosis and variable autoimmunity, with abnormal NK cell and T-lymphocyte function in vitro, but no recurrent infections or clinical immunodeficiency (Parry et al. 2016).

Gain of Function in ORAI1 and STIM1

Gain of function mutations in ORAI1 or STIM1 are not known to be associated with clinical immune deficiency (reviewed in Lacruz and Feske (2015)). Constitutive activation, increased SOCE, and impaired CRAC deactivation are instead associated with Stormoken-like syndrome, an autosomal dominant syndrome with thrombocytopenia and tubular aggregate myopathy. Clinical presentation of affected patients includes bleeding, muscle weakness, and pupilary miosis.

Diagnosis and Laboratory Testing

Combined immune deficiency associated with ORAI1 and STIM1 presents with preserved lymphocyte differentiation, but impaired activation. The absolute lymphocyte count and numbers of $CD4^+$ and $CD8^+$ T cells, NK cells, and B cells may be normal or slightly reduced. On functional testing, proliferative responses to mitogen and antigen stimulation are typically low but may be normal in some patients. Immunoglobulin levels may be normal, elevated, or slightly low, but specific antibody titers to vaccines are typically low. Some patients have been reported to have some level of residual T cell function and may intermittently have normal proliferation in vitro.

In addition, ORAI1-deficient patients have been reported to have impaired cytokine production, reduced numbers of invariant natural killer T and regulatory T cells (Tregs), and altered composition of $\gamma\delta$ T-cell and natural killer cell subsets (Lian et al. 2017). Absent iNKT (invariant NKT cells) and low MAIT (mucosal invariant T cells) have also been reported, as well as elevated soluble IL2 receptor α (CD25) (Klemann et al. 2017).

NK cell and effector T cell assays measuring cytotoxic function may show decreased effector degranulation or cell killing in vitro.

Research investigations have identified abnormal membrane potentials and calcium flux in ORAI1 and STIM1-deficient patients. In cases of suspected calcium-channel defects, confirmatory testing may require genetic testing based on clinical suspicion.

Treatment

The combined immune deficiency associated with ORAI1 or STIM1 deficiency results in recurrent and prolonged infections which greatly decrease life expectancy. Autoimmune conditions also contribute to the poor clinical prognosis.

Supportive treatment includes supplemental immunoglobulin, anti-microbial prophylaxis, and specific treatment for bacterial, viral, and fungal infections. Recombinant interleukin 2 (IL-2) has also been used in at least one case. For autoimmune cytopenias and EBV-associated lymphoproliferation, immune modulation with rituximab has been used in one patient. Supportive therapy is incompletely effective in controlling bacterial and viral infections and autoimmune disease in patients with calcium channel defects. While some patients with hypomorphic mutations may retain enough residual immune function to survive to early adulthood, few patients with calcium channel defects survive past the first decade of life. Definitive treatment with hematopoietic stem cell transplant (HSCT) has been successful in some cases but does not reverse extra-immune manifestations such as hypotonia or myopathy, which may adversely affect HSCT outcomes. Early identification may help prevent the development of uncontrolled infections, and thereby improve the likelihood of successful HSCT.

References

Feske S, et al. A mutation in Orai1 causes immune deficiency by abrogating CRAC channel function. Nature. 2006;441:179–85. https://doi.org/10.1038/nature04702.

Klemann C, et al. Hemophagocytic lymphohistiocytosis as presenting manifestation of profound combined immunodeficiency due to an ORAI1 mutation. J Allergy Clin Immunol. 2017;140:1721–4. https://doi.org/10.1016/j.jaci.2017.05.039.

Lacruz RS, Feske S. Diseases caused by mutations in ORAI1 and STIM1. Ann N Y Acad Sci. 2015;1356:45–79. https://doi.org/10.1111/nyas.12938.

Lian J, et al. ORAI1 mutations abolishing store-operated ca (2+) entry cause anhidrotic ectodermal dysplasia with immunodeficiency. J Allergy Clin Immunol. 2017; https://doi.org/10.1016/j.jaci.2017.10.031.

Parry DA, et al. A homozygous STIM1 mutation impairs store-operated calcium entry and natural killer cell effector function without clinical immunodeficiency. J Allergy Clin Immunol. 2016;137:955–957 e958. https://doi.org/10.1016/j.jaci.2015.08.051.

Picard C, et al. STIM1 mutation associated with a syndrome of immunodeficiency and autoimmunity. N Engl J Med. 2009;360:1971–80. https://doi.org/10.1056/NEJMoa0900082.

CAMPS

▶ CARD14-Mediated Psoriasis and Pityriasis Rubra Piliaris (PRP)

Candidiasis Familial 5 (CANDF5)

▶ Chronic Mucocutaneous Candidiasis: IL-17RA Deficiency

Candidiasis Familial 6 (CANDF6)

▶ Chronic Mucocutaneous Candidiasis, IL-17F Deficiency

Candidiasis Familial 7 (CANDF7)

▶ Chronic Mucocutaneous Candidiasis, STAT1 Gain of Function

CAP1

► TRAF3 Deficiency

CARD Containing Molecule Enhancing NF-kB

► B Cell Lymphoma/Leukemia 10 Deficiency

CARD12

► NLRC4-Associated Autoinflammatory Diseases

CARD14

► CARD14-Mediated Psoriasis and Pityriasis Rubra Piliaris (PRP)

CARD14-Mediated Psoriasis and Pityriasis Rubra Piliaris (PRP)

Michelle A. Lowes[1] and Anne M. Bowcock[2]
[1]The Rockefeller University, New York, NY, USA
[2]Icahn School of Medicine at Mount Sinai, New York, NY, USA

Synonyms

CARD14: Caspase recruitment domain-containing protein 14
CARMA2: CARD-containing membrane-associated guanylate kinase (MAGUK) protein 2
Bimp2: bcl10-interacting maguk protein 2
CAMPS: CARD14 mediated psoriasis
PRP: Pityriasis rubra pilaris

Michelle A. Lowes and Anne M. Bowcock equally contributed to this work.

Definition

CARD14 is an important cutaneous scaffold protein. Gain of function mutations in CARD14 lead to enhanced or sustained NF-kB activation, and up-regulation of its target genes which include pro-inflammatory cytokines. The consequence of these and downstream transcriptional alterations are seen clinically as psoriasis or pityriasis rubra pilaris (PRP).

Introduction and Background

Discovery of Disease-Causing CARD14 Mutations

Psoriasis susceptibility locus 2 (PSORS2) was mapped in 1994 to human chromosomal region 17q25-qter in a single large European family (PS1) (Tomfohrde et al. 1994). Affected members had plaque psoriasis and 30% also developed psoriatic arthritis. A second genome-wide linkage scan in a five-generation Taiwanese family further implicated PSORS2 as the site of a genetic locus that could explain some psoriasis inheritance.

In 2012, mutations in the gene caspase recruitment domain family, member 14 (CARD14), were identified as being responsible for the PSORS2 locus (Jordan et al. 2012a, b). Targeted and exome capture followed by NextGen sequencing of DNA from members of family PS1 identified a mutation in CARD14 that segregated with psoriasis (c.349G > A; p.Gly117Ser). A second CARD14 mutation at the same splice donor site was discovered in the Taiwanese family (c.349 + 5G > A). These rare pathogenic variants, explained the highly penetrant autosomal dominant inheritance of psoriasis vulgaris in these families. A de novo mutation in CARD14 was discovered in a Haitian child with sporadic, severe, generalized pustular psoriasis (c.413A > C; p.Glu138Ala). CARD14 mutations were subsequently discovered as responsible for causing pityriasis rubra pilaris (PRP), another inflammatory skin disease, in four unrelated families (Fuchs-Telem et al. 2012). Although most clinicians consider PRP and psoriasis distinct diseases, mutations in the same gene in both conditions point to shared pathogenesis.

There have now been numerous studies of these rare CARD14 mutations in patients with psoriasis (sometimes termed CARD14 mediated psoriasis, CAMPS), psoriatic arthritis, and, pityriasis rubra pilaris (Fuchs-Telem et al. 2012; Jordan et al. 2012a, b; Van Nuffel et al. 2017). In a large cohort of 6000 psoriasis patients and 4000 controls, 15 additional rare missense variants within CARD14 were identified. Each of these variants, and the familial p.G117S mutation, is rare and found in less than one in 1000 psoriasis cases. However, a common single nucleotide polymorphism in CARD14 (R820W) originally identified by Jordan et al. exceeded genome-wide significance for association with psoriasis in a large meta-genome wide association study. In this instance, the W allele confers psoriasis risk and is seen in approximately 0.56 cases versus 0.52 controls. In the case of PRP patients, with CARD14

mutations are usually familial or de-novo and include early onset, prominent facial involvement, and favorable responses to ustekinumab therapy.

Functions of CARD14 in Healthy Tissues

CARD14 is a member of the CARD-containing membrane-associated guanylate kinase (MAGUK) protein (CARMA) family of scaffolding proteins. CARD14 proteins were initially detected in the skin, thymus, aorta, and placenta. Wild-type full length CARD14 (CARD14*fl*) is a protein of 1004 amino acids consisting of an N-terminal CARD domain, followed by a coiled coil (CC) region, a linker region (LR), and a membrane-associated guanylate kinase (MAGUK) subunit composed of PDZ, SH3, and GUK subdomains (Fig. 1). The CARD14 gene also gives rise to several other splice variants, which encode a shorter CARD14 protein (CARD14*sh*) that is the most abundant in skin and consists of the CARD and CC domains, but lacks the MAGUK

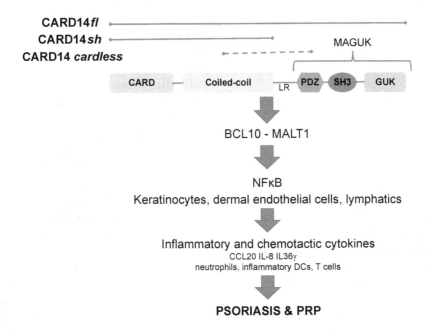

CARD14-Mediated Psoriasis and Pityriasis Rubra Piliaris (PRP), Fig. 1 Schematic diagram of caspase recruitment domain family, member 14 (CARD14) activation and pathogenic pathways for psoriasis and pityriasis rubra pilaris (PRP). CARD14 is located on chromosome 17q25.3. CARD14*fl* is the full length isoform 1. CARD14*sh* is the most abundant isoform in skin and consists of CARD and coiled-coil domains but lacks the

MAGUK domain. Assembly of CARD14- BCL10-MALT1 (CBM) complex activates NF-kB-dependent immune responses, by both CARD14*fl* and CARD14*sh* isoforms (but not CARD14*cardless*). Many CARD14 variants have been discovered along the length of the gene, which can amplify NF-kB responses leading to cutaneous diseases such as psoriasis and pityriasis rubra pilaris (PRP) domain, and a CARD14*cardless* protein that lacks the CARD domain, some of the CC domain, and the SH3 and GUK domains.

CARD proteins form intracellular scaffolds that are important in cellular activation (Van Nuffel et al. 2017). The primary function of CARD14*fl* and CARD14*sh* is to activate the transcription factor nuclear factor-kappa B (NF-kB) (Fig. 1). After an appropriate stimulus, wild-type CARD14 assembles with adapter protein B-cell lymphoma 10 (BCL10) and recruits paracaspase MALT1 to form a CARD11/BCL10/MALT1 (CBM) signaling complex (Fig. 1). This CBM complex can activate NF-kB leading to expression of proinflammatory cytokines and chemokines. CARD14 isoforms may also play a role in epidermal differentiation where CARD14*cardless* might function as a dominant-negative regulator of CARD14 signaling.

Effects of CARD14 Variants in Inflammatory Skin Disease

In vitro studies utilizing the mutated CARD14 variants indicated that one consequence of the c.349G > A mutation found in the northern European PS1 psoriasis family, and c.349 + 5G > A mutation from the Taiwanese family with psoriasis, is an in-frame insertion of 22 amino acids between exon 3 and 4 of the CARD14 protein (Jordan et al. 2012a, b). Most other CARD14 mutations lead to single amino acid substitutions.

CARD14 mutations found in psoriasis and pityriasis rubra pilaris are gain-of-function mutations, leading to amplified NF-kB responses and cutaneous inflammation (Howes et al. 2016). Cultured keratinocytes from affected individuals with psoriasis containing CARD14 mutations, as well as keratinocyte cell lines transfected with mutant CARD14, show increased psoriasis-associated cytokine transcription compared to wild-type keratinocytes, such as CXCL8 (IL-8), CCL20, and IL36γ (Jordan et al. 2012b). Van Nuffel and colleagues have listed all published CARD14 variants identified in patients with psoriasis and pityriasis rubra pilaris, located by exon and CARD

domain, as well as their effect on NF-kB activation (Van Nuffel et al. 2017).

Possible additional pathogenic signaling pathways of the CARD14 variants include direct stimulation of MALT1 paracaspase activity and activation of ERK1/2 and p38α MAP kinases (Howes et al. 2016; Van Nuffel et al. 2017). The molecular mechanism leading to CARD14 activation is similar to that identified for mutations in CARD11 that lead to diffuse large B cell lymphoma. The CARD14 linker region between the CC and PDZ domains exerts an auto-inhibitory effect due to its conformation and this is abolished in the presence of psoriasis-associated CARD14 mutations. This leads to enhanced, sustained, or constitutive levels of NF-kB activation following IkB proteosomal degradation to release NF-kB for nuclear translocation (Howes et al. 2016).

In skin biopsies from patients with familial psoriasis (PS1) and CARD14 mutations, the histological appearance is of typical psoriasis, with acanthosis (thickened epidermis), parakeratosis, dilated blood vessels, and abundant mixed inflammatory cell infiltrate. Similarly, histology of skin biopsies from patients with pityriasis rubra pilaris and CARD14 mutations is that of typical pityriasis rubra pilaris, with alternating orthokeratosis and parakeratosis, acanthosis with broadening of rete ridges, follicular plugging, and dermal lymphocytic infiltrate (Fuchs-Telem et al. 2012). However, in both psoriasis and pityriasis rubra pilaris associated with CARD14 mutations, there is less CARD14 expression in basal keratinocytes, with abundant CARD14 expression throughout the upper epidermis (Fuchs-Telem et al. 2012; Jordan et al. 2012b). CARD14 is also found in psoriatic lesional and nonlesional dermal CD31[+] endothelial cells and LYVE-1[+] lymphatics (Harden et al. 2014). Phosphorylated NF-kB colocalizes in CARD14[+] dermal endothelial cells, indicating that this pathway is active in these cells (Harden et al. 2014). Aortic endothelial cells also express CARD14 protein (Harden et al. 2014), suggesting a possible contribution of CARD14 in the cardiovascular comorbidity associated with psoriasis.

In summary, CARD14 mutations appear to augment immune responses to drive persistent cutaneous inflammation through NF-kB activation. It is not yet clear how the CARD14 mutations result in distinct clinical phenotypes such as psoriasis versus pityriasis rubra pilaris.

Clinical Presentation (History/PE)

CARD14 mutations have been described in patients with psoriasis vulgaris (the most typical presentation of psoriasis), generalized pustular psoriasis, psoriatic arthritis, palmoplantar pustulosis, and pityriasis rubra pilaris. Patients with CARD14 mutations cannot yet be easily distinguished clinically or histologically from those without CARD14 mutations.

The most common clinical presentation of psoriasis associated with CARD14 mutations is psoriasis vulgaris, which is classical large plaque psoriasis. Presentation involves well-demarcated erythematous scaly plaques usually on the extensor surfaces such as elbows and knees. Generalized pustular psoriasis can also be the presentation of CARD14 mutations, with small pustules on a widespread erythematous background. Joint symptoms associated with CARD14 mutations (seen in 30% of PS1 family members) are usually that of typical psoriatic arthritis.

Pityriasis rubra pilaris is described as follicular papules and salmon-pink erythematous plaques, with characteristic normal skin adjacent to these plaques called "islands of sparing," and often present on palms and soles as keratoderma. Type V pityriasis rubra pilaris, which is "atypical juvenile type," appears to be most commonly associated with CARD14 mutations. This type of pityriasis rubra pilaris has onset in infancy or early childhood with a chronic course.

Laboratory Findings/Diagnostic Testing

At the current time, clinicians are not able to routinely test patients with psoriasis or pityriasis rubra pilaris for CARD14 mutations.

Treatment/Prognosis

Specific recommendations for treatment options or prognosis are not yet available for patients with CARD14 mutations. The therapeutic approach includes traditional medications prescribed for moderate-to-severe psoriasis or pityriasis rubra pilaris. This can be effective in the case of psoriasis due to some CARD14 alterations, such as the p.G117S change. However, there is an impression that some patients with severe psoriasis due to CARD14 mutations, such as the p.E138A change, are more refractory to treatment and may require biologics such as anti-IL-12/23 and anti-IL-17 monoclonal antibodies. There have also been reports of anti-IL-12/23 and anti-TNF agents to treat familial pityriasis rubra pilaris (Fuchs-Telem et al. 2012; Eytan et al. 2014). Prospective studies are required to understand the clinical significance and potential therapeutic options for patients who harbor CARD14 mutations.

References

Eytan O, et al. Clinical response to us tekinumab in familial pityriasis rubra pilaris caused by a novel mutation in CARD14. Br J Dermatol. 2014;171(2): 420–2.

Fuchs-Telem D, et al. Familial pityriasis rubra pilaris is caused by mutations in CARD14. Am J Hum Genet. 2012;91(1):163–70.

Harden JL, et al. CARD14 expression in dermal endothelial cells in psoriasis. PLoS One. 2014;9(11):e111255.

Howes A, et al. Psoriasis mutations disrupt CARD14 autoinhibition promoting BCL10-MALT1-dependent NF-kappaB activation. Biochem J. 2016;473(12): 1759–68.

Jordan CT, et al. Rare and common variants in CARD14, encoding an epidermal regulator of NF-kappaB, in psoriasis. Am J Hum Genet. 2012a; 90(5):796–808.

Jordan CT, et al. PSORS2 is due to mutations in CARD14. Am J Hum Genet. 2012b;90(5):784–95.

Tomfohrde J, et al. Gene for familial psoriasis susceptibility mapped to the distal end of human chromosome 17q. Science. 1994;264(5162):1141–5.

Van Nuffel E, et al. CARD14-mediated activation of paracaspase MALT1 in keratinocytes: implications for psoriasis. J Invest Dermatol. 2017;137(3):569–75.

CARD9 Deficiency

Christina Gavino[1], Marija Landekic[1] and
Donald C. Vinh[2,3,4]
[1]Research Institute-MUHC (RI-MUHC),
Montréal, QC, Canada
[2]Infectious Disease Susceptibility Program,
McGill University Health Centre (MUHC) and
Research Institute-MUHC (RI-MUHC),
Montréal, QC, Canada
[3]Department of Medicine, Division of Infectious
Diseases & Medical Microbiology, McGill
University Health Centre, Montréal, QC,
Canada
[4]Department of Human Genetics, McGill
University, Montréal, QC, Canada

Introduction

Despite an estimated 1.5 million species of fungi, ubiquitous in distribution resulting in constant exposure, few cause human disease. Those that do reflect a defect of immunity, either inherent or acquired. Although the taxonomy of fungi and the field of medical mycology are relatively young compared to other fields of microbiology, historical reports of fungi causing nail, hair, and superficial skin infections, as well as invasive disease, can be traced back to the mid-nineteenth century, prior to the advent of advanced therapeutics accounting for modern-day iatrogenic mycoses. Further, rather than causing true epidemics like bacteria and parasites, fungi were recognized to typically cause "sporadic" disease, that is, affecting select individuals, families, or races. The study of primary immunodeficiencies (PID) has led to the identification of critical genes that account, at least in part, for this inherent basis for susceptibility.

Spontaneously occurring fungal disease is increasingly recognized as a manifestation of an underlying primary immunodeficiency (PID); further, distinct PIDs are associated with a characteristic spectrum of fungal pathogens (Vinh 2011). Fungal disease has long been categorized as being either primarily superficial (i.e., involving mucosal and/or cutaneous membranes) or invasive. Chronic mucocutaneous candidiasis (CMC) is a superficial, recurrent/recalcitrant infection due to *Candida* sp. (discussed in greater detail in chapter 9). Invasive fungal diseases (IFDs) associated with PID have previously been defined within the context of susceptibility to a broader range of microbial pathogens. For example, chronic granulomatous disease (CGD), which results from defects in the phagocyte NADPH oxidase complex, is associated with increased susceptibility not only to select bacteria but also to *Aspergillus* spp. and other hyaline filamentous fungi (Cohen et al. 1981; Winkelstein et al. 2000; Segal et al. 1998; Roilides et al. 1999; Jabado et al. 1998). Likewise, Mendelian susceptibility to mycobacterial disease (MSMD), due to defects in the interleukin (IL)-12/−23/Interferon-γ axis, predisposes not only to infections with mycobacteria and *Salmonella* sp. (Bustamante et al. 2014), but also to thermally dimorphic endemic mycoses (e.g., *Coccidiodes* sp.; *Paracoccidioides*; *Histoplasma* sp.) (Vinh et al. 2009, 2011; Sampaio et al. 2013; Moraes-Vasconcelos et al. 2005; Zerbe and Holland 2005). In contrast to these, deficiency of caspase recruitment domain-containing protein 9 (CARD9) is a recently described PID with a susceptibility that, for now, seems distinctly restricted to fungi.

Clinical Features

The central feature of CARD9 deficiency is increased susceptibility to the following fungi: *Candida*; dermatophytes; and pheohyphomycetes. Interestingly, these fungi share the common features of being pleomorphic with the natural capacity for indolent hyphal invasion into cutaneous or subcutaneous layers to produce chronic infection.

Candida

The genus *Candida* is characterized by yeast-like cells that reproduce by budding. Depending on the species, pseudohyphae and true hyphae may develop in vivo, under growth conditions routinely employed in the medical mycology diagnostic laboratory and/or under specialized conditions used in research. CARD9 deficiency is associated with two forms of candidiasis: CMC and invasive candidiasis (IC).

In the seminal discovery that recessive mutations in *CARD9* cause susceptibility to candidiasis (candidiasis familial 2, CANDF2; OMIM# 212050), four members from a single Iranian pedigree with intermittent episodes of mucocutaneous candidiasis only (oral, vaginal, and/or angular cheilitis) were found to be homozygous for a nonsense mutation (Glocker et al. 2009). Since then, a total of 38 patients with CARD9 deficiency have been reported; of these, CMC occurred in 15 (39.5%) (Lanternier et al. 2015a). Thus, it appears that a loss of CARD9 function predisposes to CMC, but apparently with variable penetrance and/or severity.

In contrast to its original association with CMC, a distinctive phenotype of CARD9 deficiency that has emerged is IC. In the original Iranian pedigree, it should be noted that three family members had previously died with anecdotal evidence of candidal infection of the central nervous system (Glocker et al. 2009): Patient 2B1 died of "candida meningitis" at the age of 19 years; Patient 5G1 died of a brain tumor with skull destruction at age 15 years; Patient 5G2 developed headache and diplopia and was suspected of having a brain tumor, but in fact, was found to have "candida meningoencephalitis" and died at age 15 years. None of these individuals had reported histopathologic or microbiologic data to corroborate the clinical diagnosis of invasive fungal disease. Understandably, none could be genetically sequenced to confirm CARD9 deficiency, although it may be reasonable to presume they were. These three cases, while incomplete, nonetheless provided an important signal that the salient phenotype of CARD9 deficiency actually extended beyond superficial candidiasis, to cause invasive disease.

Of the invasive forms of candidiasis associated with CARD9 deficiency, the most striking and consistent manifestation is that of involvement of the central nervous system (CNS), either brain parenchyma, meninges, and/or eye, in the absence of trauma (including iatrogenic bases, such as catheters, shunts, and surgeries), chemotherapeutic immunosuppression, or underlying systemic disease, which we have termed "spontaneous central nervous system candidiasis" (sCNSc) (Gavino et al. 2014). Table 1 summarizes the current published reports of sCNSc in which recessive mutations in *CARD9* have been identified or presumed by pedigree analysis. Based on available microbiologic data, the primary pathogen was *Candida albicans* (12 of 18; 67%). In one case, the phylogenetically related *C. dubliniensis* was isolated (Drewniak et al. 2013). Another patient had a history of sCNSc with *Candida* sp. (no species provided), including relapse with sino-orbital invasion (again without speciation), but subsequently developed colitis with isolation of *C. glabrata* from colonic biopsy (Lanternier et al. 2015a); thus, it is unclear if the sCNSc was caused by the same species or not. Altogether, *C. albicans* appears to be the primary cause of sCNSc due to CARD9 deficiency. Intriguingly, despite CARD9 deficiency being an inborn error of innate immunity, and despite epidemiologic surveillance data demonstrating that humans are typically colonized with *C. albicans* very early in life (e.g., ~50% before 1 year of age) (Marks et al. 1975), the age of onset that sCNSc clinically manifested was in young adulthood (mean: 21.8; median 21.5). From the reported symptomatic cases, there appears to be a female preponderance (M:F = 5:11). The presenting symptoms have been variable and related to the CNS location involved. Cerebrospinal fluid (CSF) analysis has revealed the following pattern: a mononuclear cell predominance (i.e., lymphocytes and/or mononuclear cells), with a distinct relative eosinophilic pleocytosis in multiple cases; absence of neutrophilic pleocytosis in most cases; increased protein concentration; and hypoglycorrhachia. On CNS imaging, best characterized by magnetic resonance imaging (Bertin et al. 2000), the appearance of brain abscesses has been variable, ranging from a solitary mass, to cystic lesions, to multiple nodules; in some of the cases, these have been radiologically misinterpreted as brain malignancies, but from which histopathology revealed inflammatory mass lesions with no malignancy, identified fungal elements, and complemented by microbiologic isolation of the yeast. The masses have been contrast-enhancing and surrounded by

CARD9 Deficiency, Table 1 CARD9 deficiency and sCNSc

Reference	Age of clinical disease onset/gender	Bi-allelic mutations[a]	Salient fungal disease	Features of CNS disease	Other clinical features	Outcome
Glocker et al. (2009)	18 years old/F (Iranian)	Presumed (by genetic sequencing of other family members): c.883C>T (p. Q295X)	Presumed candida meningitis	*Clinical:* seizures, loss of consciousness, complicated by hydrocephalus; *CSF:* NR; *Imaging:* NR	Intermittent thrush (since early childhood)	Deceased
	13 years old/F (Iranian)	Presumed (by genetic sequencing of other family members): c.883C>T (p. Q295X)	Presumed candida brain abscess	*Clinical:* unilateral paresthesis; *CSF:* NR; *Imaging:* NR	Ventricular septal defect (infancy); geographic tongue (presumed chronic candidiasis)	Deceased (from a brain tumor with severe skull destruction) at age 15
	15 years old/F (Iranian)	Presumed (by genetic sequencing of other family members): c.883C>T (p. Q295X)	Presumed candida meningo-encephalitis	*Clinical:* severe headache, fever, diplopia, suspected to be brain tumor; *CSF:* NR; *Imaging:* NR	Recurrent thrush (since early childhood)	Deceased 6 months later
Drewniak et al. (2013)	7 years old/F (Asian)	c.214G>A (p. G72S); c.1118G>C (p.R373P)	Recurrent *C. dubliniensis* meningo-encephalitis	*Clinical:* fevers, headaches, behavioral changes, seizures; *CSF:* eosinophilic pleocytosis; increased protein; decreased glucose; *Imaging:* infarction of left striatum; meningeal enhancement; mild ventricular dilatation	NR	Discontinuation of antifungals associated with clinical relapse
Gavino et al. (2014)	30 years old/M (French-Canadian)	c.439T>C (p. Y91H)	Recurrent *C. albicans* meningitis and brain abscess	*Clinical:* recurrent seizures; headaches; confusion/dis-orientation; *CSF:* mononuclear pleocytosis (with 11% eosinophils); increased protein; decreased glucose; *Imaging:* left parieto-occipital mass	Occasional dermatophytosis	Discontinuation of antifungals associated with clinical relapse; Alive, on antifungal and GM-CSF therapy

Reference	Patient	Mutation	Infection	Clinical/CSF/Imaging	Other	Treatment/Outcome
Lanternier et al. (2015a)	39 years old/F (P1; Turkish)	c.208C>T (p. R70W)	*C. albicans* meningitis and brain abscess	*Clinical*: fever, headache, vomiting; altered mental state; right arm paresis; facial palsy *CSF*: lymphocytic pleocytosis (with 16% eosinophils); increased protein; decreased glucose *Imaging*: frontal lesion with mass effect and contrast enhancement; ventricular dilation	Recurrent vulvo-vaginal candidiasis (since age 36)	Induction combination antifungal therapy. Required cerebral shunt. Alive on maintenance mono-therapy
	7 years old/F (P2; Turkish)	c.208C>T (p. R70W)	Recurrent *C. albicans* meningitis and brain abscess	*Clinical*: fever for weeks, headache, vomiting *CSF*: pleocytosis (20% eosinophils) *Imaging*: several enhancing lesions, including brain medulla	Thrush *Onycho-mycosis (both since age 5)*	Relapse on antifungal therapy. Alive after re-induction (for 5 months) followed by maintenance with mono-therapy
	17 years old/M (P3; Iranian)	c.104G>A (p. R35Q)	Recurrent *C. albicans* brain abscess	*Clinical*: left hemiplegia (17 years old) due to brain abscess (confirmed Candida sp. from surgical biopsy). Fever and right ptosis (20 years old) *CSF*: NR *Imaging*: for the episode at 20 years old, found to have soft tissue opacities and calcifications in the sphenoids, ethmoids, and	Bloody diarrhea and anemia (22 years old); found to have linear ulcers and polyps in colon, from which biopsy showed invasive *C. glabrata*	Surgical resection. Alive, on maintenance antifungal therapy

(continued)

CARD9 Deficiency, Table 1 (continued)

Reference	Age of clinical disease onset/gender	Bi-allelic mutations[a]	Salient fungal disease	Features of CNS disease	Other clinical features	Outcome
	37 years old/F (P4; Moroccan)	c.865C>T (p. Q289*)	C.albicans brain abscess	left maxillary and frontal sinuses, with 2 regions of bone erosion in the median wall of the right orbit adjacent to the right orbital apex *Clinical:* severe headache, vomiting, right hemiparesis; *CSF:* NR; *Imaging:* 30 × 40 mm left tempero-parietal lesion; several contrast-enhancing peripheral nodules; peri-lesional edema with mass effect	Recurrent thrush (since age 34)	Induction combination antifungal therapy (liposomal amphotericin B and 5-fluorocytosine) for 15 days, followed by fluconazole treatment. Alive
Gavino et al. (2016)	38 M (P2) *French-Canadian*	c.439T>C (p. Y91H)	C. albicans brain abscess	*Clinical:* headaches worsening over several weeks, dysphasia, left-sided weakness. Progressing to left hemiparesis and decreasing level of consciousness over next 2 months; *CSF:* NR; *Imaging:* multiple intracranial cystic masses (thought to be glioblastoma multiforme)	Onycho-mycosis	Relapse on antifungal therapy. Alive on antifungal and GM-CSF therapy
	39 F (P3) *French-Canadian*	c.439T>C (p. Y91H)	C. albicans endophthalmitis; brain abscess; vertebral osteomyelitis	*Clinical:* painless loss of vision in left eye (endophthalmitis); *CSF:* NR; *Imaging:* right parieto-temporal lesions with mass effect. Numerous, non-enhancing lesions in the basal ganglia bilaterally	Bipolar disorder (since adolescence; no imaging). Intermittent episodes of tinea versicolor (no cultures) *Found to have L4-L5 vertebral osteomyelitis (no culture; resolved with antifungal therapy)*	Alive on maintenance mono-therapy, no relapse

	39 F (P4; twin of P3)	c.439T>C (p. Y91H)	Asymptomatic	*Clinical*: intermittent episodes of migraines *CSF*: declined *Imaging*: numerous, nonenhancing lesions in the basal ganglia bilaterally; wedge-shaped encephalomalacia in left cerebral hemisphere	Intermittent episodes of tinea versicolor and oral white plaques, presumed thrush (no cultures)	On fluconazole mono-therapy
Herbst et al. (2015)	4 years old/F (Turkish)	c.883C>T (p. Q295X)	Recurrent *C. albicans* meningitis	*Clinical*: fever for 2 days, headache, fatigue (preceding 6 months of fever) *CSF*: granulocytic pleocytosis; increased protein; decreased glucose *Imaging*: MRI revealed no inflammatory process	Recurrent thrush (since age 1.5)	Difficulty to sterilize CSF, with relapse, requiring prolonged induction combination therapy, prior to maintenance with fluconazole. Alive
Celmeli et al. (2016)	25 years old/M (Turkish)	c.883C>T (p. Q295X)	*C. albicans* meningo-encephalitis	*Clinical*: headache, vomiting *CSF*: lymphocytic pleocytosis; increased protein; decreased glucose *Imaging*: NR	Recurrent mild CMC and tinea versicolor (since age 3)	Failed induction mono-therapy with fluconazole. Required induction combination therapy. Eventually, transitioned to maintenance mono-therapy with voriconazole. After 4 months, clinical relapse, requiring combination induction therapy and G-CSF
	25 years old/M (Turkish; twin of proband)	c.883C>T (p. Q295X)	Asymptomatic	*Clinical*: none *CSF*: NR *Imaging*: NR	Episode of meningitis at age 8 (no etiology provided) Episodes of tinea versicolor and tinea corporis	Alive

(continued)

CARD9 Deficiency, Table 1 (continued)

Reference	Age of clinical disease onset/gender	Bi-allelic mutations[a]	Salient fungal disease	Features of CNS disease	Other clinical features	Outcome
Drummond et al. (2015)	9 years old/F (El Salvadorian)	c.170G>A (p. R57H)	C. albicans meningitis and brain abscess; vertebral osteomyelitis	Clinical: fever, neck and back pain, headache, vomting (age 9; 15 months after completing fluconazole mono-therapy for osteomyelitis) CSF: lymphocytic pleocytosis (with 22% eosinophils); increased protein; decreased glucose Imaging: cervical spine osteomyelitis, lepto-meningeal enhancement, syrinx, obstructive hydrocephalus, brain abscesses	Recurrent oral thrush (since birth) At age 8: fever, headache, vomiting, back pain; found to have T12–L1 vertebral osteomyelitis with diskitis and paraspinal abscess. Resolved with 6 months of fluconazole mono-therapy	Alive at age 11
Jones et al. (2016)	25 years old/F	c.1138G>C (p. A38P); c.951G>A (p.R317R)	C. albicans endophthalmitis; vertebral osteomyelitis	Clinical: R eye redness and blurred vision (panuveitis with focal inflammatory mass at the right macula). Worsening over months. CSF: NR Imaging: NR	Two years and 9 months after endophthalmitis, developed left him osteomyelitis, osteonecrosis, septic arthritis with C.albicans, requiring total hip replacement	Multiple surgeries, but loss of vision in right eye
Alves de Medeiros et al. (2016)	5 years old/M (VII:3, Turkish)	Presumed (by genetic sequencing of other family members): c.208C>T (p. R70W)	C.albicans brain abscess	Clinical: right hemiparalysis CSF: pleocytosis (59% polymorphonuclear; 41% mononuclear); decreased glucose Imaging: hypodense zone in left hemisphere; internal carotid artery aneurysm with infarctio	CMC (since age 5); chronic onychomycosis; hypoparathyroidism	Induction combination antifungal therapy, but difficult to sterilize CSF; eventual good recovery

[a]Homozygous cases are indicated by the sole mutation identified. Compound heterozygous cases are indicated with both mutations identified

edema, often with mass effect, hence explaining the presentation. There has been no singular CNS zone consistently affected. When the meninges are involved, MRI has revealed leptomeningeal enhancement.

Interestingly, there have been two key reports in which there has been a set of twins bearing genetically identical *CARD9* alleles to the proband, but who were asymptomatic clinically (Gavino et al. 2016; Celmeli et al. 2016). In one, no further investigations were reported (Celmeli et al. 2016). In the other, brain MRI revealed multiple, nonenhancing hypodense lesions in the basal ganglia (similar to her affected sister, who also had active, enhancing lesions), as well as wedge-shape cerebellar encephalomalacia, suggesting a previous embolic infarction or a healed focal infection (Gavino et al. 2016). This "unaffected" twin had suffered only from intermittent episodes of headaches that were diagnosed as migraines, as well as intermittent episodes of nonrecalcitrant dermatophytosis. Because she was relatively well, she refused further investigations (e.g., lumbar puncture; brain biopsy). Whether the "unaffected" twin in the other report similarly would have abnormalities in imaging or CSF analysis would be informative. Nonetheless, these "twin studies" with genetically identical *CARD9* mutant alleles, and presumably with a relatively similar fungal exposure history (at least in early childhood), demonstrate that sCNSc from CARD9 deficiency is a phenotype of variable penetrance and/or variable expressivity.

Despite being a fungal disease of the brain, sCNSc due to CARD9 deficiency appears to frequently have a subacute course, that is, symptoms can develop and worsen over weeks-to-months (or even years), prior to the precipitous presentation. However, this should not be misinterpreted as being a benign disease. In the original report of CARD9 deficiency, the three family members with presumed sCNSc died (Glocker et al. 2009). Likewise, reports of sCNSc in French-Canadians (but without genetic confirmation of bi-allelic mutations in *CARD9*) also confirm a high mortality rate in the absence of antifungal therapy (Morris et al. 1945; Belisle et al. 1968;

Black 1970; Germain et al. 1994). Surgery may be required therapeutically; it has at least provided the means to make the diagnosis of fungal infection accurately. The sCNSc is marked by difficulty to sterilize the CSF during induction antifungal therapy, often requiring combination of agents for prolonged periods of time. Relapses appear typical and can occur during appropriate suppressive (maintenance) antifungal therapy. In two reports (Gavino et al. 2014, 2016), symptomatic relapses were accompanied by isolation of *C. albicans* that remained susceptible in vitro to antifungal agents, including the ones used during maintenance therapy. Based on an in vitro cellular phenotype of impaired granulocyte-monocyte colony stimulating factor (GM-CSF) response to fungal agonists, these two patients were treated with maintenance antifungal therapy along with adjunctive, recombinant human GM-CSF (Gavino et al. 2014, 2016). This combination resulted in sterilization of CSF, normalization of CSF parameters, and radiologic amelioration. In one of the patients, cessation of GM-CSF was followed soon after by a clinical relapse with re-worsening of CSF parameters, all of which resolved with reinitiation of GM-CSF. The temporal relation of GM-CSF to symptoms in this single case, along with the in vitro data of a defective *C. albicans*-specific GM-CSF response, buttresses a cause-and-beneficial effect of adjunctive GM-CSF therapy. No further relapse occurred in the subsequent 3 years for either patient while on adjunct GM-CSF. Subsequently, G-CSF has also been used, along with three antifungal agents (fluconazole, amphotericin B, and the non-CNS penetrating caspofungin), during the re-induction treatment for a sCNSc relapse, which led to improvement and the eventual cessation of G-CSF after 2 months (Celmeli et al. 2016). Most other patients with sCNSc due to CARD9 deficiency have not needed adjunctive colony-stimulating factor therapy and survived with aggressive antifungal therapy, apparently with no significant sequela, although the accurate evolution of many cases were censored at the time of publication. While hematopoietic stem cell transplant has been considered as potentially curative for CARD9 deficiency (Drewniak et al. 2013), no report demonstrating the efficacy or safety of this approach is available.

Dermatophytes

Dermatophytes are a group of hyalohypho-mycetous fungi that typically cause superficial diseases on humans and other mammals. By classical morphologic criteria in diagnostic mycology laboratories, the dermatophytes are composed of three genera: *Trichophyton*, *Microsporum*, and *Epidermophyton*. Superficial dermatophytosis (also called "tinea" or "ringworm") can be associated with irritative symptoms, as well as cosmetic consequences, but are not generally life-threatening.

In distinction to superficial disease, deep dermatophytosis (DD) is a rarer presentation that may be severe and even life-threatening. DD is characterized by extensive – and often destructive – dermal and subcutaneous tissue invasion, often with dissemination to lymph nodes and, occasionally, to the CNS. Cases of DD have been historically traced back to at least the 1950s, with in-depth contemporaneous characterization suggesting an autosomal recessive transmission. However, the basis for this host susceptibility to DD had remained elusive until a collaborative effort between the Casanova and Grimbacher research groups discovered that DD was due to CARD9 deficiency, in at least a subset of affected individuals (Lanternier et al. 2013). Table 2 summarizes the current published reports of DD in which recessive mutations in *CARD9* have been identified or presumed by pedigree analysis. Based on available microbiologic data, the primary pathogens causing DD associated with CARD9 deficiency are *Trichophyton violaceum* and *T. rubrum*, which are common anthrophilic dermatophytes. However, it should be noted that this conclusion is based primarily on patients from North Africa, where *T. violaceum* also happens to be the dermatophytic species most frequently isolated from patients (Lanternier et al. 2013). Whether the same or distinct *Trichophyton* species (or other dermatophytes) cause DD in CARD9 deficient patients from other parts of the world is unknown. Interestingly, *T. violaceum* and *T. rubrum* are closely related and may constitute a single clade (Graser et al. 2008); whether this translates into shared antigens relevant for CARD9-dependent host defenses remains to be addressed. Thus, it is currently unclear if the loss of CARD9 permits a species/clade-specific or genus-specific dermatophytic susceptibility.

In affected individuals, the age of onset of dermatophytosis has generally been in childhood, manifesting as superficial disease (tinea) affecting various sites of the body. However, the dermatophytosis progresses indolently to become destructive, with visible nodular/tumoral and/or ulcerative lesions in adulthood. Dissemination to regional lymph nodes, manifesting as lymphadenopathy, is common. Interestingly, multiple non-contiguous lymph node clusters may be affected in the same individual, implying a significant degree of dissemination, although it is not clear if this derives from a single port of entry or multiple ones from the vast surface area of the skin barrier. Less commonly, bone may be involved. It is particularly intriguing that one presumed case of DD due to CARD9 deficiency developed CNS involvement probably with a dermatophyte (Lanternier et al. 2013): That a loss of CARD9 function could permit a mold, which typically resides at the cutaneous interface, to invade to the brain, may reflect a common immuno-pathophysiologic mechanism with sCNSc. Further cases with definitive phenotype, microbiology, and genotype will be profoundly informative.

As with sCNSc, the DD associated with CARD9 deficiency is difficult to treat. Induction therapy, to bring cure, appears to be infrequently successful. In some cases, there is initial improvement or stabilization of lesions; however, relapse seems to be the typical natural history of the disease once antifungal therapy is stopped. In more recent cases, maintenance therapy with the extended-spectrum azole, posaconazole, seems to be adequate. Impaired GM-CSF response of PBMC to fungal stimulation has been recently demonstrated in one patient with DD due to CARD9 deficiency (Alves de Medeiros et al. 2016), reiterating the finding observed in sCNSc

C

CARD9 Deficiency, Table 2 CARD9 deficiency and DD

Reference	Age of clinical disease onset/gender	Bi-allelic mutations[a]	Sentinel fungal disease (fungal etiology if reported)	Features of deep dermatophytosis (fungal etiology if reported)	Other clinical features	Outcome
Lanternier et al. (2013)	6 years old/M (A-II-1; Algerian)	c.865C>T (p. Q289X)	*Tinea corporis; tinea capitis*; onychomycosis with pachyonychia	Lymphadenopathy in left axilla; also, submaxillary and mesenteric lymphadenopathy (at age 52)	Non-insulin-dependent diabetes mellitus (at age 50)	Treated with itraconazole. Alive
	2 year old/M (cousin of A-II-1; Algerian)	Presumed (by genetic sequencing of other family members): c.865C>T (p. Q289X)	Onychomycosis; recurrent *tinea capitis*; *tinea corporis*; lymphadenopathy	Erythrodermic cutaneous nodules and ulcers, alopecia, onychodystrophy, with iliac, inguinal, axillary, and cervical fistulizing lymphadenopathy (at age 25) with *T. violaceum*. Subsequently developed 3 cerebral abscesses (no biopsy/microbiology)	Oral thrush (at age 9)	Deceased (at age 29)
	9 years old/F (B-II-6; Algerian)	c.865C>T (p. Q289X)	Recurrent *tinea capitis*; extensive *tinea corporis*	General skin thickening, lichenification, squamous areas, pruritus, multiple erythematous nodules, palmoplantar keratotic lesions, severe nail involvement with onychogryphosis and scaly scalp. Also developed multiple lymphadenopathies with fistula formation, worsening between the ages of 12 and 17 years. (*T. rubrum*)	Insulin-dependent diabetes mellitus (at age 35)	Griseofulvin treatment (at age 17), with clear improvement, but relapse when treatment stopped. Disease controlled with itraconazole. Alive
	8 years old/M (C-II-1; Algerian)	c.865C>T (p. Q289X)	Recurrent *tinea capitis and tinea corporis*. Extensive foot and hand onychomycosis and glabrous skin lesion with lichenification. (*T. violaceum*)	Extensive foot and hand onychomycosis and glabrous skin lesion with lichenification. (*T. violaceum*)	Recurrent oral candidiasis	Griseofulvin treatment (at age 17), with some improvement, but relapses occurred when treatment stopped. Alive, treated with griseofulvin

(continued)

CARD9 Deficiency, Table 2 (continued)

Reference	Age of clinical disease onset/gender	Bi-allelic mutations[a]	Sentinel fungal disease (fungal etiology if reported)	Features of deep dermatophytosis (fungal etiology if reported)	Other clinical features	Outcome
	8 years old/M (C-II-5; brother of C-II-1; Algerian)	Presumed (by genetic sequencing of other family members): c.865C>T (p. Q289X)	Extensive *tinea capitis* and onychomycosis	Extensive keratotic and ichthyotic lesions, disseminated papules, nodules, alopecia, pachyonychia, and onycholysis; subcutaneous abscesses; peripheral lymphadenopathy that fistulized (*T. violaceum*)	Recurrent thrush with *C. albicans*	Griseofulvin (at age 15), which led to improvement initially. Deceased (at age 34); no postmortem data available
	8 years old/F (C-II-11; sister of C-II-1 and C-II-5; Algerian)	c.865C>T (p. Q289X)	Chronic onychomycosis of all nails (*T. violaceum*)	NR	None	Treated with griseofulvin
	19 years old/M (D-II-6; Algerian)	c.865C>T (p. Q289X)		Ulcerative and nodular lesions of the left thigh and scalp (at age 19). Recurrent tinea capitis, onychomycosis of the hands and feet, cervical lymphadenopathy (at age 39)		Treatment with griseofulvin and fluconazole led to temporary improvement; relapse when the antifungal drugs were stopped. Alive, maintained with griseofulvin and fluconazole
	21 years old/M (D-II-7; brother of D-II-6; Algerian)	c.865C>T (p. Q289X)		Extensive ulcerating skin lesions on the face, scalp, and perineum. Also, extensive *tinea versicolor*, onychomycosis, and inguinal lymph node involvement		Treated initially with griseofulvin, then fluconazole, with improvement. Cutaneous expansion and tissue extension when antifungal therapy stopped, leading to a stenotic anus that required surgery
	N/A/M (D-II-4; brother of D-II-7 and D-II-7; Algerian)	Presumed (by genetic sequencing of other family members): c.865C>T (p. Q289X)				Deceased from pseudotumoral and ulcerating lesions on face (at age 28)

Patient	Mutation	Clinical history	Clinical presentation	Outcome
NA/M (E-II-7; Algerian)	c.865C>T (p. Q289X)	Recurrent tinea in childhood	Erythematosquamous warty lesions with onychomycosis and giant palmo-plantar horns, with onychogryphosis (at age 27; *T. violaceum*)	Improved on griseofulvin, but relapse. Deceased (at age 39)
NA/F (E-II-10; sister of D-II-7; Algerian)	c.865C>T (p. Q289X)	Chronic onychomycosis since childhood		Alive
NA/M (F-II-6; Moroccan)	c.301C>T (p. R101C)	Recurrent thrush and tinea during childhood	Squamous hyperkeratosic skin lesions on left foot (at age 16). Worsening to vegetative and ulcerating lesions extending to feet, calves, and the left thigh (at age 35), with left inguinal lymphadenopathy, squamous pigmented lesions of the groin, left foot onychomycosis, and radiographic osteolysis of left toes. (*T. rubrum*)	Initial improvement with antifungals, but then relapse (despite multiple antifungals), requiring amputation of left foot. Alive, but disease relapsed despite voriconazole
NA/F (F-II-3; sister of F-II-6; Moroccan)	c.301C>T (p. R101C)	Recurrent severe tinea since childhood. Hand and foot onychomycosis as adult		Alive
12 years old/M (G-III-1; Tunisian)	c.865C>T (p. Q289X)	*Tinea corporis* (at age 12)	Extension of skin lesions (at age 16), with nodules and onychomycosis of all nails (T. rubrum)	Fluconazole treatment stabilized lesions, without regression. Alive
5 years old/F (G-III-4; sister of G-III-1; Tunisian)	c.865C>T (p. Q289X)	*Tinea capitis* (at age 5); *tinea corporis* and onychomycosis (at age 8). (*T. violaceum* and *T. rubrum*)	Fistulized skin nodules and axillary lymphadenopathy (at age 12)	Stabilization of skin lesions with griseofulvin, ketoconazole, and fluconazole. Alive

(continued)

C

CARD9 Deficiency, Table 2 (continued)

Reference	Age of clinical disease onset/gender	Bi-allelic mutations[a]	Sentinel fungal disease (fungal etiology if reported)	Features of deep dermatophytosis (fungal etiology if reported)	Other clinical features	Outcome
	6 years old/M (G-II-6; Tunisian)	c.865C>T (p. Q289X)	Tinea capitis (at age 6), followed by tinea corporis and onychomycosis of all nails			Deceased bed-ridden (at age 91)
	6 years old/M (H-II-1; Tunisian)		Severe tinea capitis (at age 6)	Extensive tinea corporis and numerous skin nodules, onychomycosis affecting all nails and inguinal, cervical, and axillary lymphadenopathy (at age 40). (T. rubrum and T. violaceum)		Initially required treatment with griseofulvin, fluconazole, terbinafine, and itraconazole. Alive, lesions stable on voriconazole
Grumach et al. (2015)	3 years old/M; (Italian)	c.302G>T (p. R101L)	Thrush and tinea of the mandibular area, with alopecia (at age 3)	Delineated, scaly, pruritic skin lesions on the face (at age 11). Progressed to ulcerative paiful lesions in the lips and spread to the mandibular area. Progressing to affect his back and shoulders, with alopecia and onychodystrophy. (T. mentagrophytes)		Mild improvement initially with multiple antifungal drugs, with progression during or after antifungal treatment completed. Alive, on posaconazole
Jachiet et al. (2015)	13 years old/M; (Egyptian)	c.865C>T (p. Q289X)	Erythematous lesions on his hands and lower limbs	Coalescent, annular, squamous, erythematous, and pigmented plaques scattered on his abdomen, back, gluteal region, and lower limbs. Onychomycosis. (T. rubrum)		Mild improvement initially with multiple antifungal drugs, with progression during or after antifungal treatment completed. Alive, on posaconazole
Alves de Medeiros et al. (2016)	8 years old/M (VI:5; Turkish)	c.208C>T (p. R70W)	Tinea capitis, tinea corporis, oral candidiasis, and onychomycosis (at age 8) (T. violaceum, T. verrucosum, T. rubrum, and Malassezia furfur)	Tumoral skin lesion (at age 41), failing antifungal therapy and requiring resection. Axillary lymphadenopathy (at age 45)		Treatment of lymphadenopathy with antifungals. Alive, with regression of lesions on posaconazole

[a]Homozygous cases are indicated by the sole mutation identified. Compound heterozygous cases are indicated with both mutations identified

due to CARD9 deficiency and suggesting that adjunctive cytokine therapy for DD may be an option in recalcitrant cases.

Pheohyphomyces

The pheohyphomyces, or dematiaceous fungi, are a heterogeneous group of molds with septated hyphae that are darkly pigmented due to the presence of melanin in their cell wall. These molds cause three distinct human diseases: chromoblastomycosis, eumycotic mycetoma, and phaeohyphomycosis.

The first indication that CARD9 played a central role in human susceptibility to phaeohyphomycosis was when bi-allelic mutations in the gene were identified in four patients with disfiguring subcutaneous disease due to *Phialophora verrucosa* (Wang et al. 2014; Table 3). In one of the patients, disease seemed to extend contiguously to the eye, resulting in blindness, suggesting a role for protection against deeper tissue invasion (Wang et al. 2014). Subsequently, CARD9 deficiency was identified in two patients with systemic phaeohyphomycosis due to *Exophiala* sp. (Lanternier et al. 2015b): One patient had chronically progressive invasive disease due to *E. dermatitidis*, involving the liver and, interestingly, the CNS; the other patient had musculo-skeletal, periorbital, lung, and lymph node disease due to *E. spinifera*. It is intriguing to note that historical reports of *E. (Wangiella) dermatitidis* long recognized its ability to cause fatal infections of the central nervous system in otherwise healthy subjects (Sudhadham et al. 2008). While the sporadic, neurotropic pathophysiology of *E. dermatitidis* is not well characterized, it is equally intriguing to note that human intestinal colonization with this mold is well documented (Sudhadham et al. 2011). These features are shared with *Candida* sp., which can distinctly cause sCNSc in the presence of deficient CARD9 function, raising speculation of a potentially common pathophysiologic process of dissemination. Lastly, CARD9 deficiency has been reported in a patient with subcutaneous phaeohyphomycosis due to *Corynespora*

cassiicola, a mold pathogen of grasses, cucumber, rubber tree, soybean, tomato, cacao, and other fruit and ornamental plants (Yan et al. 2016). Although this fungal etiology seems bizarre, it should be noted that *C. cassiicola* has been previously reported – albeit rarely – as a human pathogen (Mahgoub 1969; Yamada et al. 2013; Huang et al. 2010; Lv et al. 2011); it would be informative to evaluate *CARD9* in these other cases. While the number of phaeohyphomycotic cases associated with CARD9 deficiency are less numerous than sCNSc or DD, perhaps preventing a more-robust prototypical profile of associated disease, the aggregate of reports suggest that mutations in *CARD9* should be assessed in patients presenting with subcutaneous or invasive phaeohyphomycosis.

Singular Fungal Susceptibility

CARD9 deficiency has been consistently and independently shown to be associated with increased susceptibility to at least four fungal genera: *Candida* sp.; *Trichophyton* sp.; *Phialophora verrucosa*; and *Exophiala* sp. It may also account for sporadic susceptibility to unusual fungi (see *Corynespora cassiicola* above). It has recently been implicated in spontaneous extrapulmonary aspergillosis (Rieber et al. 2016); however, the identification of another subject who also had extrapulmonary aspergillosis, but who was only heterozygous for a germline *CARD9* mutation and who expressed both mutant and wild-type *CARD9* alleles (D. Vinh, unpublished data), suggests that additional definitive cases are required to firmly determine if CARD9 deficiency predisposes to invasive aspergillosis. Despite these nascent understandings of the natural history of CARD9 deficiency, it appears that these patients are not at increased risk for severe viral, bacterial or parasitic infections. Furthermore, it is intriguing that the reported CARD9 deficient patients have each displayed invasive disease with only a single fungus. The mechanistic basis for this singular fungal susceptibility remains unclear.

CARD9 Deficiency, Table 3 CARD9 deficiency and pheohyphomycosis (dematiaceous fungal disease)

Reference	Age of clinical disease onset/ gender	Bi-allelic mutations[a]	Sentinel fungal disease (fungal etiology if reported)	Other clinical features	Outcome
Wang et al. (2014)	13 years old/M (Chinese)	c.191-192insTGCT; c.472C>T (p. L64fsX59; p. Q158X)	Progressive dark red plaques and nodules on cheeks and ears bilaterally (*Phialophora verrucosa*)	NR	Induction combination antifungal therapy had limited effect. Lesions progressed with subcutaneous dissemination. Alive
	6 years old/M (Chinese)	c.819-820insG (p. D274fsX60)	Progressive enlargement of red plaques on right cheek (*Phialophora verrucosa*)	NR	Induction therapy was followed by 2 years of maintenance therapy, but recurrence with cessation of antifungal drug. Alive
	20 years old/F (Chinese)	c.819-820insG (p. D274fsX60)	Slowly enlarging plaque and nodule on right cheek (*Phialophora verrucosa*)	NR	Surgical excision of the nodule, with antifungal therapy. Alive, on antifungal maintenance
	48 years old/M (Chinese)	c.819-820insG (p. D274fsX60)	Severe biolet place on face and scalp, which involved eye to cause blindness (*Phialophora verrucosa*)	NR	Oral itraconazole combined with terbinafine for half a year. The lesions improved slightly without satisfactory response
Lanternier et al. (2015b)	5 years old/F (Angolan)	c.52C>T (uniparental disomy) (p.R18W)	Granulomatous cholestatic hepatitis (*E. dermatitidis*). Multiple cerebral abscesses on brain imaging, without neurological symptoms (presumably same *E. dermatitidis*)	None	Initial episode treated with biliary tract irrigation with AmB, L-AmB iv, and oral voriconazole for 3 months, followed by voriconazole monotherapy maintenance, with clinical and radiologic resolution of liver lesions and majority of brain lesions. Relapse on voriconazole therapy (25 months after 1st episode) with *E. dermatitidis* pachymeningitis requiring induction combination antifungal therapy
	18 years old/F (Iranian)	c.GAG967-969del (p.E323del)	Multiple small nodules in wrists bilaterally and in the right periorbital region with submental lymphadenopathy (at age 18). Lesion on the right forearm (at age 19). Subsequently found to have: abnormal bone scan with increased	None	Failure of disease control with antifungal monotherapy. After 5 years of combination antifungal therapy, she developed multiple small nodules in right periorbital region and wrists and left lung mass (*E. spinifera*)

(continued)

CARD9 Deficiency, Table 3 (continued)

Reference	Age of clinical disease onset/ gender	Bi-allelic mutations[a]	Sentinel fungal disease (fungal etiology if reported)	Other clinical features	Outcome
			activity at multiple sites consistent with osteomyelitis; submandibular lymphadenopathy; lesions on the dorsum of right foot and side of neck		
Yan et al. (2016)	35 years old/F (Chinese)	c.191–192InsTGCT	Extensive, destructive, dark red facial plaques with purulent foul-smelling discharge, and with postauricular lymphadenopathy (*Corynespora cassiicola*)	None	Induction therapy with AmB led to only slight improvement. Patient left the hospital for financial reasons

[a]Homozygous cases are indicated by the sole mutation identified. Compound heterozygous cases are indicated with both mutations identified

Genetic, Molecular, and Pathophysiologic Studies

CARD9 is located on chromosome 9 and encodes a protein of 536 amino acids. Like other CARD proteins, CARD9 has an N-terminal CARD domain that mediates binding to other CARD-domain containing molecules such as the protein B-cell lymphoma 10 (BCL10), and a C-terminal coiled-coil domain enabling protein oligomerization (Fig. 1) (Ruland 2008; Hara and Saito 2009; Roth and Ruland 2013). CARD9 is expressed primarily in myeloid cells ; consequently, CARD9 signaling is dispensable in lymphocytes but not in myeloid cells (Hara and Saito 2009; Roth and Ruland 2013).

Bi-allelic mutations in *CARD9* are required for invasive fungal disease. Several mutations in *CARD9* have been identified; they range from null alleles (i.e., loss of expression: L64 fs*59 (Wang et al. 2014), Q158X (Wang et al. 2014), D274fs*60 (Wang et al. 2014), Q289X (Lanternier et al. 2013), Q295X (Glocker et al. 2009), E323del (Lanternier et al. 2015b)) to missense mutations with detectable protein but loss of function (i.e., R57H (Drummond et al. 2015), R70W (Lanternier et al. 2015a, b), G72S

(Drewniak et al. 2013), Y91H (Gavino et al. 2014, 2016), R101C (Lanternier et al. 2013), R373P (Drewniak et al. 2013; Fig. 1)). The mutations cluster in the two functional domains of CARD9 (Fig. 1). Although CARD9 deficiency confers singular fungal susceptibility (see above), there appears to be no genotype-phenotype correlation for this phenomenon, as the exact same mutation can predispose to sCNSc in some individuals and to DD in others (e.g., R70W; Q289X; Fig. 1). In addition to mutations in coding regions, allelic imbalance resulting from nonexonic variants has been reported (Gavino et al. 2016): In a French-Canadian cohort with sCNSc, genomic DNA sequencing revealed the c.439T>C (p.Y91H) mutation in heterozygosity. However, further analysis revealed that only the p.Y91H mutant allele was expressed at the mRNA (cDNA) level. This mono-allelic expression was abnormal, as SNP analysis in unaffected family members and numerous healthy controls confirm that CARD9 is normally bi-allelically expressed. Although a private nucleotide variant in the putative promoter region upstream of *CARD9* was identified in patients and those unaffected family members with allelic imbalance (but associated with wild-type allele), reporter assay

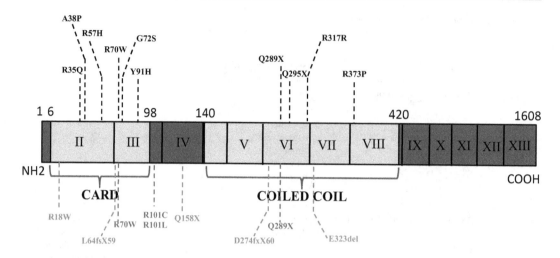

CARD9 Deficiency, Fig. 1 CARD9 protein schema with identified mutations to date. Coding exons are numbered with Roman numerals. The regions corresponding to the CARD domain and the coiled coil domain are indicated.

Mutations indicated correspond to those identified in patients with CARD9 deficiency and invasive candidiasis/spontaneous central nervous system candidiasis [*Black*], deep dermatophytosis (*blue*), or phaehyphomycosis (*orange*)

studies did not demonstrate that this variant affected transcription. Thus, the basis for the allelic imbalance in these cases remains unresolved. In a distinct patient who was not French-Canadian and who had DD, the c.439T>C (p.Y91H) was found, along with an intronic mutation (c.1435+18G>A; NM_052813) that created a novel splice acceptor site and abolished expression of the corresponding allele, again resulting in mono-allelic expression of the p.Y91H variant (D. Vinh, manuscript in preparation). These cases illustrate the diversity of mutations that affect *CARD9* and emphasize the need to comprehensively evaluate both genomic DNA and mRNA (cDNA) sequences, to ensure the detection of nonexonic variants affecting allelic expression.

The identification of humans with CARD9 deficiency provides profound insight into its immunobiology. In its seminal discovery in experimental systems, CARD9 was identified as a cytosolic adaptor molecule that signals downstream of the C-type lectin pattern recognition receptor, Dectin-1, in myeloid cells but was redundant for lymphocyte signaling (Bertin et al. 2000; Gross et al. 2006; LeibundGut-Landmann et al. 2007; Hara et al. 2007). In mice, the CARD9-null state was associated with increased death following challenge with *C. albicans*. Dissection of the cellular signaling pathway demonstrated that the recognition of β-glucan by Dectin-1 activates spleen tyrosine kinase (SYK), which triggers the assembly of CARD9 with B-cell lymphoma/leukemia 10 (BCL10) and mucosa-associated lymphoid tissue lymphoma translocation protein 1 (MALT1) to activate nuclear factor kappa-light-chain-enhancer of activated B cells (NFκB), c-Jun N-terminal kinase (JNK), and p38 to stimulate production of chemokines/cytokines (e.g., tumor necrosis factor, TNF; interleukin(IL)-6; IL-23; IL-2) and antigen presentation (Gross et al. 2006; LeibundGut-Landmann et al. 2007); of note, Dectin-1-dependent SYK activation of phagocytosis was found to be CARD9-independent. The Dectin-1-based activation of the CARD9 signaling pathway resulted in the effective generation of a CD4[+] IL-17-producing effector T cell response (Th17). Collectively, these pioneering works demonstrated that the CARD9/BCL10/MALT1 cascade was key for mammalian antifungal innate immunity.

Shortly thereafter, the discovery of CARD9 deficiency in an Iranian pedigree with familial candidiasis was reported. Glocker et al. demonstrated that the CARD9-null patients (Q295X) had significantly reduced Th17 cells ex vivo and the mutant allele failed to trigger Dectin-1-based activation of TNF production, confirming that the phenomena identified in the above fundamental work was seen in humans (Glocker et al. 2009).

CARD9/BCL10/MALT1 signaling pathway is fundamental to human host defense to invasive fungal disease, then the corollary is that loss of either BCL10 or MALT1 should phenocopy CARD9 deficiency. Herein lies the elegance – and the necessity – to study human immunodeficiencies. Pedigrees with deficiency of BCL10 or MALT1 have been subsequently identified and invasive fungal disease was notably absent (Jabara et al. 2013; Punwani et al. 2015; Torres et al. 2014). To this end, Jia et al. subsequently defined a distinct signaling axis, whereby fungal stimulation results in CARD9 interaction with Ras Protein Specific Guanine Nucleotide Releasing Factor 1 (RASGRF1) to recruit V-Ha-Ras Harvey Rat Sarcoma Viral Oncogene Homolog (H-RAS) for downstream Extracellular Signal-regulated Kinase (ERK) (Gazendam et al. 2014) activation, and that loss of this ERK activation increased the death of C. albicans-infected mice (Jia et al. 2014). As ERK plays an important role in macrophage responses (Iles and Forman 2002; Richardson et al. 2015; Valledor et al. 2000), including regulating GM-CSF responses (de Groot et al. 1998), this pathway was interrogated in the French-Canadian CARD9 deficient cohort (Gavino et al. 2016). Although the p.Y91H mutation had no demonstrable effect on CARD9's interaction with BCL10 or MALT1, it was found to decrease the ability of CARD9 to complex with RASGRF1, relative to wild-type CARD9 protein, thus reducing downstream ERK activation. While this may suggest that the CARD9/RASGRF1/ERK signalosome is important for human antifungal (at least, anti-candidal) immunity, demonstration of a similar effect due to other known

CARD9 mutations would be informative. Similarly, human diseases with loss-of-function of RASGRF1, H-RAS, or ERK, either at germline level or in acquired or iatrogenic state, have not yet been reported, but their phenotype may provide significant advances in understanding the antifungal relevance of the CARD9/RASGRF1/ERK hub. Thus, the molecular pathway(s) by which CARD9 confers susceptibility to invasive fungal disease remains to be deciphered. Further, whether the singular fungal susceptibility seen clinically reflects divergence of CARD9-dependent pathways remains to be answered.

While the molecular pathways implicating CARD9 are beginning to be deciphered, our understanding on the pathophysiology of invasive fungal disease lags behind. The typical site of human colonization with C. albicans is the gastrointestinal tract or skin, whereas for dermatophytes like Trichosporon, it is, by definition, at the skin, and for phaehyphomycetes, it is either the respiratory tract or the gastrointestinal tract. What has remained enigmatic to date is understanding not only how loss-of-function in CARD9 permits a fungus to transition from commensal to invasive pathogen at the portal of entry, but what accounts for the unusual predilection to involve the CNS? What is the process by which these fungi are able to disseminate with minimal systemic symptoms, in a clearly nonfatal process, prior to seeding distant organs, including the CNS? The demonstration of impaired neutrophilic response to C. albicans, both in capacity to migrate toward foci of fungal infection (Drummond et al. 2015) as well as in fungal handling (Drewniak et al. 2013; Gazendam et al. 2014; Liang et al. 2015), may contribute to invasion and/or dissemination. Likewise, the impaired proinflammatory response of peripheral blood mononuclear cells (Glocker et al. 2009; Lanternier et al. 2015a, b; Gavino et al. 2014, 2016; Drewniak et al. 2013) may contribute to this impaired neutrophilic response, as well as impaired handling of fungi, perhaps permitting the establishment of an intracellular latent reservoir that can escape immune recognition while serving as a nidus for subsequent reactivation, in a manner similar to that for M. tuberculosis and select other fungi (e.g., *Histoplasma*; *Cryptococcus*) (Woods 2016; Alanio et al. 2015). These processes are, however, speculative. Nonetheless, CARD9 deficiency uniquely provides a natural human model to study the pathogenesis of invasion and dissemination with respect to its spectrum of fungi.

Concluding Remarks and Future Challenges

Bi-allelic mutations in CARD9 predispose to invasive candidiasis, including sCNSc, DD, and subcutaneous/invasive phaehyphomycosis. It may also be associated with susceptibility to *Aspergillus* sp. or unusual molds. Onset of disease is variable, and select pedigrees suggest some variability in either penetrance, expressivity, or both. Natural history of disease is one of recalcitrance, with either suboptimal response to appropriate antifungal agents (as deemed by in vitro antifungal susceptibility testing) and/or relapse. Anecdotal evidence suggests potential benefit with adjunctive cytokine therapy for these cases. The investigation of more patients is clearly required to understand the clinical diseases associated with CARD9 deficiency, to dissect the mechanistic basis for unusually severe and distinctive manifestations of the various mycoses, and to explore genotype-phenotype correlations, including the enigmatic singular fungal susceptibility phenotype.

Are There Other Genes Associated with Increased Susceptibility to Fungal Diseases?

CARD9 can be added to a growing list of genes that, when lesioned, predispose to invasive fungal diseases. In distinction to other genes, mutations in *CARD9* appear to predispose only to fungal diseases. There remain patients with spontaneous, invasive fungal diseases who do not have mutations in *CARD9*. Relevant genes upstream and downstream of CARD9, as well as pathways unrelated to CARD9, are expected to broaden our understanding of those nonredundant processes that mediate human susceptibility to fungal infections.

Is There a Role for These Genes in Iatrogenic Fungal Diseases?

Invasive fungal diseases are typically not spontaneous, but rather, develop as a complication or during treatment of various underlying disorders. Whether or not CARD9, or related pathway proteins, influences susceptibility in these conditions has not been adequately explored. A single study, assessing the impact of a singular SNP in *CARD9*, found no association with the risk of candidemia in critically ill patients (Rosentul et al. 2011); however, given that the development of candida bloodstream infection in this group of patients is typically from central venous catheters or from intestinal transection (Bow et al. 2010), it would not be expected to find an effect of a gene SNP on disease biology in these conditions. Other polymorphisms, particularly those that are functional (i.e., modify the expression of a normal protein, or result in normal expression of a slightly modified protein), may ultimately impact on the development of specific syndromes. For example, the development of chronic disseminated ("hepatosplenic") candidiasis in select patients recovering from intensive cytoreductive therapy for acute myeloid leukemia remains unexplained but may be influenced by *CARD9* variants. Additionally, understanding the cellular mechanistic basis by which CARD9 mediates antifungal host resistance will likely identify nonredundant processes that may be therapeutically actionable.

References

Alanio A, Vernel-Pauillac F, Sturny-Leclere A, Dromer F (2015) Cryptococcus neoformans host adaptation: toward biological evidence of dormancy. *mBio* 6(2)

Alves de Medeiros AK, Lodewick E, Bogaert DJ, Haerynck F, Van Daele S, Lambrecht B, et al. Chronic and invasive fungal infections in a family with CARD9 deficiency. J Clin Immunol. 2016;36(3):204–9.

Belisle G, Lachance W, Leblanc G. Meningitis caused by Candida albicans. Report of a case and discussion. L'union Med Can. 1968;97(6):710–5.

Bertin J, Guo Y, Wang L, Srinivasula SM, Jacobson MD, Poyet JL, et al. CARD9 is a novel caspase recruitment domain-containing protein that interacts with BCL10/CLAP and activates NF-kappa B. J Biol Chem. 2000;275(52):41082–6.

Black JT. Cerebral candidiasis: case report of brain abscess secondary to Candida albicans, and review of literature. J Neurol Neurosurg Psychiatry. 1970;33(6): 864–70.

Bow EJ, Evans G, Fuller J, Laverdiere M, Rotstein C, Rennie R, et al. Canadian clinical practice guidelines for invasive candidiasis in adults. Can J Infect Dis Med Microbiol = J Can Mal Infect Microbiol Med. 2010;21(4):e122–50.

Bustamante J, Boisson-Dupuis S, Abel L, Casanova JL. Mendelian susceptibility to mycobacterial disease: genetic, immunological, and clinical features of inborn errors of IFN-gamma immunity. Semin Immunol. 2014;26(6):454–70.

Celmeli F, Oztoprak N, Turkkahraman D, Seyman D, Mutlu E, Frede N, et al. Successful granulocyte colony-stimulating factor treatment of relapsing Candida albicans meningoencephalitis caused by CARD9 deficiency. Pediatr Infect Dis J. 2016;35(4):428–31.

Cohen MS, Isturiz RE, Malech HL, Root RK, Wilfert CM, Gutman L, et al. Fungal infection in chronic granulomatous disease. The importance of the phagocyte in defense against fungi. Am J Med. 1981;71(1):59–66.

de Groot RP, Coffer PJ, Koenderman L. Regulation of proliferation, differentiation and survival by the IL-3/IL-5/GM-CSF receptor family. Cell Signal. 1998;10(9):619–28.

Drewniak A, Gazendam RP, Tool AT, van Houdt M, Jansen MH, van Hamme JL, et al. Invasive fungal infection and impaired neutrophil killing in human CARD9 deficiency. Blood. 2013;121(13):2385–92.

Drummond RA, Collar AL, Swamydas M, Rodriguez CA, Lim JK, Mendez LM, et al. CARD9-dependent neutrophil recruitment protects against fungal invasion of the central nervous system. PLoS Pathog. 2015;11(12): e1005293.

Gavino C, Cotter A, Lichtenstein D, Lejtenyi D, Fortin C, Legault C, et al. CARD9 deficiency and spontaneous central nervous system candidiasis: complete clinical remission with GM-CSF therapy. Clin Infect Dis: Off Publ Infect Dis Soc Am. 2014;59(1):81–4.

Gavino C, Hamel N, Zeng JB, Legault C, Guiot MC, Chankowsky J, et al. Impaired RASGRF1/ERK-mediated GM-CSF response characterizes CARD9 deficiency in French-Canadians. J Allergy Clin Immunol. 2016;137(4):1178–88.e1-7.

Gazendam RP, van Hamme JL, Tool AT, van Houdt M, Verkuijlen PJ, Herbst M, et al. Two independent killing mechanisms of Candida albicans by human neutrophils: evidence from innate immunity defects. Blood. 2014;124(4):590–7.

Germain M, Gourdeau M, Hebert J. Case report: familial chronic mucocutaneous candidiasis complicated by deep candida infection. Am J Med Sci. 1994;307(4): 282–3.

Glocker EO, Hennigs A, Nabavi M, Schaffer AA, Woellner C, Salzer U, et al. A homozygous CARD9 mutation in a family with susceptibility to fungal infections. N Engl J Med. 2009;361(18):1727–35.

Graser Y, Scott J, Summerbell R. The new species concept in dermatophytes-a polyphasic approach. Mycopathologia. 2008;166(5–6):239–56.

Gross O, Gewies A, Finger K, Schafer M, Sparwasser T, Peschel C, et al. Card9 controls a non-TLR signalling pathway for innate anti-fungal immunity. Nature. 2006;442(7103):651–6.

Grumach AS, de Queiroz-Telles F, Migaud M, Lanternier F, Filho NR, Palma SM, et al. A homozygous CARD9 mutation in a Brazilian patient with deep dermatophytosis. J Clin Immunol. 2015; 35(5):486–90.

Hara H, Saito T. CARD9 versus CARMA1 in innate and adaptive immunity. Trends Immunol. 2009; 30(5):234–42.

Hara H, Ishihara C, Takeuchi A, Imanishi T, Xue L, Morris SW, et al. The adaptor protein CARD9 is essential for the activation of myeloid cells through ITAM-associated and toll-like receptors. Nat Immunol. 2007;8(6):619–29.

Herbst M, Gazendam R, Reimnitz D, Sawalle-Belohradsky J, Groll A, Schlegel PG, et al. Chronic Candida albicans meningitis in a 4-year-old girl with a homozygous mutation in the CARD9 gene (Q295X). Pediatr Infect Dis J. 2015;34(9):999–1002.

Huang HK, Liu CE, Liou JH, Hsiue HC, Hsiao CH, Hsueh PR. Subcutaneous infection caused by Corynespora cassiicola, a plant pathogen. J Infect. 2010; 60(2):188–90.

Iles KE, Forman HJ. Macrophage signaling and respiratory burst. Immunol Res. 2002;26(1–3):95–105.

Jabado N, Casanova JL, Haddad E, Dulieu F, Fournet JC, Dupont B, et al. Invasive pulmonary infection due to Scedosporium apiospermum in two children with chronic granulomatous disease. Clin Infect Dis: Off Publ Infect Dis Soc Am. 1998;27(6):1437–41.

Jabara HH, Ohsumi T, Chou J, Massaad MJ, Benson H, Megarbane A, et al. A homozygous mucosa-associated lymphoid tissue 1 (MALT1) mutation in a family with combined immunodeficiency. J Allergy Clin Immunol. 2013;132(1):151–8.

Jachiet M, Lanternier F, Rybojad M, Bagot M, Ibrahim L, Casanova JL, et al. Posaconazole treatment of extensive skin and nail dermatophytosis due to autosomal recessive deficiency of CARD9. JAMA Dermatol. 2015;151(2):192–4.

Jia XM, Tang B, Zhu LL, Liu YH, Zhao XQ, Gorjestani S, et al. CARD9 mediates Dectin-1-induced ERK activation by linking Ras-GRF1 to H-Ras for antifungal immunity. J Exp Med. 2014;211(11):2307–21.

Jones N, Garcez T, Newman W, Denning D (2016) Endogenous Candida endophthalmitis and osteomyelitis associated with CARD9 deficiency. BMJ Case Rep 2016

Lanternier F, Pathan S, Vincent QB, Liu L, Cypowyj S, Prando C, et al. Deep dermatophytosis and inherited CARD9 deficiency. N Engl J Med. 2013; 369(18):1704–14.

Lanternier F, Mahdaviani SA, Barbati E, Chaussade H, Koumar Y, Levy R, et al. Inherited CARD9 deficiency in otherwise healthy children and adults with Candida species-induced meningoencephalitis, colitis, or both. J Allergy Clin Immunol. 2015a;135(6):1558–68.e2.

Lanternier F, Barbati E, Meinzer U, Liu L, Pedergnana V, Migaud M, et al. Inherited CARD9 deficiency in 2 unrelated patients with invasive Exophiala infection. J Infect Dis. 2015b;211(8):1241–50.

LeibundGut-Landmann S, Gross O, Robinson MJ, Osorio F, Slack EC, Tsoni SV, et al. Syk- and CARD9-dependent coupling of innate immunity to the induction of T helper cells that produce interleukin 17. Nat Immunol. 2007;8(6):630–8.

Liang P, Wang X, Wang R, Wan Z, Han W, Li R. CARD9 deficiencies linked to impaired neutrophil functions against Phialophora verrucosa. Mycopathologia. 2015;179(5–6):347–57.

Lv GX, Ge YP, Shen YN, Li M, Zhang X, Chen H, et al. Phaeohyphomycosis caused by a plant pathogen. Corynespora cassiicola. Med Mycol. 2011; 49(6):657–61.

Mahgoub E. Corynespora cassiicola, a new agent of maduromycetoma. J Trop Med Hyg. 1969;72(9): 218–21.

Marks MI, Marks S, Brazeau M. Yeast colonization in hospitalized and nonhospitalized children. J Pediatr. 1975;87(4):524–7.

Moraes-Vasconcelos D, Grumach AS, Yamaguti A, Andrade ME, Fieschi C, de Beaucoudrey L, et al. Paracoccidioides brasiliensis disseminated disease in a patient with inherited deficiency in the beta1 subunit of the interleukin (IL)-12/IL-23 receptor. Clin Infect Dis: Off Publ Infect Dis Soc Am. 2005;41(4): e31–7.

Morris AA, Kalz GG, Lotspeich ES. Ependymitis and meningitis due to Candida (Monilia) albicans. Arch Neurol Psychiatr. 1945;54:361–6.

Punwani D, Wang H, Chan AY, Cowan MJ, Mallott J, Sunderam U, et al. Combined immunodeficiency due to MALT1 mutations, treated by hematopoietic cell transplantation. J Clin Immunol. 2015;35(2): 135–46.

Richardson ET, Shukla S, Nagy N, Boom WH, Beck RC, Zhou L, et al. ERK signaling is essential for macrophage development. PLoS One. 2015;10(10): e0140064.

Rieber N, Gazendam RP, Freeman AF, Hsu AP, Collar AL, Sugui JA, et al. Extrapulmonary Aspergillus infection in patients with CARD9 deficiency. JCI Insight. 2016;1(17):e89890.

Roilides E, Sigler L, Bibashi E, Katsifa H, Flaris N, Panteliadis C. Disseminated infection due to Chrysosporium zonatum in a patient with chronic granulomatous disease and review of non-aspergillus fungal infections in patients with this disease. J Clin Microbiol. 1999;37(1):18–25.

Rosentul DC, Plantinga TS, Oosting M, Scott WK, Velez Edwards DR, Smith PB, et al. Genetic variation in the dectin-1/CARD9 recognition pathway and susceptibility to candidemia. J Infect Dis. 2011;204(7):1138–45.

Roth S, Ruland J. Caspase recruitment domain-containing protein 9 signaling in innate immunity and inflammation. Trends Immunol. 2013;34(6):243–50.

Ruland J. CARD9 signaling in the innate immune response. Ann N Y Acad Sci. 2008;1143:35–44.

Sampaio EP, Hsu AP, Pechacek J, Bax HI, Dias DL, Paulson ML, et al. Signal transducer and activator of transcription 1 (STAT1) gain-of-function mutations and disseminated coccidioidomycosis and histoplasmosis. J Allergy Clin Immunol. 2013;131(6): 1624–34.

Segal BH, DeCarlo ES, Kwon-Chung KJ, Malech HL, Gallin JI, Holland SM. Aspergillus nidulans infection in chronic granulomatous disease. Medicine. 1998;77(5):345–54.

Sudhadham M, Prakitsin S, Sivichai S, Chaiyarat R, Dorrestein GM, Menken SB, et al. The neurotropic black yeast Exophiala dermatitidis has a possible origin in the tropical rain forest. Stud Mycol. 2008; 61:145–55.

Sudhadham M, van den Gerrits EAH, Sihanonth P, Sivichai S, Chaiyarat R, Menken SB, et al. Elucidation of distribution patterns and possible infection routes of the neurotropic black yeast Exophiala dermatitidis using AFLP. Fungal Biol. 2011;115(10):1051–65.

Torres JM, Martinez-Barricarte R, Garcia-Gomez S, Mazariegos MS, Itan Y, Boisson B, et al. Inherited BCL10 deficiency impairs hematopoietic and nonhematopoietic immunity. J Clin Invest. 2014; 124(12):5239–48.

Valledor AF, Comalada M, Xaus J, Celada A. The differential time-course of extracellular-regulated kinase activity correlates with the macrophage response toward proliferation or activation. J Biol Chem. 2000;275(10):7403–9.

Vinh DC. Insights into human antifungal immunity from primary immunodeficiencies. Lancet Infect Dis. 2011;11(10):780–92.

Vinh DC, Masannat F, Dzioba RB, Galgiani JN, Holland SM. Refractory disseminated coccidioidomycosis and mycobacteriosis in interferon-gamma receptor 1 deficiency. Clin Infect Dis: Off Publ Infect Dis Soc Am. 2009;49(6):e62–5.

Vinh DC, Schwartz B, Hsu AP, Miranda DJ, Valdez PA, Fink D, et al. Interleukin-12 receptor beta1 deficiency predisposing to disseminated coccidioidomycosis. Clin Infect Dis: Off Publ Infect Dis Soc Am. 2011;52(4): e99–e102.

Wang X, Wang W, Lin Z, Wang X, Li T, Yu J, et al. CARD9 mutations linked to subcutaneous phaeohyphomycosis and TH17 cell deficiencies. J Allergy Clin Immunol. 2014;133(3):905–8.e3.

Winkelstein JA, Marino MC, Johnston RB Jr, Boyle J, Curnutte J, Gallin JI, et al. Chronic granulomatous disease. Report on a national registry of 368 patients. Medicine. 2000;79(3):155–69.

Woods JP. Revisiting old friends: developments in understanding Histoplasma capsulatum pathogenesis. J Microbiol (Seoul, Korea). 2016;54(3):265–76.

Yamada H, Takahashi N, Hori N, Asano Y, Mochizuki K, Ohkusu K, et al. Rare case of fungal keratitis caused by Corynespora cassiicola. J Infect Chemother: Off J Jpn Soc Chemother. 2013;19(6):1167–9.

Yan XX, Yu CP, Fu XA, Bao FF, Du DH, Wang C, et al. CARD9 mutation linked to Corynespora cassiicola infection in a Chinese patient. Br J Dermatol. 2016;174(1):176–9.

Zerbe CS, Holland SM. Disseminated histoplasmosis in persons with interferon-gamma receptor 1 deficiency. Clin Infect Dis: Off Publ Infect Dis Soc Am. 2005;41(4):e38–41.

CARMA2

▶ CARD14-Mediated Psoriasis and Pityriasis Rubra Piliaris (PRP)

CARMEN

▶ B Cell Lymphoma/Leukemia 10 Deficiency

Cartilage Hair Hypoplasia (RMRP)

Melissa L. Crenshaw
Division of Genetics, Johns Hopkins All Children's Hospital, St. Petersburg, FL, USA

Synonyms

CHH: Cartilage hair hypoplasia; RMRP: Ribonuclease mitochondrial RNA-processing; RNase MRP: Mitochondrial RNA-processing endoribonuclease

Definition

Cartilage hair hypoplasia (CHH) is a rare autosomal recessive condition, which uniquely combines the features of a skeletal dysplasia and immunodeficiency. These individuals are also at increased risk for autoimmune disorders such as Hirschprung's disease as well as an increased risk of malignancy, most notably lymphoma (Bordon et al. 2010). The clinical features are highly variable, and the genotype–phenotype correlations not well delineated.

The *RMRP* (RNA component of ribonuclease mitochondrial RNA-processing) gene has been identified as the causative gene for CHH (Ridanpää et al. 2001). Further study of the molecular pathways associated with this gene has elucidated the connection between the skeletal and immunologic aspects of this condition. However, much remains to be learned about RNA processing related to this gene and its contribution to CHH.

Cartilage Hair Hypoplasia

Cartilage hair hypoplasia (CHH) is a very rare condition with features of both metaphyseal chondrodysplasia and immunodeficiency. It is increased in frequency among the Amish and Finn populations with a carrier frequency of 1:19 and 1:76, respectively (Ridanpää et al. 2001). There is a great deal of intrafamilial and interfamilial variability among individuals with CHH. This is true of both the skeletal, immunologic, and autoimmune features. Some children and adults have also developed malignancies (Bordon et al. 2010). Given the rarity of CHH, there are no unifying guidelines for monitoring for these complications.

While the autosomal recessive inheritance was first described many years before, the molecular basis for CHH was finally identified in 2001. Ridanpää et al. (2001) showed the causative gene to be the ribonuclease mitochondrial RNA-processing gene (*RMRP*). They also noted that those with the same mutation have a range of severe to mild phenotype. This lack of discreet genotype-phenotype correlations makes long-term prognosis for the potential for immunodeficiency and malignancy difficult to predict. Further study revealed that the degree to which the mutation in the gene decreases ribosomal rRNA cleavage affects ribosomal construction determines the severity of skeletal features, whereas the effect on mRNA cleavage determines the degree of immunodeficiency as well as hair phenotype and risk for malignancy (Thiel et al. 2007). Susceptibility to immunodeficiency, malignancy, and autoimmune complications are the primary determinants of prognosis.

In those severely affected, these complications can be alleviated or lessened by hematopoietic stem cell transplantation. This has been studied by Bordon et al. (2010). They recommend that stem cell transplantation be performed early in those with severe immunodeficiency or autoimmunity before they develop severe infections, end organ damage, and malignancies (Bordon et al. 2010). However, it can be difficult to identify who will benefit most from stem cell transplantation and who might develop transplant-related complications.

RMRP and RNA Processing

The RMRP gene codes for the RNA component of mitochondrial RNA-processing endoribonuclease (RNase MRP) [OMIM∗157660]. This gene was first described as the cause for CHH by Ridanpää et al. (2001). This gene produces two short RNAs designated as RMRP-S1 and RMRP-S2, which function as miRNAs. Functional studies by Rogler et al. (2014) confirmed that point mutations in these subunits cause CHH. They further identified links between these subunits and the molecular pathways associated with both the skeletal and immunologic aspects of CHH including the genes SOX4 and PTCH2.

Immunological and Autoimmune Phenotype in CHH

The immunologic and autoimmune aspects of CHH vary greatly among affected individuals. Most characteristic is a variable severity of T-cell lymphocyte immunodeficiency. This leads to not only an increase in susceptibility to infections but also a greater frequency of autoimmune disorders and malignancies such as lymphoma (Bordon et al. 2010). At least two patients have also had Omenn features (Bordon et al. 2010). Bone marrow transplantation can greatly improve T cell counts but less so B cell and NKcell production with all patients showing improvement in lymphocyte function (Bordon et al. 2010).

Kostjukovits et al. (2017) evaluated a large cohort of Finnish patients with CHH all compound heterozygous or homozygous for the common g.70A>G mutation. They found deficiencies in both B and T cell lines including recent thymic emigrants as well as naïve CD4 and CD8 cells and memory B cells. This B cell pattern supported a defect in both B cell production and in maturation and survival of the B cells (Kostjukovits et al. 2017). One fourth of the CHH patients studied showed CID whereas one fourth had laboratory findings consistent with immunodeficiency but no clinical signs or symptoms (Kostjukovits et al. 2017). It is clear that some degree of genotype phenotype plays a substantial role in the variability of the immunologic complications experienced in individuals with CHH.

The cause for autoimmune abnormalities in CHH is much less well understood. A myriad of autoimmune sequelae also occur among individuals with CHH. These range from hematologic issues such as hemolytic anemia and immune thrombocytopenic purpura to hypothyroidism, arthritis, and enteropathy (Biggs et al. 2017). Broad autoantibody reactivity has been found in CHH patients suggesting a role for B cell dysregulation in this process (Biggs et al. 2017). As this process is better understood over time, this may provide for better treatment of immune and autoimmune deficiencies in CHH.

Conclusions

CHH is a rare genetic condition characterized by both features of skeletal dysplasia and immunodeficiency as well as increased tendency for autoimmune dysfunction and malignancies. This is caused by homozygous or compound heterozygous pathogenic variants in the *RMRP* gene. This gene codes for the RNA component of mitochondrial RNA-processing endoribonuclease, which is involved in both rRNA and mRNA cleavage. Its role in rRNA cleavage is thought to contribute greatly to the skeletal features and mRNA cleavage to the immunodeficiency found in these patients.

Much remains to be understood about the molecular pathways affected as well as genotype-phenotype correlations. As this becomes better elucidated, this can provide more guidance to families regarding outcome as well as to physicians in focusing medical management and monitoring of children and adults with CHH. Given the variable effects of this gene, testing of RMRP should be considered in patients with immunodeficiency, particularly those with accompanying features of a skeletal dysplasia.

When a diagnosis of CHH is made in a child with skeletal dysplasia as the presenting feature, it is important that immunologic evaluation and laboratory studies be performed promptly. A low threshold for assessment for autoimmune disorders as well as lymphoma and other malignancies should be maintained. In those with CID, hematopoietic stem cell transplantation should be considered and can offer significant improvement. It is also essential that families be well educated regarding the genetics and provided genetic counseling regarding the autosomal recessive inheritance of CHH.

References

Biggs CM, Kostjukovits S, Dobbs K, Laakso S, Klemetti P, Valta H, Taskinen M, Mäkitie O, Notarangelo LD. Diverse autoantibody reactivity in cartilage-hair hypoplasia. J Clin Immunol. 2017;37:508–10.

Bordon V, Gennery AR, Slatter MA, Vandecruys E, Laureys G, Veys P, Qasim W, Friedrich W, Wulfraat NM, Scherer F, Cant AJ, Fischer A, Cavazzana-Calvo M, Bredius RGM, Notarangelo LD, Mazzolari E, Neven B, Güngör Y. Clinical and immunologic outcome of patients with cartilage hair hypoplasia after hematopoietic stem cell transplantation. Blood. 2010;116(1):27–35.

Kostjukovits S, Klemetti P, Valta H, Martelius T, Notarangelo LD, Seppänen M, Taskinen M, Mäkitie O. Analysis of clinical and immunologic phenotype in a large cohort of children and adults with cartilage-hair hypoplasia. J Allergy Clin Immunol. 2017;140(2):612–4.

Ridanpää M, van Eenennaam H, Pelin K, Chadwick R, Johnson C, Yuan B, vanVenrooij W, Prujin G, Salmela R, Rockas S, Mäkitie O, Kaitila I, de la Chapelle A. Mutations in the RNA component of RNase MRP cause a pleiotropic human disease, cartilage-hair hypoplasia. Cell. 2001;104:195–203.

Rogler LE, Kosmyna B, Moskowitz D, Bebawee R, Rahimzadeh J, Kutchko K, Laederach A, Notarangelo LD, Giliani S, Bouhassira E, Frenette P, Roy-Chowdhury J, Rogler CE. Small RNAs derived from lncRNA *RNase MRP* have gene-silencing activity relevant to human cartilage-hair hypoplasia. Hum Molec Genet. 2014;23(2):358–82.

Thiel CT, Mortier G, Kaitila I, Reis A, Rauch A. Type and level of RMRP functional impairment predicts phenotype in the cartilage hair hypoplasia-anauxetic dysplasia spectrum. Am J Hum Genet. 2007;81:519–29.

Caspase Recruitment Domain 11, CARD11

Robert P. Nelson

Divisions of Hematology and Oncology, Stem Cell Transplant Program, Indiana University (IU) School of Medicine and the IU Bren and Simon Cancer Center, Indianapolis, IN, USA

Pediatric Immunodeficiency Clinic, Riley Hospital for Children at Indiana University Health, Indianapolis, IN, USA

Medicine and Pediatrics, Indiana University School of Medicine, Immunohematology and Transplantation, Indianapolis, IN, USA

Definition

Membrane-associated guanylate kinase.

Introduction/Background

The caspase recruitment domain (CARD) is a protein-binding module that mediates the assembly of CARD-containing proteins into apoptosis and nuclear factor kappa-light chain-enhancer of activated B cells (NF-kB) pro-inflammatory signaling complexes. Caspase recruitment and oligomerization mediated by adaptor proteins constitute one of multiple mechanisms that help coordinate immunity development, activation, cell migration, and apoptosis.

Function

The CARD domain of CARD11 associates specifically with the CARD domain of B cell lymphoma/leukemia 10 (BCL10), a signaling protein that activates NF-kB through the inhibitor of kappa B (IκB) kinase (IKK) complex. Another related paracaspase protein, mucosa-associated lymphoid tissue lymphoma-translocation gene 1 (MALT1), interacts with CARD11 and BCL10 to form the tripartite signalosome referred to as the CBM complex. The CBM bridges cell surface antigen receptor to NF-kB, mammalian target of rapamycin complex 1 and c-Jun terminal kinase signaling pathways. Mutations in CARD11 represent one of the growing number of combined T and B cell immunodeficiencies termed "CBM-opathies" (Lu et al. 2018).

Innate Defense

Apart from the receptor-mediated Rho-Rac-Cdc42 pathway, CARD11 participates in the regulation of cell migration during inflammation, by physically interacting with the carboxy-terminal WD40 propeller domain of actin interacting protein 1 (Aip1). This activates cofilin-mediated actin depolymerization. Thus, loss-of-function (LOF) mutations in CARD1 impair the migration of lymphocytes in-vitro and in-vivo (Li et al. 2007). Inflammasomes also activate CARD11 while mediating a highly inflammatory form of

programmed cell death called "pyroptosis," which is triggered by intracellular microbial pathogens. CARD11 activation is required for both IL-1α secretion and cell death and CARD11 transduces signals with Toll-like receptor 4 (TLR4) in response to virulent Gram-negative bacteria (Casson et al. 2013).

Adaptive Immunity

CARD11 is an important component of B cell development and activation of lymphocytes through T and B cell antigen receptors (TCR, BCR). This is accomplished by functioning as a molecular "scaffold" that controls entry of defined signaling components into the central cluster of molecules at the interface between the TCR and the antigen-presenting cell (APC), termed the immunological synapse. When the TCR is not bound to antigen, or binding is insufficiently strong or absent of second signal, CARD11 "autoregulates" by molecular inhibiting constitutively active transforming growth factor-beta (TGF-β) in naive T lymphocytes cells. When TCR engagement occurs with the correct specific antigen, TGF-β signaling is reduced by the downregulation of TGF-β receptor type 1, through activation of CARD11 and NF-kB (Tu et al. 2018).

The BCR-mediated activation of IKK and NF-kB requires protein kinase C β (PKCβ) and TGFβ-activated kinase 1 (TAK1), which interact with phosphorylated CARD11; IKK moves to the CBM complex and PKCβ brings TAK1 and IKK into close proximity, permitting TAK1 to phosphorylate IKK (Shinohara et al. 2005). Defects in CARD11 are also known to interrupt maturation and prevent differentiation of transitional B cells into marginal zone and follicular B cells (Pieper et al. 2013).

A single pathogenic homozygous nonsense mutation of exon 21 was shown to truncate the CARD11 protein rendering it defective in antigen receptor signaling and NF-kB activation. In particular, protein expression was abrogated after canonical NF-kB pathway activation in lymphocytes after TCR antigen or phorbol

12-myristate 13-acetate PMA stimulation (Stepensky et al. 2013).

Clinical Presentation

The clinical phenotypes associated with CARD11 range from severe combined immunodeficiency (SCID) at one end of the spectrum to selective B cell lymphocytosis, antibody production abnormalities and allergic diatheses at the other. Importantly, patients with defects in CARD11 causing "non-SCID" combined immunodeficiency can present with normal numbers of T and B cells, which may delay diagnosis if the clinician relies solely on quantitation of lymphocyte subpopulations without assessing function. They might have increased transitional B cells and decreased regulatory T cells. Stepensky et al. described the sentinel case of a 13-month-old child of consanguineous parents who presented with *Pneumocystis jirovecii* pneumonia and hypogammaglobulinemia (Stepensky et al. 2013). Greil et al. characterized a single LOF mutation in CARD11 that caused SCID (Greil et al. 2013). Dadi et al. and Ma et al. reported patients with CID, early-onset asthma, eczema, food allergies, and autoimmunity (Dadi et al. 2018). A recent screen of common variable immunodeficiency (CVID) patients found a number of variants in CARD11 in a 66 patient cohort but no disease-causing mutations (Tampella et al. 2011).

History and Physical

Combined T and B cell immunodeficiencies usually – but not always – present in persons below 18 years of age with atypical consequences of recurrent infections. A positive family history is a powerful risk factor, but de novo defects also occur, so that a negative family history does not rule out the condition. Newborn screening results will have demonstrated either normal or low T cell excision circles (TRECs). Cognitive impairment and developmental delay or failure to thrive (FTT), due to illness or consequences of

infection or inflammatory disease, may or may not have occurred. The history may include autoimmune manifestations, enteritis, or persistent or recurrent dermatological manifestations. One would not expect cardiovascular structural defects or an absent thymus. The physical exam may demonstrate small stature, severe atopic dermatitis or eczema in atypical locations, oral candidiasis, or lymphadenopathy; however, there are no specific, unusual, or unique pathognomonic physical features that distinguish CARD11 from other combined immunodeficiencies or primary immunodeficiencies affecting other pathways.

Laboratory Findings/Diagnostic Testing

Patients with homozygous LOF mutations experience hypogammaglobinemia due to impaired B-cell differentiation. Whereas B-cell production and differentiation render the patient with normal pan-B cell markers, maturation is blocked at the transitional stage. There may be decreased numbers of switched memory B cells and impaired *Inducible co-stimulator ligand* expression (Tampella et al. 2011). Although overall T cell numbers are normal, follicular helper and memory T cells may be abnormally distributed. The CARD11 defect may result in poor in vitro T cell responses to mitogens and antigens caused by reduced secretion of IFN-gamma and IL-2. Natural killer (NK) cells are decreased in number or in their capacity to form immunological synapses.

Treatment/Prognosis

The first clinical decision to make is whether to take care of the patent locally or consider referral to a center that has a multidisciplinary center for the management of these conditions, as exist for several of the classical immunodeficiency diseases. The patient and family may need input from social services regarding health care options and avenues to care that are either available or not. General treatment considerations of immunocompromised patients apply. Inactivated immunizations are indicated but live vaccines are not. Extreme isolation or avoidance of normal schooling may not be necessary or recommended, but rather prompt medical evaluation for early unusual consequences of infection is paramount to the care of patients with combined immunodeficiencies. The usual course of treatment for individual infectious episodes may require extension. Particular attention is given to address inflammatory conditions that require iatrogenic immunosuppression and anti-inflammatory therapy that exacerbate or synergistically add to the immunodeficiency's "potency" overall. Other measures include the use of prophylactic antibiotics as indicated with guidance informed by serial assessments of clinical and laboratory findings, including antibody production capacity (Ballow et al. 2018). Some patients need immunoglobulin replacement therapy. Early high-complexity care requires consideration – ideally before morbid complications ensue – as a bridge to curative therapeutic approaches such as hematopoietic cell transplantation.

Cross-References

▶ Evaluation of Suspected Immunodeficiency, Overview
▶ MALT1 Deficiency

References

Ballow M, Paris K, de la Morena M. Should antibiotic prophylaxis be routinely used in patients with antibody-mediated primary immunodeficiency? J Allergy Clin Immunol Pract. 2018;6(2):421–6.
Casson CN, Copenhaver AM, Zwack EE, Nguyen HT, Strowig T, Javdan B, et al. Caspase-11 activation in response to bacterial secretion systems that access the host cytosol. PLoS Pathog. 2013;9(6):e1003400.
Dadi H, Jones TA, Merico D, Sharfe N, Ovadia A, Schejter Y, et al. Combined immunodeficiency and atopy caused by a dominant negative mutation in caspase activation and recruitment domain family member 11 (CARD11). J Allergy Clin Immunol. 2018;141(5):1818–30.e2.
Greil J, Rausch T, Giese T, Bandapalli OR, Daniel V, Bekeredjian-Ding I, et al. Whole-exome sequencing links caspase recruitment domain 11 (CARD11) inactivation to severe combined immunodeficiency. J Allergy Clin Immunol. 2013;131(5):1376–83.e3.
Li J, Brieher WM, Scimone ML, Kang SJ, Zhu H, Yin H, et al. Caspase-11 regulates cell migration by promoting Aip1-Cofilin-mediated actin depolymerization. Nat Cell Biol. 2007;9(3):276–86.
Lu HY, Bauman BM, Arjunaraja S, Dorjbal B, Milner JD, Snow AL, et al. The CBM-opathies-a rapidly expanding spectrum of human inborn errors of immunity caused by mutations in the CARD11-BCL10-MALT1 Complex. Front Immunol. 2018;9:2078.
Pieper K, Grimbacher B, Eibel H. B-cell biology and development. J Allergy Clin Immunol. 2013;131(4):959–71.
Shinohara H, Yasuda T, Aiba Y, Sanjo H, Hamadate M, Watarai H, et al. PKC beta regulates BCR-mediated IKK activation by facilitating the interaction between TAK1 and CARMA1. J Exp Med. 2005;202(10):1423–31.
Stepensky P, Keller B, Buchta M, Kienzler AK, Elpeleg O, Somech R, et al. Deficiency of caspase recruitment domain family, member 11 (CARD11), causes profound combined immunodeficiency in human subjects. J Allergy Clin Immunol. 2013;131(2):477–85.e1.
Tampella G, Baronio M, Vitali M, Soresina A, Badolato R, Giliani S, et al. Evaluation of CARMA1/CARD11 and Bob1 as candidate genes in common variable immunodeficiency. J Investig Allergol Clin Immunol. 2011;21(5):348–53.
Tu E, Chia CPZ, Chen W, Zhang D, Park SA, Jin W, et al. T cell receptor-regulated TGF-beta type I receptor expression determines T cell quiescence and activation. Immunity. 2018;48(4):745–59.e6.

Cat Eye Syndrome Chromosome Region, Candidate 1 (CERC1)

▶ DADA2

CD134

▶ TNFRSF4 (OX40) Deficiency

CD19 Deficiency Due to Genetic Defects in the CD19 and CD81 Genes

Menno C. van Zelm[1,2,3] and Ismail Reisli[4]
[1]Department of Immunology and Pathology, Central Clinical School, Monash University, Melbourne, VIC, Australia
[2]Department of Respiratory Medicine, The Alfred Hospital, Melbourne, VIC, Australia
[3]The Jeffrey Modell Diagnostic and Research Centre for Primary Immunodeficiencies, Melbourne, VIC, Australia
[4]Meram Medical Faculty, Division of Pediatric Allergy and Immunology, Department of Pediatrics, Necmettin Erbakan University, Konya, Turkey

Definition

An immunodeficiency defined by deleterious mutations and/or deletions in CD19 or CD81 encoding CD19 and CD81 B cell surface proteins.

Prevalence

To date, 10 patients have been identified with CD19 deficiency due to mutations in CD19 and 1 patient due to a deleterious mutation in CD81.

Physiology of CD19 and the Complex Members CD21, CD81, and CD225

B-cell lineage commitment from hematopoietic stem cells is a stepwise process and critically depends on several transcription factors, including E2A, EBF, and Pax5 (Lin and Grosschedl 1995; Urbanek et al. 1994; Zhuang et al. 1994). In addition to functioning as B-cell commitment factor, Pax5 directly regulates CD19 gene expression (Kozmik et al. 1992). As a result, CD19 membrane expression – first described in 1983 (Nadler et al. 1983) – is a direct marker of committed B cells and is reflective of the expression of Pax5 (Fig. 1). CD19 is expressed prior to surface immunoglobulin (Ig) and two previously characterized markers that are now known as CD20 (Stashenko et al. 1980) and CD21 (Nadler et al. 1981) (Fig. 1).

The CD19 gene encodes a single transmembrane protein with an N-terminal extracellular domain containing 2 Ig-like domains and a C-terminal intracellular tail with conserved tyrosine residues necessary for intracellular signaling (Stamenkovic and Seed 1988; Tedder and Isaacs 1989) (Fig. 1). CD19 was found to directly bind to CD21 (complement receptor 2; CR2) (Matsumoto et al. 1991), which binds to complement fragment C3d and is the receptor for Epstein-Barr virus (EBV) (Moore et al. 1987; Tedder et al. 1984; Weis et al. 1987). Two other components of the same complex were found to be CD81 (TAPA-1) and CD225 (encoded by the *IFITM1* gene) (Bradbury et al. 1992). CD81 and CD225 had been identified before (Chen et al. 1984; Oren et al. 1990) and were found to bind each other (Takahashi et al. 1990). The proteins are not lineage-restricted and bind each other independent of CD19 or CD21. Conversely, CD19 expression does require the presence of CD81 (Maecker and Levy 1997; Miyazaki et al. 1997; Tsitsikov et al. 1997), and in turn CD19 directly binds CD21 (Matsumoto et al. 1991). The complex of CD19/CD21/CD81/CD225 is fully formed on immature and mature B cells (Fig. 1) and functions to augment signaling through surface immunoglobulins (B-cell antigen receptor; BCR) (Bradbury et al. 1992; Matsumoto et al. 1993).

Clinical Presentation

All 11 patients presented during childhood, predominantly with recurrent upper and/or lower respiratory infections (Table 1). In several cases, bacterial septicemia, meningitis, and conjunctivitis have been observed, as well as gastrointestinal problems. The severity of infections is highly variable between patients, and the benign disease course in four patients was likely the cause of

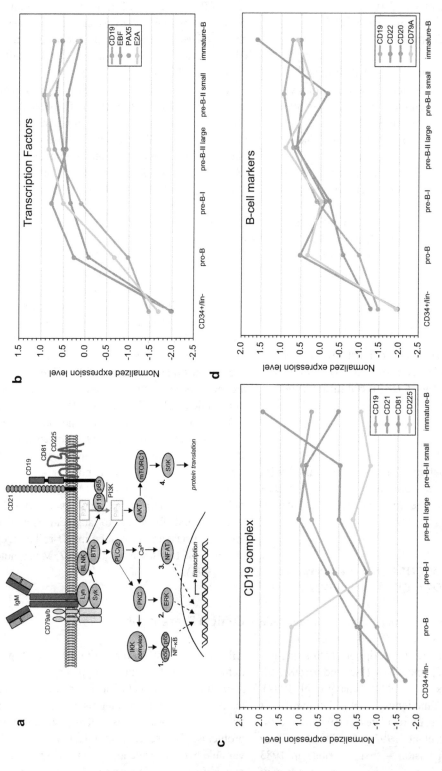

CD19 Deficiency Due to Genetic Defects in the CD19 and CD81 Genes, Fig. 1 CD19 complex function and gene expression levels in B-cell precursors. (**a**) Upon antigen recognition, the BCR induces a signaling cascade. The CD19 complex acts to lower the threshold for activation through recruitment of phosphoinositide 3-kinase (PI3K). Together, these signals induce nuclear translocation of at least three transcription factors (NF-kB, ERK, and NFAT) and stimulate protein translation. (**b–d**) Gene expression levels of CD19-complex members (**b**), other B-cell markers (**c**), and transcription factors (**d**). Data are derived from purified B-cell precursors using Affymetrix HG-U133A/B Gene Chips and data were normalized into zero mean and unit standard deviation (z-score) (van Zelm et al. 2005)

CD19 Deficiency Due to Genetic Defects in the CD19 and CD81 Genes, Table 1 Epidemiological, genetic, and clinical characteristics of all CD19 deficiency cases with genetic defects in *CD19* and *CD81* that have been reported to date

Patient	Descent	Gene	Gender	Age at onset	Age at diagnosis	Presenting manifestations	Clinical manifestations before diagnosis	Clinical manifestations at diagnosis	Treatment	Outcome	Reference
A1	Turkish	CD19	F	1	10	LRI	Recurrent LRI and meningitis	COPD, postinfectious GN	IVIG, NSAID	Mild SLE, good	(Artac et al. 2010; van Zelm et al. 2006)
A2			M	0.5	12	Recurrent URI/LRI	Recurrent LRI and otitis	Recurrent URI/LRI	IVIG	Good	
B1	Colombian	CD19	M	7	35	URI	Recurrent LRI, chronic sinusitis	LRI, bacterial conjunctivitis, gastritis	IVIG, sinus surgery	Good	(van Zelm et al. 2006)
B2			F	6	33	URI	LRI, herpes zoster, chronic sinusitis	Recurrent bacterial conjunctivitis/ dacryocystitis, diarrhea	IVIG, sinus surgery	Good	
B3			F	5	49	URI	Recurrent LRI, recurrent skin abscesses, chronic sinusitis	LRI, recurrent bacterial conjunctivitis, chronic diarrhea	IVIG, sinus surgery	Good	
C1	Japanese	CD19	M	5	8[a]	Pyelonephritis, bronchitis, gastritis, thrombocytopenia	NR	Pyelonephritis, bronchitis, gastritis, thrombocytopenia	IVIGs	Good	(Kanegane et al. 2007)
D1	Moroccan	CD19	M	NR	6	URI/LRI	Recurrent URI/LRI, *S. pneumoniae* septicemia	Recurrent URI/LRI	IVIG, SCIG	Good	(van Zelm et al. 2011)
E1	Kurdish	CD19	F	5	11	URI, giardiasis	Recurrent URI	Pneumococcal meningitis	NR	Good	(Vince et al. 2011)

(continued)

CD19 Deficiency Due to Genetic Defects in the CD19 and CD81 Genes, Table 1 (continued)

Patient	Descent	Gene	Gender	Age at onset	Age at diagnosis	Presenting manifestations	Clinical manifestations before diagnosis	Clinical manifestations at diagnosis	Treatment	Outcome	Reference
F1	Moroccan	CD19	F	13	31	Failure to thrive, microscopic hematuria, proteinuria	Chronic sinusitis, pneumococcal pneumonia	IgA nephropathy, nephrotic syndrome	Sinus surgery	Nephrotic syndrome/ ESRD	(Vince et al. 2011)
G1	French	CD19	M	3mo	11[b]	RSV bronchiolitis, asthma mimicking symptoms	Asthma resembling symptoms Recurrent URI/LRI	Bronchiectasis, lobar atelectasis, COPD	IVIG, lobectomy	Chronic lung disease	(Skendros et al. 2014)
H1	Moroccan	CD81	F	2	6[c]	NR	IgA nephropathy, Henoch-Schönlein purpura	Thrombocytopenia, hypogammaglobulinemia	IVIG, immune suppression	Nephrotic syndrome /ESRD	(van Zelm et al. 2010)

Table adapted from Skendros et al. 2014.

COPD chronic obstructive pulmonary disease, *ESRD* end-stage renal disease, *F* female, *GN* glomerulonephritis, *IVIGs* intravenous immunoglobulins, *LRI* lower respiratory infection, *M* male, *NR* non-reported, *RSV* respiratory syncytial virus, *SCIGs* subcutaneous immunoglobulins, *URI* upper respiratory infection

[a]Diagnosis of CVID and IVIG therapy at age of 5 year, genetic diagnosis of CD19 deficiency at age of 8 year

[b]Diagnosis of hypogammaglobulinemia and IVIG therapy at age of 7 year, genetic diagnosis of CD19 deficiency at age of 11 year

[c]Diagnosis of IgA nephropathy and Henoch-Schönlein purpura at age 3.5 year, genetic diagnosis of CD19 deficiency and start IVIG at age of 6 year

delayed diagnosis in adulthood, 18–44 years after onset of infections (patients B1–3 and F1).

In addition to bacterial infections, several patients experienced complications due to viral infections (herpes zoster, RSV) or parasites (giardiasis). Noninfectious complications are rare and include one patient with mild systemic lupus erythematosus (SLE). Further, two patients, one with CD19 and one with CD81 gene defects, suffered from IgA nephropathy, and 4/11 patients had specific auto antibodies and defective selection against autoreactivity in IgG and IgA transcripts (van Zelm et al. 2014), however, currently without specific organ disease.

Genetics

In total, 11 patients from 8 families have been described with a CD19 deficiency (Table 1). Ten patients have biallelic genetic defects in CD19 (Fig. 2), and all but one were homozygous.

a

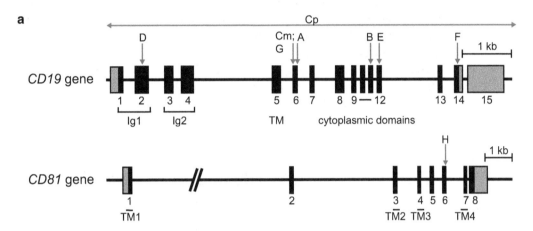

b

family	descent	patients	gene	allele	mutation	effect on protein	reference
A	Turkish	2	CD19	both	c.972insA	p.R325A fsX4	(van Zelm et al., 2006; Artac et al., 2010)
B	Colombian	3	CD19	both	c.1384delGA	p.N463R fsX3	(van Zelm et al., 2006)
C	Japanese	1	CD19	maternal paternal	c.947-1G>T deletion of entire gene	p.A316D fsX5 p.X	(Kanegane et al., 2007)
D	Moroccan	1	CD19	both	c.156G>C	p.W52C	(van Zelm et al., 2011)
E	Kurdish	1	CD19	both	c.1464delC	p.P488P fsX15	(Vince et al., 2011)
F	Moroccan	1	CD19	both	c.1653_1671+9del28ins23	G551G fsX25	(Vince et al., 2011)
G	French	1	CD19	both	c.947-1G>T *	p.A316D fsX5	(Skendros et al., 2014)
H	Moroccan	1	CD81	both	c.561+1G>A	p.E188M fsX13	(van Zelm et al., 2010)

* same mutation as maternal allele of patient from Fam C

CD19 Deficiency Due to Genetic Defects in the CD19 and CD81 Genes, Fig. 2 Overview genetic defects in CD19-deficient patients. (**a**) Schematic depiction of the human CD19 and CD81 genes with the positions of the identified genetic defects. (**b**) Overview of mutant alleles in 11 patients from 8 unrelated families

Although not all parents from patients with homozygous defects were confirmed to be relatives, taking into account the rarity of the mutant alleles, CD19 deficiency is most likely to be found in children from consanguineous parents. Remarkably, the heterozygous splice site mutation c.947-1G>T from Japanese patient C1 was also found in homozygous state in French patient G1. Considering the different genetic backgrounds, it is likely that these events occurred independently and that to date eight unique genetic lesions in CD19 have been described. These concerned four small insertions and/or deletions, one large deletion, and two splice site mutations that all resulted in complete absence of truncated CD19 proteins. In only one case, a missense mutation concerning a conserved tryptophan resulted in the complete absence of membrane CD19 (van Zelm et al. 2011). The

complete absence of CD19 membrane expression resulted in reduced CD21 expression levels but did not affect CD81 or CD225 expression (Fig. 3).

The 11th patient (H1) did not carry mutations in her CD19 alleles (Fig. 2). Instead, a homozygous splice site mutation was identified in the CD81 gene that disrupted membrane expression of both CD19 and CD81 (Fig. 3) (van Zelm et al. 2010). CD21 was only slightly reduced and CD225 normally expressed on the patient's B cells. Using in vitro complementation experiments, it was demonstrated that the defective CD81 expression resulted in absence of CD19 on the patient's B cells. These results confirmed and extended previous observations of the dependence of CD19 membrane expression in CD81 (Maecker and Levy 1997; Miyazaki et al. 1997; Tsitsikov et al. 1997).

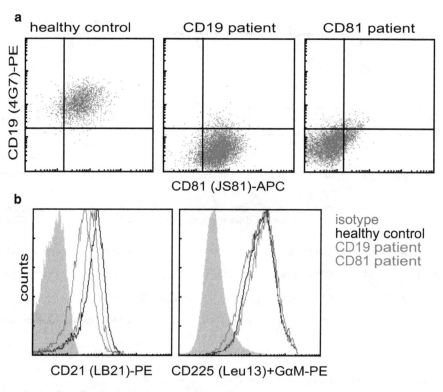

CD19 Deficiency Due to Genetic Defects in the CD19 and CD81 Genes, Fig. 3 Expression of CD19-complex members on B cells. (**a**) Dot plots showing CD19 and CD81 expression on B cells from a healthy control, patient

D1 with a CD19 gene defect and patient H1 with a CD81 gene defect. (**b**) CD21 and CD225 expression levels on B cells from the same individuals as in **a**

Immunological Phenotype

Until that time, genetic defects underlying predominantly antibody deficiencies (PAD) had only been identified in patients with agammaglobulinemia and a complete lack of B cells and in patients with a defect in germinal center responses and Ig class switch recombination (Conley et al. 2009). CD19-deficient patients differed from both groups in regards to the presence of B cells in blood and normal architecture of germinal centers in lymphoid tissue despite hypogammaglobulinemia (Artac et al. 2010; Kanegane et al. 2007; Skendros et al. 2014; van Zelm et al. 2006, 2010, 2011; Vince et al. 2011).

Immunologically, all patients show typical features of antibody deficiency with low IgG in combination with reduced serum IgA and/or IgM levels (Tables 2 and 3), and impaired responses to vaccinations (Tables 2 and 3). Only patient F1 was specifically deficient in IgG1 with normal to high levels of other IgG subclasses, IgM and IgA, and normal responses to previous vaccinations (Table 3). Thus, with the exception of patient F1, CD19-deficient patients fit the criteria of common variable immunodeficiency (CVID) (Bousfiha et al. 2015; Conley et al. 1999).

Leukocyte and lymphocyte subsets were normally present in all patients, with the exception of low total B cell numbers in one child and one adult with CD19 gene defects. The reduced IgG serum levels were accompanied by low memory B cell numbers, again with the exception of patient F1. Interestingly, most patients showed reduced numbers of transitional B cells. On the other hand, the patients did not display an expansion of $CD21^{low}$ B cells that is frequently found in patients with CVID (Warnatz et al. 2002; Wehr et al. 2008). This was irrespective of the generally lower expression levels of CD21 on patient's B cells as a result of the absence of CD19 (Fig. 3b) (van Zelm et al. 2006, 2011).

Heterozygous carriers of CD19 or CD81 gene defects have reduced expression of surface CD19 on their B cells (Fig. 3c) (Artac et al. 2010; Reisli et al. 2009; van Zelm et al. 2006, 2010, 2011). In carriers with CD19 gene defects, this is accompanied by reduced CD21 expression levels. Despite these phenotypical changes, extensive analysis of 30 carriers revealed that these were not more susceptible to infections, had normal total serum IgG, IgA and IgM levels, as well as normal responses to vaccinations and circulating memory B cells (Artac et al. 2010).

The impaired antibody responses in CD19-deficient patients seemed to result from defective activation of B cells via their BCRs. B cells from all tested patients showed impaired fluxes of intracellular Ca2+ upon stimulation with anti-IgM (van Zelm et al. 2006, 2010, 2011). CD19 is already expressed in precursor B cells in bone marrow at the stage where the pre-BCR is expressed. Signaling via the pre-BCR is crucial for developmental progression of progenitor B cells. As a result, genetic defects in genes encoding components of this pre-BCR (Igμ, CD79a, CD79b, and λ14.1) and directly downstream signaling molecules (BTK, BLNK, PLCγ2) result in a complete absence of mature B cells and hypogammaglobulinemia (Conley et al. 2009). As CD19-deficient patients do not lack mature B cells, it can be concluded that CD19 does not have a critical role in pre-BCR signaling. However, 2/11 patients presented with low total B cell numbers (Tables 2 and 3). Thus, in line with mouse models (Diamant et al. 2005; Otero and Rickert 2003), it is possible that human progenitor B cell differentiation is less efficient in absence of CD19.

Importantly, in vitro stimulation of B cells was dependent on CD19 even in the absence of complement, suggesting that the CD19-complex can be recruited to the BCR in absence of crosslinking via C3d and CD21. Indeed, CD21 is not required for B-cell activation via the BCR with large amounts of antigen (Thiel et al. 2012; Wentink et al. 2015). Only with limiting amounts of IgM, crosslinking the BCR via complement and CD21 to the CD19-complex is needed to induce a Ca2+ flux (Thiel et al. 2012). The potential of CD19 to signal independently of CD21 likely underlies the relatively mild phenotype of CD21-deficient individuals. Their B cells express normal to high levels of CD19 and are capable of mounting specific antibody responses (Thiel et al. 2012; Wentink et al. 2015).

CD19 Deficiency Due to Genetic Defects in the CD19 and CD81 Genes, Table 2   Immunological characteristics of pediatric CD19-deficient patients

	A1	A2	C1	D1	E1	G1	H1	Normal values
Gender	F	M	M	M	F	M	F	
Age (year)	10	12	8	6	11	11	4	
Blood cells (cells/µl)								
Lymphocytes	4480	1900	ND	1630	2745	ND	2195	2906 ± 1,081[a]
CD3+ T cells	3270	1700	1775	1107	2141	ND	1385	2000 ± 766
CD4+ T cells	1792	669	1064	637	1125	ND	956	1247 ± 601
CD8+ T cells	1478	1031	781	353	796	ND	345	547 ± 184
CD20+ B cells	806	**60**	538	321	300	ND	426	453 ± 265
CD16/CD56+ NK cells	313	100	ND	156	184	ND	292	266 ± 170
B-cell subsets (% of CD20)								
Transitional	ND	8	ND	3	**0**	5	**1**	6 ± 3
Naive mature	91	87	67.5	90	89	91	90	66 ± 9
CD27 + IgM + IgD+ memory	**3**	**2**	5.4	**3**	8	**2**	4	7 ± 3
CD27 + IgD- memory	**2**	**1**	7.6	**3**	**2**	**1**	**3**	11 ± 5
Ig serum levels (g/L)								
IgG	**3.25**	**0.91**	**2.49**	**3.00**	**2.30**	**4.4**	**2.40**	5.04-14.64
IgG1	ND	ND	ND	ND	**0.66**	**1.7**	ND	2.92-8.16
IgG2	ND	ND	ND	ND	**1.44**	3.4	ND	0.83-5.13
IgG3	ND	ND	ND	ND	36	**0.4**	ND	0.08-1.11
IgG4	ND	ND	ND	ND	**<0.01**	**0.002**	ND	0.01-1.21
IgA	2.92	**0.01**	**0.10**	**0.50**	1.25	Normal	0.71	0.27-1.95
IgM	**0.25**	0.59	**0.18**	**0.40**	**0.35**	**0.4**	**0.35**	0.24-2.10
IgE (IU/ml)	37	ND	9	ND	ND	ND	ND	0-100
Isohemagglutinins	**Absent**			**Low**				
Vaccination responses	Impaired	Impaired	Impaired	Impaired	Impaired	Impaired	Impaired	
Autoantibodies	SS-A, ANA	–	ND	ND	ND	ND	Anti-platelet	

M male, *F* female. Only positive tests for autoantibodies are indicated. Bold font indicates subnormal values; underlined supranormal. *ND* not determined

[a]Mean ± SD from (van Zelm et al. 2011)

CD19 Deficiency Due to Genetic Defects in the CD19 and CD81 Genes, Table 3 Immunological characteristics of adult CD19-deficient patients

	B1	B2	B3	F1	Normal values
Gender	M	F	F	F	
Age (year)	35	33	49	31	
Blood cells (cells/µl)					
Lymphocytes	2182	2508	2059	1440	1000–2800
CD3+ T cells	1520	1855	1384	1152	700–2100
CD4+ T cells	713	1070	620	590	300–1400
CD8+ T cells	720	692	696	533	200–900
CD19+ B cells	286	521	268	**61**	100–500
CD16/CD56+ NK cells	277	348	288	**23**	90–600
B-cell subsets (% of CD20)					
Transitional	ND	ND	ND	**0**	2 (1–3)[a]
Naive mature	92	96	92	59	67 (54–76)[a]
CD27 + IgM + IgD+ memory	**5**	**1**	**3**	22	15 (11–23)[a]
CD27 + IgD- memory	**1**	**0**	**2**	12	15 (10–20)[a]
Ig serum levels (g/L)					
IgG	**2.04**	**1.98**	**2.56**	**4.93**	7.51–15.6
IgG1	ND	ND	ND	**1.70**	4.9–11.4
IgG2	ND	ND	ND	3.06	1.5–6.4
IgG3	ND	ND	ND	_2.11_	0.2–1.1
IgG4	ND	ND	ND	2	0.08–1.4
IgA	**0.18**	**0.07**	**0.19**	3.50	0.82–4.53
IgM	**0.47**	**0.30**	0.60	1.35	0.46–3.04
IgE (IU/ml)	ND	ND	ND	ND	0–100
Isohemagglutinins	**Low**	**Low**	**Low**	Present	
Vaccination responses	**Impaired**	**Impaired**	**Impaired**	Normal	
Autoantibodies	–	–	Anti-DNA	ANA	

M male, *F* female. Only positive tests for autoantibodies are indicated. Bold font indicates subnormal values; underlined supranormal. *ND* not determined
[a]Median (IQR) from (Mouillot et al. 2010)

Complement-independent recruitment of the CD19-complex to the BCR is thought to be regulated via the CD81-tetraspanin network (Mattila et al. 2013). Upon antigen binding, the BCR triggers signaling and reorganization of the cytoskeleton (Freeman et al. 2015). This increases BCR mobility and diffusion (Treanor et al. 2010) to allow interactions with CD19 that is immobilized on the membrane by the CD81-tetraspanin network. Specifically, CD19-mediated recruitment of Vav, PLCγ2, and PI3K enhances BCR-induced signaling.

In addition to enhancing BCR signaling, CD19-mediated recruitment has been shown to enhance Toll-like receptor (TLR)9 and BAFFR signaling (Keppler et al. 2015; Morbach et al. 2016). Rather than a co-receptor complex that is recruited, it might be more appropriate to view the CD19-complex as a generic hub used by receptors in and on B cells to induce PI3K signaling.

Diagnosis

Currently, all identified mutations result in absence of membrane CD19 expression. This could be due to selective reporting as absence of CD19 provides the best clue for a CD19 deficiency. The conserved tyrosines in the C-terminal cytoplasmic tail of CD19 are critical for its function (Sato et al. 1997; Wang et al. 2002). Hence, mutations that affect these residues or that result in truncated forms could potentially be expressed, while still lack functional properties. Defective CD19 expression can be readily assessed by routine staining of peripheral blood lymphocytes including antibodies against CD19 for detection of B cells. It is noticed because the percentages of all lymphocyte subpopulations do not add up to 100%. The use of a CD19 antibody in combination with another broadly B-cell reactive antibody such as CD20, CD22, IgM, or IgD is suggested to prevent misdiagnosis of agammaglobulinemia.

Additional surface staining for CD81 and genetic analysis are needed for a final diagnosis and to distinguish between mutations in CD19 and CD81.

Management of CD19 Deficiency

The predominant clinical complications of CD19-deficient patients are recurrent respiratory infections (Table 1). Therefore, immunoglobulin replacement therapy is the treatment of choice. CD19-deficient patients rarely require immunosuppressive therapy. While hematopoietic stem cell transplantation is potentially curative, the prognosis of CD19 deficiency seems to be favorable in the absence of IgA nephropathy, and therefore none of the currently described patients has required this therapy.

References

Artac H, Reisli I, Kara R, Pico-Knijnenburg I, Adin-Cinar-S, Pekcan S, Jol-van der Zijde CM, van Tol MJ, Bakker-Jonges LE, van Dongen JJ, et al. B-cell maturation and antibody responses in individuals carrying a mutated CD19 allele. Genes Immun. 2010;11:523–30.

Bousfiha A, Jeddane L, Al-Herz W, Ailal F, Casanova JL, Chatila T, Conley ME, Cunningham-Rundles C, Etzioni A, Franco JL, et al. The 2015 IUIS Phenotypic Classification for Primary Immunodeficiencies. J Clin Immunol. 2015;35:727–38.

Bradbury LE, Kansas GS, Levy S, Evans RL, Tedder TF. The CD19/CD21 signal transducing complex of human B lymphocytes includes the target of antiproliferative antibody-1 and Leu-13 molecules. J Immunol. 1992;149:2841–50.

Chen YX, Welte K, Gebhard DH, Evans RL. Induction of T cell aggregation by antibody to a 16kd human leukocyte surface antigen. J Immunol. 1984;133:2496–501.

Conley ME, Notarangelo LD, Etzioni A. Diagnostic criteria for primary immunodeficiencies. Representing PAGID (Pan-American Group for Immunodeficiency) and ESID (European Society for Immunodeficiencies). Clin Immunol. 1999;93:190–7.

Conley ME, Dobbs AK, Farmer DM, Kilic S, Paris K, Grigoriadou S, Coustan-Smith E, Howard V, Campana D. Primary B cell immunodeficiencies: comparisons and contrasts. Annu Rev Immunol. 2009;27:199–227.

Diamant E, Keren Z, Melamed D. CD19 regulates positive selection and maturation in B lymphopoiesis: lack of CD19 imposes developmental arrest of immature B cells and consequential stimulation of receptor editing. Blood. 2005;105:3247–54.

Freeman SA, Jaumouille V, Choi K, Hsu BE, Wong HS, Abraham L, Graves ML, Coombs D, Roskelley CD, Das R, et al. Toll-like receptor ligands sensitize B-cell receptor signalling by reducing actin-dependent spatial confinement of the receptor. Nat Commun. 2015;6:6168.

Kanegane H, Agematsu K, Futatani T, Sira MM, Suga K, Sekiguchi T, van Zelm MC, Miyawaki T. Novel mutations in a Japanese patient with CD19 deficiency. Genes Immun. 2007;8:663–70.

Keppler SJ, Gasparrini F, Burbage M, Aggarwal S, Frederico B, Geha RS, Way M, Bruckbauer A, Batista FD. Wiskott-Aldrich syndrome interacting protein deficiency uncovers the role of the co-receptor CD19 as a generic hub for PI3 kinase signaling in B cells. Immunity. 2015;43:660–73.

Kozmik Z, Wang S, Dorfler P, Adams B, Busslinger M. The promoter of the CD19 gene is a target for the B-cell-specific transcription factor BSAP. Mol Cell Biol. 1992;12:2662–72.

Lin H, Grosschedl R. Failure of B-cell differentiation in mice lacking the transcription factor EBF. Nature. 1995;376:263–7.

Maecker HT, Levy S. Normal lymphocyte development but delayed humoral immune response in CD81-null mice. J Exp Med. 1997;185:1505–10.

Matsumoto AK, Kopicky-Burd J, Carter RH, Tuveson DA, Tedder TF, Fearon DT. Intersection of the complement and immune systems: a signal transduction complex of the B lymphocyte-containing complement receptor type 2 and CD19. J Exp Med. 1991;173:55–64.

Matsumoto AK, Martin DR, Carter RH, Klickstein LB, Ahearn JM, Fearon DT. Functional dissection of the CD21/CD19/TAPA-1/Leu-13 complex of B lymphocytes. J Exp Med. 1993;178:1407–17.

Mattila PK, Feest C, Depoil D, Treanor B, Montaner B, Otipoby KL, Carter R, Justement LB, Bruckbauer A, Batista FD. The actin and tetraspanin networks organize receptor nanoclusters to regulate B cell receptor-mediated signaling. Immunity. 2013;38:461–74.

Miyazaki T, Muller U, Campbell KS. Normal development but differentially altered proliferative responses of lymphocytes in mice lacking CD81. EMBO J. 1997;16:4217–25.

Moore MD, Cooper NR, Tack BF, Nemerow GR. Molecular cloning of the cDNA encoding the Epstein-Barr virus/C3d receptor (complement receptor type 2) of human B lymphocytes. Proc Natl Acad Sci U S A. 1987;84:9194–8.

Morbach H, Schickel JN, Cunningham-Rundles C, Conley ME, Reisli I, Franco JL, Meffre E. CD19 controls Toll-like receptor 9 responses in human B cells. J Allergy Clin Immunol. 2016;137:889–98.e6.

Mouillot G, Carmagnat M, Gerard L, Garnier JL, Fieschi C, Vince N, Karlin L, Viallard JF, Jaussaud R, Boileau J, et al. B-cell and T-cell phenotypes in CVID patients correlate with the clinical phenotype of the disease. J Clin Immunol. 2010;30:746–55.

Nadler LM, Stashenko P, Hardy R, van Agthoven A, Terhorst C, Schlossman SF. Characterization of a human B cell-specific antigen (B2) distinct from B1. J Immunol. 1981;126:1941–7.

Nadler LM, Anderson KC, Marti G, Bates M, Park E, Daley JF, Schlossman SF. B4, a human B lymphocyte-associated antigen expressed on normal, mitogen-activated, and malignant B lymphocytes. J Immunol. 1983;131:244–50.

Oren R, Takahashi S, Doss C, Levy R, Levy S. TAPA-1, the target of an antiproliferative antibody, defines a new family of transmembrane proteins. Mol Cell Biol. 1990;10:4007–15.

Otero DC, Rickert RC. CD19 function in early and late B cell development. II. CD19 facilitates the pro-B/pre-B transition. J Immunol. 2003;171:5921–30.

Reisli I, Artac H, Pekcan S, Kara R, Yumiu K, Karagol C, Cimen O, Sen M, Artac M. CD19 deficiency: a village screening study. Turk Arch Ped. 2009;44:127–30.

Sato S, Miller AS, Howard MC, Tedder TF. Regulation of B lymphocyte development and activation by the CD19/CD21/CD81/Leu 13 complex requires the cytoplasmic domain of CD19. J Immunol. 1997;159:3278–87.

Skendros P, Rondeau S, Chateil JF, Bui S, Bocly V, Moreau JF, Theodorou I, Aladjidi N. Misdiagnosed CD19 deficiency leads to severe lung disease. Pediatr Allergy Immunol. 2014;25:603–6.

Stamenkovic I, Seed B. CD19, the earliest differentiation antigen of the B cell lineage, bears three extracellular immunoglobulin-like domains and an Epstein-Barr virus-related cytoplasmic tail. J Exp Med. 1988;168:1205–10.

Stashenko P, Nadler LM, Hardy R, Schlossman SF. Characterization of a human B lymphocyte-specific antigen. J Immunol. 1980;125:1678–85.

Takahashi S, Doss C, Levy S, Levy R. TAPA-1, the target of an antiproliferative antibody, is associated on the cell surface with the Leu-13 antigen. J Immunol. 1990;145:2207–13.

Tedder TF, Isaacs CM. Isolation of cDNAs encoding the CD19 antigen of human and mouse B lymphocytes. A new member of the immunoglobulin superfamily. J Immunol. 1989;143:712–7.

Tedder TF, Clement LT, Cooper MD. Expression of C3d receptors during human B cell differentiation: immunofluorescence analysis with the HB-5 monoclonal antibody. J Immunol. 1984;133:678–83.

Thiel J, Kimmig L, Salzer U, Grudzien M, Lebrecht D, Hagena T, Draeger R, Voelxen N, Bergbreiter A, Jennings S, et al. Genetic CD21 deficiency is associated with hypogammaglobulinemia. J Allergy Clin Immunol. 2012;129:801–810.e6.

Treanor B, Depoil D, Gonzalez-Granja A, Barral P, Weber M, Dushek O, Bruckbauer A, Batista FD. The membrane skeleton controls diffusion dynamics and signaling through the B cell receptor. Immunity. 2010;32:187–99.

Tsitsikov EN, Gutierrez-Ramos JC, Geha RS. Impaired CD19 expression and signaling, enhanced antibody response to type II T independent antigen and reduction of B-1 cells in CD81-deficient mice. Proc Natl Acad Sci U S A. 1997;94:10844–9.

Urbanek P, Wang ZQ, Fetka I, Wagner EF, Busslinger M. Complete block of early B cell differentiation and altered patterning of the posterior midbrain in mice lacking Pax5/BSAP. Cell. 1994;79:901–12.

van Zelm MC, van der Burg M, de Ridder D, Barendregt BH, de Haas EF, Reinders MJ, Lankester AC, Revesz T, Staal FJ, van Dongen JJ. Ig gene rearrangement steps are initiated in early human precursor B cell subsets and correlate with specific transcription factor expression. J Immunol. 2005;175: 5912–22.

van Zelm MC, Reisli I, van der Burg M, Castaño D, van Noesel CJM, van Tol MJD, Woellner C, Grimbacher B, Patiño PJ, van Dongen JJM, Franco JL. An antibody-deficiency syndrome due to mutations in the CD19 gene. N Engl J Med. 2006;354:1901–12.

van Zelm MC, Smet J, Adams B, Mascart F, Schandene L, Janssen F, Ferster A, Kuo CC, Levy S, van Dongen JJ, van der Burg M. CD81 gene defect in humans disrupts CD19 complex formation and leads to antibody deficiency. J Clin Invest. 2010;120: 1265–74.

van Zelm MC, Smet J, van der Burg M, Ferster A, Le PQ, Schandene L, van Dongen JJ, Mascart F. Antibody deficiency due to a missense mutation in CD19 demonstrates the importance of the conserved tryptophan 41 in immunoglobulin superfamily domain formation. Hum Mol Genet. 2011;20:1854–63.

van Zelm MC, Bartol SJ, Driessen GJ, Mascart F, Reisli I, Franco JL, Wolska-Kusnierz B, Kanegane H, Boon L, van Dongen JJ, van der Burg M. Human CD19 and CD40L deficiencies impair antibody selection and differentially affect somatic hypermutation. J Allergy Clin Immunol. 2014;134:135–44.

Vince N, Boutboul D, Mouillot G, Just N, Peralta M, Casanova JL, Conley ME, Bories JC, Oksenhendler E, Malphettes M, et al. Defects in the CD19 complex predispose to glomerulonephritis, as well as IgG1 subclass deficiency. J Allergy Clin Immunol. 2011;127:538–541e1–5.

Wang Y, Brooks SR, Li X, Anzelon AN, Rickert RC, Carter RH. The physiologic role of CD19 cytoplasmic tyrosines. Immunity. 2002;17:501–14.

Warnatz K, Wehr C, Drager R, Schmidt S, Eibel H, Schlesier M, Peter HH. Expansion of CD19(hi)CD21 (lo/neg) B cells in common variable immunodeficiency (CVID) patients with autoimmune cytopenia. Immunobiology. 2002;206:502–13.

Wehr C, Kivioja T, Schmitt C, Ferry B, Witte T, Eren E, Vlkova M, Hernandez M, Detkova D, Bos PR, et al. The EUROclass trial: defining subgroups in common variable immunodeficiency. Blood. 2008;111:77–85.

Weis JH, Morton CC, Bruns GA, Weis JJ, Klickstein LB, Wong WW, Fearon DT. A complement receptor locus: genes encoding C3b/C4b receptor and C3d/Epstein-Barr virus receptor map to 1q32. J Immunol. 1987;138:312–5.

Wentink MW, Lambeck AJ, van Zelm MC, Simons E, van Dongen JJ, IJspeert H, Scholvinck EH, van der Burg M. CD21 and CD19 deficiency: Two defects in the same complex leading to different disease modalities. Clin Immunol. 2015;161:120–7.

Zhuang Y, Soriano P, Weintraub H. The helix-loop-helix gene E2A is required for B cell formation. Cell. 1994;79:875–84.

CD20 Deficiency, Lessons Related to Therapeutic Biologicals and Primary Immunodeficiency

Taco W. Kuijpers
Department of Pediatric Immunology, Rheumatology and Infectious Diseases, Emma Children's Hospital, Amsterdam University Medical Center (Amsterdam UMC), Amsterdam, The Netherlands

Background

CD20 was one of the first B-cell-specific differentiation antigens identified (Stashenko et al. 1980). Nowadays, anti-CD20 immunotherapy using chimeric monoclonal antibodies (MoAbs) is used for the treatment of B-cell neoplasia, EBV-associated immunopathology, and a growing list of diseases with presumed autoimmune origin (Franks et al. 2016; Miano 2016; Claes et al. 2015; Froissart et al. 2015).

CD20, encoded by membrane-spanning 4 domains, subfamily a, member 1 (*MS4A1*; OMIM*112210), belongs to the MS4A family of molecules with multiple membrane-spanning domains (Liang et al. 2001; Liang and Tedder 2001) and is expressed on pre-B and mature B cells but is downregulated upon differentiation into plasma cells (Tedder and Engel 1994). CD20 is unlikely to have a natural ligand, but in vitro studies with CD20, MoAbs have demonstrated its involvement in the regulation of B-cell activation and proliferation (Tedder et al. 1985, 1986).

The *CD20* gene structure and expression pattern are strongly conserved between mouse and human (Tedder et al. 1988, 1989; Uchida et al. 2004a), and CD20-knockout mice have been independently generated by two groups (Uchida et al. 2004a; O'Keefe et al. 1998). $CD20^{-/-}$ B cells develop and function normally, but spleen B cells exhibit demonstrable alterations in BCR- and CD19-induced Ca^{2+} responses (Uchida et al. 2004a). The importance of CD20 for the generation and function of human B cells has yet to be clarified.

B-Cell Development and Mechanistic Role for CD20

Peripheral B-cell survival relies on signals from the BCR and the BAFFR (O'Keefe et al. 1998). The BCR is a heterotrimeric complex consisting of Ag-binding Ig and the signaling Igα/Igβ heterodimers.

Crosslinking the BCR on mature B cells with Ag or anti-IgM Abs initiates multiple intracellular signaling cascades, which eventually lead to the activation of ERK, NF-kB, and NFAT pathways. Among these, NF-kB appears to play a prominently protective role in the survival of Ag-stimulated B cells by inducing the expression of several antiapoptotic proteins such as Bcl-2, Bcl-xL, and Bfl-1 (Mackay et al. 2010; Grumont et al. 1998, 1999). BCR signaling activates the canonical NF-kB pathway, which is characterized by the phosphorylation and ubiquitin-mediated degradation of IkB inhibitory proteins, in particular IkB-alpha. This leads to the translocation of NF-kB1 into the nucleus to activate target gene transcription. BAFFR is a member of the TNFR family.

Deficiency of BAFF or BAFFR results in an almost complete loss of follicular and marginal zone (MZ) B cells (Saijo et al. 2002; Schiemann et al. 2001; Thompson et al. 2001), demonstrating a critical role for BAFFR-mediated signaling in B-cell survival. In contrast to BCR, BAFFR activates the non-canonical NF-kB pathway, which depends on the proteolytic processing of p100 to p52 to generate p52/RelB (NF-kB2) nuclear complexes (Tedder et al. 1986, 1988, 1989; Uchida et al. 2004a; Claudio et al. 2002). Both BCR and BAFFR are required for the maintenance of peripheral B-cell homeostasis. It has been shown that signals from the BCR and BAFFR cooperate to allow B-cell survival at multiple stages of peripheral B-cell differentiation and during immune responses. BCR promotes BAFFR-mediated signals through at least two mechanisms by upregulating the expression of BAFFR and by supplying the noncanonical NF-kB pathway substrate p100 (Cancro 2009).

CD20 is a component of a multimeric cell surface complex that regulates Ca^{2+} transport across the plasma membrane (Bubien et al. 1993; Kanzaki et al. 1997). B-cell depletion using rituximab does not affect the $CD19^+CD20^-$ pro-B cell and $CD20^-CD138^+$ plasma cell populations, and within 6–8 months following treatment, the $CD20^+$ B-cell compartment begins to replenish.

Although CD20 MoAb immunotherapy depletes normal and malignant B cells in vivo by antibody-dependent activation of the innate monocytic network (Uchida et al. 2004b), crosslinking of CD20 alters Ca^{2+} homeostasis, which influences cell cycle progression and can lead to apoptosis of normal and leukemic B cells in vitro (Bubien et al. 1993; van der Kolk et al. 2002). Yet the precise functions of CD20 and the therapeutic MoAbs are still controversial issues (Okroj et al. 2013).

Clinical Presentation, Differential Diagnosis, and Treatment

To date, only a single patient has been reported that completely lacked surface CD20 expression on B cells as a result of a homozygous mutation in the *CD20* gene (Kuijpers et al. 2010). We found that the patient had a persistent hypogammaglobulinemia, normal B-cell numbers, and a strong reduction in circulating memory B cells. A decreased frequency of somatic hypermutations in IgG heavy chain genes was found. After repeated vaccinations the patient mounted proper responses to recall antigens but displayed a strongly reduced ability to respond to pneumococcal polysaccharides. In agreement with a conserved role of CD20 in the generation of T-cell-independent (TI) antibody responses, we found that CD20-deficient mice had a reduced ability to respond to TI antigens. We concluded that CD20 has a nonredundant role in the generation of optimal B-cell responses.

Human CD20 deficiency results in decreased IgG antibody levels and relatively increased IgM levels with weak responses against polysaccharides after vaccination. Importantly, we found that CD20 deficiency in mice also results in an impaired ability to make TI antibody responses. Thus, although the phenotypes of CD20-deficient humans and mice are subtly different, the current data would imply that CD20 signals are essential to enable B cells to optimally respond to antigenic stimuli.

Pathophysiology

The severe reduction of class-switched $sIgD^-CD27^+$ memory B cells might reflect suboptimal germinal center formation and is likely to cause the profound hypogammaglobulinemia. Although IgG antibodies and circulating memory B cells are not defective in the CD20-knockout mice (Uchida et al. 2004a; O'Keefe et al. 1998), the selection of naive B cells into the non-switched ($sIgD^+CD27^+$) MZ B-cell compartment seems disturbed in the patient. In healthy donors, the transition of naive B cells into MZ B cells is accompanied by a reduction of the mean IgV_H-CDR3 lengths and acquisition of IgV mutations (Tsuiji et al. 2006; Weller et al. 2004). Concomitantly, a counterselection against poly- and self-reactive antibodies and enrichment for antibodies reactive with specific bacterial polysaccharides occur (Tsuiji et al. 2006). This selection process is potentially driven by tonic BCR signals that may be assumed to be different between BCRs with longer and shorter IgV_H-CDR3 lengths. Alternatively, particular self- or commensal-related antigens, recognized with low avidity, may provide positive BCR signals, favoring the selection of B cells that have short IgV_H-CDR3 lengths in the MZ B cell compartment. In the MZ B cells of the patient, no counterselection for long IgV_H-CDR3 lengths was observed, which is in accordance with a diminished response against polysaccharide vaccination. The notion of a disturbed counterselection against poly- and self-reactive antibodies is strengthened by the observation that, in the absence of any clinical signs of autoimmunity, antinuclear antibodies in the serum of the patient were found repeatedly (Kuijpers et al. 2010).

New Avenues to Approach CD20

Apart from cell-death-inducing capacity, murine anti-CD20 MoAbs were shown to also strongly inhibit IgM and IgG secretion by B cells in vitro (Golay et al. 1985). The first therapeutic anti-CD20 MoAb rituximab and new generation anti-CD20 MoAbs are, however, widely used now to treat autoimmune diseases and organ transplant rejection. Also in this case, the mechanism of action of rituximab is still unclear, as response does not simply correlate with B-cell depletion (Townsend et al. 2010). Thus, the data together suggest that in autoimmune diseases, anti-CD20 MoAbs may be therapeutically active through both killing the autoimmune B cells and inhibition of differentiation of the residual B cells into plasma cells secreting autoimmune antibodies. Experiments are required to verify this hypothesis and to determine whether all stimuli and all B-cell

subsets may respond to such inhibition rather than cell death only.

Alternatively, low percentages of CD20-expressing T cells in human blood may be present with a pro-inflammatory role in autoimmunity as well. This minor T-cell subset was first described in 1993 (Hultin et al. 1993) and related to disease (Wilk et al. 2009), but the existence of this rather rare T-cell subset has also been disputed as an artifact (Henry et al. 2010). Others have found that CD20-expressing T cells can exhibit pro-inflammatory capacity. In rheumatoid arthritis (RA), $CD20^+$ T cells make up a larger percentage of Th17 cells when compared with healthy individuals (Eggleton et al. 2011), although the overall percentage of $CD20^+$ T cells among all T cells did not differ between RA patients and healthy individuals. Clearly, the pathological relevance, if any, of $CD20^+$ T cells in autoimmune diseases remains unknown, but these findings give new impetus for the important avenue of investigation to understand the therapeutic effects of CD20 MoAbs – in particular in disease considered to be largely caused by T cells.

References

Bubien JK, Zhou LJ, Bell PD, Frizzell RA, Tedder TF. Transfection of the CD20 cell surface molecule into ectopic cell types generates a Ca^{2+} conductance found constitutively in B lymphocytes. J Cell Biol. 1993;121(5):1121–32.

Cancro MP. Signalling crosstalk in B cells: managing worth and need. Nat Rev Immunol. 2009;9:657–61.

Claes N, Fraussen J, Stinissen P, Hupperts R, Somers V. B cells are multifunctional players in multiple sclerosis pathogenesis: insights from therapeutic interventions. Front Immunol. 2015;6:642.

Claudio E, Brown K, Park S, Wang H, Siebenlist U. BAFF-induced NEMO-independent processing of NF-kB2 in maturing B cells. Nat Immunol. 2002;3:958–65.

Eggleton P, Bremer E, Tarr JM, de Bruyn M, Helfrich W, Kendall A, Haigh RC, Viner NJ, Winyard PG. Frequency of Th17 CD20+ cells in the peripheral blood of rheumatoid arthritis patients is higher compared to healthy subjects. Arthritis Res Ther. 2011;13:R208.

Franks SE, Getahun A, Hogarth PM, Cambier JC. Targeting B cells in treatment of autoimmunity. Curr Opin Immunol. 2016;43:39–45.

Froissart A, Veyradier A, Hié M, Benhamou Y, Coppo P, French Reference Center for Thrombotic Micro-angiopathies. Rituximab in autoimmune thrombotic thrombocytopenic purpura: a success story. Eur J Intern Med. 2015;26(9):659–65.

Golay JT, Clark EA, Beverley PC. The CD20 (Bp35) antigen is involved in activation of B cells from the G0 to the G1 phase of the cell cycle. J Immunol. 1985;135:3795–801.

Grumont RJ, Rourke IJ, O'Reilly LA, Strasser A, Miyake K, Sha W, Gerondakis S. B lymphocytes differentially use the Rel and nuclear factor kB1 (NF-kB1) transcription factors to regulate cell cycle progression and apoptosis in quiescent and mitogen-activated cells. J Exp Med. 1998;187:663–74.

Grumont RJ, Rourke IJ, Gerondakis S. Rel-dependent induction of A1 transcription is required to protect B cells from antigen receptor ligation-induced apoptosis. Genes Dev. 1999;13:400–11.

Henry C, Ramadan A, Montcuquet N, Pallandre JR, Mercier-Letondal P, Deschamps M, Tiberghien P, Ferrand C, Robinet E. CD3+CD20+ cells may be an artifact of flow cytometry: comment on the article by Wilk et al. Arthritis Rheum. 2010;62:2561–3. (author reply 2563–2565)

Hultin LE, Hausner MA, Hultin PM, Giorgi JV. CD20 (pan-B cell) antigen is expressed at a low level on a subpopulation of human T lymphocytes. Cytometry. 1993;14:196–204.

Kanzaki M, Lindorfer MA, Garrison JC, Kojima I. Activation of the calcium-permeable cation channel CD20 by alpha subunits of the Gi protein. J Biol Chem. 1997;272(23):14733–9.

Kuijpers TW, Bende RJ, Baars PA, Grummels A, Derks IA, Dolman KM, Beaumont T, Tedder TF, van Noesel CJ, Eldering E, van Lier RA. CD20 deficiency in humans results in impaired T cell-independent antibody responses. J Clin Invest. 2010;120:214–22.

Liang Y, Tedder TF. Identification of a CD20-, FcepsilonRIbeta-, and HTm4-related gene family: sixteen new MS4A family members expressed in human and mouse. Genomics. 2001;72(2):119–27.

Liang Y, Buckley TR, Tu L, Langdon SD, Tedder TF. Structural organization of the human MS4A gene cluster on Chromosome 11q12. Immunogenetics. 2001;53(5):357–68.

Mackay F, Figgett WA, Saulep D, Lepage M, Hibbs ML. B-cell stage and context-dependent requirements for survival signals from BAFF and the B-cell receptor. Immunol Rev. 2010;237:205–25.

Miano M. How I manage Evans syndrome and AIHA cases in children. Br J Haematol. 2016;172(4): 524–34.

O'Keefe TL, Williams GT, Davies SL, Neuberger MS. Mice carrying a CD20 gene disruption. Immunogenetics. 1998;48(2):125–32.

Okroj M, Osterborg A, Blom AM. Effector mechanisms of anti-CD20 monoclonal antibodies in B cell malignancies. Cancer Treat Rev. 2013;39:632–6.

Saijo K, Mecklenbrauker I, Santana A, Leitger M, Schmedt C, Tarakhovsky A. Protein kinase C beta controls nuclear factor kB activation in B cells through selective regulation of the IkB kinase alpha. J Exp Med. 2002;195:1647–52.

Schiemann B, Gommerman JL, Vora K, Cachero TG, Shulga-Morskaya S, Dobles M, Frew E, Scott ML. An essential role for BAFF in the normal development of B cells through a BCMA-independent pathway. Science. 2001;293:2111–4.

Stashenko P, Nadler LM, Hardy R, Schlossman SF. Characterization of a human B lymphocyte-specific antigen. J Immunol. 1980;125(4):1678–85.

Tedder TF, Engel P. CD20: a regulator of cell-cycle progression of B lymphocytes. Immunol Today. 1994;15(9):450–4.

Tedder TF, et al. The B cell surface molecule B1 is functionally linked with B cell activation and differentiation. J Immunol. 1985;135(2):973–9.

Tedder TF, et al. Antibodies reactive with the B1 molecule inhibit cell cycle progression but not activation of human B lymphocytes. Eur J Immunol. 1986;16(8):881–7.

Tedder TF, et al. Cloning of a complementary DNA encoding a new mouse B lymphocyte differentiation antigen, homologous to the human B1 (CD20) antigen, and localization of the gene to chromosome 19. J Immunol. 1988;141(12):4388–94.

Tedder TF, Klejman G, Schlossman SF, Saito H. Structure of the gene encoding the human B lymphocyte differentiation antigen CD20 (B1). J Immunol. 1989;142(7):2560–8.

Thompson JS, Bixler SA, Qian F, Vora K, Scott ML, Cachero TG, Hession C, Schneider P, Sizing ID, Mullen C, et al. BAFF-R, a newly identified TNF receptor that specifically interacts with BAFF. Science. 2001;293:2108–11.

Townsend MJ, Monroe JG, Chan AC. B-cell targeted therapies in human autoimmune diseases: an updated perspective. Immunol Rev. 2010;237:264–83.

Tsuiji M, et al. A checkpoint for autoreactivity in human IgM+ memory B cell development. J Exp Med. 2006;203(2):393–400.

Uchida J, Lee Y, Hasegawa M, Liang Y, Bradney A, Oliver JA, Bowen K, Steeber DA, Haas KM, Poe JC, Tedder TF. Mouse CD20 expression and function. Int Immunol. 2004a;16:119–29.

Uchida J, et al. The innate mononuclear phagocyte network depletes B lymphocytes through Fc receptor-dependent mechanisms during anti-CD20 antibody immunotherapy. J Exp Med. 2004b;199(12):1659–69.

van der Kolk LE, et al. CD20-induced B cell death can bypass mitochondria and caspase activation. Leukemia. 2002;16(9):1735–44.

Weller S, et al. Human blood IgM "memory" B cells are circulating splenic marginal zone B cells harboring a prediversified immunoglobulin repertoire. Blood. 2004;104(12):3647–54.

Wilk E, Witte T, Marquardt N, Horvath T, Kalippke K, Scholz K, Wilke N, Schmidt RE, Jacobs R. Depletion of functionally active CD20+ T cells by rituximab treatment. Arthritis Rheum. 2009;60:3563–71.

CD21 Deficiency

Klaus Warnatz
Department of Rheumatology and Clinical
Immunology and Center for Chronic
Immunodeficiency, University Medical Center
and University of Freiburg, Freiburg, Germany

Definition

An immunodeficiency defined by deleterious mutations in *CD21* encoding for the complement receptor 2 (CR2).

Prevalence

Four patients with mutations in *CD21* have been reported (Wentink et al. 2018).

Clinical Presentation

The clinical presentation of CD21 deficiency seems to reflect a mild humoral immunodeficiency without signs of immune dysregulation. The first patient described with CD21 deficiency was a 28-year-old German male with recurrent upper airway infections, persistent myalgias in adulthood, and no signs of immune dysregulation. Common variable immunodeficiency (CVID) was suspected based on serum IgG levels <4 g/L, serum IgA level just below the normal range, a reduced class-switched memory B cells, and a reduced antipneumococcal polysaccharide antibody response (Thiel et al. 2012). The second patient was a 13-year-old Dutch boy who was diagnosed with hypogammaglobulinemia of all three isotypes during workup for myalgia (Wentink et al. 2015). He had no history of an increased susceptibility to infections or autoimmune manifestations. The other two patients are siblings born to consanguineous French parents and were diagnosed at the age of 14 and 11 with recurrent upper respiratory tract infections and the older sibling with one possible pneumonia at the age of 12 (Rosain et al. 2017).

Genetics

Genetic findings reported (2019) suggest autosomal recessive inheritance due to a compound heterozygous mutation consisting of a point mutation of a highly conserved splice donor site (c.1225 + 1G > C/p.W766X) and a second point mutation in exon 13 introducing a premature stop codon (c.2297G > A, p.W766X) in the German patient. The Dutch patient carried compound heterozygous point mutations (p.R142X/p.I926SfsX14) and the French family homozygous single bp deletions (c.234delC, p.T209HfsX10), leading to frameshift mutation and premature stop codons.

Immunological Phenotype

CD21 is a complement receptor binding C3d after cleavage of complement factor 3 bound to immune complexes but also other proteins including gp350/220 viral coat protein of Epstein-Barr virus (EBV) (Lowell et al. 1989). There are different splice variants which are mainly expressed on B cells and follicular dendritic cells (FDC). CD21 has been established as a co-stimulatory receptor on B cells when linked to the complex of CD19, CD225, and CD81, which are required for signaling (Matsumoto et al. 1993). Thus, immune complexes loaded with complement are shown to activate B cells by cross-linking the B-cell receptor and the costimulatory complex. It has a role in the capture of immune complexes for antigen presentation in FDC. The absence of CD21 in mice is associated with the concomitant loss of the other complement receptor CD35, since they are co-expressed. The absence of CD21 has been associated with impaired humoral immune responses (Molina et al. 1996).

In humans, all described patients had reduced switched memory B-cell numbers suggesting a role either directly on the B cell or indirectly through interference with the FDC and germinal center function or both. T-cell-dependent IgG response was normal, suggesting only a partial effect. In one patient, histopathology studies in an adenoid sample revealed a preserved and even hyperplastic structure of germinal centers despite the absence of CD21 expression on FDC network.

Diagnosis

Diagnosis is made by genetic analysis of *CD21*. All patients so far were diagnosed by the fortuitous finding of lack of CD21 when analyzing the B-cell phenotype. It is important to note that many CVID patients have so-called CD21^{low} B cells with absent CD21 expression (Rakhmanov et al. 2009), but usually there are CD21^{pos} B cells detectable in nearly all patients. This functional downregulation of CD21 needs to be clearly distinguished from the genetically determined CD21 deficiency. Suspicion should be raised in patients presenting with a rather mild infection and CVID-like clinical presentation. In the future, it is to be expected that variants in *CD21* with residual or normal expression will be discovered, requiring functional testing by co-stimulation through immune complexes (Thiel et al. 2012) which is not established in most laboratories.

Management

Management depends on the presentation of the disease and the treating center. While German and Dutch patients were treated with immunoglobulin replacement, the two French siblings were on antibiotic prophylaxis only after they were diagnosed. There are no long-term outcome reports in CD21 deficiency at this time in order to advise. Given the absence of autoimmune manifestations, the control of infection especially of the respiratory tract seems to be the main task in the management of CD21-deficient patients.

References

Lowell CA, Klickstein LB, Carter RH, Mitchell JA, Fearon DT, Ahearn JM. Mapping of the Epstein-Barr virus and C3dg binding sites to a common domain on complement receptor type 2. J Exp Med. 1989;170(6):1931–46.

Matsumoto AK, Martin DR, Carter RH, Klickstein LB, Ahearn JM, Fearon DT. Functional dissection of the CD21/CD19/TAPA-1/Leu-13 complex of B lymphocytes. J Exp Med. 1993;178(4):1407–17.

Molina H, Holers VM, Li B, Fung Y, Mariathasan S, Goellner J, et al. Markedly impaired humoral immune response in mice deficient in complement receptors 1 and 2. Proc Natl Acad Sci U S A. 1996;93(8):3357–61.

Rakhmanov M, Keller B, Gutenberger S, Foerster C, Hoenig M, Driessen G, et al. Circulating CD21low B cells in common variable immunodeficiency resemble tissue homing, innate-like B cells. Proc Natl Acad Sci USA. 2009;106(32):13451–6.

Rosain J, Miot C, Lambert N, Rousselet MC, Pellier I, Picard C. CD21 deficiency in 2 siblings with recurrent respiratory infections and hypogammaglobulinemia. J Allergy Clin Immunol Pract. 2017;5(6):1765–7.e3.

Thiel J, Kimmig L, Salzer U, Grudzien M, Lebrecht D, Hagena T, et al. Genetic CD21 deficiency is associated with hypogammaglobulinemia. J Allergy Clin Immunol. 2012;129(3):801–10.

Wentink MW, Lambeck AJ, van Zelm MC, Simons E, van Dongen JJ, H IJ, et al. CD21 and CD19 deficiency: two defects in the same complex leading to different disease modalities. Clin Immunol. 2015;161(2):120–7.

Wentink MWJ, van Zelm MC, van Dongen JJM, Warnatz K, van der Burg M. Deficiencies in the CD19 complex. Clin Immunol. 2018;195:82–7.

CD27 Deficiency

Ivan K. Chinn
Section of Immunology, Allergy, and Retrovirology, Texas Children's Hospital, Houston, TX, USA
William T. Shearer Center for Human Immunobiology, Texas Children's Hospital, Houston, TX, USA
Department of Pediatrics, Baylor College of Medicine, Houston, TX, USA

Introduction

CD27 is located at 12p13 and encodes CD27, a member of the tumor necrosis factor family that is alternately known as tumor necrosis factor receptor superfamily, member 7. The 55 kDa transmembrane molecule is constitutively expressed on the surface of naïve and memory CD4$^+$ and CD8$^+$

T cells and is downregulated by a proportion of effector T cells (Sugita et al. 1992; Hintzen et al. 1994). It is also found on CD56^{bright} natural killer (NK) cells and at low levels on CD56^{dim} NK cells (Bullock 2017; Buchan et al. 2018). CD27 is well-known as a marker for memory, but not naïve, B cells, yet its function in B lymphocytes remains poorly understood. CD27 typically resides at the cellular membrane as a disulfide-linked homodimeric receptor, but membrane-bound monomeric CD27 can also exist (Buchan et al. 2018). A smaller soluble 32 kDa form is known to be produced from the full-length, mature peptide (Hintzen et al. 1994). The role of soluble CD27 has not been established. CD70 (tumor necrosis factor ligand superfamily, member 7) represents the only identified ligand for CD27. *CD27* deficiency is inherited as an autosomal recessive Mendelian trait.

Molecular Function

CD27 signaling engages several key pathways. The receptor couples to tumor necrosis factor receptor-associated factor (TRAF) 2, TRAF3, and TRAF5 (Buchan et al. 2018). CD27-mediated activation of TRAF2 and TRAF5 drives c-Jun N-terminal kinase signaling, which modulates cell survival and promotes cytokine production (Borst et al. 2005; Nolte et al. 2009; Grant et al. 2017; Buchan et al. 2018). TRAF ubiquitination through CD27 also recruits nuclear factor kappa-light-chain-enhancer of activated B cells-inducing kinase (NIK), resulting in signaling through both the canonical and noncanonical (alternative) nuclear factor kappa-light-chain-enhancer of activated B cells pathways (Borst et al. 2005; Nolte et al. 2009; Buchan et al. 2018). CD27 further binds Siva1, which is connected to a proapoptotic pathway (Borst et al. 2005; Nolte et al. 2009). This interaction remains poorly characterized. Finally, CD27 activates a PIM1 kinase pathway (Bullock 2017).

In T cells, CD27 acts as a costimulatory molecule, and its activity is not redundant with the function of CD28 (Bullock 2017). As such, cross-linking of CD27 using agonistic monoclonal antibodies amplifies the proliferative response to mitogens (Denoeud and Moser 2011). Importantly, CD27 promotes priming, accumulation, and survival of antigen-specific T cells at sites of infection (Borst et al. 2005; Denoeud and Moser 2011; Grant et al. 2017). For CD8$^+$ T cells, CD27 stimulation leads to upregulated expression of C-X-C motif chemokine ligand 10, eomesodermin, B-cell lymphoma-extra-large protein, interleukin (IL)-2 receptor α, and IL-12 receptor β2 (Han et al. 2016; Bullock 2017; Grant et al. 2017). In this process, CD27 supports the expansion of effector CD8$^+$ T cells and survival of antigen-specific memory CD8$^+$ T cells (Bullock 2017). In CD4$^+$ T cells, CD27 contributes to T helper cell 1 (Th1) polarization and overall expansion (Nolte et al. 2009; Bullock 2017). The receptor is not necessary for thymocyte differentiation into naïve T cells or differentiation of naïve T cells into effector cells (Nolte et al. 2009; Denoeud and Moser 2011).

CD27 is known to play key roles in NK cell activity, although further work remains necessary to fully elucidate its function in these cells. Triggering of CD27 on NK cells by CD70 in the presence of IL-2 or IL-12 augments effector targets cell conjugate formation and results in its own downregulation (Nolte et al. 2009). It also induces proliferation of and interferon-γ production by NK cells while also providing the capacity to enhance their cytotoxicity (Nolte et al. 2009).

As stated earlier, CD27 function in B cells has not been extensively studied. In mice, CD27 deficiency results in delayed germinal center formation, although it remains unclear if this abnormality is due to lack of the molecule in B cells, T cells, or both (Borst et al. 2005; Denoeud and Moser 2011). In human CD27$^+$ B cells, engagement by CD70 results in immunoglobulin production together with plasma cell differentiation and survival (Nolte et al. 2009; Han et al. 2016).

Presentation

A total of 17 cases of human CD27 deficiency have been reported, first in 2012 (van Montfrans et al.

2012) and then in 2013 (Salzer et al. 2013), and subsequently summarized with additional cases in 2015 (Alkhairy et al. 2015). Of these cases, all but one carried biallelic pathogenic variants in *CD27*. In the one exception, the presence of a second pathogenic variant, not detected by the methods employed, was hypothesized. Median age at disease presentation was 6 years: for 3 cases, signs and symptoms began at 13 years of age or greater; for the remaining 14 of 17, disease manifested at 8 years of age or younger.

All reported cases have been associated with confirmed or suspected EBV-driven disease, which have resulted in notable phenotypic variability. In these patients, the virus has produced the following: lymphoproliferative disease, lymphoma, meningitis or encephalitis, uveitis, chronic viremia, pneumonia, oral or anal ulcers, hepatitis, and hemophagocytic lymphohistiocytosis. Clinical manifestations typically include signs of lymphoproliferative disease or lymphoma, such as fevers, lymphadenopathy, and hepatosplenomegaly.

Recurrent or unusual infections may develop and at times precede the EBV-driven manifestations. Such infections include gram-positive sepsis, severe varicella infection, CMV infection, recurrent sinopulmonary tract infections, toxoplasmosis, oral candidiasis, herpangina, giardiasis, and recurrent influenza infections. Although only 3 of 17 cases had primary hypogammaglobulinemia (7 others developed iatrogenic hypogammaglobulinemia), 2 of the 3 patients were initially diagnosed with common variable immunodeficiency disease.

Diagnosis

Identification of CD27 deficiency requires a high index of suspicion based upon clinical features. In all cases examined to date, absent or reduced expression of CD27 on the surface of B cells has been observed. No other immunologic feature has been consistently associated with CD27 deficiency. Expression by T cells ranges from absent to near-normal and may therefore falsely exclude the diagnosis. In the two initial cases, T-cell proliferation to mitogens was absent or reduced, but others have demonstrated normal T-cell mitogenic responses. In five of seven patients tested, NK cell function was diminished. Patients do not appear to have impaired antibody responses to immunizations. Establishment of the diagnosis therefore requires genetic testing (sequencing and copy number analysis of the *CD27* gene).

Treatment

CD27 deficiency is a condition associated with high mortality. Initial therapies typically focus upon control of EBV infection and abnormal lymphocyte proliferation. These strategies include use of chemotherapy (various protocols), corticosteroids, and rituximab (Alkhairy et al. 2015). Secondary hypogammaglobulinemia nearly invariably results from use of these agents. IgG supplementation is fully indicated in CD27-deficient patients and is linked to greater survival (Alkhairy et al. 2015). Three patients have received hematopoietic stem cell transplantation. Although all survived, one continued to experience disease- or transplantation-related complications at over 4 years posttransplantation. Overall survival for this disease stands at 71%. Causes of mortality consist of malignancy, aplastic anemia, sepsis, and respiratory failure.

References

Alkhairy OK, Perez-Becker R, Driessen GJ, et al. Novel mutations in TNFRSF7/CD27: clinical, immunologic, and genetic characterization of human CD27 deficiency. J Allergy Clin Immunol. 2015;136:703–12.e10.

Borst J, Hendriks J, Xiao Y. CD27 and CD70 in T cell and B cell activation. Curr Opin Immunol. 2005;17:275–81.

Buchan SL, Rogel A, Al-Shamkhani A. The immunobiology of CD27 and OX40 and their potential as targets for cancer immunotherapy. Blood. 2018; 131:39–48.

Bullock TNJ. Stimulating CD27 to quantitatively and qualitatively shape adaptive immunity to cancer. Curr Opin Immunol. 2017;45:82–8.

Denoeud J, Moser M. Role of CD27/CD70 pathway of activation in immunity and tolerance. J Leukoc Biol. 2011;89:195–203.

Grant EJ, Nüssing S, Sant S, Clemens EB, Kedzierska K. The role of CD27 in anti-viral T-cell immunity. Curr Opin Virol. 2017;22:77–88.

Han BK, Olsen NJ, Bottaro A. The CD27–CD70 pathway and pathogenesis of autoimmune disease. Semin Arthritis Rheum. 2016;45:496–501.

Hintzen RQ, de Jong R, Lens SMA, van Lier RW. CD27: marker and mediator of T-cell activation? Immunol Today. 1994;15:307–11.

Nolte MA, Van Olffen RW, Van Gisbergen KPJM, Van Lier RAW. Timing and tuning of CD27–CD70 interactions: the impact of signal strength in setting the balance between adaptive responses and immunopathology. Immunol Rev. 2009;229:216–31.

Salzer E, Daschkey S, Choo S, et al. Combined immuno-deficiency with life-threatening EBV-associated lymphoproliferative disorder in patients lacking func-tional CD27. Haematologica. 2013;98:473.

Sugita K, Hirose T, Rothstein DM, Donahue C, Schlossman SF, Morimoto C. CD27, a member of the nerve growth factor receptor family, is preferentially expressed on CD45RA$^+$ CD4 T cell clones and involved in distinct immunoregulatory functions. J Immunol. 1992;149:3208.

van Montfrans JM, Hoepelman AIM, Otto S, et al. CD27 deficiency is associated with combined immunodefi-ciency and persistent symptomatic EBV viremia. J Allergy Clin Immunol. 2012;129:787–93.e6.

CD283

▶ TLR3 Deficiency

CD2-Binding Protein 1

▶ Pyogenic Arthritis, Pyoderma Gangrenosum, and Acne (PAPA) Syndrome

CD3 Epsilon (ε)

▶ CD3d, e and z Deficiencies

CD3 Zeta (ζ)/CD247

▶ CD3d, e and z Deficiencies

CD3d, e and z Deficiencies

Robert P. Nelson
Divisions of Hematology and Oncology, Stem Cell Transplant Program, Indiana University (IU) School of Medicine and the IU Bren and Simon Cancer Center, Indianapolis, IN, USA
Pediatric Immunodeficiency Clinic, Riley Hospital for Children at Indiana University Health, Indianapolis, IN, USA
Medicine and Pediatrics, Indiana University School of Medicine, Immunohematology and Transplantation, Indianapolis, IN, USA

Synonyms

CD3 epsilon (ε); CD3 zeta (ζ)/CD247

Definition

Deficiency of any of the subunits that are compo-nents of the clusters of differentiation 3 (CD3) complex results in combined immunodeficiency.

Introduction/Background

The T-cell receptor (TCR) recognizes antigen peptides bound to a major histocompatibility complex (MHC) molecule presented on the cell membrane. CD3 is an accessory multiunit molecule associated with the TCR and consists of four CD3 subunits, including homologous glycoproteins CD3γ or δ, the nonglycosylated CD3ε, and the homodimer CD3ζ (Clevers et al. 1988; Reinherz et al. 1983). The invariant δ, ε, and γ chains of the TCR are closely related struc-turally and located on human chromosome 11q23.3. The ζ chain localizes to chromosome 1q24.2 and its sequences are unique in compari-son to the other CD3 chains (Weissman et al. 1988).

Molecular signals that are activated from the correct TCR-antigen engagement are transduced through the TCR-CD3 antigen receptor complex. Thus, although T lymphocyte activation begins early with binding of antigen to an α/β or γ/δ rearranged TCR, transduction of the signal is delegated to the multisubunit CD3 complex. To do this, the CD3 complex employs a transmembrane intracellular immune receptor tyrosine-based activation motif (ITAM), that recruits adaptors that enable propagation of the signal, which results in gene transcription in the nucleus (Alarcon et al. 1988a).

Functions of the CD3 Subunits

During T-cell maturation in the thymus, TCR-mediated signaling controls developmental transitions and regulates thymocyte survival. Given the conserved nature of their structure, position, and function, the CD3 subunits likely have important, nonredundant activities. The physical positions of the extracellular domains also play a role. The TCR–CD3 complex is arranged as a central core from which two TCRs project outward on the cell surface. The CD3$\epsilon\delta$ or CD3$\epsilon\gamma$ subunits reside below the TCR α-chain and β-chains, respectively (Ledbetter et al. 1986). Although there is some flexibility in the subunit stoichiometry, CD3ϵ appears central to CD3 core assembly and full complex formation (Soudais et al. 1993). CD3 δ promotes progression of early thymocytes to the double-positive stage, as illustrated by analysis of a $\delta-/-$ mouse, which expresses the α/β TCR but not the pre-TCR or $\gamma\delta$ TCR (Dave et al. 1997). In humans, the absence of CD3 δ results in a complete arrest at the double negative- to double positive transition, and the development of $\gamma\delta$ T-cells is also impaired (Roifman 2004).

The selection and activation of T lymphocytes in the thymus and periphery are also mitigated also by coreceptors CD4, CD8, and CD45 interacting with the TCR/CD3 recognition structure. Lack of the CD3 γ component impairs peripheral blood naïve CD4+ CD45RA+ and CD8+ lymphocytes long-term survival, whereas CD4 + CD45RO+, B and natural killer lymphocytes are not affected. These results suggest that

the CD3 γ of the TCR/CD3 complex is required for the peripheral presence of certain T-cell subsets.

Sussman reported on a murine T-cell hybridoma that failed to synthesize CD3 ζ (Sussman et al. 1988). The CD3-ζ deficient mice expressed small quantities of the TCR-CD3 complex. In the absence of CD3-ζ, receptor-induced phosphatidylinositol hydrolysis and interleukin-2 production occurred, but the variant failed to respond normally to antigen and mitogenic stimuli. This suggests that CD3-ζ contributes to the intracellular fate of the T cell-antigen binding and studying the consequences of its absence helps to define its role in transmembrane signaling (Sussman et al. 1988).

Clinical Manifestations

Loss-of-function mutations in CD3 subunits δ ϵ, γ, ζ may cause inherited autosomal recessive T-B + NK+ severe combined immunodeficiencies (SCID). However, SCID is only one of the phenotypes associated with CD3 subunit deficiencies.

The first reported case of a CD3 component deficiency in a human was an 11-month-old with recurrent pulmonary infections, failure to thrive, anorexia, and diarrhea (Alarcon et al. 1988b). Stool cultures grew *Salmonella enterica* and *Yersinia enterocolitica* and he experienced malabsorption unresponsive to a gluten-free diet. A small bowel biopsy revealed absent villi, but HLA typing revealed neither HLA-DR3 nor HLA-DR7. There was no history of chronic pyogenic or fungal infections, eczema, chronic moniliasis, dysmorphic features, or bony abnormalities. Normal vaccination schedules, including attenuated measles, mumps, rubella, and poliomyelitis virus, were tolerated and protective. He died at the age of 3 years secondary to autoimmune hemolytic anemia. Autopsy revealed bilateral bronchopneumonia with giant cell pneumonia, no thymus, but microscopic examination from the anterior precordium revealed thymic epithelium, severely depleted lymphocytes, and absence of Hassall's corpuscles.

Soudais et al. (1993) described defective expression of the TCR/CD3 complex in an immunodeficient child found to harbor two independent CD3-ε parental gene mutations that segregated to the patient. The gene defects impaired CD3-ε chain synthesis that prevented membrane expression of the TCR/CD3 complex. The 4-year-old boy with defective TCR-CD3 complex expression presented with recurrent chest infections and pulmonary symptoms consistent with bronchial asthma, and the authors emphasize that children with combined immunodeficiency may present with signs and symptoms of humoral immunodeficiency (Sanal et al. 1996). Hubert et al. reported two patients with CD4+T cell counts <150 cells/microliter and opportunistic infections consistent with the diagnosis of severe idiopathic CD4+ lymphocytopenia (ICL). Abnormalities of transducing molecules of the CD3-TCR pathway rendered one T lymphopenic and the other CD4+ T lymphopenic. Defects in proliferative response to CD3-TCR stimulation affected the depleted T-cell subpopulation and abnormal biochemical events and protein tyrosine phosphorylation of the CD3-TCR pathway were detected (Hubert et al. 1999).

Araniz-Villena et al. reported two siblings bearing compound heterozygous mutations in the CD3γ subunit, resulting in the lack of expression. Remarkably, one of the siblings was healthy at 10 years of age, whereas his brother had failure to thrive, diarrhea, and malabsorption since his first year of life and died of autoimmune hemolytic anemia at 3-years-old. These findings underscore the variability of clinical presentation of CD3 subunit defects (Araniz-Villena 1992).

Roifman reviewed CD3 delta deficiency in humans and emphasized profound T-cell depletion and presentation early 2–3 months with severe viral illness (Roifman 2004). Compared to the murine CD3 (−/−) δ, the δ defect in humans appears required for both αβ and γδ T-cell receptor-positive T-cell lineages. The studies also show for the first time that comparing relevant patients' with normal tissue using microarray technology can aid in the discovery of the genetic basis of inherited disorders (Roifman 2004).

Recently, multiorgan autoimmune phenomena were reported in two siblings with Evans syndrome, autoimmune hepatitis, nephrotic syndrome, and Hashimoto's thyroiditis (Tokgoz et al. 2013; Rowe et al. 2018). Patients had low TCR αβ expression, limited T-cell repertoire, decreased T-regulatory cells, and variable IgG, IgA, IgM, CD3, CD4, and CD8 T-cell counts.

Laboratory Findings and Diagnosis

CD3 subunit defects with profound immunodeficiency present as SCID. Prenatal and birth history is usually unremarkable, with delivery having occurred uncomplicated with normal birth weight. T-cell excision circles (TRECs) at birth may be low or normal. Between 3 and 12 months of age, failure to thrive ensues with symptoms appreciated retrospectively to have begun several weeks to months prior, include intermittent fevers, diarrhea, cough, and weight loss. There may have been a prior hospitalization for pneumonia. Physical exam may be remarkable for weight less than the 5th percentile. Skin exam is usually normal but a maculopapular rash may be present. Complete blood count (CBC) is remarkable for decreased numbers or percentages of lymphocytes. Comprehensive chemistry profile may show increase in liver enzymes. Screening immunological evaluation includes the measurement of total and specific antibody titers, and peripheral blood immunophenotype analysis, which demonstrate numerical and functional defects in T-cell and B-cell function. The immunophenotype for those who present as SCID is T-B + NK+ and decreases in T-cell proliferation to mitogens and/or antigens appears universal.

Patients with CD3 subunit deficiencies may also present clinically with ICL, or similar to humoral immunodeficiencies or with hematological or multiorgan autoimmune illness (Sanal et al. 1996). Most patients with non-SCID combined T and B disorders present during childhood, with adverse consequences of bacterial, viral infections, and/or opportunistic infections. A family history of PID is a strong indicator; there may be a history of consanguinity and inheritance pattern is autosomal recessive. There may be a history of autoimmune manifestations. Facial features are normal and lymph nodes likely palpable. Cognitive impairment and cardiovascular structural defects have not been reported nor would they be expected. The index patient had radiographic absence of thymus which was small but present at autopsy (Alarcon et al. 1988b). The immunophenotype for those who present as non-SCID is remarkable for CD3 lymphopenia, with normal CD2 T-cell counts. Immunoglobulins may be normal or low and decreases in T-cell proliferation to mitogens and/or antigens appears universal.

Treatment

Patients with the SCID phenotype can be cured with timely hematopoietic cell transplantation (Roifman 2004). An ideal outcome of allo-transplantation for SCID is characterized as complete immunological reconstitution, minimal transplant-related toxicity, and achievement of full lymphohematopoietic donor chimerism without graft-versus-host disease (GVHD). Important hurdles that must be overcome for healthy survival included delays in diagnosis, which permit establishment of life-threatening infections. A hematopoietic cell graft which contains HLA-suitable stem cells must be acquired in a timely fashion and referral accomplished to a transplant center expeditiously. The goal is simply the timely correction of immunological function. Potential complications include graft-versus-host disease (GVHD), conditioning toxicity, engraftment failure, peritransplant infections, delayed or partial immunological reconstitution, and secondary malignances (de la Morena and Nelson Jr. 2014).

Patients might also present with combined immunodeficiency of less severity than SCID, with recurrent infections or presenting with idiopathic T-cell lymphopenia. Antibiotic prophylaxis might be useful to reduce the frequency of infections along with surveillance for autoimmunity and inflammatory disorders.

Referral to a tertiary center with a multi-disciplinary team for the management of these conditions is recommended. The patient and family may need input from social services regarding health care options and avenues to care that are either available or not.

References

Alarcon B, Berkhout B, Breitmeyer J, Terhorst C. Assembly of the human T cell receptor-CD3 complex takes place in the endoplasmic reticulum and involves intermediary complexes between the CD3-gamma.delta.epsilon core and single T cell receptor alpha or beta chains. J Biol Chem. 1988a;263:2953–61.

Alarcon B, Regueiro JR, Arnaiz-Villena A, Terhorst C. Familial defect in the surface expression of the T-cell receptor-CD3 complex. N Engl J Med. 1988b;319:1203–8.

Arnaiz-Villena A, Timon M, Corell A, Perez-Aciego P, Martin-Villa JM, Regueiro JR. Primary immunodeficiency caused by mutations in the gene encoding the CD3-gamma subunit of the T-lymphocyte receptor. N Engl J Med. 1992;327(8):529–33.

Clevers H, Dunlap S, Terhorst C. The transmembrane orientation of the epsilon chain of the TcR/CD3 complex. Eur J Immunol. 1988;18:705–10.

Dave VP, Cao Z, Browne C, et al. CD3 delta deficiency arrests development of the alpha beta but not the gamma delta T cell lineage. EMBO J. 1997;16:1360–70.

de la Morena MT, Nelson RP Jr. Recent advances in transplantation for primary immune deficiency diseases: a comprehensive review. Clin Rev Allergy Immunol. 2014;46:131–44.

Hubert P, Bergeron F, Grenot P, et al. Deficiency of the CD3-TCR signal pathway in three patients with idiopathic CD4+ lymphocytopenia. J Soc Biol. 1999;193:11–6.

Ledbetter JA, June CH, Martin PJ, Spooner CE, Hansen JA, Meier KE. Valency of CD3 binding and internalization of the CD3 cell-surface complex control T cell responses to second signals: distinction between effects on protein kinase C, cytoplasmic free calcium, and proliferation. J Immunol. 1986;136:3945–52.

Reinherz EL, Meuer SC, Schlossman SF. The delineation of antigen receptors on human T lymphocytes. Immunol Today. 1983;4:5–8.

Roifman CM. CD3 delta immunodeficiency. Curr Opin Allergy Clin Immunol. 2004;4:479–84.

Rowe JH, Delmonte OM, Keles S, Stadinski BD, Dobbs AK, Henderson LA, Yamazaki Y, et al. Patients with CD3G mutations reveal a role for human CD3γ in Treg diversity and suppressive function. Blood. 2018;131(21):2335–44.

Sanal O, Yel L, Ersoy F, Tezcan I, Berkel AI. Low expression of T-cell receptor-CD3 complex: a case with a clinical presentation resembling humoral immunodeficiency. Turk J Pediatr. 1996;38:81–4.

Soudais C, de Villartay JP, Le Deist F, Fischer A, Lisowska-Grospierre B. Independent mutations of the human CD3-epsilon gene resulting in a T cell receptor/CD3 complex immunodeficiency. Nat Genet. 1993;3:77–81.

Sussman JJ, Bonifacino JS, Lippincott-Schwartz J, et al. Failure to synthesize the T cell CD3-zeta chain: structure and function of a partial T cell receptor complex. Cell. 1988;52:85–95.

Tokgoz H, Caliskan U, Keles S, Reisli I, Guiu IS, Morgan NV. Variable presentation of primary immune deficiency: two cases with CD3 gamma deficiency presenting with only autoimmunity. Pediatr Allergy Immunol. 2013;24:257–62.

Weissman AM, Hou D, Orloff DG, et al. Molecular cloning and chromosomal localization of the human T-cell receptor zeta chain: distinction from the molecular CD3 complex. Proc Natl Acad Sci U S A. 1988;85:9709–13.

CD40 Deficiency, Hyper-IgM Syndrome Type 3 (OMIM # 606843)

M. Teresa de la Morena
Department of Pediatrics and Division of Immunology, Seattle Children's Hospital and University of Washington, Seattle, WA, USA

Introduction/Background

Deficiency in CD40 (TNRSF5) causes an extremely rare combined immunodeficiency affecting both cellular and humoral immunity. Also called hyper-IgM type 3, the clinical phenotype is similar to X-linked hyper-IgM syndrome (XHIGM). In contrast to XHIGM, mutations in CD40 are inherited in an autosomal recessive mode. The *CD40* gene is a member of the TNF-receptor superfamily and is located on chromosome 20q13.12.

CD40 was first discovered to be constitutively expressed on B cells and then was identified on other antigen presenting cells (APC), including dendritic cells and monocytes/macrophages. Its expression on platelets suggests a role for CD40/CD40L in the pathogenesis of atherosclerosis. It is present on endothelial cells, bronchial and bile duct epithelial cells, and neurons. Analysis of proteomes suggests expression in the gallbladder, pancreas, and rectum. Therefore, CD40 is likely to play a much broader role in mammalian biology than only in the immune function (Gormand et al. 1999).

Lougaris et al. reviewed in vitro experiments that showed that in the absence of antigen and/or T cells, CD40 cross-linking on B cells promotes proliferation, differentiation, and secretion of cytokines that drive specific immunoglobulins production. In addition, B cell survival is increased by the upregulation of anti-apoptotic genes. The binding of CD40 to its ligand, CD40 ligand (CD40L) mediates T cell-dependent immunoglobulin isotype switching, memory B cell development, and germinal center formation. CD40 induces the expression of activation-induced cytidine deaminase (AID) in B cells, an enzyme that is critical for immunoglobulin isotype switching. CD40/CD40L interactions with monocytes provoke secretion of pro-inflammatory cytokines, upregulation of activation markers including CD80, CD86, and MHC class II on dendritic cells and macrophages. This contributes to T-cell dependent macrophage-mediated responses (Lougaris et al. 2005).

Clinical Presentation

Patients present with signs similar to those with Type 1 XHIGM. All affected patients reported to date were born to consanguineous parents. Recurrent sinopulmonary infections began in early infancy with pathogens including *Pseudomonas aeruginosa*, *Pneumocystis jirovecii*, and *Cryptosporidium parvum*. Chronic diarrhea is a common finding, especially in those in whom *Cryptosporidium* is identified. As with CD40L deficiency, patients may also experience sclerosing cholangitis, neutropenia, and progressive neurodegenerative deterioration of unknown etiology (Ferrari et al. 2001; Kutukculer et al. 2003; Karaca et al. 2012; Al-Saud et al. 2013).

Leven et al. reported only once case of CD40 deficiency among 145 patients with the hyper-IgM phenotype in the United States

Immunodeficiency Network (USIDNET) consortium (Leven et al. 2016). Al-Saud et al. reported that all of 11 patients from 7 families had recurrent pulmonary infections; Three patients had *Pneumocystis jirovecii* infection. Five patients had sclerosing cholangitis, and five patients had *Cryptosporidium* isolated from their stool. Fungal sinus disease occurred in two patients and eight were neutropenic (Al-Saud et al. 2013).

Diagnosis and Laboratory Testing

Laboratory findings observed include low levels of IgG, absent IgA, and elevated or normal IgM levels. The taxonomic advancements improve the accuracy of these conditions, given that "hyper" IgM is a misnomer in some patients and levels vary depending on the age of the child. In general, the younger the child, the more likely the IgM will be normal, perhaps related with transplacental transfer of maternal IgG. Patient may be neutropenic or with eosinophilia.

Antibody responses to routine childhood vaccinations are usually absent, while isohemagglutinins are usually normal or elevated. T, B, and NK enumeration and proliferation to mitogens are normal. The diagnosis is established when pathogenic mutations are found in CD40 gene sequencing, available through most commercial laboratories. If available, flow cytometry analysis of CD40 expression on B cells and monocytes provides a rapid screen.

Treatment

Patients with CD40 deficiency are treated similar to those XHIGM. Gammaglobulin replacement therapy, either intravenous (IVIG) or subcutaneous, is recommended for all patients. Treat bacterial and viral infections promptly with appropriate antimicrobial therapy; a prolonged course may be necessary. Antimicrobial prophylaxis is recommended to prevent *Pneumocystis jirovecii* pneumonia and trimethroprim-sulfamethoxazole may be used with caution, given the tendency for neutropenia. Prevention against *Cryptosporidium* spp. infection is based

in hygiene measures. The parasite is waterborn; toddlers and young children are especially vulnerable. It is important to recognize that alcohol-based sanitizers are not effective, it is recommended hand washing with soap and water. Swimming in waterparks, rivers, lakes, or drinking from water fountains should be avoided. Nitazoxanide and paramomycin have been used for treatment but do not eradicate the pathogen from immunocompromised hosts.

Neutropenia that is chronic or associated with adverse clinical consequences usually responds to human recombinant-granulocyte colony-stimulating-factor (rhG-CSF), which is available now in a less costly biosimilar formulation. The length of therapy with rhG-CSF is not established, nor is it known to be necessary in patients who have low counts but are clinically well. The risk for malignant transformation to a myeloid malignancy is not known for patients with CD40 deficiency.

To date, eight patients underwent hematopoietic cell transplantation (HCT); all of whom had matched sibling donors (Kutukculer et al. 2003; Mazzolari et al. 2007; Al-Saud et al. 2019). Seven of the eight patients who received HCT survived and developed excellent immunoreconstitution.

References

Al-Saud BK, Al-Sun Z, Alassiri H, Al-Ghonaium A, Al-Muhsen S, Al-Dhekri H, et al. Clinical, immunological, and molecular characterization of hyper –IgM syndrome due to CD40 deficiency in eleven patients. J Clin Immunol. 2013;33:1325–35.

Al-Saud B, Al-Jomaie M, Al-Ghonaium A, Al-Ahmari A, Al-Mousa H, et al. Haematopoietic stem cell transplant for hyper-IgM syndrome due to CD40 defects: a single-centre experience. Bone Marrow Transplant. 2019;54:63–7.

Ferrari S, Giliani S, Insalaco A, Al-Ghonaium A, Soresina AR, Loubser M, et al. Mutations of CD40 gene cause an autosomal recessive form of immunodeficiency with hyper IgM. Proc Natl Acad Sci U S A. 2001;98(22):12614–9.

Gormand F, Briere F, Peyrol S, Raccurt M, Durand I, Ait-Yahia S, et al. CD40 expression by human bronchial epithelial cells. Scand J Immunol. 1999;49(4):355–61.

Karaca NE, Forveille M, Aksu G, Durandy A, Kutukculer N. Hyper-immunoglobulin M syndrome type 3 with normal CD40 cell surface expression. Scand J Immunol. 2012;76(1):21–5.

Kutukculer N, Aksoylar S, Kansoy S, Cetingul N, Notarangelo LD. Outcome of hematopoietic stem cell transplantation in hyper-IgM syndrome caused by CD40 deficiency. J Pediatr. 2003a;143(1):141–2.

Kutukculer N, Moratto D, Aydinok Y, Lougaris V, Aksoylar S, Plebani A, et al. Disseminated cryptosporidium infection in an infant with hyper-IgM syndrome caused by CD40 deficiency. J Pediatr. 2003b;142(2):194–6.

Leven E, Maffucci P, Ochs H, Scholl P, Buckley R, Fuleihan R, et al. Hyper IgMsyndrome: a report from the USIDENT registry. J Clin Immunol. 2016;36:490–501.

Lougaris V, Badolato R, Ferrari S, Plebani A. Hyper immunoglobulin M syndrome due to CD40 deficiency: clinical, molecular, and immunological features. Immunol Rev. 2005;203:48–66. https://doi.org/10.1111/j.0105-2896.2005.00229.x.

Mazzolari E, Lanzi G, Forino C, Lanfranchi A, Aksu G, Ozturk C, et al. First report of successful stem cell transplantation in a child with CD40 deficiency. Bone Marrow Transplant. 2007;40(3):279–81.

CD40bp

▶ TRAF3 Deficiency

CD8 Alpha (CD8A) Deficiency

Robert P. Nelson
Divisions of Hematology and Oncology, Stem Cell Transplant Program, Indiana University (IU) School of Medicine and the IU Bren and Simon Cancer Center, Indianapolis, IN, USA
Pediatric Immunodeficiency Clinic, Riley Hospital for Children at Indiana University Health, Indianapolis, IN, USA
Medicine and Pediatrics, Indiana University School of Medicine, Immunohematology and Transplantation, Indianapolis, IN, USA

Synonyms

Alpha polypeptide; OKT8 T cell antigen; T-Cell antigen Leu2

Definition

CD8 alpha is a glycoprotein, a lymphocyte accessory molecule that regulates MHC-I restricted T-cell activation by antigen.

Introduction/Background

Kavathas et al. isolated genomic and cDNA clones encoding the Leu-2 (T8) surface molecule, later termed CD8, by combining transfection, fluorescence-activated cell-sorting, and subtractive cDNA hybridization methods (Kavathas et al. 1984). The CD8 molecule was found to have multiple forms; the most common was a dimer by the isoforms alpha (α) and beta (β), which are encoded by different genes located on the chromosome 2p11.2. Currently termed cluster of differentiation 8 (CD8), this invariant accessory molecule is expressed on MHC Class I-restricted CD3+ lymphocytes. The CD8 molecule provides the receptor for antigen-MHC I (but not antigen-MHC II) signaling to go from the outside and transmembrane area, to the internal cell space that ultimately leads to gene transcription. CD8 provides the required second signal essential for both normal interleukin 2 (IL2) production and IL2 responsiveness; the second signal may be dampened or eliminated by inhibitors of protein kinase C and cGMP or cAMP-dependent kinases (Samstag et al. 1988). Defective CD8A is one cause of congenitally determined combined immunodeficiency disease.

Function

Precisely how accessory molecules operate is not fully understood, but evidence suggests a dual role. First, they function as receptors or binding ligands; second, they are involved directly or indirectly in intracellular signaling events. Both functions are critical for immune competence. CD3/CD8-positive cells comprise approximately 3–5% of peripheral blood white blood cells; however, this percentage increases during acute and chronic viral infections including human immunodeficiency virus infections. Like CD4, CD8 molecules interact with MHC molecules not directly associated with the T cell receptor (TCR)-Ag complex and function as a co-receptor by providing a cyto-plasmic domain that binds to the protein tyrosine kinase LCK. The accessory function impacts the signaling process in the early phase of the response and does not participate with later effector functions (Lustgarten et al. 1991).

Loss-of-function (LOF) mutations in zeta-chain-associated protein kinase 70 (ZAP-70) are characterized by the absence of peripheral CD8+ T cells and the presence of normal or high levels of circulating CD4+ T lymphocytes (Elder et al. 1995; Arpaia et al. 1994; Chan et al. 1994; Elder et al. 1994). Ueno et al. quantified the clonally expanded T cells present in the memory T cell population of healthy children and found many, whereas a CD8-deficient patient had a diverse set of CD45RO+ memory T cells, but only a few clonally expanded. Interestingly, the patients CD45RO+CD4+ T cells had acquired the capacity to produce effector type cytokines in the absence of ZAP-70 (Ueno et al. 1999).

CD8 is required for effective T-cell activation the affinity or expression of antigen is low; therefore, CD8 may enhance the avidity of T cells for target cells by binding to class I antigen. CD8 participates in postbinding events that lead to cytotoxic T cells (CTL) activation and lysis of cells. The interaction between CTL and target cells precedes interaction of the TCR with its specific antigen. Although CD2 and LFA-3 on the target cell and LFA-1 with ICAM-1 are the strongest adhesion influences, CD8 may serve as adhesion molecules that binds class I MHC antigens. CD8 also participates in postbinding events leading to CTL activation and subsequent lysis of the target cells. Blocking of anti-TCR/CD3 mAb-induced CTL reactivity by anti-CD4/CD8 mAbs does not necessarily interfere the binding of CD8 to its ligands, and TCR and CD8 may form a functional complex that optimizes T-cell activation (de Vries et al. 1989).

Clinical Manifestations

Children from two different families were discovered to have absence of CD8+ T lymphocytes, normal numbers of CD4+ T lymphocytes and proliferative defects to stimulation by nonspecific mitogens, specific antibodies against T cell receptor, and specific antigens. The proliferative defects could be "bypassed" by activating agents independent of the T cell receptor. The combination of an activation defect and selective depletion of CD8+ T lymphocytes suggested that the defective pathway is important for the differentiation of immature thymocytes as well as the proliferation of mature lymphocytes (Monafo et al. 1992).

In 2001, de la Calle-Martin et al. reported an adult from a consanguineous family who had suffered repetitive bronchitis and otitis media age beginning at 5 years of age. At age 25, he developed weight loss, worsening exacerbations of respiratory symptoms, a positive sputum for Haemophilus influenza and total absence of CD8(+) cells. Genetic studies revealed that the *CD8A* gene harbored a missense mutation (p. G111S) in both alleles of the patient and his 2 two siblings. CD3+ T cells with neither CD4 nor CD8 were elevated. Chest x-ray and computed tomography (CT) revealed disseminated bronchiectasis. Pulmonary function was severely compromised. He required additional hospitalizations for respiratory infections. Although bacterial infections and bronchiectasis suggested an antibody deficiency, analysis of total immunoglobulins revealed increased IgG and IgA, consistent with polyclonal gammopathy but with normal IgM and IgG subclasses. Specific titers to tetanus, toxoplasma, *Mycoplasma pneumoniae*, cytomegalovirus (CMV), herpes zoster, herpes simplex, rubella were protective. Serologies to HIV and Epstein-Barr virus (EBV), *Legionella pneumophila*, *Aspergillus*, and *Brucella* were negative and autoantibodies, complement levels, oxidative capacity of neutrophils, and karyotype were normal. Lymphocyte phenotyping revealed normal percentages and numbers of CD4+ T cells, B cells, and natural killer (NK) cells. CD8$^+$ cells were completely absent. Two asymptomatic younger sisters also had absent

CD8$^+$ cells. CD3+CD4(−)CD8(−)TCR alpha beta (+) cells were present, while CD4+ T cells did not respond to TCR-mediated stimuli in vitro (de la Calle-Martin et al. 2001).

Katamura reported a case of CD8 deficiency, in which the patient's T cells did not respond to anti-CD3 stimulation in vitro, suggesting that they were naive. However, many CD4+ T cells with activated and memory phenotypes, which expressed CD45RO+, HLA-DR+ and CD25+, were present in the peripheral blood, and these cells were found accumulated in the perivascular area of his infiltrative erythematous skin lesions. The patient's T cells could be activated by a high concentrations of phyto-haemagglutinin (PHA), which suggested the presence of an alternate signaling pathway which bypasses ZAP-70 and activates CD4+ T cells in vivo (Katamura et al. 1999).

Dumontet et al. reported a 14-year-old boy born to consanguineous parents, who had a history of recurrent upper respiratory infections and pneumonias. Humoral immunity testing was preserved. CD8 T cells were absent. Genetic analysis of the *CD8A* gene revealed a homozygous mutation c.331G>A (p.G111S) (Dumontet et al. 2015).

Diagnoses and Laboratory Testing

Patients may present during childhood or adulthood with recurrent or persistent infections, including bacterial and viral infections and by opportunist organisms. There may be a positive family history of consanguinity or of suspected immunodeficiency. Given the normal CD4+ production, T cell excision circles (TRECs) at birth are not likely to be severely depressed. The inheritance pattern to date is autosomal recessive. Signs of failure to thrive may be present, but facial features are normal and lymph nodes likely palpable. Cognitive impairment, cardiovascular structural defects, or absent thymus are not been reported nor would they be expected. There may be erythematous skin lesions. The immunophenotype is characterized by absence of CD8+ T cells, which also occurs in patients with the autosomal recessive SCID known as ZAP-70. There may be polyclonal gammopathy. T cell proliferation to mitogens and/or antigens is likely decreased.

Treatment/Prognosis

The first clinical decision to make is whether to take care of the patient locally or consider referral to a center that has a multidisciplinary center for the management of these conditions, as exist for several of the classical immunodeficiency diseases. The patient and family may need input from social services regarding health care options and avenues to care that are either available or not.

General treatment considerations of immunocompromised patients apply. CD8A deficient patients reported to date have had normal antibody responses, but presented with frequent upper respiratory infections and pneumonias. Immunoglobulin supplementation and antibiotic prophylaxis might be used to reduce the frequency of infections. The usual course of treatment for individual infectious episodes may require extension of treatment period.

It is not yet defined whether inflammatory conditions might occur in CD8A deficiency, which might indicate the use of immunosuppression and anti-inflammatory therapy.

Data regarding the transplant management of combined (not severe) immunodeficiency secondary to CD8α deficiency is scant; however, the most recent and comprehensive retrospective for CD8 deficiency secondary to ZAP-70 deficiency were recently published. Since 1992, 3 received unconditioned bone marrow transplants from HLA-matched siblings and achieved stable mixed T cell chimerism while myeloid cells remained recipient. B cells were 4-9% but these patients had total immunoglobulin levels, were protected to post-HCT immunizations and were off exogenous immuno-globulin replacement. Five patients who received myeloablative conditioning (three T cell-depleted haploidentical and two unrelated cord blood) reconstituted donor T, B cells and myeloid lineages. One graft failed after serotherapy conditioning. T cell proliferation to phytohemagglutinin was normal in 8/8 post-HCT in 8/8 patients. Seven had discontinued immunoglobulin; this single center retrospective reveals 100% survival at 13.5 years median follow-up (Cuvelier et al. 2016).

Cross-References

▶ CD3d, e and z Deficiencies

References

Arpaia E, Shahar M, Dadi H, Cohen A, Roifman CM. Defective T cell receptor signaling and CD8+ thymic selection in humans lacking zap-70 kinase. Cell. 1994;76:947–58.

Chan AC, Kadlecek TA, Elder ME, et al. ZAP-70 deficiency in an autosomal recessive form of severe combined immunodeficiency. Science. 1994;264:1599–601.

Cuvelier GD, Rubin TS, Wall DA, Schroeder ML. Long-term outcomes of hematopoietic stem cell transplantation for ZAP70 deficiency. J Clin Immunol. 2016;36:713–24.

de la Calle-Martin O, Hernandez M, Ordi J, et al. Familial CD8 deficiency due to a mutation in the CD8 alpha gene. J Clin Invest. 2001;108:117–23.

de Vries JE, Yssel H, Spits H. Interplay between the TCR/CD3 complex and CD4 or CD8 in the activation of cytotoxic T lymphocytes. Immunol Rev. 1989;109:119–41.

Dumontet E, Osman J, Guillemont-Lambert N, Cros G, Moshous D, Picard C. Recurrent respiratory infections revealing CD8α deficiency. J Clin Immunol. 2015;35(8):692–5.

Elder ME, Lin D, Clever J, et al. Human severe combined immunodeficiency due to a defect in ZAP-70, a T cell tyrosine kinase. Science. 1994;264:1596–9.

Elder ME, Hope TJ, Parslow TG, Umetsu DT, Wara DW, Cowan MJ. Severe combined immunodeficiency with absence of peripheral blood CD8+ T cells due to ZAP-70 deficiency. Cell Immunol. 1995;165:110–7.

Katamura K, Tai G, Tachibana T, et al. Existence of activated and memory CD4+ T cells in peripheral blood and their skin infiltration in CD8 deficiency. Clin Exp Immunol. 1999;115:124–30.

Kavathas P, Sukhatme VP, Herzenberg LA, Parnes JR. Isolation of the gene encoding the human T-lymphocyte differentiation antigen Leu-2 (T8) by gene transfer and cDNA subtraction. Proc Natl Acad Sci U S A. 1984;81:7688–92.

Lustgarten J, Waks T, Eshhar Z. CD4 and CD8 accessory molecules function through interactions with major histocompatibility complex molecules which are not directly associated with the T cell receptor-antigen complex. Eur J Immunol. 1991;21:2507–15.

Monafo WJ, Polmar SH, Neudorf S, Mather A, Filipovich AH. A hereditary immunodeficiency characterized by CD8+ T lymphocyte deficiency and impaired lymphocyte activation. Clin Exp Immunol. 1992;90:390–3.

Samstag Y, Emmrich F, Staehelin T. Activation of human T lymphocytes: differential effects of CD3- and CD8-mediated signals. Proc Natl Acad Sci U S A. 1988;85:9689–93.

Ueno H, Katamura K, Yorifuji T, et al. Further characterization of memory T cells existing in a case of CD8 deficiency. Hum Immunol. 1999;60:1049–53.

CDC42 Cell Division Control Protein 42

▶ Wiskott-Aldrich Syndrome Deficiency
▶ Wiskott-Aldrich Syndrome Protein-Interacting Protein (WIP) Deficiency

c-E10

▶ B Cell Lymphoma/Leukemia 10 Deficiency

CHARGE Syndrome (CHD7, SEMA3E)

Melissa L. Crenshaw
Division of Genetics, Johns Hopkins All Children's Hospital, St. Petersburg, FL, USA

Synonyms

Hall-Hittner syndrome

Definition

CHARGE syndrome is a well-described genetic condition affecting multiple body systems and more recently noted to be associated with immunodeficiency. This is recognized as the co-occurrence of anomalies including the eyes (coloboma), heart (congenital heart defects), choanal atresia, retardation of somatic and mental development, genitourinary anomalies, and ear anomalies (Pagon et al. 1981).

The majority of individuals with CHARGE syndrome are de novo. However, rarely familiar cases are described with autosomal dominant inheritance. Over 90% of individuals with typical

CHARGE have a heterozygous pathogenic change in the gene *CHD7* (Vissers et al. 2004), which encodes the chromodomain helicase DNA-binding protein 7. *SEMA3E* has also been reported as a causative gene in at least two affected persons (Lalani et al. 2004). This produces the protein semaphorin 3E. This is an autosomal dominant condition with most cases being sporadic.

CHARGE Syndrome

CHARGE syndrome is the association of anomalies including the eyes (coloboma), heart (congenital heart defects), choanal atresia, genitourinary, and ear anomalies in conjunction with developmental defects of growth and mental abilities. It is the most common cause of congenital anomalies with prevalence of 1/15,000 to 1/17,000 live births with about 90% having pathogenic variants in *CHD7* (Janssen et al. 2012). CHARGE was first described as a unifying condition by Pagon et al. (1981). Prior to identification of a causative gene, this generally has been a clinical diagnosis based on major and minor features (Verloes 2005). The majority of individuals come to attention at birth. However, some children with milder manifestations may be diagnosed later. It is important also to distinguish CHARGE from other genetic conditions with overlapping features, most notably 22q11.2 deletion syndrome and Kallmann syndrome that is the part of the phenotypic spectrum of CHARGE (Fig. 1).

The underlying genetic cause for CHARGE was identified several years later. Most individuals are found to have a pathogenic change in the gene *CHD7* (Vissers et al. 2004). These variables are somatic or gremlin and mostly in the protein-coding exome regions, however may also occur in noncoding areas and affect splicing regulation or involve deletions or duplications (Janssen et al. 2012). Lalani et al. (2004) also have reported two children with the CHARGE phenotype related to pathogenic changes in the *SEMA3E* gene. Thus, this is thought to be a more rare cause for CHARGE syndrome. With the advent of genetic testing to confirm CHARGE, the phenotypic spectrum has widened. Further, this has contributed to our understanding of the *CHD7* gene and its effects.

Immune defects are less appreciated in CHARGE syndrome. There is significant overlap in the immunologic aspects of CHARGE and Di George syndrome. Complete DiGeorge phenotype including hypocalcemia and T-cell immune deficiency related to thymic aplasia or dysfunction has been most frequently associated with 22q11.2 deletion. However, complete DiGeorge phenotype was first described in an infant with

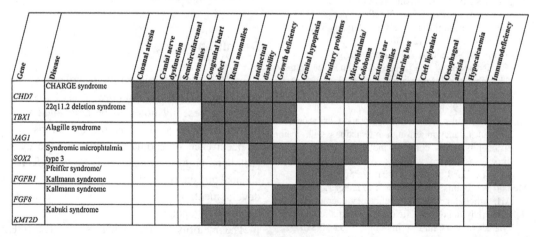

CHARGE Syndrome (CHD7, SEMA3E), Fig. 1 Adapted from Wong 2015 EJHG CHARGE syndrome – a review of the immunological aspects

a *CHD7* mutation by Sanka et al. (2007). Furthermore, in a cohort of patient with DiGeorge anomaly considered for thymus transplant, 14 of 54 cases had features consistent with CHARGE syndrome (Markert et al. 2007).

Subsequently, mutations in *CHD7* have been reported in individuals with a range of immunologic phenotypes. These include mild to severe T-cell deficiency, thymic hypoplasia or dysplasia, isolated humoral immune deficiency, and SCID (Writzl et al. 2007; Chopra et al. 2009). Additional patients had T-B+NK+ SCID, or its inflammatory phenotype, Omenn phenotype (Gennery et al. 2008). These authors further suggest a common role for *CHD7* and 22q11.2 deletion and/or the *TBX1* gene in neural crest development (Gennery et al. 2008; Wong et al. 2015b).

Children with *CHD7* mutations universally have an increase in infections including most prominently pneumonia and otitis media (Wong et al. 2015a, b). In this same cross-sectional study, 50% had decreased T-cell numbers. Decreased T cell receptor excision circle (TREC) also was suggestive that thymic function is impaired. And, while peripheral B-cell production was normal, 83% had insufficient antibody response to childhood vaccines (Wong et al. 2015a, b). Prospective study has shown that severe immune deficiencies such as SCID and DiGeorge in those with *CHD7* mutations most often present in the newborn period and are rare by school age (Hsu et al. 2016). However, a greater role for atopy was also noted in these children (Hsu et al. 2016). Thus, it is important to consider pathogenic changes in this gene in children with a variety of immunologic and atopic presentations, especially in those where there is thymic aplasia or hypoplasia or other findings suspicious for a diagnosis of 22q11.2 deletion with negative testing.

CHD7 and SEMA3A Proteins and Pathogenic Changes

CHD7 (chromodomain helicase DNA-binding protein 7) is both a positive regular of ribosomal RNA biogenesis and a transcriptional regulator, acting as a positive regulator of genes found in the nucleus and nucleoplasm (Zentner et al. 2010).

Bajpai et al. (2010) have shown an instrumental role for this protein in neural crest migration and patterning during embryonic development. It has been suggested but remains unclear whether there is a parallel in the role of *CHD7* and the *TBX1* gene responsible for neural crest progression in 22q11.2 deletion (Gennery et al. 2008; Wong et al. 2015b). The majority of individuals with a clinical diagnosis of CHARGE syndrome have a pathogenic change in this gene. Lalani et al. (2006) found that 73% of their cohort of 110 patients had truncating mutations, confirming that haploinsufficency for this protein leads to the phenotype with an increase in characteristic features such as cardiovascular defects, coloboma, and facial asymmetry among those with confirmed mutations. While most cases are the results of de novo mutations, parental somatic mosaicism has been reported, thus showing occurrence of germline mosiacism and potential for recurrence in future pregnancies for asymptomatic parents (Jongmans et al. 2006). As more individuals are found to have pathogenic changes in this gene, we may be better able to make correlations between genotype and phenotype to guide prognosis.

A mutation in *SEMA3A* has also been reported as causative in a minority of individuals with features of CHARGE. This gene codes for semaphorin 3A. This protein is a contributing factor to signaling of growth of apical dendrites as well as axonal patterning neurologic development (Polleux et al. 2000). This has also been suggested to be a component of angiogenesis in vascular development (Serini et al. 2003).

Immunologic Characteristics of CHARGE

Whether or not an individual meets the clinical diagnostic criteria for CHARGE, those with mutations in the *CHD7* gene can have significant immunologic deficiencies. The immunological aspects of this gene were noted well after the description of CHARGE syndrome and the identification of *CHD7* as the primary causative gene. The first case was reported by Sanka et al. (2007) in an infant with a *CHD7* mutation and complete DiGeorge phenotype who has initially been evaluated for the 22q11.2 deletion with negative results. This then prompted identification of additional similar cases.

The immunologic phenotype has since been assessed in more detail. Subsequent cross-sectional as well as prospective studies have elucidated a wide spectrum of immunologic abnormalities associated with this gene, the majority related to T-cell deficiencies with or without thymic aplasia/hypoplasia. Writzl et al. (2007) described 14 patients with SCID phenotype, most with severe T-cell deficiency and some patients with isolated humoral immunodeficiency. Further case study confirmed moderate to severe T-cell deficiency associated with thymic aplasia or hypoplasia as a consistent feature of CHARGE and recommended considering this as a clinical feature of CHARGE (Chopra et al. 2009). Gennery et al. (2008) expanded the phenotype to include Omenn syndrome, a highly inflammatory SCID phenotype, and strengthening the link between this gene and SCID variant. They suggested a developmental connection between CHD7 and TBX1/22q11.2 deletion. More extensive and systematic immunologic evaluation was subsequently reported (Wong et al. 2015a, b). This included complete blood counts, Ig levels, lymphocyte subpopulations, peripheral B and T-cell differentiation, TREC, T-cell functions, and vaccination responses (Wong et al. 2015b). They found all patients with increased susceptibility to infections, with upper respiratory infection (URI), pneumonia, and otitis media being the most common and a large fraction of cases (42%) required hospitalization. T cell defects included both low counts (50% of cases) and low thymic function with decreased TRECs; however, T-cell functional responses were preserved. While the majority had T-cell deficiencies, they also reported residual expression of IgM and difficulty switching to IgG in memory B cells (17%). Most patients (83%) had decreased response to at least one childhood vaccine. In contrast to preserved T cell function in the Dutch cohort of 24 patients (Wong et al. 2015a), a larger review of 59 patients (Wong et al. 2015b) confirmed similar findings with 80% of patients showing T-cell lymphopenia but a subset with reduced T-cell function. With the

finding of low TRECs, it is likely that patients with CHARGE may be diagnosed by newborn screening for SCID as cases with T cell lymphopenia.

Most recently, an additional role for atopy has been identified with 65% having at least one atopic condition (Hsu et al. 2016). While these authors found CD8+ counts were similar to those in 22q11.2 deletion syndrome, there was no correlation with hypocalcemia. The severe presentations such as SCID and recurrent infections generally present in the newborn period and if not previously diagnosed are uncommon by school age (Hsu et al. 2016). From this arises the question of evaluation in individuals newly diagnosed with CHARGE with or without associated immunologic symptoms.

Conclusions and Implications for Evaluation and Treatment

Pathogenic changes in the *CHD7* gene are associated with a variable presentation of immunodeficiency. The most severe of these such as SCID and Omenn are most often identified in the newborn period. Onset of symptoms after school age is rare. This gene should be included in the differential diagnosis of newborns and young children presenting with recurrent infections or other signs of immunodeficiency in particular if they have additional diagnostic features of CHARGE syndrome. However, mutations in this gene should also be considered in those without other anomalies. In infants and young children with a new diagnosis of CHARGE syndrome, a low threshold for immunologic evaluation is recommended. The developmental and molecular association between *CHD7* and the 22q11.2 deletion/*TBX1* gene remains to be further elucidated. However, additional evaluation of children with these genetic conditions hopefully will allow an improved understanding of these genes and their respective contributions to immunologic development. Optimally this will lead to improved diagnosis and treatment of children affected with *CHD7* mutations.

References

Bajpai R, Chen DA, Rada-Iglesias A, Zhang J, Xiong Y, Helms J, Chang CP, Zhao Y, Swigut T, Wysocka J. CHD7 cooperates with PBAF to control multipotent neural crest formation. Nature. 2010;463:958–62.

Chopra C, Baretto R, Duddridge M, Browning MJ. T-cell immunodeficiency in CHARGE syndrome. Acta Paediatr. 2009;98(2):408–10.

Gennery AR, Slatter MA, Rice J, Hoefsloot LH, Barge D, McLean-Tooke A, Montgomery T, Goodship JA, Burt AD, Flood TJ, Abinum M, Cant AJ, Johnson D. Mutations in CHD7 in patients with CHARGE syndrome cause T–B + natural killer cell + severe combined immune deficiency and may cause Omenn-like syndrome. Clin Exp Immunol. 2008;153:75–80.

Hsu P, Ma A, Barnes EH, Stat M, Wilson M, Hoefsloot LH, Rinne T, Munns C, Williams G, Wong M, Mehr S. The immune phenotype of patients with CHARGE syndrome. J Allergy Clin Immunol Pract. 2016;4(1):96–103.

Janssen N, Bergman JE, Swertz MA, Tranebjaerg L, Lodahl M, Schoots J, Hofstra RM, van Ravenswaaij-Arts CM, Hoefsloot LH. Mutation update on the CHD7 gene involved in CHARGE syndrome. Hum Mutat. 2012;33(8):1149–60.

Jongmans MC, Admiraal RJ, van der Donk KP, Vissers LE, Baas AF, Kapusta L, van Hagen JM, Donnai D, de Ravel TJ, Veltman JA, van Kessel AG, De Vries BB, Brunner HG, Hoefsloot LH, van Ravenswaaij CM. CHARGE syndrome: the phenotypic spectrum of mutations in the CHD7 gene. J Med Genet. 2006;43(4):306–14.

Lalani Lalani SR, Safiullah AM, Molinari LM, Fernbach SD, Martin DM, Belmont JW. SEMA3E mutation in a patient with CHARGE syndrome. J Med Genet. 2004; 41(7):e94.

Lalani SR, Safiullah AM, Fernbach SD, Harutyunyan KG, Thaller C, Peterson LE, McPherson JD, Gibbs RA, White LD, Hefner M, Davenport SL, Graham JM, Bacino CA, Glass NL, Towbin JA, Craigen WJ, Neish SR, Lin AE, Belmont JW. Spectrum of CHD7 mutations in 110 individuals with CHARGE syndrome and genotype-phenotype correlation. Am J Hum Genet. 2006;78(2):303–14.

Markert ML, Devlin BH, Alexieff MJ, et al. Review of 54 patients with complete DiGeorge anomaly enrolled in protocols for thymus transplantation: outcome of 44 consecutive transplants. Blood. 2007;109:4539–47.

Pagon AP, Graham JM, Siu-Li Y. Coloboma, congenital heart disease, and choanal atresia with multiple anomalies: CHARGE association. J Pediatr. 1981;99(2):223–7.

Polleux F, Morrow T, Ghosh A. Semaphorin 3A is a chemoattractant for cortical apical dendrites. Nature. 2000;404(6778):567–73.

Sanka M, Tangsinmankong N, Loscalzo M, Sleasman JW, Dorsey M. Complete DiGeorge syndrome associated with CHD7 mutation. J Allergy Clin Immunol. 2007;120(4):952–4.

Serini G, Valdembri D, Zanivan S, Morterra G, Burkhardt C, Caccavari F, Zammataro L, Primo L, Tamagnone L, Logan M, Tessier-Lavigne M, Taniguchi M, Puschel AW, Bussolino F. Class 3 semaphorins control vascular morphogenesis by inhibiting integrin function. Nature. 2003;424:391–7.

Verloes. Updated diagnostic criteria for CHARGE syndrome: a proposal. Am J Med Genet A. 2005;133A (3):303–8.

Vissers LE, Ravenswaaij RA, Hurst JA, de Vries BB, Janssen IM, van der Vliet WA, Huys EH, de Jong PJ, Hamel BC, Schoenmakers EF, Brunner HG, Veltman JA, van Kessel AG. Mutations in a new member of the chromodomain gene family cause CHARGE syndrome. Nat Genet. 2004;36(9):955–7.

Wong MT, Lambeck AJ, van der Burg M, la Bastidevan Gemert S, Hogendorf LA, van Ravenswaaij-Arts CM, Schölvinck EH. Immune dysfunction in children with CHARGE syndrome: a cross-sectional study. PLoS One. 2015a;10(11):e0142350.

Wong MT, Schölvinck EH, Lambeck AJ, van Ravenswaaij-Arts CM. CHARGE syndrome: a review of the immunological aspects. Eur J Hum Genet. 2015b;23:1451–9.

Writzl K, Cale CM, Pierce CM, Wilson LC, Hennekan RC. Immunological abnormalities in CHARGE syndrome. Eur J Med Genet. 2007;50(5):338–45.

Zentner GE, Hurd EA, Schnetz MP, Handoko L, Wang C, Wang Z, Wei C, Tesar PJ, Hatzoglou M, Martin DM, Scacheri PC. CHD7 functions in the nucleolus as a positive regulator of ribosomal RNA biogenesis. Hum Mol Genet. 2010;19(18):3491–501.

CHH

▸ Cartilage Hair Hypoplasia (RMRP)

Chromosome 7p22 Deletion

▸ B-Actin deficiency

Chromosome 11q Deletion Syndrome

▸ Jacobsen Syndrome

Chromosome 22q11.2 Deletion Syndrome

▶ DiGeorge Anomaly (del22q11)

Chronic Atypical Neutrophilic Dermatosis with Lipodystrophy and Elevated Temperature Syndrome (CANDLE)/Proteasome-Associated Autoinflammatory Syndromes (PRAAS)

Gina A. Montealegre Sanchez, Adriana A. de Jesus and Raphaela Goldbach-Mansky
Translational Autoinflammatory Diseases Section (TADS), National Institute of Allergy and Infectious Diseases (NIAID), National Institutes of Health (NIH), Bethesda, MD, USA

Synonyms

Chronic Atypical Neutrophilic Dermatosis with Lipodystrophy and Elevated temperatures (CANDLE); Joint contractures, Muscle atrophy, microcytic anemia, and Panniculitis-induced lipodystrophy (JMP); Nakajo-Nishimura Syndrome (NNS); Proteasome-Associated Auto-inflammatory Syndrome (PRAAS)

Definition

CANDLE/PRAAS is a genetically defined Type I interferonopathy caused by recessive or digenic loss-of-function (LOF) mutations in proteasome genes *PSMB8, PSMB9, PSMA3, PSMB4, and PSMG2* and dominant loss of function mutations that cause haploinsufficiency in *POMP*.

CANDLE/PRAAS patients present with recurrent fever, panniculitis-induced lipodystrophy, joint contractures, myositis, cytopenia, basal ganglia calcifications, and elevated acute phase reactants. Forty to 80% of patients develop systemic hypertension, metabolic syndrome, and hepatic steatosis often within the first decade of life. Primary pulmonary hypertension has been reported in two young patients.

Introduction and Background

In 1993 Tanaka et al. reported two Japanese patients with fever, rashes, lipodystrophy, increased intra-abdominal fat, muscular atrophy, joint contractures, hepatosplenomegaly, arrhythmias, macroglossia, low intelligence quotient (IQ), basal ganglia calcifications, hypergammaglobulinemia, and elevated sedimentation rate (ESR). He proposed that these patients in addition to 13 patients previously reported in the Japanese literature since 1939 suffered from the same syndrome, a new condition characterized by lipo-muscular atrophy, joint contractures, and skin rash (Tanaka et al. 1993).

It was not until 2010 when Garg et al. reported two Mexican siblings and a Portuguese patient and noted the similarities with the Japanese patients that the disorder was named JMP syndrome, for joint contractures, muscular atrophy, microcytic anemia, and panniculitis-induced childhood-onset lipodystrophy (Garg et al. 2010). All patients reported by Garg et al. had short stature, low HDL cholesterol, and two out of three developed seizures. The same year, Torrelo et al. proposed the acronym CANDLE for a disease described in four patients including two sisters who had early-onset recurrent fevers, lipodystrophy, and annular erythematous skin lesions with histopathologic findings consistent with atypical or immature myeloid infiltrates in the skin. These patients also presented with growth retardation, transaminitis, hypochromic anemia, and elevation of acute phase reactants (Torrelo et al. 2010). CANDLE/PRAAS is a rare disease with less than 100 cases reported worldwide most of them in Caucasian males. Untreated disease has been associated with a high mortality up to 30% (Kim et al. 2016).

Genetics

In 2011 the veil was lifted when several groups showed that autosomal recessive LOF mutations in proteasome subunit beta type (*PSMB8*) gene cause JMP syndrome (Agarwal et al. 2010), Nakajo-Nishimura syndrome or Japanese autoinflammatory syndrome with lipodystrophy (JASL) (Arima et al. 2011; Kitamura et al. 2011), and CANDLE (Liu et al. 2012) thus indicating that these disorders are the same disease (Torrelo et al. 2010; Liu et al. 2012). PRAAS1 MIM#256040 is caused by homozygous mutations in *PSMB8*; currently, eight pathogenic mutations have been described (https://infevers.umai-montpellier.fr/web). In 2015, Brehm et al. reported a digenic form of PRAAS1 caused by a heterozygous mutation in *PSMB8* and a heterozygous mutation either in *PSMA3* or in *PSMB4* (Brehm et al. 2015). Brehm et al. also reported one patient with a compound homozygous mutation in *PSMB4* and two siblings from an unrelated family with digenic inheritance caused by heterozygous mutation in *PSMB4* and a heterozygous mutation in *PSMB9*, referred as PRAAS3 MIM#617591. In 2018, Poli et al. described an autosomal dominant form denoted as PRAAS2 MIM#618048 caused by heterozygous mutations in the protein assembly protein, *POMP* (Poli et al. 2018). Most recently, de Jesus et al. described two compound heterozygous LOF mutations in *PSMG2*, as a novel genetic cause for PRAAS4 (de Jesus et al. 2019).

Pathogenesis

CANDLE is a rare disease with less than 100 cases described worldwide. However, given the likelihood that other not yet recognized proteasome mutations that cause PRAAS are not present on common screening panels, the disease is probably underdiagnosed.

Proteasomes are protein degradation systems that target intracellular polyubiquitinated proteins derived from self-structures or foreign structures for proteolytic destruction. Proteasomes are implicated in cellular processes including apoptosis, the removal of various misfolded and immature proteins, and the production of peptides for presentation by MHC class I molecules (Goldberg 2007). Gene expression profiling using whole blood microarray identified the IFN pathway as the most differentially upregulated pathway in all six CANDLE patients tested (Liu et al. 2012). Use

of Janus kinase (JAK) inhibitors in vitro resulted in the inhibition of IFN signaling and decreased IFNγ-induced IP-10 production of the patients' cells (Liu et al. 2012). Improvement of the IFN response gene signature and overall clinical improvement has proved that JAK inhibitors are an effective treatment for CANDLE/PRAAS and thus confirmed the prominent role of Type I IFN in this condition (Sanchez et al. 2018).

Clinical Manifestations

CANDLE/PRAAS patients present early in infancy with systemic inflammation (elevated acute phase reactants), recurrent fevers, nodular or plaque-like violaceous skin rash, periorbital erythema with or without eyelid inflammation, failure to thrive, and swelling of fingers and toes. Natural history of the disease is characterized by later-onset lipoatrophy affecting the face and extremities, abnormal distribution of fat with increased intra-abdominal fat deposition, development of dyslipidemia, insulin resistance, and hepatic steatosis (Figs. 1a through g and 2). Arterial hypertension is commonly seen, and 60% of patients meet criteria for metabolic syndrome during the course of their disease. Majority of patients present with severe growth delayed with heights and weights below the third percentile associated with abnormal bone age and bone mineral densities. The most common musculoskeletal manifestations are patchy myositis and non-erosive arthritis that often leads to muscular atrophy and joint contractures.

CANDLE patients should be closely monitored for pulmonary hypertension as two cases have been reported in the literature (Sanchez et al. 2018; Buchbinder et al. 2018). Disease flares are mostly characterized by worsening of underlying inflammatory manifestations (fever, rash, myositis, and synovitis) associated with elevated acute phase reactants and profound lymphopenia in some patients. Other less frequent clinical manifestations are the presence of basal ganglia calcifications, aseptic lymphocytic meningitis, alopecia areata, conjunctivitis, episcleritis, parotitis, epididymitis, and pancreatic abnormalities.

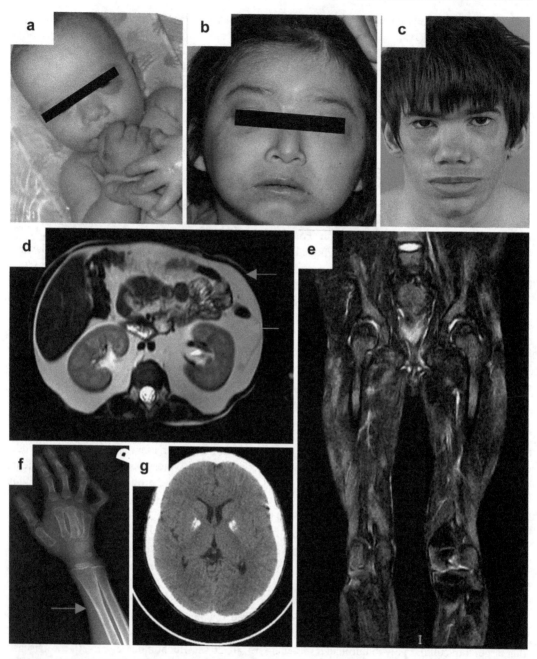

Chronic Atypical Neutrophilic Dermatosis with Lipodystrophy and Elevated Temperature Syndrome (CANDLE)/Proteasome-Associated Autoinflammatory Syndromes (PRAAS), Fig. 1 Clinical disease manifestations in CANDLE and radiological findings (**a–c**) Images of three patients with CANDLE. Images of the face show typical distribution of facial panniculitis with periorbital swelling (**b–c**) and erythema as well as characteristic lipodystrophy affecting temporal regions above and below the zygomatic bone. Lip swelling is also evident. (**d**) Abdominal MRI with absence of subcutaneous fat (red arrow) and accumulation of intraabdominal fat (blue arrow). (**e**) Bilateral thigh MRI with presence of patchy myositis. (**f**) Presence of joint contractures in small joints, fifth right proximal interphalangeal joint and presence of peripheral calcinosis (red arrow). (**g**) Brain MRI with basal ganglia calcifications

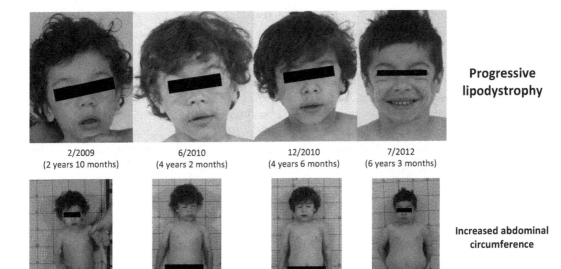

Progressive lipodystrophy

| 2/2009 | 6/2010 | 12/2010 | 7/2012 |
| (2 years 10 months) | (4 years 2 months) | (4 years 6 months) | (6 years 3 months) |

Increased abdominal circumference

Chronic Atypical Neutrophilic Dermatosis with Lipodystrophy and Elevated Temperature Syndrome (CANDLE)/Proteasome-Associated Autoinflammatory Syndromes (PRAAS),

Fig. 2 Progressive lipodystrophy, development of increased abdominal circumference, and stunted growth in a CANDLE patient over 3 years

Laboratory Testing

Elevated acute phase reactants (ESR and CRP) and microcytic anemia are seen in more than 90% of CANDLE/PRAAS patients. Elevated muscle enzymes including creatinine kinase (CK), lactate dehydrogenase (LDH), aldolase, alanine transferase (ALT), and aspartate aminotransferase (AST) are seen in the context of underlying myositis. Dyslipidemia usually precedes the development of hepatic steatosis as well as elevated insulin, and hemoglobin A1C levels precedes the development of insulin resistance. Sixty percent of patients present with transient autoantibodies (anticardiolipin antibodies, lupus anticoagulant, anti-myeloperoxidase, antinuclear antibody) during the course of their disease, autoantibodies are usually not associated with clinical pathology, and titers decreased on treatment with

JAK inhibition (Sanchez et al. 2018). Clinical flares are associated with worsening acute phase reactants and cytopenia, including lymphopenia, thrombocytopenia, and less frequently seen neutropenia.

Skin biopsies show a subcutaneous and dermal inflammatory infiltrate of immature neutrophils (Leder stain), myeloid precursors (myeloperoxidase positive), and atypical mononuclear cells, which are likely activated macrophages (positive for CD68 and CD163, negative for Leder stain) (Torrelo et al. 2015).

Diagnosis

The presence of characteristic clinical symptoms, elevated IFN score (Kim et al. 2018), and presence of pathogenic variants in a proteasome gene will confirm the diagnosis. However, the tetrad of recurrent fevers, panniculitis, lipoatrophy, and elevated acute phase reactants can misguide to the diagnosis of CANDLE as some other yet undefined interferonopathies can present with a similar clinical picture (de Jesus et al. manuscript submitted). The genetic diagnosis continues to be challenging as not all pathogenic mutations have been identified and patients continue to be undiagnosed.

Treatment

Lack of appropriate responses to available disease-modifying antirheumatic drugs (DMARDs), biologics, and other immunomodulators (Sanchez et al. 2018), associated with the mortality related to poor treatments (Kim et al. 2016), and the in vitro observations that JAK kinase inhibitors decreased STAT-1 phosphorylation and IP-10 production in mononuclear cells (PBMCs) from CANDLE patients led to the development of an Expanded Access Program with baricitinib, a JAK 1/2 inhibitor used to treat interferon-mediated diseases including CANDLE/PRAAS. Ten CANDLE/PRAAS patients were enrolled with nine of the ten receiving chronic doses of corticosteroids at the beginning of the program. After a mean follow-up of 3 years (1.5–4.9 years), 50% of CANDLE patients achieved clinical and inflammatory remission criteria with normalization of their IFN score. CANDLE patients had no disease symptoms and normalized their acute phase reactants and IFN scores. Hematological manifestations responded to the treatment with baricitinib as well. Although not all CANDLE patients achieved remission criteria, the overall response was favorable. Treatment with baricitinib resulted in amelioration and, in some cases, complete resolution of systemic and organ inflammation; however, the metabolic manifestations associated with CANDLE did not change; patients continued to develop dyslipidemia, insulin resistance, and hepatic steatosis. Most common side effects associated with baricitinib were upper respiratory infections. Of interest, the majority of these patients developed BK viremia (Sanchez et al. 2018).

Prognosis

The initial reports of CANDLE patients treated with JAK inhibitors is promising; however, long-term data needs to be collected to evaluate for the efficacy and safety. CANDLE patients should be closely monitored for the development of metabolic and vascular complications, including dyslipidemia, insulin resistance, and arterial and pulmonary hypertension. These comorbidities seem not to respond as well as the systemic manifestations to JAK inhibitors (Sanchez et al. 2018; Buchbinder et al. 2018).

Cross-References

▶ Introduction to Autoinflammatory Diseases

References

Agarwal AK, Xing C, DeMartino GN, Mizrachi D, Hernandez MD, Sousa AB, et al. PSMB8 encoding the beta5i proteasome subunit is mutated in joint contractures, muscle atrophy, microcytic anemia, and panniculitis-induced lipodystrophy syndrome. Am J Hum Genet. 2010;87(6):866–72.

Arima K, Kinoshita A, Mishima H, Kanazawa N, Kaneko T, Mizushima T, et al. Proteasome assembly defect due to a proteasome subunit beta type 8 (PSMB8) mutation causes the autoinflammatory disorder, Nakajo-Nishimura syndrome. Proc Natl Acad Sci USA. 2011;108(36):14914–9.

Brehm A, Liu Y, Sheikh A, Marrero B, Omoyinmi E, Zhou Q, et al. Additive loss-of-function proteasome subunit mutations in CANDLE/PRAAS patients promote type I IFN production. J Clin Invest. 2015;125(11):4196–211.

Buchbinder D, Montealegre Sanchez GA, Goldbach-Mansky R, Brunner H, Shulman AI. Rash, fever, and pulmonary hypertension in a 6-year-old female. Arthritis Care Res. 2018;70(5):785–90.

de Jesus AA, Brehm A, VanTries R, Pillet P, Parentelli AS, Montealegre Sanchez GA, et al. Novel proteasome assembly chaperone mutations in PSMG2/PAC2 cause the autoinflammatory interferonopathy CANDLE/PRAAS4. The Journal of allergy and clinical immunology. 2019;143(5):1939–43 e8.

Garg A, Hernandez MD, Sousa AB, Subramanyam L, Martinez de Villarreal L, dos Santos HG, et al. An autosomal recessive syndrome of joint contractures, muscular atrophy, microcytic anemia, and panniculitis-associated lipodystrophy. J Clin Endocrinol Metab. 2010;95(9):E58–63.

Goldberg AL. Functions of the proteasome: from protein degradation and immune surveillance to cancer therapy. Biochem Soc Trans. 2007;35(Pt 1):12–7.

Kim H, Sanchez GA, Goldbach-Mansky R. Insights from Mendelian Interferonopathies: comparison of CANDLE, SAVI with AGS, monogenic lupus. J Mol Med (Berl). 2016;94(10):1111–27.

Kim H, de Jesus AA, Brooks SR, Liu Y, Huang Y, VanTries R, et al. Development of a validated interferon score using NanoString technology. J Interferon Cytokine Res. 2018;38(4):171–85.

Kitamura A, Maekawa Y, Uehara H, Izumi K, Kawachi I, Nishizawa M, et al. A mutation in the immunoproteasome subunit PSMB8 causes autoinflammation and lipodystrophy in humans. J Clin Invest. 2011;121(10):4150–60.

Liu Y, Ramot Y, Torrelo A, Paller AS, Si N, Babay S, et al. Mutations in proteasome subunit beta type 8 cause chronic atypical neutrophilic dermatosis with lipodystrophy and elevated temperature with evidence of genetic and phenotypic heterogeneity. Arthritis Rheum. 2012;64(3):895–907.

Poli MC, Ebstein F, Nicholas SK, de Guzman MM, Forbes LR, Chinn IK, et al. Heterozygous truncating variants in POMP escape nonsense-mediated decay and cause a unique immune Dysregulatory syndrome. Am J Hum Genet. 2018;102(6):1126–42.

Sanchez GAM, Reinhardt A, Ramsey S, Wittkowski H, Hashkes PJ, Berkun Y, et al. JAK1/2 inhibition with baricitinib in the treatment of autoinflammatory interferonopathies. J Clin Invest. 2018;128(7):3041–3052.

Tanaka M, Miyatani N, Yamada S, Miyashita K, Toyoshima I, Sakuma K, et al. Hereditary lipomuscular atrophy with joint contracture, skin eruptions and hyper-gamma-globulinemia: a new syndrome. Intern Med. 1993;32(1):42–5.

Torrelo A, Patel S, Colmenero I, Gurbindo D, Lendinez F, Hernandez A, et al. Chronic atypical neutrophilic dermatosis with lipodystrophy and elevated temperature (CANDLE) syndrome. J Am Acad Dermatol. 2010;62(3):489–95.

Torrelo A, Colmenero I, Requena L, Paller AS, Ramot Y, Richard Lee CC, et al. Histologic and immunohistochemical features of the skin lesions in CANDLE syndrome. Am J Dermatopathol. 2015;37(7):517–22.

Chronic Atypical Neutrophilic Dermatosis with Lipodystrophy and Elevated Temperatures (CANDLE)

▶ Chronic Atypical Neutrophilic Dermatosis with Lipodystrophy and Elevated Temperature Syndrome (CANDLE)/Proteasome-Associated Autoinflammatory Syndromes (PRAAS)

Chronic Mucocutaneous Candidiasis, ACT1 Deficiency

Catherine M. Biggs[1] and Stuart E. Turvey[2,3]
[1]Department of Pediatrics, BC Children's Hospital, University of British Columbia, Vancouver, BC, Canada
[2]Division of Allergy and Clinical Immunology, Department of Pediatrics and Experimental Medicine Program, British Columbia Children's Hospital, The University of British Columbia, Vancouver, BC, Canada
[3]Willem-Alexander Children's Hospital, Leiden University Medical Center, Leiden, The Netherlands

Synonyms

TRAF3-interacting protein 2 deficiency

Definition

Nuclear factor-kappa-B activator 1 (ACT1) deficiency is an autosomal recessive disorder that leads to chronic mucocutaneous candidiasis (CMC). CMC is defined as recurrent or persistent mucocutaneous infections caused by fungi of the genus *Candida*, and primarily by the commensal organism *Candida albicans* (Kirkpatrick 2001; Puel et al. 2012). ACT1 deficiency leads to CMC through impairments in IL-17-mediated immunity.

Introduction

ACT1 was first identified in 2000 as an activating protein of NF-kappa B (NF-κB) and Jun Kinase (Awane et al. 1999; Li et al. 2000; Leonardi et al. 2000). NF-κB is a key transcription factor involved in cellular inflammatory, survival, and stress responses (Li et al. 2000; Baeuerle and Baltimore 1996). NF-κB remains latent in the cytoplasm bound to a group of inhibitor proteins that are collectively called the IκB complex (Antonio Leonardi et al. 2000). Upon stimulation of upstream signaling factors, the IκB complex undergoes ubiquitination and proteosomal degradation, leading to release of NFκB followed by its activation and translocation to the nucleus (Leonardi et al. 2000). There, NFκB mediates the transcription of a number of genes, regulating the expression of cytokines, chemokines, and cell adhesion molecules and receptors.

The *ACT1* gene (also known as *TRAF3IP2*) encodes for the ACT1 protein of 574 amino acids and is ubiquitously expressed (Li et al. 2000; Antonio Leonardi et al. 2000). It contains a helix-loop-helix domain at the N-terminus, two TRAF binding sites (EEESE and EERPA), a SEFIR domain, and a coil-coiled domain at the C-terminus (Li et al. 2000; Qian et al. 2002; Li 2008). Through its protein interactions with NFκB, ACT1 impacts both B cell and Th17 cell immunity (Li 2008). NFκB promotes B cell survival and activation by mediating signaling through CD40 and the B cell activating factor receptor (BAFFR). CD40 and BAFFR-mediated activation of the IκB complex occurs through TNF receptor associated factor (TRAF) adaptor molecules (Qian et al. 2004). ACT1 was initially hypothesized to be a positive mediator of BAFFR and CD40 signaling given its original description as a constitutive activator of NFκB. Act1-deficient mice, however, demonstrated an opposite phenotype of B cell hyperproliferation, thus uncovering Act1's role as a negative B cell regulator (Qian et al. 2004). This effect was reversed in *Cd40/Act1* and *Baff/Act1* double knockout mouse models, indicating that ACT1 exerts its inhibitory effect on B cell proliferation through both the CD40 and BAFFR pathways (Qian et al. 2004). It is hypothesized that upon stimulation of CD40 and BAFFR, ACT1 complexes with TRAF3 and targets activating proteins involved in NF-κB signaling for proteosomal degradation, thus acting in a negative feedback manner.

While ACT1 thus serves to protect against exaggerated B cell responses and B cell-mediated autoimmunity, it has also been implicated in promoting IL-17-mediated inflammation. IL-17 is a pro-inflammatory cytokine produced by T cells that results in NF-κB activation and is important in the protection against extracellular pathogens (Awane et al. 1999; Curtis and Way 2009). In addition to its protective roles in immunity, IL-17 signaling can also promote certain forms of autoimmunity, such as human and experimental models of multiple sclerosis, psoriasis, and inflammatory bowel disease (Jin et al. 2009). ACT1 is essential for signaling through the IL-17 receptor (IL-17R) and leads to the induction of pro-inflammatory cytokines through NF-kB and non-NF-kB-mediated mechanisms (Li 2008). The IL-17R and ACT1 interact through homotypic binding of their respective SEFIR domains. ACT1 then binds to and causes non-degradative ubiquitination of TRAF6, promoting downstream activation of NF-kB (Liu et al. 2009).

Clinical Presentation

ACT1 deficiency is characterized by a propensity towards chronic mucocutaneous candidiasis (CMC). CMC refers to recurrent or persistent infections involving the mucous membranes, such as skin, nails, oral and genital mucosa, and is caused primarily by the commensal fungal organism *Candida albicans* (Kirkpatrick 2001; Puel et al. 2012; Boisson et al. 2013). Patients who suffer from CMC, and who generally do not show a predisposition towards other infections, are referred to as having CMC disease (CMCD) (Boisson et al. 2013).

Patients with CMCD may also be affected by skin infections caused by the bacteria *Staphylococcus aureus*. In addition, those with CMCD have also been found to have a predisposition towards certain forms of autoimmunity, as well as cerebral aneurysms and mucocutaneous carcinomas (Boisson et al. 2013). In 2013, ACT1 deficiency was identified as a genetic cause of CMCD and was therefore added to the list of several genes that have been associated with this clinical phenotype (Boisson et al. 2013). Few cases of ACT1 deficiency have been described, with approximately only four affected patients from two families reported to date (Boisson et al. 2013; Levy et al. 2014). The clinical presentation described is in keeping with CMCD. An early feature often seen in ACT1-deficient patients is infantile seborrheic dermatitis, an inflammatory skin condition commonly affecting the scalp or face (Boisson et al. 2013). Patients with ACT1 deficiency develop persistent or recurrent mucocutaneous candidal infections, which may occur as early as infancy, or later in childhood. CMC affecting the oropharynx may cause oral thrush as well as macrocheilits (swelling and inflammation of the lip). Other affected areas may include: the genitals, the nails resulting in onychomycosis, and the skin folds causing intertrigo (Boisson et al. 2013). Superficial staphylococcal infections have also been reported in ACT1 deficiency, leading to recurrent eyelid and hair follicle infections caused by *Staphylococcus aureus* (Boisson et al. 2013; Levy et al. 2014). Despite the known importance of ACT1 as a negative B cell regulator, ACT1-deficient patients have thus far not demonstrated evidence of B cell-mediated autoimmune disorders. This is attributed to the described mutations affecting the SEFIR domain required for homotypic interactions with the IL-17 receptor, while keeping the other domains important for CD40 and BAFFR interactions intact (Boisson et al. 2013; Levy et al. 2014).

Diagnosis

CMC with or without superficial staphylococcal infections should prompt consideration of ACT1 deficiency. A standard immune workup may be largely unrevealing, therefore a high index of suspicion is required. Evaluation generally demonstrates normal white blood cell and lymphocyte subset enumeration. Immunoglobulin analysis may reveal elevated levels of IgG, variable levels of IgA and IgM, and normal levels of IgE (Boisson et al. 2013). Microbial analysis of affected sites concerning CMC often reveals *Candida albicans*, however, may reveal other candida organisms such as *Candida parapsillosis* (Boisson et al. 2013). No commercial assays to evaluate ACT1 function are currently available. Therefore, when ACT1 deficiency is suspected, targeted sequencing of the *ACT1* gene located on chromosome 6q21 should be performed. This may be performed as part of a broader genetic panel to screen for the numerous genes associated

with CMCD, such as whole exome sequencing. Sequencing of the *ACT1* gene reveals biallelic mutations.

Treatment

Treatment of ACT1 deficiency involves targeted infection prophylaxis measures as well as management of established infections (Okada et al. 2016). Oral antifungal prophylaxis with fluconazole should be considered to protect against mucocutaneous candidiasis (Okada et al. 2016). Fluconazole is also a reasonable first-line oral treatment for *Candida* infections, with alternative options including itraconazole, voriconazole, and posaconazole (Okada et al. 2016). Topical therapy with nystatin may also be considered. Patients affected by superficial staphylococcal infections may benefit from antibiotic prophylaxis with sulfamethoxazole-trimethoprim (Okada et al. 2016). Inflammatory conditions involving the skin, such as seborrheic dermatitis or scalp inflammation caused by staphylococcal infection, may also require the use of corticosteroids (Boisson et al. 2013).

References

Awane M, Andres PG, Li DJ, Reinecker HC. NF-kappa B-inducing kinase is a common mediator of IL-17-, TNF-alpha-, and IL-1 beta-induced chemokine promoter activation in intestinal epithelial cells. J Immunol. 1999;162(9):5337–44.

Baeuerle PA, Baltimore D. NF-kappa B: ten years after. Cell. 1996;87(1):13–20.

Boisson B, Wang C, Pedergnana V, Wu L, Cypowyj S, Rybojad M, et al. An ACT1 mutation selectively abolishes interleukin-17 responses in humans with chronic mucocutaneous candidiasis. Immunity. 2013;39(4): 676–86.

Curtis MM, Way SS. Interleukin-17 in host defence against bacterial, mycobacterial and fungal pathogens. Immunology. 2009;126(2):177–85.

Jin W, Zhou XF, Yu J, Cheng X, Sun SC. Regulation of Th17 cell differentiation and EAE induction by MAP3K NIK. Blood. 2009;113(26):6603–10.

Kirkpatrick CH. Chronic mucocutaneous candidiasis. Pediatr Infect Dis J. 2001;20(2):197–206.

Leonardi A, Chariot A, Claudio E, Cunningham K, Siebenlist U. CIKS, a connection to Iκ B kinase and stress-activated protein kinase. Proc Natl Acad Sci U S A. 2000;97(19):10494–99.

Levy R, Mahlaoui N, Migaud M, Casanova JL, Puel A. ACT1 deficiency: a defect in IL-17 mediated immunity underlying chronic mucocutaneous disease (CMCD) in a multiplex consanguineous kindred. J Clin Immunol. 2014;34:S272–73.

Li XX. Act1 modulates autoimmunity through its dual functions in CD40L/BAFF and IL-17 signaling. Cytokine. 2008;41(2):105–13.

Li X, Commane M, Nie H, Hua X, Chatterjee-Kishore M, Wald D, et al. Act1, an NF-kappa B-activating protein. Proc Natl Acad Sci. 2000;97(19):10489–93.

Liu C, Qian W, Qian Y, Giltiay NV, Lu Y, Swaidani S, et al. Act1, a U-box E3 ubiquitin ligase for IL-17 signaling. Sci Signal. 2009;2(92):ra63.

Okada S, Puel A, Casanova JL, Kobayashi M. Chronic mucocutaneous candidiasis disease associated with inborn errors of IL-17 immunity. Clin Transl Immunol. 2016;5(12):e114.

Puel A, Cypowyj S, Maródi L, Abel L, Picard C, Casanova J-L. Inborn errors of human IL-17 immunity underlie chronic mucocutaneous candidiasis. Curr Opin Allergy Clin Immunol. 2012;12(6):616–22.

Qian Y, Zhao Z, Jiang Z, Li X. Role of NF kappa B activator Act1 in CD40-mediated signaling in epithelial cells. Proc Natl Acad Sci U S A. 2002;99(14):9386–91.

Qian Y, Qin J, Cui G, Naramura M, Snow EC, Ware CF, et al. Act1, a negative regulator in CD40- and BAFF-mediated B cell survival. Immunity. 2004;21(4):575–87.

Chronic Mucocutaneous Candidiasis, IL-17F Deficiency

Catherine M. Biggs[1] and Stuart E. Turvey[2,3]
[1]Department of Pediatrics, BC Children's Hospital, University of British Columbia, Vancouver, BC, Canada
[2]Division of Allergy and Clinical Immunology, Department of Pediatrics and Experimental Medicine Program, British Columbia Children's Hospital, The University of British Columbia, Vancouver, BC, Canada
[3]Willem-Alexander Children's Hospital, Leiden University Medical Center, Leiden, The Netherlands

Synonyms

Candidiasis familial 6 (CANDF6)

Definition

Interleukin-17F deficiency is an autosomal dominant disorder that leads to chronic mucocutaneous candidiasis (CMC). CMC is defined as recurrent or persistent mucocutaneous infections caused by fungi of the genus *Candida* and primarily by the commensal organism *Candida albicans* (Kirkpatrick 2001; Puel et al. 2012). IL-17F deficiency leads to CMC through impairments in IL-17-mediated immunity.

Introduction

Signaling through the pro-inflammatory cytokine interleukin-17 (IL-17) plays a key role in host defense. In particular, IL-17 protects against fungal and bacterial infections occurring at sites most commonly exposed to microorganisms. These areas include the skin, the oral cavity, as well as the respiratory, gastrointestinal, and vaginal tracts (Veldhoen 2017). The IL-17 family of cytokines and receptors were first identified in the 1990s and were notable in their distinct structural appearance in comparison to other known cytokines (Aggarwal and Gurney 2002; Rouvier et al. 1993; Yao et al. 1995). Since the initial discovery of IL-17 and the IL-17R, a total of six homologous IL-17 cytokines (labeled IL-17A to IL-17F) and five homologous IL-17 receptors (labeled IL-17RA to IL-17RE) have been identified (Veldhoen 2017; Okada et al. 2016). IL-17A and IL-17RA are the founding members of the cytokine and cytokine receptor families, respectively, and are therefore also referred to as IL-17 and IL-17R (Okada et al. 2016). Linked through disulfide bonds, the IL-17 cytokines form homodimers. IL-17A and IL-17F share the most sequence homology and are also capable of forming heterodimers with each other (Okada et al. 2016). In turn, the IL-17 receptors can also form homo- and heterodimers, which bind to specific IL-17 cytokines. IL-17RA is ubiquitously expressed and binds to the inducible IL-17RC (Gaffen 2009). IL-17A and IL-17F are produced by a distinct subset of CD4$^+$ T helper cells known as

T_H17 cells and bind to the IL-17RA/C hetero-dimeric complex (Okada et al. 2016). Stimulation of IL-17 receptors present on fibroblasts, epithelial cells, osteocytes, and monocytes causes the production of pro-inflammatory cytokines and recruitment of immune cells, such as neutrophils, to the site of infection (Veldhoen 2017; Aggarwal and Gurney 2002).

The *IL-17F* gene is located on chromosome 6p12 and encodes for a protein comprised of 153 amino acids (Starnes et al. 2001). It shares 40% homology with IL-17A; however, it contains one extra disulfide bond (Starnes et al. 2001). Binding of IL-17A and IL-17F to the IL-17RA/C complex leads to recruitment of the adaptor protein Act1. Act1 interacts with the IL-17 receptor through homotypic binding of their respective SEFIR domains, leading to downstream activation of the transcription factor NF-kappa B (NF-κB) (Awane et al. 1999; Li et al. 2000). NF-κB plays an essential role in the transcription of genes important in numerous cellular processes, including inflammation and cell survival (Li et al. 2000; Baeuerle and Baltimore 1996). In its inactive form, NF-κB binds to a group of inhibitor proteins called the IκB complex located within the cytoplasm (Leonardi et al. 2000). Activation of upstream signaling factors leads to ubiquitination and degradation of the IκB complex, followed by translocation of the released NF-κB to the nucleus (Leonardi et al. 2000). This results in the transcription of several pro-inflammatory genes. Activation of the IL-17R also activates inflammatory transcriptional programs through NF-κB-independent pathways, such as the mitogen-activated protein kinase pathway (Gaffen 2009).

IL-17F deficiency leads to impairments in IL-17 receptor-mediated signaling. The condition was initially described in one family carrying a heterozygous mutation leading to a serine to leucine amino acid substitution at position 65 of the IL-17F protein (Puel et al. 2011). This mutation affects cytokine to receptor binding, leading to production of an abnormal IL-17F protein that can be secreted; however, it is unable to bind to the IL-17RA receptor. This impairs downstream signaling through the IL-17 receptor, diminishing the production of pro-inflammatory cytokines

such as interleukin-6 and growth-regulated oncogene-α (Puel et al. 2011). In addition, the heterozygous mutation confers a dominant negative effect, as wild-type IL-17A and IL-17F proteins that dimerize with the mutated form of IL-17F still exhibit impaired IL-17 receptor signaling (Puel et al. 2011).

Clinical Presentation

The clinical presentation of IL-17F deficiency is characterized by chronic mucocutaneous candidiasis (CMC). CMC is defined by persistent or recurrent infections of the mucous membranes (such as the skin, nails, and oral and genital mucosa), which are primarily caused by the commensal fungal organism *C. albicans* (Kirkpatrick 2001; Puel et al. 2012; Boisson et al. 2013). When CMC occurs without other prominent clinical abnormalities, patients are referred to as having CMC disease (CMCD) (Okada et al. 2016). Along with candidal infections, bacterial skin infections caused by *Staphylococcus aureus* have also been associated with CMCD. In addition, cerebral aneurysms and mucocutaneous carcinomas have been reported in some forms of CMCD (Boisson et al. 2013). Clinical features of IL-17F deficiency have been determined by the few cases reported in the literature (Puel et al. 2011; Bader et al. 2012). The condition has been found to display incomplete penetrance, as two individuals carrying the mutation (aged 9 months and 21 years) in the first reported family had no history of CMC and were otherwise healthy (Puel et al. 2011). Five other family members carrying the same mutation presented with recurrent mucocutaneous candidiasis beginning in the first year of life. One of those affected also suffered from recurrent bacterial infections of the hair follicle leading to furunculosis, as well as asthma and recurrent upper respiratory tract infections (Puel et al. 2011). In addition, there was another family member who died suddenly in childhood of encephalopathy of unclear etiology in the setting of extensive oral candidiasis. Although it is suspected that this family member also had IL-17F deficiency, this was not confirmed by sequencing prior to the patient's death (Puel et al. 2011).

Diagnosis

Evaluation for IL-17F deficiency should be considered in those who develop CMC with or without recurrent upper respiratory tract infections or superficial bacterial infections. A family history of autosomal dominant CMC should in particular prompt consideration for IL-17F deficiency, bearing in mind that incomplete penetrance may add some additional variability to the observed inheritance pattern. Screening immune evaluation, including CBC with differential, lymphocyte subset analysis, immunoglobulin levels, and vaccine titers may all be reassuring; therefore a high index of suspicion for IL-17F deficiency is required (Puel et al. 2011). Fungal cultures from mucocutaneous sites concerning for CMC may reveal *Candida* species. The diagnosis of IL-17F deficiency is confirmed by targeted sequencing of the *IL-17F* gene located on chromosome 6p12. This analysis could be performed as part of a broader genetic panel that would additionally evaluate for defects in other genes that have been associated with the development of CMCD, such as *IL-17RA*, *IL-17RC*, *STAT1*, and *ACT1*.

Treatment

The treatment of IL-17F deficiency involves antimicrobial measures aimed at targeted infection prophylaxis as well as management of established infections. Antifungal prophylaxis is recommended to prevent recurrent episodes of CMC. Oral fluconazole could be used for antifungal prophylaxis. Fluconazole may also be used as first-line oral treatment for *Candida* infections, with voriconazole, itraconazole, and posaconazole serving as other alternatives (Okada et al. 2016). For topical antifungal treatment, nystatin may be considered. Antibiotic prophylaxis with sulfamethoxazole-trimethoprim could be considered for those who present with recurrent superficial bacterial infections (Okada et al. 2016).

Cross-References

▶ Chronic Mucocutaneous Candidiasis, ACT1 Deficiency
▶ Chronic Mucocutaneous Candidiasis, STAT1 Gain of Function

References

Aggarwal S, Gurney AL. IL-17: prototype member of an emerging cytokine family. J Leukoc Biol. 2002;71(1):1–8.

Awane M, Andres PG, Li DJ, Reinecker HC. NF-kappa B-inducing kinase is a common mediator of IL-17-, TNF-alpha-, and IL-1 beta-induced chemokine promoter activation in intestinal epithelial cells. J Immunol. 1999;162(9):5337–44.

Bader O, Weig MS, Gross U, Schon MP, Mempel M, Buhl T. A 32-year-old man with ulcerative mucositis, skin lesions, and nail dystrophy. Clin Infect Dis. 2012;54(7):1035–6.

Baeuerle PA, Baltimore D. NF-kappa B: ten years after. Cell. 1996;87(1):13–20.

Boisson B, Wang CH, Pedergnana V, Wu L, Cypowyj S, Rybojad M, et al. An ACT1 mutation selectively abolishes interleukin-17 responses in humans with chronic mucocutaneous candidiasis. Immunity. 2013; 39(4):676–86.

Gaffen SL. Structure and signalling in the IL-17 receptor family. Nat Rev Immunol. 2009;9(8):556–67.

Kirkpatrick CH. Chronic mucocutaneous candidiasis. Pediatr Infect Dis J. 2001;20(2):10.

Leonardi A, Chariot A, Claudio E, Cunningham K, Siebenlist U. CIKS, a connection to Ikappa B kinase and stress-activated protein kinase. Proc Natl Acad Sci U S A. 2000;97(19):10494–9.

Li X, Commane M, Nie H, Hua X, Chatterjee-Kishore M, Wald D, et al. Act1, an NF-kappa B-activating protein. Proc Natl Acad Sci U S A. 2000;97(19):10489–93.

Okada S, Puel A, Casanova JL, Kobayashi M. Chronic mucocutaneous candidiasis disease associated with inborn errors of IL-17 immunity. Clin Transl Immunol. 2016;5(12):e114.

Puel A, Cypowyj S, Bustamante J, Wright JF, Liu LY, Lim HK, et al. Chronic mucocutaneous candidiasis in humans with inborn errors of interleukin-17 immunity. Science. 2011;332(6025):65–8.

Puel A, Cypowyj S, Marodi L, Abel L, Picard C, Casanova JL. Inborn errors of human IL-17 immunity underlie chronic mucocutaneous candidiasis. Curr Opin Allergy Clin Immunol. 2012;12(6):616–22.

Rouvier E, Luciani MF, Mattei MG, Denizot F, Golstein P. CTLA-8, cloned from an activated T cell, bearing AU-rich messenger RNA instability sequences, and homologous to a *Herpesvirus saimiri* gene. J Immunol. 1993;150(12):5445–56.

Starnes T, Robertson MJ, Sledge G, Kelich S, Nakshatri H, Broxmeyer HE, et al. Cutting edge: IL-17F, a novel cytokine selectively expressed in activated T cells and monocytes, regulates angiogenesis and endothelial cell cytokine production. J Immunol. 2001;167(8):4137–40.

Veldhoen M. Interleukin 17 is a chief orchestrator of immunity. Nat Immunol. 2017;18(6):612–21.

Yao ZB, Fanslow WC, Seldin MF, Rousseau AM, Painter SL, Comeau MR, et al. *Herpesvirus saimiri* encodes a new cytokine, IL-17, which binds to a novel cytokine receptor. Immunity. 1995;3(6):811–21.

Chronic Mucocutaneous Candidiasis, STAT1 Gain of Function

Catherine M. Biggs[1] and Stuart E. Turvey[2,3]
[1]Department of Pediatrics, BC Children's Hospital, University of British Columbia, Vancouver, BC, Canada
[2]Division of Allergy and Clinical Immunology, Department of Pediatrics and Experimental Medicine Program, British Columbia Children's Hospital, The University of British Columbia, Vancouver, BC, Canada
[3]Willem-Alexander Children's Hospital, Leiden University Medical Center, Leiden, The Netherlands

Synonyms

Candidiasis familial 7 (CANDF7); Immunodeficiency 31C (IMD31C)

Definition

Heterozygous *STAT1* gain-of-function (GOF) mutations lead to a broad range of clinical manifestations, including chronic mucocutaneous candidiasis (CMC). CMC is defined as recurrent or persistent mucocutaneous infections caused by fungi of the genus *Candida* and primarily by the commensal organism *Candida albicans* (Kirkpatrick 2001; Puel et al. 2012). *STAT1*

gain-of-function mutations lead to CMC through impairments in IL-17-mediated immunity.

Introduction

Signaling through the Janus kinase (JAK)–signal transducer and activator of transcription (STAT) pathway is employed by numerous cell surface receptors involved in cellular immunity and growth (O'Shea et al. 2015). The JAK family of protein kinases, of which there are four members (JAK1, JAK2, JAK3, and TYK2), associate with cytokine, colony-stimulating factor, and hormone receptors as homo- or heterodimers. Upon ligand binding, the receptor-associated JAKs become activated and phosphorylate each other and the receptor's cytoplasmic tail (O'Shea et al. 2015). Phosphorylated residues on the receptor function as docking sites for STAT proteins. After binding to the activated receptor, STAT proteins form homo- or heterodimers that subsequently translocate to the nucleus. There, they bind directly to DNA and regulate the expression of thousands of protein-coding genes, as well as long noncoding RNAs and microRNAs (O'Shea et al. 2015). There are seven known mammalian STAT proteins, identified as STAT1, STAT2, STAT3, STAT4, STAT5A, STAT5B, and STAT6 (O'Shea et al. 2015). Different receptors activate unique combinations of STAT transcription factors, and each STAT protein confers differential effects on transcriptional output and specificity (Hirahara et al. 2015). Genetic mutations causing either a loss or a gain of function in a particular STAT protein can alter the composition of STAT homo- and heterodimers that occur following receptor activation. In the absence of one STAT protein, effects of other STAT proteins may become augmented; conversely, hyperactive STATs may diminish the transcriptional effects of other STAT proteins. These mutations can therefore have broad effects on cellular transcriptional output and cell fate.

The *STAT1* gene is located on chromosome 2q32 and encodes for two isoforms (STAT1a and STAT1b) that are 91 kDa and 84 kDa in size, respectively (Haddad et al. 1998). STAT1 plays a critical role in interferon responses, and loss-of-function (LOF) mutations in *STAT1* have been associated with increased susceptibility to mycobacterial and viral infections (Weinacht et al. 2017). In turn, *STAT1* GOF mutations have been characterized by exaggerated interferon-gamma (IFN-γ) signaling, with increased susceptibility toward autoimmunity, mucocutaneous candidiasis, invasive fungal infections, cerebral aneurysms, and carcinomas (O'Shea et al. 2015; Weinacht et al. 2017). The susceptibility toward mucocutaneous candidiasis observed in patients with *STAT1* GOF mutations has been attributed to impairments in interleukin-17 (IL-17)-mediated immunity.

IL-17 is a pro-inflammatory cytokine that plays an essential role in antimicrobial defense, in particular against extracellular bacteria and fungi (Aggarwal and Gurney 2002; Rouvier et al. 1993; Yao et al. 1995). It is produced primarily by a subset of CD4$^+$ T helper cells known as T_H17 cells (Veldhoen 2017). Activation of the IL-17 receptor (IL-17R) results in pro-inflammatory cytokine production and the recruitment of other immune cells to the site of infection (Aggarwal and Gurney 2002; Veldhoen 2017). *STAT1* GOF mutations interfere with IL-17-mediated immunity via multiple mechanisms. Increased production of IFN-γ has an inhibitory effect on IL-17 transcription. Furthermore, T cells with increased STAT1 activity show impaired differentiation toward T_H17 cells, with increased percentages of the T_H1 and T follicular helper (T_{FH}) cell subsets.

Clinical Presentation

The clinical spectrum seen in patients with heterozygous *STAT1* GOF mutations is broad, ranging from susceptibility toward certain infections, as well as autoimmunity and malignancy (Toubiana et al. 2016). When first discovered in 2011, *STAT1* GOF mutations were identified as a cause of chronic mucocutaneous candidiasis (CMC) (Liu et al. 2011). CMC is defined by persistent or recurrent infections involving the mucous membranes, such as the nails, skin, and oral and genital mucosa, and is caused primarily by the commensal fungal organism *C. albicans* (Kirkpatrick 2001; Puel et al. 2012; Boisson et al.

2013). One study of 274 STAT1 GOF patients found that CMC was observed in nearly all (98%), with a median age at onset of 1 year (Toubiana et al. 2016). Bacterial infections affecting the respiratory tract and skin were also frequent, with *Staphylococcus aureus* being the most common organism. Additional infectious sequelae include viral skin infections, as well as invasive fungal and mycobacterial infections (Toubiana et al. 2016). Autoimmunity was seen in 37% of patients, ranging from hypothyroidism, type 1 diabetes, cytopenias, and systemic lupus erythematosus. Other complications included cerebral aneurysms and carcinomas (Toubiana et al. 2016). The condition is caused by heterozygous mutations conferring a GOF phenotype; therefore, family history may reveal an autosomal dominant inheritance pattern of CMC with or without other infections, autoimmunity, carcinomas, or cerebral aneurysms.

Diagnosis

GOF mutations in *STAT1* should be considered in patients who present with CMC. Because of phenotypic variability amongst those affected, CMC alone should raise concern for increased STAT1 activity; the presence of additional characteristic infections (such as invasive fungal or mycobacterial infections), autoimmunity, cerebral aneurysms, and carcinomas should further prompt evaluation. As the age of onset of CMC can vary into adulthood, STAT1 GOF can also be considered in those without CMC but other characteristic features. Lymphocyte count and proliferation are normal in the majority of patients; however, absolute lymphopenia and decreased numbers of T, B, or natural killer cells, as well as impaired lymphocyte proliferation, can also be seen. Immunoglobulin levels vary, and IgG levels may be low, normal, or elevated (Toubiana et al. 2016). Enumeration of IL-17-secreting T cells, performed by intracellular cytokine staining and flow cytometric analysis, reveals a decreased proportion of IL-17$^+$ T cells in most patients, although roughly 20% of those affected still demonstrate a normal level. Therefore, because the screening immune evaluation in STAT1 GOF patients can vary and may be largely normal, a high index of suspicion is required based on clinical concern (Toubiana et al. 2016). Clinical suspicion for a *STAT1* GOF mutation should be investigated using targeted sequencing of the *STAT1* gene located on chromosome 2q32. As mutations in several genes can lead to CMC, sequencing of *STAT1* may be performed as part of a larger panel including other potentially causative genes, such as *IL-17RA*, *IL-17RC*, *IL-17F*, and *ACT1*.

Treatment

Management of patients carrying *STAT1* GOF mutations involves infection prophylaxis, treatment of established infections, and in some cases, therapies aimed at correcting the underlying immune dysregulation. The majority of patients require long-term systemic antifungal treatment for CMC, with oral fluconazole being the most common first-line agent. Other antifungal treatment options include itraconazole and posaconazole; voriconazole, echinocandins, terbinafine, and amphotericin B may be warranted in those with fungal species demonstrating resistance to first-line agents. Antibiotic or antiviral prophylaxis could be considered in patients with recurrent bacterial or viral infections (Toubiana et al. 2016). Treatment with subcutaneous or intravenous immunoglobulin could also be considered in those with hypogammaglobulinemia and recurrent infections.

Treatments aimed at correcting the underlying immune dysregulation include hematopoietic stem cell transplantation (HSCT), as well as molecular therapies that target hyperactive STAT1 signaling. HSCT represents a potentially curative therapy; however, experience is limited and has shown significant mortality and morbidity thus far. One study of 15 patients with *STAT1* GOF mutations found that overall and event-free survival were both low, at 40% and 10%, respectively, with a high rate of secondary graft failure (Leiding et al. 2017). Another targeted treatment approach that has been employed for STAT1 GOF is the use of ruxolitinib, a combined JAK1/JAK2 tyrosine kinase inhibitor (Weinacht et al. 2017;

Toubiana et al. 2016). As interferon signaling employs the JAK1 and JAK2 kinases, ruxolitinib is believed to counteract the exaggerated STAT1 signaling that occurs following engagement of type 1 and type 2 interferons. This treatment has been employed in a small number of reported cases with encouraging results, showing amelioration of autoimmune complications as well as CMC, with in vitro data showing normalization of exaggerated T_H1 and improved T_H17 responses (Weinacht et al. 2017; Toubiana et al. 2016).

References

Aggarwal S, Gurney AL. IL-17: prototype member of an emerging cytokine family. J Leukoc Biol. 2002; 71(1):1–8.

Boisson B, Wang CH, Pedergnana V, Wu L, Cypowyj S, Rybojad M, et al. An ACT1 mutation selectively abolishes interleukin-17 responses in humans with chronic mucocutaneous candidiasis. Immunity. 2013;39(4): 676–86.

Green L, Dolen WK. Chronic candidiasis in children. Curr allergy asthma rep. 2017;17(5):31.

Haddad B, Pabon-Pena CR, Young H, Sun WH. Assignment of STAT1 to human chromosome 2q32 by FISH and radiation hybrids. Cytogenet Cell Genet. 1998;83(1–2):58–9.

Hirahara K, Onodera A, Villarino AV, Bonelli M, Sciume G, Laurence A, et al. Asymmetric action of STAT transcription factors drives transcriptional outputs and cytokine specificity. Immunity. 2015;42(5):877–89.

Kirkpatrick CH. Chronic mucocutaneous candidiasis. Pediatr Infect Dis J. 2001;20(2):10.

Leiding JW, Okada S, Hagin D, Abinun M, Shcherbina A, Balashov DN, et al. Hematopoietic stem cell transplantation in patients with gain-of-function signal transducer and activator of transcription 1 mutations. J Allergy Clin Immunol. 2017;pii: S0091-6749(17) 30916-8.

Liu LY, Okada S, Kong XF, Kreins AY, Cypowyj S, Abhyankar A, et al. Gain-of-function human STAT1 mutations impair IL-17 immunity and underlie chronic mucocutaneous candidiasis. J Exp Med. 2011;208(8):1635–48.

O'Shea JJ, Schwartz DM, Villarino AV, Gadina M, McInnes IB, Laurence A. The JAK–STAT pathway: impact on human disease and therapeutic intervention. Annu Rev Med. 2015;66:311–28.

Puel A, Cypowyj S, Marodi L, Abel L, Picard C, Casanova JL. Inborn errors of human IL-17 immunity underlie chronic mucocutaneous candidiasis. Curr Opin Allergy Clin Immunol. 2012;12(6):616–22.

Rouvier E, Luciani MF, Mattei MG, Denizot F, Golstein P. CTLA-8, cloned from an activated T cell, bearing AU-rich messenger RNA instability sequences, and homologous to a *Herpesvirus saimiri* gene. J Immunol. 1993;150(12):5445–56.

Toubiana J, Okada S, Hiller J, Oleastro M, Gomez ML, Becerra JCA, et al. Heterozygous STAT1 gain-of-function mutations underlie an unexpectedly broad clinical phenotype. Blood. 2016;127(25):3154–64.

Veldhoen M. Interleukin 17 is a chief orchestrator of immunity. Nat Immunol. 2017;18(6):612–21.

Weinacht KG, Charbonnier LM, Alroqi F, Plant A, Qiao Q, Wu H, et al. Ruxolitinib reverses dysregulated T helper cell responses and controls autoimmunity caused by a novel signal transducer and activator of transcription 1 (STAT1) gain-of-function mutation. J Allergy Clin Immunol. 2017;139(5):1629.e2–940.e2.

Yao ZB, Fanslow WC, Seldin MF, Rousseau AM, Painter SL, Comeau MR, et al. *Herpesvirus saimiri* encodes a new cytokine, IL-17, which binds to a novel cytokine receptor. Immunity. 1995;3(6):811–21.

Chronic Mucocutaneous Candidiasis: IL-17RA Deficiency

Catherine M. Biggs[1] and Stuart E. Turvey[2,3]
[1]Department of Pediatrics, BC Children's Hospital, University of British Columbia, Vancouver, BC, Canada
[2]Division of Allergy and Clinical Immunology, Department of Pediatrics and Experimental Medicine Program, British Columbia Children's Hospital, The University of British Columbia, Vancouver, BC, Canada
[3]Willem-Alexander Children's Hospital, Leiden University Medical Center, Leiden, The Netherlands

Synonyms

Candidiasis familial 5 (CANDF5); IL-17R deficiency; Immunodeficiency 51 (IMD51)

Definition

Interleukin-17 receptor A (IL-17RA) deficiency is an autosomal recessive disorder that leads to chronic mucocutaneous candidiasis (CMC). CMC is defined as recurrent or persistent mucocutaneous infections caused by fungi of the genus *Candida* and primarily by the commensal organism *Candida albicans* (Kirkpatrick 2001; Puel et al. 2012). IL-17RA deficiency leads to CMC through impairments in IL-17-mediated immunity.

Introduction

Interleukin-17 (IL-17) is a pro-inflammatory cytokine that plays a critical role in antimicrobial defense. First identified in the 1990s, both IL-17 and the IL-17 receptor were striking in their unique protein structure, bearing no resemblance to other known cytokines or cytokine receptors (Aggarwal and Gurney 2002; Rouvier et al. 1993; Yao et al. 1995). Since then, the importance of this distinct family of cytokines in immunity has become well established. IL-17 plays a key role in the protection against extracellular bacteria and fungi, in particular at body sites most commonly exposed to microorganisms (Veldhoen 2017). These areas are located at epithelial barriers, such as the skin, oral cavity, lungs, and vaginal and gastrointestinal tracts (Veldhoen 2017). IL-17 is produced by a subset of CD4$^+$ T helper cells known as T_H17 cells. Other lymphoid populations that produce IL-17 include $\gamma\delta$ T cells, group 3 innate lymphoid cells, natural killer cells, and natural killer T cells (Veldhoen 2017). IL-17 activates epithelial cells, fibroblasts, osteocytes, and monocytes; this leads to the production of pro-inflammatory cytokines and the recruitment of immune cells, such as neutrophils, to the site of infection (Aggarwal and Gurney 2002; Veldhoen 2017). Since its initial discovery, six proteins that share homology with IL-17 have been identified and are classified as IL-17A through IL-17F. The IL-17 cytokines form homodimers linked by disulfide bonds, while IL-17A and IL-17F can also form heterodimers (Veldhoen 2017; Okada et al. 2016). Furthermore, there are five IL-17 receptors, labeled IL-17RA through IL-17RE. As IL-17A and IL-17RA were the first identified members of their respective cytokine and cytokine receptor families, they are also referred to as IL-17 and IL-17R (Okada et al. 2016). The five IL-17 receptors also form homo- and hetero-dimers, which bind to distinct IL-17 cytokines (Okada et al. 2016). IL-17RA is the largest member of the receptor family and is ubiquitously expressed (Gaffen 2009).

The *IL-17RA* gene, located on chromosome 22, encodes for the IL-17RA protein of 866 amino acids. It is a type I membrane glyco-protein and contains an extracellular domain, a carboxy-proximal transmembrane domain, and a cytoplasmic tail containing a SEFIR domain (Gaffen 2009; Yao et al. 1997). Following ligand binding and activation, IL-17RA interacts with the adaptor protein Act1 through homotypic inter-actions of their respective SEFIR domains. This leads to downstream activation of NF-kappa B (NF-κB) (Awane et al. 1999; Li et al. 2000). NF-κB is a critical transcription factor for cell survival, inflammatory, and stress responses (Li et al. 2000; Baeuerle and Baltimore 1996). Prior to activation, NF-κB is located in the cyto-plasm bound to a group of inhibitor proteins called the IκB complex (Antonio Leonardi et al. 2000). Stimulation of upstream signaling factors causes ubiquitination and degradation of the IκB complex, allowing nuclear translocation of the released NF-κB (Antonio Leonardi et al. 2000). In the nucleus, NF-κB mediates the transcription of a number of pro-inflammatory genes. Signaling through IL-17RA also activates inflammatory transcriptional programs through NF-κB-independent pathways, such as the mitogen-activated protein kinase (MAPK) pathway (Gaffen 2009).

Clinical Presentation

The major clinical manifestation of IL-17RA defi-ciency is chronic mucocutaneous candidiasis (CMC). CMC is defined by persistent or recurrent infections involving the mucous membranes, such as the nails, skin, and oral and genital mucosa, and is caused primarily by the commensal fungal organism *Candida albicans* (Kirkpatrick 2001; Puel et al. 2012; Boisson et al. 2013). Patients who develop CMC but who are otherwise gener-ally healthy are referred to as having CMC disease (CMCD) (Boisson et al. 2013). In addition to mucocutaneous candidal infections, patients with CMCD may also develop skin infections caused by the bacteria *Staphylococcus aureus*. CMCD has also been associated with an increased risk of cerebral aneurysms and mucocutaneous carci-nomas (Boisson et al. 2013). Identified in 2011, IL-17RA deficiency was one of the first identified monogenic causes of CMCD (Puel et al. 2011). Development of CMC in early childhood is a characteristic feature of IL-17RA deficiency and typically occurs within the first 6 months of life. Sites affected by CMC in affected patients have included the skin, the scalp, as well as the mucosal linings of the oral and anogenital tracts (Levy et al. 2016). Early onset of staphylococcal skin infections is also seen in the majority of patients. This may cause infections of the hair follicles, as well as superficial and deep skin infections lead-ing to pustules and abscesses, respectively (Levy et al. 2016). In addition to superficial infections, a minority of patients also suffer from recurrent infections affecting the upper and lower respira-tory tracts. Seborrheic dermatitis, an inflamma-tory skin condition, was an uncommon feature seen in IL-17RA deficiency. Unlike other genetic forms of CMCD, autoimmune endocrinopathy, mucosal carcinomas, and aneurysms have not been reported in IL-17RA-deficient patients (Levy et al. 2016).

Diagnosis

The diagnosis of IL-17RA deficiency should be considered in patients who develop CMC in the presence or absence of superficial staphylococcal infections. A high index of suspicion is required based on clinical concern, as typically clinically available screening immune evaluation may be normal. Cultures obtained from sites concerning for CMC may reveal candidal fungal species. There are no commercial assays available to assess IL-17RA function. Therefore, clinical sus-picion for IL-17RA deficiency should be investi-gated using targeted sequencing of the *IL-17RA* gene located on chromosome 22q11. Sequencing could also be performed as part of a broader genetic panel that would evaluate for mutations in other genes associated with CMCD (e.g., *IL-17F*, *IL-17RC*, *STAT1*, and *ACT1*).

Treatment

Management of IL-17RA deficiency involves a combination of infection prophylaxis measures and treatment of established infections. As patients with IL-17RA are susceptible to both CMC and superficial staphylococcal infection, both fungal and antibacterial prophylaxis should be considered (Okada et al. 2016). Oral fluconazole may be utilized as a first-line agent for antifungal prophylaxis and is also a reasonable choice for oral treatment of *Candida* infections. Other antifungal treatment options include itraconazole, voriconazole, and posaconazole (Okada et al. 2016). Nystatin may be considered for topical antifungal therapy. Those suffering from superficial staphylococcal infections or recurrent sinopulmonary infections may benefit from antibiotic prophylaxis with sulfamethoxazole-trimethoprim (Okada et al. 2016).

Cross-References

▶ Chronic Mucocutaneous Candidiasis, ACT1 Deficiency
▶ Chronic Mucocutaneous Candidiasis, STAT1 Gain of Function

References

Aggarwal S, Gurney AL. IL-17: prototype member of an emerging cytokine family. J Leukoc Biol. 2002;71(1):1–8.
Antonio Leonardi AC, Claudio E, Cunningham K, Siebenlist U. CIKS, a connection to IκB kinase and stress-activated protein kinase. Proc Natl Acad Sci U S A. 2000;97(10):6.
Awane M, Andres PG, Li DJ, Reinecker HC. NF-kappa B-inducing kinase is a common mediator of IL-17-, TNF-alpha-, and IL-1 beta-induced chemokine promoter activation in intestinal epithelial cells. J Immunol. 1999;162(9):5337–44.
Baeuerle PA, Baltimore D. NF-kappa B: ten years after. Cell. 1996;87(1):13–20.
Boisson B, Wang CH, Pedergnana V, Wu L, Cypowyj S, Rybojad M, et al. An ACT1 mutation selectively abolishes interleukin-17 responses in humans with chronic mucocutaneous candidiasis. Immunity. 2013;39(4):676–86.
Gaffen SL. Structure and signalling in the IL-17 receptor family. Nat Rev Immunol. 2009;9(8):556–67.
Green L, Dolen WK. Chronic candidiasis in children. Curr allergy asthma rep. 2017;17(5):31.
Kirkpatrick CH. Chronic mucocutaneous candidiasis. Pediatr Infect Dis J. 2001;20(2):10.
Levy R, Okada S, Beziat V, Moriya K, Liu CN, Chai LYA, et al. Genetic, immunological, and clinical features of patients with bacterial and fungal infections due to inherited IL-17RA deficiency. Proc Natl Acad Sci U S A. 2016;113(51):E8277–E85.
Li X, Commane M, Nie H, Hua X, Chatterjee-Kishore M, Wald D, et al. Act1, an NF-kappa B-activating protein. Proc Natl Acad Sci U S A. 2000;97(19):10489–93.
Okada S, Puel A, Casanova JL, Kobayashi M. Chronic mucocutaneous candidiasis disease associated with inborn errors of IL-17 immunity. Clin Transl Immunol. 2016;5(12):e114.
Puel A, Cypowyj S, Bustamante J, Wright JF, Liu LY, Lim HK, et al. Chronic mucocutaneous candidiasis in humans with inborn errors of interleukin-17 immunity. Science. 2011;332(6025):65–8.
Puel A, Cypowyj S, Maródi L, Abel L, Picard C, Casanova J-L. Inborn errors of human IL-17 immunity underlie chronic mucocutaneous candidiasis. Curr Opin Allergy Clin Immunol. 2012;12(6):616–22.
Rouvier E, Luciani MF, Mattei MG, Denizot F, Golstein P. CTLA-8, cloned from an activated T-cell, bearing AU-rich messenger-RNA instability sequences, and homologous to a herpesvirus saimiri gene. J Immunol. 1993;150(12):5445–56.
Veldhoen M. Interleukin 17 is a chief orchestrator of immunity. Nat Immunol. 2017;18(6):612–21.
Yao ZB, Fanslow WC, Seldin MF, Rousseau AM, Painter SL, Comeau MR, et al. *Herpesvirus saimiri* encodes a new cytokine, IL-17, which binds to a novel cytokine receptor. Immunity. 1995;3(6):811–21.
Yao ZB, Spriggs MK, Derry JMJ, Strockbine L, Park LS, vandenBos T, et al. Molecular characterization of the human interleukin (IL)-17 receptor. Cytokine. 1997;9(11):794–800.

CINCA: Chronic Infantile Neurological Cutaneous and Articular Syndrome

▶ Neonatal-Onset Multisystem Inflammatory Disease (NOMID)

Clinical Presentation of Immunodeficiency, Overview

Elena E. Perez
Allergy Associates of the Palm Beaches,
North Palm Beach, FL, USA

Synonyms

Primary immune deficiency

Definition

Immunodeficiency refers to conditions characterized by recurrent or difficult to treat infections. These conditions can be primary, due to inherent defects in the immune system or secondary, caused by extrinsic factors that suppress the immune response. This chapter reviews the clinical presentation of immunodeficiencies.

Introduction

Immunodeficiencies are conditions that render an individual more susceptible to recurrent, severe, or unusual infections. Immunodeficiencies may be primary or secondary. Primary immunodeficiencies are typically defined by an inherited genetic defect affecting immune function (Bonilla et al. 2014). With advanced genetic sequencing techniques, primary immunodeficiency diseases are being defined at a rapid pace, numbering more than 300 (Picard et al. 2015). Secondary immunodeficiencies result in similar susceptibilities but are typically due to an external factor such as comorbid medical conditions (malnutrition, diabetes, lymphoma) and immunosuppressive medications (biologics, chemotherapies).

Clinical Presentation

The clinical presentation of immunodeficiency can be elusive at first, resulting in a significant delay between onset and diagnosis. Infection type varies depending on the part of the immune system affected. Historically, antibody disorders are characterized by recurrent bacterial sinopulmonary infections; T cell deficiencies are characterized by severe viral and fungal infections; phagocytic defects may result in granulomatous abscess formation and combined cellular and antibody deficiencies present with fungal, viral, and bacterial infections. Some classic signs of immunodeficiency in children include failure to thrive, thrush, diarrhea, lack of tonsil tissue, and recurrent respiratory infections. Autoimmunity is often a feature in primary immunodeficiencies (Todoric et al. 2013). These conditions include immune thrombocytopenic purpura (ITP), autoimmune hemolytic anemia (AHA), cytopenias, inflammatory bowel disease (IBD), thyroiditis, and vasculitis. Sometimes these are the presenting feature. Newborn screening has enabled early recognition of immunodeficiencies due to low T cell number and function before symptom onset.

Laboratory Findings/Diagnostic Testing

The laboratory evaluation of primary and secondary immune deficiencies may be directed depending on the level of suspicion and on the types of infections found (Table 1). In general, the basic immune workup often includes assessment of antibody levels (IgG, IgA, and IgM) and titers to vaccines including tetanus, diphtheria, and pneumococcus; lymphocyte enumeration for T cells, B cells, and NK cells; and a CBC with differential. Lymphocyte enumeration reveals whether there is an absence or low level of T cells, B cells, or NK cells. Vaccination with tetanus, diphtheria, and pneumococcus (among others) is used to assess specific antibody function (Orange et al. 2012). If lymphocytopenia is found, further specialized testing may be indicated, including specialized flow cytometry for other more specific lymphocyte populations and tests of lymphocyte function such as mitogen or antigen stimulation. If low T cells are found, mitogen stimulation and/or antigen stimulation testing will reveal the capacity for T cells (and B cells) to grow and divide in response to non-specific mitogen

Clinical Presentation of Immunodeficiency, Overview, Table 1 Summary of the laboratory evaluation of primary and secondary immune deficiencies based on clinical presentation

	Humoral	Cellular	Combined	Phagocytic	Secondary
Typical infections	Bacterial sinopulmonary, enteroviral	Viral, fungal	Bacterial, viral, fungal	Indolent fungal, internal organ abscess, osteomyelitis, gingivitis	Recurrent bacterial, viral, or fungal depending on underlying cause
Laboratory evaluation (commercially available)	Quantitative immunoglobulins IgG, IgA, IgM Titers to tetanus, diphtheria, pneumococcus	Lymphocyte subset panel, mitogen/ antigen stimulation	Tests for humoral and cellular	Dihydrorhodamine (test for neutrophil function) CD11/CD18 (test for lymphocyte adhesion defect)	Directed testing depending on clinical suspicion
Laboratory evaluation (specialized)	Genetic testing, detailed flow cytometry panels, functional flow cytometry testing, where indicated				Specialized flow may be helpful
Treatment	Prophylactic antibiotics, IVIG/ SCIG where indicated	Prophylactic antibiotics, possible gene therapy, or HSCT	Treatments for humoral and cellular; HSCT especially important	Prophylactic antibiotics, possible HSCT	Prophylactic antibiotics, possible IVIG/SCIG, treatment of underlying condition, removal or optimization if possible of offending drug

(including phytohemagglutinin, pokeweed mitogen, and concanavalin A) or specific antigen stimulation (such as tetanus and candida for recall response). If a phagocytic disorder is suspected (such as chronic granulomatous disease), a test of phagocyte function, also known as the dihydrorhodamine (DHR) test, is ordered. This is a specialized flow cytometry test that measures the ability of neutrophils to undergo the oxidative burst. Of note, mitogen and antigen testing as well as the DHR require that the blood specimen arrive to the laboratory via overnight shipping, as the cells need to be viable in order to have a reliable result. Other specialized flow cytometry-based testing may be used to identify subpopulations of lymphocytes including class-switched memory B cells or the presence or absence of naïve and memory T cells. Specialized flow cytometry can also be used to assess gene function. For example, expression level of CD40-ligand, aids in the diagnosis of X-linked hyper IgM, or phosphorylation of cell signaling molecules such as STAT-1, may reveal defects in the Interferon gamma/STAT-1 pathway. These specialized tests and others are often not readily available commercially and need to be sent to specialized immunology labs at academic centers or specialty labs. These are best ordered with the assistance of a clinical immunologist. Genetic testing has been increasingly employed to diagnose primary immunodeficiencies, and more than 300 genetically defined immunodeficiencies are currently known. A variety of genetic sequencing modalities exist ranging from traditional Sanger sequencing to whole exome or whole genome sequencing. Because genetic testing is becoming more available, it is important to understand the differences and expected data generated from each type of test. Some next-generation sequencing panels include all the currently known genes causing primary immunodeficiency and are convenient for screening individual suspected of having a well-described primary immunodeficiency. Whole exome sequencing may reveal novel changes in immune-related and non-related genes that are of unclear significance, which would require further study to prove causality. For the diagnosis of secondary or acquired immunodeficiency, HIV testing should be considered, where appropriate. A thorough history of HIV-related risk factors should be included in the patient's assessment. Other secondary immunodeficiencies result from treatment with immunosuppressive agents including steroids and biologics. Again, a thorough history and clinical suspicion is required in order to diagnose secondary immunodeficiencies as they are often overlooked. A similar approach to testing is recommended when there is suspicion of secondary immunodeficiency.

Treatment/Prognosis

Treatment of primary immunodeficiency is directed toward keeping the patient infection-free and controlling other complications. For milder antibody deficiencies, prophylactic antibiotics and close clinical follow-up are often employed. For more severe antibody deficiencies, for example, X-linked agammaglobulinemia or common variable immunodeficiency, gamma globulin replacement therapy via the subcutaneous or intravenous route is indicated (Perez et al 2017). Combined immunodeficiencies such as severe combined immunodeficiency require treatment with hematopoietic stem cell transplantation (HSCT) or in special cases gene therapy. Other well-described immunodeficiencies, such as Wiskott-Aldrich and chronic granulomatous disease, among others comprise a list of immunodeficiencies treated with HSCT. Aside from prophylactic antibiotics, immune globulin replacement, and HSCT where indicated, surveillance for and treatment of underlying infections should be addressed regularly. Treatment of secondary immunodeficiencies may require immune globulin replacement, and importantly the underlying reason for the secondary immunodeficiency needs to be addressed (Perez et al 2017). Other specialists including infectious disease, hematology, and rheumatology may be necessary as indicated (Table 1).

Cross-References

▶ Clinical Presentation of Immunodeficiency, Primary Immunodeficiency
▶ Clinical Presentation of Immunodeficiency, Secondary Immunodeficiency

References

Bonilla FA, Khan DA, Ballas ZK, Chinen J, Frank MM, Hsu JT, et al. Practice parameter for the diagnosis and management of primary immunodeficiency. J Allergy Clin Immunol. 2014;136(5):1187–205.

Orange O, Ballow M, Stiehm ER, Ballas ZK, Chinen J, De La Morena M, et al. IVIG use in human disease 2016 use and interpretation of diagnostic vaccination in primary immunodeficiency: a working group report of the basic and clinical immunology interest section of the American Academy of Allergy, Asthma & Immunology. J Allergy Clin Immunol. 2012;130:S1–24.

Perez EE, Orange JS, Bonilla F, Chinen J, Chinn IK, Dorsey M, et al. Work group report of the American Academy of Allergy, Asthma & Immunology: update on the use of immunoglobulin in human disease: a review of evidence. J Allergy Clin Immunol. 2017;139:S1–46.

Picard C, Al-Herz W, Bousfiha A, Casanova L, Chatila C, Conley ME, et al. Primary immunodeficiency diseases: an update on the classification from the International Union of Immunological Societies Expert Committee for primary immunodeficiency 2015. J Clin Immunol. 2015;35(8):696–726.

Todoric K, Koontz JB, Mattox D, Tarrant T. Autoimmunity in immunodeficiency. Curr Allergy Asthma Rep. 2013;13(4):361–70.

Clinical Presentation of Immunodeficiency, Primary Immunodeficiency

Elena E. Perez
Allergy Associates of the Palm Beaches, North Palm Beach, FL, USA

Synonyms

Primary immune deficiency

Introduction

The central purpose of the immune system is to recognize danger and protect us from infections and cancers. The immune system is an integral part of many other organ systems, including the skin, gastrointestinal tract, and respiratory tract, with roles in wound healing, mucosal immunity, and protection against inhaled pathogens. A complex network of cells, cytokines, antibodies, and proteins are intricately orchestrated in the development of an immune response against infection and in the resolution of the immune response. Due to the complexity of the immune system, there are often "backup" defense networks in place, such that minor defects of the immune system may not cause a great susceptibility to infections. However, defects in critical genes cause significantly increased susceptibility to recurrent, severe, or unusual infections, often accompanied by immune dysregulation or autoimmunity. The recognition of primary immunodeficiency disease dates back to 1952 with the

discovery of X-linked agammaglobulinemia (Ochs and Hitzig 2012). Historically, primary immunodeficiencies have been categorized according to phenotype: humoral, cellular, combined, innate, or phagocytic. With over 300 primary immunodeficiencies described to date, the phenotypic categories have grown to 9 (see Table 1, (Picard et al. 2015)). Phenotypic overlap among some categories exists, making the diagnosis of specific and rare primary immunodeficiencies a bit more challenging without the use of genetic sequencing.

Clinical Presentation

The clinical presentation of primary immunodeficiency varies by diagnosis. In general, the antibody deficiencies present with recurrent pyogenic infections and susceptibility to enteroviral infections or autoimmunity in some types. In X-linked agammaglobulinemia, absent tonsils are a hallmark. Cellular and combined defects may present

Clinical Presentation of Immunodeficiency, Primary Immunodeficiency, Table 1 Examples of Primary Immunodeficiency Diseases categorized by immunologic phenotype

Phenotypic category (defined by the International Union of Immunology Societies)	Examples
Combined immunodeficiencies	Severe combined immunodeficiencies: Common gamma chain deficiency, IL7Ra deficiency, ADA deficiency
Combined immunodeficiencies with associated or syndromic features	Hyper IgE syndrome, dyskeratosis congenita, DiGeorge syndrome, CHARGE, ataxia-telangiectasia
Predominantly antibody deficiencies	X-linked agammaglobulinemia, common variable immune deficiency, specific antibody deficiency, transient hypogammaglobulinemia of infancy
Diseases of immune dysregulation	Hemophagocytic lymphohistiocytosis, autoimmune lymphoproliferative syndrome, APECED, STAT3 GOF
Defects of neutrophil number, function or both	Chronic granulomatous disease, leukocyte adhesion defects, Shwachman-diamond, GATA2
Defects in innate immunity	STAT1, STAT2, IRAK4, MyD88, WHIM, CMC, Mendelian susceptibility to mycobacterial disease
Complement deficiencies	C2 deficiency C5–C9 deficiency
Autoinflammatory disorders	FMF, MKD, TRAPS, FCAS, muckle wells, CINCA, Majeed, DIRA, Blau, CANDLE, NLRC4, COPA
Phenocopies of primary immunodeficiency diseases due to somatic mutations	ALPS-SFAS, N-RAS defect, K-RAS defect, cryopyrinopathy
Phenocopies of primary immunodeficiency diseases Due to autoantibodies	CMC autoantibody to IL17, adult-onset immunodeficiency autoantibody to IFNgamma, STAT3 deficiency autoantibody to IL-6, pulmonary alveolar proteinosis autoantibody to GM-CSF, C1-INH inhibitor deficiency

with opportunistic, fungal, viral, or bacterial infections and in some cases syndromic features. Innate defects may present with severe and recurrent viral infections, mycobacterial disease, and in some cases associated physical findings such as ectodermal dysplasia. Phagocytic defects present with indolent infections often forming abscess in the lung or liver as in chronic granulomatous disease, or in leukocyte adhesion defect, severe gingivitis may be a feature. Early complement deficiencies present with autoimmune features such as lupus and soft tissue infections, while deficiencies of C5–C9 classically present with recurrent Neisseria meningitis. Periodic fever, rashes, and serositis are features of autoinflammatory syndromes. Hepatomegaly, liver dysfunction, anemia, and fevers may signal disorders of immune dysregulation such as hemophagocytic lymphohistiocytosis. Chronic cutaneous candidal infections and endocrinopathies are signs of other disorder of immune

dysregulation such as APECED. Clinical algorithms based on sentinel organisms, associated clinical features, autoimmunity, and diseases treated with hematopoietic stem cell transplant have been proposed to facilitate differential diagnoses when considering primary immunodeficiency diseases (https://www.immunodeficiencysearch.com), and other publications provide decision support based on the IUIS phenotypic categories (Bousfiha et al. 2015).

Clinical suspicion for the diagnosis of primary immunodeficiency is based on a thorough history, including family history for genetically inherited primary immunodeficiency diseases. Observed patterns of inheritance in primary immunodeficiency are autosomal recessive, X-linked, and autosomal dominant, depending on the disorder. Clinical history of recurrent respiratory infections, pneumonia, otitis, abscess, chronic diarrhea, autoimmunity, infection with unusual pathogens, or severe infections with relatively benign pathogens

Clinical Presentation of Immunodeficiency, Primary Immunodeficiency, Table 2 Initial and advanced immune evaluation based on the suspected arm of immunity affected by primary immunodeficiency diseases

Suspected primary immunodeficiency	Initial tests	Advanced tests
Antibody	Serum IgG, IgA, IgM levels Antibody levels to specific vaccines before and after vaccine boost B cell enumeration	B cell subsets Immunoglobulin production to mitogens or other stimuli Antibody response to phiX174
Cellular	TREC newborn screening T cell (CD4 and CD8), NK cell enumeration Cutaneous delayed hypersensitivity Spontaneous NK cytotoxicity	T cell subsets In vitro proliferative response to mitogens and antigens T cell cytotoxicity Specialized flow cytometry for cell surface marker expression and cytokine production in response to stimuli Cytoplasmic protein phosphorylation in response to stimuli
Phagocytic	CBC with differential Neutrophil staining, peripheral smear DHR reduction or NBT test Flow cytometry for adhesion molecules	Chemotaxis and/or phagocytosis assay Enzyme assays (MPO, G6PDH) WBC turnover Bacterial or fungal killing Bone marrow biopsy
Complement	CH50 (classic complement cascade) AH50 (alternative complement pathway) Lectin pathway function	Level or function of individual complement components
Genetic tests	Microarray for copy number variation	Target gene sequencing Whole exome/genome sequencing

should be explored carefully. Physical exam may reveal failure to thrive, rashes, lymphadenopathy or paucity of lymph tissue, hepatomegaly, splenomegaly, and unique disease-associated physical findings. Examples of primary immunodeficiencies with distinct physical findings are DiGeorge/22q11.2 deletion syndrome, hyper IgE syndrome, and ectodermal dysplasia with immunodeficiency.

Laboratory Findings/Diagnostic Testing

Depending on the suspected primary immunodeficiency, initial evaluation is directed to the relevant testing. Systematic evaluation of initial testing results may dictate further detailed evaluations as outlined in the Table 2 below (Bonilla et al. 2015).

Treatment/Prognosis

The goals for treatment of primary immunodeficiency diseases are to minimize or eliminate infections, provide curative therapies where possible, and keep underlying associated problems under control to provide a normal quality of life for patients with these diseases. Some primary immunodeficiencies are mild and have an excellent

Clinical Presentation of Immunodeficiency, Primary Immunodeficiency, Table 3 Prophylactic antibiotic regimens used in various primary immunodeficiency diseases (regimens vary by coverage needed due to infectious predisposition for given primary immunodeficiency disease) (Adapted from Kuruvilla and Morena 2013)

Immune deficiency	Prophylactic regimens
Antibody deficiencies (XLA, CVID, SAD, THI, SIgAD)	Azithromycin 5 mg/kg PO 3/wk (alternate days) or 10 mg/kg/wk SMX-TMP 5 mg/kg TMP component PO daily or 3/wk Amoxicillin 20 mg/kg PO once or twice daily
Severe combined immunodeficiency	*Pneumocystis jirovecii* prophylaxis: SMX-TMP 5 mg/kg TMP component PO once daily 3 days/wk or atovaquone 30 mg/kg once daily HSV-prophylaxis: Acyclovir 20 mg/kg/dose 3 times a day Fungal prophylaxis: Fluconazole 6 mg/kg/d PO daily Palivizumab (15 mg/kg intramuscularly) during RSV season
Hyper IgM syndrome (CD40 or CD40L deficiency)	SMX-TMP PO 5 mg/kg TMP component PO 3 days/wk; azithromycin PO
Chronic granulomatous disease	SMX-TMP 5 mg/kg TMP component PO divided twice daily plus Itraconazole 100 mg daily PO (<13 y or < 50 kg) or 200 mg daily (>13 y or > 50 kg) plus Interferon gamma: BSA ≤0.5 m^2: 1.5 mcg/kg/dose 3 times/wk or BSA >0.5 m^2: 50 mcg/m^2 (one million IU/m^2) 3 times/wk

Other primary immunodeficiencies which may benefit from antibiotic prophylactic antibiotics include congenital neutropenia, WHIM syndrome, anhidrotic ectodermal dysplasia with immune deficiency, TLR defects, IRAK4 and Myd88, MSMD, complement deficiency HIGE, WAS, DiGeorge

Primary immunodeficiencies treatable with HSCT

Severe combined immunodeficiency disease[a]

X-linked hyper IgM[a]

Wiskott-Aldrich syndrome[a]

Immunodysregulation polyendocrinopathy enteropathy X-linked syndrome

X-linked lymphoproliferative disease

Primary hemophagocytic lymphohistiocytosis

Chédiak-Higashi

Leukocyte adhesion deficiency 1[a]

Chronic granulomatous disease[a]

Interferon gamma receptor defects

DOCK8

STAT1

[a]Gene therapy for adenosine deaminase deficiency form of SCID, X-linked SCID, and CGD is available or in development

prognosis with minor treatment interventions, while others are fatal without provision of lifesaving treatments. Antibody disorders are treated with preventative antibiotics, diagnostic vaccines which may provide additional protection, and immune globulin replacement where indicated. Immune deficiencies predisposing to opportunistic, fungal, or viral infections also require more specific prophylaxis regimens. Cellular and combined defects may also require hematopoietic stem cell transplant or gene therapies. Surveillance for infections with routine lab follow-up, cultures, imaging, and biopsies if indicated is necessary due to the underlying increased susceptibilities to infection with these disorders. Prophylactic regimens are summarized in the Table 3 below (Kuruvilla and Morena 2013). With improved diagnostic tools and treatments, the prognosis for many immunodeficiencies is also improving.

Cross-References

▶ Clinical Presentation of Immunodeficiency, Overview

References

Bonilla FA, Khan DA, Ballas ZK, Chinen J, Frank MM, Hsu JT, et al. Practice parameter for the diagnosis and management of primary immunodeficiency. J Allergy Clin Immunol. 2015;136(5):1186–205.e1–78. https://doi.org/10.1016/j.jaci.2015.04.049

Bousfiha A, Jeddane L, Al-Herz W, Ailal F, Casanova JL, Chatila T, et al. The 2015 IUIS phenotypic classification for primary Immunodeficiencies. J Clin Immunol. 2015;35:727–38.

Kuruvilla M, de la Morena MT. Antibiotic prophylaxis in primary immune deficiency disorders. J Allergy Clin Immunol Pract. 2013;1(6):573–82.

Ochs HD, Hitzig WH. History of primary immunodeficiency diseases. Curr Opin Allergy Clin Immunol. 2012;12(6):577–87.

Picard C, Al-Herz W, Bousfiha A, Casanova L, Chatila C, Conley ME, et al. Primary immunodeficiency diseases: an update on the classification from the International Union of Immunological Societies Expert Committee for primary immunodeficiency 2015. J Clin Immunol. 2015;35(8):696–726.

Clinical Presentation of Immunodeficiency, Secondary Immunodeficiency

Elena E. Perez
Allergy Associates of the Palm Beaches, North Palm Beach, FL, USA

Synonyms

Secondary immune deficiency

Introduction/Background

Secondary immunodeficiency results from non-genetic factors that depress the immune response. A variety of factors can affect the diverse aspects of the immune response and result in secondary immunodeficiencies. These factors include: extremes of age; malnutrition; metabolic diseases (diabetes and uremia); genetic syndromes (as in trisomy 21); anti-inflammatory, immunomodulatory, and immunosuppressive drug therapy; surgery and trauma (including splenectomy); environmental conditions (UV light, radiation, hypoxia, space flight); and infectious diseases (HIV) (Chinen and Shearer 2010). Lymphoproliferative malignancies such as chronic lymphocytic leukemia and multiple myeloma are also associated with secondary immunodeficiency (Friman et al. 2016).

Causes of secondary immunodeficiencies
Environmental conditions
Extremes of age
Genetic syndromes
Infections
Lymphoproliferative malignancies
Medications
Immunosuppressive, anti-inflammatory, biologics
Anticonvulsants: Lamotrigine, phenytoin, valproate
Metabolic disorders
Protein-losing states
Severe malnutrition
Splenectomy
Surgery/trauma

(continued)

Medication	Effects on immune system
Anticonvulsants (lamotrigine, phenytoin, valproate)	Hypogammaglobulinemia
Steroids	Decreased cytokine production Impaired leukocyte chemotaxis, cell adhesion, phagocytosis Lymphopenia Suppressed antibody response and delayed-type hypersensitivity
Azathioprine	Inhibits B and T cell proliferation
Cyclosporine	Inhibits T cell function
Mycophenolate	Inhibits B and T cell proliferation
Tacrolimus, sirolimus, everolimus	Inhibits T cell function
Rituximab	Depletes $CD20^+$ B cells, inhibits B cell function
Alemtuzumab	Depletes mature $CD52^+$ lymphocytes, inhibits T and B cell function
Antithymocyte globulin	Depletes CD4 T cells, inhibits T cell function
Anakinra	Blocks the effects of interleukin-1 (proinflammatory cytokine with role in regulation and initiation of immune response)
Tocilizumab	Blocks the effects of interleukin-6 (proinflammatory cytokine with role in regulation and initiation of immune response)
Brodalumab	Blocks interleukin-17 receptor
Adalimumab	Blocks tumor necrosis factor alpha
Etanercept	Blocks tumor necrosis factor alpha
Infliximab	Blocks tumor necrosis factor alpha
Abatacept	Prevents costimulation of T cells (CTLA-4-Ig)
Basiliximab	Prevents IL-2R signaling, blocks T cell replication and B cell activation
Muromonab	Targets CD3 receptor on T cells; depletes T cells
Ruxolitinib	Janus kinase inhibitor; thrombocytopenia, anemia, neutropenia

Clinical Presentation

Secondary immunodeficiencies are more common than primary immunodeficiencies and can be due to underlying medical conditions or as a result of immune-suppressing therapies and certain medications. A thorough history is required to identify the underlying conditions contributing to secondary immunodeficiencies. As with primary immunodeficiencies, an increase in recurrent, severe, or difficult to treat infections indicates possible secondary immunodeficiency in the proper clinical settings:

- **Medication use:** Chronic use of steroids suppresses T cells and may affect cellular and humoral immunity. Newer biologics targeting specific receptors or pathways alter the immune response to infection and may increase susceptibility to specific infections including HSV, CMV, or pyogenic infections. Chemotherapies, cytotoxic agents, and immunomodulating drugs may also predispose to recurrent or severe infections. Certain anticonvulsants are associated with hypogammaglobulinemia. Biologics targeting B cells, such as rituximab, may result in prolonged and profound hypogammaglobulinemia and increased infections (Dhalla and Misbah 2015; Compagno et al. 2014). Prior to therapy with rituximab, baseline immunoglobulin levels should be checked and monitored for at least 6 months after the last dose, or longer in patients who present with low immunoglobulin levels prior to therapy or have increased risk factors (Compagno et al. 2014). Immune globulin replacement may be required in patients who are treated with rituximab and have hypogammaglobulinemia and severe or recurrent infections (Kaplan et al. 2014). Alemtuzumab, or anti-CD52, targets mature lymphocytes, depletes T cells, and can result in reactivation of cytomegalovirus. Clinical use of immunosuppressive therapies should be accompanied by routine surveillance for clinical signs and symptoms of secondary immunodeficiency to avoid complications.

- **Splenectomy** predisposes to poor antibody responses to polysaccharide antigens, pneumococcal sepsis as well as increased susceptibility to *H. influenza* and meningococcus. If possible, vaccination should be carried out at least 2 weeks prior to scheduled splenectomy. If this is not possible, vaccination soon after is indicated. Penicillin prophylaxis for children under age 5 is recommended.
- **Lymphoproliferative malignancies:** In chronic lymphocytic leukemia (CLL) and multiple myeloma (MM), several immune defects are found. In chronic lymphocytic leukemia, up to 85% of patients have hypogammaglobulinemia, although the mechanism is not well understood (Dhalla and Misbah 2014). In MM, B cell dysfunction leads to hypogammaglobulinemia. Abnormalities in T cell, NK cell, and dendritic cells are also a feature (Friman et al. 2016). Risk of secondary immunodeficiency in MM and CLL is increased with the use of chemotherapies and immunosuppressive medications (Friman et al. 2016). Immune assessment including history of infections and laboratory evaluation may reveal patients at risk. Along with quantitative immunoglobulins, use of diagnostic vaccines including PPSV and PCV13 may help in recognizing patients who are candidates for gamma globulin replacement therapy and/or antibiotic prophylaxis (Dhalla and Misbah 2014).
- **Other medical causes:** Many clinical factors can contribute to secondary immunodeficiency. These other possible causes including environmental conditions, extremes of age, genetic syndromes, infections including HIV, metabolic disorders, protein losing states, severe malnutrition, and surgery/trauma should be considered when secondary immunodeficiency is suspected. In some cases, such as malnutrition for example, addressing the underlying problem may relieve the immune effects. In addition to controlling underlying disease state, interventions to decrease susceptibility to infection may include prophylactic antibiotics or immune globulin replacement if indicated.

Laboratory Findings/Diagnostic Testing

Similar to the evaluation of primary immunodeficiencies, laboratory work is ordered depending on area of the immune system affected. Basic screening evaluation includes measurement of quantitative immunoglobulins (IgG, IgA, IgM), pre- and post-titers to vaccines, and lymphocyte enumeration. Specialized testing includes tests of immune function including mitogen and antigen proliferation and specialized flow cytometry. See "▶ Clinical Presentation of Immunodeficiency, Primary Immunodeficiency".

Treatment/Prognosis

As with primary immunodeficiencies, the goals for treatment of secondary immunodeficiency diseases are to minimize or eliminate infections, provide curative therapies where possible, and keep underlying associated problems under control to provide a normal quality of life for patients with these diseases. Secondary immunodeficiencies affecting antibody function may require immune globulin replacement therapy. Preventative antibiotics and diagnostic and prophylactic vaccines may provide additional protection. Surveillance for infections with routine lab follow-up, cultures, imaging, and biopsies should be considered depending on the increased susceptibilities to infection.

Cross-References

▶ Clinical Presentation of Immunodeficiency, Primary Immunodeficiency

References

Chinen J, Shearer WT. Secondary immunodeficiencies, including HIV infection. J Allergy Clin Immunol. 2010;125(Suppl 2):S195–203.

Compagno N, Malipiero G, Cinetto F, Agostini C. Immunoglobulin replacement therapy in secondary hypogammaglobulinemia. Front Immunol. 2014;5:626.

Dhalla F, Misbah SA. Secondary antibody deficiencies. Curr Opin Allergy Clin Immunol. 2015;15(6):505–13.

Friman V, Winqvist O, Blimark C, Langerbeins P, Chapel H, Dhalla F. Secondary immunodeficiency in lymphoproliferative malignancies. Hematol Oncol. 2016;34(3):121–32.

Kaplan B, Kopyltsova Y, Khokhar A, Lam F, Bonagura V. Rituximab and immune deficiency: case series and review of the literature. J Allergy Clin Immunol Pract. 2014;2(5):594–600.

Clinical Presentation of Polymerase E1 (POLE1) and Polymerase E2 (POLE2) Deficiencies

Isabelle Thiffault[1,2,4], Carol Saunders[1,2,4], Nikita Raje[3,4,5] and Nicole P. Safina[3,4,6]

[1]Center for Pediatric Genomic Medicine, Children's Mercy Hospital, Kansas City, MO, USA

[2]Department of Pathology and Laboratory Medicine, Children's Mercy Hospital, Kansas City, MO, USA

[3]Department of Pediatrics, Children's Mercy Hospital, Kansas City, MO, USA

[4]University of Missouri–Kansas City School of Medicine, Kansas City, MO, USA

[5]Pediatric Allergy, Asthma and Immunology Clinic, Children's Mercy Hospital, Kansas City, MO, USA

[6]Division of Clinical Genetics, Children's Mercy Hospital, Kansas City, MO, USA

Synonyms

FILS syndrome; POLE1; POLE2

Introduction/Background

The replicative DNA polymerases (pols) α, δ, and ε are central components in DNA replication, repair, recombination, and cell cycle control. Numerous genetic studies have provided compelling evidence to establish DNA polymerase ε (POLε/POLE) as the primary DNA polymerase responsible for leading strand synthesis during eukaryotic nuclear genome replication (Huang et al. 1999; Zahurancik et al. 2015). POLε is a highly conserved multi-subunit polymerase (heterotetramer) consisting of proteins encoded by four genes: *POLE1,* which encodes a 261 kDa protein comprising the catalytic activity complexed with the POLE2 (59 kDa) subunit, in addition to POLE3 (17 kDa) and POLE4 (12 kDa). POLE2 has no known catalytic activity, but the absence of POLE2 reduce Polε stability (Zahurancik et al. 2015). Polε is involved in several processes which include DNA replication, repair of DNA damage, control of cell cycle progression, chromatin remodeling, and epigenetic regulation of the stable transfer of information from mother to daughter cells. At this time, only two of the DNA polymerase ε subunits have been associated with Mendelian diseases; POLE1 and POLE2. POLε-deficiency patients present with immunodeficiency and other extra-immune manifestations reminiscent of chromosome instability syndromes, such as pre and/or postnatal growth retardation, microcephaly, dysmorphic features, and bone marrow failure.

Clinical Presentation

POLE1

Family 1

POLE1-related deficiency was first reported in a large consanguineous French family with three generations of affected members in which major clinical features included mild facial dysmorphism, immunodeficiency, livedo, and short stature (referred as FILS syndrome) (Pachlopnik Schmid et al. 2012). The FILS phenotype was variable but included malar hypoplasia, relative macrocephaly, recurrent infections, and short stature. Livedo on the cheeks, forearms, and/or legs was present in most patients at birth. With increasing age, telangiectasia was observed on the cheeks. Growth impairment was observed postnatally with normal growth hormone levels. Three affected individuals had bone dysplasia and suffered from pain in extremities. Patients had recurrent infections which include upper and lower respiratory tract infections, pulmonary infections, and meningitis. Allergies, autoimmunity, opportunistic infections, and malignancies were not observed in these patients. Immunological experiments showed decreased IgM and IgG2 levels, reduced isohemagglutinin titers, and a predominant lack of antibodies to polysaccharide antigens. Patients had low memory (CD27+), B cell counts, the proportion of switched B cells and non-switched memory B cells were equally affected. T lymphocytes from affected individuals showed a proliferation defect as well as impaired cell cycle progression. The phenotype was reminiscent of Bloom syndrome but with normal sister chromatid exchange. All affected patients were found to be homozygous for the same variant, *POLE1* c.4444+3A>G. This variant confers abnormal splicing of exon 34, resulting in a truncated transcript (Pachlopnik Schmid et al. 2012) and severely decreased expression of POLE1 and POLE2. Heterozygous individuals were asymptomatic. Of note, the patients did not exhibit cancer susceptibility.

Family 2

Patient CMH812 is a female infant born to healthy consanguineous Palestinian parents. The pregnancy was complicated by subchorionic bleeding in the first trimester, fetal abnormalities on ultrasound including intrauterine growth restriction, short long bones, suspected skull abnormalities, and oligohydramnios. TORCH titers were negative. Amniocentesis revealed normal 46,XX karyotype. She was delivered at 37 weeks gestation by elective C-section secondary to breech presentation. Dysmorphic features noted included malar and mandibular hypoplasia. Microcephaly and moderate growth deficiency were also noted postnatally. Initial clinical suspicion was for primordial dwarfism such as Seckel syndrome; however, molecular testing was negative. Over several months, lacy reticular pigmentation was noted on the face and extremities. She had recurrent pruritic papular eruptions and

skin findings progressed to include appearance of poikiloderma. Erupted teeth were found to be small and dysplastic. She developed a feeding aversion necessitating a gastrostomy tube. Growth remained poor postnatally. Her motor milestones were delayed but social development was normal. She suffered chronic rhinosinusitis and pulmonary infections with purulent otitis media. At age 20 months, she was admitted to the hospital with pancytopenia, splenomegaly, hepatitis, and acute cytomegalovirus (CMV) infection. Laboratory data showed mild bone marrow myelodysplasia, normal total B, T, and NK cells, low class switched and non-switched memory B cells, and high memory T cells. She had high IgA, initially normal total IgG that gradually trended down and low IgM, IgG2, and IgG4. There was no serologic response to pneumococcal vaccine despite booster dose. Lymphocyte proliferative response to mitogens was normal but absent to tetanus and candida antigens. Immunoglobulin replacement was initiated. She was found homozygous for the previously reported POLE1 splice variant (c.4444+3A>G) by trio exome-sequencing (Thiffault et al. 2015). Although she carried the same variant reported in Family 1, CMH812 seems to have had more significantly impaired growth and immunity. Re-analysis and re-interpretation of exome data did not identify additional variant that may explain the patient's more severe phenotype.

POLE2

Recently, a 5-year-old male born to consanguinous parents of Saudi origin was reported with a homozygous splicing variant (c.1074-1G>T) in POLE2 (Frugoni et al. 2016). The patient had combined immunodeficiency, facial dysmorphism, and autoimmunity. He had a history of omphalitis and erythroderma in the neonatal period, systemic Bacillus Calmette-Guerin (BCG) infection after immunization, and subsequently, multiple respiratory infections. Diabetes mellitus was diagnosed at 5 months of age. A few months later, he developed severe dyspnea with hypoxia, hepatomegaly, hypothyroidism, and recurrent respiratory infections with pulmonary atelectasis. Laboratory data showed agammaglobulinemia, absence of circulating B cells, and T cell lymphopenia and neutropenia. Replacement therapy with intravenous immunoglobulins was initiated. Later, he developed generalized lymphadenopathy. Lymph node biopsy showed abnormal architecture with lack of follicles, an increased number of CD163+ activated macrophages and activated (CD45RO+) T lymphocytes. At the time of diagnosis, his height and weight were at the 3rd percentile, and had microcephaly (−2.4 s.d.). Dysmorphic features included low anterior hairline, flat supraorbital ridges, downturned corners of the mouth, and a short philtrum. Exome sequencing identified homozygosity for a splicing variant, c.1074-1G>T, in *POLE2*. This variant confers abnormal splicing of exon 14, resulting in a truncated transcript (Frugoni et al. 2016). However, immunoblot analysis for POLE2 revealed similar levels of expression in patient and control samples. Further analysis of patient's cell lines for cell cycle progression showed reduced numbers of cells in S phase with an increased proportion of cells in G2/M, indicating a defect that was partially rescued by complementation studies (Frugoni et al. 2016).

Table 1 compares the clinical and cellular features of individuals with Polε-deficiency. Features closely matched those reported in FILS with exceptions of microcephaly and intrauterine growth restriction.

Laboratory Findings/Diagnostic Testing

Similar to the evaluation of other immunodeficiency syndromes, laboratory work is guided by the immune system defect. Basic screening includes complete blood counts and differential measurement of quantitative immunoglobulins (IgG, IgA, and IgM), pre- and post-vaccine titers, and lymphocyte enumeration. Other specialized immunological testing including lymphocyte proliferation to mitogen and antigen stimulation and T cell receptor Vβ spectratyping can be helpful.

The diagnosis of POLε-deficiency is established in a proband with the clinical findings listed above who has biallelic pathogenic variants

in *POLE1* or *POLE2*. Two approaches to molecular genetic testing should be considered; multigene panel for immunodeficiency syndromes or symptom-driven next-generation sequencing.

Treatment/Prognosis

Treatment of Manifestations: As with other immunodeficiency syndromes, the goal for treatment of immunodeficiency associated with POLE1 and POLE2 deficiencies is to minimize or eliminate infections and monitoring to control immune dysregulation with targeted therapy. Immunoglobulin replacement is useful in the patients with frequent infections and humoral immunodeficiency. Preventative antibiotics may provide additional protection. Other treatments may include Vitamin E and folic acid supplementation; standard chemotherapy protocols for malignancies (adopted to individual tolerance); growth hormone replacement therapy for individuals who have growth failure (likely needs to be used with caution in this group of patients due to potential risk of malignancy) and treatment for autoimmune complications such as autoimmune thyroid disease as described for POLE2 deficient patient. Additional supportive therapy including special education, speech and language therapy, behavioral therapy, occupational therapy, and community services for families would be beneficial.

Surveillance: For affected individuals: Periodic follow up to monitor developmental progress, physical growth, and frequency of infection and/or autoimmunity; in those with weight loss, assessment for malignancy should be considered, lifelong monitoring of immune biomarkers, and careful monitoring by an oncologist.

For carriers (heterozygotes): Parents should be monitored for malignancy, particularly colorectal and endometrial cancers.

Genetic Counselling: POLε-deficiency is inherited in an autosomal recessive manner. At conception, each siblings of an affected individual has a 25% chance of being affected, a 50% chance of being an asymptomatic carrier, and a 25% chance of being unaffected and not a carrier.

Clinical Presentation of Polymerase E1 (POLE1) and Polymerase E2 (POLE2) Deficiencies, Table 1 Comparison of clinical and immunologic features of *POLE1 and POLE2* patients

Clinical features	FILS syndrome[a]	CMH812[a]	D839	POLE2-patient[a]
MIM #	615139	615139	615139	n.a
Sex	11 affected (8 males; 6 females)	Female	Male	Male
Origin	French	Palestinian	n.a	Saudi Arabian
Age at diagnosis	3–33 years old	2 years old	25 years old	10 months
Variant	Homoz. c.4444+3A>G	Homoz. c.4444+3A>G	Het. c.1085A>GC (Tyr362Cys), no second variant detected	Homoz. c.1074-1G>T
RS ID	rs398122515	rs398122515	n.a	rs368577291
gnomAD MAF	1/30962 (0.007%)	1/30962 (0.007%)	1/246264 (0.0009%)	5/243070 (0.004%)
Microcephaly	■	■	n.a	■
Malar hypoplasia	■	■	n.a	■
Sloping head	■	■	n.a	n.a
Palpebral fissures, upslanting	■	–	n.a	n.a
Palpebral fissures, downslanting	■	■	n.a	n.a
Epicanthic folds	■	■	n.a	n.a
Micrognathia	■	–	n.a	n.a
External ear abnormalities	■	■	n.a	n.a
Short philtrum	–	–	n.a	■
Long philtrum	■	■	n.a	n.a
Clinodactily	–	■	n.a	n.a
Syndactily	–	■	n.a	n.a
Growth retardation	■	■	n.a	■
Short stature	■	■	n.a	■
Bone disease or anomalies	■	■	n.a	n.a
Skin abnormalities	■	■	n.a	■
Intellectual disability	–	–	n.a	n.a
Developmental delay	–	■	n.a	n.a
Low hairline	n.a	–	n.a	■
Recurrent infections	■	■	■	■
Brain anomalies/ degeneration	n.a	–	n.a	n.a
Dyspnea	n.a	n.a	n.a	■
Endocrine	–	–	n.a	Diabetes, hypothyroidy
Immunologic features				
Pancytopenia	–	■	n.a	n.a
Agammaglobulinemia	n.a	n.a	n.a	■
Thrombocytopenia	–	■	n.a	n.a
CID	2/14	■	■	■
SCID	n.a	-	n.a	n.a
Neutropenia	n.a	-*	n.a	■
B cell lymphocytopenia	■	■	n.a	■

(continued)

Clinical Presentation of Polymerase E1 (POLE1) and Polymerase E2 (POLE2) Deficiencies, Table 1 (continued)

Clinical features	FILS syndrome[a]	CMH812[a]	D839	POLE2-patient[a]
T cell lymphocytopenia	■	■	n.a	■
CD19	n.a	n.a	N	↓
CD3	N	n.a	↓	↓
CD4	↓	n.a	N	↓
CD8	↓	n.a	N	N
IgA	N	↑	↓	↓
IgE	N	N	n.a	↓
IgG	↓	↓**	↓	Low N
IgM	↓	↓	↓	↓
Anti-pseudomonas polysaccharide IgG	■	■	n.a	n.a
Autoimmunity	–	-	n.a	n.a
Sister chromatid	N	N	n.a	n.a
DNA breakage studies	–	N	n.a	n.a
Radiosensitivity	–	n.a.	n.a	n.a
Clinical phenotype	FILS	FILS-related disease	Polyclonal lymphoproliferation (CVI)	CVI
Gene	**POLE1**	**POLE1**	**POLE1**	**POLE2**
Mode of inheritance	**AR**	**AR**	?	**AR**

n.a, not reported/applicable; −, negative; ■, positive; N, normal range; ↓, decreased; ↑, increased; AR, autosomal recessive; CVI, common variable immunodeficiency; -*, Transient pancytopenia associated with CMV infection; ↓**, IgG2 and IgG 4 ↓. Total IgG N; Homoz, homozygous; Het., heterozygous
[a]Consanguineous family reported

Carrier testing for at-risk family members and prenatal testing are possible if both of the pathogenic variants have been identified in an affected family member.

Discussion/Summary

In summary, the clinical and immunologic features of patients with pathogenic variants in *POLE1* or *POLE2* result in variable immunodeficiency and other extra-immune manifestations. For this reason, POLε deficiency may be a more apt description of these disorders. At this time, no genotype-phenotype correlation in POLε-deficiency patients can be drawn due to the small number of patients. The impact of POLε holoenzyme deficiency causing impaired lymphocyte proliferation, altered cellular survival, and/or defective DNA repair/replication in patients with POLε defects remains to be investigated. Somatic mutations in human POLε have been demonstrated in cancers and are thought to contribute to genomic instability. Functional studies in yeast showed that heterozygosity for a pathogenic allele can cause complete Mismatch repair (MMR) deficiency, and that subsequent loss of heterozygosity is not required for the development of POLε-related tumors (Huang et al. 1999; Zahurancik et al. 2015). Taken together, longitudinal follow up studies of carrier individuals of germline POLE1 and POLE2 deficiency are needed to delineate the potential role in cancer susceptibility.

References

Frugoni F, Dobbs K, Felgentreff K, Aldhekri H, Al Saud BK, Arnaout R, Ali AA, Abhyankar A, Alroqi F, Giliani S, Ojeda MM, Tsitsikov E, Pai SY, Casanova JL, Notarangelo LD, Manis JP. A novel mutation in the POLE2 gene causing combined immunodeficiency. J Allergy Clin Immunol. 2016;137: 635–8.e631.

Huang D, Knuuti R, Palosaari H, Pospiech H, Syvaoja JE. cDNA and structural organization of the gene Pole1 for the mouse DNA polymerase epsilon catalytic subunit. Biochim Biophys Acta. 1999;1445:363–71.

Pachlopnik Schmid J, Lemoine R, Nehme N, Cormier-Daire V, Revy P, Debeurme F, Debre M, Nitschke P, Bole-Feysot C, Legeai-Mallet L, Lim A, De Villartay JP, Picard C, Durandy A, Fischer A, De Saint Basile G. Polymerase epsilon1 mutation in a human syndrome with facial dysmorphism, immuno-deficiency, livedo, and short stature ("FILS syndrome"). J Exp Med. 2012;209:2323–30.

Thiffault I, Saunders C, Jenkins J, Raje N, Canty K, Sharma M, Grote L, Welsh HI, Farrow E, Twist G, Miller N, Zwick D, Zellmer L, Kingsmore SF, Safina NP. A patient with polymerase E1 deficiency (POLE1): clinical features and overlap with DNA breakage/instability syndromes. BMC Med Genet. 2015;16:31.

Zahurancik WJ, Baranovskiy AG, Tahirov TH, Suo Z. Comparison of the kinetic parameters of the truncated catalytic subunit and holoenzyme of human DNA polymerase varepsilon. DNA Repair (Amst). 2015;29:16–22.

CNO: Chronic Non-bacterial Osteomyelitis

▶ Majeed Syndrome

Cohen Syndrome

Persio Roxo-Junior and Isabela Mina
Division of Immunology and Allergy, Department of Pediatrics, Ribeirão Preto Medical School, University of São Paulo, Ribeirão Preto, Brazil

Definition

Cohen syndrome is a rare autosomal recessive disease with diversified clinical manifestations. Patients with this syndrome may present neutropenia, hypotonia, microcephaly, mental retardation, short stature, obesity, and characteristic facial features (Rezaei et al. 2009; Duplomb et al. 2014; El Chehadeh-Djebbar et al. 2013; Chandler et al. 2003; Kolehmainen et al. 2004).

The syndrome was first described by Cohen et al. in 1973 in a few patients with hypotonia, obesity, and facial dysmorphisms (Chandler et al. 2003).

Introduction

Cohen syndrome is caused by homozygous or compound heterozygous mutations in the *COH1* gene (Rezaei et al. 2009; Duplomb et al. 2014; Chandler et al. 2003; Kolehmainen et al. 2004), also known as *VPS13B* (Duplomb et al. 2014; El Chehadeh-Djebbar et al. 2013).

COH1 gene encodes a protein whose function is unclear but that seems to be a potential transmembrane protein that may be involved in protein sorting and intracellular protein transport (Rezaei et al. 2009; Duplomb et al. 2014). Patients who suffer from Cohen syndrome have defective glycosylation, which appears by the accumulation of galactosylated fucosylated structures and asialyted fucosylated structures (Wintergerst et al. 2017).

Therefore, patients with this syndrome may present heterogeneous and variable clinical manifestations (Rezaei et al. 2009; Duplomb et al. 2014; Chandler et al. 2003).

Clinical Presentation

Cohen syndrome is a multisystem disorder. Patients may present progressive retinochoroidal dystrophy and high myopia, microcephaly, moderate to profound psychomotor retardation, hypotonia, joint hypermobility, truncal obesity, short stature, and characteristic facial features, such as smooth and short philtrum, thick hair and eyebrows, wave-shaped eyelids, long eyelashes, hypotonic appearance, prominent upper central incisors, and high nasal bridge (Rezaei et al. 2009; El Chehadeh-Djebbar et al. 2013; Chandler et al. 2003; Kolehmainen et al. 2004; Wintergerst et al. 2017).

Besides that, neutropenia is also observed in these patients, in association with recurrent infections. Severe infections are unusual in patients with Cohen syndrome; however, gingivitis, peri-odontitis, aphthous ulcers, and cutaneous infections may be seen in some patients (Rezaei et al. 2009; Chandler et al. 2003).

Laboratory Findings and Diagnostic Testing

The diagnosis of Cohen syndrome can be suspected based on the clinical phenotype of the patients (Wintergerst et al. 2017).

Therefore, the diagnosis of the syndrome is based on clinical findings and molecular genetic tests to identify mutations in *COH1* (Chandler et al. 2003; Kolehmainen et al. 2004), but there is not a consensus about clinical diagnostic criteria yet (Chandler et al. 2003).

For example, Kolehmainen et al. (2004) proposed the following criteria for diagnosis of Cohen syndrome – presence of at least six of the following eight cardinal features: retinal dystrophy and high myopia, microcephaly, developmental delay, joint hypermobility, typical Cohen syndrome facial characteristic, truncal obesity with slender extremities, overly sociable behavior, and neutropenia (Kolehmainen et al. 2004). However, Chandler et al. proposed another criteria for the diagnosis of the syndrome, such as the presence of at least two of the following features in a child with learning difficulties: facial dysmorphism (thick hair, eyelashes, and eyebrows, wave-shaped and downward slanting palpebral fissures, short and upturned philtrum with grimacing expression on smiling, prominent nose), pigmentary retinopathy, and neutropenia (Wintergerst et al. 2017).

A common laboratory finding in patients with Cohen syndrome is the neutropenia, generally intermittent (Rezaei et al. 2009; Kolehmainen et al. 2004).

Generally, the diagnosis of this syndrome is confirmed just after school age, when visual disorders are identified and the patients are forwarded to investigation because of that (El Chehadeh-Djebbar et al. 2013; Chandler et al. 2003). However, the diagnosis of certainty is only possible through genetic analysis (Wintergerst et al. 2017).

Treatment and Prognosis

A multidisciplinary intervention is important not only for the patient with Cohen syndrome but also for the family, such as physical, occupational, and speech therapy to approach psychomotor developmental delay, hypotonia, and joint hypermobility (Chandler et al. 2003).

Patients with neutropenia may use granulocyte colony-stimulating factor (GCSF), and in cases of recurrent infections, standard therapy depending on the infection may be necessary (Rezaei et al. 2009).

Some surgical procedures can also be necessary to correct facial dysmorphism (Wintergerst et al. 2017).

References

Chandler KE, Kidd A, Al-Gazali L, Kolehmainen J, Lehesjoki AE, Black GCM, Clayton-Smith J. Diagnostic criteria, clinical characteristics, and natural history of Cohen syndrome. J Med Genet. 2003;40(4):233–41.

Duplomb L, Duvet S, Picot D, Jego G, El Chehadeh-Djebbar S, Marle N, et al. Cohen syndrome is associated with major glycosylation defects. Hum Mol Genet. 2014;23(9):2391–9.

El Chehadeh-Djebbar S, Blair E, Holder-Espinasse M, Moncla A, Frances AM, Rio M, et al. Changing facial phenotype in Cohen syndrome: towards clues for an earlier diagnosis. Eur J Hum Genet. 2013;21(7):736–42.

Kolehmainen J, Wilkinson R, Lehesjoki AE, Chandler K, Kivitie-Kallio S, Clayton-Smith J, et al. Delineation of Cohen syndrome following a large-scale genotype-phenotype screen. Am J Hum Genet. 2004;75(1): 122–7.

Rezaei N, Moazzami K, Aghamohammadi A, Klein C. Neutropenia and primary immunodeficiency diseases. Int Rev Immunol. 2009;28(5):335–66.

Wintergerst U, Kuijpers TW, Rosenzweig SD, Holland SM, Abinun M, Malech HL, Rezaei N. Phagocytes defects. In: Rezaei N, Aghamohammadi A, Notarangelo LD, editors. Primary immunodeficiency diseases: definition, diagnosis, and management. 2nd ed. Springer Verlag, Berlin, Heidelberg; 2017. p. 280.

Comel-Netherton Syndrome (*SPINK5*)

Lauren Metterle and Lucia Seminario-Vidal
Department of Dermatology and Cutaneous
Surgery, University of South Florida Health
Morsani College of Medicine, Tampa, FL, USA

Synonyms

"Bamboo hair"; Ichthyosis linearis circumflexa;
Netherton syndrome; Trichorrhexis invaginata

Introduction

Netherton syndrome (NS) was first described and
defined in 1949 by Comel and in 1958 by its
namesake. It is a severe autosomal recessive
genodermatosis characterized by both dermatologic and immunologic manifestations. Its incidence has been estimated at 1–3 in 200,000
births. Over the past two decades, significant
advances have been made in understanding its
genetic basis and pathogenesis with positional
cloning and murine models.

NS results from mutations in serine protease
inhibitor kazal type 5 (*SPINK5*, OMIM*605010)
which encodes lymphoepithelial kazal-type-
related inhibitor (LEKTI). *SPINK5* is expressed
in stratified squamous epithelium and the Hassall
corpuscles of the thymus. It resides on chromosome 5 in a cluster of SPINK genes which encode
inhibitory domains that are subsequently tran-
scribed into inhibitory loops in the final protein
product. These loops form the primary mechanism of action, mimicking the substrate of
targeted proteases and inactivating them. The
distinguishing feature of *SPINK5* is that it encodes
a large number of inhibitory domains, 15. Its
protein product, LEKTI, is a "kazal-type" inhibitor which references a specific motif of six cysteine residues which interact to form three disulfide
bonds. These disulfide bonds provide rigidity to
the structure of their inhibitory loops. However,
only 2 of the 15 LEKTI inhibitory domains

possess this kazal motif (D2 and D15). LEKTI
requires proteolytic activation. It is cleaved into
active fragments that are one to six domains in
length, each fragment possessing different inhibitory functions.

More than 70 *SPINK5* mutations have been
reported in NS patients. The mutations are commonly small substitutions, insertions, or deletions
which result in premature termination codons and
complete absence of LEKTI synthesis. The
Cys297Cys mutation within exon 11 is the most
frequent mutation described in patients of
European origin (Hovnanian 2013; Hannula-
Jouppi et al. 2014; Kasparek et al. 2017).

LEKTI inhibits several proteases including
plasmin, trypsin, subtilisin A, cathepsin G, elastase, caspase-14, as well as members of the family
of kallikreins (specifically KLK5, KLK7, and
KLK14). Kallikreins (KLKs) are serine proteases
expressed in normal human skin. They are present
in lamellar bodies and are subsequently secreted
into the intercellular space of the uppermost stratum granulosum where they cleave desmosomes.
LEKTI negatively regulates KLK, maintaining
homeostasis of normal skin barrier function and
desquamation. LEKTI deficiency, therefore,
results in unopposed KLK activity which results
in stratum corneum detachment, abnormal
keratinocyte differentiation, and enhanced expression of pro-inflammatory cytokines (IL-1beta,
TNF-alpha, IL-8, and ICAM-1) and pro-allergic
mediators (TSLP, TARC, and MDC) (Hovnanian
2013). In vitro studies of the KLK proteolytic
cascade position KLK5 upstream of KLK7 and
KLK14 suggesting that its activity is pivotal both
directly and indirectly in pathogenesis. In vivo
knockout studies of KLK5 confirm this as it
results in improvement of cutaneous phenotype
and delayed mortality in NS murine models.
However, recently, it was discovered that dual
knockout of both KLK5 and KLK7 completely
rescues lethality and yields almost complete
recovery of skin barrier integrity with no major
cutaneous phenotype. This underscores the significance of KLK5 in pathogenesis, nevertheless
implicates KLK7 as a key component of pathogenesis as well, whose activity is not entirely
dependent on KLK5 (Kasparek et al. 2017).

KLK-5 is also central to the pathogenesis of atopy in NS through activation of protease-activated receptor 2 (PAR-2) on the surface of keratinocytes. PAR-2 acts via NF-kappa B to enhance thymic stromal lymphopoietin (TLSP) production, which plays a key role in the development of allergy through activation of Langerhans cells and triggering Th2 differentiation. Th2 cytokines ultimately attract and activate mast cells, eosinophils, and B cells which undergo IgE class switching to cause allergy (Hovnanian 2013). Dual KLK5 and KLK7 knockout mice, while free of typical cutaneous features, did show hair shaft defects resembling "bamboo hair." This suggests that KLK14 may be a possible candidate responsible for the trichorrhexis invaginata phenotype (Kasparek et al. 2017).

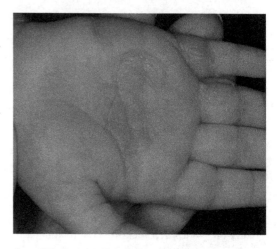

Comel-Netherton Syndrome (*SPINK5*), Fig. 1 Ichthyosis Linearis Circumflexa. Erythematous, serpiginous plaque with overlying double-edged scale. Courtesy of: Karina L. Vivar, MD and Sarah Chaplin, MD at Northwestern University

Clinical Presentation and Diagnostic Testing

NS is defined by the clinical triad of skin, hair, and immune system involvement. It initially manifests as ichthyosiform erythroderma in newborns, which consists of diffuse erythema (classically >90% body surface area) and scaling, although the extent and severity is variable. A collodion membrane is not a feature in NS, and its absence helps to differentiate it from other congenital erythrodermas. Erythroderma in neonates accounts for a significantly high risk of mortality owing to complications such as hypernatremic dehydration, sepsis, and failure to thrive secondary to increased energy expenditure. Over time, the cutaneous presentation evolves into the pathognomonic ichthyosis linearis circumflexa (ILC) which consists of pruritic, erythematous, serpiginous, or circinate plaques with overlying double-edged scale (Fig. 1), and usually presents on the trunk and extremities. ILC is intermittent with periods of flaring and clearance. Overall, cutaneous findings improve as children age, and many adults with NS may only manifest eczematous-like patches of redness and scaling or lichenified plaques. However, pruritus is a severe, constant,

and, distressing symptom for patients (Hovnanian 2013). Routine histological studies are non-diagnostic in NS. However, immunostaining with LEKTI antibodies can be used to determine the presence and distribution of LEKTI in the epidermis. In addition, ultrastructural abnormalities in the composition and organization of epidermal lipids that are not present in other erythrodermic conditions of the neonate differentiate NS from congenital ichthyosiform erythroderma (CIE) and erythrodermic psoriasis.

The second component of its clinical triad are abnormalities of the hair. If present, hair is slow to grow, thin, fragile, and spiky in gross appearance. After about 1 year of age, children may develop a specific microscopic appearance of the hair shaft referred to as trichorrhexis invaginata, otherwise known as "bamboo hair." In trichorrhexis invaginata, the distal portion of the hair shaft protrudes into an invaginated portion of the proximal shaft analogous to a "ball in cup." When hairs break, if the cup-shaped invagination remains, this is referred to as a "golf tee" hair; if the bulging end of the shaft remains, this is termed a "matchstick" hair. Electron microscopy evaluation of hair shafts demonstrates aberrant keratinization, cleavage, and electron-dense depositions in the cortex. Although specific, it is notably not present in all patients and should not exclude its diagnosis. When assessing for trichorrhexis invaginata, hair shaft anomalies are more frequently found in eyebrows and eyelashes as compared to scalp hair (Hovnanian 2013).

The final defining feature of its clinical triad consists of immune deficiencies and atopy. Patients often suffer from frequent respiratory, gastrointestinal, and systemic infections. Unlike its cutaneous features which improve with time, atopic manifestations are constant into and throughout adulthood including asthma, allergic rhinitis, food allergies, urticaria, and angioedema (Hovnanian 2013; Hannula-Jouppi et al. 2014). One patient was recently described with eosinophilic esophagitis. Laboratory studies frequently reveal peripheral blood eosinophilia and elevated serum total IgE, sometimes exceeding 10,000 IU/mL. Sequential analysis over a period of years found a trend of rapid and numerous IgE sensitization to multiple allergens with increasing age. Specific IgE antibodies are typically directed against common food allergens such as egg, cow's milk, wheat, and nuts, as well as pollens and animal proteins (Hannula-Jouppi et al. 2014).

Management

Given the rarity of NS, there are no standard management guidelines. Most of what is known is based off of case series and case reports. As such, treatment is largely symptomatic and varies based on the patient's age. In neonates, erythroderma and its associated life-threatening complications warrant monitoring in an intensive care unit where appropriate fluid, electrolyte, and nutritional support may be provided. For children and adults, cutaneous disease is often management with generous emollient use. This can be supplemented with short, conservative courses of topical therapies such as midpotency steroids or

calcineurin inhibitors. It is important to emphasize that given patient's impairment of skin barrier function, they are at increased risk for systemic absorption of such topical therapies which necessitates caution in their use. However, there is evidence in the literature that most topicals are well tolerated (Hovnanian 2013), except tacrolimus which requires monitoring of plasma drug levels. As an alternative for skin-directed therapy, there has been reported benefit for the use of narrow-band UVB in severe cutaneous diseases (Singer et al. 2015). More aggressive management with systemic treatment has also demonstrated promising results. Options which have been tried include monthly IVIG infusions, infliximab (anti-TNF alpha), and omalizumab (anti-IgE) (Hovnanian 2013; Yalcin 2016). Oral desensitization should be considered in patients with NS as severe allergic reactions are common. Decreases in specific IgE levels have been observed with desensitization, and patients have demonstrated successful induction of oral tolerance to allergens (Hannula-Jouppi et al. 2014; Pastore et al. 2012).

References

Hannula-Jouppi K, et al. IgE allergen component-based profiling and atopic manifestations in patients with Netherton syndrome. J Allergy Clin Immunol. 2014;134(4):985–8.

Hovnanian A. Netherton syndrome: skin inflammation and allergy by loss of protease inhibition. Cell Tissue Res. 2013;351(2):289–300.

Kasparek P, et al. KLK5 and KLK7 ablation fully rescues lethality of Netherton syndrome-like phenotype. PLoS Genet. 2017;13(1):e1006566.

Pastore S, Gorlato G, Berti I, Barbi E, Ventura A. Successful induction of oral tolerance in Netherton syndrome. Allergol Immunopathol. 2012;40(5):316–7.

Singer R, et al. Ichthyosis linearis circumflexa in a child. Response to narrowband UVB therapy. J Dermatol Case Rep. 2015;9(4):110–2.

Yalcin A. A case of Netherton syndrome: successful treatment with omalizumab and pulse prednisolone and its effects on cytokines and immunoglobulin levels. Immunopharmacol Immunotoxicol. 2016;38(2):162–6.

Common Variable Immunodeficiency (CVID)

Klaus Warnatz[1] and Eric Oksenhendler[2]
[1]Department of Rheumatology and Clinical Immunology and Center for Chronic Immunodeficiency, University Medical Center and University of Freiburg, Freiburg, Germany
[2]Department of Clinical Immunology, Hôpital Saint-Louis, Paris, France

Synonyms

CVID

Definition

Common variable immunodeficiency (CVID) is a heterogeneous clinical-immunological entity that represents the most common form of human primary immunodeficiency (Bonilla et al. 2016). There are several definitions of CVID. The most frequently used is the definition by the ESID/PAGID from 1999 (Conley et al. 1999) and more recently the definition by the ESID registry (Seidel et al. 2019). Alternative suggestions have been made by the group of R. Ameratunga (Ameratunga et al. 2016).

Definition according to ESID/PAGID criteria 1999 (Conley et al. 1999).

Probable: Male or female patient who has a marked decrease of IgG (at least 2 SD below the mean for age) and a marked decrease in either IgM or IgA and fulfills all of the following criteria:

(1) Onset of immunodeficiency at greater than 2 years of age.
(2) Absent isohemagglutinins and/or poor response to vaccines.
(3) Defined causes of hypogammaglobulinemia have been excluded (incl. drug induced hypogammaglobulinemia, malignancy, esp.

lymphom, protein loss and other more (for details see table 1 at the original publication)).

Definition according to ESID registry criteria 2019 (Seidel et al. 2019).

Probable: Male or female patient who is 4 years of age or older and has at least one of the following:

(1) Increased susceptibility to infection
(2) Autoimmune manifestations
(3) Granulomatous disease
(4) Unexplained polyclonal lymphoproliferation
(5) Affected family member with antibody deficiency

and marked decrease of IgG and marked decrease of IgA with or without low IgM levels (measured at least twice; <2SD of the normal levels for their age).
and at least one of the following:

(1) Poor antibody response to vaccines (and/or absent isohemagglutinins), i.e., absence of protective levels despite vaccination where defined
(2) Low switched memory B cells (<70% of age-related normal value)

and secondary causes of hypogammaglobulinemia have been excluded.
and no evidence of profound T-cell deficiency, based on absolute CD4+ T-cell numbers, percentage of naïve CD4+ T cells and T-cell proliferation.

Prevalence

The prevalence of CVID in the normal population is estimated to be about 1:25,000.

Pathogenesis

By definition, the hallmark of CVID is the reduction of the serum levels of IgG and IgA and a poor vaccine response (Conley et al. 1999; Seidel et al.

2019). Immunological characterization of CVID patients revealed that over 80% of the patients have reduced numbers of circulating switched memory B cells and long-lived plasma cells due to various intrinsic and extrinsic defects in B-cell differentiation (Wehr et al. 2008; Driessen et al. 2011). Most of these are compatible with a disturbed germinal center function, but some patients also have a disturbed differentiation or maintenance of naïve B cells or a selectively disturbed plasma cell defect. While a genetic cause of this disturbed development or output of germinal center response (Unger et al. 2018; Romberg et al. 2019) remains elusive in about 75% of patients, in up to 25% of patients, a monogenic cause can be identified (Bogaert et al. 2016; Tuijnenburg et al. 2018). These include autosomal recessive (CD19 deficiency, ICOS deficiency, and others) as well as autosomal dominant traits (CTLA4 insufficiency, NFKB1 insufficiency, and others) which may present with the clinical phenotype of CVID. More than a third of patients have additional, usually mild, T-cell abnormalities most prominently reflected in a reduction of naïve CD4 T-cell counts (Giovannetti et al. 2007). This phenotype often combined with an expansion of activated Tbet$^+$ CD21^{low} B cells (Rakhmanov et al. 2009; Isnardi et al. 2010; Mouillot et al. 2010) is usually associated with a more complex clinical presentation (see below). The current hypothesis on the pathogenesis of the immune dysregulation in these patients includes an increased Th1 shift, interferon signature, disturbed gastrointestinal barriers, and altered microbiome (Unger et al. 2018; Cols et al. 2015; Jorgensen et al. 2019; Shulzhenko et al. 2018).

Clinical Presentation

Clinically, CVID patients are classified as "infection-only" and complex CVID patients (Chapel et al. 2012; Resnick et al. 2012). The infectious profile typically includes recurrent infections of the upper and lower airways by encapsulated bacteria like *Haemophilus*

influenzae, *Streptococcus pneumoniae*, but also *Moraxella* or *Mycoplasma* species (Oksenhendler et al. 2008). Several patients suffer also from gastrointestinal infections identifying the protection of mucosal barriers as the main domain of the humoral immune defense. Typical gastrointestinal pathogens identified in CVID include *Campylobacter jejuni*, *Salmonella* species, *Giardia lamblia* but also norovirus causing a chronic enteropathy (Oksenhendler et al. 2008). Opportunistic infections are not part of the spectrum of CVID unless the patient receives immunosuppressive therapy and need to be strongly considered as signs of a combined immunodeficiency.

In complex CVID patients in addition to the increased susceptibility to infections autoimmune, inflammatory and/or lymphoproliferative manifestations are part of the clinical spectrum (Chapel et al. 2012; Gathmann et al. 2014). About 40% of patients suffer from splenomegaly and about 25% from usually generalized lymphadenopathy. In about 10–15% of patients, autoimmune cytopenias (autoimmune hemolytic anemia or autoimmune thrombocytopenia) occur usually early and even as the first manifestation during the course of the disease. As major causes of morbidity and mortality, lymphoma, interstitial lung disease, and enteropathy have been identified (Resnick et al. 2012). Lymphomas are typically of B-cell origin and include foremost BALT marginal zone type lymphoma and diffuse large B-cell lymphoma. Interstitial lung disease is part of the systemic lymphoproliferative-autoimmune spectrum and presents histologically as granuloma, lymphocytic interstitial pneumonitis, cryptic organizing pneumonia, or follicular bronchiolitis, which may lead to pulmonary fibrosis in a subgroup of patients (Prasse et al. 2013; Verma et al. 2015). The CVID-associated enteropathies include a celiac-like or more rarely a Crohn-like disease (Jorgensen et al. 2016). Some patients suffer also from hepatic disease of which the poorly understood nodular regenerative hyperplasia of the liver is the most prominent (Malamut et al. 2008). Additional clinical features include bronchiectasis, which is felt to be secondary to recurrent infections, granulomatous disease of many different organs (about 10% of patients), arthritis, autoimmune organ disease (vitiligo, thyroiditis, and others), and less frequently inflammatory CNS disease (van de Ven et al. 2020). Besides lymphoma gastric cancer is the second malignancy with increased risk among CVID patients (Quinti et al. 2012).

Genetics

While the definition of CVID isn't a genetic diagnosis, several monogenic defects may present clinically as CVID fulfilling the diagnostic criteria. Some of these defects like the autosomal recessive defects in CD19 or ICOS typically present with a CVID phenotype; others are overlapping with combined immunodeficiencies or immunodysregulatory syndromes. Depending on the CVID cohort screened, the following monogenetic defects have been frequently linked to the CVID phenotype. NFKB1 insufficiency was the most frequent in a Dutch cohort (Tuijnenburg et al. 2018), followed by CTLA4 insufficiency (Schwab et al. 2018), and mutations in *PIK3CD*, *NFKB2*, *LRBA*, and many others (Bogaert et al. 2016), but in all of the genetically defined primary immunodeficiencies it needs to be carefully evaluated whether the clinical diagnosis of CVID is justified.

Immunological Phenotype

As mentioned in the section on pathogenesis, all patients have by definition reduced IgG and nearly all IgA levels. IgM is reduced in above 50% of patients. Peripheral B-cell differentiation is disturbed in over 80% of patients resulting in reduced circulating class-switched memory B cells. About 20% of patients – mainly with a complex phenotype – have an expansion of an activated $Tbet^+CD21^{low}$ B-cell population and about 30% a reduction of naïve $CD4^+$ T cells (Mouillot et al. 2010; von Spee-Mayer et al. 2019). Similarly, a reduction of circulating regulatory T cells has been described in association with a complex course of the disease. Many other abnormalities of the immunological phenotype have been described in this heterogeneous disorder without having contributed at this time to a better

diagnosis or understanding of the pathogenesis of the disease.

Diagnosis

Diagnosis is made according to the diagnostic criteria mentioned above. The diagnosis requires the measurement of serum immunoglobulins (potentially at two different time points) and the evaluation of specific antibody responses to at least one peptide and one polysaccharide antigen. Typically, titers against tetanus and diphtheria toxoid and against pneumococcal antigens are determined. In addition, other causes of hypogammaglobulinemia as protein loss, lymphoma, drug-induced hypogammaglobulinemia, and other primary immunodeficiencies need to be excluded. A standard flow cytometric lymphocyte panel and, in most centers, a T-cell and a B-cell panel are used to screen for hints for agammaglobulinemia and combined immunodeficiencies and in order to classify CVID patients according to EUROClass (Wehr et al. 2008).

Additional tests are required to detect clinical manifestations. Thus, most centers use ultrasound and CT scan for diagnosis of lymphoproliferative disease and the latter also for diagnosis of ILD. Pulmonary function tests and blood tests are part of the surveillance. Thus many centers regard annual ultrasound of the abdomen and annual pulmonary function tests including CO diffusion test as state-of-the-art surveillance of CVID patients. There are no clear recommendations for the use and frequency of chest CT, but common standards plan follow-up low-dose chest CT scans whenever clinically indicated and otherwise every 3 years in patients with known lung involvement or every 5–10 years in patients with no known lung involvement. Genetic testing has become increasingly routine especially in patients with a complex form of disease. In patients with organ disease or suspected lymphoma, endoscopy and biopsy are regularly required to diagnose properly.

Management

Management is based on the clinical phenotype. Most patients with "infection-only" phenotype are sufficiently cared for by regular immunoglobulin replacement therapy and adequate antibiotic treatment of breakthrough infections, with a few patients especially with bronchiectasis or chronic upper-airway disease profiting from additional prophylactic antibiotic treatment (Milito et al. 2019). Patients with a complex form of disease frequently require additional treatment depending on the type of secondary complications. This entails often immunosuppressive therapy for autoimmune or inflammatory manifestations. While steroids are commonly used as a first-line therapy, there are only few evidence-based recommendations for secondary immunosuppressive treatment strategies. These treatment decisions should be taken in close collaboration with experienced immunodeficiency centers. Lymphomas are treated according to hematological guidelines, although depending on the underlying immunodeficiency, allogenic hematopoietic stem cell transplantation might be considered earlier in the course despite a currently reported poor outcome (Wehr et al. 2015). In addition, recent studies demonstrated a larger burden of reduced quality of life especially due to chronic fatigue in many patients which persists despite "optimal" treatment.

References

Ameratunga R, Gillis D, Steele R. Diagnostic criteria for common variable immunodeficiency disorders. J Allergy Clin Immunol Pract. 2016;4(5):1017–8.

Bogaert DJ, Dullaers M, Lambrecht BN, Vermaelen KY, De Baere E, Haerynck F. Genes associated with common variable immunodeficiency: one diagnosis to rule them all? J Med Genet. 2016;53(9):575–90.

Bonilla FA, Barlan I, Chapel H, Costa-Carvalho BT, Cunningham-Rundles C, de la Morena MT, et al. International consensus document (ICON): common variable immunodeficiency disorders. J Allergy Clin Immunol Pract 2016;4(1):38–59.

Chapel H, Lucas M, Patel S, Lee M, Cunningham-Rundles C, Resnick E, et al. Confirmation and improvement of criteria for clinical phenotyping in common variable immunodeficiency disorders in replicate cohorts. J Allergy Clin Immunol. 2012;130(5):1197–8.. e9

Cols M, Rahman A, Maglione PJ, Garcia-Carmona Y, Simchoni N, Ko HM, et al. Expansion of inflammatory innate lymphoid cells in patients with common variable immune deficiency. J Allergy Clin Immunol. 2015;137(4):1206–15.

Conley ME, Notarangelo LD, Etzioni A. Diagnostic criteria for primary immunodeficiencies. Representing PAGID (pan-American Group for Immunodeficiency) and ESID (European Society for Immunodeficiencies). Clin Immunol. 1999;93(3):190–7.

Driessen GJ, van Zelm MC, van Hagen PM, Hartwig NG, Trip M, Warris A, et al. B-cell replication history and somatic hypermutation status identify distinct pathophysiologic backgrounds in common variable immunodeficiency. Blood. 2011;118(26):6814–23.

Gathmann B, Mahlaoui N, Gerard L, Oksenhendler E, Warnatz K, Schulze I, et al. Clinical picture and treatment of 2212 patients with common variable immunodeficiency. J Allergy Clin Immunol. 2014;134:116.

Giovannetti A, Pierdominici M, Mazzetta F, Marziali M, Renzi C, Mileo AM, et al. Unravelling the complexity of T cell abnormalities in common variable immunodeficiency. J Immunol. 2007;178(6):3932–43.

Isnardi I, Ng YS, Menard L, Meyers G, Saadoun D, Srdanovic I, et al. Complement receptor 2/CD21-human naive B cells contain mostly autoreactive unresponsive clones. Blood. 2010;115(24):5026–36.

Jorgensen SF, Reims HM, Frydenlund D, Holm K, Paulsen V, Michelsen AE, et al. A cross-sectional study of the prevalence of gastrointestinal symptoms and pathology in patients with common variable immunodeficiency. Am J Gastroenterol. 2016;111(10):1467–75.

Jorgensen SF, Fevang B, Aukrust P. Autoimmunity and inflammation in CVID: a possible crosstalk between immune activation, gut microbiota, and epigenetic modifications. J Clin Immunol. 2019;39(1):30–6.

Malamut G, Ziol M, Suarez F, Beaugrand M, Viallard JF, Lascaux AS, et al. Nodular regenerative hyperplasia: the main liver disease in patients with primary hypogammaglobulinemia and hepatic abnormalities. J Hepatol. 2008;48(1):74–82.

Milito C, Pulvirenti F, Cinetto F, Lougaris V, Soresina A, Pecoraro A, et al. Double-blind, placebo-controlled, randomized trial on low-dose azithromycin prophylaxis in patients with primary antibody deficiencies. J Allergy Clin Immunol. 2019;144(2):584–93.

Mouillot G, Carmagnat M, Gerard L, Garnier JL, Fieschi C, Vince N, et al. B-cell and T-cell phenotypes in CVID patients correlate with the clinical phenotype of the disease. J Clin Immunol. 2010;30(5):746–55.

Oksenhendler E, Gerard L, Fieschi C, Malphettes M, Mouillot G, Jaussaud R, et al. Infections in 252 patients with common variable immunodeficiency. Clin Infect Dis. 2008;46(10):1547–54.

Prasse A, Kayser G, Warnatz K. Common variable immunodeficiency-associated granulomatous and interstitial lung disease. Curr Opin Pulm Med. 2013;19(5):503–9.

Quinti I, Agostini C, Tabolli S, Brunetti G, Cinetto F, Pecoraro A, et al. Malignancies are the major cause of death in patients with adult onset common variable immunodeficiency. Blood. 2012;120(9):1953–4.

Rakhmanov M, Keller B, Gutenberger S, Foerster C, Hoenig M, Driessen G, et al. Circulating CD21low

B cells in common variable immunodeficiency resemble tissue homing, innate-like B cells. Proc Natl Acad Sci USA. 2009;106(32):13451–6.

Resnick ES, Moshier EL, Godbold JH, Cunningham-Rundles C. Morbidity and mortality in common variable immune deficiency over 4 decades. Blood. 2012;119(7):1650–7.

Romberg N, Le Coz C, Glauzy S, Schickel JN, Trofa M, Nolan BE, et al. Patients with common variable immunodeficiency with autoimmune cytopenias exhibit hyperplastic yet inefficient germinal center responses. J Allergy Clin Immunol. 2019;143(1):258–65.

Schwab C, Gabrysch A, Olbrich P, Patino V, Warnatz K, Wolff D, et al. Phenotype, penetrance, and treatment of 133 cytotoxic T-lymphocyte antigen 4-insufficient subjects. J Allergy Clin Immunol. 2018;142:1932.

Seidel MG, Kindle G, Gathmann B, Quinti I, Buckland M, van Montfrans J, et al. The European Society for Immunodeficiencies (ESID) registry working definitions for the clinical diagnosis of inborn errors of immunity. J Allergy Clin Immunol Pract. 2019;7(6):1763–70.

Shulzhenko N, Dong X, Vyshenska D, Greer RL, Gurung M, Vasquez-Perez S, et al. CVID enteropathy is characterized by exceeding low mucosal IgA levels and interferon-driven inflammation possibly related to the presence of a pathobiont. Clin Immunol. 2018;197:139–53.

Tuijnenburg P, Lango Allen H, Burns SO, Greene D, Jansen MH, Staples E, et al. Loss-of-function nuclear factor kappaB subunit 1 (NFKB1) variants are the most common monogenic cause of common variable immunodeficiency in Europeans. J Allergy Clin Immunol. 2018;142:1285.

Unger S, Seidl M, van Schouwenburg P, Rakhmanov M, Bulashevska A, Frede N, et al. TH1 phenotype of T follicular helper cells indicates an IFNgamma-associated immune dysregulation in CD21low CVID patients. J Allergy Clin Immunol. 2018;141(2):730–40.

van de Ven A, Mader I, Wolff D, Goldacker S, Fuhrer H, Rauer S, et al. Structural noninfectious manifestations of the central nervous system in common variable immunodeficiency disorders. J Allergy Clin Immunol Pract. 2020;8(3):1047–1062.

Verma N, Grimbacher B, Hurst JR. Lung disease in primary antibody deficiency. Lancet Respir Med. 2015;3(8):651–660.

von Spee-Mayer C, Koemm V, Wehr C, Goldacker S, Kindle G, Bulashevska A, et al. Evaluating laboratory criteria for combined immunodeficiency in adult patients diagnosed with common variable immunodeficiency. Clin Immunol. 2019;203:59–62.

Wehr C, Kivioja T, Schmitt C, Ferry B, Witte T, Eren E, et al. The EUROclass trial: defining subgroups in common variable immunodeficiency. Blood 2008;111(1):77–85.

Wehr C, Gennery AR, Lindemans C, Schulz A, Hoenig M, Marks R, et al. Multicenter experience in hematopoietic stem cell transplantation for serious complications of common variable immunodeficiency. J Allergy Clin Immunol. 2015;135(4):988–97.

Complement C3 Deficiency

Arije Ghannam[1,2] and Christian Drouet[1]
[1]GREPI EA7408, University Grenoble Alpes, Grenoble, France
[2]KininX SAS, Grenoble, France

Definition

Genetic C3 deficiency is a rare primary immunodeficiency disorder in cases of complete loss of C3 production with both affected alleles; it may be associated with inflammatory disorders in monoallelic defects. Secondary C3consumptions are associated with renal diseases.

Introduction

Complement is a crucial network for both innate and adaptive immune responses. The third component of complement (C3) plays a pivotal role in the complement pathway; it is one of the sources of these biologically active fragments that induce pro-inflammatory responses and mark the particles for clearance by cell lysis or phagocytosis and for activation and control of adaptive immunity (Ricklin et al. 2010).

Given the importance of C3 in the immune response, it is not surprising that its deficiency has been associated with clinical phenotypes. Complete C3 deficiency is a rare disorder with severe recurrent bacterial infections and immune complex-mediated diseases, particularly glomerulonephritis. Heterozygous individuals with missense mutations are at risk for noninfectious diseases, such as membranoproliferative glomerulonephritis, age-related macular degeneration, atypical hemolytic and uremic syndrome, and dense deposit disease as well as with the clinical outcome of certain organ transplantation and vaccination procedures (Sfyroera et al. 2015).

Complement C3

C3 is a member of the C3/α2-macroglobulin protein family of host-defense molecules with an intramolecular thioester bond, which are large proteins of 1400–1800 amino acid residues in length. Human C3 is encoded by a 42-kb gene (41 exons) located on chromosome 19. C3 is synthesized as a single-chain pro-molecule (Mr 185,000), the mature C3 molecule results from a C3 precursor is composed of two disulfide-linked chains, the first 16 exons code for the β-chain (645 aa and 70 kDa), and the second 25 exons code for the α chain (992 aa and 71 kDa) (Fong et al. 1990). Before being secreted as a mature protein, C3 forms a rare internal thioester bond and is split into the two chains. C3 is the most abundant complement protein in serum (0.8–1.8 mg/ml in normal adults) (Ritchie et al. 2004). It normally undergoes low levels of continuous autoactivation by vulnerability to nucleophilic attack of its thioester. C3 is proteolytically cleaved by C3 convertase into C3a and C3b, with concomitant reaction with nucleophilic groups, e.g., hydroxyl groups on complex carbohydrates, cell surfaces, immune complexes, and free IgG. This reaction operates within a radius of approximately 60 nm from the point of its generation.

C3 is synthesized mainly by hepatocytes and also by cells at extrahepatic sites including monocytes and macrophages, fibroblasts, endothelial cells, dendritic cells, and smooth muscle cells.

C3 split products issued from in vivo sequential proteolytic cleavages result in complement amplification. These products are important mediators signaling for inflammatory responses, with C3b/iC3b acting as an opsonin that enhances phagocytosis and C3d,g/C3d as a B-cell stimulator and C3a as an anaphylatoxin and an essential supervisor of cytokine and chemokine expression.

Inherited C3 Deficiency: Clinical Presentation

Primary Immunodeficiency
Inherited C3 deficiency (OMIM: 120700) is a rare primary immunodeficiency; total deficiency of C3 predisposes to recurrent pyogenic infections at an early age. It is characterized by susceptibility to invasive infections by encapsulated bacteria such as *S. pneumoniae*, *H. influenzae*, *N. meningitidis*, and *E. aerogenes*. Recurrent pyogenic infections begin shortly after birth. The clinical symptoms are similar to that observed in hypogammaglobulinemia (Lewis and Botto 2006). Respiratory tract infections are prominent, including pneumonia, tonsillitis, sinusitis, and otitis. Severe conditions are frequent with ethmoiditis and meningitis. Unlike inherited deficiency of the classical pathway components, the incidence of SLE among the C3-deficient patients reported in the literature is low. Membranoproliferative glomerulonephritis and purpura have been described in a few cases. An SLE-like syndrome with fever, vasculitis skin lesions, and arthritis has been seen in only three patients from two Japanese families without detectable autoantibodies. However this condition can be observed later in the childhood (Reis et al. 2006). In cases with glomerulonephritis, ANAs are usually undetectable, and other systemic signs of SLE-like disease are missing.

The first subject with homozygous C3 deficiency had been identified by (Alper et al. in 1972). A variety of molecular defects responsible for primary C3 deficiency have been described including homozygous mutations in the *C3* gene leading to the formation of premature stop codons, exon deletions, and aberrant splicing (reviewed by Reis et al. 2006). In addition, compound heterozygotes have been reported that result in impaired C3 secretion (reviewed by Reis et al. 2006; Ghannam et al. 2008) and missense mutations in the *C3* gene are described that predispose to the development of atypical hemolytic uremic syndrome (aHUS; see below). Functional differences among C3 allotypes were associated with an increased risk for age-related macular degeneration (AMD; see below).

Important observations reported that $C3^{-/-}$ patients exhibit a defective B-cell memory, with compromised vaccine response, in addition to functional defects of dendritic and regulatory T cells (Ghannam et al. 2008). These data highlight the importance of C3 as a key regulator of cell-mediated immunity. It has been evaluated whether the CD46-mediated costimulatory function could be retained in $C3^{-/-}$ human T cells. $C3^{-/-}$ $CD4^+$ T submitted to activation by CD3, CD46, and IL-2, resulted in much lower IL-10 secretion relative to C3-sufficient control T cells; i.e., $C3^{-/-}$ patients were also $Tr1^{-/-}$ (Ghannam et al. 2008). As the patient's T cells exhibited normal CD46 expression levels, it was hypothesized that the lack of Tr1 induction could have resulted from other impaired signalling in $C3^{-/-}$ (Ghannam et al. 2008). In a follow-up study of two $C3^{-/-}$ patients, it was found that Th1, but not Th2, responses were impaired in both $C3^{-/-}$ individuals (Ghannam et al. 2014). However, when $C3^{-/-}$ T cell cultures were reconstituted with C3a and IL-2, Th1 and Tr1 induction was restored. These data, combined with the defective Th1 induction in $CD46^{-/-}$ individuals, suggest that engagement of C3aR and CD46 is required for the CD46-mediated regulation of human Th1 cells and subsequent Tr1 induction (Ghannam et al. 2014).

Presently, 35 patients from 25 families with inherited C3 deficiency have been reported; the molecular genetic basis causing C3 deficiency is known in only 17 families. Table 1 shows the reported cases with clinical phenotypes, molecular identification, and biological abnormalities. Primary C3 deficiency is caused by defects directly related to the biosynthesis, protein expression, or C3 secretion.

It is worth to consider that C3-deficient patient management remains uncertain. The standard therapeutic strategies (prophylactic antibiotics, active immunization, and C3 substitution therapy) have been adopted with variable results. The majority of the patients receive prophylactic antibiotics, and this may help to reduce the incidence of infection. Even if the B-cell response to vaccine is impaired, the rationale to use vaccines directed against encapsulated pathogens has been advocated as shortly beneficial, and it is usually adopted in these patients.

Atypical Hemolytic Uremic Syndrome (aHUS)

Hemolytic uremic syndrome (HUS) is characterized by microangiopathic hemolytic anemia, thrombocytopenia, and renal impairment. It most frequently occurs in children under 5 years of age, with an annual incidence of 6.1 cases per 100,000 children under 5 years, 3 times more than the overall incidence, regardless of age. Most childhood cases are caused by Shiga toxin-producing bacteria and several other bacteria, e.g., *S pneumoniae*. Ten percent of atypical HUS (aHUS) forms are not associated with Shiga-like toxin-producing bacteria or streptococci and have a worse outcome, i.e. up to 50% of cases progressing to end-stage renal failure and 10–15% dying during the acute phase. The histologic lesions of Shiga toxin-related HUS are indistinguishable from those of its atypical form. They are characterized by thickening of arterioles and capillaries, endothelial swelling and detachment, and subendothelial accumulation of proteins and cell debris. Less than 20% of cases, aHUS occurs in a familial context (Matsumoto et al. 2014); developed in patients who do not have a family history, the disease is classified as sporadic. Complement plays an important role in the pathophysiology of aHUS. Producing irreversible renal damage, the disease appears prototypically induced by overactivation of the alternative pathway of complement with impaired regulation. This leads to the excessive liberation of cleavage fragments of C3, e.g., C3a and C5a, and to the formation of the C5b9 complex. These components generate endothelial damage and microangiopathic lesions. Complement genes associated with aHUS have been described (Noris et al. 2010; *Fremeaux*-Bacchi et al. 2013). The great majority of aHUS cases associate with the loss of function mutations in complement regulatory proteins (encoded by *CFH*, *CFI*, and *MCP* genes). Gain-of-function mutations have also been reported in the genes encoding key proteins of the alternative pathway, C3 (*C3*), and complement factor B (*CFB*). In this condition, the increased C3bBb convertase stability leads to permanent activation of the alternative pathway with low peripheral C3, while factor B levels are normal. Many C3 mutations, with nearly half are associated with a gain of function, have been identified in heterozygous conditions as responsible for aHUS at the positions shown in Fig. 1a (Noris et al. 2010; Bresin et al. 2013). The penetrance of aHUS-associated

Complement C3 Deficiency, Table 1 Reported cases of C3 deficiency with clinical presentation, laboratory data, and molecular analysis of the *C3* gene. The laboratory data are expressed using conventional units and sometimes using percentage of a normal control. *C3* nucleotide sequence numbering is according to NM_000064.2. The intron/exon organization is according to Vik et al., *Biochemistry* 1991; 30:1080–1085. *F* Female, *M* male, *bp* base pair, *nt* nucleotide

Patients	Clinical presentation	Laboratory data	Molecular defect	References
South Africa, F, 16 years, consanguineous parents	Recurrent meningitis at 5–6 years of age, from the age of 6 to 18 years pneumonia episodes, erythema multiforme following infections, Sweet syndrome	C3 1/1000 of the control	An 800-bp deletion in exons 22 and 23, resulting in a frameshift and a stop codon 19-bp downstream from the deletion	Alper et al. (1972), Botto et al. (1992)
United Kingdom, M, 10 years, consanguineous parents	Frequent pyogenic infections of the upper respiratory tract, erythema multiform following infection	CH50 42 U/ml (normal control 2512 U/ml) AP < 10% Functional fB 112% of NHS C1q 75%, C2 57%, C4 55%, undetectable C3, the addition of purified C3 to patient's serum restored CH50 to 2010 U/ml	2415G > A mutation with impact at the 5′ donor splice site of intron 18 resulting in 61-bp deletion in exon 18, subsequent from splicing of a cryptic 5′ donor splice site in exon 18 with the normal 3′ splice site in exon 19, generating a stop codon 17-bp downstream of the abnormal splice in exon 19	Botto et al. (1990)
Taïwan, F, 22 years, nonconsanguineous parents	Episodic attacks of pneumonia, otitis media, septic arthritis, and skin infection	Undetectable C3	1181 + 1G > T mutation at the 5′ donor splice site of intron 10, with a subsequent premature termination in exon 11, resulting in a shorter β-chain	Huang (1994), Hsieh et al. (1981)
Laos, M, 10 years, nonconsanguineous parents	Recurrent episodes of pneumonia, membranoproliferative glomerulonephritis	CH50 < 1% C3 4 mg/l	Normal size but decreased levels of C3-specific mRNA	Borzy et al. (1988), Singer et al. (1996)
Brazil, M, 19 years, consanguineous parents	Recurrent infections including bronchopneumonia, meningococcal meningitis, otitis media, osteomyelitis, pyodermitis, urinary tract infection, arthritis, and fever of unknown origin	Undetectable C3	(a) Silent missense mutation 972G > A in exon 9 (b) Missense mutation 1001 T > C in exon 9 (Leu314Pro ; MG3 domain) (c) Nonsense mutation 1716G > A in exon 13	Reis et al. (2002), Grumach et al. (1988)
New Zealand, M, 19 years + his sister	Periorbital cellulitis, recurrent pneumonia	C3 7 mg/l, CH50 < 200 U/ml, AP50 < 20 U/ml Normal size of mRNA, Pro C3 is synthesized in normal amounts	Missense mutation 1705G > A in exon 13 (Asp549Asn; MG5 domain) with defect of C3 secretion (suspected as being caused by compound heterozygous mutations)	Singer et al. (1994), Katz et al. (1995)

(continued)

Complement C3 Deficiency, Table 1 (continued)

Patients	Clinical presentation	Laboratory data	Molecular defect	References
Brazil, M, 8 years, consanguineous parents	Recurrent bacterial infections, severe adenitis and maxillary sinusitis, tonsillitis, bronchopneumonia, *Giardia lamblia* infection, vasculitis Post-infectious purpura	C3 0.15 mg/l, C4 602 mg/l, fI 55 mg/l, fH 448 mg/l, undetectable CH50, undetectable AP50 LPS-stimulated blood leukocytes from the proband also showed impairment in the synthesis/secretory defect of C3	Nonsense mutation 2602C > T in exon 20 (Arg848Stop) decreased C3 transcription with (1) a Leu314Pro (MG3 domain); (2) silent mutations at codons P577, S798, and A1437; and (3) a substitution that results in the production of a truncated protein	Ulbrich et al. (2001), Reis et al. (2004)
(a) Japan, F, 36 years (b) Japan, F, 34 years	At 16 years, SLE-like symptoms, vasculitis	Undetectable C3	Nonsense mutation 3303C > G in exon 26 (Tyr1081Stop)	Matsuyama et al. (2000)
Japan, M, 23 years, consanguineous parents	SLE, recurrent tonsillitis and pneumonia	Undetectable C3 CH50 0.1%	Homozygous 84-bp deletion at exon 39: a single base substitution AG to GG in the 3′ splice acceptor site of intron 38	Tsukamoto et al. (2005)
Japan, M, 2 years, nonconsanguineous parents	Meningitis, bronchitis, and pneumonia	Undetectable C3, CH50 < 12 U/ml	Compound heterozygous mutations: (a) Insertion 3176insT in exon 24 resulting in a frameshift and a premature downstream stop codon (Lys1105Stop) (b) Nonsense mutation 3303C > G in exon 26 (Tyr1081Stop)	Kida et al. (2008)
France, M, 5 years, nonconsanguineous parents	Meningitis, otitis, and pneumonia	Undetectable C3, CH50 < 10%	Compound heterozygous mutations: (a) Missense mutation 1648 T > C in exon 13 (Ser550Pro; MG5 domain) (b) Null allele	Ghannam et al. (2008)
Japan, M, 4 years, nonconsanguineous parents	Bacteremia caused by *S. pneumoniae*, pneumonia, acute otitis media, and gastroenterocolitis	C3 3 mg/l, CH50 4.7 U/ml	Compound heterozygous mutations: (a) Nonsense mutation 1432C > T in exon 12 (Arg478Stop) (b) 1066-2A > T transition at intron 9	Okura et al. (2011)

(continued)

Complement C3 Deficiency, Table 1 (continued)

Patients	Clinical presentation	Laboratory data	Molecular defect	References
Arab M, 4 years, consanguineous parents	Invasive pneumococcal disease	C3 < 100 mg/l	Homozygous 1-nt deletion 3997delA in exon 31 with frameshift and a stop signal 13 codons downstream of the deletion	Goldberg et al. (2011)
Turkey, M, 16 years, consanguineous parents	Recurrent airway infections caused by *S. pneumoniae* and bronchiectasis	C3 80–190 mg/l, undetectable CH50, selective IgA deficiency	Homozygous missense mutation 4554C > G in exon 38 (Cys1518Trp; first position of the C345C domain)	Santos-Valente et al. (2013)
France, M, 9 years	Recurrent otitis and pneumonia	Undetectable C3, CH50 < 22%, decreased IgG4	Compound heterozygous mutations: (a) Nonsense mutation 2290C > T in exon 18 (Arg764Stop) (b) 1-nt deletion 2002Cdel in exon 16 resulting in a frameshift Arg668AlafsX35	Ghannam et al. (2014)
Sweden, F, 42 years, + her sister	Systemic lupus erythematosus-like syndrome associated with several autoimmune manifestations, including fatigue, swollen fingers, arthralgia, and the presence of antinuclear, anti-dsDNA, anti-SSA, and anti-centromere Abs	C3 400–700 mg/l lack of alternative pathway-mediated complement activity ($\leq$14%)	Heterozygous missense mutation 1180 T > C in exon 10 (Met373Thr; MG4 domain)	Sfyroera et al. (2015)
Spain, 2 patients found in independent families	Purpura and membranoproliferative glomerulonephritis for both patients	Undetectable C3 for both patients	Homozygous deletion 168_169del in exon 2 (56YfsX15) Homozygous 1682G > A in exon 13 (Gly561Asp)	Jimenez-Reinoso et al. (2015)

mutations is incomplete. The explanation could be that other risk factors or environmental hits act as modifiers of disease penetrance. This is consistent with the observation that at least 10% of patients have combined mutations, especially of *CFI* mutation with either *CFH* or *MCP* or *CFB* or *C3*.

Age-Related Macular Degeneration AMD

Age-related macular degeneration (AMD) is the leading cause of blindness in developed countries for those over the age of 55 years with approximately 50 million sufferers worldwide. AMD disease associates with yellow deposits lying within the ocular Bruch's membrane, beneath the retinal

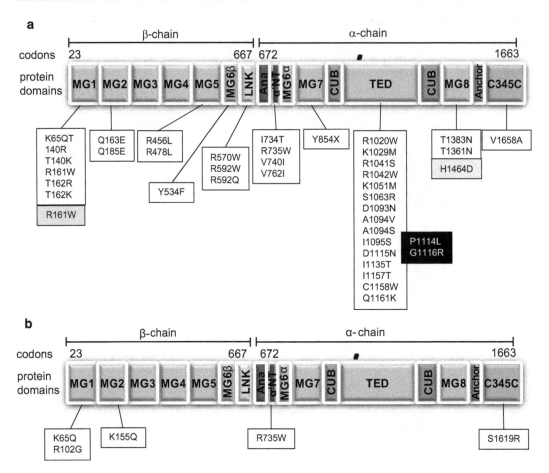

Complement C3 Deficiency, Fig. 1 Summary of the mutations in the C3 protein identified by the different groups within patient cohorts. The amino acid numbering refers to the pro-C3 protein (codons), and the 17 C3 domains are identified. (**a**) Patients with atypical hemolytic uremic syndrome (aHUS), including the International Registry of Recurrent and Familial HUS/TTP. C3 variants and combined mutations are spread all over the gene; a hot spot is evidenced in the thioester-containing domain (TED) with 17 independent mutations (42.5%). Changes found only combined with other mutations are in a *black square*, and changes found both as single or combined mutations are in *light gray squares*. (**b**) Patients with age-related macular degeneration (AMD). Locations of the variants are indicated. MG, macroglobulin domain; LNK, linker domain (residues 578–645); Ana, anaphylatoxin domain; CUB, CUB domain; TED, thioester-containing domain; anchor, anchor domain; C345C, netrin module of an about 130-residue domain found in the C-terminal parts of complement proteins C3, C4, and C5

pigment epithelium. These extracellular deposits are called drusen, naturally occurring with age. Drusen contain cellular debris, lipids, and various protein components including a number from the innate immune system. They are believed to be the result of the eye's failure to eliminate waste products produced in the cells of the eye. This accumulation disrupts the nutrient flow from the choroid to the retinal pigment epithelium cells, leading to cell disruption and death, subsequently affecting the adjacent photoreceptor cells. Due to localized inflammation and ultimately

neurodegeneration, the disease appears with the loss of photoreceptor cells in the central region of the retina (macula) with subsequent loss of central and sharp vision. There are two types of AMD: dry (atrophic) and wet (neovascular or exudative). Most AMD starts as the dry type, and in 10–20% of individuals, it progresses to the wet type. AMD is always bilateral (i.e., occurs in both eyes), but does not necessarily progress at the same extent in both eyes. Rare and highly penetrant variants in the genes encoding complement factor H (*CFH*), complement factor I (*CFI*), complement component 3 (*C3*), and complement component 9 (*C9*) have recently been found to be associated with AMD. Rare variants (K65Q, K155Q, R735W, and S1619R) in C3 were shown to be associated with AMD disease risk (Schramm et al. 2015). The K65Q variant resides in the macroglobulin 1 (MG1) domain of C3 and was shown to cause decreased binding to CFH (Schramm et al. 2014). The R161Q variant was shown to cause hyperactive C3 convertase due to increased binding to factor B (CFB) and reduced binding to CFH and membrane cofactor protein (MCP; CD46), resulting in higher complement activity. In addition, a common SNP in *C3* results in a R102G substitution is associated with risk of AMD (Yates et al. 2007). This polymorphism results in reduced FH binding to the R102G variant and subsequent decreased factor I-mediated cofactor activity, with subsequent enhanced alternative convertase amplification. This effect on FH cofactor activity is specific, as the decay-accelerating activities of FH, decay-accelerating factor (DAF), and MCP are not affected (Heurich et al. 2011). The R102G polymorphism is also associated with other diseases such as the kidney condition dense deposit disease (DDD, see below). Interestingly, recent studies suggested a genetic overlap between AMD and aHUS (K65Q, R735W, and S1619R). *C3* mutations have been identified in heterozygous conditions as responsible for AMD at the positions shown in Fig. 1b. As already highlighted by the group of Atkinson, these two distinct diseases, in which pathogenesis is sometimes due to the same innate immune defect, are overreacting to tissue injury. The genetics of C3 contributes to the genetic variance of AMD; this may have implications for predictive testing of AMD patients (Seddon et al. 2013). Based on the genetic evidence for a role of the alternative pathway in AMD, manipulation of complement activity systemically or locally could be a promising therapeutic option in the future.

Dense Deposit Disease (DDD)

Dense deposit disease (DDD) is characterized by isolated C3 deposits (and associated with dysregulation of the complement alternative pathway). Its primary feature is the presence of electron dense transformation of the glomerular basement membrane, and not the membranoproliferative pattern. Components of the alternative pathway including C3b and its breakdown products iC3b, C3dg, or C3c and C5b-C9 complex are contained in the dense deposits. The alternative pathway dysregulation in DDD is commonly induced by C3 nephritic factor (C3Nef), an autoantibody stabilizing the C3 convertase. Few patients with homozygous or heterozygous mutations in the *CFH, CFI,* and *C3* genes have been identified. From etiological consideration, DDD is classified as complement-mediated disease. Few clinical cases with complement analysis have been reported. No frequencies of acquired or genetic abnormalities are available, and no biological or genetic markers influencing the location of the dense deposits have been identified.

Acquired C3 Deficiency

Acquired or secondary C3 deficiency is observed in patients with a normal C3 biosynthesis but with an excessive consumption leading to a marked reduction or complete absence of serum C3 protein. For example, impairment in the complement regulatory proteins factor H or factor I leads to uncontrolled amplification of C3 cleavage by an uncontrolled alternative C3 convertase. Another example is given by C3 nephritic factor (C3Nef) where an autoantibody that increases the half-life of the alternative C3 convertase leads to excessive C3 turnover. Patients with acquired C3 deficiency predispose the same risks: susceptibilities to infections by *S. pneumoniae* and *N. meningitidis* or immune complex deposition-mediated diseases such as SLE-like syndrome and membranoproliferative glomerulonephritis type II (MPGN II). In these examples the patients also exhibit low levels of C3, associated with impaired factor H activity or C3Nef autoantibodies. Unlike primary C3 deficiency conditions, where the patients present with complete lack of C3, acquired or secondary C3 deficiency patients may present with a residual concentration of intact circulating C3 with C3 split products. Acquired C3 deficiency results in higher susceptibility to recurrent infections, meningitis, and kidney impairment.

MPGN II is a rare disease (<20% of cases of MPGN in children and only a fractional percentage of cases in adults); it is characterized by the deposition of abnormal electron dense material within the glomerular basement membrane of the kidney and often within Bruch's membrane in the eye. It has no known association with immune complexes, in contrast to MPGN I and III variants of immune complex-mediated disease. MPGN II affects both genders equally and is usually diagnosed in children between 5 and 15 year of age and present with one of five symptoms: hematuria, proteinuria, hematuria and proteinuria, acute nephritic syndrome, or nephrotic syndrome. Although these findings are nonspecific, >80% of patients are positive for serum C3Nef, an autoantibody which stabilizes the C3bBb convertase by protecting it from factor I inactivation. The native convertase is labile (half-life of 4 min), and binding of C3Nef increases the half-life to 45–60 min. As a consequence a C3Nef-stabilized convertase consumes C3b, with subsequent amplified C3 cleavage, enhanced local complement activation, and increased C3b deposition. Because C3Nef is also present in individuals with MPGN types I and III (nearly 50%), the definitive diagnosis of MPGN II depends on the demonstration of dense deposits in the glomerular basement membrane (Appel et al. 2005).

MPGN II patients can develop drusen. As above described for AMD, these deposits lie under the retina; in this condition, they occur at an early age and often are detectable in the second decade of life, in contrast to AMD where drusen form after 55 year of age. The distribution of these deposits varies among patients and initially has little impact on visual acuity and fields. Over time, however, specialized tests of retinal function, such as dark adaptation, electroretinography, and electrooculography, can become abnormal. Vision can deteriorate as subretinal neovascular membranes, macular detachment,

and central serous retinopathy develop. The long-term risk for visual problems is approximately 10%. There is no correlation between disease severity in the kidney and the eye; and an ophthalmologic examination at the time of diagnosis and periodic funduscopic assessments should be part of patient treatment.

MPGN II can be associated with acquired partial lipodystrophy. The loss of subcutaneous fat in the upper half of the body usually precedes the onset of kidney disease by several years and can result in a strikingly haggard facial appearance. It has been reported that approximately 83% of acquired partial lipodystrophy patients have low C3 levels and polyclonal C3Nef and that approximately 20% go on to develop MPGN after a median of approximately 8 year after the onset of lipodystrophy. Compared with acquired lipodystrophy patients without renal disease, those with MPGN have an earlier age of onset of lipodystrophy and a higher prevalence of C3 hypocomplementemia. The deposition of activated components of complement in adipose tissue results in the destruction of adipocytes in areas high in factor D content (otherwise referred to as adipsin).

Spontaneous remission of MPGN II is uncommon. The more probable outcome is chronic deterioration of renal function leading to end-stage renal disease in approximately half of patients within 10 year of diagnosis. In >50% of patients with MPGN II, serum C3Nef persists throughout the disease course. C3Nef is nearly always associated with biological evidence of complement activation such as a decrease in CH50 and C3 levels and an increase in C3dg/C3d.

Comparing the clinical features between the primary and secondary C3-deficient patients, primary C3 deficiency results in higher susceptibility to recurrent infections, meningitis, and kidney impairment. In the case of factor I or factor H deficiencies, a severe depletion of C3 and other alternative pathway proteins is observed. In the secondary C3-deficient patients, C3 depletion may be the direct cause for the infections. Kidney impairment was observed in 13% of patients and autoimmune diseases in 6% of patients.

Biological Diagnostic of Primary and Secondary C3 Deficiencies

Complement Laboratory Analysis of C3 Deficiencies

As recently and extensively described by the international group (www.IUIS.org; Grumach and Kirschfink 2014), the identification of a complement deficiency involves a multistep process starting with hemolytic testing of each activation pathway (or with functional ELISA or liposome-based assays) and proceeds in specialized laboratories with the characterization of the defect at functional, protein, and molecular level. The laboratory must distinguish between a deficiency, a functional disorder, or the activation state of complement. It is essential that blood samples are processed as quickly as possible to serum and citrate/EDTA platelet-poor plasma. Samples can be frozen at $-80\ °C$ until assayed or shipped on dry ice if needed. Repeated freezing and thawing should be avoided because of the risk of in vitro activation. Serum is used for the analysis of the hemolytic function, of complement proteins and regulators, as well as of autoantibodies; a quantitation of activation products requires the use of citrate/EDTA plasma. The soluble activation product of the terminal complement cascade, SC5b-9, has received more attention as unrestricted progression to its final steps was linked to specific pathology as in aHUS, and the efficacy of the recently introduced C5 antibody eculizumab in treating aHUS patients is reflected by SC5b-9 suppression. Patients under eculizumab therapy are monitored using plasma C3adesArg, C3d, or SC5b-C9 as global markers of complement activation.

Complement Profile of Primary C3 Deficiencies

C3 deficiency patients present with a very low hemolytic activity of the classical and alternative pathway targets, associated with dramatically decreased C3 and normal C4 levels. With the absence of C3Nef and a normal factor B level, these features are in favor of a C3 deficiency. Selective immunoglobulin deficiency could be observed, in agreement with the decrease of memory B-cells.

Complement Profile of Secondary Deficiencies

Reduced serum levels of complement C3 with normal levels of C4 have been reported in patients with aHUS, AMD, and MPGN. A low C3 level reflects complement activation and consumption, with subsequent reduced CH50. Patients with the HUS who have low C3 levels have high levels of activated complement components, including C3b, C3c, and C3d. Most C3 gain-of-function mutations reduce C3b binding to CFH and MCP, which severely impairs degradation of mutant C3b. Granular C3 deposits in glomeruli and arterioles during acute disease are consistent with the activation of complement and local C3 consumption. C9 staining in glomeruli and small arteries with intimal proliferation and thrombosis documents activation up to the final lytic C5b-9 membrane attack complex.

Nearly 10% of patients with aHUS develop anti-CFH autoantibodies. These antibodies bind to the CFH C-terminal, reduce CFH binding to C3b, and enhance alternative pathway-dependent lysis of unsensitized sheep erythrocytes, supporting the factor H testing, without influencing fluid-phase cofactor activity. The lack of complement control on cells, despite control in the fluid phase, mimics the course of the disease in patients with CFH mutations.

Only occasionally AMD is associated with alterations in routine complement analysis, and C3 levels are nearly normal when a C3 abnormality is associated with AMD. Serum of AMD patients could present with reduced hemolysis of rabbit erythrocytes with a decreased C3 level, indicating an activation of the alternative pathway, when a decreased function of factor H is responsible for AMD. Accumulation in drusen of alternative and terminal complement components has been observed, demonstrating complement activation in AMD (Mullins et al. 2000).

The serum autoantibody C3Nef is demonstrated after mixing equal volumes from the patient serum with normal human serum and C3 consumption next determined by hemolytic testing, specific C3 titration, estimation of C3 split products, or loss of factor B antigen from C3. Stabilization of cell C3bBb convertase by the precipitated IgG is the gold standard for measuring C3Nef. An ELISA assay utilizing plate-bound C3bBb and a microassay based on peroxidase-like activity of heme groups are available.

Cross-References

► Complement Deficiencies Associated with Atypical Hemolytic Uremic Syndrome

References

Alper CA, Colten HR, Rosen FS, Rabson AR, Macnab GM, Gear JS. Homozygous deficiency of C3 in a patient with repeated infections. Lancet. 1972;2 (7788):1179–81.

Appel GB, Cook HT, Hageman G, Jennette JC, Kashgarian M, Kirschfink M, Lambris JD, Lanning L, Lutz HU, Meri S, Rose NR, Salant DJ, Sethi S, Smith RJ, Smoyer W, Tully HF, Tully SP, Walker P, Welsh M, Würzner R, Zipfel PF. Membranoproliferative glomerulonephritis type II (dense deposit disease): an update. J Am Soc Nephrol. 2005;16(5):1392–403.

Borzy MS1, Gewurz A, Wolff L, Houghton D, Lovrien E. Inherited C3 deficiency with recurrent infections and glomerulonephritis. Am J Dis Child. 1988;142(1):79–83.

Botto M, Fong KY, So AK, Rudge A, Walport MJ. Molecular basis of hereditary C3 deficiency. J Clin Invest. 1990;86(4):1158–63.

Botto M, Fong KY, So AK, Barlow R, Routier R, Morley BJ, Walport MJ. Homozygous hereditary C3 deficiency due to a partial gene deletion. Proc Natl Acad Sci U S A. 1992;89(11):4957–61.

Bresin E, Rurali E, Caprioli J, Sanchez-Corral P, Fremeaux-Bacchi V, Rodriguez de Cordoba S, Pinto S, Goodship TH, Alberti M, Ribes D, Valoti E, Remuzzi G, Noris M, European Working Party on Complement Genetics in Renal Diseases. Combined complement gene mutations in atypical hemolytic uremic syndrome influence clinical phenotype. J Am Soc Nephrol. 2013;24(3):475–86.

Da Silva Reis E, Baracho GV, Sousa Lima A, Farah CS, Isaac L. Homozygous hereditary C3 deficiency due to a premature stop codon. J Clin Immunol. 2002;22 (6):321–30.

Fong KY, Botto M, Walport MJ, So AK. Genomic organization of human complement component C3. Genomics. 1990;7(4):579–86.

Fremeaux-Bacchi V, Fakhouri F, Garnier A, Bienaimé F, Dragon-Durey M-A, Ngo S, Moulin B, Servais A, Provot F, Rostaing L, Burtey S, Niaudet P, Deschênes G, Lebranchu Y, Zuber J, Loirat C. Genetics and outcome of atypical hemolytic uremic syndrome: a nationwide French series comparing children and adults. Clin J Am Soc Nephrol. 2013;8(4):554–62.

Ghannam A, Pernollet M, Fauquert J-L, Monnier N, Ponard D, Villiers M-B, Péguet-Navarro J, Tridon A, Lunardi J, Gerlier D, Drouet C. Human C3 deficiency associated with impairments in dendritic cell differentiation, memory B cells, and regulatory T cells. J Immunol. 2008;181(7):5158–66.

Ghannam A, Fauquert J-L, Thomas C, Kemper C, Drouet C. Human complement C3 deficiency: Th1 induction requires T cell-derived complement C3a and CD46 activation. Mol Immunol. 2014;58(1):98–107.

Goldberg M, Fremeaux-Bacchi V, Koch P, Fishelson Z, Katz Y. A novel mutation in the C3 gene and recurrent invasive pneumococcal infection: a clue for vaccine development. Mol Immunol. 2011;48(15–16):1926–31.

Grumach AS, Vilela MM, Gonzalez CH, Starobinas N, Pereira AB, Dias-da-Silva W, Carneiro-Sampaio MM. Inherited C3 deficiency of the complement system. Braz J Med Biol Res. 1988;21(2):247–57.

Grumach AS, Kirschfink M. Are complement deficiencies really rare? Overview on prevalence, clinical importance and modern diagnostic approach. Mol Immunol. 2014;61(2):110–7.

Heurich M, Martínez-Barricarte R, Francis NJ, Roberts DL, Rodríguez de Córdoba S, Morgan BP. Common polymorphisms in C3, factor B, and factor H collaborate to determine systemic complement activity and disease risk. Proc Natl Acad Sci U S A. 2011;108(21):8761–6.

Hsieh KH, Lin CY, Lee TC. Complete absence of the third component of complement in a patient with repeated infections. Clin Immunol Immunopathol. 1981;20(3):305–12.

Huang JL, Lin CY. A hereditary C3 deficiency due to aberrant splicing of exon 10. Clin Immunol Immunopathol. 1994;73(2):267–73.

Jiménez-Reinoso A, López-Lera A, Marin AVM, López-Rela J, Martínez-Naves E, de Córdoba SR, Román-Ortiz E, López-Trascasa M, Regueiro JR. Differential impairment of dendritic, B and T cell differentiation in congenital primary (C3-deficient) as opposed to secondary (factor I-deficient) human plasma C3 deficiencies. Mol Immunol. 2015;67(1):147–8 [abstract].

Katz Y, Wetsel RA, Schlesinger M, Fishelson Z. Compound heterozygous complement C3 deficiency. Immunology. 1995;84(1):5–7.

Kida M, Fujioka H, Kosaka Y, Hayashi K, Sakiyama Y, Ariga T. The first confirmed case with C3 deficiency caused by compound heterozygous mutations in the C3 gene; a new aspect of pathogenesis for C3 deficiency. Blood Cells Mol Dis. 2008;40(3):410–3.

Lewis MJ, Botto M. Complement deficiencies in humans and animals: links to autoimmunity. Autoimmunity. 2006;39(5):367–78.

Matsuyama W, Nakagawa M, Takashima H, Muranaga F, Sano Y, Osame M. Identification of a novel mutation (Tyr1081Ter) in sisters with hereditary component C3 deficiency and SLE-like symptoms. Hum Mutat. 2001;17(1):79.

Matsumoto T, Fan X, Ishikawa E, Ito M, Amano K, Toyoda H, Komada Y, Ohishi K, Katayama N, Yoshida Y, Matsumoto M, Fujimura Y, Ikejiri M, Wada H, Miyata T. Analysis of patients with atypical hemolytic uremic syndrome treated at the Mie University Hospital: concentration of C3 p.I1157T mutation. Int J Hematol. 2014;100(5):437–42.

Mullins RF, Russell SR, Anderson DH, Hageman GS. Drusen associated with aging and age-related macular degeneration contain proteins common to extracellular deposits associated with atherosclerosis, elastosis, amyloidosis, and dense deposit disease. FASEB J. 2000;14(7):835–46.

Noris M, Caprioli J, Bresin E, Mossali C, Pianetti G, Gamba S, Daina E, Fenili C, Castelletti F, Sorosina A, Piras R, Donadelli R, Maranta R, van der Meer I, Conway EM, Zipfel PF, Goodship TH, Remuzzi G. Relative role of genetic complement abnormalities in sporadic and familial aHUS and their impact on clinical phenotype. Clin J Am Soc Nephrol. 2010;5(10):1844–59.

Okura Y, Yamada M, Takezaki S, Nawate M, Takahashi Y, Kida M, Kawamura N, Ariga T. Novel compound heterozygous mutations in the C3 gene: hereditary C3 deficiency. Pediatr Int. 2011;53(2):e16–9.

Reis ES, Falcão DA, Isaac L. Clinical aspects and molecular basis of primary deficiencies of complement component C3 and its regulatory proteins factor I and factor H. Scand J Immunol. 2006;68(4):445–55.

Ricklin D, Hajishengallis G, Yang K, Lambris JD. Complement: a key system for immune surveillance and homeostasis. Nat Immunol. 2010;11(9):785–97.

Ritchie RF, Palomaki GE, Neveux LM, Navolotskaia O, Ledue TB, Craig WY. Reference distributions for complement proteins C3 and C4: a practical, simple and clinically relevant approach in a large cohort. J Clin Lab Anal. 2004;18(1):1–8.

Santos-Valente E, Reisli I, Artaç H, Ott R, Sanal Ö, Boztug K. A novel mutation in the complement component 3 gene in a patient with selective IgA deficiency. J Clin Immunol. 2013;33(1):127–33.

Schramm EC, Clark SJ, Triebwasser MP, Raychaudhuri S, Seddon JM, Atkinson JP. Genetic variants in the complement system predisposing to age-related macular degeneration: a review. Mol Immunol. 2014;61(2):118–25.

Schramm EC, Roumenina LT, Rybkine T, Chauvet S, Vieira-Martins P, Hue C, Maga T, Valoti E, Wilson V, Jokiranta S, Smith RJ, Noris M, Goodship T, Atkinson JP, Fremeaux-Bacchi V. Functional mapping of the interactions between complement C3 and regulatory proteins using atypical hemolytic uremic syndrome-associated mutations. Blood. 2015;125(15):2359–69.

Seddon JM, Yu Y, Miller EC, Reynolds R, Tan PL, Gowrisankar S, Goldstein JI, Triebwasser M, Anderson HE, Zerbib J, Kavanagh D, Souied E, Katsanis N, Daly MJ, Atkinson JP, Raychaudhuri S. Rare variants in CFI, C3 and C9 are associated with high risk of advanced age-related macular degeneration. Nat Genet. 2013;45(11):1366–70.

Sfyroera G, Ricklin D, Reis ES, Chen H, Wu EL, Kaznessis YN, Ekdahl KN, Nilsson B, Lambris JD. Rare loss-of-function mutation in complement component C3 provides insight into molecular and pathophysiological determinants of complement activity. J Immunol. 2015;194(7):3305–16.

Singer L, Whitehead WT, Akama H, Katz Y, Fishelson Z, Wetsel RA. Inherited human complement C3 deficiency. An amino acid substitution in the betachain (ASP549 to ASN) impairs C3 secretion. J Biol Chem. 1994;269(45):28494–9.

Singer L, Van Hee ML, Lokki ML, Kramer J, Borzy MS, Wetsel RA. Inherited complement C3 deficiency: reduced C3 mRNA and protein levels in a Laotian kindred. Clin Immunol Immunopathol. 1996;81(3):244–52.

Tsukamoto H, Horiuchi T, Kokuba H, Nagae S, Nishizaka H, Sawabe T, Harashima S, Himeji D, Koyama T, Otsuka J, Mitoma H, Kimoto Y, Hashimura C, Kitano E, Kitamura H, Furue M, Harada M. Molecular analysis of a novel hereditary C3 deficiency with systemic lupus erythematosus. Biochem Biophys Res Commun. 2005;330(1):298–304.

Ulbrich AG, Florido MP, Nudelman V, Reis ES, Baracho GV, Isaac L. Hereditary human complement C3 deficiency owing to reduced levels of C3 mRNA. Scand J Immunol. 2001;53(6):622–6.

Yates JRW, Sepp T, Matharu BK, Khan JC, Thurlby DA, Shahid H, Clayton DG, Hayward C, Morgan J, Wright AF, Armbrecht AM, Dhillon B, Deary IJ, Redmond E, Bird AC, Moore AT, Genetic Factors in AMD Study Group. Complement C3 variant and the risk of age-related macular degeneration. N Engl J Med. 2007;357(6):553–61.

Complement Component C2 Deficiency

Gunnar Sturfelt[1] and Lennart Truedsson[2]
[1]Department of Rheumatology, University Hospital of Skåne, Lund, Sweden
[2]Dept. of Laboratory Medicine, Section of Microbiology, Immunology and Glycobiology, Lund University, Lund, Sweden

Definition

C2 deficiency is a relatively common complement deficiency with an estimated prevalence of 1/20,000 in the Caucasian population. In the

Gunner Sturfelt: deceased.

great majority of cases, the deficiency is caused by homozygosity for a 28-base pair deletion in the C2 gene, which is located in the MHC haplotype HLA-B*18, S042, DRB1*15. Major disease associations are increased susceptibility for infections with encapsulated bacteria, development of SLE or SLE-like disease, and slightly increased risk for atherosclerosis. The SLE disease is generally mild with skin symptoms and the autoantibody profile differs from that in SLE in general since positivity for anti-dsDNA antibodies is rare. From the prevalence it is concluded that many CD2 individuals are apparently healthy. A probable explanation is that complement activation may go through bypass mechanisms involving C1q or MBL, C4, and the alternative pathway. In addition C2D individuals show good response in antibody production after vaccination although for some antigens not quite as good as in normal individuals.

Introduction

Complement deficiency is a primary immunodeficiency which according to the classic definition predisposes to infections and immune dysregulation with autoimmune disease and also malignancy. Complement deficiency states can be either primary (hereditary) or secondary (acquired). Primary C2 deficiency (C2D) is fairly common and has been estimated to occur in about 1 in 20,000 individuals in Caucasian population. Secondary deficiency can be caused by complement consumption, for instance, induced by immune complexes, autoantibodies, reduced synthesis, or increased catabolism of complement components, but then there is not a low level of C2 alone. The first report of C2D was in 1960 when Silverstein described a clinically healthy adult male with a selective deficiency of C2 (Silverstein 1960). Later C2D has been shown to be associated with disease although apparently healthy individuals with C2D also are seen, which is discussed further in this article.

Diagnostic Procedures

When clinical symptoms such as recurrent bacterial infections or development of SLE is found, analyses of complement should be performed. The initial analyses should include screening for deficiencies. This has since long been done by hemolytic methods, such as CH50 for the classical pathway of complement activation and AP50 for the alternative pathway. The absence of activity in CH50 should lead to further analysis of individual components in the classical pathway to show which factor is missing. Other similar methods are hemolysis in gel (HIG) assays which are described and in use for both the classical and the alternative pathways.

A more recent approach to screen for complement deficiencies is with ELISAs for complement function. Assays for all three pathways, the classical, alternative, and lectin pathway, are developed (Mollnes et al. 2007). These are also commercially available, and the more widespread use of complement screening assays appears to increase the number of identified deficiency cases. One such example is the first case of complete factor B deficiency, which recently was detected by the use of these ELISA assays. In the case of C2D, like in C4 deficiency, there is no activity in either the classical or the lectin pathway. Thus, the use of these screening assays is a very effective way to determine which components that may be missing.

C2 serum concentration can be measured by several immunochemical methods such as electro-immunoassay or ELISA. In rare cases when a nonfunctional C2 molecule is expected to be produced, the immunochemical assay has to be supplemented with a functional assay for C2. This can be done by adding purified functionally active C2 to the sample and then check for functional activity in an assay for complement activation (Mollnes et al. 2007).

Genetics of C2 Deficiency

The gene for C2 is located within the MHC class III region together with the genes for factor B and

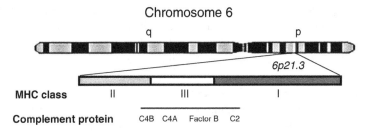

Complement Component C2 Deficiency, Fig. 1 Schematic presentation of the location of the genes for complement components C2, C4 isotypes (C4A and C4B) and factor B within the MHC class III region on the human chromosome 6p

the two C4 isotypes C4A and C4B (Fig. 1). These complement genes exist in a number of genetic variants, and the combination of these complement variants have been described as complotypes and are part of the MHC haplotypes. C2D, in more than 90% of Caucasian cases, is explained by a 28-base pair deletion in the C2 gene, and this is stated as C2D type I. This non-expressed C2 gene is located in the MHC haplotype HLA-B*18, S042, DRB1*15 (Johnson et al. 1992). In addition, this haplotype is associated with a specific HLA-C allele. Thus, C2D has a homogeneous genetic background regarding MHC association. Based on the analyses of microsatellite markers, the mutation has been estimated to have occurred within the last 242 generations (Carrington et al. 1999). With a generation of 20 years, this dates the mutation to have occurred about 5000 years ago, thus a relatively recent event.

Other mutations can cause C2D and are stated as C2D type II. In the first described case, two missense mutations both causing a selective block in C2 secretion was found (Wetsel et al. 1996). In another case heterozygous for the type I C2D gene, the other C2 gene was found to have a mutation that affected the secretion from transfected COS cells thus being a C2D type II mutation. In these cases there is no association to a specific MHC haplotype.

Prevalence of C2 Deficiency

In the Caucasian population the prevalence of complete C2 deficiency is about 1 in 20,000

individuals (Pickering et al. 2000). The estimation is based on the fact that the great majority of C2D individuals are homozygous for the same deletion in a specific MHC haplotype. Heterozygous carriers of the deletion are found in about 1.4% of the Caucasian population and from that the prevalence of total deficiency is calculated. Thus C2D is the most common of deficiencies within the classical pathway and, if MBL deficiency not is included, the most common of all complement deficiencies in the Caucasian population. In the Japanese population C9 deficiency is more common, approximate prevalence 1/1000 but other complement deficiencies are rare (Skattum et al. 2011).

Infections in C2 Deficiency

C2D is associated with bacterial infections, particularly invasive infection by encapsulated bacteria, but also with development of SLE or SLE-like disease. Based on RFLP analysis, there was no evidence of that MHC class II genes linked to the C2 gene carrying the mutation determine different clinical consequences of C2 deficiency (Truedsson et al. 1993). However, C2D is associated with abnormalities in serum immunoglobulin concentrations, such as lower levels of IgG2 and IgG4 which also may contribute to increased infection susceptibility.

More than half (57%) of C2D patients in a study including 40 patients had suffered from invasive infection mainly meningitis or septicemia caused by *Streptococcus* (*S.*) *pneumoniae* (Jönsson et al. 2005). Other infections seen in

C2D are with *Haemophilus* (*H.*) *influenzae* type b and *Neisseria* (*N.*) *meningitidis*. The association of C2D and infection has been shown to depend on the IgG2 subclass allotype, and homozygosity for G2M(n) protects against severe infection (Jönsson et al. 2006). In the same study, a weak association with MBL deficiency resulting in increased infection susceptibility was noted. Thus, based on the prevalence of C2D, a portion of these individuals have no susceptibility for infections that make them known in the healthcare system.

The capacity to produce specific antibodies in response to infection or vaccination is important. It has been shown that vaccination in C2D individuals against pneumococci and *H. influenzae* type b results in antibody responses that are lower or similar to normal depending on the antigen (Jönsson et al. 2012). Also vaccination against meningococci gave rise to antibody responses in the C2D patients equal to healthy controls (Brodszki et al. 2015). In this study, the response rate was lower to serogroup A and among C2D patients with history of invasive infections. In accordance with previous findings, the presence of *G2M*n/G2M*n* genotype was associated with higher production of specific antibodies after immunization.

Autoimmune Diseases in C2 Deficiency

Deficiency states of the components of the classical pathway, C1q, C1r, C1s, C2, and C4, are all associated with an increased risk to develop autoimmune disease. There is a hierarchy regarding risk to develop autoimmune disease among the early components within the classical pathway (C1q,r,s and C4 and C2) with highest risk in individuals with C1q deficiency, somewhat less risk in C4 deficiency and lowest risk in C2D. Of autoimmune disorders seen in individuals with C2D, systemic lupus erythematosus (SLE) or SLE-like disease is most common. SLE is a complex autoimmune disorder characterized by the production of autoantibodies against nuclear, cytoplasmic, and other cellular components leading to chronic inflammation with involvement of multiple organs. It was shown about 1960 that the complement system appeared to be involved in the pathogenesis in SLE. Somewhat later it was found that complement deficiency did not protect but was rather associated with an increased risk for SLE, and this was called the lupus paradox.

It has been estimated that 10–20% of homozygous C2-deficient individuals develop SLE. The disease usually develops at similar age interval as in general, i.e., at 30–50 years of age, and there is also a clear female preponderance (Jönsson et al. 2007). In comparison with C1q, C1r/C1s, and C4 deficiency states, SLE associated with C2D is considered less severe. Skin and joint involvement is common in SLE patients with C2D, and severe chronic cutaneous and/or subacute cutaneous lupus erythematosus may occur. Renal and neuropsychiatric disease, however, is generally thought to be rare in these SLE patients, but there are a few reports from C2D cohorts of relatively high frequency of kidney involvement. In Table 1 (data modified from Jönsson et al. 2007) a comparison between SLE patients with C2D and control SLE patients from the same area in Southern Sweden (Lund cohort) is given regarding prevalence of ACR classification criteria.

Complement Component C2 Deficiency, Table 1 Clinical manifestations/ACR classification criteria in SLE patients with C2D (C2D SLE) compared to control SLE patients (c-SLE) in the Lund cohort

ACR criterium fulfilled	C2D SLE (%)	c-SLE (%)
ACR 1 (malar rash)	92	38
ACR 2 (discoid rash)	67	25
ACR 3 (photosensitivity)	67	64
ACR 4 (oral ulcers)	25	10
ACR 5 (arthritis)	83	71
ACR 6 (serositis)	42	48
ACR 7 (renal disorder)	8	30
ACR 8 (neurologic disorder)	8	13
ACR 9 (hematologic disorder)	25	57
ACR 10 (immunologic disorder)	50	71
ACR 11 (antinuclear antibody)	50	100

Jönsson et al. (2007)

Complement Component C2 Deficiency, Table 2 Frequencies of some autoantibodies in SLE patients with C2D (C2D SLE) in comparison with control SLE patients (c-SLE) in the Lund cohort

Autoantibody	C2D SLE (%)	c-SLE (%)
ANA (HEP-2)	50	100
Anti-RNP	45	24
Anti-SSA 60	18	40
Anti-C1q	42	17
Anti-CL	83	38
Anti-dsDNA	8	78

Jönsson et al. (2007)

The autoantibody profile in SLE patients with C2D differs from that generally seen in SLE patients. In Table 2 the autoantibody profile in the C2D SLE cohort in Lund is compared with a control SLE cohort from the same area, i.e., non-C2D SLE patients. A positive ANA as estimated by the HEp-2 cell assay is found at a lower frequency in SLE patients with C2D than in other SLE patients. Furthermore anti-dsDNA antibodies (Crithidia luciliae test) are seen at a low frequency in C2D SLE which is in accordance to the findings in other reports. Anti-RNP and anti-SSA antibodies are from our and others' experience seen in C2D SLE at least as common as in SLE in general (Jönsson et al. 2007). Interestingly, anti-C1q and anti-cardiolipin antibodies were quite common in the Lund cohort of C2D SLE (Jönsson et al. 2007). Notably anti-C1q antibodies were found without clinical relationship to kidney involvement. Of interest is also that anti-cardiolipin antibodies were found in C2D SLE apparently without relation to antiphospholipid syndrome. Whether complement deficiency protects from the antiphospholipid syndrome might be possible but must be confirmed from other cohorts.

These patients also have problems with infections with encapsulated bacteria not least in childhood prior to development of SLE. The long-term prognosis of patients with C2D SLE is characterized by a high frequency of cardiovascular disease (Jönsson et al. 2005). Organ damage after 10 years duration of disease using the SLICC organ damage index was compared between SLE patients with C2D and ordinary age-matched SLE patients

(Jönsson et al. 2007). In this study there was a clear increase in the frequency of cardiovascular and skin damage in the SLE patients with C2D.

The reason why individuals with deficiency of components within the classical pathway have a very high risk for development of SLE has been discussed for several years and includes the importance of C1q,r,s, C4, and C2 for solubilization and clearance of immune complexes (Sturfelt et al. 1992) and apoptotic debris (Gullstrand et al. 2009). MBL may have a role in clearance of circulating immune complexes in C2D individuals as suggested by a study from Iceland (Saevarsdottir et al. 2007). This is in accordance with findings suggesting that MBL can bypass C2 directly and activate C3 (Selander et al. 2006). Another hypothesis that has been discussed is the possibility that complement may play a role in the activation of lymphocytes and in the mechanisms for induction of tolerance (Carroll 2000). Furthermore C1q, but not C2 and C4, appears to be of importance for the regulation of immune complex-induced production of type-1 interferons by plasmacytoid dendritic cells which probably is of importance for the very high risk of SLE development in C1q deficiency (Lood et al. 2009).

Complement Activation Mechanisms Overcoming C2 Deficiency

There may be several reasons why many C2D individuals do not suffer from increased infection susceptibility and the weak association to autoimmune disease compared to other classical pathway deficiencies. One point is that the lack of C2 does not hinder formation of C4b which has some opsonizing capacity. There are also C2 bypass mechanisms described where complement activation may proceed in the deficient serum (Fig. 2). It was shown several years ago that in C2D complement activation may take place by a mechanism involving high concentration of specific antibodies, C1q, and the alternative pathway components, a phenomenon referred to as the C2 bypass pathway (Knutzen Steuer et al. 1989). It has been demonstrated that C2D sera with increased antibody titers after vaccination could support an

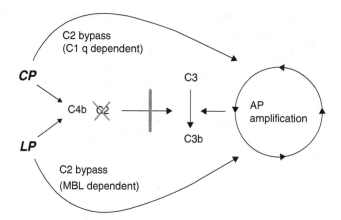

Complement Component C2 Deficiency, Fig. 2 In C2 deficiency complement activation through both the classical (CP) and the lectin pathway (LP) is prevented. Activation of C3 and the subsequent terminal sequence may still take place through activation of C2 bypass mechanisms depending on C1q or MBL, respectively, C4, and the alternative pathway (AP) components

increased opsonization of a *S. pneumoniae* serotype by increased deposition of both C3 and C4 fragments in the presence of a functional alternative pathway (Jönsson et al. 2012). Thus, there is evidence for the existence of this mechanism. In line with these results, studies of immune complex opsonization in vitro indicate that individuals with C2D could retain some immune complex opsonizing activity via the alternative pathway. Still, another mechanism may work through MBL where activation of C3 and the alternative pathway without involvement of C2 has been described (Selander et al. 2006).

Treatment in C2 Deficiency

Specific treatment to correct for the deficiency by gene therapy or by infusion of C2 protein is so far not available. However, to restore the deficiency, therapy with fresh frozen plasma has been tried. In at least two cases, regular infusions of plasma were beneficial in patients with C2D and SLE, and positive effect was ascribed to the C2 in the plasma. Recombinant human complement factor C2 (rhC2) has been produced by using a human cell line. The rhC2 was shown to restore classical pathway activation in vitro in serum from C2D patients. Whether this protein can be administered in vivo and improve the condition of C2D patients

is so far not known since no clinical trials are reported.

Thus, in the absence of specific treatment for C2D, individuals with SLE and C2D are treated as regular SLE patients, and especially antimalarial drugs are recommended. Furthermore coxinhibitors, glucocorticoids, and rarely cytostatic and biologic drugs can be used. As previously mentioned, infections are often the greatest clinical problem, and prophylactic treatment especially with proper vaccinations are recommended to C2D SLE patients.

References

Brodszki N, Skattum L, Bai X, Findlow H, Borrow R, Jönsson G. Immune responses following meningococcal serogroups a, C, Y and W polysaccharide vaccination in C2-deficient persons: evidence for increased levels of serum bactericidal antibodies. Vaccine. 2015;33(15):1839–45.

Carrington M, Marti D, Kissner T, Malasky M, Wade J, Klitz W, Barcellos L, Thomson G, Chen J, Truedsson L, Sturfelt G, Alper C, Awdeh Z, Huttley G. Microsatellite markers in complex disease: mapping of disease-associated regions within major histocompatibility complex. In: Goldstein DB, Schlötterer C, editors. Microsatellites Evolution and Application. Oxford: Oxford University Press; 1999.

Carroll MC. The role of complement in B cell activation and tolerance. Adv Immunol. 2000;74:61–88.

Gullstrand B, Mårtensson U, Sturfelt G, Bengtsson AA, Truedsson L. Complement classical pathway components are all important in clearance of apoptotic and secondary necrotic cells. Clin Exp Immunol. 2009;156(2):303–11.

Johnson CA, Densen P, Hurford Jr RK, Colten HR. Wetsel RA. Type I human complement C2 deficiency. A 28-base pair gene deletion causes skipping of exon 6 during RNA splicing. J Biol Chem. 1992;267(13):9347–53.

Jönsson G, Truedsson L, Sturfelt G, Oxelius VA, Braconier JH, Sjöholm AG. Hereditary C2 deficiency in Sweden: frequent occurrence of invasive infection, atherosclerosis, and rheumatic disease. Medicine (Baltimore). 2005;84(1):23–34.

Jönsson G, Oxelius VA, Truedsson L, Braconier JH, Sturfelt G, Sjöholm AG. Homozygosity for the IgG2 subclass allotype G2 M(n) protects against severe infection in hereditary C2 deficiency. J Immunol. 2006;177(1):722–8.

Jönsson G, Sjöholm AG, Truedsson L, Bengtsson AA, Braconier JH, Sturfelt G. Rheumatological manifestations, organ damage and autoimmunity in hereditary C2 deficiency. Rheumatology (Oxford). 2007;46(7):1133–9.

Jönsson G, Lood C, Gullstrand B, Holmström E, Selander B, Braconier JH, Sturfelt G, Bengtsson AA, Truedsson L. Vaccination against encapsulated bacteria in hereditary C2 deficiency results in antibody response and opsonization due to antibody-dependent complement activation. Clin Immunol. 2012;144(3):214–27.

Knutzen Steuer KL, Sloan LB, Oglesby TJ, Farries TC, Nickells MW, Densen P, Harley JB, Atkinson JP. Lysis of sensitized sheep erythrocytes in human sera deficient in the second component of complement. J Immunol. 1989;143(7):2256–61.

Lood C, Gullstrand B, Truedsson L, Olin AI, Alm GV, Rönnblom L, Sturfelt G, Eloranta ML, Bengtsson AA. C1q inhibits immune complex induced interferon-α production in plasmacytoid dendritic cells – a novel link between C1q deficiency and systemic lupus erythematosus pathogenesis. Arthritis Rheum. 2009;60(10):3081–90.

Mollnes TE, Jokiranta TS, Truedsson L, Nilsson B, Rodriguez de Cordoba S, Kirschfink M. Complement analysis in the 21st century. Mol Immunol. 2007;44(16):3838–49.

Pickering MC, Botto M, Taylor PR, Lachmann PJ, Walport MJ. Systemic lupus erythematosus, complement deficiency, and apoptosis. Adv Immunol. 2000;76:227–324.

Saevarsdottir S, Steinsson K, Ludviksson BR, Grondal G, Valdimarsson H. Mannan-binding lectin may facilitate the clearance of circulating immune complexes – implications from a study on C2 deficient individuals. Clin Exp Immunol. 2007 May;148(2):248–53.

Selander B, Mårtensson U, Weintraub A, Holmström E, Matsushita M, Thiel S, Jensenius JC, Truedsson L, Sjöholm AG. Mannan binding lectin activates C3 and

the alternative complement pathway without involvement of C2. J Clin Invest. 2006;116(5):1425–34.

Silverstein AM. Essential hypocomplementemia: report of a case. Blood. 1960;16:1338–41.

Skattum L, van Deuren M, van der Poll T, Truedsson L. Complement deficiency states and associated infections. Mol Immunol. 2011;48(14):1643–55.

Sturfelt G, Nived O, Sjöholm AG. Kinetic analysis of immune complex solubilisation: complement function in relation to disease activity in SLE. Clin Exp Rheumatol. 1992;10(3):241–7.

Truedsson L, Alper CA, Awdeh ZL, Johansen P, Sjöholm AG, Sturfelt G. Characterization of type I complement C2 deficiency MHC haplotypes. Strong conservation of the complotype/HLA-B-region and absence of disease association due to linked class II genes. J Immunol. 1993;151(10):5856–63.

Wetsel RA, Kulics J, Lokki ML, Kiepiela P, Akama H, Johnson CA, Densen P, Colten HR. Type II human complement C2 deficiency. Allele-specific amino acid substitutions (Ser189 – > Phe; Gly444 – > Arg) cause impaired C2 secretion. J Biol Chem. 1996;271(10):5824–31.

Complement Deficiencies Associated with Atypical Hemolytic Uremic Syndrome

Elizabeth C. Schramm[1], Anuja Java[2],
M. Kathryn Liszewski[3] and John P. Atkinson[3]
[1]Sevion Inc, Anthro Bio Inc, St. Louis, MO, USA
[2]Division of Nephrology, Department of Medicine, Washington University School of Medicine, St. Louis, MO, USA
[3]Division of Rheumatology, Department of Medicine, Washington University School of Medicine, St. Louis, MO, USA

Definition

Atypical hemolytic uremic syndrome (aHUS) is a thrombotic microangiopathy characterized by a triad of thrombocytopenia, microangiopathic hemolytic anemia, and acute renal failure in the absence of an infection with Shiga toxin-producing bacteria.

Introduction

The complement system is a major component of innate immunity and an effector arm and instructor of the adaptive immune response (Walport 2001a, b). It plays a key role in immune complex handling and clearance of apoptotic cells. Because of the potency of the system, strict regulation is required in time and space. Dysregulation of complement is increasingly recognized as a predisposing factor to human disease such as in aHUS (Holers 2008). Inherited defects in complement genes and acquired autoantibodies against a regulatory protein have been linked to development of aHUS. Until recently, the prognosis for aHUS patients was poor, but a novel complement inhibitory monoclonal antibody (mAb) has revolutionized treatment.

aHUS

There are two forms of HUS, typical (diarrheal positive) and atypical (diarrheal negative) (Kavanagh et al. 2013). While typical or enteropathic HUS is associated with an *E. coli* infection, aHUS is associated with genetic alterations in regulatory and activating proteins of the complement system and could be referred to as "complement-mediated HUS (C-HUS)." Acute mortality for aHUS occurs in up to 25% of patients (many of whom are children). For patients who survive, morbidity is substantial with about 50% requiring long-term dialysis. Thus, the kidney is the main target organ, although in ~20% of cases there are clinically important extrarenal manifestations (Noris et al. 2010). Why these changes primarily affect the glomerulus is not fully understood but may be in part related to the unique vascular anatomy of this filtering structure, which includes a fenestrated endothelium (Kerr and Richards 2012). Additionally, a lack of endogenous regulators on the kidney basement membrane may make it particularly vulnerable to complement attack (Atkinson et al. 2005).

Complement System

The complement system is an ancient branch of the innate immune system, composed of approximately 60 components, regulators, and receptors. There are three activating pathways or cascades, the classical, lectin, and alternative (reviewed in Walport (2001a, b)). The classical pathway (CP) is commonly activated by the C1q subcomponent of the C1 complex binding to the Fc region of IgG- and IgM-containing immune complexes. The lectin pathway (LP) is initiated when sugar-binding proteins (lectins) bind to carbohydrate moieties on a target (such as bacteria). The alternative pathway (AP) is continuously activated at low levels by a spontaneous tickover of the central component C3 to form the AP C3 convertase. The three pathways converge at a central step, the activation of C3 to C3b followed by the formation of the membrane attack complex. The AP also serves as a powerful feedback loop that can become engaged any time (Fig. 1). Further, dysregulation (inadequate control) of this potent amplification loop contributes to multiple human diseases including aHUS (Holers 2008).

Following activation of C3 to C3b, there are four potential outcomes for the generated C3b.

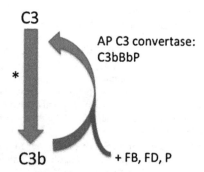

Complement Deficiencies Associated with Atypical Hemolytic Uremic Syndrome, Fig. 1 Schematic representation of the amplification or feedback loop of the complement system. * The generation of the initial C3b which covalently attaches to the target (i.e., bacteria, viruses, immune complexes, debris, etc.) can be via the classical pathway, lectin, or alternative (spontaneous tickover) pathway. Once generated, C3b binds to the protease factor B which is then activated to Bb by the protease factor D. The C3bBb complex is a C3 convertase that can efficiently generate more C3b. Properdin (P) stabilizes the AP C3 convertase. Depending largely upon the presence of regulators, the feedback loop shown will be variably engaged

First, it can function as an opsonin. Multiple clustered copies of C3b on a surface lead to immune adherence, which is commonly followed by internalization by phagocytic cells. *Second*, C3b can participate in the potent feedback loop of the AP. Once generated, C3b binds factor B (FB), which is then proteolytically activated by factor D (FD) to form the AP C3 convertase, C3bBb. This convertase rapidly generates more C3b, thereby feeding the amplification loop (Fig. 1). *Third*, C3b can be inactivated by the serine protease factor I (FI) to generate iC3b (Fig. 2), which does not participate in the amplification loop. This reaction requires a cofactor protein such as the plasma protein factor H (FH) or a membrane cofactor protein (MCP; CD46) to first engage the C3b before FI can act. This cleavage event is critical to protect healthy host membranes from undesirable complement activation (wrong target) and excessive fluid-phase turnover in blood (no target). *Fourth*, as the AP C3 convertase generates more C3b, it attaches to the C3 convertase, forming the C5 convertase (C3b$_2$Bb). The C5 convertase cleaves C5 into C5a and C5b, the latter being the initiating protein of the terminal pathway. The generation of C5b leads to downstream formation of the membrane attack complex (MAC; C5b-9), which causes membrane perturbation including target cell lysis. C5b binds C6 and C7, and this complex can insert into lipid-protein bilayers. This is followed by attachment of C8, and then multiple (12–16) molecules of C9 are engaged to form a pore in the membrane.

The amplification loop of the AP can deposit several million copies of C3b on a single bacterium in less than 5 min. Therefore, strict regulation of the complement system is required to prevent collateral damage to host cells and tissues. The regulatory proteins that protect against undesirable AP activation include two in plasma, FH and FI, and four membrane proteins, namely, CD46, decay-accelerating factor (DAF; CD55), the membrane attack inhibitor CD59, and complement receptor 1 (CR1; CD35; immune adherence receptor). By disassociating the C3 and C5 convertases (decay-accelerating activity, DAA) and irreversibly cleaving the activation fragments C3b and C4b (cofactor activity, CA), the regulatory proteins play key roles in maintaining homeostasis. Numerous genetic and functional studies have demonstrated that a defect or alteration in the cofactor activity capacity (FH, FI, MCP) leads to a hyperfunctional AP (Kavanagh et al. 2013). The basic underlying defect is inadequate CA for C3b leading to excessive generation of C3a, C3b, C5a, and C5b-9.

Mouse studies have demonstrated that terminal pathway activation is essential for development of the endothelial lesion that is the hallmark of aHUS (de Jorge et al. 2011). When an aHUS-susceptible mouse was bred to a C5-deficient strain, there was complete protection from this thrombotic microangiopathy. These data strongly implicate the terminal pathway in aHUS pathogenesis, consistent with the positive clinical results employing a mAb to C5 (eculizumab).

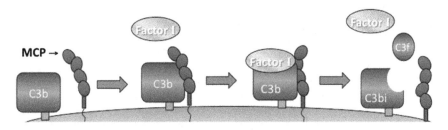

Complement Deficiencies Associated with Atypical Hemolytic Uremic Syndrome, Fig. 2 Cofactor activity is an essential regulatory mechanism of the complement system. In healthy tissue, C3b is inactivated by host regulatory proteins. A cofactor protein such as MCP (shown here) or factor H (not shown) will bind to C3b and allow the serine protease factor I to cleave C3b. C3bi cannot participate in the application loop shown in Fig. 1. Published by BioMed Central © 2015 and with permission of Liszewski and Atkinson 2015a

Complement Proteins and aHUS

Two types of mutations have been identified: activating mutations (i.e., gain of function (GOF)) in the complement components C3 and FB and, more commonly, loss of function (LOF) mutations in the regulatory proteins FH, FI, MCP, and thrombomodulin (THBD) (Kavanagh et al. 2013; Nester et al. 2015) (Table 1). Mutations in the activating components usually lead to reduced regulation by at least one of the regulatory proteins and thus represent a secondary GOF.

The primary LOF mutations either lead to a defect in protein secretion or are present in normal antigenic quantities but are dysfunctional. In the latter case, the protein fails to regulate the amplification loop adequately. In either scenario, the end result is haploinsufficiency relative to cofactor activity.

Factor H

Mutations in FH are the most common, being identified in 20–30% of aHUS patients (Noris et al. 2010). FH is a 150 kDa linear plasma protein composed entirely of 20 repeating homologous domains of approximately 60 amino acids each [complement control protein (CCPs) repeats] (Fig. 3). The CCPs house the sites for the interactions with C3b. The mutations in aHUS are primarily clustered in domains 19 and 20 that facilitate FH's binding to damaged cell membranes and debris such as via an interaction with

glycosaminoglycans (GAGs) and also contain sites for C3b/C3d binding. Many mutations identified in aHUS patients disrupt GAG interactions or C3b binding, resulting in impairment of AP homeostasis at the target surface. Mutations have also been identified in FH 1–4 (Kavanagh et al. 2013). This region is responsible for the cofactor activity of the protein and leads to impaired regulation in the fluid phase and at the cell surface.

MCP

Mutations in MCP account for 10–15% of aHUS cases (Kavanagh et al. 2013). Most mutations are missense, but nonsense and splice site variants have been observed (Liszewski and Atkinson 2015a). MCP is a type 1 transmembrane regulator composed of four amino terminal CCPs, with CCPs 2, 3, and 4 being critical for C3b binding and cofactor activity (Fig. 3). Most mutations in MCP are associated with aHUS, but other disease states have been implicated (Liszewski and Atkinson 2015a). Overall, two mutations have been identified in the promoter, 4 in the signal peptide, 13 in CCP1, 9 in CCP2, 14 in CCP3, 12 in CCP4, 1 in the STP region, 4 in the transmembrane domain, and 1 in cytoplasmic tail one (Liszewski and Atkinson 2015b) (Fig. 3). While 51 mutations are associated with the development of aHUS, 12 may be associated with other diseases [systemic sclerosis, systemic lupus erythematosus, hemolysis, elevated liver enzymes, low platelets (HELLP) syndrome, thrombotic

Complement Deficiencies Associated with Atypical Hemolytic Uremic Syndrome, Table 1 Complement proteins associated with aHUS

Protein	Size (kDa)	Location	Function	Plasma concentration
Factor H	150	Plasma	Regulator – binds C3b[a], decays convertase	250–750 µg/ml
Factor I	95	Plasma	Regulator – serine protease, cleaves C3b	15–30 µg/ml
MCP (CD46)	45–68	Membrane	Regulator – binds C3b[a]	NA
C3	180	Plasma	Activator: binds to cells; part of convertases[b]	0.8–1.2 mg/ml
Factor B	90	Plasma	Activator – binds to C3b to form C3 convertase[c]	180 µg/ml
Thrombomodulin	74	Membrane	Regulator – cofactor activity	NA

NA not applicable

[a]This allows factor I to then cleave C3b

[b]Covalently binds to targets via cleavage of its thioester bond which then forms an ester linkage with hydroxyl groups; C3b also participates in C5 convertases and the C3 convertase of CP

[c]Then serves as the protease to cleave C3 to C3b

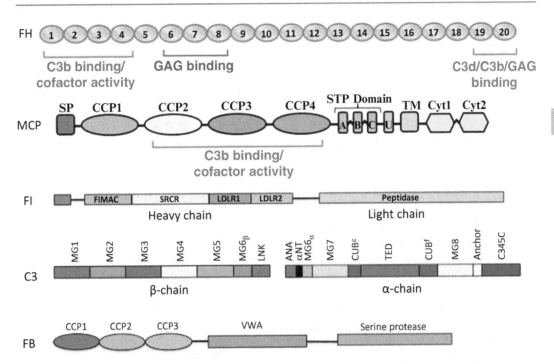

Complement Deficiencies Associated with Atypical Hemolytic Uremic Syndrome, Fig. 3 Schematic representation of the major complement proteins implicated in aHUS. Mutations have been identified in FH, FI, MCP, C3, and FB. FH, FI, C3, and FB are plasma proteins derived primarily from the liver. MCP is an alternatively spliced type 1 transmembrane protein. FI and C3 are two chain proteins that are held together by a disulphate bond *ANA*, anaphylatoxin; *CCP*, complement control protein (repeat); *FB*, factor B; *FH*, factor H; *FI*, factor I; *FIMAC*, factor I membrane attack complex domain; *LDLR*, low-density lipoprotein receptor domain; *MCP*, membrane cofactor protein; *MG*, macroglobulin; *SP*, signal peptide; *SRCR*, scavenger receptor cysteine-rich domain; *STP*, serine-, threonine-, proline-rich domain; *TED*, thioester domain; *TM*, transmembrane; *VWA*, von Willebrand factor type A domain

thrombocytopenia purpura, glomerulonephritis, C3 glomerulonephritis, preeclampsia, and miscarriage], and three mutations have been described in several diseases (Liszewski and Atkinson 2015b). Approximately 75% of MCP mutations result in decreased surface expression. The remaining are expressed normally, but are defective in C3b/C4b binding and cofactor activity.

Factor I

FI is a serine protease that cleaves C3b in the presence of a cofactor protein. Mutations in FI are observed in 5–10% of patients (Noris et al. 2010). FI is a composed of two chains (Fig. 3), with mutations in aHUS being equally distributed between the light chain serine protease domain and the heavy chain domains. In the few mutations for which functional analyses have been performed, the primary defect is a loss of regulatory activity in the fluid phase (plasma) and on the cell surface (Kavanagh et al. 2013).

C3

C3 is the central protein of the complement system. All three pathways converge at the step of C3 cleavage. It is a relatively large protein of 180 kDa, composed of an alpha- and a beta-chain (Fig. 3). Mutations in C3 account for 5–10% of aHUS patients (Schramm et al. 2015). The majority of these mutations lead to a secondary gain of function, being less susceptible to inactivation by one or more of the regulatory protein(s). A few of the C3 mutations demonstrate increased binding to FB that serve to stabilize the convertases and result in excessive complement activation (Schramm et al. 2015).

Factor B

Factor B contains the serine protease domain (Bb) that becomes part of the AP C3 convertase. Gain-of-function mutations have also been identified in FB, but they are rare (~1% of mutations in aHUS). These mutations lead to increased convertase function either due to increased C3b affinity for FB or resistance to DAA (Roumenina et al. 2009).

Thrombomodulin

Mutations in the thrombomodulin, a protein of the clotting cascade, have also been associated with aHUS in two reports (Delvaeye et al. 2009; Maga et al. 2010). Thrombomodulin facilitates activation of protein C by thrombin and enhances thrombin-mediated activation of plasma procarboxypeptidase B, an inhibitor of fibrinolysis. It has also been shown to accelerate FI-mediated cofactor cleavage of C3b. The thrombomodulin mutations identified in aHUS are heterozygous missense mutations. The few that have been functionally characterized resulted in a decrease in cofactor activity (Delvaeye et al. 2009). Thrombomodulin mutations have been described in just two cohorts, while several large cohorts have yet to report any mutations (Kavanagh et al. 2013).

Anti-factor H Antibodies

An informative cause of dysregulated complement activity in 10–15% of aHUS cases is inhibition of FH function by autoantibodies (Noris et al. 2010). About 90% of these cases are associated with a homozygous deletion of the complement FH-related genes, *CFHR1* and *CFHR3* (Kavanagh et al. 2013). Alternatively, in some patients, there are point mutations in *CFHR1*, while in others there is no detectable mutation in the *CFHR1* or *CFHR3* genes. Functionally, these autoantibodies reduce FH binding to C3b, block attachment of FH to cell surfaces, and/or interfere with CA and/or DAA. Patients with FH autoantibodies often have low serum C3 levels, reflecting a systemic dysregulation of the AP.

Clinical Features

Onset of aHUS is usually sudden although some patients exhibit a slowly progressive relapsing and remitting course (Loirat and Frémeaux-Bacchi 2011). Children may present with non-specific symptoms such as decreased appetite, vomiting, and drowsiness. Adults often report generalized fatigue and malaise associated with severe hypertension. More than 50% of patients progress to end-stage renal disease requiring renal replacement therapy. Extrarenal manifestations are observed in about 20% of patients and can include central nervous system involvement with symptoms such as headache and confusion and cardiovascular system problems including myocardial infarction, arrhythmia, or sudden cardiac death (Noris et al. 2010).

Epidemiology

aHUS represents 5–10% of HUS in children and the majority of HUS in adults. It is equally common in boys and girls during childhood, but a female preponderance is observed in adults (Loirat and Frémeaux-Bacchi 2011). Incomplete penetrance (~50%) has been reported for the genes associated with aHUS. This suggests that a secondary trigger is necessary. Often an event, such as an upper respiratory tract infection, gastroenteritis, or pregnancy, will trigger onset of disease in those with a genetic predisposition (Loirat and Frémeaux-Bacchi 2011).

Diagnosis

Laboratory evaluation reveals anemia, thrombocytopenia, and renal failure. Evidence for intravascular hemolysis can be confirmed by schistocytes on peripheral blood smear, an undetectable haptoglobin level, and a high serum lactate dehydrogenase (LDH) (Java et al. 2013). Reduced ADAMTS13 activity should be ruled out to exclude the diagnosis of the related disease, thrombotic thrombocytopenic purpura. Serum concentration of C3, C4, FH, FB, and FI should be determined and presence of anti-FH antibodies ascertained. Surface expression

Complement Deficiencies Associated with Atypical Hemolytic Uremic Syndrome, Fig. 4 Diagnostic algorithm for aHUS. The diagram describes an approach for evaluation of patients presenting with a thrombotic microangiopathy

DIAGNOSTIC ALGORITHM FOR aHUS

- Medical history/Physical examination
- Labs (Thrombocytopenia, Microangiopathic hemolytic anemia
  + one or more of the following:
  Renal failure/Neurological symptoms/Gastrointestinal symptoms)

Evaluate ADAMTS13 activity/STEC-toxin

≤10% ADAMTS 13 activity → TTP

>10% ADAMTS 13 activity

STEC toxin positive → STEC-HUS

aHUS

Genetic testing (FH. FI. MCP. C3. FB)

Anti-FH autoantibodies

Antigenic levels (FH. FI. MCP. C3. FB)

Variant identified

In-silico prediction models

Known mutation

Novel variant or Known variant but never studied

Prepare mutant in lab to study function

Low (candidate)   Normal

Functional assays (FH. FI. MCP)

Low (candidate)

Combine Genetic and Protein data to define variant

of MCP should be evaluated. In addition, genetic testing of FH, FI, MCP, FB, C3, and THBD should be carried out in all patients with a clinical diagnosis of aHUS (Fig. 4).

Treatment

Plasma Therapy

Plasma exchange or plasma infusion has traditionally been the first line of treatment (Kavanagh et al. 2013; Nester et al. 2015). However, there are no randomized controlled trials of plasma therapy in aHUS, and the efficacy is poor. The rationale behind this treatment is related presumably to the removal of mutant protein and the ability to deliver normal levels of the functional protein. Plasma exchange should be initiated within 24 hours of diagnosis and performed daily until platelet count, hemoglobin, and LDH normalize. Lack of improvement in these parameters should be considered a nonresponse to therapy, and plasma exchange should be discontinued.

Eculizumab

Eculizumab is a humanized mAb directed against the terminal complement protein C5 that prevents C5 activation by the C5 convertase (Hillmen et al. 2006). The drug was originally approved by US Food and Drug Administration (FDA) to treat paroxysmal nocturnal hemoglobinuria. Later (in 2011) it was approved to treat aHUS. Several small clinical trials have reported successful treatment with eculizumab especially in patients with plasmapheresis-resistant disease (Licht et al. 2015). However, early initiation of the mAb therapy offers the best chance to recover renal function. Eculizumab is administered intravenously (IV) and has a half-life of ~11 days. The recommended dosage regimen for a patient with aHUS is 900 mg IV weekly for four doses and then 1200 mg at week 5 followed by 1200 mg every 2 weeks. In patients receiving plasmapheresis, a supplemental dose should be administered after each plasma exchange.

The predominant side effects include potentially life-threatening infection with *Neisseria meningitidis* (due to blockage of the terminal complement pathway) and infusion reactions. A meningococcal vaccination should be administered to everyone undergoing treatment with eculizumab. Physicians need to be aware that the standard vaccine does not protect against the B serotype of the bacteria nor many infrequent serotypes. The CDC now recommends serotype B *Neisseria* vaccine in patients receiving eculizumab in addition to the usual *Neisseria* vaccine. In addition, appropriate antibiotics should be used for 14 days if there is not enough time to wait for the immune response. Moreover, any suggestive symptoms should necessitate urgent investigation and antibiotic therapy. Overall, though, eculizumab is well tolerated and relatively safe. The optimal therapeutic regimen for this drug remains unclear as well as the duration of therapy. These remaining questions underscore the necessity to continue therapeutic studies, in particular, to employ large-scale, prospective randomized trials.

Renal Transplantation

Patients with aHUS who progress to end-stage renal disease are candidates for renal transplantation. However, there is a recurrence risk of >50% with graft loss occurring in 80–90% of cases. The time from transplantation to recurrence of aHUS may vary between a few days and 2 years, although the majority (60%) of recurrences occur within the first month. The outcome is also dependent on the complement abnormality. The risk of recurrence is 70–90% with a FH mutation,

50–80% with a FI mutation, and 40–70% with a C3 mutation (Noris et al. 2010). Recurrence rate is low in patients with MCP mutations since the allograft will express the normal protein. Intensive plasma therapy before and after transplantation has shown modest benefit in preventing disease recurrence (Java et al. 2013). However, the graft outcome has been poor with plasmapheresis alone for treatment of a recurrence. Since FH, FI, and C3 are primarily synthesized in the liver, combined liver-kidney transplantation has been performed in a few pediatric patients with mixed results and therefore requires careful assessment of individual risk/benefit (Forbes et al. 2013). Emerging data show promising results for eculizumab in preventing and treating posttransplant aHUS recurrence (Licht et al. 2015). Prophylactic therapy should be initiated preoperatively and continued indefinitely, especially for high-risk mutations (FH, FI, C3), until more data become available.

Conclusions

aHUS is a disease of dysregulated complement activation. Genetic- and functionally based studies have firmly linked alterations in the regulatory capacity of the complement system with a predisposition to developing aHUS. Mutations in the regulatory proteins FI, FH, and MCP result in haploinsufficiency, leading to dysregulation of the AP. Secondary gain-of-function mutations in the activating component C3 lead to increased activation usually due to an impairment in regulatory protein binding. Gain-of-function mutations in FB and in C3 give rise to increased C3 convertase function.

Until recently, treatment options for aHUS were poor, and aHUS was associated with up to 25% mortality, and 50% of cases resulted in end-stage renal disease. However, with the introduction of eculizumab, treatment of aHUS is much improved.

Cross-References

▶ Complement System, C5, C6, C7, C8, C9, Component

References

Atkinson JP, Liszewski MK, Richards A, Kavanagh D, Moulton EA. Hemolytic uremic syndrome: an example of insufficient complement regulation on self-tissue. Ann N Y Acad Sci. 2005;1056:144–52.

de Jorge EG, Macor P, Paixão-Cavalcante D, Rose KL, Tedesco F, Cook HT, et al. The development of atypical hemolytic uremic syndrome depends on complement C5. J Am Soc Nephrol JASN. 2011;22(1):137–45.

Delvaeye M, Noris M, De Vriese A, Esmon CT, Esmon NL, Ferrell G, et al. Thrombomodulin mutations in atypical hemolytic-uremic syndrome. N Engl J Med. 2009;361(4):345–57.

Forbes TA, Bradbury MG, Goodship THJ, McKiernan PJ, Milford DV. Changing strategies for organ transplantation in atypical haemolytic uraemic syndrome: a tertiary case series. Pediatr Transplant. 2013;17(3):E93–9.

Hillmen P, Young NS, Schubert J, Brodsky RA, Socié G, Muus P, et al. The complement inhibitor eculizumab in paroxysmal nocturnal hemoglobinuria. N Engl J Med. 2006;355(12):1233–43.

Holers VM. The spectrum of complement alternative pathway-mediated diseases. Immunol Rev. 2008;223:300–16.

Java A, Atkinson J, Salmon J. Defective complement inhibitory function predisposes to renal disease. Annu Rev Med. 2013;64:307–24.

Kavanagh D, Goodship TH, Richards A. Atypical hemolytic uremic syndrome. Semin Nephrol. 2013;33(6):508–30.

Kerr H, Richards A. Complement-mediated injury and protection of endothelium: lessons from atypical haemolytic uraemic syndrome. Immunobiology. 2012;217(2):195–203.

Licht C, Greenbaum LA, Muus P, Babu S, Bedrosian CL, Cohen DJ, et al. Efficacy and safety of eculizumab in atypical hemolytic uremic syndrome from 2-year extensions of phase 2 studies. Kidney Int. 2015;87(5):1061–73.

Liszewski MK, Atkinson JP. Complement regulator CD46: genetic variants and disease associations. Hum Genomics. 2015a;9:7.

Liszewski MK, Atkinson JP. Complement regulators in human disease: lessons from modern genetics. J Intern Med. 2015b;277(3):294–305.

Loirat C, Frémeaux-Bacchi V. Atypical hemolytic uremic syndrome. Orphanet J Rare Dis. 2011;6(1):60.

Maga TK, Nishimura CJ, Weaver AE, Frees KL, Smith RJH. Mutations in alternative pathway complement proteins in American patients with atypical hemolytic uremic syndrome. Hum Mutat. 2010;31(6):E1445–60.

Nester CM, Barbour T, de Cordoba SR, Dragon-Durey MA, Fremeaux-Bacchi V, Goodship THJ, et al. Atypical aHUS: state of the art. Mol Immunol. 2015;67(1):31–42.

Noris M, Caprioli J, Bresin E, Mossali C, Pianetti G, Gamba S, et al. Relative role of genetic complement abnormalities in sporadic and familial aHUS and their impact on clinical phenotype. Clin J Am Soc Nephrol. 2010;5(10):1844–59.

Roumenina LT, Jablonski M, Hue C, Blouin J, Dimitrov JD, Dragon-Durey M-A, et al. Hyperfunctional C3 convertase leads to complement deposition on endothelial cells and contributes to atypical hemolytic uremic syndrome. Blood. 2009;114(13):2837–45.

Schramm EC, Roumenina LT, Rybkine T, Chauvet S, Vieira-Martins P, Hue C, et al. Mapping interactions between complement C3 and regulators using mutations in atypical hemolytic uremic syndrome. Blood. 2015;125(15):2359–69.

Walport MJ. Complement. First of two parts. N Engl J Med. 2001a;344(14):1058–66.

Walport MJ. Complement. Second of two parts. N Engl J Med. 2001b;344(15):1140–4.

Complement Factor P (CFP) Deficiency

▸ Properdin Deficiency

Complement System, C5, C6, C7, C8, C9, Component

▸ C5b-C9 Deficiency

Complete Deficiency of Complement C4

Karine R. Mayilyan, Armenuhi A. Hyusyan and Jack Farah
Institute of Molecular Biology, Armenian National Academy of Sciences, Yerevan, Republic of Armenia

Definition

C4 is an important component of the complement system and operates as an early effector of the classical and the lectin pathways, assisting in elimination of cellular debris and infectious microbes. It is also involved in bridging innate and adaptive branches of immunity. This entry intended to provide a summary of current knowledge (1) on versatile functions of C4 component within the complement network, (2) its genetic and protein polymorphisms and their peculiarities, (3) and the disease association of the C4 complete deficiency.

C4 as a Major Component of the Complement System

The fourth component discovered in the complement system and hence stated by its name was C4 (Gordon et al. 1926). C4 arose early in vertebrate evolution at the time of cartilaginous fish along with the proteins involved in adaptive immunity. Human C4 is a three-chain (α, 93 kD; β, 78 kD; and γ, 33 kD) glycoprotein derived from a single-chain precursor. It is a major protein of the complement lectin and the classical pathways. In the complement cascades, pattern recognition molecules (in the classical pathway C1q, and in the lectin pathway mannan-binding lectin (MBL)) and ficolins bind to target surface and activate their associated serine proteases (reviewed in Mayilyan et al. 2008a; Mayilyan 2012). In the classical pathway, C1q bound to the protein surface activates C1r, then C1s, which then cleaves C4 followed by C2. Activated C4b either binds to targets and opsonizes them, promoting their transportation, and/or clearance by phagocytosis (e.g., C4b binds immune complexes and attaches them to the membrane of erythrocytes promoting their transportation within circulation and subsequent clearance in liver and spleen), or binds covalently to C2a forming C4b2a complex (C3 convertase), which is able to cleave C3. One nascent C3b binds to C4b2a complex and forms a binding site for C5 (C5 convertase). The cleavage of C5 culminates in the assembly of C5b678(C9)n complex (membrane attack complex), which causes membrane damage of a target cell (e.g., bacterial). A similar scenario works for the lectin pathway but with activation by MBL–MASPs (MBL associated serine proteases) and ficolin–MASPs complexes. Thus, in the both cascades, C4 activation is required after activation of the complement initiator complexes, prior to C2 activation (Wallis et al. 2007), indicating its crucial role in

activation of this system with broad spectrum of duties (Mayilyan et al. 2008b; Ricklin et al. 2010).

Polymorphism of C4

C4 is the only protein of the complement system, which is coded by two genes showing 99% sequence identity (i.e., *C4A*, MIM 120810; and *C4B*, MIM 120820). C4 genes are located at the third region of the major histocompatibility complex of chromosome 6 (MHC-III; Chr.6p21.3). Together with genes of the serine/threonine nuclear kinase RP (or *STK19*, MIM604977), the steroid 21-hydroxylase *CYP21* (MIM 201910), and the extracellular matrix protein tenascin *TNX* (MIM 600985), C4 genes form a genetic unit, the *RP-C4-CYP21-TNX* (RCCX; Fig. 1). The number of the RCCX units on each chromosome typically varies from 1 to 4, and hence the number of C4 genes within the human genome ranges from 2 to 8. About 70% of C4 genes in Caucasians have the endogenous retrovirus HERV-K(C4) in intron nine and are longer than the genes without it, thus referred to as "long" (C4L; 20.6 kb) and "short" (C4S; 14.3 kb) C4 genes. Within the RCCX structure, C4 displays almost inconceivable genetic diversity. The frequent inter-individual variation in the copy number, size, and isotypes of C4 genes is extraordinary (reviewed in Yu et al. 2003). More than 200 SNPs, among which 81 are in exons of each gene (23 nonsynonymous, 9 frame-shifts, and 49 synonymous) (data provided by UCSC genome browser, 2015), supplement the C4 gene polymorphism peculiarities. However, only five SNPs are responsible for C4A and C4B isotype specific aminoacid substitutions at residues 1101–1106 (*PCPVPD*, C4A; and *LSPVIH*, C4B), resulting in distinct physicochemical properties, propensities to react with specific nucleophilic groups, functional activities and preferences. Thus, C4A is thought to have a greater role in opsonization and clearance of immune complexes, while C4B considered being more important in further activation of complement cascade and neutralization of pathogens (reviewed in Yu et al. 2003).

Human serum C4 protein levels are determined by the dosage and size of C4 genes, and strangely, by the body mass index (BMI) of an individual. An average serum C4 level in Caucasians is about 0.40 g/l, while in CSF its concentration more than 100-folds less. However, as C4 is acute phase protein, its expression level can rapidly change under different stressful or diseased conditions.

Molecular Basis of C4 Null Alleles

Partial deficiency of C4 is quite common with ethnic and international bias. While of about 20% and 27% healthy Caucasians are at least heterozygous for *C4A* and *C4B* deficiency (Yang et al. 2007), in Oriental population (Chinese) only

9% and 18% have *C4A**Q0 and *C4B**Q0, respectively (Hou et al. 2014). C4 null alleles can occur due to point mutations leading to either frame shifts and premature termination of transcription (Rupert et al. 2002) or C4B gene conversion to C4A. However, about half of null alleles for both genes have developed due to deletions of about 28 kb DNA fragment involving C4 and CYP21 genes, as a result of copy number variation process (Fig. 1) (reviewed in Campbell et al. 2008). However, deletions of *C4A* and *CYP21A2* or *C4A* and *C4B* together have never been observed; thus, complete deficiency of C4 is not a result of both C4 genes deletion and requires the presence of mutations associated with protein nonexpression. Therefore, RCCX units carrying null alleles for both *C4A* and *C4B* (*C4A**Q0-*C4B**Q0) are extremely infrequent.

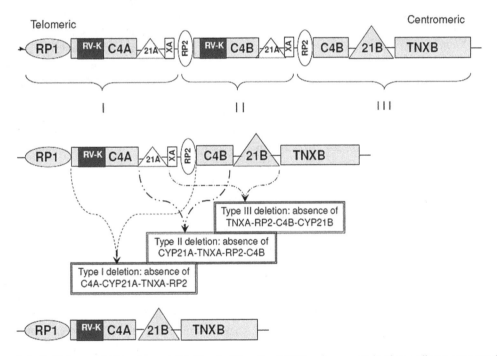

Complete Deficiency of Complement C4, Fig. 1 C4 genes within the RCCX units. *C4* genes together with the serine/threonine nuclear kinase gene *RP*, the steroid 21-hydroxylase *CYP21A2/A1*, and the extracellular matrix protein *TNXB/A* form a genetic unit, the *RP-C4-CYP21-TNX* (RCCX) module. The functional genes of RCCX modules are highlighted. The first diagram shows trimodular RCCX with one long *C4A*, one long and one short *C4B*. The second diagram presents bi-modular RCCX indicating three types of C4 gene deletion within

the RCCX unit as a result of an ordinary copy number variation process. The third diagram expresses composition of mono-modular RCCX with one long *C4A*. RP1 – serine/threonine nuclear kinase gene RP; RP2 – pseudogene of RP; RV-K – gene of human endogenous retrovirus K (HERV-K(C4)); 21A – pseudogene of the steroid 21-hydroxylase *CYP21A1*; XA – pseudogene of the extracellular matrix protein TNX; 21B – gene of the steroid 21-hydroxylase *CYP21A2*; *TNXB* – gene of the extracellular matrix protein TNX

C4 Complete Deficiency and Disease Association

Thus, C4 total deficiency (C4A*Q0 + C4B*Q0) is very rare. The first case with the C4 total deficiency was documented in 1974 (Hauptmann et al. 1974). An 18-year-old French female with an elevated erythrocyte sedimentation rate, photosensitivity, facial erythema, alopecia, oral ulcers, serositis, and proteinuria was diagnosed with SLE and found to have complete C4 deficiency. Since then, only 28 C4-deficient cases from 19 families have been reported so far (Table 1). The majority of C4-deficient subjects (20 cases) were homozygous for a given extended MHC haplotypes, and for some cases it was caused by consanguinity of the parents (Hauptmann et al. 1988). Exceptionally, in one case, the homozygosity in MHC haplotype resulted from auniparental isodisomy (Welch et al. 1990).

Only two out of 28 C4-defficient subjects were healthy at the time of reporting, and one had only photosensitivity. Nevertheless, 75% of C4-deficient subjects had either severe discoid lupus and systemic lupus erythematosus (SLE) or lupus-like disorder at infancy. Antinuclear antibodies, the major serological hallmark of SLE disease, were positive in 16 of 21 cases tested. Thus, according to the known hierarchy of severity and susceptibility of SLE (Pickering et al. 2000; Yu et al. 2007), from the entire complement spectra, total lack of C4 is second only to C1q deficiency, the most SLE-associated complement factor (>90% of total $C1q$*Q0 cases). The reason for this is the classical pathway activation sequence in which the C4 component is only downstream of C1. It is evident that the deposition of immune-complexes in tissues, leading to leukocyte activation, underlies the pathogenesis of the tissue injury in SLE. Therefore, it is likely that C4A nonexpression is the main immune challenge of C4-deficient SLE patients, due to the crucial role of C4A isotype in tagging and immunoclearance of those complexes. Confirmatory to this notion, in Caucasian population the odds ratio for carriers of only $C4A$ null alleles to develop SLE was found to be more

than 5, while the same for carriers of $C4B$*Q0 was equal to that of general population (Yang et al. 2007). And according to the recent review, the relative risk of $C4A$*Q0 in SLE varies between 2.3 and 5.3 among different ethnic groups (Yang et al. 2004a).

Although disruption in clearance of immune complexes is a reasonable explanation for a contribution of either C1q or C4 deficiency to the effector phase of autoimmunity, the link between C4 deficiency and generation of self-reactive antibodies in SLE is not readily apparent. It is noteworthy that mechanistic information on C4 deficiency and its role in SLE came from model experiments. C4 knockout (C4KO) mice developed autoantibodies and lupus-like immune abnormalities with a concomitant glomerulonephritis (Carroll 2008). The mice had a profound defect in the antibody response to T cell antigen, while B cell signalling was seemingly normal. Moreover, by 6 months, C4KO mice had relatively high titer of IgM anti double-strand DNA (anti-dsDNA) antibodies than controls. Three months later, IgG anti-dsDNA antibodies were developed in those mice as well. Notably, mice heterozygous for C4*Q0 also develop autoantibodies, reminiscent of the high incidence of partial C4 deficiency observed in human SLE. Further experiments with chimeric mice bearing the anti Hel Ig transgene (MD4 line) and complete lack of complement C4 or its B cell receptors CD21/CD35 demonstrated impairments in negative selection of the self-reactive B cells (Carroll 2008). The results from this and similar models led to current understanding that B cells pass through multiple checkpoints during early differentiation. Cells that engage self-antigen undergo clone deletion in which the complement has a significant role. Thus, the complement classical pathway early components, particularly C4, have a major contribution in the development of the B cell tolerance to self-antigens. Hence, C4-deficency paired with other genetic risk factors may contribute to SLE disease (Carroll 2008).

Nonetheless, lupus-like illness in C4-deficient subjects, often developing at an early age, is also associated with increased

Complete Deficiency of Complement C4, Table 1 A list of individuals with complete C4 deficiency in chronological order of documentation

Family/ subject	Age (years) at onset, gender, race/ethnicity, nationality	Disease, clinical feature (remarks)	MHC/HLA haplotype	C4L and C4S genes on each Chr.6	References
1	18, F, CAUC, French	SLE; rash, alopecia, photosensitivity, hematuria, proteinuria at 2 months gestation	A2 Cw3 B40 DRw19	C4L/C4L	Hauptmann et al. (1974)
2	1.5, M, CAUC, US	SLE nephritis; diffuse interstitial pneumonitis, disseminated vascular coagulation, herpes simplex and cytomegalovirus infection (died at age 7½)	A2 B12 Dw2/A2 Bw15 Dw8	ND	Schaller et al. (1977)
3a	17, M, CAUC, Austrian	Severe mesangio-proliferative GN, recurrent Henoch-Schönleinpurpura (hemodialysis at 24, kidney transplant at 25, hemodialysis since 29, the end stage of renal failure)	A30 B18 DR7	C4S-C4S/ C4S-C4S	Tappeiner et al. (1978) and Yang et al. (2004b)
3b	21, M, CAUC, Austrian	Asymptomatic, healthy	A30 B18 DR7	ND	Tappeiner et al. (1978)
4	24, F, CAUC, US	Discoid lupus; oral ulceration, leukopenia, malaise	A26 B49 DR2	ND	Ballow et al. (1979)
5	19, F, CAUC, Dutch-Canadian	SLE; photosensitivity, thrombocytopenia, arthralgia, proteinuria (splenectomy; two sisters died of SLE at ages 17 and 14 and a third died at age 3 months of unknown cause)	A2 Cw3 B40 DR1	ND	Minta et al. (1981)
6a	2, F, CAUC, Austrian	SLE; severe growth retardation	A24 Cw7 B38 DR13	C4L/C4L	Tappeiner et al. (1982) and Yang et al. (2004b)
6b	2.5, M, CAUC, Austrian	SLE; septicemia and cerebral vasculitis (died at age ~3)	A24 Cw7 B38 DR13	C4L/C4L	Tappeiner et al. 1982
6c	5, M, CAUC, Austrian	GN; healthy at age 10 (treated with prednisolone)	A24 Cw7 B38 DR13	C4L/C4L	Tappeiner et al. (1982) and Yang et al. (2004b)
7a	6, F, CAUC, Italian/German	Lupus-like, mesangial and endocapillary proliferative GN; rash, proteinuria, hematuria, hypertension	A30 B18 DR7	C4S-C4S/ C4S-C4S	Tappeiner et al. (1982) and Yang et al. (2004b)
7b	5, M, CAUC, Italian/German	Mesangial and endocapillary proliferative GN; minor rash, proteinuria, hematuria, hypertension	A30 B18 DR7	C4S-C4S/ C4S-C4S	Tappeiner et al. (1982) and Yang et al. (2004b)
7c	5/22, F, CAUC, Italian/German	Mesangial and endocapillary proliferative GN, SLE at 22 (cerebral vasculitis since 23)	A30 B18 DR7	C4S-C4S/ C4S-C4S	Tappeiner et al. (1982) and Yang et al. (2004b)
8a	2.5, F, North African, Moroccan	Recurrent pulmonary infections (since 3 months), lupus-like; photosensitive severe cutaneous lesions (consanguineous parents)	A11 Cw4 B35 DR1	C4L/C4L	Mascart-Lemone et al. (1983)

(continued)

Complete Deficiency of Complement C4, Table 1   (continued)

Family/ subject	Age (years) at onset, gender, race/ethnicity, nationality	Disease, clinical feature (remarks)	MHC/HLA haplotype	C4L and C4S genes on each Chr.6	References
8b	1.5, F, North African, Moroccan	Recurrent pulmonary infections, lupus-like (skin lesions); pneumonia with pleurisy (consanguineous parents)	*A11 Cw4 B35 DR1*	C4L/C4L	Mascart-Lemone et al. (1983)
9	6/27, F, CAUC, Austrian	Lupus like, SLE at age 27, infections; Raynaud's phenomenon	*A30 B18 DR7*	ND	Klein et al. (1984)
10	26, M, Sioux Indian, US	SLE (blood transfusion led to generation of anti-C4 antibodies)	*A2 B15 DR2/A2 B15 DR3*	ND	Giles and Swanson (1984)
11	44, F, CAUC, US	SLE; hemolytic anemia (positive test at 17 treated at age 23, developed photosensitivity rash at age 41; one sister died of fulminating lupus, nephritis, familial trend to multiple autoimmune disease)	*A11 Cw5 B18 DR2/A1 Cw7 B7 DR2*	ND	Reveille et al. (1985)
12	2, F, CAUC, Swedish	SLE and GN; atypical rash, recurrent otitis media and purulent parotitis, polyarthritis	*A2 Cw3 B40 DR6/A30 B18 DR3*	C4L/C4L	Reveille et al. (1985)
13	2, F, North African, Algerian	Lupus-like, bacterial meningitidis; recurrent pulmonary infections (died of cardiopulmonary complications)	*A1 B17 DR13*	C4L-C4S/ C4L-C4S	Meyer et al. (1985) and Wu et al. (2009)
14	9, F, –, US	SLE; malar and vasculitic rash, photosensitivity (uniparentalisodisomy, without maternal chromosome)	*A28 Cw3 B40 DR6*	C4L/C4L	Welch et al. (1990)
15	15, M, Oriental, Japanese	SLE	*A31 B51 DRw9/A24 B52 DR2*	ND	Komine et al. (1992)
16a	16, M, North African, Algerian	SLE; malar rash at age 6, hematuria, photosensitivity, polyarthralgia	*A2, B17, DR7*	C4L/C4L	Fremeaux-Bacchi et al. (1994)
16b	12, M, North African, Algerian	Asymptomatic, healthy	*A2, B17, DR7*	C4L/C4L	Fremeaux-Bacchi et al. (1994)
17[a]	10, M, CAUC, Austrian/Italian	Recurrent hematuria, mesangioproliferative GN; nephropathy (related to family #6)	*A24 Cw7 B38 DR13DQ6*	C4L/C4L	Lhotta et al. (1996)
18a	30, F, CAUC, Finnish	SLE; malar rash, photosensitivity, polyarthritis, leukopenia	*A2 Cw3 B40 DR6/A2 Cw7 B39 DR15*	C4L/C4L-C4S	Lokki et al. (1999)
18b	<30, M, CAUC, Finnish	Photosensitivity	*A2 Cw3 B40 DR6/A2 Cw7 B39 DR15*	C4L/C4L-C4S	Lokki et al. (1999)

(continued)

Complete Deficiency of Complement C4, Table 1 (continued)

Family/ subject	Age (years) at onset, gender, race/ethnicity, nationality	Disease, clinical feature (remarks)	MHC/HLA haplotype	C4L and C4S genes on each Chr.6	References
19a	10, M, CAUC, US	SLE; class III nephritis, CNS vasculitis (died at age 25)	A2 B12 DR6	C4L-C4S/ C4L-C4S	Rupert et al. (2002)
19b	21, M, CAUC, US	Discoid lupus; photosensitivity	A2 B12 DR6	C4L-C4S/ C4L-C4S	Rupert et al. (2002)

CAUC Caucasian, *C4L* C4 long gene, *C4S* C4 short gene, *GN* glomerulonephritis, *ND* not determined
[a]Related to family number 6

pyogenic infections, indicating the negative impact of C4B nonexpression on the immune defense mechanisms of those subjects. Eleven of the C4*Q0 established cases had clinical features of nephritis, such as hematuria and proteinuria, or developed mesangio-proliferative glomerulonephritis (Table 1), a severe autoimmune disease characterized by deposition of immune-complexes either in the glomeruli or small blood vessels of kidneys. One subject in conjunction with mesangio-proliferative glomerulonephritis suffered from recurrent Henoch-Schönleinpurpura (Tappeiner et al. 1978), another immune-complex related disorder. Thus, given the high prevalence of immune-complex mediated diseases in C4-deficient cases (89%), it is evident that the complete lack of C4A is the indispensable pre-requisite to develop those autoimmune disor-ders, while the lack of C4B is secondary. On the other hand, a relatively small burden of infectious diseases (21%) denotes a consider-able caution of the complement system in host-defense mechanisms involving all three, often functionally overlapping, activation pathways. In C4-deficient cases, for neutralization of invaded pathogens, the complete lack of C4B (important for further activation of the comple-ment via the classical and the lectin pathways) can be compensated by the activation of the alternative pathway. In addition, pattern recog-nition molecules (i.e., C1q, MBL and ficolins) still can efficiently recognize and tag the micro-organisms and process their clearance by phagocytosis.

Diagnosis and Treatment

Clinically, C4 complete deficiency is easily detected during low complement diagnosis procedure, which is based on the combination of C3, C4, and total complement activity, CH50, levels. While for the complement activity Wieslab® Complement System Screen kits are currently preferentially used, for C3 and C4 protein concentration in body fluids a number of single radial immunodiffusion (RIA) and enzyme linked immunosorbent assay (ELISA) kits are commercially available. More-over, some of those are able to distinguish C4 occurred (due to high consumption of the protein) deficiency based on detection of its activated com-ponents (e.g., C4a). However, for an ascertainment of C4 hereditary deficiency, DNA screening and, perhaps, mRNA expression investigation are required by C4-specialized research laboratories.

As C4 complete deficiency is very rare and manifests in different phenotypes, the treatment of clinical cases therefore varied, depending on the diagnosis.

Conclusion

The C4 total deficiency may severely impair human innate and adaptive immunity, and may serve as a strong risk factor for susceptibility to lupus-like illnesses, and particularly, to SLE. At an early age of C4-deficent individuals, pyogenic infections may assist in the development of lupus-like disorders. It is likely that depending on genetic and epigenetic profile of an individual, the generated SLE can have different phenotypes with manifestation of the other immune-complex mediated autoimmune diseases, such as glomerulonephritis and polyarthritis.

Cross-References

▶ Complement Component C2 Deficiency
▶ C1 Deficiency and Associated Disorders

References

Ballow M, McLean RH, Einarson M, Martin S, Yunis EJ, DuPont B, O'Neill GJ. Hereditary C4 deficiency: genetic studies and linkage to HLA. Transplant Proc. 1979;11:260–3.

Campbell RD, Thomson W, Morley B. Molecular genetics of the major histocompatibility complex class III region. In: Ried KBM, Sim RB, editors. Molecular aspects of innate and adaptive immunity. Cambridge: RSC; 2008. p. 219–37.

Carroll MC. Biology and genetics of C4. In: Ried KBM, Sim RB, editors. Molecular aspects of innate and adaptive immunity. Cambridge, UK: RSC; 2008. p. 105–17.

Fremeaux-Bacchi V, Uring-Lambert B, Weiss L, Brun P, Blouin J, Hartmann D, Loirat C, Hauptmann G, Kazatchkine MD. Complete inherited deficiency of the fourth complement component in a child with systemic lupus erythematosus and his disease-free brother in a North African family. J Clin Immunol. 1994;14:273–9.

Giles CM, Swanson JL. Anti-C4 in the serum of a transfused C4-deficient patient with systemic lupus erythematosus. Vox Sang. 1984;46:291–9.

Gordon J, Whitehead HR, Wormall A. The action of ammonia on complement. The fourth component. Biochem J. 1926;20:1028–35.

Hauptmann G, Grosshans E, Heid E. Systemic lupus erythematosus and hereditary complement deficiency: a case of with total C4 defect. Ann Dermatol Syphiligr. 1974;101:479–96.

Hauptmann G, Tappeiner G, Schifferli JA. Inherited deficiency of the fourth component of human complement. Immunodefic Rev. 1988;1:3–22.

Hou S, Qi J, Liao D, Fang J, Chen L, Kijlstra A, Yang P. High C4 gene copy numbers protects against Vogt–Koyanagi–Harada syndrome in Chinese Han. Br J Ophthalmol. 2014;98:1733–7.

Klein G, Tappeiner G, Hinter H, Scholz S, Wolff K. Systemischer lupus erythematodes bei hereditärer Defizienz der vierten Komplementkomponente. Hautarzt. 1984;35:27–32.

Komine M, Matsuyama T, Nojima Y, Minoda S, Furue M, Tsuchida T, Sakai S, Ishibashi Y. Systemic lupus erythematosus with hereditary deficiency of the fourth

component of complement. Int J Dermatol. 1992;31:653–6.

Lhotta K, Neunhauserer M, Solder B, Uring-Lambert B, Wurzner R, Rumpelt HJ, Konig P. Recurrent hematuria: a novel clinical presentation of hereditary complete complement C4 deficiency. Am J Kidney Dis. 1996;27:424–7.

Lokki M-L, Circolo A, Ahokas P, Rupert KL, Yu CY, Colten HR. Deficiency of complement protein C4 due to identical frameshift mutations in the *C4A* and *C4B* genes. J Immunol. 1999;162:3687–93.

Mascart-Lemone F, Hauptmann G, Goetz J, Duchateau J, Delespesse G, Vray B, Dab I. Genetic deficiency of C4 presenting with recurrent infections and SLE-like disease. Am J Med. 1983;75:295–304.

Mayilyan KR. Complement genetics, deficiencies, and disease associations. Protein Cell. 2012;3:487–96.

Mayilyan KR, Kang YH, Dodds AW, Sim RB. The complement system in innate immunity. In: Heine H, editor. Innate immunity of plants, animals and humans, Nucleic acids and molecular biology, vol. 21. Heidelberg: Springer; 2008a. p. 219–36.

Mayilyan KR, Weinberger DR, Sim RB. The complement system in schizophrenia. Drug News Perspect. 2008b;21:200–10.

Meyer O, Hauptmann G, Tappeiner G, Ochs HD, Mascart-Lemone F. Genetic deficiency of C4, C2 or C1q and lupus syndromes. Association with anti-Ro (SS-A) antibodies. Clin Exp Immunol. 1985;62:678–84.

Minta JO, Urowitz MB, Gladman DD, Irizawa T, Biggar WD. Selective deficiency of the fourth component of complement in a patient with systemic lupus erythematosus (SLE): immunological studies. Clin Exp Immunol. 1981;45:72–80.

Pickering MC, Botto M, Taylor PR, Lachmann PJ, Walport MJ. Systemic lupus erythematosus, complement deficiency, and apoptosis. Adv Immunol. 2000;76:227–324.

Reveille JD, Arnett FC, Wilson RW, Bias WB, McLean RH. Null alleles of the fourth component of complement and HLA haplotypes in familial systemic lupus erythematosus. Immunogenetics. 1985;21:299–311.

Ricklin D, Hajishengallis G, Yang K, Lambris JD. Complement: a key system for immune surveillance and homeostasis. Nat Immunol. 2010;11:785–97.

Rupert KL, Moulds JM, Yang Y, Arnett FC, Warren RW, Reveille JD, Myones BL, Blanchong CA, Yu CY. The molecular basis of complete C4A and C4B deficiencies in a systemic lupus erythematosus (SLE) patient with homozygous C4A and C4B mutant genes. J Immunol. 2002;169:1570–8.

Schaller JG, Gilliland BG, Ochs HD, Leddy JP, Agodoa LCY, Rosenfeld SI. Severe systemic lupus erythematosus with nephritis in a boy with deficiency of the fourth component of complement. Arthritis Rheum. 1977;20:1519–25.

Tappeiner G, Scholz S, Linert J, Albert ED, Wolff K. Hereditary deficiency of the fourth component (C4): study of a family. Colloq INSERM Cutan Immunopathol. 1978;80:399–404.

Tappeiner G, Hintner H, Scholz S, Albert E, Linert J, Wolff K. Systemic lupus erythematosus in hereditary deficiency of the fourth component of complement. J Am Acad Dermatol. 1982;7:66–79.

Wallis R, Dodds AW, Mitchell DA, Sim RB, Reid KB, Schwaeble WJ. Molecular interactions between MASP-2, C4, and C2 and their activation fragments leading to complement activation via the lectin pathway. J Biol Chem. 2007;282:7844–51.

Welch TR, Beischel LS, Choi E, Balakrishnan K, Bishof NA. Uniparental isodisomy 6 associated with deficiency of the fourth component of complement. J Clin Invest. 1990;86:675–8.

Wu YL, Hauptmann G, Viguier M, Yu CY. Molecular basis of complete complement C4 deficiency in two North-African families with systemic lupus erythematosus. Genes Immun. 2009;10:433–45.

Yang Y, Chung EK, Zhou B, Lhotta K, Hebert LA, Birmingham DJ, Rovin BH, Yu CY. The intricate role of complement component C4 in human systemic lupus erythematosus. Curr Dir Autoimmun. 2004a;7:98–132.

Yang Y, Lhotta K, Chung EK, Eder P, Neumair F, Yu CY. Complete complement components C4A and C4B deficiencies in human kidney diseases and systemic lupus erythematosus. J Immunol. 2004b;173:2803–14.

Yang Y, Chung EK, Wu YL, Savelli SL, Nagaraja HN, Zhou B, Hebert M, Jones KN, Shu Y, Kitzmiller K, Blanchong CA, McBride KL, Higgins GC, Rennebohm RM, Rice RR, Hackshaw KV, Roubey RA, Grossman JM, Tsao BP, Birmingham DJ, Rovin BH, Hebert LA, Yu CY. Gene copy-number variation and associated polymorphisms of complement component C4 in human systemic lupus erythematosus (SLE): low copy number is a risk factor for and high copy number is a protective factor against SLE susceptibility in European Americans. Am J Hum Genet. 2007;80:1037–54.

Yu CY, Chung EK, Yang Y, Blanchong CA, Jacobsen N, Saxena K, Yang Z, Miller W, Varga L, Fust G. Dancing with complement C4 and the RP-C4-CYP21-TNX (RCCX) modules of the major histocompatibility complex. Prog Nucleic Acid Res Mol Biol. 2003;75:217–92.

Yu CY, Hauptmann G, Yang Y, Wu YL, Birmingham DJ, Rovin BH, Hebert LA. Complement deficiencies in human systemic lupus erythematosus (SLE) and SLE nephritis: epidemiology and pathogenesis. In: Tsokos GC, Gordon C, Smolen JS, editors. Systemic lupus erythematosus: a companion to rheumatology. Elsevier: Philadelphia; 2007. p. 203–13.

Congenital Telangiectatic Erythema

▶ Bloom Syndrome

COPA Syndrome

Levi B. Watkin[1] and Jordan Scott Orange[2]
[1]Department of Pediatrics, Baylor College of Medicine, Center for Human Immunobiology, Division of Allergy, Immunology, and Rheumatology, Texas Children's Hospital, Houston, TX, USA
[2]Department of Pediatrics, Columbia University Vagelos College of Physicians and Surgeons, New York-Presbyterian Morgan Stanley Children's Hospital, New York, NY, USA

Synonyms

AILJK – autoimmune interstitial lung, joint, and kidney disease

Definition

COPA syndrome is an inherited autosomal dominant immuno-dysregulatory disease presenting with interstitial lung disease, pulmonary hemorrhage, and arthritis as the most prominent presentations. It is caused by autosomal dominant loss-of-function mutations in the gene *COPA* (MIM# 601923.).

Introduction

The immune system is a tightly regulated system harnessing the power to control and/or eliminate infections. COPA syndrome represents clinical manifestations suggesting sterile inflammation due to inherent defects in innate and adaptive immunity. Here we provide a brief synopsis of our current understanding of this novel disease, which is named for the defective gene underlying the disease; COPA syndrome was reported in 2015 in five unrelated families, probands in these families presented with similar histories and shared clinical features (Watkin et al. 2015).

Genetics

COPA syndrome is caused by mutations in the *COPA* gene. Single-heterozygous non-synonymous disease-causing variants were identified by whole-exome sequencing and found to encode amino acid changes in COPα positions K230N, R233H, E241K, and D243G. These mutations are restricted to exons 8 and 9 which encode the sixth WD40 repeat domains within the N-terminal portion of the protein, which are responsible for the binding of coatomer cargo. These positions are highly conserved all the way down to *Saccharomyces cerevisiae* with prediction algorithms indicating potential to be highly damaging. Additionally, when the LOD scores of the five unrelated families are combined, the resulting score is >5 thus indicating disease linkage to the gene. The disease-causing COPA mutations have variable penetrance. Families carrying the K230N and R233H mutation show a near complete penetrance of disease with only one member of each family carrying the variant not having symptoms of disease, and family members without disease are both male and under 5 years of age, which does not exclude disease development later in life. In families harboring the D243G mutation, all female carriers present with disease, and all male carriers are unaffected. The E241K mutation also had variable penetrance with a higher preponderance of females with disease. Interestingly, the two variants with variable penetrance are encoded on exon 9. The preponderance in women suggests the possibility of sex hormones modifying the disease, or a gene dosage effect from an interacting partner from the X chromosome. Further investigation is needed to elucidate the mechanism of variable penetrance in COPA syndrome.

Pathogenesis

COPA is part of the seven-member coatomer-I (COP-I) complex which is responsible for transporting proteins in a retrograde fashion from the Golgi apparatus to the endoplasmic reticulum (ER) (Schekman and Orci 1996). COPA is responsible for binding dilysine motif-containing-proteins and retention in the complex for transport (Jackson et al. 2012; Letourneur et al. 1994). Mutations identified in COPA syndrome result in decreased binding of coatomer cargo (Watkin et al. 2015) and some affect the binding ability of COPA to dilysine motifs in yeast, predicting decreased transport of cargo from the Golgi to the ER. Supporting this function, patient-derived cells and cell lines carrying the identified mutations show an increase in ER stress as measured by an increase of BiP and CHOP expression (Watkin et al. 2015). ER stress can activate transcription of pro-inflammatory cytokines through NF-κB by way of Ca^{++} leakage from the ER (Deniaud et al. 2008; Pahl and Baeuerle 1996). ER stress is also known to induce the unfolded protein response (UPR) (Diehl et al. 2011) which in itself can lead to a pro-inflammatory environment.

In an effort to relieve ER stress, the cell will engage the cellular, catabolic process of autophagy (Yorimitsu et al. 2006). In COPA syndrome, this process is amplified with an increase in the size and number of autophagosomes within the cell and an increase of catabolism determined by a decrease in the catabolic substrate p62 (Watkin et al. 2015). The cell then senses this increase in autophagy by an unknown mechanism and attempts to dampen it with increased activation of mTOR which cannot even be dampened with torin treatment (unpublished observation). Interestingly, increased mTOR activity has been associated with increased Th17 frequencies (Almeida et al. 2016; Kurebayashi et al. 2012; Sasaki et al. 2016) of which there is a significant increase in COPA syndrome.

Clinical Manifestations

Pulmonary Manifestations
COPA syndrome is primarily a disease of pulmonary and articular involvement typically presenting before the age of 5 and as early as 6 months of age. Initial presentation often is either chronic cough and tachypnea followed by joint pain or vice versa. Patients develop progressive

lung disease and decreased pulmonary function in the context of interstitial lung disease and hemoptysis. Often joint pain worsens with pulmonary exacerbations.

Musculoskeletal Manifestations

Of the studied patients, 95% had physician-diagnosed arthritis. Of these, half tested positive for rheumatoid factor (RF) and some had anti-cyclic citrullinated peptide (CCP) antibodies which have been correlated with joint destruction. The joints most commonly showing signs of arthritis are the knees and interphalangeal joints of the hand. Osteonecrosis was reported in two patients with one requiring bilateral knee replacement; however, it is unclear whether this was caused by the disease or chronic steroid use.

Renal Manifestations

COPA patients have an increased risk for renal disease with an average age of onset in the mid to late teen years. Of the patients studied, approximately 40% had clinical features of glomerular disease indicated by either proteinuria and/or decreased renal function. Of those with renal biopsies, all had histological evidence of glomerulopathy. Unlike other systemic autoimmune diseases such as SLE and ANCA vasculitis, there are no defined distinct patterns of renal injury. The pathological features of the glomerular lesions varied between crescentic disease with immune complexes and crescentic disease with focal segmental glomerulonephritis without immune deposits, mesangial hypercellularity without immune deposits, and IgA nephropathy with necrotizing lesions. Necrotizing lesions and cellular crescents were identified in three quarters of the individuals with renal disease, with one patient progressing to end-stage renal disease necessitating renal transplant.

Laboratory Findings

Patients have an elevated level of serum inflammatory markers including C-reactive protein and erythrocyte sedimentation rate. Nearly 80% of affected individuals have positive anti-nuclear antigen (ANA) titer with homogenous, speckled, and diffuse patterns of staining being reported with titers as high as 1:1280. Other autoantibodies reported include both anti-proteinase-3 (or cANCA) and anti-myeloperoxidase (or pANCA), RF and anti-CCP antibodies. While the presence and titer of inflammatory markers and autoantibodies fluctuate with time and disease severity, there appears to be no definitive single marker of disease activity, severity, or progression. COPA patients had increased pro-inflammatory cytokine production. Patient-derived B-cells had increased pro-IL-1β, IL-6, and IL-23 transcription. Increased serum TNF and type I and type III interferon levels were reported. This pro-inflammatory cytokine environment primes highly inflammatory IL-17A producing CD4 T-cells (Th17 cells) which were drastically increased in COPA patients.

Treatment

In the absence of treatment recommendations for COPA, patients are managed similarly to other patients with pulmonary hemorrhages and autoimmune/autoinflammatory syndromes. During acute exacerbations, patients are treated with cyclophosphamide or rituximab in addition to systemic corticosteroids. The steroids offer beneficial results to the other autoimmune components such as arthritis. Maintenance therapies usually include methotrexate or azathioprine with pulse steroids and gradual tapering. Other therapies have included hydroxychloroquine, etanercept, and IVIG. However, unlike other pulmonary hemorrhage syndromes, the optimal treatment options and durations of therapy are unknown. To date, no patients have received hematopoietic stem cell transplantation, and it is unclear as to if this would be of benefit given the wide tissue expression of COPA.

Prognosis

Due to the progressive nature of the disease, patients ultimately succumb to acute exacerbations suggesting any present management of the disease is suboptimal. A number of patients diagnosed or suspected to have COPA from family genetics have had premature and pathology-related deaths. Most of these have occurred in the fourth decade and beyond and some from complications of disease-related interventions such as lung transplantation. Collection of full patient details from many newly diagnosed families of which the authors are anecdotally aware of should allow for an appropriate picture of prognosis to be created. Most patients had arthritis/arthralgia at presentation and features of pulmonary disease. The presence of one should prompt more careful consideration of the other and with an effort to prevent what would appear to otherwise be an inevitable progression of these clinical features. While the disease pattern can be severe, the heterogeneity of the pathological features of renal disease does not point toward a single immune-mediated injury, and thus it is likely that a multimodal approach to diagnosis and treatment will be most effective. Presently, it is unknown if early detection and treatment could or would reduce the development of renal injury. Currently new treatment options are being considered and tested in vitro based upon the physiological and immunological stress points identified in the disease to be caused by the described mutations.

Cross-References

▶ AILJK – Autoimmune Interstitial Lung, Joint, and Kidney Disease
▶ Introduction to Autoinflammatory Diseases
▶ Primary Immune Deficiency

References

Almeida L, Lochner M, Berod L, Sparwasser T. Metabolic pathways in T cell activation and lineage differentiation. Semin Immunol. 2016. https://doi.org/10.1016/j.smim.2016.10.009.

Deniaud A, Sharaf el dein O, Maillier E, Poncet D, Kroemer G, Lemaire C, Brenner C. Endoplasmic reticulum stress induces calcium-dependent permeability transition, mitochondrial outer membrane permeabilization and apoptosis. Oncogene. 2008;27:285–99. https://doi.org/10.1038/sj.onc.1210638.

Diehl JA, Fuchs SY, Koumenis C. The cell biology of the unfolded protein response. Gastroenterology. 2011;141:38–41.e2. https://doi.org/10.1053/j.gastro.2011.05.018.

Jackson LPL, Lewis MM, Kent HMH, Edeling MAM, Evans PRP, Duden RR, Owen DJD. Molecular basis for recognition of Dilysine trafficking motifs by COPI. Dev Cell. 2012;23:1255–62. https://doi.org/10.1016/j.devcel.2012.10.017.

Kurebayashi Y, Nagai S, Ikejiri A, Ohtani M, Ichiyama K, Baba Y, Yamada T, Egami S, Hoshii T, Hirao A, Matsuda S, Koyasu S. PI3K-Akt-mTORC1-S6K1/2 axis controls Th17 differentiation by regulating Gfi1 expression and nuclear translocation of RORγ. Cell Rep. 2012;1:360–73. https://doi.org/10.1016/j.celrep.2012.02.007.

Letourneur F, Gaynor EC, Hennecke S, Démollière C, Duden R, Emr SD, Riezman H, Cosson P. Coatomer is essential for retrieval of dilysine-tagged proteins to the endoplasmic reticulum. Cell. 1994;79:1199–207.

Pahl HL, Baeuerle PA. Activation of NF-kappa B by ER stress requires both Ca^{2+} and reactive oxygen intermediates as messengers. FEBS Lett. 1996;392:129–36.

Sasaki CY, Chen G, Munk R, Eitan E, Martindale J, Longo DL, Ghosh P. p70S6K1 in the TORC1 pathway is essential for the differentiation of Th17 cells, but not Th1, Th2, or Treg cells in mice. Eur J Immunol. 2016;46:212–22. https://doi.org/10.1002/eji.201445422.

Schekman R, Orci L. Coat proteins and vesicle budding. Science. 1996;271:1526–33.

Watkin LB, Jessen B, Wiszniewski W, Vece TJ, Jan M, Sha Y, Thamsen M, Santos-Cortez RLP, Lee K, Gambin T, Forbes LR, Law CS, Stray-Pedersen A, Cheng MH, Mace EM, Anderson MS, Liu D, Tang LF, Nicholas SK, Nahmod K, Makedonas G, Canter DL, Kwok P-Y, Hicks J, Jones KD, Penney S, Jhangiani SN, Rosenblum MD, Dell SD, Waterfield MR, Papa FR, Muzny DM, Zaitlen N, Leal SM, Gonzaga-Jauregui C, Baylor-Hopkins Center for Mendelian Genomics, Boerwinkle E, Eissa NT, Gibbs RA, Lupski JR, Orange JS, Shum AK. COPA mutations impair ER-Golgi transport and cause hereditary autoimmune-mediated lung disease and arthritis. Nat Genet. 2015;47:654–60. https://doi.org/10.1038/ng.3279.

Yorimitsu T, Nair U, Yang Z, Klionsky DJ. Endoplasmic reticulum stress triggers autophagy. J Biol Chem. 2006;281:30299–304. https://doi.org/10.1074/jbc.M607007200.

CRAC Channelopathy

▶ Calcium Channel Defects (STIM1 and ORAI1)

CRAF1

▶ TRAF3 Deficiency

Cranial Developmental Disorder Cherubism

Yoshinori Matsumoto[1,2] and Robert Rottapel[1,3,4]
[1]Princess Margaret Cancer Center, University
Health Network, University of Toronto, Toronto,
ON, Canada
[2]Department of Nephrology, Rheumatology,
Endocrinology and Metabolism, Okayama
University Graduate School of Medicine,
Dentistry and Pharmaceutical Sciences,
Okayama, Japan
[3]Department of Medicine, Department of Medical
Biophysics and Department of Immunology,
University of Toronto, Toronto, ON, Canada
[4]Division of Rheumatology, St. Michael's
Hospital, Toronto, ON, Canada

Synonyms

SH3 domain-binding protein 2; SH3BP2

Definition

Cherubism is a rare autosomal dominant disorder
which is characterized by progressive, painless
facial bone destruction in children at age 2–5 years
(MIM#118400).

Introduction and Background

The craniofacial disorder known as cherubism was
first described by Jones et al. (1950) and named
because the facial changes of some affected children is reminiscent of the cherubs famously
depicted in Raphael's Sistine Madonna. Cherubism
manifests as bilateral and symmetric enlargement
of the mandible and/or maxilla due to rapid bone

resorption, bony cyst formation, displacement of
the position of the permanent teeth, and upturned
tilting eyes due to involvement of the infraorbital
rim and orbital floor. Some patients develop cervical and submandibular lymphadenopathy. The
clinical features of cherubism usually progress
until puberty, followed by spontaneous regression.
Penetrance is close to 100% in males and 50–75%
in females. Males tend to manifest more severe
phenotypic features than females. The basis of
this gender dimorphism is not known.

Genetics

The gene associated with cherubism was mapped
to chromosome 4p16.3 by linkage analysis
(Tiziani et al. 1999; Mangion et al. 1999). Further
linkage and haplotype analysis of 12 affected families defined the cherubism locus to a 1.5 mega-
base interval (Ueki et al. 2001). Direct sequencing
of this region detected point mutations causing
amino acid substitutions in *SH3BP2*, encoding
the adapter SH3 binding protein 3BP2. 3BP2
was originally identified as an ABL kinase SH3
domain binding protein (Ren et al. 1993). The
domain organization of the 3BP2 protein consists
of an N-terminal phospholipid-binding pleckstrin
homology (PH) domain, a central proline-rich
(PR) region and a C-terminal phosphotyrosine-
binding Src-homology 2 (SH2) domain. Most of
the documented gene mutations reported to date
are clustered in exon nine of *SH3BP2* and affect
one of the three amino acids within the hexapeptide sequence (RSPPDG) residing in the disordered region between the PH and SH2 domains
(Fig. 1) (Ueki et al. 2001). Mutations in Pro
418 (to Leu, Arg, or His) are the most common,
while other mutations result in Arg 415 being
replaced by Pro or Gln and in Gly 420 being
replaced by Glu or Arg. Mutations in other
exons of *SH3BP2* have been reported (Carvalho
et al. 2009), while the biochemical function of
these alterations has not been established.
Although *SH3BP2* is the only gene whose mutation is known to cause cherubism, single allele
mutations in *SH3BP2* are detected in 80% of
cherubism patients diagnosed on the presence of

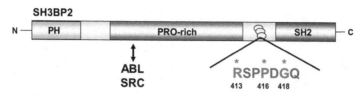

Cranial Developmental Disorder Cherubism, Fig. 1 Domain structure of SH3BP2. The proteins known to interact with specific domain and residues subjected to tyrosine and serine phosphorylation. The cherubism mutations are located within a hexapeptide interval (RSPPDG) in the PR domain

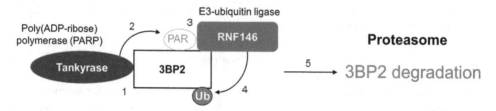

Cranial Developmental Disorder Cherubism, Fig. 2 Schematic model of the SH3BP2 degradation pathway controlled by tankyrase and RNF146. 3BP2 binds to tankyrase through a hexapeptide interval in the PR domain (Jones et al. 1950). Tankyrase-mediated 3BP2 ribosylation (Tiziani et al. 1999) creates a recognition site for the E3-ubiquitin ligase RNF146 (Mangion et al. 1999), leading to its ubiquitylation (Ueki et al. 2001) and proteasomal degradation (Ren et al. 1993)

clinical manifestations and radiographic and histologic findings, leaving approximately 20% of patients who present with clinical features of cherubism with mutations in other genes possibly involved in the 3BP2 signaling pathway.

Pathogenesis

We and others have found that 3BP2 functions as a docking protein that binds to VAV, SYK, and SRC in osteoclasts required for integrin-mediated formation of the actin-containing sealing zone. 3BP2 binds to and activates the SRC tyrosine kinase by engagement of its SH3 domain and recruits the SRC substrates VAV and SYK for tyrosine phosphorylation and activation (Fig. 1). We have shown in 3BP2 knockout studies in mice that 3BP2 is required for the normal function of multiple immune cell lineages including macrophages, marginal zone B cells, and granulocytes.

3BP2 is subject to tight negative regulation by tankyrase, a poly(ADP-ribose) polymerase (PARP) family member (Fig. 2) (Levaot et al. 2011). Tankyrase-mediated 3BP2 ribosylation

creates a recognition site for the E3-ubiquitin ligase RNF146, leading to its ubiquitylation and proteasomal degradation (Fig. 2) (Levaot et al. 2011).

All the mutations in exon 9 of the *SH3BP2* gene found to be associated to cherubism are located precisely in the tankyrase-binding hexapeptide sequence that serve to uncouple 3BP2 from tankyrase-mediated negative regulation (Fig. 2). Thus, these pathogenic exon 9 mutations serve to stabilize the steady protein levels of 3BP2 and cause hyperactivation of the downstream signaling pathway including SRC, SYK, and VAV, leading to increased osteoclastogenesis and osteoclast activity and hyperactivation of macrophage-mediated TNF-α production (Fig. 2) (Levaot et al. 2011). These data confirmed that cherubism mutations resulting in 3BP2 gain of function are thus hypermorphic and explain the autosomal dominant mode of inheritance of the syndrome.

Cherubism has been modeled in mice using the P418R in humans and P416R in mice, knocked into the mouse *Sh3bp2* gene (Ueki et al. 2007). The cherubism mice carry a single *Sh3pb2* mutant allele phenocopy, which has many features of the human syndrome. Mutant mice are osteoporotic with increased numbers of osteoclasts in bone. Of significance is that these homozygous mice die from an inflammatory wasting syndrome associated with high levels of serum TNF-α and myelomonocytic infiltration of the skin and visceral organs, a phenotype that is rescued by eliminating TNF-α expression. 3BP2 is involved in LPS-mediated TNF-α production in murine primary macrophages (Prod'Homme et al. 2015). These data show that 3BP2 is a key regulator of TNF-α production (Ueki et al. 2007). Moreover, the phenotype of the cherubism mouse model points to the broader clinical features of cherubism in humans that have not yet been fully investigated including elevated cytokine levels, osteoporosis, and innate and adaptive immune activation.

Clinical Manifestations

The clinical manifestations of cherubism are characterized by erosion of maxillar and mandibular bone with severe pain as a consequence of replacement of bone with multilocular cysts composed of fibrotic stromal cells and osteoclast-like multinucleated giant cells. These lesions usually appear between 2 years and 5 years of age and increase in size until puberty. The patients display dental abnormalities, which include premature exfoliation of the deciduous teeth and displacement of permanent teeth. In advanced stages, upturned tilting of the eyes is also observed because of enlargement of the maxilla and penetration of the stromal mass into the orbital floor, leading to visual loss due to optic atrophy. Affected patients often suffer from difficulty in mastication and speech.

Laboratory Findings

Cherubism is diagnosed on the basis of the distinct clinical findings, radiographic features, and tissue histopathology from affected areas. No set of specific clinical criteria nor any biochemical markers have been established, although elevation of alkaline phosphatase levels and other

indicators of bone resorption and osteoclast activity might be observed in some of the patients. Radiographic findings show well-defined, radiolucent, and often extensive bilateral multilocular cystic areas in the mandible and/or maxilla. The multiloculated areas of reduced radiodensity become replaced by sclerosis and progressive calcification. Numerous multinucleated osteoclast-like giant cells and fibrosis are observed by histopathology.

Diagnosis

Since no diagnostic criteria have been established, diagnosis of cherubism is made based on the presence of clinical manifestations and radiographic and histologic findings. Genetic testing exon 9 in the *SH3BP2* gene has been helpful to confirm the diagnosis for approximately 80% of the clinically diagnosed cherubism patients.

Treatment

No standard therapeutic strategy for cherubism has been established. Many children are followed conservatively until puberty when the disease often stabilizes and occasionally spontaneously regresses, followed by tooth extraction and cosmetic osteoplasty and dental reconstruction of the affected jaws. Based on the efficacy of TNF-α blockade in the cherubism mouse model, Hero et al. reported the utility of anti-TNF-α treatment in two cherubism children and described a significant reduction in the number of multinucleated giant cells and TNF-α staining positivity in both patients (Hero et al. 2013).

Additional therapeutic options, which target the signaling pathway activated by 3BP2, may have clinical utility including SYK or SRC small molecule inhibitors in treating Cherubism (Levaot et al. 2011). Other strategies may include the use of biologics which block osteoclast function such as the RANKL-neutralizing antibody denosumab, CSF-1 blocking antibodies, or CSF-1R small-molecule inhibitors which are currently in clinical development. Further studies will be required to establish the timing and mode of the optimal therapeutic strategy for the cherubism patients.

Prognosis

Cherubism patients are mentally and otherwise physically normal aside from the facial bone destruction. Cherubism manifests in children at age 2–5 years and progresses until puberty while the disease will spontaneously regress after puberty.

References

Carvalho VM, Perdigao PF, Amaral FR, de Souza PE, De Marco L, Gomez RS. Novel mutations in the SH3BP2 gene associated with sporadic central giant cell lesions and cherubism. Oral Dis. 2009;15(1):106–10.

Hero M, Suomalainen A, Hagström J, Stoor P, Kontio R, Alapulli H, et al. Anti-tumor necrosis factor treatment in cherubism–clinical, radiological and histological findings in two children. Bone. 2013;52(1):347–53.

Jones WA, Gerrie J, Pritchard J. Cherubism–familial fibrous dysplasia of the jaws. J Bone Joint Surg Br. 1950;32-B(3):334–47.

Levaot N, Voytyuk O, Dimitriou I, Sircoulomb F, Chandrakumar A, Deckert M, et al. Loss of Tankyrase-mediated destruction of 3BP2 is the underlying pathogenic mechanism of cherubism. Cell. 2011;147(6):1324–39.

Mangion J, Rahman N, Edkins S, Barfoot R, Nguyen T, Sigurdsson A, et al. The gene for cherubism maps to chromosome 4p16.3. Am J Hum Genet. 1999;65(1):151–7.

Prod'Homme V, Boyer L, Dubois N, Mallavialle A, Munro P, Mouska X, et al. Cherubism allele heterozygosity amplifies microbe-induced inflammatory responses in murine macrophages. J Clin Invest. 2015;125(4):1396–400.

Ren R, Mayer BJ, Cicchetti P, Baltimore D. Identification of a ten-amino acid proline-rich SH3 binding site. Science. 1993;259(5098):1157–61.

Tiziani V, Reichenberger E, Buzzo CL, Niazi S, Fukai N, Stiller M, et al. The gene for cherubism maps to chromosome 4p16. Am J Hum Genet. 1999;65(1):158–66.

Ueki Y, Tiziani V, Santanna C, Fukai N, Maulik C, Garfinkle J, et al. Mutations in the gene encoding c-Abl-binding protein SH3BP2 cause cherubism. Nat Genet. 2001;28(2):125–6.

Ueki Y, Lin CY, Senoo M, Ebihara T, Agata N, Onji M, et al. Increased myeloid cell responses to M-CSF and RANKL cause bone loss and inflammation in SH3BP2 "cherubism" mice. Cell. 2007;128(1):71–83.

CRMO: Chronic Recurrent Multifocal Osteomyelitis

▶ Majeed Syndrome

Cryopyrin-Associated Periodic Syndromes (CAPS)

▶ Familial Cold Autoinflammatory Syndrome (FCAS) and Muckle-Wells Syndrome (MWS)

Cryopyrinopathies

▶ Familial Cold Autoinflammatory Syndrome (FCAS) and Muckle-Wells Syndrome (MWS)

CTSC Deficiency

▶ Localized Juvenile Periodontitis

CVID

▶ Common Variable Immunodeficiency (CVID)

CVID-Like

▶ Unclassified Primary Antibody Deficiency (unPAD)

CXCL12 – Cysteine-X-Cysteine Chemokine Ligand 12

▶ Warts, Hypogammaglobulinemia, Infections, Myelokathexis (WHIM) Syndrome

CXCR4 – Cysteine-X-Cysteine Chemokine Receptor 4

▶ Warts, Hypogammaglobulinemia, Infections, Myelokathexis (WHIM) Syndrome

CYBB X-Linked Chronic Granulomatous Disease (CGD)

Antonio Condino-Neto[1] and Peter E. Newburger[2]
[1]Department of Immunology, Institute of Biomedical Sciences – University of São Paulo, São Paulo, SP, Brazil
[2]Department of Pediatrics, Division of Hematology/Oncology, University of Massachusetts Medical School, Worcester, MA, USA

Chronic granulomatous disease (CGD) is a primary immunodeficiency which was originally characterized in the 1950s as a clinical entity affecting male infants and termed "fatal granulomatous disease of childhood." CGD is characterized by early onset of severe recurrent infections affecting mainly the natural barriers of the organism such as the respiratory tract and lymph nodes, and eventually internal structures such as the liver, spleen, bones, and brain. The estimated incidence of this disease is approximately 1/250,000 live births per year. CGD can also present with abnormal inflammatory responses, which often result in the dysregulated granuloma formation in inflamed tissues (Arnold and Heimall 2017; Roos 2016; Holland 2013).

Phagocytes, such as monocytes/macrophages, contain a membrane-associated nicotinamide adenine dinucleotide phosphate (NADPH) oxidase that produces superoxide and other reactive oxygen intermediates involved in microbicidal, tumoricidal, and inflammatory activities. Defects in NADPH oxidase activity lead to defective superoxide production and predispose the patient to severe, life-threatening infections, generally by catalase-positive pathogens, which demonstrate the importance of the oxygen-dependent microbicidal system in host defense (Arnold and Heimall 2017; Roos 2016; Holland 2013). Phagocyte NADPH oxidase activation results in conversion of molecular oxygen to superoxide anion. Superoxide dismutase converts superoxide anion to hydrogen peroxide. In neutrophils, myeloperoxidase (MPO) catalyzes the production of hypochlorous acid from hydrogen peroxide and chloride ions (Arnold and Heimall 2017; Roos 2016; Holland 2013). The terminal electron donor to oxygen is a unique low-midpoint-potential flavocytochrome b, cytochrome b_{558}, a heterodimer composed of a 91 kDa glycoprotein (termed gp91-$phox$, for glycoprotein 91 kDa of $phagocyte$ $oxidase$) and a 22 kDa non-glycosylated polypeptide (p22-$phox$). Upon activation, the cytoplasmic subunits p47$phox$, p67$phox$, p40$phox$, and rac protein translocate to the membrane-bound cytochrome b_{558}.

The X-linked form of the disease is caused by mutations in the *CYBB* gene encoding the heavy chain of the flavocytochrome b (also called cytochrome b_{558}) component (gp91-phox) and accounts approximately 60% of the cases in the western world. *CYBB* is fully expressed in differentiated phagocytes and is induced by various cytokines, including interferon-gamma (IFN-γ) (Arnold and Heimall 2017; Roos 2016; Holland 2013; Rae et al. 1998). In the X-linked form, the defective component is represented by the molecular weight of the protein, "91"; and the level of expression of such protein is designated as "0" for absent, "+" for present, and "- "for reduced. The X91^0 phenotype is the most frequent and results in the absence of cytochrome b_{558} and absent NADPH oxidase activity. The X91$^-$ phenotype designates the mild variant form of CGD. The X91$^+$ phenotype has normal levels of cytochrome b_{558}; however, the NADPH oxidase activity is decreased or absent (Arnold and Heimall 2017; Roos 2016; Holland 2013; Rae et al. 1998). The *CYBB* gene was localized to the short arm of the X chromosome at segment Xp21.1. The complete *CYBB* gene spans approximately 30 kb and contains 13 exons (Arnold and Heimall 2017; Roos 2016; Holland 2013; Rae et al. 1998). Gene mutations leading to X-linked CGD have been identified in a similar frequency in the coding region, introns, and (rarely) 5' flanking regulatory regions of the *CYBB* gene. These mutations include large multigenic deletions, minor deletions and insertions, missense or nonsense substitutions, and splicing defects (Arnold and Heimall 2017; Roos 2016; Holland 2013; Rae et al. 1998).

Clinical Presentation

X-linked CGD should be suspected in boys with failure to thrive, early onset of recurrent pneumonias, lymphadenitis, liver abscess, osteomyelitis, and skin infections (pyoderma, abscesses, or cellulitis). Other clinical manifestations include granuloma formation, especially genitourinary and gastrointestinal (often initially pyloric and later esophageal, jejunal, ileal, cecal, rectal, and perirectal), and colitis, presenting as frequent stooling and fistulae or fissures. This may be the sole finding in some individuals. Abnormal wound healing caused by excessive granulation may also occur. A single infection by a characteristic organism – e.g., BCG, *Serratia* spp., *Burkholderia cepacia*, or *Chromobacterium violaceum* – should raise immediate suspicion of CGD (Roos and de Boer 2014; Thomsen et al. 2016).

The types of infections seen in CGD vary widely in different geographical regions. In the USA and Europe, the most frequent causative agents are *Staphylococcus aureus*, *Burkholderia cepacia*, *Serratia marcescens*, *Nocardia*, and *Aspergillus*. In other parts of the world, *Salmonella*, Bacillus Calmette-Guerin (BCG), *Mycobacterium tuberculosis*, *Burkholderia pseudomallei*, and *Chromobacterium violaceum* are also important (Marciano et al. 2015; de Oliveira-Junior et al. 2015; Winkelstein et al. 2000; van den Berg et al. 2009; Lee and Lau 2017). In a US registry of 368 patients with CGD, pneumonia was the most frequent infection, with *Aspergillus* spp. being the most common pathogens. Other major infections included suppurative adenitis, soft tissue abscesses, and liver abscesses with *Staphylococcus aureus* being

the most common cause. *Serratia* spp. infection (commonly manifesting as osteomyelitis), *Burkholderia cepacia* (commonly manifesting as pneumonia and sepsis), and *Salmonella* sepsis were common complications (Winkelstein et al. 2000). The median age at death has increased from 15 years before 1990 to 28 years after year 2000. Analysis of clinical data from 429 European patients with CGD showed that the most frequent pathogens per episode were *Staphylococcus aureus* (30%) and *Aspergillus* spp. (26%). Clinical outcomes and occurrences were similar compared to US data (8). Analysis of the Latin American Society of Primary Immunodeficiencies (LASID) database shows 71 patients with CGD with a confirmed genetic diagnosis. Fifty-six patients had genetically confirmed X-linked CGD. Within this cohort of patients, 26% of the cases had a family history of recurrent or unusual infections. Recurrent pneumonia (76.8%) was the most frequent clinical condition, from which 13% of the cases presented with concomitant pleural effusion. Other clinical manifestations included lymphadenopathy (59.4%), granulomata (49.3%), skin infections (42%), chronic diarrhea (41.9%), otitis (29%), sepsis (23.2%), liver abscesses (21.7%), recurrent urinary tract infections (20.3%), and osteomyelitis (15.9%). A broad range of etiologic organisms were involved: *Staphylococcus aureus*, *Escherichia coli*, *Aspergillus* spp., *Serratia marcescens*, *Candida* spp., *Klebsiella* spp., *Salmonella* spp., and *Nocardia* spp. Other pathogens isolated from this cohort included *Acinetobacter* spp., *Pseudomonas* spp., H1N1 virus, rotavirus, adenovirus, *Trichophyton*, *Ascaris* spp., and *Giardia* spp. Approximately 85% of the X-linked CGD patients presented with significant adverse reactions to BCG vaccination (de Oliveira-Junior et al. 2015).

Clinicians should be familiar with local epidemiology and be aware of unusual microorganisms as causative pathogens when evaluating CGD patients with infections. Special attention to these pathogens should be given to CGD patients after returning from endemic regions. Microbiological confirmation must be pursued, and appropriate antimicrobial regimen should be given. BCG vaccine is contraindicated in CGD and should be withheld for neonates who have a family history of CGD or suspected primary immunodeficiency disease until excluded by appropriate investigations (de Oliveira-Junior et al. 2015; Lee and Lau 2017).

Patients with X-linked CGD typically have a greater risk for infectious complications than autosomal recessive forms of CGD. This increased risk likely reflects the complete absence of NADPH oxidase activity with mutations that completely disable gp91*phox* function. Residual NADPH oxidase activity in neutrophils from CGD patients is associated with less severe illness and a greater likelihood of long-term survival than for patients with little or no NADPH oxidase function, demonstrating that even low residual levels of ROS formation in neutrophils are protective (Kuhns et al. 2010).

Laboratory Findings/Diagnostic Testing

Laboratory diagnosis of CGD is made by direct measurement of superoxide or peroxide production by ferricytochrome c reduction, chemiluminescence, nitroblue tetrazolium (NBT) reduction, or dihydrorhodamine oxidation (DHR). DHR is currently the most popular test because of its relative ease of use, its ability to distinguish X-linked from autosomal forms of CGD, and its sensitivity to even very low numbers of functional neutrophils. The DHR test uses flow cytometry to measure fluorescence emitted during the oxidation of dihydrorhodamine 123 to rhodamine 123 in phorbol myristate acetate (PMA)-stimulated neutrophils, as a marker for cellular NADPH oxidase activity. Mean fluorescence intensity of the activated cells correlates directly with (and thus serves as a reliable surrogate for) superoxide production (Roos and de Boer 2014; Thomsen et al. 2016). Female carriers of X-linked CGD have two populations of phagocytes due to X-chromosomal inactivation: one population produces superoxide and one does not, giving carriers a characteristic bimodal pattern on oxidase testing. Infections are not usually seen in female carriers unless the proportion of normal neutrophils is below 5–10%. The NBT reduction test

relies on light microscopy to provide a qualitative determination of phagocyte NADPH oxidase activity. When stimulated in vitro, normal phagocytes produce superoxide that reduces yellow NBT to blue/black formazan, forming a precipitate in cells. The NBT test is typically performed on a microscope slide, which is read manually to distinguish reducing (blue-black) from non-reducing (unstained) cells. In normal individuals, more than 95% of cells produce superoxide that reduces NBT to formazan. In individuals with CGD, production of superoxide is absent or greatly diminished. In female carriers of X-linked CGD (who have two populations of leukocytes), superoxide is typically produced in 20–80% of cells (Roos and de Boer 2014; Thomsen et al. 2016). Early-onset, more severe infections and male sex suggest X-linked CGD, and *CYBB* gene analysis may be considered first as a target for direct sequencing after establishment of the diagnosis by DHR or NBT testing.

Treatment/Prognosis

Prophylaxis in CGD
Standard infection prophylaxis for CGD includes an antibacterial agent, a mold-active antifungal agent, and recombinant interferon-γ (Thomsen et al. 2016).

Antibacterial Prophylaxis
Trimethoprim-sulfamethoxazole has been used for decades in CGD. This agent has been proven to be safe and effective in reducing bacterial infections. -Trimethoprim-sulfamethoxazole is active against most of bacterial pathogens that cause infection in CGD, including *S. aureus*, *Burkholderia* spp., and *Nocardia* spp. In CGD patients who are allergic or intolerant of trimethoprim-sulfamethoxazole, alternative agents (e.g., cephalexin or doxycycline) with anti-staphylococcal activity should be used as prophylaxis (Arnold and Heimall 2017; Roos 2016; Holland 2013; Thomsen et al. 2016).

Antifungal Prophylaxis
Prevention of invasive aspergillosis and other filamentous fungal diseases relies on avoiding

environments where high levels of fungal spores are expected (e.g., playing on mulch or wood chips, gardening, and building renovations) and mold-active antifungal prophylaxis. Itraconazole prophylaxis has been shown to be safe and effective in patients with CGD. Other mold-active azoles are voriconazole and posaconazole (Arnold and Heimall 2017; Roos 2016; Holland 2013; Thomsen et al. 2016).

Recombinant Interferon-γ

Recombinant interferon-γ has been widely used as prophylaxis in patients with CGD for approximately 25 years. In a randomized trial, recombinant interferon-γ reduced in 70% the incidence of serious infections and was beneficial regardless of age, the use of prophylactic antibiotics, or the type of CGD (X-linked or autosomal recessive). The benefit of prophylactic recombinant interferon-γ may result from augmentation of oxidant-independent pathways, as well as an increase in oxidase activity in variant CGD cases with residual NADPH oxidase function. Long-term recombinant interferon-γ has been generally well tolerated in CGD, with fever being the most frequent side effect (Arnold and Heimall 2017; Roos 2016; Holland 2013; Thomsen et al. 2016).

Treatment of Infections in CGD

Invasive bacterial infections (e.g., pneumonia, osteomyelitis, and deep soft tissue infections) require prolonged antibiotic therapy. Bacterial infections involving bone or viscera frequently require surgery. Decisions about surgical intervention must be individualized based on the pathogen, location and extent of disease, and likelihood of response to antibacterial treatment alone (Arnold and Heimall 2017; Roos 2016; Holland 2013; Thomsen et al. 2016).

Voriconazole was shown to be superior to conventional amphotericin B as primary therapy for aspergillosis. Lipid formulations of amphotericin B, posaconazole, isavuconazole, and echinocandins are additional options for therapy of invasive aspergillosis in patients who are intolerant to voriconazole or who have refractory disease. In addition to antifungal therapy,

debridement or resection of infected tissue may be required. This is particularly the case for refractory aspergillosis or extension of fungal disease to vertebrae or chest wall (Arnold and Heimall 2017; Roos 2016; Holland 2013; Thomsen et al. 2016).

Granulocyte Transfusions

Adjunctive granulocyte transfusions have been used for severe or refractory infections in CGD patients, based on the likelihood that a proportion of normal neutrophils can augment host defense in CGD neutrophils by providing a source of diffusible ROS. Hydrogen peroxide generated by normal neutrophils can diffuse into CGD neutrophils and provide the necessary substrate to generate hypochlorous acid and hydroxyl anion in vitro. Alloimmunization is a potential complication when performing granulocyte transfusion, as this can be a major stumbling block to allogeneic stem cell transplantation (Arnold and Heimall 2017; Roos 2016; Holland 2013; Thomsen et al. 2016).

Hematopoietic Stem Cell Transplantation and Gene Therapy

Allogeneic hematopoietic stem cell transplantation is usually curative in CGD and is becoming accepted as a standard of care for those cases with severe recurrent infections, intensive inflammatory disease and no residual oxidative respiratory burst infection. The major risk is graft-versus-host disease. There are gene therapy approaches under current development to treat CGD with variable success rates (Arnold and Heimall 2017; Roos 2016; Holland 2013; Thomsen et al. 2016).

Prognosis

Since the advent of prophylactic antibiotics, antifungals, and recombinant interferon-γ, the prognosis for patients with CGD has improved. Patients living to their 30s and 40s are now common (Arnold and Heimall 2017; Roos 2016; Holland 2013). The production of residual ROS is predicted by the specific NADPH oxidase mutation and is a predictor of survival in patients with CGD (Arnold and Heimall 2017; Roos 2016; Holland 2013).

Survival rates are variable but improving; approximately 50% of patients survive to age 30–40 years. Infections are less common in adults than in children, but the propensity for severe life-threatening bacterial infections persists throughout life. Fungal infections remain a major determinant of survival in CGD (Arnold and Heimall 2017; Roos 2016; Holland 2013). Currently, the annual mortality rate is 1.5% per year for persons with autosomal recessive CGD and 5% for those with X-linked CGD (Arnold and Heimall 2017; Roos 2016; Holland 2013). Morbidity secondary to infection or granulomatous complications remains significant for many patients, particularly those with the X-linked form.

Cross-References

▶ Autosomal Recessive CGD (NCF-1, NCF-2, CYBA, NCF4)

References

Arnold DE, Heimall JR. A review of chronic granulomatous disease. Adv Ther. 2017;34(12):2543–57. https://doi.org/10.1007/s12325-017-0636-2.

de Oliveira-Junior EB, Zurro NB, Prando C, Cabral-Marques O, Pereira PV, Schimke LF, Klaver S, Buzolin M, Blancas-Galicia L, Santos-Argumedo L, Pietropaolo-Cienfuegos DR, Espinosa-Rosales F, King A, Sorensen R, Porras O, Roxo-Junior P, Forte WC, Orellana JC, Lozano A, Galicchio M, Regairaz L, Grumach AS, Costa-Carvalho BT, Bustamante J, Bezrodnik L, Oleastro M, Danielian S, Condino-Neto A. Clinical and genotypic spectrum of chronic granulomatous disease in 71 Latin American patients: first report from the LASID registry. Pediatr Blood Cancer. 2015;62(12):2101–7. https://doi.org/10.1002/pbc.25674.

Holland SM. Chronic granulomatous disease. Hematol Oncol Clin North Am. 2013;27(1):89–99. https://doi.org/10.1016/j.hoc.2012.11.002, viii

Kuhns DB, Alvord WG, Heller T, Feld JJ, Pike KM, Marciano BE, Uzel G, DeRavin SS, Priel DA, Soule BP, Zarember KA, Malech HL, Holland SM, Gallin JI. Residual NADPH oxidase and survival in chronic granulomatous disease. N Engl J Med. 2010;363(27):2600–10. https://doi.org/10.1056/NEJMoa1007097.

Lee P, Lau Y-L. Endemic infections in chronic granulomatous disease. In: Seger RA, Roos D, Segal BH, Kuijpers TW, editors. Immunology and immune system disorders. Chronic granulomatous disease genetics, biology and clinical management. Nova Science Publishers; 2017. p. 125–61.

Marciano BE, Spalding C, Fitzgerald A, Mann D, Brown T, Osgood S, Yockey L, Darnell DN, Barnhart L, Daub J, Boris L, Rump AP, Anderson VL, Haney C, Kuhns DB, Rosenzweig SD, Kelly C, Zelazny A, Mason T, DeRavin SS, Kang E, Gallin JI, Malech HL, Olivier KN, Uzel G, Freeman AF, Heller T, Zerbe CS, Holland SM. Common severe infections in chronic granulomatous disease. Clin Infect Dis. 2015;60(8):1176–83. https://doi.org/10.1093/cid/ciu1154.

Rae J, Newburger PE, Dinauer MC, Noack D, Hopkins PJ, Kuruto R, Curnutte JT. X-linked chronic granulomatous disease: mutations in the CYBB gene encoding the gp91-phox component of respiratory-burst oxidase. Am J Hum Genet. 1998;62(6):1320–31.

Roos D. Chronic granulomatous disease. Br Med Bull. 2016;118(1):50–63. https://doi.org/10.1093/bmb/ldw009.

Roos D, de Boer M. Molecular diagnosis of chronic granulomatous disease. Clin Exp Immunol. 2014;175(2):139–49. https://doi.org/10.1111/cei.12202.

Thomsen IP, Smith MA, Holland SM, Creech CB. A comprehensive approach to the management of children and adults with chronic granulomatous disease. J Allergy Clin Immunol Pract. 2016;4(6):1082–8. https://doi.org/10.1016/j.jaip.2016.03.021.

van den Berg JM, van Koppen E, Ahlin A, Belohradsky BH, Bernatowska E, Corbeel L, Español T, Fischer A, Kurenko-Deptuch M, Mouy R, Petropoulou T, Roesler J, Seger R, Stasia MJ, Valerius NH, Weening RS, Wolach B, Roos D, Kuijpers TW. Chronic granulomatous disease: the European experience. PLoS One. 2009;4(4):e5234. https://doi.org/10.1371/journal.pone.0005234.

Winkelstein JA, Marino MC, Johnston RB Jr, Boyle J, Curnutte J, Gallin JI, Malech HL, Holland SM, Ochs H, Quie P, Buckley RH, Foster CB, Chanock SJ, Dickler H. Chronic granulomatous disease. Report on a national registry of 368 patients. Medicine (Baltimore). 2000;79(3):155–69.

Cyclic Hematopoiesis

▶ Cyclic Neutropenia

Cyclic Neutropenia

Eli Mansour and Bruna Bombassaro
Division of Clinical Immunology and Allergy,
Department of Clinical Medicine, State
University of Campinas (UNICAMP), Campinas,
Brazil

Synonyms

Cyclic hematopoiesis; Periodic neutropenia

Definition

Cyclic neutropenia (OMIM #162800) is an auto-somal dominant or de novo autosomal disease caused by mutations on the *ELANE* (formerly known as *ELA2*) gene that encodes for neutrophil elastase. *ELANE* gene localization is 19p13.3.

Introduction

Cyclic neutropenia was first mentioned by Reimann and DeBerardinis in the 1940s as they observed a cyclic phenomenon of increase and decrease in neutrophil counts within 18–21 days (Donadieu et al. 2017). In 1999, Horwitz and colleagues identified mutations in the neutrophil elastase gene (*ELANE*), which were also found in patients with severe congenital neutropenia 1 (SCN1, OMIM #202700). As the same mutation is observed in patients with cyclic neutropenia and permanent SCN and the cyclic aspect is rarely seen in clinical practice, some authors believe that there is a continuum between SCN and intermittent/cyclic neutropenia (Donadieu et al. 2017). Additionally, intermittent neutropenia can occur in other inborn errors of immunity such as Shwachman-Diamond syndrome (Costa-Carvalho et al. 2014) or mutation *HAX1* (Cipe et al. 2018).

Pathogenesis and Genetics

Neutrophil elastase (NE) is a cytotoxic serine protease stored in granules of neutrophils and macrophages. NE is produced during the promyelocyte stage, and the newly formed protein goes to the endoplasmic reticulum where it can be folded and packaged in granules. The NE is released during inflammation to destroy microorganisms and contribute to tissue damage (Skokowa et al. 2017; Spoor et al. 2019). Cyclic neutropenia is of an autosomal dominant inheritance due to mutations in the *ELANE* gene, most of them being missense mutations (around 80%) (Xia and Link 2008). There is a substantial overlap in the mutations causing SCN and those causing cyclic neutropenia. *ELANE* mutations lead to the synthesis of nonfunctional and misfolded NE proteins which accumulate in the endoplasmic reticulum (ER). This process leads to ER stress that triggers an unfold protein response (UPR) to reduce ER stress, reestablish ER homeostasis, and prevent cell death. Prolonged ER stress, however, leads to apoptosis of neutrophils in the bone marrow. Why the same *ELANE* mutations activate UPR in SCN and not in cyclic neutropenia is still an open question. Recent findings suggest the presence of an UPR inhibitor in cyclic neutropenia, protecting the cell from the apoptosis seen in SCN and accounting for a milder disease (Donadieu et al. 2017; Skokowa et al. 2017; Spoor et al. 2019).

Clinical Presentation

Cyclic neutropenia has a characteristic periodic oscillation in peripheral neutrophil counts varying from normal to very low ($<500/mm^3$). In general, this oscillation occurs in a 21-day cycle; this period is not always seen, but rather an intermittent neutropenia may be found. There is an inverse relation between neutropenia and monocytes. During neutropenia, monocytosis can be observed and return to normal with reversion of neutropenia. Eosinophilia and hypergammaglobulinemia are also frequently associated with neutropenia (Donadieu et al. 2017; Spoor et al. 2019).

Cyclic neutropenia is considered a more benign disorder. Infections occur during periods of neutropenia. Patients may present recurrent bacterial infections of mucous membranes and the skin. The most common manifestations are fever, oral ulcerations, gingivitis and secondary teeth damage, skin infections, and respiratory tract infections. Mortality from sepsis or acute myeloid leukemia (AML) or myelodysplastic syndrome (MDS) is less common than with SCN. The most frequent infectious agents are *Staphylococcus aureus*, *S. epidermidis*, streptococci, enterococci, pneumococci, *Pseudomonas aeruginosa*, and Gram-negative bacilli (Donadieu et al. 2017; Spoor et al. 2019).

Diagnosis

Medical and family history and a careful exam are important, and if possible previous exams can be helpful to determine if neutropenia is acute or chronic, permanent or intermittent (Dale 2016). For the diagnosis of cyclic neutropenia, classically, two to three complete peripheral blood counts per week for 6 consecutive weeks are needed (Cipe et al. 2018). Bone marrow examination is important for the evaluation of SCN but can be considered, exceptionally, in cyclic neutropenia patients to rule out leukemia, myelodysplasia, or aplastic anemia (Skokowa et al. 2017).

Genetic analysis is increasingly important in confirming the diagnosis in most primary immunodeficiency diseases. As *ELANE* mutation is the most common cause of cyclic neutropenia as well as SCN, *ELANE* sequencing is the first step. If negative, other genes associated with neutropenia, like *HAX1*, *G6PC3*, *WAS*, and *SBD*S, can be analyzed (Dale 2016; Skokowa et al. 2017).

Treatment

The only treatment modalities available in the past were general measures such as skin and oral hygiene, supportive care, and aggressive broad-spectrum antibiotics to treat infections. Antibiotic prophylaxis with sulfamethoxazole-trimethoprim (SMX-TMP) decreases the frequency of infection but is now considered secondary to G-CSF. Although important, these measures alone are insufficient (Kuruvilla and de la Morena 2013; Dale 2016; Spoor et al. 2019). Therefore, recombinant granulocyte colony-stimulating factor (G-CSF), a myeloid growth factor, is considered as first treatment as it stimulates the development and function of neutrophils. G-CSF is given subcutaneously, daily, on alternate days, or three times per week. For cyclic neutropenia the median starting dose is 2.4 mcg/kg/day (1–3 μg/kg per day). The most common adverse events are related to the initiation of G-CSF: bone pain, headache, and myalgias. Splenomegaly, thrombocytopenia, and osteopenia/osteoporosis may occur. While controversial, AML and MDS were reported as secondary effects of G-CSF use. Hematopoietic stem cell transplantation (HSCT) is recommended for severe cases, such as SCN, unresponsive to G-CSF or for the treatment of AML or MDS. The administration of neutrophil elastase inhibitors and vector-mediated gene therapy for *ELANE*-positive SCN is under investigation. Whether these new treatment modalities will be applied to cyclic neutropenia remains to be seen (Dale 2016; Skokowa et al. 2017; Spoor et al. 2019).

Cyclic neutropenia patients should receive all inactivated vaccines, and annual inactivated influenza vaccine can be considered. Live viral vaccines are also recommended. Live bacterial vaccines, like BCG, should be avoided (Sobh and Bonilla 2016).

References

Cipe FE, Celiksoy MH, Erturk B, Aydogmus Ç. Cyclic manner of neutropenia in a patient with HAX-1 mutation. Pediatr Hematol Oncol. 2018;35:181–5.

Costa-Carvalho BT, Grumach AS, Franco JL, Espinosa-Rosales FJ, et al. Attending to warning signs of primary immunodeficiency diseases across the range of clinical practice. J Clin Immunol. 2014;34:10–22.

Dale DC. How I diagnose and treat neutropenia. Curr Opin Hematol. 2016;23:1–4.

Donadieu J, Beaupain B, Fenneteau O, Bellanné-Chantelot C. Congenital neutropenia in the era of genomics: classification, diagnosis, and natural history. Br J Haematol. 2017;179:557–74.

Kuruvilla M, de la Morena MT. Antibiotic prophylaxis in primary immune deficiency disorders. J Allergy Clin Immunol Pract. 2013;1:573–82.

Skokowa J, Dale DC, Touw IP, et al. Severe congenital neutropenias. Nat Rev Dis Primers. 2017;3:17032.

Sobh A, Bonilla FA. Vaccination in primary immunodeficiency disorders. J Allergy Clin Immunol Pract. 2016;4:1066–75.

Spoor J, Farajifard H, Rezaei N. Congenital neutropenia and primary immunodeficiency diseases. Crit Rev Oncol Hematol. 2019;133:149–62.

Xia J, Link DC. Severe congenital neutropenia and the unfolded protein response. Curr Opin Hematol. 2008;15:1–7.

Cytidine 5-Prime Triphosphate Synthase 1 (CTPS1) Deficiency (OMIM # 615897)

Thomas G. Fox

Department of Pediatrics, Section of Pediatric Infectious Diseases, Indiana University School of Medicine, Riley Hospital for Children, Indianapolis, IN, USA

Department of Pediatrics, Division of Pediatric Infectious Disease, Emory University School of Medicine, Atlanta, GA, USA

Introduction/Background

Deficiency in cytidine 5-prime triphosphate synthase 1 (CTPS1) causes a combined immunodeficiency affecting both cellular and humoral immunity. CTPS1, one of two mammalian CTP synthases (the other being CTPS2), catalyzes the formation of CTP, an essential nucleotide for DNA and RNA synthesis (Veillette and Davidson 2014). The *CTPS1* gene is located on chromosome 1p34.2. CPTS1 is expressed in lymphocytes at very low levels, but marked upregulation in T cells occurs upon activation. Lymphocytes from patients with CTPS1 deficiency have reduced intracellular levels of CTP but not the mRNA transcript product, which suggests a defect in protein stability (Martin et al. 2014). Lymphocytes arrest in G1 phase of cellular replication, severely limiting lymphocyte expansion following activation.

The diagnosis of CTPS1 deficiency is difficult. Patients can have a relatively normal immunologic workup, especially in the absence of chronic EBV infection (Truck et al. 2016). Humoral immunity can appear normal despite susceptibility to invasive bacterial disease (Truck et al. 2016). It is noteworthy that all cases to date have been diagnosed using whole exome sequencing (WES). The ultimate prognosis is unclear, and the clinical severity and disease course is variable. Hematopoietic stem cell transplantation (HCT) can be curative.

Clinical Presentation

This immunodeficiency manifests in early childhood and is associated with chronic infection with Epstein-Barr virus (EBV), severe viral infections, and invasive infection with encapsulated bacteria. Although lymphoproliferative disease is common, extrahematopoietic manifestations have not been reported.

Martin et al. provided the first report of CTPS1 deficiency in 2014 with a description of eight cases from five unrelated families in northwest England (Martin et al. 2014). The investigators identified a common homozygous guanine to cytosine (G > C) mutation in the *CTPS1* gene in affected individuals; parents were found to be heterozygous. As a proof of concept, the group replicated the conditions in vitro by reducing CTPS1 expression in normal lymphocytes using lentiviral transduction of short hairpin RNA's. They showed that CTPS1 expression could be restored through retrovirus-mediated gene transfer.

The age at onset varied from birth to age 5 years. Most patients had a history of recurrent bacterial respiratory tract infections with encapsulated organisms. Two patients had invasive bacterial infection, one with pneumococcal sepsis and meningitis and the other with meningococcal meningitis. All patients suffered from chronic EBV infection. Additional viral infections seen in this cohort included varicella, adenovirus, human herpesvirus 6 (HHV-6), and cytomegalovirus. Gastrointestinal disease with rotavirus and norovirus was reported in four patients. One patient died from disseminated varicella. Two patients had EBV-driven B cell non-Hodgkin lymphoma (Martin et al. 2014).

Following the initial report, two independent groups reported sibling pairs (two patients in each study; four total) with the disorder bringing the total number of cases in the literature to twelve. Interestingly, all patients with the disorder reported to date resided in or had ancestors from northwest England. DNA sequencing of a healthy cohort from this region of England revealed an estimated frequency of homozygosity of 1:560,000, tenfold higher than that estimated from other exome databases, suggesting a founder effect (Martin et al. 2014).

Kucuk et al. reported the first cases from the USA (Kucuk et al. 2016). They describe two sisters born to nonconsanguineous parents with ancestry from northern England who presented with recurrent sinopulmonary infections, chronic EBV, and cutaneous varicella. At 18 months of age, the index patient developed recurrent cutaneous varicella with varicella zoster viremia and presumed varicella hepatitis. She later suffered an acute ischemic stroke at which time she was discovered to have acute EBV. Her sister had parvovirus infection with anemia requiring red blood cell transfusions at age 2.5. She had a history of recurrent pneumonia and at age three had pneumococcal pneumonia with effusion. At age 3.5 years, she had severe tonsillitis and was diagnosed with acute EBV. Both siblings had chronic EBV viremia. They also had abdominal lymphadenopathy with EBV+ biopsies without evidence of malignancy. The siblings had previously undergone HCT ten and eleven years prior the report, respectively, and were alive and well without evidence of persistent immunologic derangement. The investigators used WES from saved fibroblast genomic DNA to identify the same homozygous G- > C mutation in *CTPS1* in both children.

Truck et al. used WES to identify CTPS1 deficiency in two siblings (male and female) from northern England born to nonconsanguineous parents (Truck et al. 2016). The index patient (male) had a history of recurrent otitis media and lower respiratory tract infections starting in infancy. He had a culture-negative sepsis episode at age

2 months and invasive pneumococcal disease at 7 months due to serotype 19A, despite having received two doses of 13-valent pneumococcal conjugate vaccine. He experienced acute EBV at 34 months and subsequently developed persistent EBV viremia. His sister had an episode of aseptic meningitis at 8 months and at 12 months began suffering from recurrent upper and lower respiratory tract infections. However, she did not have recurrent otitis media and had no invasive bacterial infections. She also had no evidence of EBV infection and remained EBV naïve at the time of study publication. Both children suffered from chronic diarrhea and eczema, symptoms not previously described with CTPS1 deficiency.

Despite the variation in clinical presentation, age of onset, and severity of disease, common themes emerge from the twelve patients reported thus far with CTPS1 deficiency. A combined cellular and humoral immune deficiency pattern is observed, with severe and chronic viral infections and susceptibility to invasive bacterial infections. Chronic EBV infection with persistent viremia is nearly universal following acute infection. There are no reports of growth abnormalities or dysmorphic facial features. Lymphoproliferative disease is reported, likely a consequence of unchecked EBV infection. Despite repeated respiratory infections, bronchiectasis has been notably absent. It is also interesting that hemophagocytic lymphohistiocytosis has not been seen with CTPS1 deficiency. See Table 1 for a summary of the clinical phenotypes, immunologic profiles, and outcomes of the twelve reported cases.

Diagnosis and Laboratory Testing

An important consideration is that the initial immunological evaluation in patients with CTPS1 deficiency can be normal. Important to consider is that chronic infection with viruses, especially EBV, likely has a significant impact on the degree of lymphopenia and T cell disturbance (Truck et al. 2016). Chronic EBV can substantially impact B cell populations, particularly memory B cells. Complete blood counts are often normal. Impairment of T cell proliferative

Cytidine 5-Prime Triphosphate Synthase 1 (CTPS1) Deficiency (OMIM # 615897), **Table 1** Clinical, immunologic profile, and outcome of twelve patients with CTPS1 deficiency

Patient	Age at onset of symptoms	Bacterial infections	Viral infections	Other clinical findings	Summary of immunologic findings	HSCT	Outcome
1*	18 months	Recurrent sinopulmonary	Chronic EBV; recurrent VZV with hepatitis and viremia	Ischemic stroke; EBV+ abdominal lymphadenopathy	Decreased IgM, IgA, IgG2; decreased vaccine titers; decreased T cell proliferation to mitogens/antigens	MUD BMT 8/8 donor EBV+, CMV-; RIC; engrafted +10	Alive and well
2*	2.5 years	Recurrent pneumonia	Chronic EBV; parvovirus with anemia requiring transfusion	EBV+ abdominal lymphadenopathy	—	MUD BMT 7/8 donor EBV+, CMV-; RIC; engrafted +14	Alive and well
3**	2 months	Pneumococcal sepsis; recurrent otitis media	Chronic EBV	Chronic diarrhea	Poor persistence of vaccine titers; lymphopenia and B cell deficiency from chronic EBV; low naïve B cells; normal CD4; low memory and terminally differentiated CD8	MUD peripheral SCT; RIC with in vivo T cell depletion	Alive and well
4**	8 months	Recurrent sinopulmonary	Aseptic meningitis; EBV naïve	Eczema	Poor response to booster PCV and Hib boosters; low memory and terminally differentiated CD8	Considered	Alive
5***	1 year	Recurrent sinopulmonary	Chronic EBV; CMV, rotavirus	—	—	HSCT (8y)	Died (GVHD)
6***	1 month	None	Chronic EBV; adenovirus, HHV-6, norovirus	—	Naïve CD4 lymphopenia; increased effector memory T; low memory CD27 B; absence of invariant T cell populations; impaired mitogen/antigen responses	No	Alive

			Varicella	CNS LPD		HSCT	Alive and well
7#	5 years	Recurrent sinopulmonary		–	–	HSCT (9y)	Alive and well
8#	2 years	Recurrent sinopulmonary	Chronic EBV	–	–	HSCT (7y)	Alive and well
9^	1 year	Invasive pneumococcal (sepsis, meningitis)	EBV; VZV (disseminated)	–	–	No	Died (disseminated VZV)
10^	3 months	None	Chronic EBV; VZV; HHV-6	–	–	HSCT (8y)	Alive and well
11	Birth	None	EBV; VZV; CMV, adenovirus, rotavirus	CNS LPD (NHL; EBV)	–	HSCT (6y)	Died (LPD)
12	3 months	Invasive meningococcal (meningitis)	Chronic EBV; norovirus, adenovirus	CNS LPD (NHL; EBV)	–	HSCT (1y)	Alive

*, **, *** #, ^ denote sibling pairs

Abbreviations: *MUD* matched unrelated donor, *BMT* bone marrow transplant, *RIC* reduced intensity conditioning, *PCV* pneumococcal conjugate vaccine, *GVHD* graft versus host disease, *CNS LPD* central nervous system lymphoproliferative disease, *VZV* varicella zoster virus, *CMV* cytomegalovirus

Sources: Kucuk et al. 2016 (patients 1, 2); Truck et al. 2016 (patients 3, 4); Martin et al. 2014 (patients 5–12)

responses to mitogens and antigens is common, but not universal. Similarly, reduced serologic responses to vaccine antigens are not uniformly observed. Serum immunoglobulin levels are usually normal or only modestly reduced (See Table 1).

The eight patients from Martin et al. shared common immunologic features: variable lymphopenia that correlated with viral infections; inversed CD4:CD8 ratio; normal blood counts and immunoglobulin levels; and low titers to pneumococcal antigens. More detailed immunological results are available from the second patient. This child suffered infections from EBV, adenovirus, and HHV-6 starting at 1 month of age. Specific immunologic findings included naïve CD4 lymphopenia, with increased effector memory T cells; low CD27 memory B cells; absence of invariant T cell populations (mucosal associated invariant T cells and invariant natural killer T cells); and impaired mitogen and antigen proliferative T cell responses.

Kucuk et al. provide detailed results from the immunologic workup of the index patient, a 3-year-old girl with recurrent sinopulmonary infections, persistent EBV, and recurrent varicella infections (including varicella viremia and hepatitis). She had decreased levels of IgM, IgA, and IgG2; decreased diphtheria, tetanus, and pneumococcal titers; decreased T cell responses to mitogens and antigens; decreased naïve CD8 T cells; and decreased CD3CD8αβ with increased CD3CD8γδ T cells (during EBV viremia).

The index patient from Truck et al. had normal serum immunoglobulins. However, this patient had moderate responses to the 13-valent pneumococcal conjugate vaccine and antibodies to *Haemophilus influenzae* and tetanus toxoid waned quickly over time. Lymphopenia and low B cell numbers were observed, attributable to chronic EBV. The index patient's sister, also with recurrent respiratory tract infections but naïve to EBV, had poor responses to pneumococcal conjugate and *Haemophilus influenzae* b vaccines. Both children had elevated transitional B cells, low naïve B cells, and normal CD4 populations but decreased numbers of different CD8 subpopulations.

Treatment and Prognosis

The optimal treatment and ultimate prognosis in patients with CTPS1 deficiency is unknown. Of the eight patients in the original study, six underwent HCT (Martin et al. 2016). There were three deaths: two children died soon after HCT from complications of graft-versus-host disease and lymphoproliferative disease (LPD) of the central nervous system, respectively. One child not transplanted (no HCT) succumbed to disseminated varicella infection. Overall, three patients developed LPD, two of whom had EBV driven B cell non-Hodgkin lymphoma.

There were no deaths in the four children reported from the two most recent studies (Kucuk et al. 2016; Truck et al. 2016). Three of four children underwent successful HCT and were alive and well. Two patients were 10 and 11 years posttransplant. The fourth child was being considered for transplantation. Of note, this child had relatively mild disease and remained EBV uninfected. Transplant methods are described in these two studies. All patients underwent reduced intensity conditioning regimens and received matched, unrelated bone marrow (Kucuk et al. 2016) and peripheral stem cell (Truck et al. 2016) grafts. The donor for each patient in the Kucuk study was EBV-positive, and the authors highlight the potential role of selecting EBV positive donors in patients with CTPS1 deficiency and chronic EBV infection. The rationale would be to provide immediate adoptive immune response by transplanted lymphocytes in the hematopoietic cell graft. Following HCT, the index patient from Kucuk et al. had EBV reactivation and adenovirus infection treated with rituximab and intravenous immune globulin (IVIG) respectively, with complete resolution of both. Her sister required a donor lymphocyte infusion 134 days after transplant and developed autoimmune thrombocytopenia that was treated successfully with rituximab and IVIG. Both patients from Kucuk et al. had normal T cell and cytotoxic function within 2 years of transplant. Thus, with this particular combined immunodeficiency there does not appear to be a good rationale for in- or ex-vivo T cell depletion and should be avoided.

References

Kucuk ZY, Zhang K, Filipovich L, Bleesing JJH. CTP Synthase 1 Deficiency in Successfully Transplanted Siblings with Combined Immune Deficiency and Chronic Active EBV Infection. J Clin Immunol. 2016;36(8):750–3.

Martin E, Palmic N, Sanquer S, Lenoir C, Hauck F, Mongellaz C, et al. CTP synthase 1 deficiency in humans reveals its central role in lymphocyte proliferation. Nature. 2014;510(7504):288–92.

Martin E, et al. First report establishing link between CTPS1 mutation and immune deficiency in eight patients with severe EBV disease. 2016.

Trück J, Kelly DF, Taylor JM, Kienzler AK, Lester T, Seller A, et al. Variable phenotype and discrete alterations of immune phenotypes in CTP synthase 1 deficiency: Report of 2 siblings. J Allergy Clin Immunol. 2016;138(6):1722–25.

Veillette ACA, Davidson D. Immunology: When lymphocytes run out of steam. Nature. 2014;510(7504):222–3.

D

DADA2

Amanda K. Ombrello
National Human Genome Research Institute,
National Institutes of Health, Bethesda, MD, USA

Synonyms

Cat eye syndrome chromosome region, candidate 1 (CERC1); Deficiency of adenosine deaminase type 2 (DADA2)

Definition

The deficiency of adenosine deaminase type 2 (DADA2) is an autosomal recessive disease resulting from biallelic, loss-of-function mutations in *ADA2* (formerly known as *CECR1*), located in chromosome 22q11.1. DADA2 is characterized by systemic vasculitis and features of both autoinflammation and immunodeficiency (MIM#615688).

Introduction and Background

DADA2 was initially reported in 2014 in patients who presented with inflammatory phenotypes that resembled vasculitis and polyarteritis nodosa (PAN) and recurrent ischemic and/or hemorrhagic strokes (Zhou et al. 2014; Navon Elkan et al. 2014). Since the initial publications, the clinical phenotype has expanded significantly to include additional disease manifestations. The identification of DADA2 expands the family of adenosine deaminase-related diseases from the most commonly known severe combined immune deficiency (SCID) due to deficiency of adenosine deaminase 1 (ADA1). ADA1 and ADA2 have partial structural homology, and both are involved in the purine metabolism pathway, converting adenosine to inosine and $2'$-deoxyadenosine to $2'$-deoxyinosine (Zavialov and Engstrom 2005). ADA1-deficient patients present with profound lymphopenia and immunodeficiency associated with toxic intracellular deoxyadenosine nucleotides due to the lack of effective conversion to deoxyinosine. ADA2-deficient patients do not accumulate deoxyadenosine nucleotides and have a mild form of immunodeficiency (Zhou et al. 2014).

Genetics

DADA2 is an autosomal recessive disease resulting from biallelic mutations in *ADA2*. To date, there are over 60 reported mutations in the literature. Genotype-phenotype correlation is not significant. Families with multiple affected sib-

© Springer Science+Business Media LLC, part of Springer Nature 2020
I. R. Mackay et al. (eds.), *Encyclopedia of Medical Immunology*,
https://doi.org/10.1007/978-1-4614-8678-7

lings and identical genotype have been described with one sibling may have a vascular phenotype and another with a hematologic phenotype. It has been postulated that epigenetic or environmental factors may influence the disease expression in individuals.

Pathogenesis

ADA2 encodes the adenosine deaminase 2 protein (ADA2). ADA2 is dimeric and expressed mainly in myeloid cells. ADA2 is secreted by monocytes, macrophages, and dendritic cells into the extracellular environment and highly expressed in plasma. It has two known functions: ADA2 catalyzes the extracellular degradation of adenosine and acts as growth factor for endothelial cells and leukocytes. In contrast, ADA1 is intracellular, monomeric, and its affinity for adenosine is 100-fold greater than ADA2.

The endothelium represents a major target of inflammation in DADA2 patients. Both skin and brain biopsies from ADA2-deficient patients have demonstrated substantial endothelial damage. These biopsies also have increased staining for interleukin (IL)-1β, inducible nitric oxide synthase, and tumor necrosis factor (TNF) which implicates an inflammatory component to DADA2 (Zhou et al. 2014). There is evidence that ADA2 acts as a growth factor for endothelial cells, and, in a deficient state, endothelial cells do not develop normally resulting in friability of the endothelial cells. Additionally, ADA2 increases the proliferation of monocyte-activated CD4+ T cells and induces T-cell-dependent differentiation of monocytes into macrophages. In a deficient state, there is skewing of macrophage development away from the anti-inflammatory, M2, macrophage, toward the inflammatory, M1, macrophage (Zavialov et al. 2010).

Patients with DADA2 have significantly decreased ADA2 activity in the plasma compared to heterozygote relatives and healthy adult and pediatric controls. When measured, ADA1 activity was indistinguishable in DADA2 patients compared to healthy control (Zhou et al. 2014).

Clinical Manifestations

Although initially described as a disease that promoted inflammation, early-onset ischemic strokes, livedo racemosa, and vasculopathy, the clinical presentation of DADA2 has expanded significantly. Now, in addition to the originally described neurologic, inflammatory, and vascular phenotypes, there exist phenotypes that include varying forms of hematologic and immunologic involvement and, in some patients, significant overlap of the phenotypes. Although the disease presents primarily in childhood (Zhou et al. 2014; Navon Elkan et al. 2014), there are multiple reports of patients who have their initial presenting symptom in adulthood.

Patients with DADA2 can have periods of intense disease activity followed by long periods of symptoms remission. During an inflammatory episode, patients can manifest fever with marked elevation of their acute phase reactants. Other inflammatory symptoms such as strokes, worsening cutaneous disease, systemic features of active vasculitis such as ischemic bowel, mesenteric aneurysmal disease, muscle inflammation, and renal involvement can be associated with these fevers.

Neurologic Manifestations
The neurologic manifestations are the most devastating to the patient. Patients with ADA2 deficiency might develop lacunar strokes in small terminal vessels located deep in the brain (Zhou et al. 2014). The brainstem, thalamus, internal capsule, corpus callosum, basal ganglia, and cerebellum are the most frequently affected areas (Fig. 1). DADA2 patients are at increased risk for ischemic and hemorrhagic strokes. The affected vessels are usually very small, and magnetic resonance angiography (MRA) of the brain is not sensitive enough to detect small lacunar strokes in affected patients. There can also be infarcts of the spinal cord that result in bilateral limb involvement as well as bowel and bladder dysfunction. Hemorrhagic strokes can occur at the site of an infarct or in a separate location; sometimes involving large vessels, the subdural, and

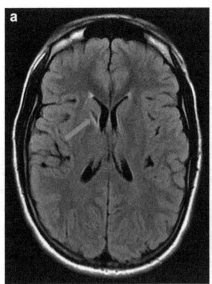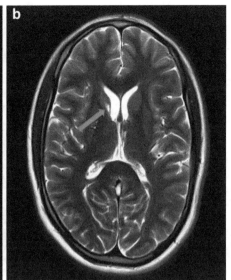

DADA2, Fig. 1 Characteristic MRI Findings in DADA2. The ischemic strokes in DADA2 occur in terminal vessels and are termed lacunar infarcts. This MRI identifies a cystic lesion in the right caudate head (blue arrow) that is representative of an old lacunar stroke visualized on both T1 (left) and T2 (right). The caudate nucleus is part of the basal ganglia which is a commonly affected location for stroke in patients with DADA2

subarachnoid space (Zhou et al. 2014; Nanthapisal et al. 2016). Patients also develop peripheral nervous system manifestations, including mononeuritis multiplex, carpal tunnel, or reflex sympathetic dystrophy.

Cutaneous Manifestations

The initial DADA2 reports highlighted the occurrence of livedo reticularis and livedo racemosa (Zhou et al. 2014; Navon Elkan et al. 2014; Pichard et al. 2016) (Fig. 2a and b). The livedo can be faint and present only on the extremities or become very pronounced with extension to the abdomen, back, and, in some cases, the face. Other dermatologic manifestations include subcutaneous nodules that resemble cutaneous polyarteritis nodosa, urticarial rashes, and panniculitis-like lesions (Fig. 2c). Biopsies can show signs of vasculopathy and, in some cases, small and medium vessel vasculitis. Patients with compromised peripheral vasculature can present with pronounced Raynaud's phenomenon, digital necrosis, and cutaneous ulcers. Autoamputation may occur in patients with profound peripheral vascular involvement.

Gastrointestinal Manifestations

The gastrointestinal involvement in patients with ADA2 deficiency is mainly associated with the inflammatory and vascular features of disease. Patients can develop with ischemic bowel and, in some cases, bowel perforation. Nonspecific abdominal pain is commonly reported, and there have been cases of ulcerative bowel disease (Caorsi et al. 2016). Hepatomegaly is frequently reported, and liver biopsies from DADA2 patients show nodular regenerative hyperplasia and hepatoportal sclerosis. Non-cirrhotic portal hypertension has been reported resulting, at times, in splenomegaly and esophageal varices (Zhou et al. 2014).

Immunological Manifestations

The immunodeficiency in ADA2 deficiency is milder than in ADA1-deficient patients. Most commonly, there are defects in B cells with low numbers of transitional and memory-switched B cells. Immunoglobulin deficiencies can range from a mild IgM deficiency to profound hypogammaglobulinemia (Zhou et al. 2014; Schepp et al. 2017). Patients might have a diagnosis of selective antibody deficiency or common variable

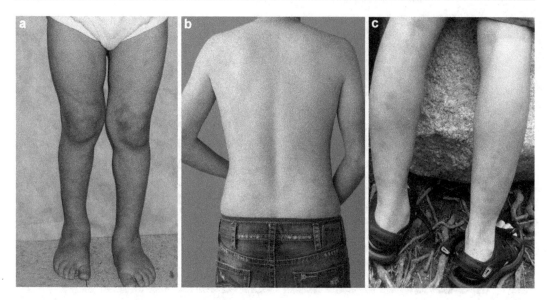

DADA2, Fig. 2 Cutaneous manifestations of DADA2. (**a**) This patient presents with prominent livedo racemosa over his bilateral extremities. (**b**) This patient presents with significant livedo racemosa over all four extremities and extending onto the bilateral flanks, back, and abdomen. (**c**) The tender, raised, erythematous lesions over the bilateral lower extremities were biopsied and had lymphocytic infiltrate of the blood vessels. This patient was diagnosed with erythema nodosum and subsequently polyarteritis nodosa prior to genetic testing revealing the two mutations in *ADA2*

immunodeficiency. T-cell studies show normal naïve T cells as well as normal short-term T-cell activation and proliferative responses to anti-CD3 antibodies (Zhou et al. 2014). There are also T-cell-reported deficiencies such as CD4+ and/or CD8+ lymphopenia, and some patients presented with infections caused by herpes viruses or verrucous warts (Schepp et al. 2017; Trotta et al. 2018).

Hematologic Manifestations

Patients with *ADA2* mutations can present with anemia that resembles Diamond-Blackfan anemia or pure red cell aplasia (Trotta et al. 2018; Michniacki et al. 2018; Schepp et al. 2017). Patients can also have thrombocytopenia and varying forms of leukopenia. These hematologic features can present independently or in conjunction with one another. Bone marrow biopsies might have variable findings, from profound hypocellularity to a hypercellular marrow. T-cell large granular lymphocytes infiltrating the marrow indicates possible immune-mediated effects (Trotta et al. 2018; Hashem et al. 2017).

Musculoskeletal, Renal, and Ophthalmologic Manifestations

DADA2 patients might develop arthralgias and myalgias as well as synovitis and myositis (Zhou et al. 2014; Schepp et al. 2017). Renal manifestations can include hypertension and hematuria. Patients with histories of stroke can present with strabismus and ptosis. Panuveitis, episcleritis, and optic neuritis have also been described (Sahin et al. 2018; Caorsi et al. 2017; Schepp et al. 2017). As the spectrum of disease continues to expand, it is important that the clinicians caring for these patients remain attuned to potential new manifestations of disease and to promptly evaluate any new findings.

Laboratory Findings

There are varying reference ranges for ADA2 depending on the assay used. DADA2 patients have very low or undetectable ADA2 levels, carriers have midrange values, and healthy controls are significantly higher than both the affected patients and the heterozygotes (Zhou et al. 2014; Trotta et al. 2018; Ben-Ami et al. 2016).

Diagnosis

The diagnosis of DADA2 can be made by demonstrating biallelic mutations in *ADA2* or by a low serum ADA2 levels. In some of these patients, only one *ADA2* affected allele can be demonstrated. If a patient with a single mutation has low serum ADA2 level consistent with levels seen in DADA2 patients with biallelic mutations, a diagnosis of DADA2 should be made. If a patient is identified with ADA2 deficiency, genetic testing should be offered to all siblings as there have been multiple cases of seemingly "unaffected" siblings who carry two mutations. As DADA2 can have a delayed presentation in adulthood, early diagnosis could prevent some of the sequelae of disease (Trotta et al. 2018; Michniacki et al. 2018; Schepp et al. 2017).

Patients with DADA2 should undergo a comprehensive evaluation to assess for clinically apparent (and non-apparent) disease-related features (Table 1). Baseline laboratory studies should include a complete blood count (CBC) with differential to assess for cytopenias as well as signs of inflammation such as thrombocytosis. Serum electrolytes should be analyzed to assess for kidney function as should a urinalysis. A hepatic function panel and coagulation studies should be drawn to evaluate for liver involvement. If a patient has a history of muscle pain, muscle enzymes (creatine kinase, lactose dehydrogenase, and aldolase) should be assessed. To evaluate for potential immunodeficiencies, serum immunoglobulins and a lymphocyte phenotype panel assessing T, B, and NK cells is recommended. Acute phase reactants should be evaluated routinely to quantify clinically apparent and subclinical inflammation. In preparation for potential anti-TNF medication, a tuberculosis screen to evaluate for active or latent tuberculosis such as a purified protein derivative (PPD) skin test or QuantiFERON test should be conducted.

Baseline imaging should include an MRI of the brain to assess for strokes. There are cases of clinically silent strokes that have been observed on imaging thus the need to have a baseline MRI even in those patients without clear evidence of stroke. In general, magnetic resonance angiography (MRA) is not sensitive to detect lacunar infarcts and is not a useful screening tool (Vu et al. 2006). Patients presenting with symptoms concerning for spinal cord involvement such

DADA2, Table 1 Recommended laboratory and imaging for DADA2 patients

Laboratory evaluation	Imaging/testing	Optional tests	Possible consultants
Complete blood count with differential	MRI brain	Echocardiogram	Neurology
Serum chemistries	Abdominal ultrasound with Doppler	MRI/MRA abdomen	Hepatology
Hepatic panel	Electrocardiogram	Renal ultrasound	Dermatology
Erythrocyte sedimentation rate		Nerve conduction study/electromyogram	Ophthalmology
C-reactive protein		MRA extremities/angiogram	Immunology
Immunoglobulins		Esophagogastroduodenoscopy/colonoscopy	Hematology
Lymphocyte phenotype panel		Fibroscan	Nephrology
Urinalysis			Cardiology
Creatine kinase			
Lactate dehydrogenase			
Aldolase			
Purified protein derivative (PPD) test/QuantiFERON			

as bilateral limb involvement and/or bowel or bladder incontinence should have an MRI of the spine.

Medically indicated screening procedures and subspecialty follow-up are needed for patients who have signs and symptoms of other organ involvement such as hepatic disease non-cirrhotic portal hypertension, abdominal claudication, mononeuritis multiplex, evidence of bone marrow dysfunction, and Raynaud's phenomenon.

Treatment

The treatment of DADA2 patients has largely focused on a) the correction of the ADA2 deficiency and b) treatment of the specific disease manifestations.

Fresh frozen plasma (FFP) infusion to correct ADA2 levels were administered in a Phase I trial (Ombrello et al. 2019). FFP infusions were well tolerated and serum ADA2 level increased on serial ADA2 level measurements. Pharmacokinetic analysis showed rapid clearance of the infused ADA2, indicating that large volume infusions of FFP are needed to maintain serum ADA2 levels in the range of the unaffected heterozygote individuals. Hematopoietic stem cell transplant (HSCT) was curative in 14 patients undergoing 20 transplants with 100% survival rate (Hashem et al. 2017). Posttransplant complications included acute graft versus host disease (GvHD) in six patients, chronic GvHD in one patient, veno-occlusive disease in two patients, and viral reactivations in ten patients. Autoimmune complications posttransplant included idiopathic thrombocytopenic purpura, autoimmune hemolytic anemia, and neutropenia with immune-mediated pure red cell aplasia.

Therapeutic success has been reported with anti-TNF treatments (Navon Elkan et al. 2014). In a recent trial, 15 consecutive DADA2 patients with a history of stroke were treated with 1 of 4 anti-TNF agents: etanercept (at a dose of 0.8 to 1.2 mg per kilogram of body weight to a maximum of 50 mg weekly), adalimumab (40 mg

every 1 to 2 weeks), infliximab (4 to 5 mg per kilogram every 6 weeks), or golimumab (50 mg weekly). Before anti-TNF treatment, patients had 55 strokes in 733 patient-months, compared to no strokes in 583 patient-months on anti-TNF treatment (Ombrello et al. 2019). All patients were weaned entirely off their glucocorticoids. Based on these data, anti-TNF agents are recommended in DADA2 to reduce the risk of stroke. It remains unclear whether anti-TNF agents are effective in treating other clinical manifestations in DADA2. Given the risk of hemorrhagic stroke antiplatelet, antithrombotic, or anticoagulation agents should not routinely be given.

Prognosis

The prognosis for DADA2 patients is currently not well defined. The lack of apparent genotype, phenotype correlation and the varying clinical presentation among genotypically identical family members, highlights the importance of comprehensive evaluation of DADA2 patients. There can be serious clinical complications and sequelae arising from some of the disease manifestations (strokes, portal hypertension, bone marrow failure) that can only be prevented by careful assessment and screening.

Cross-References

▶ Barth Syndrome
▶ Comel-Netherton Syndrome (*SPINK5*)
▶ Hepatic Veno-Occlusive Disease with Immunodeficiency (VODI)

References

Ben-Ami T, Revel-Vilk S, Brooks R, et al. Extending the clinical phenotype of adenosine deaminase 2 deficiency. J Pediatr. 2016;177:316–320.
Caorsi R, Penco F, Schena F, Gattorno M. Monogenic polyarteritis: the lesson of ADA2 deficiency. Pediatr Rheumatol Online J. 2016;14:51.

Caorsi R, Penco F, Grossi A, et al. ADA2 deficiency (DADA2) as an unrecognized cause of early onset polyarteritis nodosa and stroke: a multicenter national study. Ann Rheum Dis. 2017;76:1648–56.

Hashem H, Kumar AR, Müller I, et al. Hematopoietic stem cell transplantation rescues the hematological, immunological and vascular phenotype in DADA2. Blood. 2017;130:2682–8.

Michniacki TF, Hannibal M, Ross CW, et al. Hematologic manifestations of deficiency of adenosine deaminase 2 (DADA2) and response to tumor necrosis factor inhibition in DADA2-associated bone marrow failure. J Clin Immunol. 2018;38:166–73.

Nanthapisal S, Murphy C, Omoyinmi E, et al. Deficiency of adenosine deaminase type 2: a description of phenotype and genotype in fifteen cases. Arthritis Rheumatol. 2016;68:2314–22.

Navon Elkan P, Pierce SB, Segel R, et al. Mutant adenosine deaminase 2 in a polyarteritis nodosa vasculopathy. N Engl J Med. 2014;370:921–31.

Ombrello AK, Qin J, Hoffmann P, et al. Treatment strategies for the deficiency of adenosine deaminase 2. N Engl J Med. 2019;380:1582–4.

Pichard DC, Ombrello AK, Hoffmann P, Stone DL, Cowen EW. Early-onset stroke, polyarteritis nodosa (PAN), and livedo racemosa. J Am Acad Dermatol. 2016;75:449–53.

Sahin S, Adrovic A, Barut K, Ugurlu S, Turanli E, Ozdogan H, Kasapcopur O. Clinical, imaging and genotypical features of three deceased and fiver surviving cases with ADA2 deficiency. Rheumatol Int. 2018;38(1):129–136.

Schepp J, Proietti M, Frede N, et al. Screening of 181 patients with antibody deficiency for deficiency of adenosine deaminase 2 sheds new light on the disease in adulthood. Arthritis Rheumatol. 2017;69:1689–700.

Trotta L, Martelius T, Siitonen T, et al. ADA2 deficiency: clonal lymphoproliferation in a subset of patients. J Allergy Clin Immunol. 2018;141:1534–7.

Vu D, Gonzalez RG, Schaefer PW. Conventional MRI and MR angiography of stroke. In: Gonzalez RG, Hirsch JA, Koroshetz WJ, Lev MH, Schaefer P, editors. Acute ischemic stroke: imaging and intervention. Berlin: Springer; 2006. p. 115–37.

Zavialov AV, Engstrom A. Human ADA2 belongs to a new family of growth factors with adenosine deaminase activity. Biochem J. 2005;391:51–7.

Zavialov AV, Garcia E, Glaichenhaus N, et al. Human adenosine deaminase 2 induces differentiation of monocytes into macrophages and stimulates proliferation of T helper cells and macrophages. J Leukoc Biol. 2010;88:279–90.

Zhou Q, Yang D, Ombrello AK, et al. Early-onset stroke and vasculopathy associated with mutations in ADA2. N Engl J Med. 2014;370:911–20.

Dedicator of Cytokinesis 2: DOCK2 Deficiency

Robert P. Nelson

Divisions of Hematology and Oncology, Stem Cell Transplant Program, Indiana University (IU) School of Medicine and the IU Bren and Simon Cancer Center, Indianapolis, IN, USA
Pediatric Immunodeficiency Clinic, Riley Hospital for Children at Indiana University Health, Indianapolis, IN, USA
Medicine and Pediatrics, Indiana University School of Medicine, Immunohematology and Transplantation, Indianapolis, IN, USA

Synonyms

DOCK2

Introduction/Background

The Rho families GTPases regulate membrane polarization and cytoskeletal dynamics fundamental to cell migration. The protein families *Caenorhabditis elegans* CED-5 and *Drosophila melanogaster* Myoblast City (CDM), associated with the gene product of avian sarcoma virus CT10 (CRK), function to extend cell membranes (Nishihara et al. 1999). A mammalian homologue to the CDM family, dedicator of cytokinesis 2 (DOCK2) binds and activates Rac family small GTPase 1 (Rac1) and associates with engulfment and cell motility (ELMO1) through its Src-homology 3 (SH3) domain (Sanui et al. 2003). This signaling matrix regulates cytoskeletal reorganization through Ras-related C3 botulinum toxin substrate (Rac) that generates actin-rich lamelli-podial protrusions that drive movement. DOCK2 is expressed predominantly in peripheral blood cells, less in the spleen and thymus, and enables T- and B-lymphocytes to migrate in the search for antigens in lymphoid tissues (Fukui et al. 2001). DOCK2 is also essential for T cell receptor (TCR)-mediated Rac activation required for creation of immunological synapses.

Function

Innate Host Defense

DOCK2 regulates neutrophil chemotaxis via formation of the leading edge through phosphatidylinositol 3-kinase (PI3K)-dependent phosphatidylinositol triphosphate (PIP3)-dependent membrane translocation and Rac activation (Kunisaki et al. 2006a). Murine DOCK2 mutations result in defective integrin activation in B cells but not T cells and DOCK2 and DOCK5 regulate formation of neutrophil extracellular traps (NETs) that are involved in vascular inflammation and autoimmune reactivity (Watanabe et al. 2014). DOCK2 is essential for Toll-like receptor (TLR) 7- and TLR9-mediated IFN-alpha induction in plasmacytoid DCs, where it acts in parallel with TLR engagement to regulate IKK-α-mediated induction of type-1 interferons. DOCK2 is required for the migration of plasmacytoid dendritic cells (DCs) but not myeloid DCs (Gotoh et al. 2010). DOCK2 contributes to the positive selection of Valpha14 natural killer T (NKT) cells, a unique subset of lymphocytes that provides tumor surveillance and regulates adaptive immunity function and innate defense (Kunisaki et al. 2006b). The DOCK2-Rac axis also controls NK cell-mediated cytotoxicity by facilitating lytic synapse formation. Dobbs et al. demonstrated that during viral infection, peripheral-blood mononuclear cells from a patient with a defect failed to increase interferon-alpha and interferon-lambda production normally. Viral replication in fibroblasts was increased and cell death enhanced, conditions that normalized with interferon alfa-2b administration or wild-type DOCK2 expression (Dobbs et al. 2015).

Hematopoiesis, Adaptive Immunity, and Cancer

Chemokine-induced actin polymerization and migration are defective, as Dobbs et al. reported with studies of human DOCK2-deficient T cells, B cells, and NK cells. After viral infection, peripheral-blood mononuclear cells failed to increase interferon-alpha and interferon-lambda production normally. Moreover, in DOCK2-deficient fibroblasts, viral replication was increased and virus-induced cell death enhanced; these conditions normalized with interferon alfa-2b administration or wild-type DOCK2 expression.

CD8 (+) TCR (−) graft facilitating cells (FCs) enhance the engraftment of hematopoietic stem cells (HSCs) in allogeneic and syngeneic recipients; DOCK2 appears to play a critical role in optimizing the function. Wen et al demonstrated this with DOCK2 (−/−) FCs that lost capacity for enhancing c- Kit (+) Sca-1(+) lineage (−) homing and lodgment in hematopoietic niches. Deletion of DOCK2 in FCs also impairs naive CD4 (+) CD25 (−) T cells into FoxP3 (+) regulatory T cells and interleukin-10-producing type 1 regulatory T cells in vitro, which suggests its importance in immunoregulation. (Wen, 2014).

Chemokine-induced actin polymerization and migration were defective in T cells, B cells, and NK cells. After viral infection, peripheral-blood mononuclear cells failed to increase interferon-alpha and interferon-lambda production normally. Moreover, in DOCK2-deficient fibroblasts, viral replication was increased and virus-induced cell death enhanced; these conditions normalized with interferon alfa-2b administration or wild-type DOCK2 expression. DOCK2 regulates the survival of leukemia cells with elevated FLT3 activity and sensitizes FLT3/ITD leukemic cells to conventional antileukemic agents.

Other

DOCK2 also functions as a regulator of vascular smooth muscle cells (SMC) and vascular lesion formation after vascular injury and influences vascular remodeling in proliferative vascular diseases. DOCK2 deficiency protects mice from high-fat diet-induced obesity, at least in part, by stimulating brown adipocyte differentiation. DOCK2 regulates the survival of leukemia cells with elevated FLT3 activity and sensitizes FLT3/ITD leukemic cells to conventional antileukemic agents. Targeting DOCK2 may be a potential therapeutic strategy for treating obesity-associated diseases or leukemia, in which case, the clinical phenotypes seen with the inborn errors of immunity may predict iatrogenic DOCK2-deficiency consequences in the future.

Clinical Presentation

History

To date, there has been only one publication describing DOCK2 deficiency (Dobbs et al. 2015). Five cases reported comprehensively by Dobbs et al. presented with early-onset, invasive infections associated with lymphopenia and history of consanguinity. All patients presented during childhood with recurrent persistent and/or severe mixed infections, including encapsulated bacterial, chronic viral infections, and opportunistic pathogens. Vaccine strain-related, life-threatening varicella infections, and meningoencephalitis due to mumps virus were also documented. Additional features are similar to those of DOCK8 deficiency, an autosomal recessive immunodeficiency characterized by elevated IgE, atopy, cutaneous viral infections, and cancer. However, cognitive impairment, developmental delay, cardiovascular structural defects, facial dysmorphia, and absent thymus were not reported.

Physical

Signs of failure to thrive were present, but facial features were normal and lymph nodes palpable. One patient at 1 year of age had growth failure (body weight: 4.5 kg, 3.5 kg below third percentile; length: 64 cm, 9 cm below third percentile), a nodular erythematous lesion at the site of BCG vaccination, and hepatomegaly. There were no specific, unusual or unique pathognomonic sign that distinguishes this defect from other combined T and B cell deficiencies.

Laboratory Findings/Diagnostic Testing

Screening Labs

Screening immunological evaluation demonstrated a normal complete blood count (CBC) or lymphopenia and/or signs of autoimmune cytopenias. One case had recurrent thrombocytopenia that resolved spontaneously. T-cell receptor excision circles (TRECs), a marker of active thymopoiesis, are likely to be low. IgA and IgM levels are normal and IgE levels normal or elevated. Total lymphocytes percentages may be normal or decreased; however, patients had T-cell lymphopenia and low levels of CD4 and CD8 expression on T-cells. Natural killer (NK) cells were normal or decreased in number or function. Complement levels were normal and B cells likely present.

Immunological Assessments

At 5 months of age, one patient presented with severe T-cell lymphopenia and markedly impaired in-vitro T-cell activation in response to phytohemagglutinin (PHA). Maternal T-cell engraftment was not detected. Naïve (CD45RA+CCR7+) CD4+ and CD8+ lymphocytes were reduced and associated with an increased proportion of effector memory (CD45RA−CCR7−) CD4+ T lymphocytes and either effector memory or CD45RA+CCR7− CD8+. Although total immunoglobulins were normal, patients failed to produce specific antibodies. Natural killer (NK)-cell responses were normal or low. Dobbs et al. demonstrated chemokine-induced actin polymerization and migration defective in DOCK2-deficient T cells, B cells, and NK cells. After viral infection, peripheral-blood mononuclear cells failed to increase interferon-α and interferon-ι production normally. Viral replication and viral-induced cell death was enhanced and reversible following wild-type DOCK2 expression and interferon administration. A liver biopsy in one patient at 3 months of age revealed macrovesicular steatosis, non-necrotic eosinophilic granuloma-like lesions and lobular inflammation. A colon biopsy in the same patient revealed focal active colitis with few B and plasma cells and to a lesser extent of T cells in the lamina propria of the gut and a restricted repertoire (oligoclonality). A lung biopsy from one patient revealed granulomatous inflammation, acid-fast bacilli, and positive Mycobacterium avium culture. Herpes virus-6 DNA was detected and at autopsy, nuclear inclusion bodies were observed within pneumocytes, consistent with viral pneumonitis.

Treatment/Prognosis

Practical considerations for management are similar to those of any other severe T and B cell combined immunodeficiencies. Immunizations with killed vaccines can be administered, but the child may not respond. Live viral vaccines should be avoided. Children may go to school with recognition of the need for prompt evaluation for unusual consequences of infection. These measures may include prolonged courses of antibiotics for bacterial infections and appropriate antimicrobials for herpetic, fungal, and pneumocystis prophylaxis require consideration, depending on the degree of immunological compromise. Immunoglobulin replacement therapy is indicated for those whose functional antibody production is demonstrably low.

For consideration of definitive therapy and attempt to cure the disease, the first decision to make is whether to take care of the patient locally or consider referral to a multidisciplinary clinic engaged in research related to the disease. Input from the family is paramount with this process, as risk and benefits related to traveling or staying local may depend on the resources of the family and type of health care support that is available. Social services play an important role in connecting with support and advocacy groups for PIDD may be informative to the family.

Two patients died of infections at age 20 months and 3 years before receiving HCT. Three HCT recipients experienced normalization of T-cell function and clinical improvement. One child received a matched unrelated donor conditioned with treosulfan, fludarabine, and alemtuzumab at 3.8 years of age and was well 8 months post-transplant. A second received a T-cell-depleted haploidentical HCT from his father at 9 months of age, following myeloablative conditioning with busulfan and fludarabine. He is well without IVIG at 13 months post. A third patient received HCT from his HLA-identical brother following myeloablative busulfan/cyclophosphamide and is alive, well, and off IVIG 17.5 years posttransplant. At the time of this publication, there are no gene therapy trials open for this disorder.

Cross-References

▶ Evaluation of Suspected Immunodeficiency, Overview

References

Dobbs K, Dominguez Conde C, Zhang SY, et al. Inherited DOCK2 deficiency in patients with early-onset invasive infections. N Engl J Med. 2015;372:2409–22.

Fukui Y, Hashimoto O, Sanui T, et al. Haematopoietic cell-specific CDM family protein DOCK2 is essential for lymphocyte migration. Nature. 2001;412:826–31.

Gotoh K, Tanaka Y, Nishikimi A, et al. Selective control of type I IFN induction by the Rac activator DOCK2 during TLR-mediated plasmacytoid dendritic cell activation. J Exp Med. 2010;207:721–30.

Kunisaki Y, Nishikimi A, Tanaka Y, et al. DOCK2 is a Rac activator that regulates motility and polarity during neutrophil chemotaxis. J Cell Biol. 2006a;174:647–52.

Kunisaki Y, Tanaka Y, Sanui T, et al. DOCK2 is required in T cell precursors for development of Valpha14 NK T cells. J Immunol. 2006b;176:4640–5.

Nishihara H, Kobayashi S, Hashimoto Y, et al. Non-adherent cell-specific expression of DOCK2, a member of the human CDM-family proteins. Biochim Biophys Acta. 1999;1452:179–87.

Sanui T, Inayoshi A, Noda M, et al. DOCK2 regulates Rac activation and cytoskeletal reorganization through interaction with ELMO1. Blood. 2003;102:2948–50.

Watanabe M, Terasawa M, Miyano K, et al. DOCK2 and DOCK5 act additively in neutrophils to regulate chemotaxis, superoxide production, and extracellular trap formation. J Immunol. 2014;193:5660–7.

Wen Y, Elliott MJ, Huang Y, et al. DOCK2 is critical for CD8(+) TCR(−) graft facilitating cells to enhance engraftment of hematopoietic stem and progenitor cells. Stem Cells. 2014;32:2732–43.

Defects in B12 and Folate Metabolism (TCN2, SLC46A1 (PCFT Deficiency), MTHFD1)

Arturo Borzutzky and Rodrigo Hoyos-Bachiloglu
Department of Pediatric Infectious Diseases and Immunology, School of Medicine, Pontificia Universidad Católica de Chile, Santiago, Chile

Synonyms

FOCM: Folate-mediated one-carbon metabolism; HFM: Hereditary folate malabsorption; MTHFD1: Methylenetetrahydrofolate dehydrogenase 1; PCFT: Proton-coupled folate transporter; SLC46A1: Solute carrier family 46, member 1; TCN2: Transcobalamin II

The interplay between cellular metabolism and immune function has been highlighted by the occurrence of severe combined immunodeficiency (SCID) in patients with defective mitochondrial function and purine metabolism, as reported in reticular dysgenesis, adenosine deaminase (ADA), and purine nucleoside phosphorylase (PNP) deficiency. Besides these well-established associations, only a few other metabolic defects have been reported to present with combined immunodeficiency. However, the list of metabolism-related genes causing abnormalities in the immune system is likely to grow in the coming years as a consequence of the use of next-generation sequencing technologies in patients with suspected immunodeficiency.

Folate and vitamin B12 (cobalamin) are essential nutrients that have a key role in formation of purine and pyrimidine nucleotides for synthesizing DNA and RNA, production of methionine, and other cellular processes. Although their deficiency is best known for abnormalities in erythropoiesis that lead to megaloblastic anemia, these cofactors are also central to lymphocyte development and function. As such, profound deficiencies of folate or vitamin B12 or alterations in their metabolism are associated with immunodeficiency of varying severity. In this chapter, defects in three genes involved in folate-mediated one-carbon metabolism (FOCM), leading to immunodeficiency are presented.

FOCM refers to serial highly regulated metabolic reactions that utilize folate for the methylation of homocysteine to methionine and the synthesis of adenosine, guanosine, and thymidylate. Folate-dependent metabolic pathways have access to limited amounts of folate-derived substrates and compete for the usage of 5,10-methylenetetrahydrofolate (5,10-methyleneTHF) to synthesize thymidylate or methionine. MethyleneTHF dehydrogenase 1 (MTHFD1) is a key enzyme in FOCM that acts as the primary source of one-carbon units for the synthesis of 5,10-methyleneTHF and regulates the use of this cofactor for homocysteine remethylation or thymidylate synthesis through nuclear localization. Vitamin B12 availability also plays an important role in regulating FOCM since vitamin B12 deficiency causes folate metabolites to accumulate as 5-methylTHF and lead to impaired DNA synthesis. Genetic defects affecting vitamin B12 availability (TCN2), the gastrointestinal absorption, and CNS transport of folate (SLC46A1) and FOCM (MTHFD1) have been reported in patients presenting with combined immunodeficiency and will be described in this chapter.

Transcobalamin Deficiency

Transcobalamin deficiency (OMIM #275350) is a rare autosomal recessive disease caused by homozygous or compound heterozygous mutations affecting the TCN2 gene. Most of the disease-causing mutations in TCN2 reported to date are insertions or deletions that result in frameshifts leading to expression of a truncated protein; however, nonsense mutations and point mutations that activate the expression of cryptic splice sites have also been reported. To date, no genotype-phenotype correlation has been described this group of patients.

Patients with transcobalamin deficiency begin to manifest a diverse constellation of symptoms during the first year of life, including glossitis, mucosal ulcerations, failure to thrive, purpura, vomiting, diarrhea, megaloblastic anemia, neutropenia, and pancytopenia. A recently published cohort of 30 patients (Trakadis et al. 2014) reports that the most common complication of transcobalamin deficiency is the development of hematological abnormalities (87% of patients), followed by gastrointestinal symptoms (37% of patients) and neurological findings such as weakness, hypotonia, myoclonic like movements, and neurodevelopmental delay (29% of patients). Although transcobalamin deficiency has been associated with granulocyte dysfunction and infections, this series of patients report that only 8% of the cohort suffered from recurrent or opportunistic infections, while immunological abnormalities like agammaglobulinemia, hypogammaglobulinemia, and T or B cell lymphopenia were found in 17% of patients.

Laboratory evaluation of patients with transcobalamin deficiency is characterized by elevated serum levels of homocysteine, normal serum levels of folate, megaloblastic anemia, and methylmalonic aciduria. Serum levels of cobalamin are usually within normal range as most of the circulating cobalamin pool is bound to haptocorrin, a protein of unknown function, and not to transcobalamin. In this patient group, evaluation of cobalamin absorption from the gastrointestinal tract with a Schilling test is typically abnormal and cannot be corrected by the administration of intrinsic factor. Bone marrow evaluation of patients with this condition shows megaloblastic changes and may exhibit features suggestive of a myelodysplatic syndrome or leukemia (Trakadis et al. 2014). It has been reported that decreased levels of transcobalamin in cord blood and decreased transcobalamin production by amniotic cells in at-risk pregnancies could be used to screen for the disease. The diagnosis of transcobalamin deficiency is confirmed by protein expression analysis in skin-derived fibroblasts or by sequencing of the TCN2 gene.

Transcobalamin deficiency can be treated with cobalamin supplementation. Currently, there are two cobalamin formulations clinically available: hydroxycobalamin and cyanocobalamin; however, data to support the use of a specific formulation is lacking. There is no consensus regarding the optimal route of cobalamin administration, although the Trakadis' series suggests that intramuscular cobalamin could be safer as significant neurological deficits (retinopathy and intellectual disability) were observed in the only patient in this report that received oral cobalamin. There is also a lack of consensus regarding the frequency of cobalamin administration, but weekly supplementation is needed in most cases to achieve an optimal response. Early treatment with cobalamin is recommended, as patients diagnosed in the neonatal period due to a family history of cobalamin deficiency, who received early supplementation did not develop long-term complications. The most common complications observed in TCN2-deficient patients receiving cobalamin supplementation are speech and attention deficits, late onset complications reported in this series included tremors, chorea, anemia, and visual problems, which appear to be reversible with optimization of their treatment regimen.

SLC46A1 (PCFT) Deficiency

Autosomal recessive mutations in the *SLC46A1* gene, which encodes the proton-coupled folate transporter (PCFT), lead to a rare inborn error of metabolism called "hereditary folate malabsorption" (HFM, OMIM 229050) or PCFT deficiency (Qiu et al. 2006). The PCFT is essential for intestinal folate absorption as it is highly expressed in the brush border of the proximal small intestine but is also essential for the transport of folates across the choroid plexus into the cerebrospinal fluid (CSF). This disease is particularly frequent in a specific region of Puerto Rico called Villalba or in infants of Puerto Rican ancestry, likely due to a founder's effect.

The clinical presentation of PCFT deficiency usually begins at about 3 months of age, when transplacentally acquired folate reserves are depleted. At this age, infants usually develop protracted diarrhea or severe infections, including most frequently Pneumocystis jirovecii pneumonia (PJP) and systemic cytomegalovirus infection. In addition, patients have anemia, which is frequently megaloblastic, neutrophil hypersegmentation and occasional neutropenia, poor growth, and severe neurologic involvement with microcephaly, hypotonia, developmental delay, and seizures. It is important to note that if the patient is also iron deficient, anemia may not be macrocytic, which could confound or delay the diagnosis.

From an immunological standpoint, absence of folates profoundly affects lymphocyte function, leading to hypogammaglobulinemia and cellular immunodeficiency (Borzutzky et al. 2009). In this context, lymphocyte subsets can be normal in numbers, including recent thymic emigrants, but may have severely impaired lymphocyte function, with abrogated T cell proliferation and activation.

These alterations are partially corrected by folate supplementation.

Diagnosis is usually suspected by typical opportunistic infections accompanied by megaloblastic anemia and/or neurologic symptoms, with confirmation of HFM being done by measuring serum, red blood cell, and cerebrospinal fluid folate concentrations, which are extremely reduced or undetectable. The folinic acid (5-methylTHF) levels in CSF are also low and have been shown to be a good parameter to serially monitor to adjust therapy and prevent neurological disease.

Unlike most other primary immunodeficiencies that are not amenable to pharmacologic treatment, early treatment with intramuscular folinic acid (5-formylTHF) restores immune function and may prevent devastating neurological disease. The intramuscular route of administration is key. Due to the fact that the PCFT is essential for intestinal absorption of folates, affected patients fail to absorb enterally administered folate supplements. In addition, even if blood folate levels are restored, CSF folate concentrations are still greatly reduced as the PCFT is necessary for transport across the choroid plexus, eventually leading to devastating neurological disease. Folinic acid accesses the CSF across the blood-brain barrier (instead of the blood-choroid plexus epithelial cell-CSF barrier), and thus, daily parenteral folinic acid is the treatment of choice for PCFT deficiency. Treatment with pharmacologic doses of intramuscular folinic acid has been shown to reverse anemia and immunodeficiency, preventing opportunistic and other serious infections, by restoring folate availability. In addition, early initiation of this therapy may prevent severe neurological complications that if not treated in a timely fashion would lead to permanent brain damage. Thus, this therapy should be instituted upon suspicion of HFM given its safety and efficacy profile with life-changing consequences.

Defects in B12 and Folate Metabolism (TCN2, SLC46A1 (PCFT Deficiency), MTHFD1), Table 1 Comparison of typical genetic, metabolic, and clinical features of *TCN2*, *SLC46A1*, and *MTHFD1* deficiency before vitamin replacement therapy is instituted

	TCN2 deficiency	*SLC46A1* deficiency	*MTHFD1* deficiency
Inheritance	Autosomal recessive	Autosomal recessive	Autosomal recessive
Clinical features			
Neurological abnormalities	30%	100%	Frequent
Failure to thrive	60–70%	100%	Frequent
Gastrointestinal symptoms (vomiting/diarrhea)	30–40%	Frequent	Frequent
Severe or recurrent infections	<10%	100%	80%
Opportunistic infections	<10%	Frequent	Frequent
Macrocytic/megaloblastic anemia	Yes	Yes	Yes
Neutropenia/pancytopenia	>60%	Frequent	Infrequent
Cellular immunodeficiency	Infrequent	100%	100%
Humoral immunodeficiency	No	Frequent	Frequent
Atypical hemolytic uremic syndrome	No	No	40–50%
Metabolic features			
Serum folate	Normal	Low	Normal
Serum cobalamin	Normal	Normal	Normal
CNS 5-methyltetrahydrofolate	Normal	Low	Low
Homocysteine	High	Normal/high	Normal/high
Methylmalonic acid	High		Normal/high

MTHFD1 Deficiency

MTHFD1 encodes an essential trifunctional enzyme that interconverts several THF metabolites. Less than 10 cases of MTHFD1 deficiency due to biallelic mutations have been described. All the affected patients reported to date have had macrocytic or megaloblastic anemia and most have had a combined immunodeficiency, with a SCID phenotype in several cases (Ramakrishnan et al. 2016). Affected patients frequently suffer from pyogenic bacterial infections, sepsis, and opportunistic infections including pneumocystis jirovecii pneumonia, with several early deaths due to infections occurring in affected patients or siblings. In addition, atypical hemolytic uremic syndrome with kidney failure has been reported in several patients. Although the pathogenesis of this complication is unclear, it may be related to hyperhomocysteinemia as occurs in some vitamin B12 metabolic defects. Neurological manifestations of MTHFD1 deficiency include mild mental retardation, epilepsy, retinopathy, and sensorineural hearing loss but do not uniformly affect all MTHFD1-deficient patients.

Immune phenotype in these patients is variable, including severe lymphopenia, hypogammaglobulinemia, and poor response to conjugated polysaccharide immunizations. As in PCFT deficiency, lymphocyte proliferation is decreased in absence of adequate folic acid replacement but improves upon therapy (Keller et al. 2013). As shown in Table 1, affected patients frequently have elevated serum and urine homocysteine and methylmalonic acid but normal folate and vitamin B12 levels. Diagnostic confirmation in all cases has been made through Sanger or high-throughput sequencing demonstrating biallelic mutations in the *MTHFD1* gene, revealing the autosomal recessive nature of this condition. Studies performed in fibroblasts harboring *MTHFD1* mutations have defective methionine formation that is rescued by folic or folinic acid, but not by vitamin B12.

Initially, patients are treated with parenteral immunoglobulin and trimethoprim/sulfamethoxazole prophylaxis. As soon as a folate metabolism alteration is suspected, treatment with folic or folinic acid supplementation must be started. Several patients have also been treated with

vitamin B12 and betaine, particularly before genetic confirmation. Anemia and immunodeficiency appear to be folate responsive, although reports show that some patients have continued to present with recurrent infections despite supplementation and immunoglobulin replacement. Neurological complications have shown variable response to vitamin replacement, probably related to early damage that occurred before therapy was instituted, highlighting the importance of early diagnosis and aggressive replacement therapy in defects of B12 and folate metabolism.

References

Borzutzky A, Crompton B, Bergmann AK, et al. Reversible severe combined immunodeficiency phenotype secondary to a mutation in the proton-coupled folate transporter. Clin Immunol. 2009;133:287–94.

Keller MD, Ganesh J, Heltzer M, et al. Severe combined immunodeficiency resulting from mutations in MTHFD1. Pediatrics. 2013;131:e629–34.

Qiu A, Jansen M, Sakaris A, et al. Identification of an intestinal folate transporter and the molecular basis for hereditary folate malabsorption. Cell. 2006;127: 917–28.

Ramakrishnan KA, Pengelly RJ, Gao Y, et al. Precision molecular diagnosis defines specific therapy in combined immunodeficiency with megaloblastic anemia secondary to MTHFD1 deficiency. J Allergy Clin Immunol Pract. 2016;4(6):1160–1166.e10.

Trakadis YJ, Alfares A, Bodamer OA, et al. Update on transcobalamin deficiency: clinical presentation, treatment and outcome. J Inherit Metab Dis. 2014;37(3):461–73.

λ5 Deficiency

Vassilios Lougaris and Alessandro Plebani
Pediatrics Clinic and Institute for Molecular Medicine A. Nocivelli, Department of Clinical and Experimental Sciences,
University of Brescia and ASST-Spedali Civili of Brescia, Brescia, Italy

Definition

λ5 deficiency (OMIM #613500) is a rare primary immunodeficiency characterized by reduced serum levels of all immunoglobulin classes and very low numbers of peripheral B cells (peripheral B cells <2%). To date, one patient has been well described, and in addition two siblings in a cohort of patients with antibody deficiency were reported to present with homozygous defects in *IGLL1*. λ5 deficiency is caused by biallelic pathogenic mutations in the *IGLL1* gene encoding for λ5, located in chromosome 22q11.23.

Pathogenesis

Early B cell development takes place in the bone marrow. An important maturational step is the progression from the pro-B to the pre-B stage (Espeli et al. 2006; Rudin and Thompson 1998; Bartholdy and Matthias 2004). This passage depends on the expression of a functional B cell receptor composed of the μ heavy chain (*IGHM*; OMIM∗147020), Igα (CD79A; OMIM∗112205), Igβ (CD79B; OMIM∗147245), and surrogate chains VpreB and λ5 (*IGLL1*; OMIM∗146770) that initiates downstream signalling necessary for early B cell differentiation through kinases such as BTK and BLNK. Animal models and in vitro studies over the years have underlined the importance of each of the pre-BCR components and associated transcription factors for the transition from pro-B to pre-B stage of maturation, suggesting that these genes may be responsible for agammaglobulinemia in humans (Conley and Cooper 1998).

Clinical Presentation

The clinical history of the only patient with λ5 deficiency reported in detail presented at the age of 2 months with recurrent otitis media was found to be hypogammaglobulinemic and with absence of peripheral B cells at the age of 3 years, when he was hospitalized for *Haemophilus* meningitis and arthritis (Minegishi et al. 1998). He did not have protective antibodies developed against tetanus and diphtheria toxoids and *Haemophilus influenzae* vaccines, which he had received. Peripheral B cell analysis demonstrated less than 0.06% of B cells. Bone marrow studies showed a specific block at the pro-B to pre-B stage of differentiation. At follow-up at 5 years of age, he was on immunoglobulin supplementation and had no detectable IgA and IgM. T cell numbers and proliferative responses were normal.

Diagnosis

Immunological work-up in affected patients is expected to find undetectable levels of serum immunoglobulins in the complete absence of peripheral B cells. BTK mutations might first be considered in male patients, and then genetic screening for autosomal recessive gene mutations should be performed. Lambda 5 chain sequence is variable, in part due to gene conversion from the λ5 pseudogenes: 16.1, 16.2, and lambda1 (Moens et al. 2014).

Management

As in other forms of humoral immunodeficiencies, immunoglobulin replacement treatment should be started as soon as the immunological diagnosis of agammaglobulinemia is established. Currently two options are available: intravenous or subcutaneous. Normally, a dose of 400 mg/kg/dose every 3–4 weeks is sufficient to maintain pre-infusion IgG levels >500 mg/dl that should be able to reduce the number of infectious episodes, especially that of invasive infections.

Antibiotic treatment should be strongly considered for every infectious episode, and in some cases, prophylactic antibiotic regimen may be added to help reduce the frequency of infections.

The spectrum of disease and long-term prognosis are not well defined, in light of having only one case reported.

References

Bartholdy B, Matthias P. Transcriptional control of B cell development and function. Gene. 2004;327:1–23.

Conley ME, Cooper MD. Genetic basis of abnormal B cell development. Curr Opin Immunol. 1998;10(4):339–406.

Espeli M, Rossi B, Mancini SJ, Roche P, Gauthier L, Schiff C. Initiation of pre-B cell receptor signaling: common and distinctive features in human and mouse. Semin Immunol. 2006;18:56–66.

Minegishi Y, Coustan-Smith E, Wang YH, Cooper MD, Campana D, Conley ME. Mutations in the human lambda5/14.1 gene result in B cell deficiency and agammaglobulinemia. J Exp Med. 1998;187:71–7.

Moens LN, Falk-Sorqvist E, Asplund AC, Bernatowska E, Smith CIE, Nilsson M. Diagnostics of primary immunodeficiency diseases: a sequencing capture approach. PLoS One. 2014;9:e114901.

Rudin CM, Thompson CB. B-cell development and maturation. Semin Oncol. 1998;25:435–46.

Deficiency of Adenosine Deaminase Type 2 (DADA2)

► DADA2

Deficiency of Interleukin 36 Receptor Antagonist (DITRA)

Suzanne C. Ward and Edward W. Cowen
Dermatology Branch, National Institute of Arthritis and Musculoskeletal and Skin Diseases, National Institutes of Health, Bethesda, MD, USA

Synonyms

DITRA: Deficiency of interleukin 36 receptor antagonist; GPP: Generalized pustular psoriasis

Definition

Deficiency of interleukin 36 receptor antagonist (DITRA) is a monogenic autoinflammatory disease caused by loss-of-function mutations in the interleukin 36 receptor antagonist (*IL36RN*) gene. The disease is characterized by recurrent episodes of generalized pustular psoriasis (GPP) and systemic inflammation (MIM#614204).

Introduction and Background

Interleukin 36 (IL-36) and its isoforms are interleukin-1 (IL-1) family members, although their functions are less well characterized than the IL-1 signaling pathway proteins. DITRA was first described in 2011 (Marrakchi et al. 2011; Onoufriadis et al. 2011). Since then, affected families have been reported in Europe, Asia, North America, and Africa. To date, 16 distinct, disease-causing mutations have been identified (Navarini et al. 2017).

Genetics

DITRA follows an autosomal recessive inheritance pattern; however, recent data suggests a single heterozygous *IL36RN* mutation may lead to GPP in a subset of patients. Hussain et al. identified homozygous or compound heterozygous *IL36RN* mutations in 49/233 (21%) of patients with GPP and a single mutation in 18/233 (7.7%) of patients with GPP (Hussain et al. 2015).

Pathogenesis

The interleukin (IL) 36 pathway is thought to play an important role in innate immunity of the skin. IL-36α, IL-36β, and IL-36γ are richly expressed in keratinocytes, macrophages, and monocytes. Ligand binding of IL-36 leads to interaction between the IL-36 receptor and its co-receptor, the IL-1 receptor accessory protein (IL1RAcP), followed by activation of the nuclear factor NF-κB and mitogen-activated protein kinase (MAPK) pathways. This results in local recruitment of immune cells and release of additional cytokines (Fig. 1). *IL36RN* encodes the IL-36 receptor antagonist (IL-36Ra). In the presence of IL-36Ra, the IL-36 receptor is unable to associate

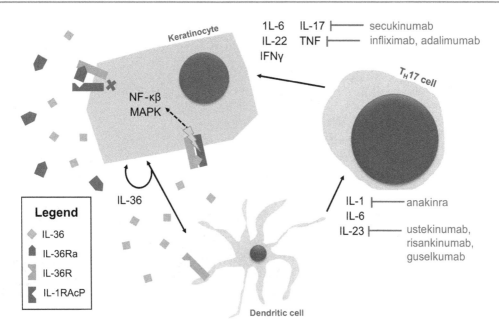

Deficiency of Interleukin 36 Receptor Antagonist (DITRA), Fig. 1 The IL-36 pathway. Schematic of selected inflammatory processes mediated by IL-36 (α, β, and γ) and role of IL-36Ra as an antagonist. Proposed treatments for DITRA are shown in red. *IL* interleukin,

IL-36Ra IL-36 receptor antagonist, *IL-36R* IL-36 receptor, *IL-1RAcP* IL-1 receptor accessory protein, *NF-κB* nuclear factor κB, *MAPK* mitogen-activated protein kinase, *IFNγ* interferon gamma, *TNF* tumor necrosis factor, *T_H17* T helper 17 cell

with IL1RAcP, thus halting the inflammatory response. In DITRA, absence of functional IL-36Ra leads to loss of this negative feedback mechanism, resulting in a self-perpetuating cycle of auto-inflammation.

Clinical Manifestations

Cutaneous Manifestations

DITRA most often presents as a diffuse pustular eruption similar to GPP. Individual pustules may coalesce into larger plaques with an erythematous base (Fig. 2). Many patients present in childhood, but the age of onset is variable. Whereas non-DITRA pediatric GPP tends to have a benign course with high rates of spontaneous resolution (compared to adult-onset GPP), the majority of patients with DITRA have severe disease characterized by systemic inflammation and a recalcitrant disease course. Systemic symptoms include fever (>38 °C) and asthenia coinciding with

disease flares. As in typical GPP, skin lesions in patients with DITRA may become secondarily infected and progress to septicemia.

The initial onset of GPP and subsequent disease flares in patients with DITRA may be triggered by a variety of stressors. Commonly cited triggers include bacterial or viral infection, withdrawal of anti-inflammatory medication, and hormonal changes such as menstruation or pregnancy (Tauber et al. 2016).

Although most commonly associated with generalized pustular disease, disease-causing mutations in *IL36RN* have been associated with other forms of pustular disease, including acrodermatitis continua of Hallopeau (pustular disease localized to the digits and nail apparatus), acute generalized exanthematous pustulosis (a generalized pustular reaction following certain drug exposures), impetigo herpetiformis (pustular psoriasis occurring during pregnancy), and palmoplantar pustulosis (pustular disease primarily of the palms and soles) (Navarini et al. 2017).

Deficiency of Interleukin 36 Receptor Antagonist (DITRA), Fig. 2 DITRA. (**a**) Pustules coalescing into plaques on the chest with superficial skin sloughing. (**b**) Geographic pustular plaques on the forearm and hand. (Photos courtesy of Kelly M. Cordoro, MD)

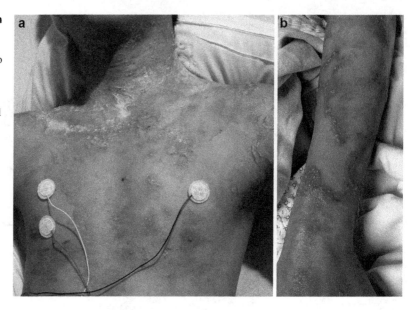

Although advances in our understanding of the genetic basis of psoriasis have improved dramatically in recent years, most cases of both plaque psoriasis (psoriasis vulgaris, PV) and pustular psoriasis (PP) still do not appear to have a monogenic origin. Nonetheless, certain clinical factors may suggest DITRA in patients who present with pustular psoriasis. Whereas GPP skin lesions often occur in the presence of PV, DITRA is much less likely to be associated with typical plaque psoriasis. In fact, Sugiura et al. identified mutations in *IL36RN* in 82% (9/11) of patients who presented with GPP in the absence of PV compared to only 10% (3/29) of patients with GPP and concomitant PV (Sugiura et al. 2013). DITRA is also associated with earlier onset of disease and a markedly increased risk of systemic inflammation compared to *IL36RN* mutation negative PP. Geographic tongue has been associated with mutations in *IL36RN*, both in patients with DITRA and unaffected family members who are carriers of the mutation. DITRA should be suspected in patients who have PP with the clinical triad of early-onset disease (median age of onset of 17 $\pm$ 2.4 years for DITRA patients compared to 33 $\pm$ 1.5 years for patients with non-DITRA GPP), systemic inflammation, and absence of concurrent PV (Hussain et al. 2015).

Laboratory Findings

During an episode of pustulosis, patients develop laboratory abnormalities consistent with systemic inflammation, including leukocytosis (white blood cell count $>12 \times 10^9$/L) and elevated C-reactive protein (CRP). Between flares, laboratory values may return to normal. Skin biopsy shows typical signs of pustular psoriasis: spongiform pustules of Kogoj with a neutrophilic inflammatory infiltrate are present in the epidermis, along with acanthosis, parakeratosis, and elongation of the rete ridges.

Diagnosis

When DITRA is suspected, it may be definitively diagnosed by genetic analysis of the *IL36RN* gene. Loss-of-function mutations responsible for DITRA may be inherited or arise de novo.

Treatment

To date, there have been no clinical trials specifically for the treatment of DITRA. Case reports detail the successful use of anakinra, infliximab, ustekinumab, secukinumab, and granulocyte and monocyte apheresis (Cordoro et al. 2017). Anakinra, a recombinant form of the IL-1 receptor antagonist, is the most studied treatment for DITRA in both adults and children. Anakinra is FDA approved for rheumatoid arthritis and cryopyrin-associated periodic syndromes (CAPS, a group of IL-1-mediated autoinflammatory diseases), but the results have been mixed in patients with DITRA, and the precise mechanism for improvement of DITRA symptoms is not well understood. Infliximab, ustekinumab, and secukinumab are monoclonal antibodies against TNF, IL-12/23, and IL-17, respectively (Fig. 1). These biologic therapies are thought to decrease inflammation in DITRA through modifying effects on T helper 17 (T_H17) cells.

Clinical trials are currently underway for the use of anakinra, secukinumab, adalimumab (anti-TNF monoclonal antibody), alitretinoin (a first-generation retinoid), and risankizumab and guselkumab (anti-IL-23 monoclonal antibodies) for the treatment of GPP. Patients with DITRA are currently managed on an individual basis, as a uniformly effective treatment has yet to be identified.

Prognosis

Patients experiencing an acute episode of GPP may require hospitalization for management of systemic inflammation, fluid balance, and possible complications such as septicemia. Once stabilized, systemic medications are often required to control GPP. The long-term prognosis of DITRA compared to non-DITRA GPP is unknown.

References

Cordoro KM, Ucmak D, Hitraya-Low M, Rosenblum MD, Liao W. Response to interleukin (IL)-17 inhibition in an adolescent with severe manifestations of IL-36 receptor antagonist deficiency (DITRA). JAMA Dermatol. 2017;153(1):106–8.

Hussain S, Berki DM, Choon SE, Burden AD, Allen MH, Arostegui JI, et al. IL36RN mutations define a severe autoinflammatory phenotype of generalized pustular psoriasis. J Allergy Clin Immunol. 2015;135(4): 1067–70.e9.

Marrakchi S, Guigue P, Renshaw BR, Puel A, Pei XY, Fraitag S, et al. Interleukin-36-receptor antagonist deficiency and generalized pustular psoriasis. N Engl J Med. 2011;365(7):620–8.

Navarini AA, Burden AD, Capon F, Mrowietz U, Puig L, Koks S, et al. European consensus statement on phenotypes of pustular psoriasis. J Eur Acad Dermatol Venereol. 2017;31(11):1792–9.

Onoufriadis A, Simpson MA, Pink AE, Di Meglio P, Smith CH, Pullabhatla V, et al. Mutations in IL36RN/ IL1F5 are associated with the severe episodic inflammatory skin disease known as generalized pustular psoriasis. Am J Hum Genet. 2011;89(3):432–7.

Sugiura K, Takemoto A, Yamaguchi M, Takahashi H, Shoda Y, Mitsuma T, et al. The majority of generalized pustular psoriasis without psoriasis vulgaris is caused by deficiency of interleukin-36 receptor antagonist. J Invest Dermatol. 2013;133(11):2514–21.

Tauber M, Bal E, Pei XY, Madrange M, Khelil A, Sahel H, et al. IL36RN mutations affect protein expression and function: a basis for genotype-phenotype correlation in pustular diseases. J Invest Dermatol. 2016;136(9):1811–9.

Deficiency of the IL-1 Receptor Antagonist

▶ Deficiency of the IL-1 Receptor Antagonist (DIRA)

Deficiency of the IL-1 Receptor Antagonist (DIRA)

Megha Garg and Adriana A. de Jesus
Translational Autoinflammatory Diseases Section (TADS), National Institute of Allergy and Infectious Diseases (NIAID), National Institutes of Health (NIH), Bethesda, MD, USA

Synonyms

DIRA; Deficiency of the IL-1 Receptor Antagonist; IL-1Ra; IL-1 receptor antagonist

Definition

DIRA, deficiency of the IL-1 receptor antagonist, is a monogenic autosomal recessive autoinflammatory disease that presents with systemic inflammation, pustulosis, sterile osteomyelitis, and osteolytic lesions and is caused by loss-of-function mutations in *IL1RN*, the gene that encodes the IL-1 receptor antagonist (IL-1Ra) (MIM#612852).

Introduction and Background

At a time when whole exome sequencing was not yet available, the diagnosis of sporadic diseases required a candidate gene approach. DIRA was in fact discovered in two patients who had complete responses to empirically administered IL-1 blocking treatments with recombinant IL-1 receptor antagonist, anakinra, which strongly suggested an IL-1-mediated disease, and resulted in a candidate screen of genes in the IL-1/inflammasome pathway that eventually led to finding "the needle in the haystack" (Reddy et al. 2009; Aksentijevich et al. 2009). Historic descriptions of patients with pustulosis and sterile bone lesions point to a pathogenic connection between neutrophilic pustulosis and osteomyelitis. However, the majority of these patients do not have *IL1RN* mutations, and most are not monogenic. These conditions are referred to as chronic recurrent multifocal osteomyelitis (CRMO), a group of autoinflammatory bone diseases that also include the monogenic disease Majeed syndrome (Stern and Ferguson 2013). Two historical descriptions of patients who likely had DIRA illustrate the poor outcomes of young undiagnosed patients who are not receiving IL-1 blocking therapies (Leung and Lee 1985; Ivker et al. 1993).

Genetics

In 2009, two groups led by Verbsky and Goldbach-Mansky identified a homozygous 175-kb deletion in two patients of Puerto Rican descent who presented with systemic inflammation, pustulosis, and aseptic osteomyelitis. The deletion on the long arm of chromosome 2 included the locus for *IL1RN* as well as five adjacent genes; all are agonists and antagonists of the IL-36 receptor (encoded by *IL1RL2*). The IL-36 receptor agonists are *IL36A, IL36B, IL36G*, and the *IL36RN* which encodes the IL-36 receptor antagonist (IL-36Ra), and *IL38* encodes the second IL-36 receptor antagonist, IL-38 (Reddy et al. 2009; Aksentijevich et al. 2009) (Fig. 1). The latter group also found damaging mutations affecting *IL1RN* exclusively, thus confining the clinical phenotype to complete loss of function of IL1Ra, the protein encoded by IL1RN (Aksentijevich et al. 2009). Eleven different disease-causing mutations in *IL1RN* in 22 patients with DIRA have been reported to date (Mendonca et al. 2017; Kuemmerle-Deschner et al. 2018; Schnellbacher et al. 2013; Infevers 2019). These include five nonsense mutations, one in-frame deletion, three frameshift deletions, the genomic 175-kb deletion on chromosome 2, and a recently reported 22-kb deletion in an Indian patient with DIRA (Reddy et al. 2009; Aksentijevich et al. 2009; Mendonca et al. 2017; Stenerson et al. 2011; Ulusoy et al. 2015; Jesus et al. 2011; Schnellbacher et al. 2013; Altiok et al. 2012; Kuemmerle-Deschner et al. 2018; Infevers 2019). Most mutations identified are thought to be rare founder mutations in the Netherlands, Newfoundland (Aksentijevich et al. 2009), Puerto Rico (Reddy et al. 2009; Aksentijevich et al. 2009; Schnellbacher et al. 2013), Brazil (Jesus et al. 2011), India (Mendonca et al. 2017), Turkey (Altiok et al. 2012; Ulusoy et al. 2015; Infevers 2019) and Germany (Kuemmerle-Deschner et al. 2018).

Pathogenesis

DIRA is caused by loss-of-function mutations in *IL1RN*, which encodes the endogenous interleukin-1 (IL-1) receptor antagonist (IL1Ra). Most of the DIRA-causing mutations are nonsense or frameshift mutations that lead to either no expression of protein or to expression of truncated nonfunctional protein, IL-1Ra. Loss of

Pathogenesis of DIRA

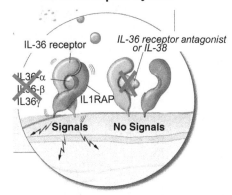

Deficiency of the IL-1 Receptor Antagonist (DIRA), Fig. 1 Pathogenesis of DIRA. (a) Loss of IL-1 receptor antagonist (IL-1Ra) caused by *IL1RN* recessive loss-of-function mutations results in unopposed IL-1 action through the IL-1 receptor. **(b)** The large genomic deletion on chromosome 2 in Puerto Rican patients with DIRA includes gene loci for *IL1RN* and five adjacent members of the *IL-1* gene family. The five adjacent genes include the agonists and antagonists of the IL-36 receptor. The agonists include *IL36A*, *IL36B*, and *IL36G*, and the antagonists include *IL36RN* and *IL38*. These genes likely do not contribute to the DIRA inflammatory phenotype. Common aliases: *IL36A* or *IL-1F6* encodes IL-36α, *IL36B* or *IL-1F8* encodes IL-36β, *IL36G* or *IL-1F9* encodes IL-36γ, *IL36RN* or *IL-1F5* encodes the IL-36 receptor antagonist, *IL38* or *IL-1F10* encodes IL-38, *IL1RL2* encodes the IL-36 receptor, *IL1RAP* encodes IL-1 receptor accessory protein which is a co-receptor in the IL-1 receptor and the IL-36 receptor system

IL-1Ra results in unopposed IL-1 action leading to escalation of IL-1-driven systemic and organ-specific inflammation involving the skin and bone (Fig. 1).

Clinical Manifestations

DIRA presents in early childhood with marked skin and bone involvement and systemic inflammation with elevation of acute-phase reactants. The age of onset is around 2 to 2.5 weeks of life.

Cutaneous Manifestations
DIRA skin manifestations are characterized by perinatal-onset pustular dermatitis resembling pustular psoriasis (Fig. 2a–c). Nail changes in the form of onychomadesis (splitting of the nail bed) and nail pitting can also be seen.

Musculoskeletal Manifestations
Inflammatory bone disease includes osteomyelitis of ribs with rib widening (Fig. 2e), periostitis affecting several long bones, and multifocal osteolytic lesions (Fig. 2d) (Aksentijevich et al. 2009). Sequela of sterile osteomyelitis includes odontoid destruction leading to atlantoaxial joint instability and requiring cervical spine surgery, kyphotic deformities in the form of gibbus formation from vertebral collapse from vertebral osteomyelitis (Fig. 2f), and limb length discrepancy. Osteopenia and osteoporosis are other common findings in untreated patients.

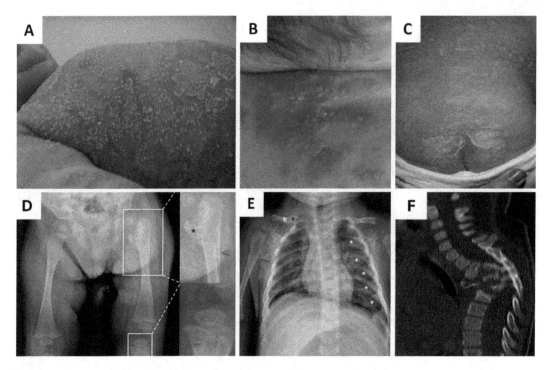

Deficiency of the IL-1 Receptor Antagonist (DIRA), Fig. 2 **Skin and bone manifestations in patients with DIRA. (a–c)** Generalized pustular dermatitis in patients with DIRA. **(d)** Hip x-ray shows a mixed lytic/sclerotic bone lesion (black star) in the left proximal femur with adjacent periosteal reaction (red arrow head) and lytic bone lesion (blue arrow head) with mild periosteal reaction in the left proximal tibia. **(e)** Anteroposterior chest x-ray showing expansion of the ribs in the left at 5–7 levels (white stars) and widening of the right clavicle (black star). There is an osteolytic lesion with periosteal reaction on the right humerus (red arrow head). **(f)** Gibbus formation secondary to osteolytic vertebral lesions and collapse of vertebral bodies

Vascular Manifestations

Untreated patients could have a hypercoagulable state manifesting in the form of deep vein thrombosis or thrombosis at the catheter site, CNS vasculitis, or vasculopathy. Carotid arteritis has also been seen in one patient of Puerto Rican descent.

Laboratory Findings

Leukocytosis, thrombocytosis, and elevated acute-phase reactants are present with active disease (Aksentijevich et al. 2009). Anemia can be severe requiring blood transfusions in untreated patients. If available, the absence of IL-1 receptor antagonist by ELISA can aide in making a diagnosis, as endogenous serum IL-1 receptor antagonist levels are undetectable in DIRA (serum needs to be assessed before initiation of treatment

with recombinant IL-1 receptor antagonist, anakinra). The severity of escalating inflammation in an infant in critical condition with a clinically suggestive phenotype should prompt empiric treatment with an IL-1 blocking agent rapidly. A rapid response to a therapeutic challenge with the short-acting IL-1 receptor antagonist, anakinra, can be diagnostic.

Diagnosis

The diagnosis of DIRA is made based on clinical features as treatment should be started in patients with a suspicion of DIRA even before a genetic diagnosis is made. However, detection of mutations in *IL1RN* is mandatory for a definitive diagnosis. Specific primers that facilitate the identification of two founder mutations, 175-kb deletion described in two Puerto Rican patients and a the recently described homozygous 22-kb deletion found in an Indian patient, are published and can aid in making a diagnosis (Aksentijevich et al. 2009; Mendonca et al. 2017).

rilonacept, maintained patients with DIRA in clinical remission by providing sustained control of symptoms and inflammatory markers. The weekly injections of rilonacept were preferred over the daily anakinra injections (Garg et al. 2017).

Treatment

Rapid response to treatment with recombinant IL-1Ra, anakinra, validates the key role of IL-1 in causing the severe phenotype of DIRA. IL-1 blockade with anakinra results in complete disease remission (Fig. 3) (Reddy et al. 2009; Aksentijevich et al. 2009; Jesus et al. 2011). One report used canakinumab, targeting IL-1β only (Ulusoy et al. 2015). Given the fact that IL-1 receptor antagonist, anakinra, which is recombinant IL-1 receptor antagonist, antagonizes IL-1α and IL-1β, treatments that would restore the IL-1α and IL-1β blocking activity have historically been used. While anakinra causes complete remission, a recent pilot study of six DIRA patients using the longer-acting soluble IL-1 receptor molecule,

Prognosis

The prognosis of untreated patients with DIRA is historically poor. So far, no adult patients who are homozygous for the disease-causing mutations have been identified. The mortality of untreated DIRA based on published reports is over 25% and occurred at 2, 4, and 21 months and 9.5 years of age. One case of intrauterine demise at 27 weeks of gestational age has also been reported (Aksentijevich et al. 2009; Altiok et al. 2012). In families with an affected child, and in populations where DIRA has been reported, genetic counseling and testing should be recommended. If both patients carry a heterozygous mutation, they have a 25% chance of having an affected child. Prenatal diagnosis can be made

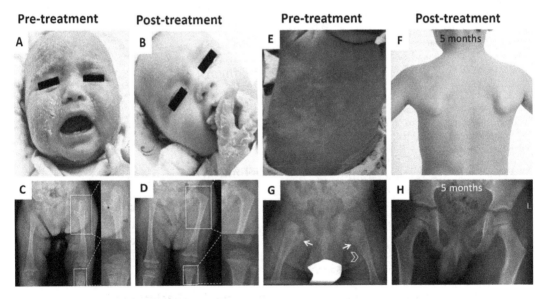

Pre-treatment   Post-treatment   Pre-treatment   Post-treatment

Deficiency of the IL-1 Receptor Antagonist (DIRA), Fig. 3 Clinical response to IL-1 inhibition in patients with DIRA. (a, b) Improvement of skin rash 7 days after anakinra was started. **(c, d)** Hip x-ray shows resolution of osteolytic lesion on the right humerus and improvement of the left femur and left tibia bone lesions after treatment with anakinra. **(e, f)** Persistence of clinical remission of skin lesions 5 months after discontinuation of anakinra and initiation of rilonacept. **(g, h)** Persistence of clinical remission of osteomyelitis 5 months after discontinuation of anakinra and initiation of rilonacept through diagnostic techniques like chorionic villous sampling or amniocentesis.

Cross-References

▶ DITRA: Deficiency of Interleukin 36 Receptor Antagonist
▶ Majeed Syndrome

References

Aksentijevich I, Masters SL, Ferguson PJ, Dancey P, Frenkel J, van Royen-Kerkhoff A, et al. An autoinflammatory disease with deficiency of the interleukin-1-receptor antagonist. N Engl J Med. 2009;360(23):2426–37.

Altiok E, Aksoy F, Perk Y, Taylan F, Kim PW, Ilikkan B, et al. A novel mutation in the interleukin-1 receptor antagonist associated with intrauterine disease onset. Clin Immunol. 2012;145(1):77–81.

Garg M, de Jesus AA, Chapelle D, Dancey P, Herzog R, Rivas-Chacon R, et al. Rilonacept maintains long-term inflammatory remission in patients with deficiency of the IL-1 receptor antagonist. JCI Insight. 2017;2(16): e94838. https://doi.org/10.1172/jci.insight.94838

Infevers: an online database for autoinflammatory mutations. Copyright. Available at http://fmf.igh.cnrs.fr/ISSAID/infevers/. Accessed 12 Mar 2019. [Internet].

Ivker RA, Grin-Jorgensen CM, Vega VK, Hoss DM, Grant-Kels JM. Infantile generalized pustular psoriasis associated with lytic lesions of the bone. Pediatr Dermatol. 1993;10(3):277–82.

Jesus AA, Osman M, Silva CA, Kim PW, Pham TH, Gadina M, et al. A novel mutation of IL1RN in the deficiency of interleukin-1 receptor antagonist syndrome: description of two unrelated cases from Brazil. Arthritis Rheum. 2011;63(12):4007–17.

Kuemmerle-Deschner JB, Hoertnagel K, Schlipf S, Hansmann S, Hospach T, Tsiflikas I, et al. Expanding the Phenotype: New Variant in the IL1RN-Gene Associated with Late Onset and Atypical Presentation of Dira [abstract]. Arthritis Rheumatol. 2018; 70 (suppl 10).

Leung VC, Lee KE. Infantile cortical hyperostosis with intramedullary lesions. J Pediatr Orthop. 1985; 5(3):354–7.

Mendonca LO, Malle L, Donovan FX, Chandrasekharappa SC, Montealegre Sanchez GA, Garg M, et al. Deficiency of Interleukin-1 receptor antagonist (DIRA): report of the first Indian patient and a novel deletion affecting IL1RN. J Clin Immunol. 2017;37(5):445–51.

Reddy S, Jia S, Geoffrey R, Lorier R, Suchi M, Broeckel U, et al. An autoinflammatory disease due to homozygous deletion of the IL1RN locus. N Engl J Med. 2009;360(23):2438–44.

Schnellbacher C, Ciocca G, Menendez R, Aksentijevich I, Golbach-Mansky R, Duarte A, et al. Deficiency of interleukin-1 receptor antagonist responsive to anakinra. Pediatr Dermatol. 2013;30(6):758–760.

Stenerson M, Dufendach K, Aksentijevich I, Brady J, Austin J, Reed AM. The first reported case of compound heterozygous IL1RN mutations causing deficiency of the interleukin-1 receptor antagonist. Arthritis Rheum. 2011;63(12):4018–22.

Stern SM, Ferguson PJ. Autoinflammatory bone diseases. Rheum Dis Clin N Am. 2013;39(4):735–49.

Ulusoy E, Karaca NE, El-Shanti H, Kilicoglu E, Aksu G, Kutukculer N. Interleukin-1 receptor antagonist deficiency with a novel mutation; late onset and successful treatment with canakinumab: a case report. J Med Case Rep. 2015;9:145.

DiGeorge Anomaly (del22q11)

Sonia Joychan[1] and Panida Sriaroon[2]
[1]Division of Allergy and Immunology, University of South Florida/Johns Hopkins All Children's Hospital, Tampa, FL, USA
[2]Department of Pediatrics, Division of Allergy and Immunology, University of South Florida/ Johns Hopkins All Children's Hospital, Tampa, FL, USA

Synonyms

Chromosome 22q11.2 deletion syndrome; DiGeorge syndrome; Velocardiofacial syndrome

Definition

DiGeorge syndrome is a primary immunodeficiency caused by a defect in chromosome 22, often resulting in T cell lymphopenia, congenital heart disease, hypocalcemia, and characteristic facies.

Introduction/Background

DiGeorge anomaly, also known as DiGeorge syndrome (DGS), or 22q11.2 deletion syndrome, arises from failure of differentiation and migration of neural crest cells into the third and fourth pharyngeal arches during early embryogenesis, resulting in hypoplasia or aplasia of the thymus and parathyroid glands as well as other structures that are derived from the pharyngeal arch system, including craniofacial structures, the aortic arch, and cardiac outflow tract (McDonald-McGinn et al. 2015). The syndrome, first described by Dr. Angelo DiGeorge in 1965, originally included infants with thymic aplasia and hypoparathyroidism. The definition was later expanded to include congenital heart diseases (McDonald-McGinn et al. 2015). Chromosome 22q11.2 microdeletions in one allele are identified in the majority of patients and, in about 90%, the deletion occurs as a de novo mutation (McDonald-McGinn et al. 1993). DGS presents with wide phenotypic heterogeneity, irrespective of gene deletion size, leading to some confusion regarding the nomenclature. In general, the term DGS encompasses a wide range of defects including chromosome 22q11.2 deletion syndrome and velocardiofacial syndrome and can also be associated with CHARGE syndrome (coloboma, heart, atresia, retardation of growth, genitourinary problems, ear abnormalities), chromosome 10p deletions, or mutations in a T-box transcription family member, *TBX1*, which is located in the region of 22q11 (Pai and Notarangelo 2018).

The prevalence of DGS is estimated to be between 1 in 3,000 and 1 in 6,000 live births based on epidemiologic studies conducted in the early 1990s and 2000s using fluorescence in situ hybridization (FISH) (McDonald-McGinn et al. 2015). Although DGS can affect individuals regardless of sex and ethnicity, it is less commonly diagnosed in nonwhite patients, which could be due to less recognizable craniofacial features in these populations. The 22q11.2 gene deletion appears to originate more often from maternal versus paternal source.

Clinical Presentation

DGS can have multiple organ system involvement including congenital heart defects, palatal abnormalities, immunodeficiency with complete or partial defects, developmental and speech delay and learning disabilities, neonatal hypocalcemia, renal anomalies, and gastrointestinal disorders (McDonald-McGinn et al. 1993). As noted above, the pharyngeal arch system is the common embryonic precursor for the thymus, parathyroid glands, and cardiac outflow tract. For this reason, cardiac defects in DGS are predominantly conotruncal abnormalities, such as tetralogy of Fallot (with or without pulmonary atresia), truncus arteriosus, interrupted aortic arch type B, and ventricular septal defects (McDonald-McGinn et al. 2015). Patients are at increased risk of atopy and autoimmunity, such as juvenile rheumatoid arthritis, immune cytopenias, and thyroid disease (McDonald-McGinn et al. 2015; Pai and Notarangelo 2018). Autoimmune hemolytic anemia, thrombocytopenia, or Evan's syndrome can be chronic and sometimes difficult to treat. Neurobehavioral problems are common, including bipolar disorder, autism spectrum disorders, and schizophrenia later in life (McDonald-McGinn et al. 1993). Characteristic facial features include a long face, malar flatness, upslanting palpebral fissures, "hooded eyelids," hypertelorism, prominent nasal root, bulbous nasal tip, short philtrum, downturned mouth, micrognathia, and low-set malformed ears with overfolded or squared-off helices. Patients may also have asymmetric crying facies.

Based on T cell counts, patients might be diagnosed with "partial" DGS, characterized by mild decrease of T cell counts (Pai and Notarangelo 2018), usually thrive well, or only have minor infections. They have little trouble with severe, life-threatening infections; however, cardiac defects, dysmorphic features, and cognitive developmental delay are common (Adkinson and Middleton 2014).

Approximately 1% of patients with 22q11 microdeletion have "complete" DGS characterized by an absent or severely hypoplastic thymus resulting in profound T cell lymphopenia (Pai and Notarangelo 2018). B cells are present, but specific antibody production is impaired due to poor T cell help. Patients with complete DGS may resemble patients with severe combined immunodeficiency (SCID) in their susceptibility to opportunistic infections with organisms such as fungi, viruses, and *Pneumocystis jiroveci* (Adkinson and Middleton 2014). There is also an atypical DGS variant, in which patients develop oligoclonal T-cell populations causing rash, liver dysfunction, and lymphadenopathy, phenotypically similar to Omenn syndrome (Pai and Notarangelo 2018).

In partial DGS, T cell counts are often within normal range by 5 years of age. The mechanism is unknown and could be due to the presence of some thymic tissue or maturation of T cells at extrathymic sites yet to be discovered (Abbas et al. 2015). Naïve T cells are generally low. Conversely, T cell counts in complete DGS do not improve with age. The degree of immunodeficiency does not correlate with any phenotypic features except for thymic size; however, thymic size correlates poorly with peripheral T lymphocyte counts, suggesting the presence of extrathymic T-cell production (Kobrynski and Sullivan 2007).

Laboratory Findings/Diagnostic Testing

The clinical findings noted above, particularly conotruncal heart anomalies, palatal defects, neonatal hypocalcemia, and characteristic facial features, should prompt diagnostic testing for DGS. Diagnosis is typically made using FISH, multiplex ligation-dependent probe amplification, or chromosomal microarray (McDonald-McGinn et al. 1993). The syndrome most often results from submicroscopic deletions (approximately 0.7–3 million base pairs in size) in the long arm of chromosome 22 (McDonald-McGinn et al. 2015). The region encompasses nearly 40 genes although many are not well characterized (McDonald-McGinn et al. 1993). The most common deletion involves *TBX1* (McDonald-McGinn et al. 1993), which is likely responsible for the cardiovascular, thymic, parathyroid, and craniofacial phenotypes observed in DGS (Kobrynski and Sullivan 2007). The loss of another gene, *COMT*, mapped to the same region of chromosome 22, may account for the increased risk of behavioral

and psychiatric problems (McDonald-McGinn et al. 2015). Deletion of additional genes within this region probably contributes to the heterogeneous clinical presentation.

Patients with complete DGS may be detected at birth during newborn screening for SCID based on a low number of T cell receptor excision circles. The initial laboratory evaluation in patients with confirmed DGS should include a complete blood count, chemistry profile, and lymphocyte subset analysis by flow cytometry (T cells, naïve T cells, memory T cells, B cells, and natural killer cells). As a result of accelerated conversion, the ratio of naïve to memory T cells is usually reduced (Adkinson and Middleton 2014). Patients with partial DGS are generally only mildly lymphopenic (Adkinson and Middleton 2014) and their humoral immunity is usually intact. Serum immunoglobulin (Ig) concentrations, particularly IgG and IgM, are generally normal but may be decreased in severely affected patients (Kobrynski and Sullivan 2007). Selective IgA deficiency is more common than in the general population, with estimates ranging from 2% to 30%. IgE levels are sometimes elevated (Adkinson and Middleton 2014), especially in cases with atopic manifestations.

Treatment/Prognosis

Management of DGS should involve an individualized and multidisciplinary approach. Early diagnosis is essential in modifying disease course and optimizing outcomes for these patients. Treatment involves surgical correction of severe congenital heart malformations, cleft palate repair, as well as correction of hypocalcemia via calcium and vitamin D supplementation. To maximize their learning ability, modifications in school environment are often required, and most patients benefit from educationally related services, such as speech and language therapy, cognitive therapy, physical therapy, behavioral counseling, and occupational and vocational counseling.

In patients with profound T cell dysfunction, trimethoprim-sulfamethoxazole is indicated for *Pneumocystis jiroveci* pneumonia prophylaxis. Live-attenuated vaccines are contraindicated in patients with complete DGS but might be safely administered to patients with partial DGS who have intact cellular immunity (Pai and Notarangelo 2018). Immunosuppressive agents and systemic corticosteroids may be indicated in DGS patients presenting with Omenn syndrome features or autoimmune cytopenias.

The profound immunodeficiency associated with complete DGS can be corrected with thymic transplantation or hematopoietic stem cell transplantation (HSCT). Reconstitution of T-cell immunity via thymic transplantation is the corrective treatment of choice for individuals with complete DGS (Pai and Notarangelo 2018). Thymic tissue from unrelated infants undergoing cardiac surgery is cultured in vitro and then implanted in the quadriceps muscles of the infants with DGS. Typically, naïve T cells are produced around 4–7 months of age. These cells have normal proliferative capacity, are tolerant to donor thymic cells, and display a polyclonal repertoire. The number of CD3+ T cells is usually lower in transplanted patients, but these cells maintain the functionality and diversity needed to prevent life-threatening infections. Compared to thymic transplantation, HSCT is a less preferred T cell reconstitution treatment option for patients with complete DGS. Unlike in other forms of SCID, the donor's T cells may be engrafted into the bone marrow of patients with complete DGS; however, most do not demonstrate ongoing T cell lymphopoiesis due to the lack of thymic tissue and patients may remain vulnerable to pathogens not recognized by the donor-derived T cells (Pai and Notarangelo 2018).

DGS is inherited via an autosomal dominant pattern. Patients with DGS have a 50% chance of having an affected child with each pregnancy, so genetic counseling is crucial (Kobrynski and Sullivan 2007). The long-term prognosis of patients depends on the nature of their underlying medical issues and involvement of different organs. For most, the immune defect is mild and life expectancy is not significantly affected, but the risk of autoimmunity increases with age.

References

Abbas AK, Lichtman AH, Pillai S. Cellular and molecular immunology. 8th ed. Philadelphia: Elsevier Saunders; 2015. viii, 535 pages.

Adkinson NF, Middleton E. Middleton's allergy: principles and practice. 8th ed. Philadelphia: Elsevier/Saunders; 2014. 2 volumes (xxvii, 1690, I–74 pages).

Kobrynski LJ, Sullivan KE. Velocardiofacial syndrome, DiGeorge syndrome: the chromosome 22q11.2 deletion syndromes. Lancet. 2007;370(9596):1443–52.

McDonald-McGinn DM, Emanuel BS, Zackai EH. 22q11.2 deletion syndrome. In: Adam MP, Ardinger HH, Pagon RA, Wallace SE, Bean LJH, Stephens K, et al., editors. GeneReviews((R)). Seattle: University of Washington; 1993. https://www.ncbi.nlm.nih.gov/books/NBK1523/

McDonald-McGinn DM, Sullivan KE, Marino B, Philip N, Swillen A, Vorstman JA, et al. 22q11.2 deletion syndrome. Nat Rev Dis Primers. 2015;1:15071.

Pai S, Notarangelo L. In: Hoffman R, Benz E, Silberstein L, Heslop H, Weitz J, Anastasi J, editors. Hematology: basic principles and practice. 7th ed. Philadelphia: Elsevier; 2018. p. 710–23.

DiGeorge Syndrome

▶ DiGeorge Anomaly (del22q11)

DIRA

▶ Deficiency of the IL-1 Receptor Antagonist (DIRA)

DITRA: Deficiency of Interleukin 36 Receptor Antagonist

▶ Deficiency of Interleukin 36 Receptor Antagonist (DITRA)

DKC1, Dyskeratosis Congenita/Hoyeraal-Hreidarsson Syndrome

Nicholas L. Rider
Section of Immunology, Allergy and
Retrovirology, Department of Pediatrics, Baylor
College of Medicine, Texas Children's Hospital,
Houston, TX, USA

Introduction

DKC1 encodes the dyskerin protein, a member of the human telomerase complex (Mochizuki et al. 2004). The gene is comprised by 15 exons spanning approximately 16 kb, located at Xq28 (Hassock et al. 1999). Human telomerase is a ribonucleoprotein complex which functions to maintain telomere length during normal cell division through controlled elongation thereby preventing shortening and ensuing cell cycle arrest and cell death (Du et al. 2009). Hemizygous pathogenic variants in *DKC1* lead to dyskeratosis congenita and the Hoyeraal-Hreidarsson syndrome (Knight et al. 1999a, b).

Clinical Relevance

Defects of human telomerase biology lead principally to dyskeratosis congenita (DC) (Mitchell et al. 1999). Patients with DC often present with progressive bone marrow failure and a triad of mucocutaneous findings which includes abnormal skin pigmentation, dystrophic nails, and leukoplakia of the oral mucosa (Dokal 2000). It is important to note that a minority of DC patients present with mucocutaneous features; thus, the disease must be suspected in their absence by signs of marrow failure (Du et al. 2009). Both *DKC1* and *TERT* mutations have been found to underlie the particularly severe form of DC, Hoyeraal-Hreidarsson (HH) syndrome which is noted

phenotypically by intrauterine growth restriction, cerebellar hypoplasia, microcephaly, severe immunodeficiency, and early-life marrow failure (Khincha and Savage 2016).

Diagnosis

A diagnosis of DC should be suspected in anyone with aplastic anemia (AA) or hypoplastic myelodysplastic syndrome (Townsley et al. 2014). Also, chronic cytopenias, unexplained thrombocytopenia, or an unexplained hypocellular marrow may also warrant consideration of a general telomeropathy. As mentioned above, nail dystrophy or tongue leukoplakia in children may suggest the disease (Dokal 2000). Additionally, premature graying of hair in adults could prompt consideration. Laboratory assessment of mean telomere length (MTL) is available via flow-FISH, a technique for measuring telomere length (Aubert et al. 2012). A finding of <1% MTL in peripheral blood lymphocytes compared to age-matched controls strongly suggests an underlying telomerase gene mutation (Alter et al. 2012). Since shortened telomeres may be secondarily affected by chronic inflammation, DNA oxidative stress, or a host of other environmental stressors, gene sequencing of telomerase genes (*DKC1*, *TERT, TERC,* and *TINF2*) is warranted (Houben et al. 2008).

Treatment and Prognosis

The telomeropathies are a clinically severe set of monogenic disorders which dramatically affect life span. Average age at death is presently noted to be 49 years (Shimamura and Alter 2010). Given the severe phenotype and dominantly inherited nature of DC, all family members of the proband should be assessed for disease via careful history, genomic testing for the variant, and/or telomere length measurement. Presently, only hematopoietic stem cell transplantation (HSCT) is curative;

however, supportive therapies such as red cell and platelet transfusions may be utilized for marrow failure management, and androgen therapy can aid in maintaining telomere length (Dietz et al. 2011; Townsley et al. 2016).

References

Alter BP, Rosenberg PS, Giri N, Baerlocher GM, Lansdorp PM, Savage SA. Telomere length is associated with disease severity and declines with age in dyskeratosis congenita. Haematologica. 2012;97(3):353–9.

Aubert G, Hills M, Lansdorp PM. Telomere length measurement-caveats and a critical assessment of the available technologies and tools. Mutat Res. 2012;730(1–2):59–67.

Dietz AC, Orchard PJ, Baker KS, et al. Disease-specific hematopoietic cell transplantation: nonmyeloablative conditioning regimen for dyskeratosis congenita. Bone Marrow Transplant. 2011;46(1):98–104.

Dokal I. Dyskeratosis congenita in all its forms. Br J Haematol. 2000;110(4):768–79.

Du HY, Pumbo E, Ivanovich J, et al. TERC and TERT gene mutations in patients with bone marrow failure and the significance of telomere length measurements. Blood. 2009;113(2):309–16.

Hassock S, Vetrie D, Giannelli F. Mapping and characterization of the X-linked dyskeratosis congenita (DKC) gene. Genomics. 1999;55(1):21–7.

Houben JM, Moonen HJ, van Schooten FJ, Hageman GJ. Telomere length assessment: biomarker of chronic oxidative stress? Free Radic Biol Med. 2008;44(3): 235–46.

Khincha PP, Savage SA. Neonatal manifestations of inherited bone marrow failure syndromes. Semin Fetal Neonatal Med. 2016;21(1):57–65.

Knight SW, Heiss NS, Vulliamy TJ, et al. Unexplained aplastic anaemia, immunodeficiency, and cerebellar hypoplasia (Hoyeraal-Hreidarsson syndrome) due to mutations in the dyskeratosis congenita gene, DKC1. Br J Haematol. 1999a;107(2):335–9.

Knight SW, Heiss NS, Vulliamy TJ, et al. X-linked dyskeratosis congenita is predominantly caused by missense mutations in the DKC1 gene. Am J Hum Genet. 1999b;65(1):50–8.

Mitchell JR, Wood E, Collins K. A telomerase component is defective in the human disease dyskeratosis congenita. Nature. 1999;402(6761):551–5.

Mochizuki Y, He J, Kulkarni S, Bessler M, Mason PJ. Mouse dyskerin mutations affect accumulation of telomerase RNA and small nucleolar RNA, telomerase activity, and ribosomal RNA processing. Proc Natl Acad Sci U S A. 2004;101(29):10756–61.

Shimamura A, Alter BP. Pathophysiology and management of inherited bone marrow failure syndromes. Blood Rev. 2010;24(3):101–22.

Townsley DM, Dumitriu B, Young NS. Bone marrow failure and the telomeropathies. Blood. 2014;124(18):2775–83.

Townsley DM, Dumitriu B, Liu D, et al. Danazol treatment for telomere diseases. N Engl J Med. 2016; 374(20):1922–31.

D

DOCK2

▸ Dedicator of Cytokinesis 2: DOCK2 Deficiency

DOCK8 Deficiency

Robert P. Nelson
Divisions of Hematology and Oncology, Stem Cell Transplant Program, Indiana University (IU) School of Medicine and the IU Bren and Simon Cancer Center, Indianapolis, IN, USA
Pediatric Immunodeficiency Clinic, Riley Hospital for Children at Indiana University Health, Indianapolis, IN, USA
Medicine and Pediatrics, Indiana University School of Medicine, Immunohematology and Transplantation, Indianapolis, IN, USA

Definition

One member of the CrkII-binding protein family DOCK180

Introduction/Background

Cell division control protein 42 homolog (Cdc42) participates in a broad range of fundamental cellular processes. While screening Cdc42-interacting proteins in a yeast two-hybrid system, Ruusala et al. identified a protein similar to the

CrkII-binding protein DOCK180 and designated the clone "dedicator of cytokinesis 8" (DOCK8) (Ruusala and Aspenstrom 2004). DOCK8 encodes a guanine nucleotide exchange factor highly expressed lymphocytes. The encoded protein consists of 1701 amino acids and localizes to the edges of cells undergoing lamellipodia formation that occurs with movement. A C-terminal fragment forms vesicles that contain filamentous actin that drives leukocyte cell motility (Ruusala and Aspenstrom 2004).

The multi-system disorder Job's syndrome, later termed hyper-IgE syndrome (HIES), causes defects in neutrophil chemotaxis and is an autosomal dominant form of HIES mediated by defective signal transducer and activation of transcription 3 (STAT3) function (Coles 1950; Davis et al. 1966; Hill et al. 1974). Loss-of-function (LOF) mutations in *DOCK8* were found associated with an autosomal recessive-inherited illness that exhibited certain common immunological and clinical symptoms, but without the nonimmune features observed with HIES secondary to STAT3 defects (Zhang et al. 2009). Over the recent 20 years, remarkably cohesive and effective global cooperative group efforts have crystalized the molecular, clinical, immunological, and therapeutic aspects of this disabling combined immunodeficiency, also known as DOCK8 immunodeficiency syndrome (DIDS). Many new insights regarding the relationships between host defense and the microbial environment are brought to light and were comprehensively summarized recently (Su et al. 2019).

Function

Innate Defense

Abnormal function of DOCK8 in mice causes the selective loss of group 3 innate lymphoid cells (ILC3). In humans, DOCK8 regulates ILC3 cytokine signaling after IL-7, IL-23, and IL-12 stimulation, and defective DOCK8 (but not STAT3) results in a profound depletion of ILC3s, and to a lesser extent ILC2s, in their peripheral blood. ILC1–3 subsets had defective

proliferation and expressed lower levels of IL-7R and were prone to apoptosis. The authors suggest lack of ILC expansion as one of the mechanisms that make patients prone to infections (Eken et al. 2019). Actin cytoskeletal function is critical for leukocyte cell migration through skin and subcutaneous tissues, which alters immune surveillance and increases eukaryotic viral representation and diversity. Novel viral genomes are created that expand the viral colonial diversity and promote the severe and sustained infections observed in DOCK8-deficient patients (Tirosh et al. 2018).

Adaptive Immunity

Humoral Immunity

Antibody production requires a certain organization of the immunological synapse that promotes the survival of B-cell subsets required for generating plasma cells and humoral memory (Randall et al. 2009). Randall et al. screened mutations in mice that disrupted humoral responses and discovered a LOF mutation in *DOCK8* that prevents B cells from forming marginal zone B cells and truncate normal affinity maturation. Accumulation of integrin ligand ICAM-1 in B cells is prevented, and imaging of the cytoskeleton reveals ezrin-defined actin networks that shape BCR diffusion and signaling in both resting and activated cells. Pathogenic mutations in *DOCK8* appear to impair sustained antibody production, and some patients with DOCK8 immunodeficiency syndrome (DIDS) experience skewing of the BCR repertoire, reduce the frequency of somatic hypermutations in the IGHV3 gene, and weaken antibody avidity (Batista et al. 2010).

Cellular Immunity

Mice with splice site mutations in DOCK8 fail to produce a humoral immune response due to the loss of germinal center B cells. They also experience T-cell lymphopenia secondary to decreased survival and diminished thymic egress of mature CD4+ thymocytes. The primary

CD8 + immune responses to viruses appear intact, despite the twofold reduction in peripheral naive T cells. Thus, DOCK8-deficient mice survive acute influenza infection, but produce low levels of CD8 (+) memory T cells following infection. These findings implicate DOCK8 as an important component that contributes to the establishment of sustained T-cell memory (Lambe et al. 2011).

Clinical Manifestations

The clinical description of a large number of patients with HIES was characterized prior to the molecular era (Donabedian and Gallin 1983). With the advent of genetic sequencing analysis and its capacity to sometimes predict certain clinical details, autosomal recessive hyper-IgE variants secondary to DOCK8 deficiencies were described and identified to lack the nonimmune manifestations that characterize autosomal dominantly-inherited defects in STAT3 deficiency. Immune abnormalities are similar, particularly the elevated serum IgE levels, eosinophilia, and absent Th17 cells.

Zhang et al. performed genetic studies in 11 patients from 8 families with sinopulmonary and cutaneous viral infections and found novel mutations in *DOCK8* and patient lymphocytes with absent DOCK8 protein. These patients experienced recurrent otitis, sinusitis, pneumonias, *Staphylococcus aureus* skin infections, severe herpes simplex or zoster infections, molluscum contagiosum, and human papillomavirus infections. Severe atopy with anaphylaxis and squamous cell carcinomas were common. One patient experienced T-cell lymphoma-leukemia (Zhang et al. 2009). Engelhardt et al. performed genetic studies in a total of 27 patients with autosomal-recessive *DOCK8* mutations and found CD4+ and CD8 + T activation defects, as well as defective T(h)17 cell differentiation and impaired eosinophil homeostasis (Engelhardt et al. 2009).

With respect to skin manifestations, 21 patients from 14 families with confirmed homozygous or compound heterozygous mutations in *DOCK8* had frequent skin viral infections. Recalcitrant, widespread cutaneous viral infections, food and environmental allergies, and absence of newborn rash and coarse facies point toward DOCK8 over STAT3 deficiency. Malignancies were extremely common and included aggressive cutaneous T-cell lymphoma, anal and vulvar squamous cell carcinomas, and diffuse large B-cell lymphoma, which developed in five patients during adolescence and young adulthood (Chu et al. 2012).

Sixty-two patients with AR-HIES DOCK8 deficiency had a median IgE level of 5201 IU, eosinophil counts of at least 800/muL (92% of patients), and usually low IgM levels (62%). Lymphopenia occurred in 20% of patient primarily because of low CD4(+) and CD8(+) T-cell counts. Over half of patients made protective specific antibody responses to recall antigens. Skin abscesses and allergies were common; however, there were few pneumatoceles, bone fractures, or teething problems, and mortality was high (34%). The authors suggest that DOCK8 deficiency is likely in patients with severe viral infections, allergies, low IgM levels, hypereosinophilia, and upper respiratory tract infections who lack parenchymal lung abnormalities, retained primary teeth, or minimal trauma fractures that are more likely HIES due to defects in STAT3 (Engelhardt et al. 2015).

Diagnosis and Laboratory Findings

Patients may present during childhood or as adults, with recurrent persistent and/or severe mixed infections, including high-grade encapsulated bacterial pathogens and/or chronic viral infections. There may be a positive family history of PID or consanguinity. Low T-cell receptor excision circles (TRECs), a marker of active thymopoiesis, has not been reported in DOCK8 deficiency. Facial features are normal and lymph nodes likely palpable. A child may have experienced growth failure or failure to thrive. Atopic dermatitis may be particularly severe, secondarily infected, and of an atypical distribution. Cognitive impairment, developmental delay, cardiovascular structural defects, facial dysmorphia, and absent thymus are not part of the syndrome. Genetic sequencing of *DOCK8* gene might reveal pathogenic mutations. Microdeletions of several exons of the *DOCK8* gene have also been described.

Screening immunological evaluation may demonstrate a complete blood count (CBC) with reduced lymphocyte percentages and increased eosinophil percentages. IgA and IgG are likely normal, but IgM may be low and IgE levels elevated. Elevated serum IgE levels, hypereosinophilia, low numbers of T cells and B cells, low serum IgM levels, and variable IgG antibody responses are common, and expansion in vitro of activated CD8 T cells may be impaired (Zhang et al. 2009). T(h)17 cells are absent. Natural killer (NK) cells are normal or decreased in number. Complement levels would be normal and B cells present (Zhang et al. 2010).

Treatment

Currently, the definitive therapy for DOCK8 deficiency is hematopoietic stem cell transplantation (HCT). There is not a standard conditioning regimen for HCT, and the transplant methods take into account the state of disease and degree of inflammation.

One 5-year-old boy with combined immunodeficiency characterized by severe eczema, multiple food allergies, excessively elevated serum IgE levels, and eosinophilia underwent HCT prior to the genetic definition of the condition. Although full donor chimerism was not achieved, the authors reported that mixed chimeric engraftment completely corrected the immunological defect. Skin manifestations disappeared, severe infections resolved, pulmonary function improved, and IgE levels declined. She was found later to carry a homozygous nonsense mutation in the *DOCK8* gene (Bittner et al. 2010). McDonald et al. reported an 8-year-old girl, who presented with pneumococcal meningitis at 11 months of age, complicated by chorda tendinae rupture, flail mitral valve, and isolated asplenia. She had deletions of exons 28 to 35 in *DOCK8*. She received conditioning treatment with busulfan and cyclophosphamide

and received an unaffected sibling bone marrow graft and cyclosporine and methotrexate graft-versus-host prophylaxis. She engrafted neutrophils on day +16 and lymphopenia resolved. After discharge, she suffered a lethal *Klebsiella* sepsis day +58 (McDonald et al. 2010).

Cuellar-Rodriguez J et al. performed HCT in six patients with DOCK8 deficiency using myeloablative busulfan/fludarabine and matched peripheral blood or marrow cell grafts, with tacrolimus/methotrexate GVHD prophylaxis. All patients were alive a median of 22.5 months, having experienced complete reversal of the clinical and immunologic phenotype. One patient with pre-transplant lung disease developed bronchiectasis post-transplant (Cuellar-Rodriguez et al. 2015). Reduced intensity conditioning and donor sources have expanded application of HCT to the management of DOCK8, and the global experience is uniquely broad and well documented compared to most other combined immunodeficiencies. A total of 81 patients from 22 centers were reported in a large retrospective analysis, and 84% of transplanted patients were living at the time of the publication. Eczema, infections, and mollusca appears to resolve rapidly compared to food allergies or failure to thrive (Aydin et al. 2019).

Clinicians should consider referral to a multidisciplinary center for the management of this complex condition. Dermatology expertise is essential for the management of challenging skin manifestations (Chu et al. 2012). Patients who receive immunoglobulin supplementation experience fewer and less severe infections despite normal IgG levels, given the defective antibody repertoire and reduced avidity (Tang et al. 2019).

Other considerations to reduce the risk of infections in immunocompromised patients are indicated; inactivated immunizations are indicated, but live vaccines might be avoided.

Cross-References

▶ DOCK2
▶ STAT Signal Transducer and Activator of Transcription

References

Aydin SE, Freeman AF, Al-Herz W, et al. Hematopoietic stem cell transplantation as treatment for patients with DOCK8 deficiency. J Allergy Clin Immunol Pract. 2019;7:848–55.

Batista FD, Treanor B, Harwood NE. Visualizing a role for the actin cytoskeleton in the regulation of B-cell activation. Immunol Rev. 2010;237:191–204.

Bittner TC, Pannicke U, Renner ED, et al. Successful long-term correction of autosomal recessive hyper-IgE syndrome due to DOCK8 deficiency by hematopoietic stem cell transplantation. Klin Padiatr. 2010;222:351–5.

Chu EY, Freeman AF, Jing H, et al. Cutaneous manifestations of DOCK8 deficiency syndrome. Arch Dermatol. 2012;148:79–84.

Coles HM. Staphylococcal pyaemia with pulmonary and cold subcutaneous abscesses. Arch Dis Child. 1950;25:280–1.

Cuellar-Rodriguez J, Freeman AF, Grossman J, et al. Matched related and unrelated donor hematopoietic stem cell transplantation for DOCK8 deficiency. Biol Blood Marrow Transplant. 2015;21:1037–45.

Davis SD, Schaller J, Wedgwood RJ. Job's syndrome. Recurrent, "cold", staphylococcal abscesses. Lancet. 1966;1:1013–5.

Donabedian H, Gallin JI. The hyperimmunoglobulin E recurrent-infection (Job's) syndrome. A review of the NIH experience and the literature. Medicine (Baltimore). 1983;62:195–208.

Eken A, Cansever M, Okus FZ, et al. ILC3 deficiency and generalized ILC abnormalities in DOCK8-deficient patients. Allergy. 2019;00:1–12.

Engelhardt KR, McGhee S, Winkler S, et al. Large deletions and point mutations involving the dedicator of cytokinesis 8 (DOCK8) in the autosomal-recessive form of hyper-IgE syndrome. J Allergy Clin Immunol. 2009;124:1289–302.e4.

Engelhardt KR, Gertz ME, Keles S, et al. The extended clinical phenotype of 64 patients with dedicator of cytokinesis 8 deficiency. J Allergy Clin Immunol. 2015;136:402–12.

Hill HR, Ochs HD, Quie PG, et al. Defect in neutrophil granulocyte chemotaxis in Job's syndrome of recurrent "cold" staphylococcal abscesses. Lancet. 1974;2:617–9.

Lambe T, Crawford G, Johnson AL, et al. DOCK8 is essential for T-cell survival and the maintenance of CD8+ T-cell memory. Eur J Immunol. 2011;41:3423–35.

McDonald DR, Massaad MJ, Johnston A, et al. Successful engraftment of donor marrow after allogeneic hematopoietic cell transplantation in autosomal-recessive hyper-IgE syndrome caused by dedicator of cytokinesis 8 deficiency. J Allergy Clin Immunol. 2010;126:1304–5.e3.

Randall KL, Lambe T, Johnson AL, et al. Dock8 mutations cripple B cell immunological synapses, germinal centers and long-lived antibody production. Nat Immunol. 2009;10:1283–91.

Ruusala A, Aspenstrom P. Isolation and characterisation of DOCK8, a member of the DOCK180-related regulators of cell morphology. FEBS Lett. 2004;572:159–66.

Su HC, Jing H, Angelus P, Freeman AF. Insights into immunity from clinical and basic science studies of DOCK8 immunodeficiency syndrome. Immunol Rev. 2019;287:9–19.

Tang W, Dou Y, Qin T, et al. Skewed B cell receptor repertoire and reduced antibody avidity in patients with DOCK8 deficiency. Scand J Immunol. 2019;89:e12759.

Tirosh O, Conlan S, Deming C, et al. Expanded skin virome in DOCK8-deficient patients. Nat Med. 2018;24:1815–21.

Zhang Q, Davis JC, Lamborn IT, et al. Combined immunodeficiency associated with DOCK8 mutations. N Engl J Med. 2009;361:2046–55.

Zhang Q, Davis JC, Dove CG, Su HC. Genetic, clinical, and laboratory markers for DOCK8 immunodeficiency syndrome. Dis Markers. 2010;29:131–9.

Down Syndrome

Luke A. Wall[1,3] and Regina M. Zambrano[2,3]
[1]Section of Allergy Immunology, New Orleans, LA, USA
[2]Section of Clinical Genetics, New Orleans, LA, USA
[3]Department of Pediatrics, Louisiana State University Health Sciences Center and Children's Hospital, New Orleans, LA, USA

Definition

Down syndrome results from a trisomy of the 21st chromosome. The syndrome encompasses a recognizable, yet highly variable, pattern of clinical features including abnormal facies, intellectual disability, and involvement of multiple organ systems.

Introduction

Down syndrome (DS) is the most common chromosome aneuploidy. According to the Centers for Disease Control and Prevention, approximately 1 in every 700 babies in the

United States is born with Down syndrome (Parker et al. 2010). This is a recognizable disorder with variable phenotype and clinical features in multiple organ systems. The majority of patients present with intellectual disability and findings in the cardiovascular (CV), gastrointestinal (GI), neurologic, endocrinologic, hematologic, orthopedic, and immunologic systems are typically described.

Patients with DS have increased susceptibility to infections. Otitis media is one of the most frequently encountered health problems. Bacterial sinusitis and lower respiratory tract infections such as pneumonia, bronchiolitis, and croup are also common. The course of illness due to infection may be longer and more severe compared to general population. Patients with DS have higher incidence of acute lung injury secondary to pneumonia. Among children requiring mechanical ventilation, acute respiratory distress syndrome (ARDS) is much higher among children with DS. In addition, DS may be a risk factor for death due to sepsis (Ram and Chinen 2011). Numerous specific factors, both immunologic and nonimmunologic, place patients with DS at increased risk for infections. Such factors may show significant variability among individuals.

Many immunologic derangements occur in patients with DS including tendency for infections with immune deficiency and for immune dysregulation resulting in autoimmunity, lymphoproliferation, and/or malignancy. Specifically, immune dysregulation includes autoimmune conditions such as hypothyroidism, diabetes (Anwar et al. 1998), and celiac disease (Carnicer et al. 2001), as well as hematologic conditions such as leukemia and transient myeloproliferative disorders.

Nonimmunologic Abnormalities

Essentially, all patients with DS have craniofacial anatomical abnormalities, a major contributing factor to chronic and recurrent bacterial otitis media and sinusitis. Some patients also have

Down Syndrome, Table 1 Anatomical and functional factors which may contribute to increased frequency, severity, or duration of infections in individuals with Down syndrome

Nonimmunologic factors
Craniofacial abnormalities
• Tonsil and adenoid hypertrophy
• Midface hypoplasia
• Mandibular hypoplasia
• Small otic canals and eustachian tubes
Lower airway abnormalities
• Laryngomalacia
• Tracheomalacia
• Tracheal stenosis
• Pulmonary hypoplasia
Functional abnormalities
• Gastroesophageal reflux and aspiration
• Hypotonia
• Eustachian tube dysfunction
• Obstructive sleep apnea
Other factors allowing portals for infection
• Chronic dermatitis
• Periodontal disease

abnormalities of the lower airway which can lead to difficulty clearing secretions and increased risk for pulmonary infections. While airway abnormalities may be severe enough to warrant tracheostomy, in the majority of patients, such alterations are at the milder end of the spectrum and may be an occult factor contributing to infections. Functional abnormalities such as gastroesophageal reflux and aspiration (compounded by hypotonia, abnormal anatomical relationships and obstructive sleep apnea) increase the risk for sinopulmonary infections. A list of such nonimmunologic factors is summarized in Table 1.

Immunologic Abnormalities

Primary immune defects may contribute to the higher incidence and prolonged course of infections observed in patients with DS (Ram and Chinen 2011). Intrinsic abnormalities of the immune system are numerous, involving the T and B cell compartment, and neutrophils as summarized in Table 2. In addition, Natural Killer (NK) cell abnormalities have been investigated but its clinical relevance is unclear. The reason

Down Syndrome, Table 2 Immunologic factors which may be abnormal in patients with Down syndrome

Immunologic factors
T cell abnormalities
• Reduced T cell numbers
• Reduced naïve T cell percentage
• Impaired T cell proliferation with mitogens
• Limited T cell repertoire
• Small thymus size with decreased AIRE expression
• Abnormal regulatory T cell function
B cell abnormalities
• Reduced B cell numbers
• Impaired vaccine response
• Decreased IgG2
• Impaired Memory B cells
Neutrophil abnormalities
• Decreased neutrophil chemotaxis

why trisomy of chromosome 21 leads to immune alterations remains largely a mystery. Theories which attributed weak immunity to the premature aging process known to occur in DS have fallen out of favor. Recent analyses of the circulating proteome in patients with DS demonstrated higher levels of pro-inflammatory cytokines and pronounced complement consumption. In addition, recent transcriptome analyses by the same group of investigators revealed consistent activation of the interferon transcriptional response. These findings all support a new theory that DS may be variant of type I interferonopathy. Increased gene dosage of the four interferon receptors encoded on chromosome 21 is proposed to play a major role (Sullivan et al. 2017). Autoimmune complications may be related to dysfunction of a central T cell tolerance mechanism, dependent on autoimmune regulator (AIRE) (Giménez-Barcons et al. 2014). *AIRE* is encoded by AIRE, which is located in 21q22.3. Although allele-specific quantification of *AIRE* showed that three copies are expressed, overall level of expression was lower. This can compromise tissue-specific antigen presentation and negative selection of autoreactive T cells. Furthermore, autoreactive T cells serve as pool for natural regulatory T cell (nTreg) generation. It has been observed that although nTregs expand in DS patients, they have less inhibitory activity and therefore allow autoreactivity to occur.

T Cell Abnormalities

T cell count and in-vitro proliferation with mitogen are often moderately reduced in children with DS. While T cell counts often increase with age, the T cell receptor diversity may remain limited. The thymic size is small and the percentage of naïve T cells is reduced in infants, corresponding with low T cell receptor excision circle (TREC) counts (Ram and Chinen 2011; Joshi et al. 2011). Therefore, DS should be included in differential diagnosis for patients with T cell lymphopenia identified by newborn screening for severe combined immune deficiency (SCID). While patients with DS do not typically contract opportunistic infections, any patient found to have an extremely impaired T cell compartment could be considered at risk. This would be unusual among patients with DS.

B Cell Abnormalities

B cell numbers are typically reduced. In addition, antibody response to polysaccharide vaccines may be sub-optimal (Joshi et al. 2011). While immunoglobulin levels are normal or elevated in most patients, hypogammaglobulinemia may occur. Reduced IgG2 subclass has been documented (Ram and Chinen 2011; Saha et al. 2017). Patients with DS are less able to produce and maintain switched memory B cells, the main player in the antibody recall response (Joshi et al. 2011).

Neutrophil Abnormalities

While respiratory burst capacity is typically normal in DS, neutrophil chemotaxis is impaired (Ram and Chinen 2011). Patients with DS do not typically manifest the type of infections generally thought to be associated with neutrophil defects. However, the impaired chemotaxis could be a contributing factor in the susceptibility to infections, in general.

Diagnostic and Treatment Approach

Regarding the diagnostic approach and treatment interventions, there are no specific guidelines regarding infections in DS. Certainly, any child, especially one with underlying DS, deserves to be evaluated by an immunologist if infections are occurring at increased frequency or severity compared to the general population. Immunologic evaluation in patients with DS should encompass B and T cell enumeration, including naïve T cell and switched memory B cell percentage. Immunoglobulins and vaccine titers to common immunizations are also necessary. If protection to vaccines is low, additional boosters should be administered, and postvaccine titers measured. Reevaluation every 6–12 months, depending on the clinical progress of the patient, should be considered. Daily prophylactic antibiotics may be a viable treatment option in select patients and may reduce the frequency of sinopulmonary, periodontal, and skin infections. The risks and benefits of daily antibiotics should be weighed carefully. Some patients may benefit from immunoglobulin replacement, especially those with low immunoglobulin levels, weak vaccine response, and a pattern of severe infections.

The Complexity of Care

In addition to the factors mentioned above surrounding the approach to patients with DS and an abnormal pattern of infections, the complexity goes much deeper. Some patients have complex congenital abnormalities which may require repeated surgeries and hospital admissions with frequent exposure to nosocomial pathogens. Apart from this, patients with DS are often highly affectionate and may closely encounter other individuals, even strangers, with hugs and handshakes much more than the average person. This contact increases exposure to bacteria and viruses. Hygiene may present a challenge due to factors such as limited cognitive ability and limited coordination to proceed through multiple steps required to effectively perform tasks such as cleansing one's hands.

Behavioral and psychological aspects of DS impact all angles of the disorder. Repetitive scratching and picking at wounds lead to delayed healing and increased contamination. Anxiety regarding medical interventions and impaired capacity to understand the procedures are factors which should always be considered by the medical team. The care of patients with DS who experience increased frequency or severity of infections requires a multidisciplinary approach involving pulmonology, otolaryngology, immunology, dentistry, dermatology, genetics, and psychology. Good communication with, and involvement of, the patient's family is an absolute necessity.

References

Anwar AJ, Walker JD, Frier BM. Type 1 Diabetes mellitus and Down's syndrome: prevalence, management and diabetic complications. Diabet Med. 1998;15:160–3.

Carnicer J, Farré C, Varea V, Vilar P, Moreno J, Artigas J. Prevalence of coeliac disease in Down's syndrome. Eur J Gastroenterol Hepatol. 2001;13:263–7.

Giménez-Barcons M, Casteràs A, Armengol Mdel P, Porta E, Correa PA, Marín A, Pujol-Borrell R, Colobran R. Autoimmune predisposition in Down syndrome may result from a partial central tolerance failure due to insufficient intrathymic expression of AIRE and peripheral antigens. J Immunol. 2014;193(8):3872–9.

Joshi AY, Abraham RS, Snyder MR, Boyce TG. Immune evaluation and vaccine responses in Down syndrome: evidence of immunodeficiency? Vaccine. 2011;29(31):5040–6.

Parker SE, Mai CT, Canfield MA, Rickard R, Wang Y, Meyer RE, Anderson P, Mason CA, Collins JS, Kirby RS, Correa A, National Birth Defects Prevention Network. Updated National Birth. Prevalence estimates for selected birth defects in the United States, 2004–2006. Birth Defects Res A Clin Mol Teratol. 2010;88(12):1008–16. https://doi.org/10.1002/bdra.20735. Epub 2010 Sep 28

Ram G, Chinen J. Infections and immunodeficiency in Down syndrome. Clin Exp Immunol. 2011;164(1):9–16.

Saha SP, Khan M, Chowdhury AK. Immunoglobulin G1 and G2 profile in children with Down syndrome. IMC J Med Sci. 2017;11(1):1–4.

Sullivan KD, Evans D, Pandey A, Hraha TH, Smith KP, Markham N, Rachubinski AL, Wolter-Warmerdam K, Hickey F, Espinosa JM, Blumenthal T. Trisomy 21 causes changes in the circulating proteome indicative of chronic autoinflammation. Sci Rep. 2017;7(1):14818.

Dysgammaglobulinemia

▶ Unclassified Primary Antibody Deficiency (unPAD)

E

E47 Transcription Factor Deficiency

Vassilios Lougaris and Alessandro Plebani
Pediatrics Clinic and Institute for Molecular
Medicine A. Nocivelli, Department of Clinical
and Experimental Sciences, University of Brescia
and ASST-Spedali Civili of Brescia, Brescia, Italy

Definition

E47 transcription factor deficiency or autosomal dominant TCF3 deficiency (OMIM # 616941) is a rare primary immunodeficiency characterized by reduced serum levels of all immunoglobulin classes and the absence of peripheral B cells (peripheral B cells<2%). To date, a very small number of patients have been described. TCF3 deficiency is caused by monoallelic autosomal dominant mutations in the TCF3 gene, coding for the transcription factor E47. TCF3 is located in chromosome 19p13.3.

Pathogenesis

Early B cell development takes place in the bone marrow. An important maturational step is the progression from the pro-B to the pre-B stage (Espeli et al. 2006; Rudin and Thompson 1998;

Bartholdy and Matthias 2004). This step depends on the expression of a functional B cell receptor composed of the μ heavy chain (*IGHM*; OMIM∗147020), Igα (CD79A; OMIM∗112205), Igβ (CD79B; OMIM∗147245), VpreB, and λ5 (*IGLL1*; OMIM∗146770) that initiates downstream signaling necessary for early B cell differentiation through kinases such as *BTK* and *BLNK* (OMIM∗604615). Animal models and in vitro studies over the years have underlined the importance of each of the pre-BCR components and associated transcription factors for the transition from pro-B to pre-B stage of maturation, suggesting that these genes may be responsible for agammaglobulinemia in humans (Conley and Cooper 1998).

Numerous transcription factors are important for early B cell development. In particular, the E2A family of transcription factors, which includes E47, was shown to play an essential role in early B cell development (Bain et al. 1994). In fact, reported on a recurrent dominant E47 mutation (p.E555K) responsible for agammaglobulinemia in four unrelated patients, characterized by BCR negative B cells and enhanced expression of CD19 (Dobbs et al. 2011; Boisson et al. 2013). Bone marrow evaluation showed reduction of both pro-B and pre-B cells, without immunoglobulin expression. The mutant E47 protein localized to the nucleus, however had impaired DNA binding and had dominant negative action over wild-type E47 protein.

© Springer Science+Business Media LLC, part of Springer Nature 2020
I. R. Mackay et al. (eds.), *Encyclopedia of Medical Immunology*,
https://doi.org/10.1007/978-1-4614-8678-7

Clinical Presentation

The four unrelated patients described by Dobbs et al. and Boisson et al. presented in the 1st years of life with severe infections, including pneumococcal meningitis, recurrent otitis, vaccine-associated polio, and arthritis. Associated clinical features included eosinophilic dermatitis and hepatomegaly. Laboratory studies showed severely decreased levels of serum immunoglobulins and less than 3% of CD19+ circulating B cells. B cells did not express surface immunoglobulins.

Diagnosis

Immunological work-up in affected patients shows very low levels of serum immunoglobulins and complete absence of peripheral B cells. Once BTK mutations are excluded for male patients, genetic screening for mutations in components of the pre-BCR and downstream signaling molecules such as BLNK and p85α should be performed. Detection of pathogenic mutations in TCF3, encoding E47, makes the diagnosis.

Management

As in other forms of primary humoral immunodeficiencies, immunoglobulin replacement treatment should be undertaken once the immunological diagnosis of agammaglobulinemia is established. Currently two options are available: intravenous or subcutaneous. Normally, a dose of 400 mg/kg/dose every 3–4 weeks is sufficient to maintain pre-infusion IgG levels >500 mg/dl that should be able to reduce the number of infectious episodes, especially that of invasive infections.

Antibiotic usage should be undertaken for every infectious episode, and in some case, prophylactic regimen may also be prescribed.

Considering the limited number of affected patients, long-term disease progression is not well known.

References

Bain G, Robanus Maandag EC, Izon DJ, Amsen D, Kruisbeek AM, Weintraub BC, Krop I, Schlissel MS, Feeney AJ, van Roon M, van der Valk M, te Riele HPJ, Berns A, Murre C. E2A proteins are required for proper B cell development and initiation of immunoglobulin gene rearrangement. Cell. 1994;79:885–1994.

Bartholdy B, Matthias P. Transcriptional control of B cell development and function. Gene. 2004;327:1–23.

Boisson B, Wang YD, Bosompem A, Lim A, Kochetkov T, Tangye SG, Casanova JL, Conley ME. A recurrent dominant negative E47 mutation causes agammaglobulinemia and BCR-B cells. J Clin Invest. 2013;123:4781–5.

Conley ME, Cooper MD. Genetic basis of abnormal B cell development. Curr Opin Immunol. 1998;10(4):339–406.

Dobbs AK, Bosompem A, Coustan-Smith E, Tyerman G, Saulsburry FT, Conley ME. Agammaglobulinemia associated with BCR-Bcells and enhanced expression of CD19. J Clin Invest. 2011;118:1828–37.

Espeli M, Rossi B, Mancini SJ, Roche P, Gauthier L, Schiff C. Initiation of pre-B cell receptor signaling: common and distinctive features in human and mouse. Semin Immunol. 2006;18:56–66.

Rudin CM, Thompson CB. B-cell development and maturation. Semin Oncol. 1998;25:435–46.

Early Onset Sarcoidosis

▶ Blau Syndrome

EBV-Associated Autosomal Lymphoproliferative Syndrome

▶ ITK Deficiency

EDA-ID

▶ Autosomal Dominant Anhidrotic Ectodermal Dysplasia with Immunodeficiency (AD-EDA-ID)

Elastase Deficiency, Severe Congenital Neutropenia (SCN) 1

Anders Fasth
Department of Pediatrics, Institute of Clinical Sciences, Sahlgrenska Academy at University of Gothenburg, Gothenburg, Sweden

Synonyms

Severe congenital neutropenia 1(SCN1)

Definition

Severe congenital neutropenia is by the European Society for Immunodeficiencies (ESID, www.esid.org) defined as neutropenia $<0.5 \times 10^9$/L (500/µL) measured on at least three occasions *or* neutropenia $<1.0 \times 10^9$/L (1000/µL) measured on at least three occasions with at least one of the following: deep-seated infection due to bacteria and/or fungi, recurrent pneumonia, buccal and/or genital aphthous lesions, omphalitis and affected family members, *and* exclusion of secondary causes of neutropenia (ESID Registry).

In elastase deficiency, mutations are found in the *ELANE* gene at 19p13. Inheritance is autosomal dominant.

Introduction/Background

Cyclic and severe neutropenias have in common mutations in *ELANE*. Some mutations are responsible for the cyclic form, others are for severe neutropenia, but several mutations can give both forms. Certain mutations are associated with milder disease, while others carry a higher risk for malignant transformation.

The protein formed as the result of the mutations causes endoplasmatic stress misfolded protein response and apoptosis. Elastase deficiency accounts for close to half of all cases of severe congenital neutropenias. The estimated incidence is less than 1 per 100,000 newborns (Makaryan et al. 2015).

Clinical Presentation (History/PE)

- First manifestation is often omphalitis and/or delayed detachment of the umbilical stump, later recurrent bacterial infections of the skin and the respiratory tract, and also serious infections such as septicemia, meningitis, and osteomyelitis.
- Typical is painful recurrent non-herpetic oral cavity aphthae and inflamed gingiva and periodontitis leading to premature tooth loss (Skokowa et al. 2017).

Laboratory Findings/Diagnostic Testing

- Severe neutropenia, usually $<0.2 \times 10^9$/L.
- Bone marrow with typical maturation arrest at the level of promyelocytes.
- Diagnostic testing should verify severe neutropenia at at least three occasions followed by DNA analysis to diagnose mutation in *ELANE*.

Treatment/Prognosis

- Vigorous treatment of any infection. Consider treatment/prophylaxis until normalization of neutrophils upon G-CSF treatment.
- Recombinant human G-CSF in doses 3–10 (60) µg/Kg restores neutrophil count and normalizes infection rate. Without G-CSF treatment, mortality is very high, 80–90%.
- Periodontitis and aphthae usually do not respond to G-CSF, which makes professional dental care important.
- The disorder carries a 15–20% lifetime risk for MDS/AML, and yearly bone marrow aspirations including cytogenetics and analysis of somatic mutations in *GCSFR* and *RUNX1* are mandatory.
- In case of resistance to G-CSF and/or development of MDS/AML hematopoietic stem cell transplantation (Skokowa et al. 2017).

References

ESID Registry. Clinical criteria. https://esid.org/content/download/15478/424246/file/ESIDRegistry_Clinical Criteria.pdf. Retrieved October, 2017.

Makaryan V, Zeidler C, Bolyard AA, Skokowa J, Rodger E, Kelley ML, Boxer LA, Bonilla MA, Newburger PE, Shimamura A, Zhu B, Rosenberg PS, Link DC, Welte K, Dale DC. The diversity of mutations and clinical outcomes for ELANE-associated neutropenia. Curr Opin Hematol. 2015;22:3–11.

Skokowa J, Dale DC, Touw IP, Zeidler C, Welte K. Severe congenital neutropenias. Nat Rev Dis Prim. 2017;3:17032.

Epidermodysplasia Verruciformis/Lewandowsky-Lutz Dysplasia

▶ *EVER1* and *EVER2* Mutations in Epidermodysplasia Verruciformis

Evaluation of Suspected Immunodeficiency, Cellular

Panida Sriaroon
Department of Pediatrics, Division of Allergy and Immunology, University of South Florida/Johns Hopkins All Children's Hospital, Tampa, FL, USA

Introduction

Cellular immunodeficiency (T cell immunodeficiency) is a group of disorders caused by decreased number or function of T cells. Unusual infections or severe complications of common infections, are often seen in patients with a defect in cellular immunity. The condition can be either a primary defect of the thymus, T cell progenitors, T cell signaling, or a combined immunodeficiency with or without syndromic features (Picard et al. 2015). Severe cellular immune defects, such as severe combined immunodeficiency (SCID), complete DiGeorge syndrome (DGS), and Wiskott-Aldrich syndrome (WAS), usually manifest in infancy and can be fatal if untreated. SCID is characterized by defects in T cell number and function. Complete DGS is characterized by severe T cell lymphopenia due to thymic hypoplasia. Although presentation varies, the historic triad of DGS includes hypocalcemia, conotruncal cardiac anomaly, and hypoplastic thymus. In WAS, the classic clinical triad found in about one third of patients includes eczema, thrombocytopenia, and recurrent infections. Commonly encountered infections in patients with defective cellular immunity include chronic mucocutaneous candidiasis, warts, invasive fungal infections, persistent infections with cytomegalovirus, and other herpes viruses such as simplex or zoster, *Pneumocystis jiroveci* pneumonia, infections with atypical mycobacteria species, and other opportunistic infections. There is also an increased risk for malignancy, particularly B-cell lymphoma or lymphoproliferative diseases, driven by Epstein-Barr virus. Some classic clinical features of cellular immune defects include failure to thrive, chronic diarrhea, and dermatitis.

Diagnostic Testing

A summary of the tests for evaluation of cellular immunodeficiency is listed in the Table 1. One of the most basic and useful screening tests is the complete blood count (CBC) with absolute lymphocyte count (ALC). Total lymphocyte counts below 1500/mm^3 in an adult or below 4000/mm^3 in an infant should raise the suspicion of a T cell immunodeficiency. Patients with WAS have thrombocytopenia and small platelets evident on CBC. Almost all states in the United States use the T cell receptor excision circle (TREC) assay, which detects T cell lymphopenia prior to clinical symptoms of T cell deficiency, as part of routine newborn screening programs (Kwan and Puck 2015). So far, TREC screening has identified infants with various forms of SCID and infants with T cell lymphopenia due to other immunodeficiency or other conditions (Jyonouchi et al. 2017).

When T cell immunodeficiency is suspected, HIV testing and lymphocyte subset analysis for quantitative assessment of T cells, B cells, and NK cells should be performed. Healthy infants are known to have a natural lymphocytosis at birth, which gradually declines over time. Therefore, all values from lymphocyte subset analysis must be compared to age-appropriate reference ranges. In healthy individuals, CD3 T cells make up 60–70% of the total lymphocyte count. These CD3 T cells are subdivided into CD4 T helper cells and CD8 T suppressor cells in a ratio that is typically greater than 1.0. Inverted CD4 to CD8 T ratios with low total CD4 T cell numbers are seen in patients with acquired immunodeficiency syndrome (AIDS), some common variable immunodeficiency (CVID) subtypes, and idiopathic CD4 T cell lymphopenia, and in some cases post-transplant. In some specialized laboratories, the percentages of the naïve CD45RA and the memory CD45RO T cells can also be measured for evaluation of T cell output by the thymus and memory phenotype T cells, respectively. Additional testing of T cell function can be performed by delayed type hypersensitivity (DTH) skin testing to recall antigens and by in vitro mitogen- and antigen-induced lymphocyte proliferation assays (Bonilla et al. 2015). Mitogens, including phytohemagglutinin (PHA), concanavalin A (Con A), and pokeweed mitogen (PWM), can stimulate lymphocyte proliferation nonspecifically and are used to evaluate cellular immune responsiveness. Lymphocyte proliferation response to antigens, such as

Candida, Tetanus toxoid, and tuberculin purified protein derivative (PPD), are used to evaluate memory function of cell-mediated immune response in older children and adults. The mitogen and antigen-induced proliferation assays are highly sensitive to specimen handling and require sufficient numbers of viable lymphocytes to reach the laboratory in order to conduct the assay reliably. Taken together, lymphocyte subset analysis and tests of lymphocyte function help direct the clinical diagnosis of SCID and focus on the most likely genetic defects responsible (Bousfiha et al. 2013). Some of the genetic defects causing SCID are presented in Table 2, along with the respective lymphocyte phenotype.

Alpha-fetoprotein levels are usually elevated in patients with ataxia-telangiectasia. In neonates, chest radiograph with absence of the thymic shadow may indicate SCID or complete DGS. When classic DGS is suspected, the diagnosis can be confirmed by a fluorescent in situ hybridization (FISH) test for chromosomal deletions at 22q11.2. Additional tests, such as chromosome microarray and gene sequencing, should be performed in patients with clinical phenotypes resembling DGS and negative result of FISH for 22q11.2 deletions.

More advanced analysis for T cell function, signaling pathways, or cytokine production may be required for investigation of cellular immunity. Identification of genetic mutations by single or multiple gene sequencing and whole exome sequencing can help confirm the diagnosis for cellular immune disorders. These assays are now

Evaluation of Suspected Immunodeficiency, Cellular, Table 1 Laboratory evaluation of suspected cellular immunodeficiency

General screening tests: CBC for ALC, newborn screening for TREC assay (not available in all states)
Screening tests for T cell defects: HIV testing, T cell subset enumeration by flow cytometry, DTH, chest radiograph for thymic shadow in neonates
Advanced tests: Mitogen- and antigen-induced lymphocyte proliferation responses, signal transduction studies, production of cytokines, FISH analysis for chromosome 22q11.2 deletion, gene sequencing for specific defects, whole exome sequencing
Abbreviations: CBC, complete blood count; ALC, absolute lymphocyte count; TREC, T cell receptor excision circle; HIV, human immunodeficiency virus; DTH, delayed type hypersensitivity; FISH, fluorescent in situ hybridization

Evaluation of Suspected Immunodeficiency, Cellular, Table 2 Severe combined immunodeficiency (SCID) phenotypes

Lymphocyte profile	Genetic defect causing SCID
$T^- B^+ NK^+$	IL7R-α deficiency, CD3D, CD3E, PTPRC, CD247, FOXN1, CORO1A, complete DiGeorge
$T^- B^- NK^+$	RAG1/RAG2; Artemis (DCLRE1C), PRKCD, *Cernunnos* (NHEJ1), DNA Ligase4 deficiency (LIG4)
$T^- B^+ NK^-$	γc deficiency (IL2Rγ), Jak3 deficiency
$T^- B^- NK^-$	Reticular dysgenesis (AK2), adenosine deaminase deficiency (ADA)

available commercially and at major immunology research laboratories, but at relatively high cost. Moreover, clinicians must be aware of the limitations of each assay and interpret results within the context of clinical presentation.

References

Bonilla FA, Khan DA, Ballas ZK, Chinen J, Frank MM, Hsu JT, et al. Practice parameter for the diagnosis and management of primary immunodeficiency. J Allergy Clin Immunol. 2015;136(5):1186.

Bousfiha A, Jeddane L, Ailal F. A phenotypic approach for IUIS PID classification and diagnosis: guidelines for clinicians at the bedside. J Clin Immunol. 2013;33(6):1078–87.

Jyonouchi S, Jongco AM, Puck J, Sullivan KE. Immunodeficiencies associated with abnormal newborn screening for T cell and B cell lymphopenia. J Clin Immunol. 2017;37(4):363–74.

Kwan A, Puck JM. History and current status of newborn screening for severe combined immunodeficiency. Semin Perinatol. 2015;39(3):194–205.

Picard C, Al-Herz W, Bousfiha A, Casanova JL, Chatila T, Conley ME, et al. Primary immunodeficiency diseases: an update on the classification from the International Union of Immunological Societies Expert Committee for primary immunodeficiency 2015. J Clin Immunol. 2015;35(8):696–726.

Evaluation of Suspected Immunodeficiency, Flow Cytometry

Jennifer W. Leiding
Department of Pediatrics, Division of Allergy and Immunology, University of South Florida at Johns Hopkins – All Children's Hospital, St. Petersburg, FL, USA

Flow cytometry is a laboratory tool that has become standard in the evaluation of hematopoietic cell subpopulations. The application of flow cytometry allows for the detailed assessment of cell surface markers, intracellular protein expression, cellular activation, and cell death that characterize all immunodeficiencies. A flow cytometer analyzes the physical and chemical characteristics of cells in a fluid status that pass through a laser in single file. Cells are labeled with florescent markers that emit light at varying wavelengths.

The components of a flow cytometer are the light source, optical bench, fluidic system, and computer. Stained cells enter in single file through the fluidic system, are interrogated by the light source, then generated light signals are directed by the optical system to the photodetectors, and light is converted into an electronic signal. Analysis programs often evaluate the number and percentage of events, detect the mean or median channel florescence, and have statistical measures for identified cell populations.

Florescent reagents consist of standard monoclonal antibodies that bind to cell surface or intracellular markers. The monoclonal antibody is conjugated with a flourochrome, a dye that absorbs and emits light of different wavelengths.

The proper assessment of specific cell types within a mixture of cells requires initial identification of specific white blood cells separating lymphocytes from non-lymphocytes through a process termed gating. Gating initially focuses on specific leukocyte populations by using forward and side light scatter. Forward scatter is a measurement of cellular cross-sectional area that directly correlates with cell size and side scatter is a reflection of cell granularity (Fig. 1). The combination of forward and side light scatter separates leukocytes into three distinct populations:

- Lymphocytes – are the smallest and least granular cells and have the lowest side and forward scatter.
- Neutrophils – are the largest and highly granular cells and exhibit high side and forward scatter.
- Monocytes – are large but less granular and show similar forward scatter as that of neutrophils but lower side scatter.

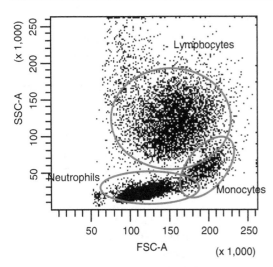

Evaluation of Suspected Immunodeficiency, Flow Cytometry, Fig. 1 Leukocyte subpopulations separated with forward and side scatter. Lymphocyte, neutrophil, and monocyte populations are separated within the flow cytometer based on size and granularity (Figure provided by Matt Morrow, MS, Johns Hopkins-All Children's Hospital)

Flow cytometry data is most simply displayed in a single parameter histogram. The cell number is expressed on the y axis and the light intensity from a single flourochrome on the x axis.

Quantification of cell populations is easily accomplished with flow cytometry and is important in the evaluation of a patient with a suspected immunodeficiency. In addition to determining quantity, clonality can also be evaluated. Cell populations such as B cells are a heterogenous population of cells with κ and λ light chains. In the case of B cells, the disruption of the κ:λ ratio is indicative of malignancy or diseases of lymphoproliferation. Flow cytometry can also be utilized to test for the presence or absence of a particular cell surface antigen. The pattern of surface antigen expression can provide information regarding cell ontogeny, differentiation, activation, and death. Lymphoid activation is studied by staining for cell surface markers that are upregulated upon cell activation.

Another way to assess lymphoid function is with intracellular cytokine staining. Cells can be stained with surface markers first, then fixed and permeabilized and re-stained for presence of intracellular cytokines. There is little to no presence of intracellular cytokines present at baseline in lymphocytes, so an activating event must take place to up-regulate the expression of these cytokines (Oliveira and Fleisher 2010).

Functional assessment of certain cell populations can also be investigated with flow cytometry. Carboxyfluorescein succinimidyl ester (CFSE) is a fluorescent stain that is taken up by proliferating lymphocytes and is used to monitor lymphocyte proliferation and migration. The florescence of CFSE decreases by half with every cell division cycle directly correlates with the proliferation capacity of lymphocytes. The neutrophil oxidative burst can be assessed using the dihydrorhodamine (DHR) assay. Following activation with phorbol myrisate acetate (PMA), granulocytes tagged with dihydrorhodamine fluoresce in the presence of reactive oxygen species directly correlates with NADPH function within granulocytes. In contrast, when components of the NADPH oxidase are mutated, little to no ROS is produced leading to little or no florescence in the DHR assay (Vowells et al. 1995).

The use of flow cytometry has emerged as a very useful tool in the evaluation of patients with or suspected to have primary immunodeficiency diseases. In many cases, the specific immune defect can be diagnosed with flow cytometry, while in others the immune defect can be better characterized.

References

Oliveira JB, Fleisher TA. Molecular- and flow cytometry-based diagnosis of primary immunodeficiency disorders. Curr Allergy Asthma Rep. 2010;10(6):460–7.

Vowells SJ, Sekhsaria S, Malech HL, Shalit M, Fleisher TA. Flow cytometric analysis of the granulocyte respiratory burst: a comparison study of fluorescent probes. J Immunol Methods. 1995;178(1):89–97.

Evaluation of Suspected Immunodeficiency, Genetic Testing

Jennifer W. Leiding
Department of Pediatrics, Division of Allergy and Immunology, University of South Florida at Johns Hopkins – All Children's Hospital, St. Petersburg, FL, USA

Primary immunodeficiency diseases (PIDDs) are a heterogenous group of disorders that have been linked to mutations in more than 300 different genes. Clinical presentation and immunophenotyping can be distinct but, more often, overlap with many other primary immune defects, complicating investigation into the correct diagnosis. Determining the genetic defect can be prognostic and can help tailor therapy. Most PIDDs have variable expressivity and often incomplete penetrance. In the past 20 years, advances in gene sequencing have improved our capabilities of finding a genetic mutation that is causative of disease.

Sanger sequencing of clinically suspected individual disease causing genes initiated the era of genetic investigation of primary immunodeficiency diseases. The method of Sanger sequencing involves using polymerase chain reactions (PCR) to amplify desired genomic regions. A second PCR is performed with normal and modified nucleotides that terminate the reaction leading to the generation of DNA fragments of all sizes. DNA is then separated by gel electrophoresis and individual mutations are identified. Using a candidate gene approach can be successful but most often requires full penetrance and expressivity of the disease in order to identify the correct patient and gene to sequence. Therefore, this approach can be very costly and time consuming. For these reasons, Sanger sequencing of candidate genes has become obsolete except in isolated cases. Next-generation sequencing (NGS)

based gene panel sequencing, whole exome sequencing (WES), and whole genome sequencing (WGS) are ideal and have become standard in the identification of genetic causes of PIDDs (Conley and Casanova 2014; Stray-Pedersen et al. 2017).

NGS, also referred to as deep sequencing, second-generation sequencing, or massive parallel sequencing, sequences hundreds of millions of DNA fragments in parallel. It can be used to sequence specific gene panels associated with a certain disease phenotype, whole exome sequencing (WES), or the entire genome with whole genome sequencing (WGS) (Yu et al. 2016). The details of each method are described in Table 1.

The targeting and coverage of coding regions within a gene differ substantially between gene panel sequencing and WES and WGS. Identification and capture of exons in WES is subject to bias: the primers are designed from known coding sequences and therefore do not recognize unknown exons. WES also cannot capture and identify intronic mutations which can contain disease causing mutations (Meyts et al. 2016; Raje et al. 2014).

NGS identifies up to 50,000 variants per exome. Analysis of the variant for pathogenicity includes analysis of how often the variant is found in the general population (allele frequency) and the potential functional effect that the variant may have on the gene and protein expression (Yu et al. 2016). An allele with an allele frequency >1% is considered common. Public databases of variants contain data from thousands of healthy subjects from various ethnicities. Variants that are nonsense, affect splice sites, deletions, and insertions, and mutations within the start or stop codon are the most likely to be deleterious. The pathogenicity of missense mutations is harder to predict and so multiple software programs have been developed to predict the pathogenicity of mutations (Sorting Intolerant from Tolerant (SIFT) and Polymorphism Phenotyping v2 (PolyPhen2)). A combined annotation-dependent depletion (CADD) score is determined using these methods, scoring both protein altering and regulatory variants. The characteristics of the gene and the

Evaluation of Suspected Immunodeficiency, Genetic Testing, Table 1 Methods of genetic testing to evaluate for primary immunodeficiency diseases

| Sanger sequencing | Next-generation sequencing | | |
	gene panel	WES	WGS
High sequencing depth	Several to hundreds of genes	Covers the entire exome	Covers entire genome
One gene at a time	High sequencing depth	Less coverage than sequencing individual genes	High sequencing depth
Expensive	Not cost effective	Cost efficient	Expensive but getting more cost efficient
Will not identify novel genetic defects	Will not identify novel genetic defects	Will identify novel genes	Will identify novel genes
Does not include introns	Does not include introns	Does not include introns	Includes introns and regulatory domains

impact of the variant at the gene level are also taken into account when prioritizing the importance or likely pathogenicity of variants. Criteria used include whether the gene encodes for a protein that acts in a pathway that relates to the clinical phenotype; knowledge about how the gene is expressed in human cells, tissues, and organs; and knowledge about the preservation and therefore the importance of the gene across species and human evolution. The gene damage index (GDI) takes into account evolutionary pressure and protein complexity to determine the degree of damage of a variant on the gene (Stray-Pedersen et al. 2017).

Once a candidate gene has been determined through targeted gene sequencing, WES, or WGS, experimental validation of the mutation is necessary to prove that the mutation is in fact pathogenic and the cause of the patient's disease. These studies usually show that the variant affects the expression or function of the encoded protein. Validation studies also show that the phenotype can be rescued with transduction of the wild-type or normal allele into cell culture (Stray-Pedersen et al. 2017).

Determining which whether a candidate gene, gene panel, or WES approach of genetic testing to be performed can be difficult. When the clinical manifestations and immunophenotyping of the patient points to one specific disease, then candidate sequencing may be most appropriate. An example of this would be in the case of X-linked agammaglobulinemia with a boy with low or absent B cells, hypogammaglobulinemia, recurrent infections, and a mutation in Bruton's tyrosine kinase (*BTK*). In the case of severe combined immunodeficiency, mutations in one of more than 30 different genes can cause SCID. In this case a NGS gene panel may be more appropriate. The panel chosen should consist of SCID associated genes to be sequenced. WES and WGS often are reserved for cases in which the clinical and immune phenotype are unclear and the differential genetic diagnosis cannot be narrowed.

Over the last two decades, genetic sequencing has become standard in the evaluation of patients with primary immunodeficiency diseases. Determining the specific mutation is important for guiding treatment and for preventing or recognizing disease-related complications. Technologies for the evaluation of genetic variants are improving at a remarkable pace and becoming much more cost effective, giving clinicians the necessary tools to fully evaluate their patients.

Cross-References

► Evaluation of Suspected Immunodeficiency, Overview
► Management of Immunodeficiency: Gene Therapy

References

Conley ME, Casanova JL. Discovery of single-gene inborn errors of immunity by next generation sequencing. Curr Opin Immunol. 2014;30:17–23.

Meyts I, Bosch B, Bolze A, Boisson B, et al. Exome and genome sequencing for inborn errors of immunity. J Allergy Clin Immunol. 2016;138(4):957–69.

Raje N, Soden S, Swanson D, Ciaccio CE, et al. Utility of Next Generation Sequencing in Clinical Primary Immunodeficiencies. Allergy Asthma Rep. 2014;14 (10): 468.

Stray-Pedersen A, Sorte HS, Samarakoon P, Gambin T, et al. Primary immunodeficiency diseases: genomic approaches delineate heterogeneous Mendelian disorders. J Allergy Clin Immunol. 2017;139(1):232–45.

Yu H, Zhang VW, Stray-Pedersen A, Hanson IC, et al. Rapid molecular diagnostics of severe primary immunodeficiency determined by using targeted next-generation sequencing. J Allergy Clin Immunol. 2016;138(4):1142–51.

Evaluation of Suspected Immunodeficiency, Humoral

Panida Sriaroon
Department of Pediatrics, Division of Allergy and Immunology, University of South Florida/Johns Hopkins All Children's Hospital, Tampa, FL, USA

Humoral or antibody immunodeficiencies are the most common forms of primary immunodeficiency disease (PID), accounting for over half of all cases. Examples of antibody deficiencies are X-linked agammaglobulinemia (XLA or Bruton's agammaglobulinemia), common variable immunodeficiency (CVID), transient hypogammaglobulinemia of infancy (THI), IgG subclass deficiency, selective IgA deficiency, and specific antibody deficiency (SAD) (Picard et al. 2015). Secondary antibody deficiency results from chronic conditions such as B-cell chronic lymphocytic leukemia, protein-losing enteropathies, nephrosis, or after chemotherapy or treatment with B cell depleting agents such as rituximab, an anti-CD20 biologic drug.

A comprehensive clinical and laboratory evaluation and a detailed family history should be part of the evaluation of all patients with suspected humoral immunodeficiency. Clinical manifestations are primarily recurrent bacterial sinopulmonary infections, including pneumonia and sinusitis, although bacterial sepsis and meningitis have been frequently described. Infections with *Streptococcus pneumoniae*, *Haemophilus influenzae*, and other encapsulated bacterial organisms are most common. Patients are also at greater risk of developing enteroviral infections and chronic gastrointestinal giardiasis. Manifestations are not only limited to recurrent infections, however. Patients with XLA are prone to have juvenile idiopathic arthritis and a dermatomyositis-like syndrome. Approximately 20–30% of patients with CVID have autoimmune disease. The most common autoimmune manifestations in CVID are hematologic, such as idiopathic thrombocytopenic purpura and hemolytic anemia. Gastrointestinal lymphoid hyperplasia, inflammatory bowel-like disease, celiac disease, or autoimmune endocrinopathies also occur in patients with CVID.

To optimize the use of the clinical laboratory, initial testing should include quantitative and qualitative screening evaluations, with more costly and complex testing used to identify the precise nature of the defect and confirm the suspected diagnosis. A summary of the screening tests for evaluation of antibody immunodeficiency is provided in Table 1. Initial laboratory investigation should include complete blood count (CBC) and comprehensive metabolic

Evaluation of Suspected Immunodeficiency, Humoral, Table 1 Laboratory evaluation of suspected humoral immunodeficiency

General screening tests: CBC, CMP, UA
Screening tests for B cell function: Serum IgG, IgA, IgM levels, isohemagglutinins, antibodies to infectious agent, antibody titers to vaccines, B cell enumeration by flow cytometry
Advanced tests: Extended B cell phenotyping, gene sequencing analysis for specific defects

CBC complete blood count, *CMP* comprehensive metabolic profile, *Ig* immunoglobulin, *UA* urinalysis profile. Screening laboratory tests to evaluate humoral immunity include quantitative serum immunoglobulins IgG, IgA, IgM, isohemagglutinins, antibody titers to vaccine or infectious pathogens, and B cell numbers by flow cytometry (Bonilla et al. 2015). Urinalysis for evaluation of secondary IgG loss through the kidneys should be obtained in all patients with low serum IgG level. In healthy individuals, the predominant immunoglobulin in the blood is IgG. Serum IgA may be low or absent in young children. Values for children must be compared with age-matched laboratory values. Isohemagglutinins (anti-A and/or anti-B IgM) are natural antibodies to blood group A or B antigens found in all individuals except those with type AB red blood cells. In children greater than 6 months of age and adults who have A, B, or O blood group, the absence of isohemagglutinins may suggest antibody deficiency.

Specific antibody titers measured prior to and 30 days after immunization is an accepted means to measure functional immunity to T-dependent (tetanus and diphtheria) and T-independent (different serotypes of pneumococcal polysaccharide) antigens (Orange et al. 2012). Alternatively, serum can be tested for the presence of antibodies to previous infection with pathogens such as influenza A and B, mycoplasma, and some respiratory viruses and bacteria. Some patients may have normal value of serum IgG but low levels of specific antibodies. In these cases, IgG subclass measurements may be helpful. However, the significance of IgG subclass deficiency in the presence of normal antibody responses to protein and polysaccharide antigen is not known. Up to 5% of healthy adults have low or absent IgG4, and its deficiency is not considered to be clinically relevant. Elevation in serum IgE can be helpful in differentiating patients who have IgE-mediated allergic rhinosinusitis, allergic asthma, and other allergic diseases from those who have antibody defects.

In more than 90% of healthy individuals, typical postimmunization protective response to T-dependent antigens such as tetanus and diphtheria exceeds 1.0 IU/ml. However, the protective level of antibody following pneumococcal polysaccharide vaccination for assessment of T-independent response is poorly defined (Perez et al. 2017). The American Academy of Allergy, Asthma, and Immunology (AAAAI) and the American College of Allergy, Asthma, and Immunology (ACAAI) practice parameters define a normal response to be titers over 1.3 μg/ml with a twofold rise in at least 70% of the immunizing serotypes in adults or 50% of serotypes in children (Bonilla et al. 2015). However, some experts believe this definition is too broad as many healthy individuals do not achieve this level of response following immunization.

It is crucial that humoral immunity, including measurement of IgG levels and specific antibodies to prior vaccination or infections, be assessed before initiating IgG replacement therapy (Orange et al. 2012). Once IgG treatment is initiated, some IgG antibody-based tests can be falsely positive due to antibodies in IgG preparations, and thus cannot be used to accurately measure a patient's antibody function. In a patient with a previously confirmed antibody deficiency, stopping IgG therapy to remeasure antibody levels and vaccine response is unnecessary and may place the patient at risk of developing infection during the period when the IgG therapy is stopped. Nevertheless, in a patient whose diagnosis of antibody deficiency is unclear, it may be necessary to stop IgG therapy for at least 3 months so that the patient's humoral immunity can be adequately evaluated.

Diagnostic testing should also focus on distinguishing between PID and secondary causes of antibody deficiency. Evaluation of recurrent sinopulmonary infections should include, where necessary, a detailed radiographic assessment of the sinuses and high resolution imaging of the lungs to detect occult bronchiectasis, hilar adenopathy, and granulomas. The findings should be interpreted in the context of other laboratory and clinical findings.

Enumeration of B cells using flow cytometry can differentiate congenital agammaglobulinemia in which CD20+ or CD19+ B cells are low or absent, from CVID where total B cell numbers are generally normal. Extended B cell phenotyping assay can be used in the diagnosis of antibody deficiency as some conditions are associated with aberrant switched memory B cells. Molecular analysis for genetic abnormalities, especially those that involve the early stages of B cell maturation in patients who present without B cells (e.g., XLA), can aid diagnostic evaluations.

References

Bonilla FA, Khan DA, Ballas ZK, Chinen J, Frank MM, Hsu JT, et al. Practice parameter for the diagnosis and management of primary immunodeficiency. J Allergy Clin Immunol. 2015;136(5):1186–205.e1-78.

Orange JS, Ballow M, Stiehm ER, Ballas ZK, Chinen J, De La Morena M, et al. Use and interpretation of diagnostic vaccination in primary immunodeficiency: a working group report of the Basic and Clinical Immunology Interest Section of the American Academy of Allergy, Asthma & Immunology. J Allergy Clin Immunol. 2012;130(3 Suppl):S1–24.

Perez E, Bonilla FA, Orange JS, Ballow M. Specific antibody deficiency: controversies in diagnosis and management. Front Immunol. 2017;8:586.

Picard C, Al-Herz W, Bousfiha A, Casanova JL, Chatila T, Conley ME, et al. Primary immunodeficiency diseases: an update on the classification from the International Union of Immunological Societies expert committee for primary immunodeficiency 2015. J Clin Immunol. 2015;35(8):696–726.

Evaluation of Suspected Immunodeficiency, Internet Resources

Elena E. Perez
Allergy Associates of the Palm Beaches, North Palm Beach, FL, USA

Definition

Resources and links available on the internet to aid in the diagnosis, management, and understanding of primary immunodeficiencies

Many Internet resources regarding varying aspects of primary immunodeficiencies are now available for clinicians, patients, and researchers. Resources include professional organizations, registries, clinical/diagnostic tools, research, and advocacy/patient organizations. These websites often share links with each other and point to other important and useful resources. Clinical features, genetic defects, algorithms, and testing resources are available on several sites. Websites are summarized in the table, and features of several selected resources are discussed below.

Professional Organizations

- **Clinical Immunology Society.** The Clinical Immunology Society is a professional society whose mission is "to facilitate education, translational research and novel approaches to therapy in clinical immunology to promote excellence in the care of patients with immunologic/inflammatory disorders." The webpage provides educational resources including webinars, links to CME, a WEBbook of biologic therapies, links to clinical practice guidelines, clinical pearls, journal club, a lab directory, and links to many other resources.

Clinical/Diagnostic

A few of the diagnostic resources for evaluation of suspected immunodeficiency are summarized below.

- **Immunodeficiencysearch.com** is a searchable interactive database of primary immunodeficiency diseases. It provides algorithms for evaluation of primary immunodeficiency diseases as well as overview of cases, and resources for testing.
- **Eurogentest.org** provides user-friendly tools to locate genetic tests available in Europe. General patient information regarding genetic testing is also available in more than 27 languages. Furthermore, disease specific clinical utility gene cards (CUGCs) are disease-

specific guidelines regarding the clinical utility of genetic testing and are available online at the *European Journal of Human Genetics* and EuroGentest. This is a particularly useful resource when needing to justify coverage for genetic testing.

- **The Genetic Testing Registry (GTR®)** is a central location for voluntary submission of genetic test information by providers. Information regarding the test's purpose, methodology, validity, evidence of the test's usefulness, and laboratory contacts and credentials are provided. The website includes links to GeneReviews, a collection of expert-authored peer reviewed disease descriptions, an international directory of genetic testing laboratories, an international directory of genetics and prenatal diagnosis clinics, educational materials including an illustrated glossary, power point presentations, and links to an annotated Internet resources guide.

Patient Education and Advocacy

- **Immune Deficiency Foundation.** The Immune Deficiency Foundation (IDF) is a national nonprofit patient organization dedicated to improving the diagnosis, treatment and quality of life of persons with PI through advocacy, education, and research. The website is a comprehensive collection of information regarding primary immunodeficiency that is useful for patients and clinicians. There are numerous educational publications available to download including the *IDF Patient and Family Handbook for Primary Immunodeficiency Diseases*.
- **Jeffrey Modell Foundation.** The Jeffrey Modell Foundation is a public charity devoted to early and precise diagnosis, meaningful treatments, and cures – through clinical and basic research, physician education, patient support, advocacy, public awareness, and newborn screening. The interactive website features resource links for patients, families, clinicians, and researchers (Table 1).

Evaluation of Suspected Immunodeficiency, Internet Resources, Table 1 Resources available for clinicians, researchers, and patients

Resource	Website address
Professional organizations	
American Academy of Allergy Asthma and Immunology (AAAAI)	www.aaaai.org
American College of Allergy Asthma and Immunology (ACAAI)	www.acaai.org
European Society for Immunodeficiencies (ESID)	www.esid.org
Latin American Society for Immunodeficiencies (LASID)	www.lasid.org
Clinical Immunology Society (CIS)	www.clinimmsoc.org
The J Project	http://jprojectnetwork.org
Registries	
United States Immunodeficiency Network (USIDET)	https://usidnet.org/usidnet-registry/
ESID registry	https://esid.org/Working-Parties/Registry
Primary Immunodeficiency Database in Japan (PIDJ)	http://pidj.rcai.riken.jp/en/index.html
Clinical/diagnostic	
Immunodeficiency search	http://www.immunodeficiencysearch.com
EuroGentest	http://www.eurogentest.org
Clinical Utility Gene Cards (CUGC)	http://www.eurogentest.org/index.php?id=668
Gene Cards (Weizmann Institute of Science)	http://www.genecards.org
IPID (Immune Phenotyping in Primary Immunodeficiency)	http://www.ipidnet.org/index.html
Genetic testing registry	https://www.ncbi.nlm.nih.gov/gtr/
Research	
Riken	http://www.riken.go.jp/en/
NIAID	http://www.niaid.nih.gov
European Research Council	http://erc.europa.eu
Pharmaceutical companies	Various manufacturers of immune globulin

(continued)

Reproduced with permission from Perez (2014) and Bonilla et al. (2014) JACI (Table V in this document has internet resources)

Cross-References

▶ Evaluation of Suspected Immunodeficiency, Overview

References

Bonilla FA, Khan DA, Ballas ZK, Chinen J, Frank MM, Hsu JT, et al. Practice parameter for the diagnosis and management of primary immunodeficiency. J Allergy Clin Immunol. 2014;136(5):1187–205.

Perez E. Chapter 62: Resources for clinicians. In: Stiehm's immune deficiencies. Amsterdam: Academic; 2014. p. 1075–83.

Evaluation of Suspected Immunodeficiency, Overview

Elena E. Perez
Allergy Associates of the Palm Beaches, North Palm Beach, FL, USA

Introduction

Patients with recurrent infections, autoimmune disease, malignancy, or a combination of these merit a high index of suspicion for underlying immunodeficiencies (Bonilla et al. 2015). While distinct, primary and secondary immunodeficiencies can have similar presentations including increased susceptibility to frequent, severe, or unusual infections, immune dysregulation, autoimmune disease, and malignancy. The overall incidence of symptomatic primary immunodeficiency diseases ranges from 1:10,000 to 1:2,000 live births and a prevalence of 1:10,0000 to 1:12,000 in the general population (Bonilla et al. 2015). Severe combined immunodeficiency has an incidence of approximately 1:58,000 live births in the USA (Bonilla et al. 2015). Antibody deficiency is the most common type of primary immunodeficiency (Bonilla et al. 2015). Historically, primary immunodeficiencies were characterized according to the immune effector mechanism affected including cellular, humoral, combined, or innate and the typical infections seen with each. Now there are nine phenotypic categories of primary immunodeficiency to consider according to the International Union of Immunologic Society (Picard et al. 2015). Secondary immunodeficiencies result from a variety of factors affecting diverse aspects of the immune response. These factors include extremes of age; malnutrition; metabolic diseases (diabetes and uremia); genetic syndromes; anti-inflammatory, immunomodulatory, and immunosuppressive drug therapy; surgery and trauma; environmental conditions (UV light, radiation, hypoxia, space flight); infectious diseases (HIV); and lymphoproliferative malignancies (Chinen and Shearer 2010). Evaluation of suspected immunodeficiency involves a careful history and physical exam looking for defining characteristics in some cases and laboratory and genetic evaluation where warranted.

Other conditions associated with recurrent infections
Adenoid hypertrophy
Allergic inflammation
Asplenia
Ciliary dyskinesia
Cystic fibrosis
Daycare
Extremes of age
Extreme stress

(continued)

Other conditions associated with recurrent infections
Immunosuppressive therapies
Infectious disease (HIV)
Lung malformation
Malignancy
Malnutrition
Passive exposure to smoking
Protein losing disorders
Radiation
Sleep deprivation
Trauma/surgery

History/Physical Exam

Evaluation of suspected immunodeficiency is carried out in a stepwise approach according to clinical presentation and suspicion of the underlying defect. Several algorithms to aid in diagnosis have been published (de Vries and European Society for Immunodeficiencies 2011; Bousfiha et al. 2015), and the "Practice parameter for the diagnosis and management of primary immunodeficiency" (Bonilla et al. 2015) is a valuable resource for clinicians that is updated regularly. Evaluation of immunodeficiency begins with a thorough history including frequency, severity, and nature of recurrent infections, early childhood history, family history of diagnosed immunodeficiency, or early childhood death. Primary immunodeficiency diseases can be inherited as autosomal recessive, autosomal dominant, and X-linked.

Examples of X-linked primary immunodeficiencies
X-linked agammaglobulinemia (Bruton's tyrosine kinase)
Wiskott-Aldrich syndrome
X-linked severe combined immune deficiency (common gamma chain)
X-linked hyper IgM syndrome (CD40 ligand)
X-linked lymphoproliferative disease (SH2D1A and XIAP)
X-linked chronic granulomatous disease (gp91)

Certain immunodeficiency diseases present with characteristic features (Bonilla et al. 2015). For example, combined immunodeficiencies (if not diagnosed while asymptomatic by newborn screening) may present with failure to thrive, diarrhea, opportunistic infections, and rashes. Wiskott-Aldrich presents with a clinical triad of thrombocytopenia, eczema, and recurrent infections with encapsulated organisms. Cerebellar ataxia, oculocutaneous telangiectasia, and malignancy are features of ataxia telangiectasia. DiGeorge syndrome also may present with characteristic features including hypocalcemia due to hypoparathyroidism, cardiac disease, abnormal facial features, and recurrent infections. Antibody deficiencies often present with recurrent sinopulmonary infections, viral respiratory tract infections, and gastrointestinal infections. Abscess of the liver or lung with granuloma formation and indolent infections with catalase positive organisms are hallmarks of chronic granulomatous disease. Delayed separation of the umbilical cord, poor wound healing, and leukocytosis are found in leukocyte adhesion deficiency. Recurrent infections with N. meningitides may indicate terminal complement deficiencies. Pneumatoceles, eczema, and skin infections as well as failure to shed primary teeth are features of autosomal dominant hyper IgE syndrome. Other innate immune defects such as NEMO and IRAK-4 deficiency are, respectively, characterized by severe bacterial infections, opportunistic infections and anhidrotic ectodermal dysplasia, or severe Gram-positive invasive bacterial infections in early childhood. Familiarity with these and other characteristic features seen in particular primary immunodeficiencies may improve timely diagnosis.

Diagnostic Testing

First-line laboratory evaluation for primary immunodeficiency consists of readily available commercial tests that are accessible to most clinicians. Advanced testing may require commercial specialty labs or immunology labs located at major medical centers. Initial tests of antibody function include quantitative immunoglobulins and titers to vaccines (usually tetanus, diphtheria, and pneumococcus) before and after vaccine boost if baseline titers are non-protective. B cell enumeration via flow cytometry is helpful in ruling out X-linked agammaglobulinemia

Evaluation of Suspected Immunodeficiency, Overview, Table 1 Initial and advanced testing is listed on the table according to the immune defect suspected

Suspected primary immunodeficiency	Initial tests	Advanced tests
Antibody	Serum IgG, IgA, IgM levels Antibody levels to specific vaccines before and after vaccine boost B cell enumeration	B cell subsets Immunoglobulin production to mitogens or other stimuli Antibody response to phiX174
Cellular	TREC newborn screening T cell (CD4 and CD8), NK cell enumeration Cutaneous delayed hypersensitivity Spontaneous NK cytotoxicity	T cell subsets In vitro proliferative response to mitogens and antigens T cell cytotoxicity Specialized flow cytometry for cell surface marker expression and cytokine production in response to stimuli Cytoplasmic protein phosphorylation in response to stimuli
Phagocytic	CBC with differential Neutrophil staining, peripheral smear DHR reduction or NBT test Flow cytometry for adhesion molecules	Chemotaxis and/or phagocytosis assay Enzyme assays (MPO, G6PDH) WBC turnover Bacterial or fungal killing Bone marrow biopsy
Complement	CH50 (classic complement cascade) AH50 (alternative complement pathway) Lectin pathway function	Level or function of individual complement components
Genetic tests	Targeted gene sequencing Gene panels for defined immunodeficiencies	Microarray for copy number variation Whole exome/genome sequencing

which is marked by absence of B cells. Newborn screening for T cell lymphopenia identifies babies at risk for SCID and other disorders characterized by low T cells, prior to onset of infections. Forty-four states in the USA are currently screening, and four additional states are conducting pilot screening programs in 2017. Louisiana and Indiana are not currently screening as of June 2017. First-line tests for suspected cellular deficiencies include T cell and NK cell enumeration via flow cytometry, cutaneous-delayed hypersensitivity, and NK cell cytotoxicity. For complement deficiencies, a CH50 and AH50 are markers of the classical and alternative complement cascades, respectively. There is now a wide variety of genetic testing platforms for investigating disease-causing mutations in genes associated with primary immunodeficiency diseases; however, access to these tests can be more challenging due to the need for insurance authorization. Advanced tests for each category are discussed further in their respective sections (Table 1).

Cross-References

▶ Clinical Presentation of Immunodeficiency, Overview

▶ Clinical Presentation of Immunodeficiency, Primary Immunodeficiency

▶ Clinical Presentation of Immunodeficiency, Secondary Immunodeficiency

▶ Evaluation of Suspected Immunodeficiency, Cellular

▶ Evaluation of Suspected Immunodeficiency, Flow Cytometry

▶ Evaluation of Suspected Immunodeficiency, Genetic Testing

▶ Evaluation of Suspected Immunodeficiency, Internet Resources

▶ Unclassified Primary Antibody Deficiency (unPAD)

References

Bonilla FA, Khan DA, Ballas ZK, Chinen J, Frank MM, Hsu JT, et al. Practice parameter for the diagnosis and management of primary immunodeficiency. JACI. 2015;136(5):1187–205.

Bousfiha A, Jeddane L, Al-Herz W, Ailal F, Casanova JL, Chatila T, et al. The 2015 IUIS phenotypic classification for primary Immunodeficiencies. J Clin Immunol. 2015;35:727–38.

Chinen J, Shearer WT. Secondary immunodeficiencies, including HIV infection. J Allergy Clin Immunol. 2010;125(2 Suppl 2):S195–203.

de Vries E, European Society for Immunodeficiencies. Patient-centered screening for primary immunodeficiency, a multi-stage diagnostic protocol designed for non-immunologists: 2011 update. Clin Exp Immunol. 2011;167:108–19.

Picard C, Al-Herz W, Bousfiha A, Casanova L, Chatila C, Conley ME, et al. Primary immunodeficiency diseases: an update on the classification from the International Union of Immunological Societies Expert Committee for primary immunodeficiency 2015. J Clin Immunol. 2015;35(8):696–726.

EVER1 and EVER2 Mutations in Epidermodysplasia Verruciformis

Robert J. Ragotte[1] and Stuart E. Turvey[2,3]
[1]Nuffield Department of Medicine, University of Oxford, Oxford, UK
[2]Division of Allergy and Clinical Immunology, Department of Pediatrics and Experimental Medicine Program, British Columbia Children's Hospital, The University of British Columbia, Vancouver, BC, Canada
[3]Willem-Alexander Children's Hospital, Leiden University Medical Center, Leiden, The Netherlands

Synonyms

Epidermodysplasia verruciformis/Lewandowsky-Lutz dysplasia; EVER1/TMC6; EVER2/TMC8

Definition

Papillomavirus: double stranded DNA virus of the family Papillomaviridae macule: a flat region of discoloured skin monogenic: a disease caused by an abnormality in a single gene biallelic mutations: mutations in both copies of a gene in a diploid organism, but not necessarily the exact same mutation (compound heterozygosity) consanguinous: families where the parents are related as second cousins or closer EV-HPV: the subtypes of HPV specifically associated with epidermodysplasia verruciformis.

Epidermodysplasia verruciformis (EV) is a rare condition caused by increased susceptibility to betapapillomaviruses. First described in 1922 by Lewandowsky and Lutz, the disease presents early in life with discolored flat warts or macules on the neck, abdomen, and extremities. These lesions can be red, brown, or grey and are typically scaly with irregular borders (Orth 2008). Over the long term, the disease results in epithelial proliferations and nonmelanoma skin cancer (NMSC) (Orth 2008). Approximately, half of EV patients will go on to develop NMSC (Gewirtzman et al. 2008). Among the betapapillomaviruses, HPV-5, HPV-8, and HPV-14d are known oncogenic viruses and their proliferation within the cutaneous lesions likely causes malignancy (Lazarczyk et al. 2009; Gewirtzman et al. 2008). Importantly, EV patients do not suffer from increased susceptibility to other types of infection. This includes bacterial, viral, fungal, or other types of HPV infection, such as genital warts where the causative agent is alphapapillomaviruses.

Human papillomaviruses associated with EV (EV-HPV) are widespread among healthy individuals. EV-HPV DNA is often detected on the skin of immunocompetent individuals (de Koning et al. 2007; Harwood et al. 2004). However, only in patients with EV does this colonization result in the growth of lesions and subsequent malignant transformation. EV-associated NMSCs generally develop in sun-exposed regions of the skin, indicative of a role of UV radiation in malignant transformation (Majewski; Jablonska 1995).

EV is thought to be an unconventional primary immune deficiency (Casanova et al. 2005). It is significantly different from severe combined immune deficiency and other monogenic impairments of immunity that generally confer susceptibility to a wide range of infections (Casanova et al. 2005). Further, primary immune deficiencies are generally defined by a clear immunological phenotype in the form hematopoietic abnormalities (Casanova and Abel 2007). EV patients lack a stark hematopoietic signature and manage to retain most normal immune function. As a result, EV patients experience increased susceptibility to a remarkably narrow range of HPV subtypes.

Genetics and Diagnostics

Biallelic mutations in *EVER1* and *EVER2* have been identified as the most common genetic etiology for EV, accounting for approximately 75% of EV cases (Ramoz et al. 2002; Orth 2008). A significant portion (~10%) of cases occur in consanguineous families, which is consistent with an autosomal recessive mode of inheritance (Orth 2008). Reported mutations in *EVER1* and *EVER2* that cause EV are summarized in Table 1.

Despite these well-established causal mutations, a subset of EV cases lack a clear monogenic explanation. This suggests that there are other impairments that result in increased EV-HPV susceptibility, indicative of genetic heterogeneity. For instance, there are case studies of autosomal dominant and X-linked recessive transmission, which differs from the typical mode of inheritance (Androphy et al. 1985; McDermott et al. 2009). Additionally, there are other examples of mutations that confer susceptibility to the EV-HPV family of viruses that fall beyond the traditional definition of EV (Crequer et al. 2012a; Li et al. 2016). These diseases appear to be distinct from conventional EV in that they result in increased susceptibility to other bacterial, viral and/or fungal infection, which is not observed in typical EV (Parvaneh et al. 2013).

Taken together, these cases demonstrate EV exhibits a pattern genetic heterogeneity that extends beyond EVER1 and EVER2. In a clinical setting, this means that even the absence of EVER1 and EVER2 mutations, EV is still a diagnostic possibility. Still, EVER1 and EVER2 mutations remain the most common and best-defined etiologies of EV.

Disease Mechanism

EVER1 and EVER2 belong to the transmembrane channel-like family of proteins (TMC) (Keresztes et al. 2003). EVER1 (TMC6) and EVER2 (TMC8) are expressed in the endoplasmic reticulum and have been implicated in zinc homeostasis, through their known interactions with ZnT-1 (Lazarczyk et al. 2009). ZnT-1 is involved in zinc efflux. Cells lacking functional ZnT-1 have higher cellular levels of zinc and are more susceptible to zinc toxicity (Palmiter and Findley 1995). The

EVER1 and EVER2 Mutations in Epidermodysplasia Verruciformis, Table 1 Summary of known *EVER1* and *EVER2* mutations that cause EV

	Mutation	Classification	Reference
EVER1	c.220C > T	Nonsense	(Aochi et al. 2007)
	c.280C > T	Nonsense	(Ramoz et al. 2002)
	c.744C > A	Nonsense	(Tate et al. 2004)
	c.1726G > T	Nonsense	(Ramoz et al. 2002)
	IVS8-2A > T	Splice site	(Tate et al. 2004)
	c.916insCAGT	Frame shift	(Zuo et al. 2006)
	c.968delT	Frame shift	(Gober et al. 2007)
EVER2	c.917A > T	Missense	(Arnold et al. 2011)
	c.568C > T	Nonsense	(sun et al. 2005)
	c.1084G > T	Nonsense	(Ramoz et al. 2002)
	c.188G > A	Nonsense	(Rady et al. 2007)
	c.561-583del	Frame shift	(Berthelot et al. 2007)
	c.754/755delT	Frame shift	(Ramoz et al. 2002)
	g.6609-6621del	Frame shift	(Landini et al. 2012)
	g.7668delG	Frame shift	(Landini et al. 2012)

Zn-T1:EVER complex has been shown to affect zinc distribution within keratinocytes, including the inhibition of zinc transport into the nucleus and down regulation of zinc-inducible gene expression (Lazarczyk et al. 2008, 2009). The impact of changes in intracellular zinc distribution via EVER loss-of-function is far reaching; this includes inhibition of JNK and Elk-1 signaling cascades, which have important roles in the immune system (Lazarczyk et al. 2008).

EVER1/2 expression is not limited to keratinocytes, as they are also highly expressed among cells of the adaptive immune system. As a result, it cannot be assumed that susceptibility to EV-HPV infection of the skin is rooted in keratinocytes defects. Rather it may be caused by immunological abnormalities that prevent an effective immune response to EV-HPV (Majewski et al. 1986; Cooper et al. 1990).

Controlling intracellular zinc distribution is an essential process in cellular homeostasis. It is well established that zinc plays an important structural and catalytic role across a range of metalloproteins. As a result of *EVER1/2* mutations, perturbations in zinc homeostasis are thought to impair immune function. Minor immunological abnormalities have been observed in EV patients, though the clinical significance of these findings remains unclear. In small studies of EV patients, changes in T cell subtype frequency have been described (Crequer et al. 2013). Further, there is some evidence supporting impaired T cell activation in the presence of elevated zinc concentrations, which may point to a mechanism by which EV patients' immune response is impaired. Zn^{2+} accumulates in T cells upon activation, which is accompanied by a decrease in EVER expression (Lazarczyk et al. 2012). The inability to effectively regulate this process may result in immunological impairments that confer susceptibility to EV-HPV.

To understand the mechanism of the disease, some insight can be gained from the non-*EVER1/2* mutations that confer susceptibility to EV-HPV. In a study of two individuals who presented with EV-HPV infection, but lacked mutations in *EVER1* or *EVER2*, *RHOH* deficiency was identified as the cause (Crequer et al. 2012b). Deficiencies in *RHOH* resulted in T cell defects, including altered T cell subtype frequency with an overrepresentation of effector memory T cells and the lack of β7 integrin, an important homing protein (Crequer et al. 2012b). These lines of evidence lend support to the hypothesis that defects in the adaptive immune system may be the mechanism by which EVER1/2 deficits cause disease. However, it remains possible that these immunological abnormalities are the result of the chronic HPV infection rather than its cause (Orth 2006).

Interestingly, alphapapillomaviruses, which are able to cause disease in immunocompetent individuals, have an E5 protein, including HPV16, which carries with it a high risk of malignancy (Chan et al. 1995; Bravo and Alonso 2004). The E5 protein binds to the ZnT-1 and the EVER proteins (Lazarczyk et al. 2008). The E5 protein is missing from betapapillomaviruses (Bravo and Alonso 2004). This suggests that the E5 protein is necessary to evade the host immune response and without it, the virus is unable to cause disease. In the case of EV patients, the loss of EVER1/2 function compensates for the lack of an E5 protein. There are two possible explanations for this observation. One is that EVER1 and EVER2 act as viral restriction factors against EV-HPV. In their absence EV-HPV gene expression and replication is unconstrained by the immune system, resulting in disease that is not observed in healthy patients harboring the same virus (Orth 2008). Alternatively, EVER1 and EVER2 may be necessary for an effective adaptive immune response against EV-HPV infected cells, as supported by the observed T cell abnormalities in EVER1/2 deficient cells.

EV as a Result of Immunosuppression

Increasingly, there have been reports of the development of EV upon immunosuppression, either intentionally through drug treatment regimen or unintentionally via HIV infection (Cowan et al.

2013; Lowe et al. 2012; Fernandez et al. 2014; Rogers et al. 2009). These reports are consistent with a model of EV wherein immunological abnormalities result in greater susceptibility to certain HPV infections. However, in the cases reported, the immunological deficits are more pronounced than in conventional EV, leading to widespread immunosuppression and susceptibility to a greater range of infections. Similar cases have been reported in the context of severe combined immunodeficiency where patients with Υc or JAK3 deficiency go on to develop EV following hematopoietic stem cell transplantation (Laffort et al. 2004).

Treatment

Treatment options of individuals with EV remain limited. Surgery is often required to remove malignant growths. However, this is not effective in addressing smaller EV lesions, which remain intractable. Nonsurgical treatments have had limited and inconsistent success in treating EV. There has been a report of successfully using imiquimod to treat and eliminate EV lesions (Berthelot et al. 2007). In another small study 5-aminolevulinic acid photodynamic therapy eliminated EV lesions though they rapidly returned after the cessation of therapy (Karrer et al. 1999). Other approaches that have been met with some limited success in individual cases include retinoids, retinoids in combination with interferon therapy and 5-fluorouracil (Orth et al. 1979; Kanerva et al. 1985; Majewski et al. 1994). However, since the success of these approaches has been mixed, none have been widely adopted. As a result, treatment is typically limited to management of the condition with a specific focus on surgical removal of malignancies.

References

Androphy EJ, Dvoretzky I, Lowy DR. X-linked inheritance of epidermodysplasia verruciformis. Genetic

and virologic studies of a kindred. Arch Dermatol. 1985;121(7):864–8.

Aochi S, Nakanishi G, Suzuki N, Setsu N, Suzuki D, Aya K, et al. A novel homozygous mutation of the EVER1/TMC6 gene in a Japanese patient with epidermodysplasia verruciformis. Br J Dermatol. 2007;157(6):1265–6.

Arnold AW, Burger B, Kump E, Rufle A, Tyring SK, Kempf W, et al. Homozygosity for the c.917A → T (p.N306l) polymorphism in the EVER2/TMC8 gene of two sisters with Epidermodysplasia Verruciformis Lewandowsky-Lutz originally described by Wilhelm Lutz. Dermatology. 2011;222(1):81–6.

Berthelot C, Dickerson MC, Rady P, He Q, Niroomand F, Tyring SK, et al. Treatment of a patient with epidermodysplasia verruciformis carrying a novel EVER2 mutation with imiquimod. J Am Acad Dermatol. 2007;56(5):882–6.

Bravo IG, Alonso A. Mucosal human papillomaviruses encode four different E5 proteins whose chemistry and phylogeny correlate with malignant or benign growth. J Virol. 2004;78(24):13613–26.

Casanova J-L, Abel L. Primary Immunodeficiencies: a field in its infancy. Science. 2007;317(5838):617–9.

Casanova JL, Fieschi C, Bustamante J, Reichenbach J, Remus N, Von Bernuth H, et al. From idiopathic infectious diseases to novel primary immunodeficiencies. J Allergy Clin Immunol. 2005;116(2):426–30.

Chan S-Y, Delius H, Halpern AL, Bernard H-U. Analysis of genomic sequences of 95 papillomavirus types: uniting typing, phylogeny, and taxonomy. J Virol. 1995;69(5):3074–83.

Cooper KD, Androphy EJ, Lowy D, Katz SI. Antigen presentation and T-cell activation in epidermodysplasia verruciformis. J Inves Dermatol. 1990;94:769–76.

Cowan KR, Gonzalez Santiago TM, Tollefson MM. Acquired epidermodysplasia verruciformis in a child with the human immunodeficiency virus. Pediatr Dermatol. 2013;30(6):252–4

Crequer A, Picard C, Patin E, D'Amico A, Abhyankar A, Munzer M, et al. Inherited MST1 deficiency underlies susceptibility to EV-HPV infections. PLoS One. 2012a;7(8):e44010

Crequer A, Troeger A, Patin E, Ma CS, Picard C, Pedergnana V, et al. Human RHOH deficiency causes T cell defects and susceptibility to EV-HPV infections. J Clin Invest. 2012b;122(9):3239–47.

Crequer A, Picard C, Pedergnana V, Lim A, Zhang SY, Abel L, et al. EVER2 deficiency is associated with mild T-cell abnormalities. J Clin Immunol. 2013;33(1):14–21.

de Koning MNC, Struijk L, Bouwes Bavinck JN, Kleter B, ter Schegget J, Quint WGV, et al. Betapapillomaviruses frequently persist in the skin of healthy individuals. J Gen Virol. 2007;88(5):1489–95.

Fernandez KH, Rady P, Tyring S, Stone MS. Acquired epidermodysplasia verruciformis in a child with atopic dermatitis. Pediatr Dermatol. 2014;31(3):400–2.

Gewirtzman A, Bartlett B, Tyring S. Epidermodysplasia verruciformis and human papilloma virus. Curr Opin Infect Dis. 2008;21(2):141–6.

Gober MD, Rady PL, He Q, Tucker SB, Tyring SK, Gaspari AA. Novel homozygous Frameshift mutation of EVER1 gene in an Epidermodysplasia Verruciformis patient. J Invest Dermatol. 2007;127(4):817–20.

Harwood CA, Surentheran T, Sasieni P, Proby CM, Bordea C, Leigh IM, et al. Increased risk of skin cancer associated with the presence of epidermodysplasia verruciformis human papillomavirus types in normal skin. Br J Dermatol. 2004;150(5):949–57.

Kanerva LO, Johansson E, Niemi K-M, Lauharanta J, Salo OP. Epidermodysplasia verruciformis. Clinical and light-and electron-microscopic observations during etretinate therapy. Arch Dermatol Res. 1985;278(2):153–60.

Karrer S, Szeimies RM, Abels C, Wlotzke U, Stolz W, Landthaler M. Epidermodysplasia verruciformis treated using topical 5-aminolaevulinic acid photodynamic therapy. Br J Dermatol. 1999;140(5):935–8.

Keresztes G, Mutai H, Heller S, Venter J, Adams M, Myers E, et al. TMC and EVER genes belong to a larger novel family, the TMC gene family encoding transmembrane proteins. BMC Genomics. 2003;4(1):1304–51.

Laffort C, Le Deist F, Favre M, Caillat-Zucman S, Radford-Weiss I, Debré M, et al. Severe cutaneous papillomavirus disease after haemopoietic stem-cell transplantation in patients with severe combined immune deficiency caused by common γc cytokine receptor subunit or JAK-3 deficiency. Lancet. 2004;363(9426):2051–4.

Landini MM, Zavattaro E, Borgogna C, Azzimonti B, De Andrea M, Colombo E, et al. Lack of EVER2 protein in two Epidermodysplasia Verruciformis patients with skin cancer presenting previously unreported homozygous genetic deletions in the EVER2 gene. J Invest Dermatol. 2012;132(4):1305–8.

Lazarczyk M, Pons C, Mendoza J-A, Cassonnet P, Jacob Y, Favre M. Regulation of cellular zinc balance as a potential mechanism of EVER-mediated protection against pathogenesis by cutaneous oncogenic human papillomaviruses. J Exp Med. 2008;205(1):35–42.

Lazarczyk M, Cassonnet P, Pons C, Jacob Y, Favre M. The EVER proteins as a natural barrier against papillomaviruses: a new insight into the pathogenesis of human papillomavirus infections. Microbiol Mol Biol Rev. 2009;73(2):348–70.

Lazarczyk M, Dalard C, Hayder M, Dupre L, Pignolet B, Majewski S, et al. EVER proteins, key elements of the natural anti-human papillomavirus barrier, are regulated upon T-cell activation. PLoS One. 2012;7(6): e39995

Li S-L, Duo L-N, Wang H-J, Dai W, Zhou E-YH XY-N, et al. Identification of the LCK mutation in an atypical epidermodysplasia verruciformis family with T cell defects and virus-induced squamous cell carcinoma. Br J Dermatol. 2016;175(6):1204–9.

Lowe SM, Katsidzira L, Meys R, Sterling JC, De Koning M, Quint W, et al. Acquired epidermodysplasia verruciformis due to multiple and unusual HPV infection among vertically-infected, HIV-positive adolescents in Zimbabwe. Clin Infect Dis. 2012;54(10):119–123

Majewski S, Skopinska-Rozewska E, Jahłonska S, Wasik M, Misiewicz J, Orth G. Partial defects of cell-mediated immunity in patients with epidermodysplasia verruciformis. J Am Acad Dermatol. 1986;15:966–73.

Majewski S, Szmurlo A, Marczak M, Jablonska S, Bollag W. Synergistic effect of retinoids and interferon α on tumor-induced angiogenesis: anti-angiogenic effect on HPV-harboring tumor-cell lines. Int J Cancer. 1994;57(1):81–5.

Majewsi S, Jablonska S. Epidermodyslplasia verruciformis is a model of human papillomavirus induced genetic cancer of the skin. Arch Dermatol. 1995;131 (11):1312–1318

McDermott DF, Gammon B, Snijders PJ, Mbata I, Phifer B, Howland Hartley A, et al. Autosomal dominant epidermodysplasia verruciformis lacking a known EVER1 or EVER2 mutation. Pediatr Dermatol. 2009;26(3):306–10.

Orth G. Genetics of epidermodysplasia verruciformis: Insights into host defense against papillomaviruses. Semin Immunol. 2006;18:362–74.

Orth G. Host defenses against human papillomaviruses: Lessons from epidermodysplasia verruciformis. Curr Top Microbiol Immunol. 2008;321:59–83.

Orth G, Jablonska S, Jarzabek-Chorzelska M, Obalek S, Rzesa G, Favre M, et al. Characteristics of the lesions and risk of malignant conversion associated with the type of human papillomavirus involved in Epidermodysplasia Verruciformis. Cancer Res. 1979;39(3):1074–82.

Palmiter RD, Findley SD. Cloning and functional characterization of a mammalian zinc transporter that confers resistance to zinc. EMBO J. 1995;14(4):639–49.

Parvaneh N, Casanova JL, Notarangelo LD, Conley ME. Primary immunodeficiencies: a rapidly evolving story. J Allergy Clin Immunol. 2013;131:314–23.

Rady PL, De Oliveira WRP, He Q, Festa C, Rivitti EA, Tucker SB, et al. Novel homozygous nonsense TMC8 mutation detected in patients with epidermodysplasia verruciformis from a Brazilian family. Br J Dermatol. 2007;157(4):831–3.

Ramoz N, Rueda L-A, Bouadjar B, Montoya L-S, Orth G, Favre M. Mutations in two adjacent novel genes are associated with epidermodysplasia verruciformis. Nat Genet. 2002;32:1–3.

E

Rogers HD, MacGregor JL, Nord KM, Tyring S, Rady P, Engler DE, et al. Acquired epidermodysplasia verruciformis. J Am Acad Dermatol. 2009;60(2):315–20.

Sun X-K, Chen J-F, Xu A-E. A homozygous nonsense mutation in the EVER2 gene leads to epidermodysplasia verruciformis. Clin Exp Dermatol. 2005;30(5):573–4.

Tate G, Suzuki T, Kishimoto K, Mitsuya T. Novel mutations of EVER1/TMC6 gene in a Japanese patient with epidermodysplasia verruciformis. J Hum Genet. 2004;49(4):223–5.

Zuo YG, Ma D, Zhang Y, Qiao J, Wang B. Identification of a novel mutation and a genetic polymorphism of EVER1 gene in two families with epidermodysplasia verruciformis. J Dermatol Sci. 2006;44(3):153–9.

EVER1/TMC6

▶ *EVER1* and *EVER2* Mutations in Epidermodysplasia Verruciformis

EVER2/TMC8

▶ *EVER1* and *EVER2* Mutations in Epidermodysplasia Verruciformis

FAAP24 Deficiency

Ivan K. Chinn
Section of Immunology, Allergy, and
Retrovirology, Texas Children's Hospital,
Houston, TX, USA
William T. Shearer Center for Human
Immunobiology, Texas Children's Hospital,
Houston, TX, USA
Department of Pediatrics, Baylor College of
Medicine, Houston, TX, USA

Introduction

FAAP24 is located at 19q13 and encodes a 24 kDa, 215 amino acid molecule that is a member of the xeroderma pigmentosum complementation group F family of proteins (Ciccia et al. 2007, 2008).

Molecular Function

Fanconi anemia-associated protein of 24 kDa (FAAP24) forms a heterodimer with the C-terminal region of Fanconi anemia complementation group M protein (FANCM) and directs its binding to single-stranded DNA (Ciccia et al. 2007; Niedernhofer 2007; Wang et al. 2013). FANCM-FAAP24 does not appear to have inherent endonuclease activity (Ciccia et al. 2008). Instead, it is recruited to stalled replication forks in response to DNA damage, particularly at interstrand crosslinks (Ciccia et al. 2007; Wang et al. 2013). The dimer is not required for formation of the Fanconi anemia core complex but may target it toward sites of DNA damage (Wang et al. 2013; Thompson and Hinz 2009). Loss of FAAP24 results in defective mono-ubiquitination of Fanconi anemia complementation group D2 protein (FANCD2), which represents an integral function of the Fanconi anemia core complex in initiation of DNA repair (Ciccia et al. 2007). The FANCM-FAAP24 heterodimer also exhibits adenosine triphosphate-dependent translocase activity and interactions with human homolog of the *Caenorhabditis elegans* biological clock protein Clk-2 that are both critical for ataxia telangiectasia and Rad3-related (ATR)-checkpoint kinase 1 (Chk1) checkpoint activation in response to replication stress (Thompson and Hinz 2009; Hořejší et al. 2009). The dimer further suppresses sister chromatid exchange formation (Wang et al. 2013). FAAP24 therefore plays a key role in maintaining genomic integrity.

Presentation

FAAP24 deficiency has been reported in only one family consisting of two siblings (ages 15 years and 30 months) who carried a homozygous pathogenic variant in *FAAP24* that resulted in c.635C>T,

© Springer Science+Business Media LLC, part of Springer Nature 2020
I. R. Mackay et al. (eds.), *Encyclopedia of Medical Immunology*,
https://doi.org/10.1007/978-1-4614-8678-7

p.T212M (Daschkey et al. 2016). They were children of healthy, consanguineous Turkish parents. The clinical presentation was characterized by EBV-associated lymphoproliferative disease (fever, lymphadenopathy, and hepatosplenomegaly). The younger sibling also developed encephalopathy and recurrent thigh abscesses. The presentation was complicated by the detection of an Epstein-Barr virus (EBV) strain that carried its own gain-of-function variant in EBNA2, resulting in increased virulent activity. The siblings did not have dysmorphic features, developmental delay, or bone marrow failure.

Diagnosis

Only the younger sibling was immunologically characterized (Daschkey et al. 2016). Standard test results were reported to be normal, including the following: serum immunoglobulin levels, specific antibody response to immunization, numbers of CD4$^+$ and CD8$^+$ T cells and total B cells, and T-cell proliferative responses to mitogens. Upon development of EBV-associated lymphoproliferative disease, the child was noted to have hypogammaglobulinemia, decreased CD4$^+$ T-cell count, expansion of CD8$^+$ T cells, and increased T-cell expression of HLA-DR. Patient T cells demonstrated impaired cytotoxicity toward autologous EBV-transformed B cells, while NK cell function was reported to be normal. Research testing confirmed decreased ubiquitination of FANCD2 and delayed activation of Chk1/2 in response to DNA damage. These tests are not generally available on a clinical basis. Diagnosis therefore requires a high index of suspicion and genetic testing for pathogenic variants in *FAAP24*.

Treatment

The optimal treatment strategy for FAAP24 deficiency remains unclear. Both affected siblings were treated with acyclovir, corticosteroids, and cyclophosphamide and failed to survive.

Mortality resulted from progressive lymphoproliferative disease.

References

Ciccia A, Ling C, Coulthard R, et al. Identification of FAAP24, a Fanconi anemia core complex protein that interacts with FANCM. Mol Cell. 2007;25:331–43.

Ciccia A, McDonald N, West SC. Structural and functional relationships of the XPF/MUS81 family of proteins. Annu Rev Biochem. 2008;77:259–87.

Daschkey S, Bienemann K, Schuster V, et al. Fatal lymphoproliferative disease in two siblings lacking functional FAAP24. J Clin Immunol. 2016;36:684–92.

Hořejší Z, Collis SJ, Boulton SJ. FANCM-FAAP24 and HCLK2: roles in ATR signalling and the Fanconi anemia pathway. Cell Cycle. 2009;8:1133–7.

Niedernhofer LJ. The Fanconi anemia signalosome anchor. Mol Cell. 2007;25:487–90.

Thompson LH, Hinz JM. Cellular and molecular consequences of defective Fanconi anemia proteins in replication-coupled DNA repair: mechanistic insights. Mutation Research/Fundamental and Molecular Mechanisms of Mutagenesis. 2009;668:54–72.

Wang Y, Han X, Wu F, et al. Structure analysis of FAAP24 reveals single-stranded DNA-binding activity and domain functions in DNA damage response. Cell Res. 2013;23:1215–28.

Familial Cold Autoinflammatory Syndrome (FCAS) and Muckle-Wells Syndrome (MWS)

Hal M. Hoffman

Division of Pediatric Allergy, Immunology, and Rheumatology, University of California, San Diego and Rady Children's Hospital, San Diego, CA, USA

Synonyms

Cryopyrin-associated periodic syndromes (CAPS); Cryopyrinopathies; Familial cold urticaria; (FCAS); Muckle-wells syndrome (MWS); Neonatal-onset multisystem inflammatory disease (NOMID); Nod, Leucine-rich Repeat, Pyrin 3 (NLRP3)

Definition

Familial cold autoinflammatory syndrome and Muckle-Wells syndrome are autoinflammatory diseases presenting with urticarial-like rash, limb pain, and other systemic inflammatory manifestations due to autosomal dominant gain-of-function mutations in *NLRP3* (MIM MWS #191900, MIM FCAS #120100).

Introduction and Background

The cryopyrin-associated periodic syndromes (CAPS) are a spectrum of genetically determined autoinflammatory disorders including familial cold autoinflammatory syndrome (FCAS), Muckle-Wells syndrome (MWS), and neonatal-onset multisystem inflammatory disease (NOMID) (Aksentijevich et al. 2007). This monograph will focus on FCAS and MWS, the milder end of the disease continuum, while a discussion of NOMID appears elsewhere. In 1940, Kile and Rusk described a multigenerational North American family with recurrent episodes of urticarial-like rash, fever, and arthralgia associated with generalized cold exposure. The syndrome was referred as cold hypersensitivity and classified as a rare form of cold urticaria. Since that time numerous reports of similar patients and families from around the world have been published, and the disorder was commonly referred to as familial cold urticaria but later renamed FCAS to capture the systemic nature of the disease. In 1960, Muckle and Wells described patients with recurrent episodes of urticarial-like rash, fever, and arthralgia, but symptoms were not cold triggered. Several patients from their cohort also developed progressive neurosensory hearing loss and AA renal amyloidosis. Several additional families with similar clinical presentation were reported since that initial report and the disease was then referred to as MWS.

Estimated prevalence of CAPS ranges from 1:300,000 to 1:1,000,000. CAPS has been reported from all continents of the world which is consistent with de novo mutations or autosomal dominant inheritance. In North America, the most common CAPS subtype is FCAS due to a founder effect traced back to the seventeenth century. However, MWS is the most common CAPS subtype in other parts of the world including Europe. Many patients with FCAS in the USA avoid living in cooler climates or hotter climates where air conditioning, a common trigger, is prevalent.

Genetics

Using DNA collected from large families with autosomal dominant inheritance, both FCAS and MWS were genetically linked to chromosome 1q44 providing evidence that these two diseases with similar phenotype may be due to mutations in the same gene. In 2001, heterozygous missense mutations were discovered in FCAS and MWS patients in a single novel gene, initially termed as *cold-induced autoinflammatory syndrome 1* (*CIAS1*) but later given the official name *Nod, leucine-rich repeat, pyrin 3* (*NLRP3*) based on shared domain structures of a family of NLR proteins. Since that time more than 90 pathogenic *NLRP3* mutations have been described in patients with FCAS, MWS, and NOMID. Most disease mutations are found in the Nod domain, although a few are described in the leucine-rich repeat or pyrin domains. *NLRP3* codes for the protein cryopyrin, which is why the disease spectrum is now referred to as CAPS. Some CAPS patients or families have clinical features of both FCAS and MWS or MWS and NOMID, which is consistent with a disease continuum. There is strong genotype-phenotype correlation in that each mutation is usually associated with only one of the three disease subtypes except in patients with clinical overlap where specific mutations can be associated with two subtypes.

There are some patients with a typical clinical presentation of CAPS who do not have readily identifiable mutations on standard genetic testing. Many of these patients have somatic mosaicism, where the mutation is only present in a small percentage of cells or limited to specific cells or tissues. More advanced testing such as deep sequencing or testing of tissues or cells other than blood may be required to detect these mutations. Rarely, there are patients with an FCAS-like phenotype who have mutations in other NLR genes including *NLRP12* and *NLRC4*. There are also some patients with atypical clinical presentations who possess low penetrance mutations (V198M, R488K, Q703K). These variants are also identified in a small percentage of the normal population making it challenging to confirm the clinical significance of these mutations.

Pathogenesis

Cryopyrin, an intracellular pattern recognition receptor in the NLR family of innate immune proteins, forms a protein complex known as the NLRP3 inflammasome that is expressed primarily in myeloid cells. Normally, the NLRP3 inflammasome is activated by several danger signals or pathogens to oligomerize with the adaptor ASC and cleave and activate caspase 1 (Fig. 1). Activated caspase 1 subsequently cleaves pro-IL-1β and pro-IL-18 to their active pro-inflammatory and releasable forms and also regulates pyroptosis, a form of inflammatory cell death (Doherty et al. 2011). There is some evidence that the NLRP3 inflammasome regulates or is regulated by the microbiome, which might have implications for human disease including CAPS. Heterozygous CAPS-associated mutations in *NLRP3* are gain of function in that they lead to an inflammasome that is constitutively active or has a lower threshold for activation resulting in cytokine release and systemic and tissue inflammation responsible for CAPS symptoms. This is apparent when peripheral blood monocytes from CAPS patients are isolated and cultured and then stimulated with various innate immune triggers such as LPS. Interestingly, monocytes from FCAS patients are unique in that they release IL-1β when cultured at 32 °C instead of 37 °C in the absence of other triggers.

Knock-in mice have been developed in which CAPS-associated mutations are engineered into the

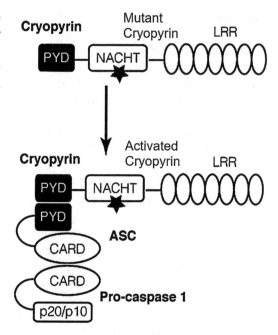

Familial Cold Autoinflammatory Syndrome (FCAS) and Muckle-Wells Syndrome (MWS), Fig. 1 Cryopyrin structure. Gain-of-function mutations in NLRP3 result in a constitutively active or hyperactive inflammasome leading to caspase 1 activation and IL-1β release

mouse *Nlrp3* gene. These mouse models mimic the clinical features of human CAPS in that the skin, joints, and conjunctiva are affected. Additionally, myeloid cells derived from these mice are also hyper-responsive to LPS in that they release IL-1β at a lower threshold. Cells from FCAS mice also release IL-1β when cultured at 32 °C similar to FCAS human monocytes. These mice have been used to elucidate the important proteins involved in the pathophysiology of CAPS. Specifically, the mouse phenotype is dependent on ASC and caspase 1, partially dependent on IL-1β, IL-18, TNF and pyroptosis, and not dependent on IL-6 or IL-17. These mouse models have also been used to test various therapies for CAPS.

Clinical Manifestations

FCAS, MWS, and NOMID were described as three distinct diseases, but advances in genetics and overlapping signs and symptoms support the concept of a common disease continuum. However, the distinction between the three sub-phenotypes is still useful due to differences in symptom severity and long-term morbidity. CAPS is a systemic inflammatory disease similar to other autoinflammatory diseases and can affect multiple tissues including the skin, muscles, joints, bones, eyes, ears, and the central nervous system. Age of onset is often at birth or early infancy, but some patients with somatic mosaicism may present as late as adulthood. CAPS symptoms can be due to acute tissue inflammation during flares such as rash and limb pain but also result from chronic inflammation such as fatigue or renal failure from amyloidosis. Common triggers for flares include stress or infection, but FCAS is unique in that episodes are triggered by generalized mild cold exposure. Many FCAS and MWS patients have some symptoms on a daily basis in the absence of triggers and experience worse symptoms at the end of the day. Many FCAS episodes resolve within 12–24 h, but MWS flares may last for 1–2 days (Hawkins et al. 2004; Hoffman et al. 2001).

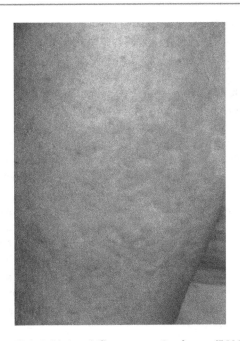

Familial Cold Autoinflammatory Syndrome (FCAS) and Muckle-Wells Syndrome (MWS), Fig. 2 Urticaria-like rash observed in FCAS and MWS

Cutaneous Involvement

Patients present clinically with "urticaria-like" lesions that start as small erythematous and edematous papules and progress to wheals. The rash typically occurs on the trunk and limbs, less commonly on the face, but spares palms and soles. In some patients there is predisposition to the skin overlying the fatty areas including upper arms, thighs, and abdomen (Fig. 2). Patients usually complain of burning pain or tenderness, but pruritus is sometimes present. If untreated, most patients have some limited rash on a daily basis with more generalized distribution during flares. Specific lesions usually persist for several hours unlike classic fleeting urticaria. Some patients may also experience painful extremity swelling similar to angioedema. In FCAS, rashes often appear 1–4 h after cold exposure in areas not necessarily subjected directly to cold air and are not induced by direct immediate contact with cold

objects or water (negative ice cube test) (Hawkins et al. 2004; Hoffman et al. 2001).

Musculoskeletal Involvement

Patients complain of arm or leg pain (myalgia and arthralgia) that often localizes to specific joints, and sometimes this can be associated with obvious swelling around the joints (periarthritis). FCAS patients rarely have true arthritis, but patients suffering from MWS can have frank arthritis with wrists, knees, and ankles most commonly affected. Chronic polyarticular arthritis with bone and joint deformation can be seen in severe forms of MWS.

Ocular Involvement

A variety of inflammatory eye diseases have been reported in FCAS and MWS patients including conjunctivitis, keratitis, episcleritis, and anterior or posterior uveitis. The most common inflammatory eye manifestation is conjunctivitis occurring during flares in many CAPS patients. Patients often complain of burning pain and redness without significant discharge. Ocular exam may show stromal corneal scarring, opacification, or infiltrates as well as uveitis.

Otologic Involvement

A significant number of MWS patients and small percentage of FCAS patients develop progressive sensorineural hearing loss. Onset can be early in life but commonly occurs in adolescence and early adulthood. Primarily high frequencies (4–10 kHz) are affected early, but broader frequencies become affected later with progressive worsening with age. Unlike more common diseases of hearing loss, the pathogenesis is due to ongoing cochlear inflammation. Therefore, prevention of progression of hearing loss and even sometimes reversal of hearing loss may be achieved with targeted anti-inflammatory treatment.

Amyloidosis

MWS patients and some FCAS patients are at risk for the development of secondary AA amyloidosis due to chronic inflammation. Kidneys are the most commonly affected tissue often leading to end-stage renal disease (Hawkins et al. 2004). Therefore, proteinuria is often the first indicator of systemic amyloidosis. While disease severity and persistently elevated serum amyloid A levels appear to be important predictors for the development of amyloidosis, the most important risk factor is a family history of amyloidosis, suggesting heritable components other than specific disease gene mutations.

Other Symptoms

Fatigue or malaise is commonly reported by FCAS and MWS patients and is associated with severely compromised quality of life. Headache without significantly increased intracranial pressure is also a common symptom and may be associated with low-grade sterile meningeal inflammation. Fever is not a common presenting complaint, and objective measurement of body temperature is only significantly elevated in severe flares. For example, in FCAS patients

undergoing cold challenge, body temperature increased less than 1 °C. Chills or shivers, sweating, excessive thirst, and dizziness are often reported by many FCAS patients.

Laboratory Findings

Blood leukocytosis with neutrophilia, thrombocytosis, and anemia are commonly seen at baseline, and neutrophilia increases rapidly during flares. Elevated inflammatory markers such as erythrocyte sedimentation rate (ESR), C-reactive protein (CRP), and serum amyloid A (SAA) are observed at baseline in almost all patients with CAPS, and levels decrease with effective therapy. The phagocytic-specific S100 proteins S100 A12 and MRP 8/14 are increased in serum of CAPS patients, and a good correlation to treatment response has also been demonstrated. As described above, elevated protein levels in urine are usually the first sign of systemic amyloidosis.

Diagnosis

In most cases FCAS and MWS become apparent during early childhood, but because the disease is rare and some patients present with only mild symptoms, the diagnosis of CAPS also has to be considered in adults. The suspected diagnosis is frequently supported by the patient's history, family history, physical examination, and additional tests such as inflammatory markers and audiograms. Patient symptom diaries and in some cases diagnostic therapeutic trials can also be used to establish the correct diagnosis.

Diagnostic Criteria for CAPS

Diagnostic criteria for CAPS have been validated using different cohorts of patients with CAPS and other autoinflammatory and autoimmune diseases. The following criteria are based on the finding that most patients have detectable systemic inflammation and on uniquely CAPS-specific clinical features to achieve reasonable specificity and sensitivity. The last two signs are common features of NOMID.

Raised Inflammatory Markers (CRP/SAA) (Mandatory Criterion) Plus
≥ 2 of 6 **CAPS typical signs/symptoms**:

- Urticaria-like rash
- Cold/stress-triggered episodes
- Sensorineural hearing loss
- Musculoskeletal symptoms (arthralgia/arthritis/myalgia)
- Chronic aseptic meningitis
- Skeletal abnormalities (epiphyseal overgrowth/frontal bossing) Kuemmerle-Deschner et al. (2017)

Genetic Testing
Genetic testing for mutations in the *NLRP3* gene may help to confirm the diagnosis as the majority of patients with CAPS carry germ line mutations in *NLRP3*. However, the diagnosis can often be made on clinical basis alone, as there are patients with clinical features that are consistent with CAPS who do not have easily identifiable mutations (approximately 25% of MWS patients and 10% of FCAS patients). Often this is due to somatic mosaicism. Therefore, the presence of *NLRP3* mutations is not necessary to make the diagnosis, and a genetic diagnosis should not be required prior to initiation of appropriate therapy.

Pathology and Imaging
Skin biopsies show dermal edema and a neutrophilic infiltrate in the dermis often near the sweat glands.

Patients with amyloidosis have AA amyloid deposits in various tissues including kidneys, heart, and gut. Inner ear FLAIR MRI may demonstrate inner ear inflammation as a cause for sensorineural hearing loss in CAPS patients.

Differential Diagnosis
The diagnosis of FCAS or MWS should be suspected in any patient with recurrent episodes of urticarial-like rash, unexplained systemic inflammation, a positive family history, and early onset of symptoms. Differential diagnosis includes disorders such as tumor necrosis factor (TNF) receptor-associated periodic syndrome (TRAPS), hyper-immunoglobulinemia D with periodic fever syndrome (HIDS), familial Mediterranean fever, Behcet's disease, Schnitzler's disease, and juvenile idiopathic arthritis. While patients with acquired cold urticaria also have cold-induced rash, they have immediate pruritic urticaria with direct cold exposure (positive ice cube test) and can develop anaphylaxis with significant cold water exposure. PLAID patients with phospholipase C gamma 2 mutations develop antihistamine-responsive urticaria immediately with evaporative cooling but may also have hypogammaglobulinemia or autoimmune disease. Patients with chilblains have itching, red patches, swelling, and blistering primarily on hands and feet with cold exposure.

Treatment

Nonsteroidal anti-inflammatory drugs and steroids have limited benefit for FCAS and MWS patients. There are three injectable IL-1-blocking therapies approved for the treatment of CAPS: anakinra (Kineret®, recombinant IL-1 receptor antagonist), rilonacept (Arcalyst®, IL-1 Trap, a fusion protein of the IL-1 receptor and the Fc portion of IgG), and canakinumab (Ilaris®, IL-1-β-blocking antibody). The pharmacokinetics of each is very different resulting in different dosing recommendations. Anakinra has a short half-life and therefore usually dosed daily. Rilonacept has a longer half-life resulting in recommended dosing once weekly. Canakinumab has a long half-life and unique pharmacokinetic profile in CAPS patients allowing for dosing every 2 months. Some milder FCAS patients are able to maintain symptom control with decreased dosing frequency, while patients with more severe disease require more frequent dosing (Doherty et al. 2011). For anakinra, the typical dosing regimen varies from 1–2 mg/kg/day for FCAS patients and up to 4–5 mg/kg/day for MWS patients to achieve optimal clinical responses. The rilonacept doses vary between 2.2 mg/kg/week and 4.4 mg/kg/week. Canakinumab is administered at 150 mg for MWS and FCAS patients with body weights greater than 40 kg and at 2 mg/kg for CAPS patients with body weight greater than or equal to 15 kg and less than or equal to 40 kg every 8 weeks. For children 15–40 kg with an inadequate response, the dose can be increased (see package inserts). Dose requirements are often higher in younger and more severe patients.

Successful treatment with IL-1-blocking agents leads to complete resolution of symptoms in most cases and is therefore the standard of care. Some FCAS patients choose to avoid therapy as some patients can limit symptoms by controlling their environment. Patients with more severe forms of MWS or FCAS patients with a family history of amyloidosis or hearing loss are likely to develop organ damage from untreated disease, so optimal IL-1-targeted therapy should be initiated early to prevent the development and progression of organ damage. All three IL-1-targeted drugs appear to control symptoms, hearing loss, and eye disease in a similar fashion if dosed appropriately.

The most common side effect of IL-1-targeted therapies in CAPS patients is an increased risk of common non-opportunistic, but sometimes serious, infections. This is a particular problem since these drugs may blunt some of the clinical signs of infection including fever and leukocytosis. Therefore, early and aggressive use of antimicrobial agents in CAPS patients on therapy should be considered. Other side effects include local injection site reactions. Vertigo has also been observed in some CAPS patients on canakinumab (Doherty et al. 2011). Additional IL-1-blocking agents are currently under development, which could be used to treat CAPS in the future. However, biologic therapies have some disadvantages including high cost, requirement for injection, and storage restrictions. There are also several small molecule inhibitors under development that target NLRP3 directly and may be useful for the treatment of CAPS in the future.

Prognosis

Clinical outcomes and quality of life for CAPS patients vary by disease severity. In the past, many MWS patients had increased morbidity and mortality due to organ damage or side effects from ineffective therapies. The prognosis of CAPS patients has changed considerably since the widespread use of IL-1-targeted therapy. However, early and aggressive treatment is crucial to improve quality of life and to avoid end-organ damage.

Cross-References

▶ Neonatal-Onset Multisystem Inflammatory Disease (NOMID)
▶ PLAID and APLAID

References

Aksentijevich I, DP C, Remmers EF, Mueller JL, Le J, Kolodner RD, et al. The clinical continuum of cryopyrinopathies: novel CIAS1 mutations in North American patients and a new cryopyrin model. Arthritis Rheum. 2007;56(4):1273–85.

Doherty TA, Brydges SD, Hoffman HM. Autoinflammation: translating mechanism to therapy. J Leukoc Biol. 2011;90(1):37–47.

Hawkins PN, Lachmann HJ, Aganna E, McDermott MF. Spectrum of clinical features in muckle-wells syndrome and response to anakinra. Arthritis Rheum. 2004;50(2):607–12.

Hoffman HM, Wanderer AA, Broide DH. Familial cold autoinflammatory syndrome: phenotype and genotype of an autosomal dominant periodic fever. J Allergy Clin Immunol. 2001;108(4):615–20.

Kuemmerle-Deschner JB, Ozen S, Tyrrell PN, Kone-Paut I, Goldbach-Mansky R, et al. Diagnostic criteria for cryopyrin-associated periodic syndrome (CAPS). Ann Rheum Dis. 2017;76(6):942–947.

Familial Cold Urticaria

▶ Familial Cold Autoinflammatory Syndrome (FCAS) and Muckle-Wells Syndrome (MWS)

Familial Infantile, with Intracranial Calcification and Chronic Cerebrospinal Fluid Lymphocytosis

▶ Aicardi-Goutières Syndrome (AGS1–AGS7)

Familial Mediterranean Fever and Pyrin-Associated Autoinflammatory Syndromes

Seza Ozen and Hafize Emine Sönmez
Department of Pediatric Rheumatology, Faculty of Medicine, Hacettepe University, Ankara, Turkey

Acronyms

FMF   Familial Mediterranean Fever
MEFV   MEditerranean FeVer
PAAS   Pyrin-associated autoinflammatory syndromes
PAAND   Pyrin-associated autoinflammation with neutrophilic dermatosis

Definition

Familial Mediterranean Fever (FMF) is an autosomal recessive inherited disorder which is caused by mutations in the *MEditerranean FeVer (MEFV)* gene on chromosome 16p13.3 (MIM # 608107). It is the most common monogenic autoinflammatory disease (Kastner et al. 2010).

Introduction and Background

FMF is a condition characterized by recurrent fever and inflammatory manifestations. It is most frequent among the Eastern Mediterranean populations: non-Ashkenazi Jews, Armenians, Turks, and Arabs. The prevalence of FMF is estimated to be 1 in 500 to 1 in 1000 in these populations. The carrier frequency of *MEFV* mutation has been estimated as high as 1 in 5 in these populations. Although rarely, FMF has been reported in other populations all over the world (Kastner et al. 2010). FMF affects both sexes at a similar rate.

Genetics

FMF is caused by mutations in *MEFV,* a 10 exon gene encoding a 781 amino acid protein which is called pyrin or marenostrin. Although FMF follows autosomal recessive inheritance, individuals with only monoallelic mutation in the *MEFV* gene may display signs of FMF phenotype. Studies have suggested that this may be associated with the penetrance of the gene, modifier genes and/or environmental factors.

Pathogenesis

Pyrin is expressed in granulocytes, monocytes, and dendritic cells and in peritoneal, synovial, and dermal fibroblasts. Pyrin interacts with the inflammasome adaptor protein (ASC) which results in increased caspase-1 activation, subsequently converting the pro-IL-1β into the biologically active pro-inflammatory cytokine, IL-1β. Recent work suggests that pyrin is regulated by Rho GTPase (RhoA). Bacterial toxins or intracellular cAMP inactivate RhoA, which disrupts the phosphorylation of the serine-threonine protein kinase N1 (PKN1) and protein kinase N2 (PKN2) which bind and phosphorylate pyrin, preventing the assembly of the pyrin inflammasome (Park et al. 2016).

Clinical Manifestations

Systemic Manifestations

Familial Mediterranean Fever is an autoinflammatory disease characterized by recurring, self-limited febrile attacks. The first febrile attack usually manifests during childhood, and approximately 90% of patients present the first attacks under 20 years. FMF attacks last between 6 h to 3 days. They are accompanied with polyserositis and elevated acute phase reactants. Most of the patients appear clinically well during attack-free periods; however elevated inflammatory markers may be seen in-between the attacks. The attack frequency is not regular.

In infants, fever may be the only symptom. Abdominal pain (95%) is the most common symptom during the attacks and is caused by acute peritonitis. Abdominal pain ranges from mild discomfort to severe pain mimicking appendicitis or other surgical pathologies. Constipation may occur; on the other hand pediatric patients may also have diarrhea. Pleuritis may occur in 34–45% of patients and is presented with unilateral chest pain. Recurrent pericarditis is another rare manifestation of FMF, and it is observed in 0.5% of patients.

Musculoskeletal Manifestations

Joint involvement (75%) is a common manifestation of the disease. Patients usually present with acute monoarthritis which affect large joints such as knee, ankles, and wrist. However, approximately 5% of patients have been reported to have chronic arthritis, mostly in hips or knees. Mild muscle pain may occur in about 20% of patients, affects usually lower extremities, improves with exercise, and resolves with rest. However, protracted febrile myalgia is a rare, severe manifestation of FMF and characterized by paralyzing myalgia and high fever. Patients with protracted febrile myalgia require treatment with corticosteroids. It is imported to distinguish protracted febrile myalgia from colchicine myopathy. High fever, elevated acute phase reactants, and normal levels of serum creatine kinase are typical findings of protracted febrile myalgia.

Cutaneous Manifestations

The most common skin finding of FMF is erysipelas-like erythema, which mostly appears on the extensor surface of lower extremities and resembles cellulitis (Kastner et al. 2010).

FMF is associated with increased risk for other inflammatory diseases such as vasculitis (polyarteritis nodosa, immunoglobulin A vasculitis/ Henoch Schönlein purpura, and Behcet's disease), inflammatory bowel diseases, and chronic arthritis.

Pyrin-associated autoinflammation with neutrophilic dermatosis (PAAND) is a pyrin-associated autoinflammatory syndrome (PAAS), a term used to combine FMF and PAAND based on their shared pathogenesis involving the pyrin inflammasome, which presents with a clinical phenotype that is different from FMF. It is characterized by neutrophilic dermatosis, childhood-onset recurrent episodes of fever lasting several weeks, increased levels of acute-phase reactants, arthralgia, and myalgia/myositis. The disease is caused by a specific mutation in *MEFV*, the gene encoding pyrin, at amino acid residue 242 changing a serine to arginine (p.S242R). Increased IL-1β production was described in affected individuals. Thus, anti-IL1 treatment may be an effective treatment for these patients.

Laboratory Findings

During the attacks, leukocytosis, increased erythrocyte sedimentation rate, elevated acute phase reactants such as CRP, and serum amyloid A may occur; and in the attack-free period, they may not return to normal in untreated patients. Inflammatory markers remain elevated between the attacks in patients who have an increased risk of developing systemic amyloidosis.

The EULAR recommendations for the management of FMF suggest to perform urinalysis periodically to detect the proteinuria which may be the first evidence of amyloidosis (Ozen et al. 2016).

Diagnosis

The diagnosis of FMF depends on clinical findings. Different sets of classification and diagnostic criteria were created. Firstly, adult criteria were established (Table 1) (Livneh et al. 1997). Finally, pediatric FMF criteria was developed by a Turkish group in 2009 which included the following five criteria: (1) fever (axillary, >38 °C, ≥3 attacks of 6–72 h duration), (2) abdominal pain (≥3 attacks of 6–72 h duration), (3) chest pain (≥3 attacks of 6–72 h duration),(4) arthritis (oligoarthritis, ≥3 attacks of 6–72 h duration), and (5) family history of FMF (Table 1) (Yalcinkaya et al. 2009). According to this criteria, in the presence of two or more criteria, the sensitivity and specificity of diagnosis FMF were 86.5% and 93.6%, respectively (Yalcinkaya et al. 2009).

Genetic testing helps to diagnosis of the disease, especially in areas where the clinicians are not familiar with this disease. To date, more than 300 disease-associated *MEFV* mutations have been identified, but most of them are extremely rare (http://fmf.igh.cnrs.fr/infevers). Finally, a consensus guideline for genetic diagnostic testing of hereditary recurrent fevers (HRFs) including FMF was established in 2012 (Shinar et al. 2012). According to this guideline, testing of a total of 14 variants is recommended (9 variants are defined as clearly pathogenic, M694V, M694I, M680I, V726A, R761H, A744S, E167D, T267I, I692del, and five variants defined as unknown significance, K695R, E148Q, P369S, F479L, and I591T) (Shinar et al. 2012).

Genetic testing for *MEFV* mutations is not recommended in siblings of FMF patients. However, it is necessary to inform the parents or siblings about the clinical signs of FMF. On the other hand, genetic testing is recommended if there is a rise in the acute phase reactants (Ozen et al. 2016).

Treatment

Colchicine is effective in controlling the inflammation, in decreasing the attack frequency, and also in preventing secondary amyloidosis. Colchicine binds to tubulin and depolymerizes microtubules, resulting in the release of the RhoA activator guanine-nucleotide-exchange factor (GEF)-H1 (Heck et al. 2012). RhoA activation inactivates the pyrin inflammasome.

Colchicine is a safe, well-tolerated drug, even in infancy and pregnancy. However, 5–10% of the

Familial Mediterranean Fever and Pyrin-Associated Autoinflammatory Syndromes, Table 1 The clinical criteria sets for Familial Mediterranean Fever (FMF) diagnosis

Tel Hashomer criteria (long version) (Livneh et al. 1997)

Major criteria

Typical attacks (≥3 of the same type, rectal temperature ≥ 38 °C, attacks lasting 12 h to 3 days)
- Peritonitis
- Pleuritis (unilateral) or pericarditis
- Monoarthritis (hip, knee, ankle)
- Fever alone

Minor criteria
- Incomplete attacks (typical attacks including one of the following sites: Abdomen, chest, or joint with 1 or 2 of the following exception: (1) temperature <38 °C, (2) attacks lasting 6–12 h or 3–7 days, (3) no signs of peritonitis during abdominal attacks, (4) localized abdominal pain, (5) arthritis in joints other than hip, knee, or ankle
- Exertional leg pain
- Favorable response to colchicine

Supportive criteria
- Family history of FMF
- Appropriate ethnic origin
- Age <20 years at disease onset
(Four criteria below are related to the features of attacks)
- Severe, requiring bed rest
- Spontaneous remission
- Symptom-free interval
- Transient inflammatory response with one or more abnormal test result(s) for white blood cell count, erythrocyte sedimentation rate, serum amyloid A, and/or fibrinogen
- Episodic proteinuria/hematuria
- Unproductive laparotomy or removal of "white" appendix
- Consanguinity of parents

Diagnosis:
≥1 major OR ≥ 2 minor criteria OR 1 minor+ ≥ 5 supportive criteria OR
1 minor+ ≥ 4 of the first 5 supportive criteria

Tel Hashomer criteria (short version) (Livneh et al. 1997)

Major criteria
- Recurrent febrile episodes accompanied by peritonitis, synovitis, or pleuritis
- Favorable response to continuous colchicine treatment
- AA type amyloidosis without predisposing disease

Minor criteria
- Recurrent febrile episodes
- Erysipelas-like erythema
- FMF in a 1° relative

(continued)

Familial Mediterranean Fever and Pyrin-Associated Autoinflammatory Syndromes, Table 1 (continued)

Diagnosis: 2 major OR 1 major+2 minor criteria
Livneh criteria (simplified) (Livneh et al. 1997)
Major criteria

• Typical attacks of (recurrent [=3 of the same type], febrile [rectal, ≥38 °C], and short [12 h–3 days])
   - Generalized peritonitis
   - Unilateral chest pain (pleuritis or pericarditis)
   - Hip, knee, or ankle monoarthritis
   - Fever alone
 • Incomplete abdominal attacks

Minor criteria
• 1–2 incomplete attacks involving ≥1 of the following: • Chest   • Joint   • Exertional leg pain   • Favorable response to colchicine
Diagnosis: 1 major OR 2 minor criteria
Turkish FMF pediatric criteria (Yalcinkaya et al. 2009)
• Fever (axillary, >38 °C, ≥3 attacks of 6–72 h duration)   • Abdominal pain (≥3 attacks of 6–72 h duration)   • Chest pain (≥3 attacks of 6–72 h duration)   • Arthritis (oligoarthritis, ≥3 attacks of 6–72 h duration)   • Family history of FMF
Diagnosis: 2 out of 5 criteria

patients suffer from side effects at recommended doses. Gastrointestinal symptoms such as nausea, vomiting, transient elevation of transaminases, and especially diarrhea are the most common side effects. Dose reduction may resolve these symptoms, and lactose-free diet may help to control gastrointestinal symptoms as some patients develop lactose intolerance due to colchicine. Colchicine-induced myopathy, bone marrow depression (e.g., hemolytic or aplastic anemia, pancytopenia, neutropenia, and thrombocytopenia) may rarely be observed at recommended doses (Ozen et al. 2016).

Drug interactions and toxicity may occur when drugs (such as macrolides, cyclosporine, cimetidine) are given together with colchicine as they are metabolized by the same enzyme (CYP3A4) (Ozen et al. 2016).

Colchicine prevents FMF attacks and subclinical inflammation in most patients, although a small percentage of patients do not respond to colchicine therapy. Drug compliance has to be attentively evaluated in patients non-responsive to colchicine therapy. If a patient suffers of an attack at least a month or has persistent elevated acute-phase reactants (APRs) during the attack-free periods, this patient should be considered as non-responsive to colchicine therapy. Biologic agents may be used in unresponsive patients. With the improvement of knowledge about the pathogenesis of FMF, inhibition of IL-1 became an alternative treatment for colchicine-resistant FMF patients. There are three forms of anti-IL-1 therapy: anakinra, canakinumab, and rilonacept.

Prognosis

There are limited data on long-term comorbidities and mortality among patients with FMF. Secondary amyloidosis is the most serious complication that presents with proteinuria and may lead to end-stage renal disease. However, due to advances in the early diagnosis and effective treatment, this complication is now very rare. Some predisposing factors associated with increased risk of developing amyloidosis have been found in patients with FMF: such as positive family history of amyloidosis, male gender, M694V homozygosity, and SAA1.1α/α genotype. Previous studies concluded that FMF patients homozygous for M694V have an increased risk of severe phenotype and early disease onset.

In conclusion FMF should be suspected in patients with recurrent fever and polyserositis attacks lasting less than 3 days, especially in certain ethnic groups. The goal of treatment is to control attacks and to suppress the subclinical inflammation to prevent complications such as secondary amyloidosis.

Cross-References

▶ Introduction to Autoinflammatory Diseases

References

Heck JN, Ponik SM, Garcia-Mendoza MG, Pehlke CA, Inman DR, Eliceiri KW, Keely PJ. Microtubules regulate GEF-H1 in response to extracellular matrix stiffness. Mol Biol Cell. 2012;23(13):2583–92.

Kastner DL, Aksentijevich I, Goldbach-Mansky R. Autoinflammatory disease reloaded: a clinical perspective. Cell. 2010;140(6):784–90.

Livneh A, Langevitz P, Zemer D, Zaks N, Kees S, Lidar T, Migdal A, Padeh S, Pras M. Criteria for the diagnosis of familial Mediterranean fever. Arthritis Rheum. 1997; 40(10):1879–85.

Ozen S, Demirkaya E, Erer B, Livneh A, Ben-Chetrit E, Giancane G, Ozdogan H, Abu I, Gattorno M, Hawkins PN, Yuce S, Kallinich T, Bilginer Y, Kastner D, Carmona L. EULAR recommendations for the management of familial Mediterranean fever. Ann Rheum Dis. 2016;75(4):644–51.

Park YH, Wood G, Kastner DL, Chae JJ. Pyrin inflammasome activation and RhoA signaling in the autoinflammatory diseases FMF and HIDS. Nat Immunol. 2016;17:914–21.

Shinar Y, Obici L, Aksentijevich I, et al. Guidelines for the genetic diagnosis of hereditary recurrent fevers. Ann Rheum Dis. 2012;71(10):1599–605.

Yalcinkaya F, Ozen S, Ozcakar ZB, Aktay N, Cakar N, Duzova A, Kasapcopur O, Elhan AH, Doganay B, Ekim M, Kara N, Uncu N, Bakkaloglu A. A new set of criteria for the diagnosis of familial Mediterranean fever in childhood. Rheumatology (Oxford). 2009; 48(4):395–8.

FCAS – Familial Cold Autoinflammatory Syndrome

▶ PLAID and APLAID

(FCAS)

▶ Familial Cold Autoinflammatory Syndrome (FCAS) and Muckle-Wells Syndrome (MWS)

Ficolin-1: M-Ficolin

▶ Ficolin-3

Ficolin-2: L-Ficolin

▶ Ficolin-3

Ficolin-3

Ninette Genster and Peter Garred
Laboratory of Molecular Medicine, Department of Clinical Immunology, Section 7631
Rigshospitalet, Faculty of Health and Medical Sciences, University of Copenhagen, Copenhagen, Denmark

Synonyms

Ficolin-1: M-ficolin; Ficolin-2: L-ficolin; Ficolin-3: Hakata antigen or H-ficolin

Definition

Ficolin-3 is a recognition molecule of the lectin pathway of complement. The lectin pathway of the complement system is initiated when pattern-recognition molecules bind to invading pathogens or damaged host cells. This leads to activation of MBL-/ficolin-/collectin-associated serine proteases (MASPs), which in turn activate downstream complement components, ultimately leading to elimination of pathogens. A rare frameshift mutation in the gene encoding ficolin-3 has been reported: a mutation resulting in no detectable ficolin-3 protein.

Lectin Pathway of Complement

The complement system is a part of the innate immune system responsible for initiation of inflammation and elimination of invading pathogens or altered host cells (Ricklin et al. 2010). Three pathways initiate the complement cascade: the classical, alternative, and lectin pathways. The initiators of the lectin pathway include mannose-binding lectin (MBL), collectin-10, collectin-11, and the three ficolins -1, -2, and -3 (Endo et al. 2015). The lectin pathway is initiated when the pattern recognition molecules bind to pathogen-associated molecular patterns on the surface of microorganisms or altered host cells, promoting the activation of associated serine proteases, which lead to subsequent cleavage of C4 and C2 to form the C3 convertase (Fig. 1). All three pathways fuse at formation of the C3 convertase and cleavage of C3 into C3a and C3b, followed by the formation of the C5 convertase and cleavage of C5 into C5a and C5b. C5b can interact with C6, followed by interaction with C7, C8, and multiple C9 units to form the lytic terminal complement complex C5b-9 (also named the membrane attack complex). This cascade of events leads to the formation of cleavage products that function in opsonization, generation of the inflammatory response and cell lysis. Numerous soluble or surface bound regulatory molecules protect the host from collateral damage mediated via complement activation.

Genetics and Structure of Ficolins

In 1973, the first ficolin was shown to exist as a thermolabile macro protein in human serum. This protein later turned out to be ficolin-3 (Hakata antigen). In 1991, a porcine ficolin known as transforming growth factor-β1-binding protein was isolated from pig uterus membranes, and subsequently a human homologue of the protein (ficolin-2) was isolated from plasma. In addition, a third human ficolin (ficolin-1) was identified. Accordingly, three human ficolin genes have been identified: *FCN1*, *FCN2*, and *FCN3*, encoding ficolin-1(M-ficolin), ficolin-2 (L-ficolin), and ficolin-3 (H-ficolin), respectively (Garred et al. 2010). Ficolin-2 is expressed in the liver; ficolin-3 is expressed in the liver and the lungs, whereas ficolin-1 is predominantly expressed in bone marrow cells and human peripheral blood leukocytes. All three human ficolins are present in serum. An overview of the human ficolins is provided in Table 1.

The ficolin genes encode similar polypeptides containing a collagen-like domain and a C-terminal fibrinogen-like (FBG) domain (Fig. 2) (Endo et al. 2015; Garred et al. 2010). The *FCN3* gene is located on chromosome 1p36, whereas *FCN1* and *FCN2* are located on

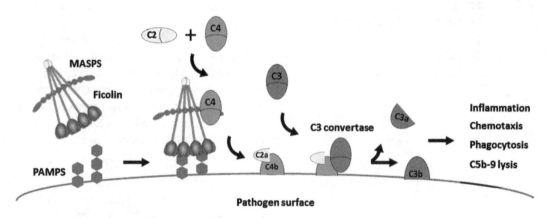

Ficolin-3, Fig. 1 Ficolin-mediated initiation of the lectin pathway of complement. Ficolins associated with serine proteases (*MASPs*) initiate the lectin pathway of complement by the binding to pathogen-associated molecular patterns (*PAMPs*) – an array of carbohydrate groups on the pathogen surface. Activated *MASPs* cleave C4 to *C4a* and *C4b*, and some *C4b* binds covalently to the pathogen surface. Activated *MASPs* also cleave C2 to *C2a* and *C2b*; *C2a* binds to surface *C4b* forming the *C3* convertase (*C4bC2a*). The *C3* convertase binds *C3* and cleaves it to *C3a* and *C3b*; *C3b* binds covalently to the pathogen surface promoting phagocytosis and lysis of pathogens or endogenous waste material. *C3a* is a mediator of inflammation and phagocyte recruitment chromosome 9q34. Exon 1 of the *FCN* genes encodes a signal peptide and the N-terminal region. Exons 2 and 3 encode the collagen-like domain, exon 4 encodes a linker region, and exons 5–8 encode the FBG domain. The ficolins exist as multimeric proteins consisting of 34–35 kDa subunits. Ficolin-1 and ficolin-2 are 79% identical at the amino acid level, whereas ficolin-3 is 48% homologous with ficolin-1 and ficolin-2. Three identical polypeptides are assembled into structural subunits through the collagen-like domain. These trimers are further assembled into higher oligomeric forms that resemble the bouquet-like structures of MBL and C1q. The collagen-like domain interacts with the MASPs, and the FBG domain is involved in ligand recognition. The

Ficolin-3, Table 1 Overview of the human ficolins

Ficolin	Gene	Site of expression	Serum level (μg/ml)	Microbial specificity
Ficolin-1	*FCN1*	Peripheral leukocytes Lung Spleen	0.3	*E. coli* *S. aureus* *S. agalactiae*
Ficolin-2	*FCN2*	Liver	5	*S. aureus* *S. pneumoniae* *S. typhimurium* *E. coli* *P. aeruginosa* *M. bovis* *G. lamblia* *T. cruzi* *A. fumigatus*
Ficolin-3	*FCN3*	Liver Lung	25	*A. viridans* *T. cruzi*

Ficolin-3, Fig. 2 Exon organization of *FCN* genes and oligomeric structure of ficolins. The ficolin genes encode a polypeptide consisting of an N-terminal region followed by a collagen-like domain, a short linker region, and a C-terminal fibrinogen-like (*FBG*) domain. Three identical polypeptides are assembled into trimeric structural subunits that are further assembled into higher oligomeric forms through formation of disulfide bridges between the polypeptides. The fibrinogen-like domain is the recognition unit, whereas the collagen-like domain interacts with the associated serine proteases (MASPs)

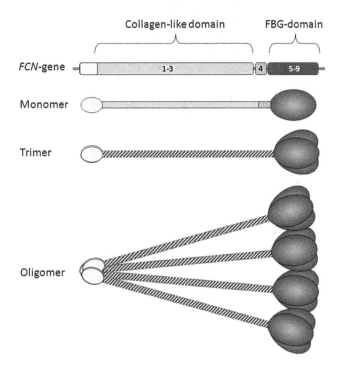

ficolins exhibit individual binding properties, and their microbial specificity differs (Table 1). Taken together the ficolins recognize a broad spectrum of microorganisms, including bacterial, viral, and fungal pathogens (Ren et al. 2014). In addition the ficolins play a role in tissue homeostasis as they bind to and help eliminate endogenous debris.

Clinical Significance of Ficolins

During the past decades, it has become evident that abnormal function or expression of ficolins is involved in the development/progression of infectious diseases and inflammation. Various nucleotide polymorphisms of all three human ficolin genes have been identified, including single nucleotide polymorphisms (SNPs), and some of these variants are related to the structure and function of ficolin, affecting the serum concentration and ligand-binding activities (Garred et al. 2010; Endo et al. 2015). Accordingly, certain functional SNPs are also associated with disease. An overview of known associations between SNPs and ficolin levels, and disease is provided in Table 2.

A large number of genetic variants with race-related differences have been observed in the *FCN1* gene, and several SNPs have been associated with the level of ficolin-1 in serum (Garred et al. 2010). Some of these variants are associated with fatal outcomes from systemic inflammation (Munthe-Fog et al. 2012) and leprosy (Boldt et al. 2013). Other SNPs in *FCN1* have been associated with rheumatoid arthritis (Vander et al. 2007) or an earlier colonization of *P. aeruginosa* in cystic fibrosis patients (Haerynck et al. 2012).

FCN2 is polymorphic, and several SNPs are associated with the serum concentration of ficolin-2 (Garred et al. 2010). Certain SNPs give rise to an altered binding activity of ficolin-2, and one such SNP representing low ficolin-2 level and increased binding activity is associated with chronic Chagas disease (Luz et al. 2013) and leprosy (Zhang et al. 2013). In addition, an improved outcome of renal transplantation has been reported if the donor carries this SNP (Eikmans et al. 2012).

FCN3 is the most conserved among the *FCN* genes since only a few variations in *FCN3* have been detected and these are present in low frequencies (Garred et al. 2010). Thus, ficolin-3 deficiency is a rare condition, and only a few cases have been reported. The first patient with ficolin-3 deficiency to be reported was a 32-year-old male homozygous for at frameshift mutation (1637delC) in exon 5 of *FCN3* (rs28357092) (Munthe-Fog et al. 2009). The frameshift mutation results in an altered amino acid composition of the C-terminal end of ficolin-3, spanning from amino acid position 117 to position 180, where the nonsense protein sequence is terminated due to an early stop codon (Fig. 3). Therefore, this ficolin-3 lacks most of the FBG domain, and experiments utilizing a recombinant version of the protein reveal that it cannot be expressed (Munthe-Fog et al. 2008). Accordingly, no ficolin-3 was detected in the patient's serum, and no complement activation via the ficolin-3-mediated pathway was detected in the serum. The activities of the MBL, the classical, and the alternative pathways were normal. The patient was suffering from recurrent bacterial pulmonary infections, leading to development of bronchiectasis, pulmonary fibrosis, and cerebral abscesses. At the time of discovery, no other abnormalities of the immune system were found, thus it was interpreted that inherited deficiency of ficolin-3 may be associated with chronic and/or recurrent infections and lung damage. However, recently the patient in question with ficolin-3 deficiency has been diagnosed with Wiskott-Aldrich syndrome due to a mutation in the *WASP* gene, which partly may explain his symptoms. Thus, it is difficult to determine which aspects of the clinical phenotype that may relate to the mutation in *WASP* gene alone and what may relate to frameshift variant in *FCN3* gene. However, in relation to Wiskott-Aldrich syndrome, the case was very unusual. Nevertheless an infant cousin of the patient revealed classical Wiskott-Aldrich symptoms leading to the suspicion and genetic screening showing that both carried the same mutation. As described, the mutation in the homozygous state results in total lack of ficolin-3 in serum, whereas the

Ficolin-3, Table 2 Disease associations of ficolin insufficiency/deficiency (Table modified from Endo et al. (2015))

Disease	Associated with
Systemic inflammation	*FCN1* SNPs → ↓ Serum ficolin-1
Leprosy	*FCN1* SNPs
Cystic fibrosis	*FCN1* SNPs
RA	*FCN1* SNPs
Head and neck squamous cell carcinoma	↑ Ficolin-1
RA	↑/↓ Ficolin-1
Microscopic polyangitis	↑ ficolin-1
Neonatal sepsis	↑ Ficolin-1
Severe infection in patients with hematological cancer	↓ Ficolin-1
Necrotizing enterocolitis	↓ Ficolin-1
Increased need for ventilation and increased mortality in babies	↓ Serum ficolin-1
Chronic fatigue syndrome	↑ Ficolin-1
Staphylococcal peritonitis	*FCN2* SNPs
Recurrent infection in children	*FCN2* SNPs
Chronic Chagas disease	*FCN2* SNPs
Leprosy	*FCN2* SNPs
Cystic fibrosis	*FCN2* SNPs
Renal transplant outcome	*FCN2* SNP
Schistosomiasis	*FCN2* SNPs
Cutaneous leishmaniasis	*FCN2* SNPs
Hepatitis B infection outcome	*FCN2* SNPs
Cytomegalovirus infection after orthotopic liver transplantation	*FCN2* SNPs
Malaria infection	*FCN2* SNPs
S. peritonitis	*FCN2* SNPs
Rheumatic fever and rheumatic heart disease	*FCN2* SNPs
SLE	↑ Ficolin-2
Ovarian cancer	↑ Ficolin-2
Chronic Chagas disease	↓ Ficolin-2
Hereditary angiodema	↓ Ficolin-2
Preclampsia	↓ Ficolin-2
Combined allergic and infectious respiratory disease	↓ Ficolin-2
Bronchiectasis	↓ Ficolin-2
IgA nephropathy	↓ Ficolin-2
Recurrent infection	
Perinatal infections	↓ Serum ficolin-2
S. peritonitis	↓ Serum ficolin-2

(continued)

Ficolin-3, Table 2 (continued)

Disease	Associated with
Severe recurrent infection	FCN3 SNP (defect)
Necrotizing enterocolitis	FCN3 SNP (defect)
Essential hypertension	FCN3 SNP
Ovarian cancer	↑/↓ Ficolin-3
Advanced heart failure	↓ Ficolin-3
RA	↑ Ficolin-3
Type-2 diabetes	↑/↓ Ficolin-3
Recurrent infection	No Ficolin-3
Necrotizing enterocolitis	No Ficolin-3
Neonatal sepsis	↓ Ficolin-3
Chemotherapy-related infections	↓ Ficolin-3
SLE	↑ Ficolin-3
Sarcoidosis	↓ Ficolin-3
Hepatocellular carcinoma	↓ Ficolin-3

heterozygous state results in ficolin-3 levels approximately half of the wild-type ficolin-3 (Munthe-Fog et al. 2009). The allele frequency of the *FCN3 + 1637delC* variant was estimated to be 0.01 in Caucasians (Munthe-Fog et al. 2008). However, ficolin-3 has been detected in the sera of 100% of healthy Japanese blood donors (*n* >10,000) as well as 99.99% of Japanese patients (*n* >100,000) (Inaba et al. 1990). The second patient with congenital ficolin-3 deficiency to be reported was a premature infant diagnosed with necrotizing enterocolitis shown to be homozygous for the *FCN3 + 1637delC* mutation (Schlapbach et al. 2011). A third patient was another premature baby but with a perinatal infection caused by *Streptococcus agalactiae* (Michalski et al. 2012). In this patient, in addition to ficolin-3 deficiency (1637delC homozygote with no detectable protein), several other abnormalities of the innate immune system were found; making it difficult to draw a conclusion whether the lack of ficolin-3 was decisive. Recently, further two examples of primary ficolin-3 deficiency have been reported (Michalski et al. 2015).

In addition to gene polymorphisms, the ficolin protein levels are associated with several diseases (Table 2) (Endo et al. 2015). As described, the gene polymorphisms could be partly responsible

Ficolin-3, Fig. 3 Effect of the *FCN3* + *1637delC* frameshift mutation on the ficolin-3 structure. The exonic regions of both the wild type and the *L117fs* mutant of *FCN3* are shown. The *FCN3* + *1637delC*_/ L117*fs*) frameshift mutation is indicated as a *red star*. The frameshift mutation results in an altered amino acid composition of the C-terminal end of ficolin-3, spanning from amino acid position 117 to position 180, where the nonsense protein sequence is terminated due to an early stop codon

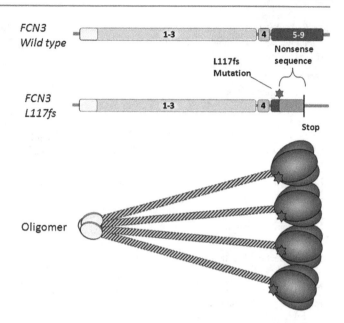

for the increase or decrease of the ficolin levels. Seemingly, infectious and inflammatory diseases are associated with low ficolin levels, whereas autoimmune disorders are associated with high ficolin levels (Endo et al. 2015).

Ficolin Knockout Mice

Two ficolins, termed ficolin-A and ficolin-B, have been identified in mice. The primary structure of ficolin-A is approximately 80% identical to human ficolin-2 and ficolin-1 and mouse ficolin-B, suggesting that these four ficolins are closely related (Garred et al. 2010). In terms of distribution and function, it appears that murine ficolin-A and human ficolin-2 resemble each other and may be regarded as functional equivalents. The same apply to murine ficolin-B and human ficolin-1. Ficolin-3 has been identified only in human and primates, and the mouse homologue exists as a pseudogene. The investigation of ficolin-deficient mice is merely initiated, and at present only a limited number of reports have been published (Genster et al. 2014). The general

phenotypes of ficolin-deficient mice were first described in 2012 (Endo et al. 2012).Three strains of ficolin-deficient mice were generated: ficolin-A knockout, ficolin-B knockout, and ficolin double knockout. None of the ficolin-deficient strains display abnormalities in their general state of health. The role of ficolins in host defense was evaluated by infection with *Streptococcus pneumonia*, and all three strains of ficolin-deficient mice showed reduced survival rates compared to WT mice, suggesting that ficolins play a crucial role in immunity against pneumococcal infection. The animal studies, although sparse, have confirmed the importance of ficolins in protection against certain pathogens in vivo, and indeed the ficolin-deficient mice will be an important tool in future investigations of the clinical consequences of ficolin deficiency.

Concluding Remarks

The ficolins might be involved in the pathophysiology of different infectious and inflammatory diseases, and polymorphisms or haplotypes in the FCN genes may be associated with different diseases. To date, deficiencies of ficolin-1 or ficolin-2 have not been reported, and only a few cases of ficolin-3 have been reported. Presumably, the low frequency of ficolin deficiency indicates an important role of ficolins in humans. The real clinical consequences of ficolin-3 deficiency are still unclear, and it remains to be elucidated whether ficolin-3 deficiency is indeed a primary immune deficiency or rather acts as a disease modifier.

References

Boldt AB, Sanchez MI, Stahlke ER, Steffensen R, Thiel S, Jensenius JC, Prevedello FC, Mira MT, Kun JF, Messias-Reason IJ. Susceptibility to leprosy is associated with M-ficolin polymorphisms. J Clin Immunol. 2013;33:210–9.

Eikmans M, De CI, van der Pol P, Baan CC, Haasnoot GW, Mallat MJ, Vergunst M, De Meester E, Roodnat JI, Anholts JD, Van Thielen M, Doxiadis II, de Fijter JW, van der Linden PJ, van Beelen E, van Kooten C, Kalvan Gestel JA, Peeters AM, Weimar W, Roelen DL, Rossau R, Claas FH. The functional polymorphism Ala258Ser in the innate receptor gene ficolin-2 in the donor predicts improved renal transplant outcome. Transplantation. 2012;94:478–85.

Endo Y, Takahashi M, Iwaki D, Ishida Y, Nakazawa N, Kodama T, Matsuzaka T, Kanno K, Liu Y, Tsuchiya K, Kawamura I, Ikawa M, Waguri S, Wada I, Matsushita M, Schwaeble WJ, Fujita T. Mice deficient in ficolin, a lectin complement pathway recognition molecule, are susceptible to Streptococcus pneumoniae infection. J Immunol. 2012;189:5860–6.

Endo Y, Matsushita M, Fujita T. New insights into the role of ficolins in the lectin pathway of innate immunity. Int Rev Cell Mol Biol. 2015;316:49–110.

Garred P, Honore C, Ma YJ, Rorvig S, Cowland J, Borregaard N, Hummelshoj T. The genetics of ficolins. J Innate Immun. 2010;2:3–16.

Genster N, Takahashi M, Sekine H, Endo Y, Garred P, Fujita T. Lessons learned from mice deficient in lectin complement pathway molecules. Mol Immunol. 2014;61:59–68.

Haerynck F, Van SK, Cattaert T, Loeys B, Van DS, Schelstraete P, Claes K, Van TM, De CI, Mahachie John JM, De BF. Polymorphisms in the lectin pathway genes as a possible cause of early chronic *Pseudomonas aeruginosa* colonization in cystic fibrosis patients. Hum Immunol. 2012;73:1175–83.

Inaba S, Okochi K, Yae Y, Niklasson F, de Verder CH. Serological studies of an SLE-associated antigen-antibody system discovered as a precipitation reaction in agarose gel: the HAKATA antigen-antibody system. Fukuoka Igaku Zasshi. 1990;81:284–91.

Luz PR, Boldt AB, Grisbach C, Kun JF, Velavan TP, Messias-Reason IJ. Association of L-ficolin levels and FCN2 genotypes with chronic Chagas disease. PLoS One. 2013;8:e60237.

Michalski M, Szala A, St SA, Lukasiewicz J, Maciejewska A, Kilpatrick DC, Matsushita M, Domzalska-Popadiuk I, Borkowska-Klos M, Sokolowska A, Szczapa J, Lugowski C, Cedzynski M. H-ficolin (ficolin-3) concentrations and FCN3 gene polymorphism in neonates. Immunobiology. 2012;217:730–7.

Michalski M, Swierzko AS, Pagowska-Klimek I, Niemir ZI, Mazerant K, Domzalska-Popadiuk I, Moll M, Cedzynski M. Primary ficolin-3 deficiency – is it associated with increased susceptibility to infections? Immunobiology. 2015;220(6):711–3.

Munthe-Fog L, Hummelshoj T, Ma YJ, Hansen BE, Koch C, Madsen HO, Skjodt K, Garred P. Characterization of a polymorphism in the coding sequence of FCN3 resulting in a ficolin-3 (Hakata antigen) deficiency state. Mol Immunol. 2008;45:2660–6.

Munthe-Fog L, Hummelshoj T, Honore C, Madsen HO, Permin H, Garred P. Immunodeficiency associated with FCN3 mutation and ficolin-3 deficiency. N Engl J Med. 2009;360:2637–44.

Munthe-Fog L, Hummelshoj T, Honore C, Moller ME, Skjoedt MO, Palsgaard I, Borregaard N, Madsen HO, Garred P. Variation in FCN1 affects biosynthesis of ficolin-1 and is associated with outcome of systemic inflammation. Genes Immun. 2012;13:515–22.

Ren Y, Ding Q, Zhang X. Ficolins and infectious diseases. Virol Sin. 2014;29:25–32.

Ricklin D, Hajishengallis G, Yang K, Lambris JD. Complement: a key system for immune surveillance and homeostasis. Nat Immunol. 2010;11:785–97.

Schlapbach LJ, Thiel S, Kessler U, Ammann RA, Aebi C, Jensenius JC. Congenital H-ficolin deficiency in premature infants with severe necrotising enterocolitis. Gut. 2011;60:1438–9.

Vander CB, Nuytinck L, Boullart L, Elewaut D, Waegeman W, Van TM, De ME, Lebeer K, Rossau R, De KF. Polymorphisms in the ficolin 1 gene (FCN1) are associated with susceptibility to the development of rheumatoid arthritis. Rheumatology (Oxford). 2007;46:1792–5.

Zhang DF, Huang XQ, Wang D, Li YY, Yao YG. Genetic variants of complement genes ficolin-2, mannose-binding lectin and complement factor H are associated with leprosy in Han Chinese from Southwest China. Hum Genet. 2013;132:629–40.

Ficolin-3: Hakata Antigen or H-Ficolin

► Ficolin-3

FILS Syndrome

► Clinical Presentation of Polymerase E1 (POLE1) and Polymerase E2 (POLE2) Deficiencies

FOCM: Folate-Mediated One-Carbon Metabolism

► Defects in B12 and Folate Metabolism (TCN2, SLC46A1 (PCFT Deficiency), MTHFD1)

FOXN1 Deficiency

► Winged Helix Deficiency (FOXN1)

G

G-CSF Receptor Deficiency

Gesmar Rodrigues Silva Segundo
Pediatrics Allergy and Immunology,
Universidade Federal de Uberlandia, Uberlandia,
Brazil

Introduction

Granulocyte colony-stimulating factor (G-CSF) is a hematopoietic cytokine that stimulates neutrophil production and hematopoietic stem cell mobilization by starting the dimerization of homodimeric granulocyte colony-stimulating factor receptor. G-CSF receptor (G-CSFR) is member of type I cytokine receptor superfamily, encoded by CSF3R. G-CSFR is a transmembrane protein consisting of 813 amino acids: 604 as an extracellular domain, 26 in the transmembrane domain, and 184 in the intracellular cytoplasmic domain. The extracellular domain of the receptor contains an immunoglobulin-like (Ig-like) domain, a cytokine receptor homology domain (CRH domains), and three fibronectins type III (FN III) domains, and four highly conserved cysteine residues and a WSXWS motif of the CRH domains are required for ligand binding and receptor activation. The cytoplasmic region has no intrinsic kinase activity, but the receptor suffers a conformational change leading to the activation of several different pathways including JAK/STAT, PI3K/AKT, and MAPK/ERK (Dwivedi and Greis 2017).

Mutations on CSF3R can affect the G-CSFR in different regions leading to diverse clinical manifestations. In general, extracellular domains mutations are related with severe congenital neutropenia (SCN) and chronic idiopathic neutropenia; transmembrane proximal mutations are associated with chronic neutrophilic leukemia and acute myeloid leukemia (AML); and intracellular truncated mutations are correlated with myelodysplastic syndrome and AML (Dwivedi and Greis 2017; Klimiankou et al. 2016).

In 2014, Triot et al. identified recessively inherited, loss-of-function CSF3R mutations in four affected children with SCN from two unrelated families, with morphologic evidence of full myeloid cell maturation in bone marrow. The novel monogenic disorder associated with congenital neutropenia was identified as SCN type 7 (SCN7). Other inherited heterozygous CSF3R mutation had been reported earlier leading to neutrophilia.

Most of the mutations located in transmembrane proximal domains and the truncated intracellular mutations of G-CSFR are somatic. The mutants of intracellular area exhibit a normal affinity for G-CSF but intermediate a higher proliferation and lower differentiation in response to G-CSF. Intracellular truncation mutations have not been found to cause SCN; however, SCN patients carrying this class of mutations have a strong predisposition to MDS or AML (Ward et al. 2008).

In this chapter we will discuss the disease caused by germline biallelic loss-of-function mutations in the extracellular domain of CSF3R leading to the presence of severe congenital neutropenia recognized as a primary immunodeficiency.

Clinical and Laboratorial Presentation

Patients with G-CSFR deficiency presented onset of recurrent infections in infancy or early childhood associated with peripheral neutropenia. The absolute neutrophils count (ANC) varies from 200 to 2180 cells/μl. Bone marrow aspiration in the first report showed no maturation arrest and the presence of mature granulocytes in all patients; a subsequent report showed one patient that presented bone marrow examination showing a granulopoietic hypoplasia with reduction of all stages, but also without maturation arrest (Triot et al. 2014; Klimiankou et al. 2016).

The use of G-CSF in the other SCN types showed a good recovery on the ANC in the peripheral blood, and SCN patients who do not respond to G-CSF should be screened for germline biallelic CSF3R mutations to confirm the G-CSFR deficiency (Klimiankou et al. 2015).

Treatment and Prognosis

Klimiankou et al. (2015) reported one patient with SCN treated with G-CSF without response that started GM-CSF at a dose of 3 μg/kg twice a week to maintain the patient's ANC above 1000 cells per microliter and kept her free from infections last 12 years without adverse events. Recently, after the G-CSFR deficiency description, researchers sequence the patient and confirm loss-of-function biallelic heterozygous CSF3R mutations. For these reason, the authors suggest the treatment with GM-CSF should be considered in patients with G-CSFR deficiency.

There is no enough data concerning the development of hematologic malignancies in the long term and the follow-up of these patients is important to demonstrate their progression.

References

Dwivedi P, Greis KD. Granulocyte colony-stimulating factor receptor signaling in severe congenital neutropenia, chronic neutrophilic leukemia, and related malignancies. Exp Hematol. 2017;46:9–20.

Klimiankou M, Klimenkova O, Uenalan M, Zeidler A, Mellor-Heineke S, Kandabarau S, et al. GM-CSF stimulates granulopoiesis in a congenital neutropenia patient with loss-of-function biallelic heterozygous CSF3R mutations. Blood. 2015;126:1865–7.

Klimiankou M, Mellor-Heineke S, Zeidler C, Welte K, Skokowa J. Role of CSF3R mutations in the pathomechanism of congenital neutropenia and secondary acute myeloid leukemia. Ann N Y Acad Sci. 2016;1370:119–25.

Triot A, Järvinen PM, Arostegui JI, Murugan D, Kohistani N, Dapena Díaz JL, et al. Inherited biallelic CSF3R mutations in severe congenital neutropenia. Blood. 2014;123:3811–7.

Ward AC, Gits J, Majeed F, Aprikyan AA, Lewis RS, O'Sullivan LA, et al. Functional interaction between mutations in the granulocyte colony-stimulating factor receptor in severe congenital neutropenia. Br J Haematol. 2008;142:653–6.

Glucose-6-Phosphate Transport Defect

▶ Glycogen Storage Disease Type 1b

Glycogen Storage Disease Type 1b

Eli Mansour and Ana Flavia Bernardes Sousa
Division of Clinical Immunology and Allergy, Department of Clinical Medicine, State University of Campinas (UNICAMP), Campinas, Brazil

Synonyms

Glucose-6-phosphate transport defect; GSD1B

Definition

Glycogen storage disease type 1b (GSD1b) (OMIM #232220) is an autosomal recessive inborn error of metabolism caused by mutations in the glucose-6-phosphate transporter 1 gene (*SLC37A4*) crucial for glycogen/glucose homeostasis and located in the long arm of chromosome 11q23.3 (Melis et al. 2017; Annabi et al. 1998).

Introduction

Glycogen storage disease type 1b (GSD1b), first described as a separate entity in 1978, is an inborn disorder of metabolism. GSD1b is a subtype of GSD1 with an incidence of 1/100,000, and 20% of these are estimated as having GSD1b. The inherited defects in the microsomal glucose-6-phosphate transporter (G6PT) lead to clinical features characteristic of GSD1b, such as hepatomegaly, growth retardation, osteopenia, kidney enlargement, hypoglycemia, hyperlactacidemia, hyperlipidemia, and hyperuricemia. The majority of patients have intermittent severe neutropenia and neutrophil dysfunction and as a consequence recurrent infections and inflammatory bowel disease (IBD) (Visser et al. 2002; Melis et al. 2005; Chou et al. 2018; Mehyar et al. 2018).

Pathogenesis and Genetics

GSD1b is an autosomal recessive inborn disorder of metabolism due to homozygous or compound heterozygous mutations causing stop codons or missense mutations in the gene encoding for the microsomal glucose-6-phosphate transporter (G6PT) (SLC37A4, also known as *G6PT1* gene), in chromosome 11q23.3 (Annabi et al. 1998; Melis et al. 2005).

G6PT is important to translocate glucose-6-phosphate (G6P) from the cytoplasm to the endoplasmic reticulum (ER) lumen, where it is hydrolyzed by glucose-6-phosphatase (G6Pase) to glucose and inorganic phosphate. G6PT function is dependent on its ability to complex with G6Pase (Melis et al. 2017; Chou et al. 2018).

In gluconeogenic organs such as the liver, kidney, and gut, the G6PT/G6Pase complex is important in interprandial glucose homeostasis. In non-gluconeogenic tissues, such as neutrophils, G6PT/G6Pase complex maintains energy homeostasis and function. The loss of neutrophil energy homeostasis results in ER stress and consequently neutrophil apoptosis and neutropenia. Dysfunctional neutrophils exhibit impaired chemotaxis, migration and adhesion, calcium mobilization, phagocytosis, and respiratory burst. Excess of glycogen and fat accumulation in the liver and kidney are the main causes of organ enlargement (Chou et al. 2010, 2018; Kim et al. 2017; Mehyar et al. 2018).

GSD1b patients have increased risk of developing autoimmune disorders, explained by alterations in glucose metabolism in T cells with impaired regulatory T cell (Treg) function and the loss of self-immune tolerance. The expression of the transcription factor FOXP3 was reduced in patients' Tregs (Melis et al. 2017).

Clinical Presentation

Affected persons typically have round face and full cheeks, impaired glucose homeostasis signs with fasting hypoglycemia, lactic acidosis, hyperlipidemia, hepatomegaly, growth retardation with short stature, osteopenia, nephromegaly, and hyperuricemia. Hypoglycemia may appear soon after birth. Other long-term manifestations include liver adenomas with increased risk of malignancy, renal failure, and polycystic ovaries. Splenomegaly is not uncommon either. Most patients have neutropenia, ranging from severe to intermittent, and neutrophil dysfunction predisposing them to recurrent bacterial infections. The most common are upper and lower respiratory tract infections, gastrointestinal tract infections, pyogenic skin infections, urinary tract infections, and deep abscesses. The most common pathogens are *Staphylococcus aureus*, *Streptococcus pneumoniae*, and *Escherichia coli*. Neutropenia may cause IBD, and up to 75% of neutropenic persons have IBD which may manifest as perioral or perianal infections and protracted diarrhea.

Dental caries, periodontitis, gingivitis, oral ulcers, and dental maturation and eruption delay may occur. GSD1b patients have increased risk of developing autoimmune disorders, such as IBD, Crohn's disease, thyroid autoimmunity, and myasthenia gravis (Visser et al. 2002; Melis et al. 2005; Chou et al. 2010, 2018; Kishnani et al. 2014).

Diagnosis and Follow-Up

Diagnosis is based on clinical history, biochemical abnormalities, genetic testing, or liver biopsy if the latter is unavailable. Patient history of frequent infections and antibiotic use, hospitalization, and diarrhea, associated with physical examination for the presence of oral and bowel inflammatory diseases, must be assessed. On physical examination short stature and protuberant abdomen due to hepatomegaly may help in the diagnosis, as well as abdominal ultrasound for hepatomegaly and nephromegaly. Biochemical abnormalities such as hypoglycemia, lactic acidosis, hypercholesterolemia, hypertriglyceridemia, and hyperuricemia are typical findings of GSD1. Neutropenia is seen in GSD1b (Visser et al. 2002; Kishnani et al. 2014).

Diagnosis is confirmed by full gene sequencing of *SLC37A4*. G6Pase enzyme activity on a liver biopsy specimen establishes the diagnosis if molecular genetic testing is inconclusive or not available (Kishnani et al. 2014).

For follow-up, total blood count with differential, abdominal ultrasound to check for spleen, kidney, and liver enlargement, with fecal alfa-1-antitrypsin as a marker for IBD, must be routinely performed. Colonoscopy with biopsy and contrast radiology may be indicated. Bone marrow studies must be carried out only with suspicion of leukemia, such as worsening of neutropenia, unexplained fever, and lymphadenopathy (Visser et al. 2002).

Treatment

Dietary and pharmacological therapies may help control the metabolic abnormalities (Kishnani et al. 2014).

Liver transplant (LT) or combined liver and renal transplantation may be needed. Hepatic transplantation can restore metabolic homeostasis and reduction in malignancy risks. LT is indicated mostly in patients refractory to medical treatment. As LT does not correct neutropenia and myeloid abnormalities, recombinant granulocyte colony-stimulating factor (G-CSF) is often needed. G-CSF, a myeloid growth factor, stimulates the development and function of neutrophils. G-CSF use shows reduction in the number and severity of infections and in the manifestations of IBD. G-CSF is given subcutaneously, daily, on alternate days, or three times per week, and the dose used is approximately 2 mcg/kg/day. G-CSF treatment can cause bone pain, splenomegaly, and hepatomegaly, and for that reason, the lowest effective dose should be used. While controversial, myeloid malignancy was reported as a secondary effect of G-CSF use. In severe refractory forms of GSD1b, hematopoietic cell transplantation (HCT) was shown to improve neutropenia, decreasing infections and indirectly improving metabolic control (Visser et al. 2002; Kishnani et al. 2014; Mehyar et al. 2018).

Bone marrow-targeted, to correct neutropenia and myeloid abnormalities, and liver-targeted vector-mediated gene therapies are promising approaches (Kishnani et al. 2014; Chou et al. 2018).

Antibiotic prophylaxis with sulfamethoxazole-trimethoprim (SMX-TMP) can be indicated in symptomatic patients or those with severe neutropenia ($<500/mm^3$) (Visser et al. 2002).

All inactivated vaccines are indicated for GSD1b patients. Live bacterial vaccines, such as BCG and oral salmonella vaccine, should be avoided in severely neutropenic patients. Live viral vaccines are also recommended. Immunization may prevent hypoglycemia caused by the infection process (Kishnani et al. 2014; Sobh and Bonilla 2016).

References

Annabi B, Hiraiwa H, Mansfield BC, Lei KJ, et al. The gene for glycogen-storage disease type 1b maps to chromosome 11q23. Am J Hum Genet. 1998;62:400–5.

Chou JY, Jun HS, Mansfield BC. Neutropenia in type Ib glycogen storage disease. Curr Opin Hematol. 2010;17:36–42.

Chou JY, Cho JH, Kim GY, et al. Molecular biology and gene therapy for glycogen storage disease type Ib. J Inherit Metab Dis. 2018;41:1007–14.

Kim GY, Lee YM, Kwon JH, et al. Glycogen storage disease type Ib neutrophils exhibit impaired cell adhesion and migration. Biochem Biophys Res Commun. 2017;482:569–74.

Kishnani PS, Austin SL, Abdenur JE, et al. Diagnosis and management of glycogen storage disease type I: a practice guideline of the American College of Medical Genetics and Genomics. Genet Med. 2014;16:e1.

Mehyar LS, Abu-Arja R, Rangarajan HG, et al. Matched unrelated donor transplantation in glycogen storage disease type 1b patient corrects severe neutropenia and recurrent infections. Bone Marrow Transplant. 2018;53:1076–8.

Melis D, Fulceri R, Parenti G, et al. Genotype/phenotype correlation in glycogen storage disease type 1b: a multicentre study and review of the literature. Eur J Pediatr. 2005;164:501–8.

Melis D, Carbone F, Minopoli G, et al. Cutting edge: increased autoimmunity risk in glycogen storage disease type 1b is associated with a reduced engagement of glycolysis in T cells and an impaired regulatory T cell function. J Immunol. 2017;198:3803–8.

Sobh A, Bonilla FA. Vaccination in primary immunodeficiency disorders. J Allergy Clin Immunol Pract. 2016;4:1066–75.

Visser G, Rake JP, Labrune P, et al. Consensus guidelines for management of glycogen storage disease type 1b – European Study on Glycogen Storage Disease Type 1. Eur J Pediatr. 2002;161(Suppl 1):S120–3.

Good Syndrome

Eric Oksenhendler
Department of Clinical Immunology, Hôpital Saint-Louis, Paris, France

Synonyms

Thymoma with hypogammaglobulinemia

Definition and Epidemiology

Good syndrome (GS) is defined by the association of thymoma and hypogammaglobulinemia. GS is a rare adult-onset immunodeficiency with less than 300 cases reported in the literature and an incidence evaluated around 0.15 per 100,000 population per year (Engels 2010). Most cases have been described as sporadic cases occurring in the elderly without any evidence for an hereditary genetic disease.

Introduction

Good syndrome (GS) was first reported by Dr. Good as an association of thymoma and hypogammaglobulinemia (Good et al. 1956). Once immunophenotyping became available, it was found that low to absent B cells in peripheral blood was very frequent if not constant. Defects in T-cell-mediated immunity are also frequent, while autoimmunity is also reported (Kelleher and Misbah 2003; Montella et al. 2003). Thymoma is the most common neoplasm arising from the thymus and consists of neoplastic thymic epithelial cells and nonneoplastic maturing thymocytes (Thomas et al. 1999). Patients with thymoma frequently present with autoimmune disorders, mostly myasthenia gravis (30–50%) (Souadjian et al. 1974; Marx et al. 2010; Holbro et al. 2012). Less frequently, hypogammaglobulinemia develops to form the so-called Good syndrome (1–6% of thymomas) (Filosso et al. 2014). The pathogenesis of this immunodeficiency remains elusive. Notably, hypogammaglobulinemia is not corrected following thymus removal.

Clinical Spectrum

Patients

Good syndrome is usually diagnosed in patients in their 50s or 60s, with the exception of a single reported pediatric case. The sex ratio is close to 1:1. The first symptom leading to the diagnosis can be thymoma, infection, autoimmune manifestation, or hypogammaglobulinemia (Tarr et al. 2001; Kelesidis and Yang 2010; Malphettes et al. 2015).

Thymoma

The diagnosis of thymoma precedes the diagnosis of hypogammaglobulinemia in about 40% of the patients. All types of thymoma have been described in GS with a majority of spindle cell thymomas and types AB or B2 in the WHO classification.

Infections

Based on a review of 152 cases reported in the literature in 2010 and a recent single center series of 21 patients, the infectious complications appear as the major complication of GS as more than 80% of the patients present with severe, recurrent, or unusual infections (Kelesidis and Yang 2010; Malphettes et al. 2015).

Most commonly reported infections are recurrent infections of the upper and lower respiratory tract. Pneumonia is the most frequent invasive infection with a pathogen documentation in half of the cases, most frequently with *S. pneumonia* and *H. influenzae*. Bacteremia is reported in about 40% of the cases. Besides these invasive infections, most patients develop recurrent bronchitis and sinusitis, and 15–38% develop bronchiectasis. A majority of patients deserves immunoglobulin therapy. In addition to these complications that can be directly related to hypogammaglobulinemia, a large number of patients present with infections suggestive of a cellular immune defect: CMV infection, *P. jirovecii (carinii)* pneumonia, mucocutaneous candidiasis or candidemia, invasive fungal infection, mycobacterial infection, invasive HSV and VZV infections, viral encephalitis, mycoplasma infection, toxoplasma chorioretinitis, and Kaposi sarcoma. In addition, yellow fever vaccine associated disease has also been reported in 4 patients. The prevalence of these "opportunistic" infections may have been biased and overestimated in the early cases reports. However, the large spectrum of infectious complications has been confirmed in a recent series (Malphettes et al. 2015).

Around 40% of the patients present with recurrent or chronic diarrhea. Documented infections mainly involve *Campylobacter, Giardia, Salmonella,* and *Shigella* species as well as CMV and fungal infections.

Gastrointestinal Disease

Diarrhea is present in almost 50% of the patients with GS, and in most cases it is chronic. It has rarely been associated with malabsorption due to villous atrophy. Although enteric bacteria or viruses are occasionally isolated, in the majority of cases no definite pathogens can be identified. The presence of inflammatory lesions similar to that observed in inflammatory bowel diseases is observed in some patients and are considered as autoimmune or autoinflammatory colitis. However, in most cases the cause of chronic diarrhea in GS remains unknown.

Autoimmunity

Around 60% of the patients with GS will present with at least one autoimmune complication. The major autoimmune complication observed in classic thymoma is myasthenia gravis, reported in 30–40%, followed by pure red cell aplasia and thymoma associated multiorgan autoimmunity (TAMA). The spectrum of autoimmune diseases observed in GS is slightly different. The most frequent autoimmune complication is pure red cell aplasia (PRCA) with a 30–35% prevalence followed by oral lichen planus (15–40%), myasthenia gravis (5–15%), and inflammatory bowel disease (5–20%); aplastic anemia or autoimmune cytopenia (thrombocytopenia, hemolytic anemia, neutropenia) have also been reported in a few percent of the patients.

Immunological Characteristics

According to the definition, all patients present with hypogammaglobulinemia. Most patients (>70%) disclose a CVID-like phenotype with a global hypogammaglobulinemia with reduced levels of serum IgG, IgA, and IgM. However, some patients may disclose only a partial immunoglobulin production deficiency but usually associated with a defect in vaccine responses. Global lymphocytopenia is observed in around one third of the patients, while low or absent peripheral B cells is almost constant (>85%). Low T-cell count is reported in 15% of the patients, while low CD4 cell count and increased

CD8 cell count are frequent with a CD4/CD8 ratio below 1 in more than 70% of the patients (Kelleher and Misbah 2003; Montella et al. 2003; Kelesidis and Yang 2010; Malphettes et al. 2015).

Pathophysiology

The late onset and the absence of familial cases suggest that GS may be an acquired disorder and not a genetically defined hereditary disease. Given the particular spectrum of autoimmune complications, one could speculate that hypogammaglobulinemia might be another autoimmune features. Pathogenic autoantibodies are common in thymoma, mostly anti-acetylcholine receptor antibodies causing myasthenia gravis but also a wide range of anti-cytokine autoantibodies (Meager et al. 2003; Scarpino et al. 2007; Kisand et al. 2011). In a study of 17 patients with thymoma, all patients with opportunistic infection showed multiple anticytokine autoantibodies (IFNα, IFNβ, IL-1α, IL-12, IL-17A) with blocking activity in vitro, suggesting that these autoantibodies may be important in the pathogenesis of adult-onset immunodeficiency associated with thymoma in these patients (Burbelo et al. 2010). A similar feature of adult-onset immunodeficiency has been described in association with anti-interferon-gamma autoantibodies in the Asian population (Browne et al. 2012; Jansen et al. 2016).

Diagnosis

The diagnosis is based on the association of thymoma and hypogammaglobulinemia. Therefore, an evaluation of serum immunoglobulin levels should be performed in every patient with a thymoma, and conversely, all patients with a CVID-like phenotype should have a CT scan looking for a possible thymic tumor with a specific attention for patients diagnosed after 40 years or exhibiting a very low B-cell count. The diagnosis can also be suggested while exploring unusual autoimmune diseases such as PRCA or lichen planus as well as in patients with an atypical chronic intestinal disease. Currently no specific immunologic and no genetic tests are available to confirm the diagnosis.

Management and Outcome

Treatment starts with the treatment of thymoma, which is surgical removal or debulking when possible and radiotherapy in combination with chemotherapy in advanced disease. Thymectomy usually has a favorable effect on associated conditions such as PRCA or myasthenia gravis but does not usually reverse the immunological abnormalities.

Immunoglobulin replacement therapy has been reported to improve infection control. According to the associated T-cell defect, additional measures in diagnosis of infectious complications, prophylaxis, and treatment may be considered. Immunosuppressive treatments are often used to control the autoimmune complications of GS.

The prognosis in patients with GS is believed to be worse than in other patients with primary immunodeficiencies mainly characterized by an antibody production defect such as CVID. In a single center, the estimate survival at 10 years was 33%, and the overall mortality in a review of the literature cases was 46% (Hermaszewski and Webster 1993; Kelesidis and Yang 2010). However, the prognosis has probably improved in the last two decades with a 10-year overall survival at 84% in a more recent short series (Malphettes et al. 2015) LIT.

Conclusion

Good syndrome strikingly differs from CVID in terms of its very late onset, lack of familial cases, and the usual absence of lymphoid hyperplasia, suggesting that GS might be an acquired immunodeficiency, part of an increasingly recognized group of adult-onset immunodeficiency disorders associated with thymoma. However, given the high frequency of invasive bacterial infections and the particular autoimmune spectrum, it is relevant to keep on distinguishing this puzzling entity.

G

References

Browne SK, Burbelo PD, Chetchotisakd P, Suputtamongkol Y, Kiertiburanakul S, Shaw PA, Kirk JL, et al. Adult-onset immunodeficiency in Thailand and Taiwan. N Engl J Med. 2012;367(8):725–34.

Burbelo PD, Browne SK, Sampaio EP, Giaccone G, Zaman R, Kristosturyan E, Rajan A, et al. Anti-cytokine autoantibodies are associated with opportunistic infection in patients with thymic neoplasia. Blood. 2010;116(23):4848–58.

Engels EA. Epidemiology of thymoma and associated malignancies. J Thorac Oncol. 2010;5(10 Suppl 4): S260–5.

Filosso PL, Venuta F, Oliaro A, Ruffini E, Rendina EA, Margaritora S, Casadio C, et al. Thymoma and inter-relationships between clinical variables: a multicentre study in 537 patients. Eur J Cardiothorac Surg. 2014;45(6):1020–7.

Good RA, Maclean LD, Varco RL, Zak SJ. Thymic tumor and acquired agammaglobulinemia: a clinical and experimental study of the immune response. Surgery. 1956;40(6):1010–7.

Hermaszewski RA, Webster AD. Primary hypo-gammaglobulinaemia: a survey of clinical manifestations and complications. Q J Med. 1993;86(1):31–42.

Holbro A, Jauch A, Lardinois D, Tzankov A, Dirnhofer S, Hess C. High prevalence of infections and autoimmunity in patients with thymoma. Hum Immunol. 2012;73(3):287–90.

Jansen A, van Deuren M, Miller J, Litzman J, de Gracia J, Sáenz-Cuesta M, Szaflarska A, et al. Prognosis of good syndrome: mortality and morbidity of thymoma associated immunodeficiency in perspective. Clin Immunol. 2016;171:12–7.

Kelesidis T, Yang O. Good's syndrome remains a mystery after 55 years: a systematic review of the scientific evidence. Clin Immunol. 2010;135(3):347–63.

Kelleher P, Misbah SA. What is good's syndrome? Immunological abnormalities in patients with thymoma. J Clin Pathol. 2003;56(1):12–6.

Kisand K, Lilic D, Casanova J-L, Peterson P, Meager A, Willcox N. Mucocutaneous candidiasis and autoimmunity against cytokines in APECED and thymoma patients: clinical and pathogenetic implications. Eur J Immunol. 2011;41(6):1517–27.

Malphettes M, Gérard L, Galicier L, Boutboul D, Asli B, Szalat R, Perlat A, et al. Good syndrome: an adult-onset immunodeficiency remarkable for its high incidence of invasive infections and autoimmune complications. Clin Infect Dis. 2015;61(2):e13–9.

Marx A, Willcox N, Leite MI, Chuang W-Y, Schalke B, Nix W, Ströbel P. Thymoma and paraneoplastic myasthenia gravis. Autoimmunity. 2010;43(5–6):413–27.

Meager A, Wadhwa M, Dilger P, Bird C, Thorpe R, Newsom-Davis J, Willcox N. Anti-cytokine autoantibodies in autoimmunity: preponderance of neutralizing autoantibodies against interferon-alpha, interferon-omega and interleukin-12 in patients with thymoma and/or myasthenia gravis. Clin Exp Immunol. 2003;132(1):128–36.

Montella L, Masci AM, Merkabaoui G, Perna F, Vitiello L, Racioppi L, Palmieri G. B-cell lymphopenia and hypo-gammaglobulinemia in thymoma patients. Ann Hematol. 2003;82(6):343–7.

Scarpino S, Di Napoli A, Stoppacciaro A, Antonelli M, Pilozzi E, Chiarle R, Palestro G, et al. Expression of autoimmune regulator gene (AIRE) and T regulatory cells in human thymomas. Clin Exp Immunol. 2007;149(3):504–12.

Souadjian JV, Enriquez P, Silverstein MN, Pépin JM. The spectrum of diseases associated with thymoma. Coincidence or syndrome? Arch Intern Med. 1974;134(2):374–9.

Tarr PE, Sneller MC, Mechanic LJ, Economides A, Eger CM, Strober W, Cunningham-Rundles C, Lucey DR. Infections in patients with immunodeficiency with thymoma (good syndrome). Report of 5 cases and review of the literature. Medicine. 2001;80(2):123–33.

Thomas CR, Wright CD, Loehrer PJ. Thymoma: state of the art. J Clin Oncol. 1999;17(7):2280–9.

GPP: Generalized Pustular Psoriasis

▶ Deficiency of Interleukin 36 Receptor Antagonist (DITRA)

Growth Hormone Insensitivity Due to Post-Receptor Defect

▶ STAT5b Deficiency, AR

Growth Hormone Insensitivity with Immunodeficiency (MIM #245590)

▶ STAT5b Deficiency, AR

GSD1B

▶ Glycogen Storage Disease Type 1b

H

Hall-Hittner Syndrome

▶ CHARGE Syndrome (CHD7, SEMA3E)

HED-ID

▶ Autosomal Dominant Anhidrotic Ectodermal Dysplasia with Immunodeficiency (AD-EDA-ID)

Hepatic Veno-occlusive Disease with Immunodeficiency (VODI)

Donald B. Bloch[1] and Mike Recher[2]
[1]Division of Rheumatology, Allergy and Immunology, Department of Medicine and the Anesthesia Center for Critical Care Research of the Department of Anesthesia, Critical Care, and Pain Medicine, Harvard Medical School and Massachusetts General Hospital, Boston, MA, USA
[2]Immunodeficiency laboratory and Immunodeficiency Clinic, Medical Outpatient Unit and Department Biomedicine, University Basel Hospital, Basel, Switzerland

Synonyms

Sp110 deficiency

Definition

Hepatic veno-occlusive disease with immunodeficiency (VODI) is a rare, combined immunodeficiency caused by homozygous mutations in the gene encoding nuclear body protein Sp110.

Introduction/Background

In 1976, Mellis and Bale described five infants from three families who had hepatomegaly caused by veno-occlusive disease of the liver and evidence of immunodeficiency (Mellis and Bale 1976). The children experienced a variety of infections including those caused by *Pneumocystis jiroveci*, cytomegalovirus, enterovirus, and *Staphylococcus aureus*. Because all of the children died within the first year of life and there was a history of consanguinity in two of the three families, Mellis and Bale suggested that there was a congenital cause for this new syndrome (Mellis and Bale 1976).

Thirty years later, Roscioli and colleagues identified six patients from five consanguineous families of Lebanese origin who met the clinical criteria used to diagnose veno-occlusive disease with immunodeficiency syndrome (VODI) (Roscioli et al. 2006). Using homozygosity mapping in four of the affected individuals and their parents, from three different families, the VODI gene was mapped to chromosome 2q36.3-37.1. Fine-mapping studies further narrowed the

© Springer Science+Business Media LLC, part of Springer Nature 2020
I. R. Mackay et al. (eds.), *Encyclopedia of Medical Immunology*,
https://doi.org/10.1007/978-1-4614-8678-7

genomic interval, which was found to contain the gene encoding Sp110. Nucleotide sequencing of *SP110* coding exons revealed a homozygous single base pair deletion (642delC) in exon 5 in affected individuals from the initial three families (Roscioli et al. 2006). Members of the fourth family carried the same *SP110* gene mutation. A fifth family was found to have a single base pair deletion in Sp110 exon 2 (40delC). The product of the *SP110* gene was not detected in EBV-transformed B cells from affected individuals by either indirect immunofluorescence or immunoblot. The results indicated that homozygous mutations in *SP110* and the absence of this protein are associated with VODI (Roscioli et al. 2006). Cliffe and colleagues subsequently described nine additional VODI patients with four additional disease-associated alleles, further confirming that pathogenic mutations in *SP110* are the cause of VODI (Cliffe et al. 2012).

Sp110 is a member of the Sp100 family of proteins, which includes Sp110, Sp140, and Sp100 (Bloch et al. 1999). The names of these proteins derive from the apparent molecular weights of the proteins as determined by immunoblot and the nuclear speckled distribution of the proteins within the nucleus. Sp100 was the first member of this family to be described and the gene was originally expression-cloned using autoantibodies in serum from patients with primary

biliary cirrhosis, an autoimmune disease that destroys biliary ductule cells. Sp100 was subsequently shown to be a component of the promyelocytic leukemia (PML) protein-containing nuclear structure, now known as the PML-Sp100 nuclear body. Under resting conditions, there are 5–20 PML-Sp100 nuclear bodies in each nucleus (Fig. 1). Although the precise function of PML-Sp100 nuclear bodies is not yet known, components of the structure are involved in a wide variety of cellular processes, including regulation of the cell cycle, apoptosis, cellular senescence, cellular stress response, and DNA repair. Components of the PML-Sp100 nuclear body also have critical roles in host defense. Genomes of herpesviruses, including HSV and CMV, become associated with PML-Sp100 nuclear bodies shortly after entering the cell and the interaction results in epigenetic silencing of the viral genomes. PML-Sp100 nuclear bodies also restrict the activity of other DNA as well as RNA viruses.

The longest isoform of human Sp110 (designated Sp110C) has 713 amino acids and at least four important domains: (1) an alpha helical, N-terminal, "HSR1" or "Sp100-like" domain; (2) a "SAND" domain, which is a motif that has been shown to bind to the minor groove of DNA; (3) a plant homeobox domain, which is a zinc finger motif that interacts with DNA; and

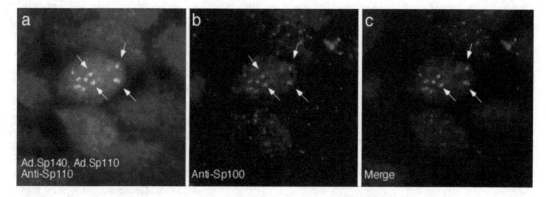

Hepatic Veno-occlusive Disease with Immunodeficiency (VODI), Fig. 1 Co-expression of Sp140 and Sp110, using adenovirus (Ad) vectors, in HEp-2 cells results in co-localization of the two proteins in nuclear dots. Rabbit anti-Sp110 antibodies indicate the location of Sp110 in a transfected cell (panel **a**, green). Sp110 co-localizes with Sp100 in nuclear bodies (panel **b**, red). White arrows indicate the location of representative nuclear bodies. Merge of panels **a** and **b** is shown in **c**. DAPI staining in **c** indicates the location of nuclei. Note that Sp110 is not normally expressed in HEp-2 cells, while Sp100 nuclear bodies can be detected in all of the cells

(4) a bromodomain motif, which binds to histone proteins (Bloch et al. 2000). The structural domains in Sp110, and additional experimental evidence, suggest that Sp110 has a role in the regulation of gene transcription. Sp110 localizes to Sp100-containing nuclear bodies by interacting, via its N-terminal domain, with Sp140 (Fig. 1). In the absence of Sp140, Sp110 localizes to hundreds of smaller speckles distributed throughout the nucleus (Marquardsen et al. 2017). Sp100, in the absence of Sp140, is unable to recruit Sp110 to PML-Sp100 nuclear bodies. Sp110 is expressed in a wide variety of cell types and tissues and its expression is increased in the setting of interferon-induced inflammation. Expression of Sp140 is also increased by interferons; however, in contrast to Sp110, expression of Sp140 is limited to leukocytes. Because localization of Sp110 to nuclear bodies is dependent on Sp140, the location of Sp110 would be expected to vary, depending on the cell type. Whether the different cellular locations of Sp110 (nuclear bodies vs. nuclear speckles) imply that the protein has more than one function has not yet been explored.

A murine orthologue of human Sp110 (designated "*lpr1*") was reported to have a role in the innate immune control of tuberculosis in mice (Pan et al. 2005). However, in *Mus musculus*, the genes encoding Sp100, Sp140, and Sp110 localize together in a "homogeneous staining region" (HSR) on chromosome 1. HSRs are chromosomal segments that have uniform staining intensity after treatment with Giemsa stain. HSRs often indicate a location in the genome that contains genes that are highly amplified. Because the individual exons of murine Sp100, Sp140, and Sp110 are highly amplified, it is difficult to know which, if any, of the transcripts are translated into protein. The longest identified transcript potentially encoding Sp110 in *Mus musculus* has 445 amino acids (compared with 713 for human Sp110). A high degree of sequence identity between murine and human Sp110 is limited to the first 195 amino acids of the protein. None of the reported murine *SP110* transcripts encode the PHD and bromodomain that are present in human Sp110.

Following the reported link between *lpr1* and tuberculosis in mice, several genetic studies were conducted to determine whether there is an association between variants in the human *SP110* gene and susceptibility to tuberculosis. While some studies showed an association, other studies did not. Because of the widely divergent structures of murine and human Sp110, it is difficult to determine the significance of the reported association between variations in murine *lpr1* and tuberculosis. Of note, susceptibility to tuberculosis is not a known clinical feature of VODI (see section "Clinical Presentation" below).

Clinical Presentation

Children with VODI develop the initial manifestations of the disease within the first 6 months of life. Initial symptoms may be related to hepatic disease caused by vascular occlusion and subsequent fibrosis. Children may also develop a variety of infections, including infections with *Pneumocystis jirovecii*, cytomegalovirus, enterovirus, or candida (mucocutaneous candidiasis).

Laboratory Testing

Laboratory tests that may be used to diagnose other immunodeficiency disorders may fail to identify patients with VODI. Despite the fact that VODI patients have a severe combined immunodeficiency, they usually have normal numbers of peripheral B and T lymphocytes. Therefore, neonatal screening for primary immunodeficiencies that are based on the number of T cell receptor excision circles (TREC) will fail to detect VODI.

Although patients with VODI are unable to produce normal amounts of immunoglobulins, initially, the level of immunoglobulins in VODI patients may be normal, because of placentally transferred maternal antibodies. Therefore testing immunoglobulin levels is not helpful for the early diagnosis of this disease (before 6 months of age). Furthermore, even if immunoglobulins are found to be decreased later in infancy, the diagnosis of

VODI might be confounded by the known physiologic transitional hypogammaglobulinemia of infancy.

The absolute number of differentiated B cells (e.g., memory IgD$^-$CD27$^+$ B cells) is decreased in patients with VODI (Cliffe et al. 2012). However, the number of differentiated memory B cells is physiologically decreased in a healthy child during the first year of life.

Until recently, DNA sequencing and identification of homozygous or compound disease-causing *SP110* mutations was the only clinically available approach to diagnose or exclude VODI. However, in 2017, a novel, easy to perform, flow-cytometric assay for quantification of Sp110 expression in blood-derived T cells was reported (Marquardsen et al. 2017). This method will permit testing for the effect of Sp110 mutations on the level of Sp110 protein. It should be noted that this assay will fail to detect mutations in Sp110 that do not decrease protein level. However, missense mutations that alter the function, but not the level, of Sp110 have not yet been described in patients with VODI.

Treatment

Prophylactic treatment with intravenous immunoglobulins and Trimethoprim/Sulfamethoxazole (TMP/SMX) has greatly prolonged the lifespan of children with VODI. Appropriate additional supportive care includes the use of antimicrobial and antiviral therapy as needed. Hematopoietic stem cell transplantation (HSCT) as treatment for VODI is complicated by the risk of hepatic veno-occlusive disease. Conditioning regimens that do not include potentially hepatotoxic drugs and the prophylactic use of defibrotide may improve the outcome of HSCT in these patients.

Any drugs with potential liver-toxic side effects, including over-the-counter medication such as nonsteroidal anti-inflammatory drugs, should be avoided in VODI patients or require very close monitoring of serum liver enzymes.

As in other immunosuppressed patients, live vaccines should be avoided while inactivated vaccines can be administered as recommended by the countries' health organization.

It is important to state that in case of infection, serologic diagnosis is not reliable due to the administration of intravenous immunoglobulins. Thus, direct detection of the infectious agent either by PCR, culture, or direct detection of pathogen-derived antigen (e.g., immunofluorescence) should be pursued.

Because early prophylactic treatment of patients with VODI with immunoglobulin replacement and TMP/SMX remains the cornerstone of therapy, it is critical to diagnose this disorder as early as possible. The presence of a family history of a severe immunodeficiency disorder, liver disease, and consanguinity should serve as clues to this diagnosis. The use of flow cytometry, and the increasing availability of genetic testing, will facilitate the early diagnosis of VODI and thereby improve outcomes.

Cross-References

▶ Evaluation of Suspected Immunodeficiency, Humoral
▶ Evaluation of Suspected Immunodeficiency, Overview
▶ Immunoglobulin Class Switch Recombination Defects
▶ Thymoma with Hypogammaglobulinemia

References

Bloch DB, et al. Structural and functional heterogeneity of nuclear bodies. Mol Cell Biol. 1999;19:4423–30.
Bloch DB, et al. Sp110 localizes to the PML-Sp100 nuclear body and may function as a nuclear hormone receptor transcriptional coactivator. Mol Cell Biol. 2000;20:6138–46.
Cliffe ST, et al. Clinical, molecular, and cellular immunologic findings in patients with SP110-associated veno-occlusive disease with immunodeficiency syndrome. J Allergy Clin Immunol. 2012;130:735–42.e736.
Marquardsen FA, et al. Detection of Sp110 by flow cytometry and application to screening patients for veno-occlusive disease with immunodeficiency. J Clin Immunol. 2017;37:707–14.

Mellis C, Bale PM. Familial hepatic venoocclusive disease with probable immune deficiency. J Pediatr. 1976;88:236–42.

Pan H, et al. Ipr1 gene mediates innate immunity to tuberculosis. Nature. 2005;434:767–72.

Roscioli T, et al. Mutations in the gene encoding the PML nuclear body protein Sp110 are associated with immunodeficiency and hepatic veno-occlusive disease. Nat Genet. 2006;38:620–2.

Hereditary Deficiency of C1 Inhibitor and Angioedema

Marco Cicardi[1,2], Andrea Zanichelli[1,2], Chiara Suffritti[1,2], Maddalena Wu[1,2] and Sonia Caccia[3]
[1]Department of Biomedical and Clinical Sciences Luigi Sacco, University of Milan, Milan, Italy
[2]ASST Fatebenefratelli Sacco, Milan, Italy
[3]"Luigi Sacco" Department of Biomedical and Clinical Sciences, University of Milan, Milan, Italy

Definition

C1 inhibitor (C1-INH) is a serine protease inhibitor intimately involved in the regulation of the complement cascade and the contact system. Heterozygous deficiency of C1-INH is the most common cause of hereditary angioedema.

The Deficiency of C1 Inhibitor

C1-INH was first identified in the late 1950s as the serum inhibitor of C1 esterase (Levy and Lepow 1959). Today we know that it inhibits other serine proteases in various enzymatic systems. When the levels of C1-INH fall below 50% of normal, the contact system is exposed to inappropriate activation with local release of bradykinin, increase of endothelial permeability, fluid extravasation, and edema formation (Fig. 1). The most common cause of C1-INH deficiency are mutations in its coding gene SERPING1. An acquired deficiency of C1-INH, with identical clinical features, has also been described (Caccia et al. 2014). Genetic deficiency of C1-INH with angioedema symptoms (C1-INH-HAE) has a prevalence around 1:50,000 subjects in the general population (Zanichelli et al. 2015).

SERPING1 is located in the chromosome 11 (locus 11q11-q13.1). The database of SERPING1 mutations found in patients with hereditary angioedema (HAE) (http://hae.enzim.hu/; last update 2014-12-04) lists 252 micromutations and 45 gross mutations. On the other hand, one single variant affecting the primary protein structure, Val458Met, is common in healthy subjects and can be considered as a protein polymorphism (Cumming et al. 2003).

HAE occurs in individuals carrying one SERPING1 mutated allele and represents an autosomal dominant trait. Three families with homozygous patients have also been described (Bafunno et al. 2013). Interestingly, members carrying the heterozygous defect in these families were asymptomatic, suggesting that some SERPING1 mutations can be responsible for a recessive form of HAE due to C1-INH deficiency. Another characteristic aspect of C1-INH genetic defect is the high frequency of de novo mutations. In a series of families, it has been proved that up to 25% of the cases have parents without SERPING1 mutations and normal plasma levels of C1-INH (Tosi et al. 1998).

C1-INH-HAE exists in two phenotypic variants. The most frequent, C1-INH-HAE type I, has levels of functional and antigenic C1-INH equally reduced in plasma. About 15% of families carry mutations that allow nonfunctional protein products to be secreted in plasma. These patients present with normal to elevated antigenic plasma levels of C1-INH, and function below 50%, they are identified as C1-INH-HAE type II. The two phenotypes are clinically indistinguishable. In both, functional C1-INH deficiency leads to a marked decrease of plasma C4, which reflects an increased activation of the classical complement pathway deprived of its major inhibitor. Nevertheless, C1s and C1r, direct target proteases of C1-INH in this system, remain normal in patients' plasma, and the same is true for C1q, the third subcomponent of the C1 complex. C1q is instead frequently reduced in the acquired form of C1-INH deficiency, and this can help in distinguishing the two forms.

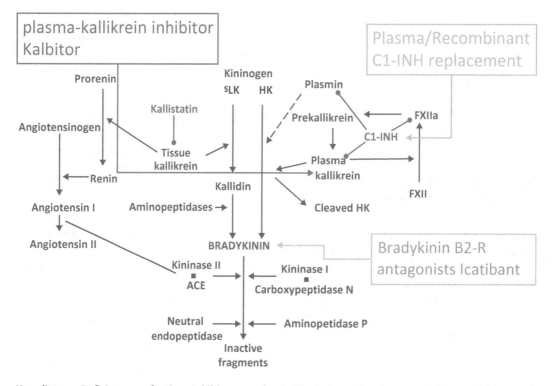

Hereditary Deficiency of C1 Inhibitor and Angioedema, Fig. 1 Bradykinin formation and bradykinin-targeted treatments approved for C1-INH-HAE. Bradykinin mainly derives from cleavage of high molecular weight kininogen (HK) by plasma kallikrein. Tissue kallikrein may contribute in part to bradykinin formation through the cleavage of kallikrein by aminopeptidase. C1-INH prevents kallikrein formation inhibiting factor XII (FXII) and directly inhibits plasma kallikrein preventing cleavage of HK. Bradykinin is rapidly inactivated by several degrading enzymes. Among them kininase II-angiotensin-converting enzyme is able to act on the renin-angiotensin system converting angiotensin I in angiotensin II. C1-INH-based treatments prevent bradykinin release acting at several point replacing the physiologic protein. Kalbitor is a small recombinant protein that specifically inhibits plasma kallikrein. Icatibant is a synthetic antagonist of bradykinin B2 receptors

Patients with C1-INH-HAE do not exhibit reductions in plasma levels of components of the contact system, but its activation is pivotal to generate angioedema symptoms (Kaplan and Joseph 2014). The components of this system bind to specific receptors on endothelial cells and upon stimulation generate the inflammatory peptide bradykinin (Nussberger et al. 2002). Although the mechanisms of initiation of contact system activation in angioedema is still unclear, the role of local bradykinin generation is well proved and has been successfully used to develop specific therapies (Bhardwaj and Craig 2014).

The Clinical Picture of the Genetic Deficiency of C1 Inhibitor

Episodic accumulation of bradykinin at specific sites causes angioedema symptoms that present as recurrent nonpitting, nonpruritic, self-limiting edema of the subcutaneous and submucosal tissues (Table 1) (Longhurst and Cicardi 2012). Almost all subjects with genetic C1-INH deficiency manifest recurrent angioedema of the limbs, trunk, and face and recurrent abdominal pain with edema of the gastrointestinal mucosa. Recurrent upper airway obstruction is present only in 50% of the subjects

Hereditary Deficiency of C1 Inhibitor and Angioedema, Table 1 Clinical picture of hereditary angioedema with C1-inhibitor deficiency

• Clinical symptoms are recurrent, noninflammatory, nonpitting, self-limiting edema located in
– Subcutaneous tissue
– Gastrointestinal mucosa
– Oro-pharyngo-laryngeal mucosa
• Duration of each angioedema attack ranges between 1 and 5 days
• Frequency of recurrences varies among patients and also within the same patient
– From life-long asymptomatic to 3 attacks/week
• Mortality for HAE is >25% in undiagnosed patients

with C1-INH-HAE but can be the cause of death for more than 25% of carriers of this disease when it goes undiagnosed and untreated (Bork et al. 2012). The large majority of patients become symptomatic within the second decade of life, with a peak around puberty. Symptoms recur with highly variable frequency. Less than 5% of carriers remain asymptomatic lifelong, and average frequency of symptoms is around once per month. There is little consistency in angioedema frequency throughout life and we have no tools for predicting attack recurrences. Even if micro-trauma, psychological stress, infections and menstruation are known to facilitate the appearance of angioedema, the majority of attacks remain unexplained.

Unpredictability, frequency and direct complications of recurrences determine the burden of C1-INH-HAE. Cutaneous locations have direct impact on patients' appearance and performance status. Angioedema of the face impedes social life, while involvement of limbs may impair walking and manual activities. The gastrointestinal location may be highly insidious when the disease is not properly identified and sometimes even after appropriate diagnosis. The clinical presentation is undistinguishable from many conditions causing gastrointestinal symptoms with pain, vomiting, and diarrhea. The laboratory studies show mild neutrophilic leukocytosis and increase in C-reactive protein. Ultrasounds and CT scan can show nonspecific mild peritoneal fluid and bowel wall thickness. The only clear distinguishing criterion is the response to treatments known to reverse attacks in C1-INH-HAE. Absence of response within 2 h makes the diagnosis of angioedema of the gastrointestinal mucosa highly unlikely.

Historically, C1-INH-HAE related mortality could exceed 25% of affected subjects. Edema of the larynx usually progress slowly, and several hours are necessary before respiratory impairment start manifesting, but the time gap from initial respiratory distress and complete asphyxia can be in terms of minutes. Moreover, unresponsiveness to traditional anti-allergic drugs as epinephrine, corticosteroids, and antihistamine renders invasive management unavoidable. In the presence of massive pharyngeal edema, oro-laryngeal intubation is difficult, and fiber-optic-guided nasopharyngeal intubation is recommended. Concomitant massive edema of the neck may impair emergency tracheostomy. For all these reasons, an accurate educational program should be undertaken enabling patients to carry specific effective treatments at all times and to use them as soon as symptoms start.

The Diagnosis of Hereditary Angioedema Due to C1 Inhibitor Deficiency

The diagnosis of C1-INH-HAE starts from the presence of abovementioned symptoms in the absence of urticarial eruptions. HAE patients may present erithema marginatum as prodome of upcoming attack. This cutaneous symptoms should not be cofused with urticarial wheals. Absence of wheals is a feature typical of this and other forms of angioedema that have been recently characterized (Mansi et al. 2015). The presence of a family history is a distinguishing feature, but when absent, the diagnosis remains possible considering the high number of de novo mutations. Antigenic and/or functional C1-INH plasma levels below 50% is the biochemical diagnostic test that confirms diagnosis. The levels of C4 are usually reduced. In a recent, large survey, C1-INH-HAE patients with C4 above 50% of normal were less than 4%, giving to this simple measurement a relevant negative predictive value (Zanichelli et al. 2015).

The value of SERPING1 genotyping for C1-INH-HAE diagnosis is minimal. In the absence of family history, it may represent a confirmatory test to be used for genetic counseling. In the presence of ambiguous C1-INH plasma levels, genotyping confirms diagnosis when it detects the same disease-causing mutation that has been already identified within the family. In the presence of C1-INH functional plasma levels above 50%, diagnosis of C1-INH-HAE cannot be based on the presence of a mutation in SERPING1. Attempts to correlate different genotypes to the phenotypic expression of the disease have not been informative.

The Treatment of Hereditary Angioedema Due to C1 Inhibitor Deficiency

Soon after identifying that C1-INH deficiency was the genetic defect underlying HAE, replacement of the deficiency became the obvious therapeutic target. This approach, initially used just to revert ongoing attacks, is now employed also in long-term prevention of symptoms. The first C1-INH replacement was performed using fresh frozen plasma, which is still a therapeutic option where more refined products are not available. Starting from the 1970s, C1 inhibitor concentrates were prepared from pooled human plasma. Use of one of the initial products, and before virucidal methods started to be adopted for plasma derived products, resulted in high rate of hepatitis C transmission. Virus-inactivated products became commercially available in Europe starting from 1985. Post-marketing surveillance of the most widely used C1-INH concentrate shows no reported transmission of infectious agents in more than 30 years (Bork 2014). Despite such a long clinical

experience, controlled studies on efficacy of replacing C1-INH in patients with C1-INH-HAE are recent. Two plasma-derived and one recombinant product are now available for intravenous treatment of acute attacks. Safety profiles appear extremely good, efficacy depends on the dose, and time elapsed from attack onset and treatment administration: early administration significantly shortens posttreatment attack duration. One plasma-derived C1-INH is approved for long-term prevention of attacks. Its registration relies on a single controlled study showing 50% reduction of angioedema attacks with infusions of 1000 units every 3–4 days. Open-label extension phases of this study confirmed efficacy and safety of this approach. A major warning is to avoid use of indwelling catheters for intravenous infusions due to the risk of thrombosis and infections. Long-term replacement therapy with another plasma-derived C1-INH given subcutaneously has just been developped (Longhurst et al. 2017).

Slightly before the discovery of C1-INH as genetic defect underlying HAE, methyltestosterone was found to be effective in long-term prevention of symptoms in these patients. Analogs of testosterone with attenuated androgenic activity have largely been used in severe C1-INH-HAE patients, demonstrating high efficacy and an acceptable safety profile under careful monitoring and wise dosing and patients' selection (Riedl 2015). Alternative therapies have been developed targeting the release and the activity of bradykinin. Two drugs with these characteristics are now available in United States: the plasma kallikrein inhibitor Kalbitor and the bradykinin receptor 2 antagonist icatibant, the last one available also in Europe. Both treatments are for on demand use during attacks and demonstrated their efficacy in several controlled blind and open-label studies. Both products are administered subcutaneously with license for self-administration limited to icatibant (Farkas 2013).

Due to the apparent benign clinical phenotype of the genetic deficiency of plasma kallikrein, long-term prophylaxis of C1-INH-HAE is now approached with different technologies aimed at precluding formation of active plasma kallikrein or blocking its activity. The goal is to prevent cleavage of high molecular weight kininogen and formation of bradykinin. Several such products, with subcutaneous or oral formulations, are in early or advanced phase of human study. Their arrival may further change the treatment of C1-INH-HAE in the near future (Banerji et al. 2017).

References

Bafunno V, Divella C, Sessa F, Tiscia GL, Castellano G, Gesualdo L, et al. De novo homozygous mutation of the C1 inhibitor gene in a patient with hereditary angioedema. J Allergy Clin Immunol. 2013;132:748.

Banerji et al. Inhibiting plasma kallikrein for hereditary angioedema prophylaxis. N Engl J Med. 2017;376:717–28.

Bhardwaj N, Craig TJ. Treatment of hereditary angioedema: a review. Transfusion. 2014;54:2989.

Bork K, Hardt J, Witzke G. Fatal laryngeal attacks and mortality in hereditary angioedema due to C1-INH deficiency. J Allergy Clin Immunol. 2012;130(3):692–7.

Bork K. Pasteurized and nanofiltered, plasma-derived C1 esterase inhibitor concentrate for the treatment of hereditary angioedema. Immunotherapy. 2014;6(5):533–51.

Caccia S, Suffritti C, Cicardi M. Pathophysiology of hereditary angioedema. Pediatr Allergy Immunol Pulmonol. 2014;27(4):159–63.

Cumming SA, Halsall DJ, Ewan PW, Lomas DA. The effect of sequence variations within the coding region of the C1 inhibitor gene on disease expression and protein function in families with hereditary angiooedema. J Med Genet. 2003;40(10):e114.

Farkas H. Current pharmacotherapy of bradykinin-mediated angioedema. Expert Opin Pharmacother. 2013;14(5):571–86.

Kaplan AP, Joseph K. Pathogenic mechanisms of bradykinin mediated diseases: dysregulation of an innate inflammatory pathway. Adv Immunol. 2014;121:41–89.

Levy LR, Lepow IH. Assay and properties of serum inhibitor of C'1-esterase. Proc Soc Exp Biol Med. 1959;101:608–11.

Longhurst H, Cicardi M. Hereditary angio-oedema. Lancet. 2012;379(9814):474–81.

Longhurst et al. Prevention of hereditary angioedema attacks with subcutaneous C1 inhibitor. N Engl J Med. 2017;376:1131–40.

Mansi M, Zanichelli A, Coerezza A, Suffritti C, Wu MA, Vacchini R, et al. Presentation, diagnosis and treatment of angioedema without wheals: a retrospective analysis of a cohort of 1058 patients. J Intern Med. 2015;277(5):585–93.

Nussberger J, Cugno M, Cicardi M. Bradykinin-mediated angioedema. N Engl J Med. 2002;347(8):621–2.

Riedl MA. Critical appraisal of androgen use in hereditary angioedema: a systematic review. Ann Allergy Asthma Immunol. 2015;114(4):281–8. e7

Tosi M, Carugati A, Hernandez C, Boucontet L, Pappalardo E, Agostoni A, et al. De novo C1 inhibitor mutations in hereditary angioedema. Mol Immunol. 1998;35(6–7):406.

Zanichelli A, Arcoleo F, Barca MP, Borrelli P, Bova M, Cancian M, et al. A nationwide survey of hereditary angioedema due to C1 inhibitor deficiency in Italy. Orphanet J Rare Dis. 2015;10:11.

Zuraw BL, Cicardi M, Longhurst HJ, Bernstein JA, Li HH, Magerl M, et al. Phase II study results of a replacement therapy for hereditary angioedema (HAE) with subcutaneous C1-inhibitor concentrate. Allergy. 2015;70:1319.

HFM: Hereditary Folate Malabsorption

▶ Defects in B12 and Folate Metabolism (TCN2, SLC46A1 (PCFT Deficiency), MTHFD1)

HLA Class I Deficiency

▶ MHC Class I, A Deficiency of

HOIL1 Deficiency

▶ TIR Signaling Pathway Deficiency, HOIL1 Deficiency

HOIL-1 Deficiency

▶ LUBAC Deficiencies

HOIL-1 Heme-Oxidized IRP2 Ubiquitin Ligase 1

▶ OTULIN Deficiency-Associated Disease Spectrum

HOIP Deficiency

▶ LUBAC Deficiencies

HOIP HOIL1 Interacting Protein

▶ OTULIN Deficiency-Associated Disease Spectrum

HPV – Human Papillomavirus

▶ Warts, Hypogammaglobulinemia, Infections, Myelokathexis (WHIM) Syndrome

Human IkB-Alpha Gain of Function

▶ Anhidrotic Ectodermal Dysplasia with Immunodeficiency (EDA-ID), Autosomal-Dominant

Human Serum's Trypanosome-Killing Component

▶ APOL-1 Variants, Susceptibility and Resistance to Trypanosomiasis

Hypohidrotic Ectodermal Dysplasia with Immunodeficiency

▶ Autosomal Dominant Anhidrotic Ectodermal Dysplasia with Immunodeficiency (AD-EDA-ID)

I

ICA

▶ Isolated Congenital Asplenia (ICA) and Mutations in RPSA

ICE-Protease Converting Factor

▶ NLRC4-Associated Autoinflammatory Diseases

Ichthyosis Linearis Circumflexa

▶ Comel-Netherton Syndrome (*SPINK5*)

ICOS (Inducible T-Cell Costimulatory) Deficiency (OMIM # 607594)

Lisa J. Kobrynski
Children's Healthcare of Atlanta, Department of Pediatrics, Emory University School of Medicine, Atlanta, GA, USA

Introduction/Background

Deficiency in I **inducible T-cell costimulatory** (ICOS) causes a combined immunodeficiency affecting both cellular and humoral immunity. ICOS (CD278) is an immunoglobulin-like costimulatory receptor belonging to the same family as CD28 and CTLA4 = cytotoxic T-lymphocyte associated protein 4. The *ICOS* gene contains five exons encoding a 199 amino acid protein, which is a disulfide-linked homodimer. The *ICOS* gene is located close to the genes for CTLA4 and CD28, on the long arm of chromosome 2q33.2. ICOS is expressed on the surface of activated or memory T-cells and its only ligand is ICOSL (CD275), which is found on the surface of B cells, dendritic cells, monocytes, macrophages, endothelial cells, fibroblasts, and renal epithelial cells. (Alcher et al. 2000).

ICOS expression is not constitutive. Its expression is induced after T cell activation through TCR = T cell receptor and CD28 signaling. ICOS expression is seen on CD4+, Th1, Th2, Th17, Treg, and Tfh cells (Burmeister et al. 2008). Expression of ICOS is upregulated through NFATc2 and ERK in activated T cells, by NFATc2 and T-bet in Th1 cells and by NFATc2 and GATA3 binding in Th2 cells. In Treg cells, IRF4 binds to the ICOS promoter region and appears to upregulate expression (Tan et al. 2008). In addition, ICOS expression is controlled post-transcriptionally by one of the RING-type ubiquitin ligases, which stimulate degradation of ICOS mRNA (Vinuesa et al. 2005).

After binding ICOSL, ICOS signaling occurs through binding of the intracellular tail of ICOS to the p85α catalytic subunit and the regulatory p50α

© Springer Science+Business Media LLC, part of Springer Nature 2020
I. R. Mackay et al. (eds.), *Encyclopedia of Medical Immunology*,
https://doi.org/10.1007/978-1-4614-8678-7

isoform of phosphatidyl-inositol-3-kinase (PI3K). The cytoplasmic domain contains a conserved YMNM motif, which binds the SH2 domains of PI3K. This domain is similar to that found in CTLA4 and CD28, although ICOS activation results in greater production of PI3K compared to CTLA4 and CD28. Binding causes activation and signaling through phosphorylation of serine/ threonine kinase (Akt) (Fos et al. 2008). ICOS is not known to signal through other pathways such as Lck, Itk, or Tek. ICOS binding of ICOSL can upregulate production of IL4, IL5, IL6, IFNγ, TNFα, GM-CSF, and IL10, but does not stimulate IL-2 secretion. Activation of ICOS also inhibits T-cell apoptosis following T cell activation (Yoshinaga et al. 1999).

T cells in the light zones of lymphoid germinal centers, the medulla of fetal thymi, and the germinal centers in the spleen, lymph nodes and Peyer's patches have the highest levels of ICOS expression. ICOS is also expressed on a subset of FOXP3+ T cells.

ICOS Function

ICOS is critical for germinal center formation, as evidenced by the impaired germinal center formation seen in ICOS −/− knock out (KO) mice and humans with common variable immunodeficiency (CVID) and no ICOS expression (Burmeister et al. 2008). This may be a consequence of the important role of ICOS in follicular helper T cell (TFH) cell development. ICOS −/− mice demonstrate a loss of TFH cells with a reduction in c-Maf transcription and IL-21 (Bauquest et al. 2009). ICOS is important in maintaining the TFH cell pool in germinal centers; without ICOS signaling, TFH cells leave the germinal center and return to the T cell zone (Weber et al. 2015). ICOS causes a reduction in the expansion of CD4+ T cells and creation of the memory CD4+ T cell pool. Loss of either ICOS or ICOS-L results in impairment of the memory CD4+ T cell pool and a decrease in both central (Tcm) and effector (Tem) T-cell memory populations (Marriott et al. 2015). ICOS −/− and ICOSL −/− mice have defects in isotype class switching, suggesting that ICOS plays an important role in antibody isotype switching (Wong et al. 2003).

Clinical Presentation

Most ICOS deficient patients experience adult-onset of respiratory infections; however, disease onset in childhood does occur. Patients present with upper and lower respiratory infections, gastrointestinal problems with giardiasis, lymphonodular hyperplasia, and hepatosplenomegaly. Autoimmune diseases, such as autoimmune neutropenia and rheumatoid arthritis, are reported. One patient in the original cohort of ICOS patients developed autoimmune neutropenia and one developed human papilloma virus (HPV) driven malignancy (Grimbacher et al. 2003).

The first description of an ICOS mutation in patients with CVID identified an identical homozygous deletion of a region encompassing intron 1, Exon 1, intron 2, exon 2, exon 3, and part of intron 3. The resulting premature stop codon resulted in the production of a nonfunctional truncated protein. The original cohort was all from the Black Forest area of Germany (Grimbacher et al. 2003).

Two siblings born to nonconsanguineous parents were found to have a novel homozygous 10 base pair frameshift deletion in exon 2, discovered by whole exome sequencing. Both siblings presented at age 2 years with chronic diarrhea, weight loss, abdominal pain, and fevers. Stool samples from one of the siblings were positive for norovirus, adenovirus, and *Cryptosporidium*. Liver biopsy showed mild chronic hepatitis and gastrointestinal biopsy specimens showed severe active chronic enteritis. In addition, human herpesvirus 6 (HHV6) was identified by PCR in the sigmoid colon, duodenum, and liver (Robertson et al. 2015).

Opportunistic infection with *Pneumocystis jirovecii* and hypogammaglobulinemia was described in a child born to consanguineous parents from Kuwait. A homozygous ICOS mutation: c.90delG; NM_012092, and p.M30 fs*26, that leads to a frameshift and premature truncation of the ICOS protein in exon 2 was described (Chou et al. 2015).

Diagnosis and Laboratory Testing

A defect in ICOS should be considered in patients with a CVID phenotype, particularly those with a family history suggesting autosomal recessive inheritance. Current criteria for a diagnosis of CVID include: age >4 years, a serum IgG level >2 SD below the mean for age, plus a low IgA or IgM, abnormal specific antibody response measured after immunization, and a history of infections consistent with CVID. Confirmation of ICOS deficiency is demonstrated by the absence of ICOS expression on the surface of activated T cells. Genetic sequencing confirms the diagnosis (Warnatz et al. 2006).

Patients with a homozygous mutation in ICOS have severely decreased serum IgG and IgA, variable levels of IgM, and decreased the production of specific IgG to T cell-dependent antigens. Switched memory B cells in peripheral blood are reduced markedly or absent. Most patients have decreases in the marginal zone IgM memory (CD27+IgM+IgD+) B cell subset. In contrast, absolute numbers of T cell subsets in peripheral blood are generally normal and proliferation in response to mitogens is normal. The proportion of naïve to memory T cells is also normal. T cells may show a reduction in IL10 and IL17 production after simulation, but production of other cytokines (IFNγ, IL2, IL4, IL13, and TNFα) is normal. There is the poor development of lymphoid germinal centers (Warnatz et al. 2006).

Treatment/Prognosis

Treatment is directed at providing adequate immunoglobulin replacement, through regular infusions of gamma globulin. Some patients are reported to benefit from prophylactic therapy with antibiotics. One patient is described as receiving an unrelated 11/12 HLA-matched hematopoietic cell transplant (HCT) following reduced intensity conditioning. The patient died from posttransplant complications including capillary leak syndrome on day 5 with respiratory distress followed by toxic epidermal necrolysis (Robertson et al. 2015). A second patient was reported to receive a matched related donor following myeloablative conditioning. Importantly, duodenal villous atrophy and diarrhea resolved posttransplant, total parental nutrition was discontinued and the patient gained weight (Chou et al. 2015).

References

Aicher A, Hayden-Ledbetter M, Brady WA. Characterization of human inducible costimulatory ligand expression and function. J Immunol. 2000;164:4689–96.

Bauquet AT, Jin H, Paterson AM, et al. The co-stimulatory molecule ICOS regulates the expression of c-Maf and IL-21 in the development of follicular T helper cells and TH-17 cells. Nat Immunol. 2009;10:167–75.

Burmeister Y, Lischke T, Dahler AC, et al. ICOS controls the pool size of effector-memory and regulatory T cells. J Immunol. 2008;180:774–82.

Chou J, Massad MJ, Cangemi B, et al. A novel mutation in ICOS presenting as hypogammaglobulinemia with susceptibility to opportunistic pathogens. J Allergy Clin Immunol. 2015;136(3):794–797.e1. https://doi.org/10.1016/j.jaci.2014.12.1940. Epub 2015 Feb 10. No abstract available. PMID:25678089

Fos C, salles A, Lang V, et al. ICOS ligation recruits the p50alpha PI3K regulatory subunit to the immunological synapse. J Immunol. 2008;181:1969–77.

Grimbacher B, Hutloff A, Schlesier M, et al. Homozygous loss of ICOS is associated with adult onset common variable immune deficiency. Nat Immunol. 2003;4:261–8.

Marriott CL, Carlesso G, Herbst R, Withers DR. ICOS is required for the generation of both central and effector memory T-cell populations following acute bacterial infection. Eur J Immunol. 2015;45:1706–15.

Robertson N, Engelhardt KR, Morgan NV et al. Astute Clinician Report: A Novel 10 bp Frameshift Deletion in Exon 2 of ICOS Causes a Combined Immunodeficiency Associated with an Enteritis and Hepatitis. J Clin Immunol. 2015;35(7):598–603. https://doi.org/10.1007/s10875-015-0193-x. Epub 2015 Sep 23. PMID: 26399252

Tan AM, Goh SYP, Wong SC, Lam KP. T helper cell-specific regulation of inducible costimulatory expression via distinct mechanisms mediated by T-bet and GATA3. J Biol Chem. 2008;283:128–36.

Vineusa CG, Cook MC, Angelucci C, et al. A RING-type ubiquitin ligase family member required to repress follicular helper T cells and autoimmunity. Nature. 2005;435:452–8.

Warnatz K, Bossaller L, Salzer U et al. Homozygous ICOS deficiency abrogates the germinal center reaction and provides a monogeneic model for common variable deficiency. Blood. 2006;107:3045–52.

Weber JP, Fuhrmann F, Feist RK, et al. ICOS maintains the T follicular helper cell phenotype by down-regulating Kruppel-like factor 2. J Exp Med. 2015;212:217–33.

Wong SC, Oh E, Ng CH, Lam KP. Impaired germinal center formation and recall T-cell dependent immune responses in mice lacking the costimulatory ligand B7-H2. Blood. 2003;102:1381–8.

Yoshinaga SK, Whoriskey JS, Khare SD, et al. T-cell co-stimulation through B7RP-1 and ICOS. Nature. 1999;402:827–32.

ICOS Deficiency

Klaus Warnatz
Department of Rheumatology and Clinical Immunology and Center for Chronic Immunodeficiency, University Medical Center and University of Freiburg, Freiburg, Germany

Definition

An immunodeficiency defined by deleterious mutations in *ICOS* encoding for the inducible co-stimulator.

Prevalence

So far (2017), 15 patients with mutations in *ICOS* have been published (Schepp et al. 2017).

Clinical presentation: The first published nine cases from four families presented with a phenotype compatible with common variable immunodeficiency (Grimbacher et al. 2003; Warnatz et al. 2006). This included recurrent bacterial infections of the respiratory tract in all but two patients who were put prophylactically on IgG replacement therapy because of the diagnosis, hypogammaglobulinemia, and positive family history. Subsequently six additional patients were identified with a different clinical phenotype. Two Japanese patients presented with psoriasis, arthritis,

and recurrent herpes simplex infection (Takahashi et al. 2009). The last four patients of two families with consanguineous background presented early in childhood with enteropathy (Robertson et al. 2015) and one patient with an opportunistic infection (pneumocystis jirovecii) (Chou et al. 2015). The most common form of secondary complications among patients with ICOS deficiency was enteropathy in 9/15 patients. Other clinical manifestations observed in CVID-like ICOS-deficient patients, including autoimmune cytopenia, splenomegaly, and lymphadenopathy, have been diagnosed only in single patients. While most CVID-like patients presented during adolescence or adulthood, childhood onset has been observed. CID-like patients presented early in life.

Genetics

Genetic findings reported so far (2017) include autosomal recessive inheritance due to homozygous deletions of 1815 bp comprising exons two and three in the first four reported families (c.126–568.del) and different single bp deletions in the remaining three families, leading to frame shift mutations or premature stop codons (c.285delT, c.90delG, c.321_330del).

Immunological Phenotype

Inducible costimulator (ICOS) belongs to the CD28 costimulatory receptor family. It is expressed exclusively on activated T cells. It has a crucial role during the T-B cell interaction at the initiation and maintenance of the germinal center (GC) response. Therefore, ICOS-deficient mice present with a poor GC formation and severely disturbed humoral memory response (Hutloff et al. 1999). Correspondingly, the first nine human ICOS deficient patients presented with hypogammaglobulinemia with reduced IgG and IgA (100%) and severely impaired specific antibody responses while IgM was less regularly affected. All patients had (severely) reduced class-switched memory B cells. In several patients, an increasing B lymphopenia was observed beyond the expected reduction of the memory B cells. Among T cells, no consistent abnormality was observed except the reduction of circulating T follicular helper (Tfh) cells (Bossaller et al. 2006). Further analysis of T cell function revealed impaired cytokine production of IL-10 and IL-17, while other cytokines were less consistently affected (Warnatz et al. 2006) reflecting a role of ICOS in the induction of different memory T cell populations. The reduction of regulatory T cells described in mice was not a consistent finding in humans.

Diagnosis

Diagnosis is made by genetic analysis of *ICOS*. Suspicion should be raised in patients presenting with a CVID-like clinical presentation (which may include infections and/or auto-immunity) with strongly reduced IgG and IgA levels and nearly absent class-switched memory B cells. So far, all patients with ICOS deficiency examined for protein expression had absent ICOS expression on T cells after in vitro stimulation of PBMCs, so flowcytometric evaluation is a helpful diagnostic tool. Additional awareness is necessary in patients with combined immunodeficiency or immune dysregulation, extending the clinical picture and rendering next generation sequencing especially in patients with consanguineous background necessary.

Management

Management depends on the presentation of the disease. While most patients with a CVID-like disease were adequately treated by IgG replacement therapy, 40% of the patients received systemic steroids for different reasons but rarely required additional immunosuppressive drugs. Only one patient required hematopoietic stem cell transplantation (HSCT) for severe secondary cytopenia of unknown origin at age 53. In contrast, both patients presenting with combined immunodeficiency during early childhood underwent HSCT, with favorable outcome in one and death in the other.

References

Bossaller L, Burger J, Draeger R, Grimbacher B, Knoth R, Plebani A, et al. ICOS deficiency is associated with a severe reduction of CXCR5+CD4 germinal center Th cells. J Immunol. 2006;177(7):4927–32.

Chou J, Massaad MJ, Cangemi B, Bainter W, Platt C, Badran YR, et al. A novel mutation in ICOS presenting as hypogammaglobulinemia with susceptibility to opportunistic pathogens. J Allergy Clin Immunol. 2015;136(3):794–7.e1.

Grimbacher B, Hutloff A, Schlesier M, Glocker E, Warnatz K, Drager R, et al. Homozygous loss of ICOS is associated with adult-onset common variable immunodeficiency. Nat Immunol. 2003;4(3):261–8.

Hutloff A, Dittrich AM, Beier KC, Eljaschewitsch B, Kraft R, Anagnostopoulos I, et al. ICOS is an inducible T-cell co-stimulator structurally and functionally related to CD28. Nature. 1999;397(6716):263–6.

Robertson N, Engelhardt KR, Morgan NV, Barge D, Cant AJ, Hughes SM, et al. Astute clinician report: a Novel 10 bp frameshift deletion in Exon 2 of ICOS causes a combined immunodeficiency associated with an enteritis and hepatitis. J Clin Immunol. 2015;35(7):598–603.

Schepp J, Chou J, Skrabl-Baumgartner A, Arkwright PD, Engelhardt KR, Hambleton S, et al. 14 years after discovery: clinical follow-up on 15 patients with inducible co-stimulator deficiency. Front Immunol. 2017;8:964.

Takahashi N, Matsumoto K, Saito H, Nanki T, Miyasaka N, Kobata T, et al. Impaired CD4 and CD8 effector function and decreased memory T cell populations in ICOS-deficient patients. J Immunol. 2009;182(9):5515–27.

Warnatz K, Bossaller L, Salzer U, Skrabl-Baumgartner A, Schwinger W, van der BM, et al. Human ICOS deficiency abrogates the germinal center reaction and provides a monogenic model for common variable immunodeficiency. Blood. 2006;107(8):3045–52.

Ig Heavy Chain Deletions

Mirjam van der Burg

Department of Pediatrics, Willem-Alexander Children's Hospital, Leiden University Medical Center, Leiden, the Netherlands

Synonyms

Immunoglobulin heavy chain deficiency

Definition

Patients with Ig heavy chain deletions lack one or more IgG, IgA, and/or IgE classes due to a genetic deletion. In this disorder deletion of IgM is not involved, because deletions of the *IGHM* gene, which are mediated by transposable elements, (van Zelm et al. 2008) give rise to agammaglobulinemia, because the lack of IgM expression leads to a block of the precursor B-cell differentiation at the pre-B-II cell stage and no mature B cells can be formed (Yel et al. 1996).

Genetics

Ig heavy chain deletion is an autosomal recessive disorder, caused by chromosomal deletions of a cluster of genes, the constant regions of the IgG and/or IgA and IgE genes (OMIM 147100). Deletion of the IgG locus has first been described by Lefranc et al. in (1982). Homologous recombination is involved in the deletion process and several deletion haplotypes have been described (Lefranc et al. 1991; Olsson et al. 1991).

Immunological Phenotype

Ig heavy chain deletions present immunologically as hypogammaglobulinemia with isotype or IgG subclass deficiency depending on the deleted part of the Ig locus. No reports on the B-cell phenotype of the affected patients exist.

Clinical Presentation and Therapy

Ig heavy chain deletions are generally asymptomatic and do not require treatment. For specific deletions involving one or more classes or isotypes (IgG and/or IgA) giving rise to partial IgA deficiency and/or IgG subclass deficiency, treatment might be necessary.

References

Lefranc G, Lefranc MP, Helal AN, et al. Unusual heavy chains of human IgG immunoglobulins: rearrangements of the ch domain exons. J Immunogenet. 1982;9(1):1–9.

Lefranc MP, Hammarstrom L, Smith CI, et al. Gene deletions in the human immunoglobulin heavy chain constant region locus: molecular and immunological analysis. Immunodefic Rev. 1991;2(4):265–81.

Olsson PG, Hofker MH, Walter MA, et al. Ig H chain variable and C region genes in common variable immunodeficiency. Characterization of two new deletion haplotypes. J Immunol. 1991;147(8):2540–6.

van Zelm MC, Geertsema C, Nieuwenhuis N, et al. Gross deletions involving IGHM, BTK, or Artemis: a model for genomic lesions mediated by transposable elements. Am J Hum Genet. 2008;82(2):320–32.

Yel L, Minegishi Y, Coustan-Smith E, et al. Mutations in the mu heavy-chain gene in patients with agammaglobulinemia. N Engl J Med. 1996;335(20):1486–93.

IgA Deficiency With or Without IgG Subclass Deficiencies

Lilly M. Verhagen[1] and Lennart Hammarström[2]
[1]Department of Pediatric Immunoloy and Infectious Diseases, Wilhelmina Children's Hospital, Utrecht, The Netherlands
[2]Karolinska Institute, Stockholm, Sweden

Definitions

Selective immunoglobulin A (IgA) deficiency is defined by the European Society for Immunodeficiencies (ESID) and the Pan-American Group for Immunodeficiency (PAGID) as an IgA serum concentration below 0.07 g/l in male or female patients over 4 years of age. In addition, patients show normal values of other immunoglobulins and normal IgG antibody responses to vaccines. The threshold of 4 years is chosen because delayed production of IgA in children is common due to maturation of the immune system. The term *partial* IgA deficiency is reserved for those patients with serum IgA levels ≥0.07 g/l but below minus two standard deviations compared with age-normalized levels. *Transient* IgA deficiency refers to those IgA-deficient children that reach normal IgA levels over time. Around 20% of children diagnosed between 4 and 13 years of age reach a normalized level of IgA with age (Lim et al. 2015).

Selective IgA deficiency is believed to be one end of a spectrum of an immunodeficiency disease with common variable immunodeficiency (CVID) at the most severe end, where both serum IgA and total IgG levels are decreased. In this spectrum, there are patients with a combination of IgA and IgG subclass deficiency. IgG subclass deficiency is defined as a deficiency in one or more IgG subclasses (<-2 SD below age-matched reference values) with normal or near normal total IgG serum concentration.

Immunobiology of IgA and IgG Subclass Production

IgA is by far the most abundant antibody isotype produced in non-deficient individuals. Circulating IgA is in a monomeric form, whereas secretory IgA (sIgA), which protects the surfaces of the respiratory, gastrointestinal, and genitourinary tract, is dimeric. Dimerization includes the addition of a polypeptide termed "J chain." Both IgA and the J chain are produced by lymphocytes in organized germinal centers of mucosa-associated lymphoid tissues such as Peyer's patches. The induction and secretion of IgA as well as the size of the Peyer's patches seem to be driven by microbial communities at the mucosal surfaces, also called the microbiome (Macpherson et al. 2015). Transport of dimeric IgA from the basolateral to the apical/luminal side of mucosal epithelial cells occurs with the aid of a membrane-associated polymeric Ig receptor (pIgR). Proteolytic cleavage of pIgR on the luminal side generates the so-called secretory component, which remains associated with dimeric IgA, forming sIgA. While pIgR is critical for transport of IgA into mucosal secretions, receptors for the Fc portion of IgA, in particular the IgA-Fc alpha receptor, are present on circulating blood cell types including neutrophils, macrophages, monocytes, and eosinophils. Binding of IgA to Fc-alpha receptors on these cells can lead to several different outcomes, depending on the cytokine milieu and the nature of the stimulus. Serum IgA in the human bloodstream is thought to be involved in both the dampening of an excessive immune response and the initiation of protective immunity. Whereas monomeric interaction of IgA with its Fc-alpha receptor on circulating leukocytes and monocytes triggers inhibitory signals that block activation of other receptors, multimeric IgA-Fc-alpha receptor cross-linking induces a pro-inflammatory response including phagocytosis and antigen presentation. While the function of serum IgA in the systemic immune response is ambivalent, sIgA, which is found in saliva, tears, gastrointestinal fluids, nasal bronchial secretions, and urine, plays a major protective anti-inflammatory role in maintaining the epithelial barrier and limiting penetration of mucosal surfaces by microorganisms and foreign proteins. In addition, sIgA neutralizes toxins.

In human serum, IgG is the most abundant immunoglobulin class and one of the most abundant proteins. The four IgG subclasses in order of decreasing abundance, IgG1, IgG2, IgG3, and IgG4, differ in their constant region and have different effector functions. Typically, IgG antibody responses to different types of antigens lead to skewed production of one of the subclasses. In general, protein antigens that trigger B-cells receiving T-cell help lead to the production of IgG1 or IgG3 which are efficient activators of the classical complement pathway. In the absence of T-cell help, polysaccharide antigens may induce class switching to IgG2 in particular. IgG4 responses tend to occur after repeated antigen exposure, but their clinical significance is thought to be limited.

Prevalence of IgA Deficiency With or Without IgG Subclass Deficiency

IgA deficiency is the most common primary immune deficiency. Since many individuals with IgA deficiency are asymptomatic, blood donor studies may provide the most reliable estimate of population prevalence rates. Based on these reports, IgA deficiency in adults is most commonly observed in the Caucasian populations with prevalence rates around 1:500, while Mongoloid populations show much lower rates of around 1:2000 up to 1:20,000 (Kanoh et al. 1986; Litzman et al. 2000; Lu et al. 2016). While blood donor studies provide estimates of the adult prevalence rate, reports from healthy pediatric populations show higher IgA deficiency prevalences of 1:200–1:400 (Basturk et al. 2011). Rates in pediatric populations are probably higher than in adults because of the occurrence of transient IgA deficiency in childhood that resolves upon maturation. In non-healthy patient populations, most notably those patients referred for recurrent infections, high rates of IgA deficiency (varying from 1% in adults to 25% in children) are observed (Litzman et al. 2000; Aldirmaz et al. 2014).

IgA deficiency co-occurs in up to 10–20% of the patients with a deficiency in one or more IgG subclasses, mainly IgG2 or IG4. The prevalence of IgG2 or IgG4 deficiency does not differ significantly between those with complete or partial IgA deficiency (Litzman et al. 2000; Ozkan et al. 2005; Roberton et al. 1990). Patients with IgA deficiency with one or more IgG subclass deficiencies may be more likely to evolve into CVID over time.

Pathophysiology

The etiology of IgA deficiency with or without IgG subclass deficiency represents a heterogeneous group of abnormalities. An intrinsic B-cell defect, T helper cell dysfunction, and suppressor T cells have all been suggested to play a role. In addition, cytokine abnormalities have also been associated with IgA deficiency. In particular,

IL-21 has been proposed to play a role in both IgA and IgG (subclass) deficiency. In ex vivo studies, immunoglobulin production in patients with IgA deficiency and common variable immunodeficiency (CVID) was partially restored after IL-21 stimulation (Borte et al. 2009).

There are numerous reports of familial cases of IgA deficiency with or without IgG (subclass) deficiencies. In line with the view of the two defects being ends of a spectrum of diseases, in multiple case families, usually both CVID and IgA deficiency are present (Rezaei et al. 2013). Although this suggests a genetic basis of IgA deficiency, no clear-cut pattern of inheritance has been observed, and DNA testing is currently not part of the routine diagnostic work-up for IgA-deficient patients. Several types of defects have been considered as the main genetic contributors. Large chromosomal aberrations and associations with the human major histocompatibility complex (MHC) locus, in particular with HLA class II loci, have frequently been described. For specific HLA-DQB and HLA-DRB alleles, this link is well established. The strongest association observed in a genome-wide association study (GWAS) meta-analysis of 1635 cases with IgA deficiency and 4852 controls was with the MHC region 2.7 kb upstream of HLA-DQA1 (Bronson et al. 2016). Several autoimmune diseases including rheumatoid arthritis, systemic lupus erythematosus, and multiple sclerosis also have associations reported at this locus, suggesting a link between IgA deficiency and autoimmunity on a genetic level.

A role for polymorphisms in non-HLA loci in the development of IgA deficiency has also been suggested (Abolhassani et al. 2016). A number of genes affecting various aspects of immune function, including humoral but also innate and cellular immunity as well as complement deficiencies, seem to play a role. Furthermore, key cell surface molecules on B and T cells also seem to be involved. For example, mutations in the gene TNFRSF13B which encodes the TACI (transmembrane activator and calcium modulator and cyclophilin ligand interactor), a member of the tumor necrosis factor superfamily receptors, were observed in IgA-deficient patients. Similar to MHC loci, overlap with autoimmune markers was also noted for non-MHC polymorphisms, such as for the newly identified variants in PVT1, ATG13-AMBRA, AHI1, and CLEC16A in the abovementioned GWAS analysis (Bronson et al. 2016). Some defects, such as gene deletions involving various chromosome 14 segments and loss of function variants in encoding TACI, have been described in both IgA and IgG subclass deficiencies and CVID, which underscores the relationship between these defects also on a genetic level. However, the relationship of genotype to phenotype for IgA with or without IgG subclass deficiency is only partially understood. Pathway analysis suggests that the intestinal immune network is essential for IgA production. This includes genes encoding inflammatory and immune regulatory cytokines (such as APRIL and BAFF) and molecules essential for the homing of lymphocytes to the gut (Bronson et al. 2016). In addition to genetic factors, immunoregulatory mechanisms modifiable by exogenous factors or the endogenous gut microflora may affect IgA production and the development of IgA deficiency.

Although primary IgA deficiency is the most prevalent form, secondary deficiencies due to the effects of drugs or the result of other conditions are recognized. Diseases such as viral infections (most notably Epstein-Barr virus or hepatitis C) but also nephrotic syndrome and hematological malignancies can play a role in developing IgA and/or IgG subclass deficiency. In addition, the use of anticonvulsants, nonsteroidal anti-inflammatory drugs (NSAIDs), disease-modifying antirheumatic drugs (DMARDs), and chemotherapeutics may cause an iatrogenic decrease of IgA and/or IgG subclass levels (Duraisingham et al. 2014). Drug-induced deficiencies typically resolve spontaneously after cessation of treatment in approximately half of the patients.

Clinical Presentation

There is a discrepancy between the critical role sIgA is thought to play in the mucosal immune response and the absence of symptoms in most people with an IgA deficiency. The reason why patients with IgA deficiency are asymptomatic is still unclear. It has been suggested that a compensatory increase in IgM and/or IgG makes up for the lack of IgA to prevent mucosal infiltration of microorganisms. The latter may be the explanation that (infectious) symptoms are more prevalent and severe in patients with combined IgA and IgG subclass deficiencies. On the other hand, the high percentage of asymptomatic IgA deficient patients could be an overestimation. Long-term follow-up studies of asymptomatic individuals revealed an increased prevalence of respiratory tract infections and autoimmune diseases later in life (Koskinen 1996).

Because of the relative high frequency of IgA deficiency and its prevalence in asymptomatic individuals, care must be taken in the assessment of an association of IgA deficiency with clinical diseases. Recurrent infections, allergies, and autoimmune diseases are among the most commonly reported diseases in symptomatic IgA-deficient patients. The respiratory and gastrointestinal tracts are the main site of infections (Ludvigsson et al. 2016). In addition to gastrointestinal infections, IgA-deficient patients have an increased frequency of other gastrointestinal disorders such as malabsorption, lactose intolerance, celiac disease, and inflammatory bowel disease. Allergic diseases also appear to be common in IgA-deficient patients. The most common allergic conditions reported are allergic rhinoconjunctivitis, urticaria, atopic dermatitis, and asthma. Rheumatoid arthritis, autoimmune thyroiditis, idiopathic thrombocytopenic purpura, systemic lupus erythematosus, and diabetes mellitus are examples of autoimmune diseases observed in IgA-deficient patients. Even in the absence of clinical disease, autoantibodies have been found in some IgA-deficient patients (Aytekin et al. 2012). It is not entirely clear what the pathophysiological substrate for the relationship between IgA deficiency and allergic conditions or autoimmunity is. Impaired mucosal immunity may result in inflammatory conditions, loss of mucosal homeostasis with diminished mucosal barrier function, and increased exposure to food and microbial components. Furthermore, decreased serum monomeric IgA levels may diminish the IgA-Fc-alpha receptor-mediated downregulation of pro-inflammatory responses paving the way for allergies and autoimmunity.

In addition to infectious, allergic, and autoimmune diseases, a recently performed nationwide population-based cohort study from Sweden suggests that individuals with IgA deficiency carry a moderately increased risk to develop cancer, mainly gastrointestinal cancer (Ludvigsson et al. 2015). Another concern in IgA-deficient patients is the reported adverse reaction to blood products as a result of anti-IgA antibodies. Around 25% of IgA-deficient individuals have anti-IgA antibodies. In these patients, infusion with blood products may lead to a severe allergic reaction. However, these reactions are quite rare. This may be related to the current widespread use of washed erythrocytes instead of complete blood, which do not contain more than trace amounts of IgA.

IgA deficiency combined with a deficiency of one or more IgG subclasses is associated with an increased prevalence and severity of infections compared with IgA deficiency alone. Typically, deficiency of IgG1 results in low levels of total IgG and is often associated with susceptibility to bacterial infections. IgG2 is particularly important in the immune response against respiratory pathogens such as *Streptococcus pneumoniae* and *Haemophilus influenzae*, making IgG2-deficient individuals more prone to respiratory tract infections (Bossuyt et al. 2007). The IgG3 subclass is mainly composed of antibodies directed to viral antigens. The clinical relevance of IgG4 evaluation and undetectable IgG4 subclass levels are still unclear. Recurrent respiratory tract infections in patients with IgA with or without IgG subclass deficiencies can lead to chronic pulmonary damage, such as bronchiectasis and bronchiolitis obliterans (Ozkan et al. 2005).

For children, it is not known how to predict which child with IgA deficiency with or without IgG subclass deficiency is just showing delayed maturation of the immune system, and in which child it is the first sign of a lasting primary antibody deficiency, or maybe even a development toward CVID. A retrospective study from a tertiary hospital in the Netherlands suggests that children with transient antibody deficiencies can be identified by their increased pneumococcal polysaccharide vaccine-induced IgA response compared with children that remain deficient for 3–5 years after diagnosis (Janssen et al. 2015).

Diagnosis

The diagnosis of IgA and IgG subclass deficiencies depends on the measurement of these antibodies in serum. In newly presenting patients with IgA with or without IgG subclass deficiency, a familial history and, if indicated, immunological screening of relatives is warranted. In addition, a complete blood count, optionally also including lymphocyte and B- and T-cell subset phenotyping should be performed. Furthermore, antibody responses to routine vaccinations can be measured to determine if there is a concomitant functional antibody deficiency. Finally, the response to pneumococcal polysaccharide vaccination may be determined in children aged 3 years or more. Impaired polysaccharide responsiveness indicates a decreased ability to produce protective IgG molecules against polysaccharide-coated bacteria. Several major airway pathogens, such as *S. pneumoniae* and *H. influenzae*, belong to this group of bacteria, and problems with specific antibody production may lead to an increased frequency of respiratory infections. Tests of cellular immunity, complement activity, and phagocytic function should be considered if necessary. Particularly, in those patients with a history of recurrent respiratory tract infections, chest X-ray or CT, sinus imaging, and pulmonary function studies should be considered.

A UK national audit revealed that patients with primary antibody deficiencies present to a wide variety of clinical specialties other than clinical immunology. This leads to a diagnostic delay because recurrent infections are regarded as normal variation or mistaken for more common conditions, such as secondary to asthma or chronic obstructive pulmonary disease (COPD). The delay in diagnosis depends on the type of antibody deficiency and occurs more often in "milder" antibody deficiencies such as IgA deficiency and IgG subclass deficiencies, where delays of up to 10 years are reported (Wood et al. 2007). Diagnostic delays are potentially associated with higher rates of structural lung damage.

Treatment

There is no curative treatment for primary IgA deficiency, whether or not combined with IgG subclass deficiencies. The cornerstone of therapy is the treatment of associated diseases. For patients with acute infections, antibiotics are generally prescribed. Those with recurrent respiratory tract infections may benefit from antibiotic prophylaxis. The choice of drug and doses vary between hospitals and countries, and there are no consensus guidelines on this matter. In case of associated IgG subclass deficiency and a high rate of infections, immunoglobulin treatment via venous or subcutaneous route may be given. Gamma globulin substitution may also be given to IgA-deficient patients without IgG subclass deficiency. Although the preparations hardly contain IgA, improvement of IgG antibody levels may positively affect the infectious burden. Secondary IgA and/or IgG (subclass) deficiencies as a result of (hematological) malignancies or medication may also be treated with immunoglobulin replacement therapy to reduce infections during the period of low antibody levels.

Additional immunization with conjugate vaccines against *S. pneumoniae* and *H. influenzae* type B has been suggested by some for improved protection of IgA-deficient patients. This seems particularly useful in patients with a decreased ability to make anti-polysaccharide antibodies. Multiple doses of conjugate vaccines are typically required. Management of allergies and autoimmune disorders in IgA-deficient patients is similar to the management of these diseases in non-IgA-deficient individuals.

Conclusions

- Primary IgA deficiency is a multifactorial disease where genetic, environmental, and possible microbiome triggers lead to impaired production of IgA. Secondary IgA deficiency can occur following diseases such as viral infections and hematological malignancies or the use of anti-epileptics, NSAIDs, DMARDs, or chemotherapeutics.
- The genetic base of IgA deficiency, with or without IgG subclass deficiency, is multifactorial. Large chromosomal aberrations, associations with the MHC locus, as well as non-MHC polymorphisms have been suggested to play a role.
- Despite the presumed critical role of IgA in the mucosal immune response, many people with an IgA deficiency are asymptomatic.
- Patients with a combined IgA and IgG subclass deficiency suffer from more (severe) infections and carry an increased risk of pulmonary damage compared with selective IgA-deficient patients.
- In addition to infections of the respiratory or gastrointestinal tract, IgA-deficient patients experience allergic and autoimmune diseases.
- Treatment of IgA with or without IgG subclass deficiency consists of antibiotic prophylaxis which may be combined with gamma globulin substitution. Although this decreases the frequency and severity of infections, no therapies to restore endogenous IgA or IgG subclass production are currently available.

References

Abolhassani H, Aghamohammadi A, Hammarstrom L. Monogenic mutations associated with IgA deficiency. Expert Rev Clin Immunol. 2016:1–15. https://doi.org/10.1080/1744666X.2016.1198696.

Aldirmaz S, Yucel E, Kiykim A, Cokugras H, Akcakaya N, Camcioglu Y. Profile of the patients who present to immunology outpatient clinics because of frequent infections. Turk Pediatri Ars. 2014;49:210–216.

Aytekin C, Tuygun N, Gokce S, Dogu F, Ikinciogullari A. Selective IgA deficiency: clinical and laboratory features of 118 children in Turkey. J Clin Immunol.

2012;32:961–6. https://doi.org/10.1007/s10875-012-9702-3.

Basturk B, Sari S, Aral A, Dalgic B. Prevalence of selective immunoglobulin A deficiency in healthy Turkish school children. Turk J Pediatr. 2011;53:364–8.

Borte S, et al. Interleukin-21 restores immunoglobulin production ex vivo in patients with common variable immunodeficiency and selective IgA deficiency. Blood. 2009;114:4089–98. https://doi.org/10.1182/blood-2009-02-207423.

Bossuyt X, et al. Coexistence of (partial) immune defects and risk of recurrent respiratory infections. Clin Chem. 2007;53:124–30. https://doi.org/10.1373/clinchem.2007.075861.

Bronson PG, et al. Common variants at PVT1, ATG13-AMBRA1, AHI1 and CLEC16A are associated with selective IgA deficiency. Nat Genet. 2016;48:1425–9. https://doi.org/10.1038/ng.3675.

Duraisingham SS, Buckland M, Dempster J, Lorenzo L, Grigoriadou S, Longhurst HJ. Primary vs. secondary antibody deficiency: clinical features and infection outcomes of immunoglobulin replacement. PLoS One. 2014;9:e100324. https://doi.org/10.1371/journal.pone.0100324.

Janssen WJ, Nierkens S, Sanders EA, Boes M, van Montfrans JM. Antigen-specific IgA titres after 23-valent pneumococcal vaccine indicate transient antibody deficiency disease in children. Vaccine. 2015;33:6320–6. https://doi.org/10.1016/j.vaccine.2015.09.041.

Kanoh T, et al. Selective IgA deficiency in Japanese blood donors: frequency and statistical analysis. Vox Sang. 1986;50:81–6.

Koskinen S. Long-term follow-up of health in blood donors with primary selective IgA deficiency. J Clin Immunol. 1996;16:165–70.

Lim CK, et al. Reversal of immunoglobulin a deficiency in children. J Clin Immunol. 2015;35:87–91. https://doi.org/10.1007/s10875-014-0112-6.

Litzman J, Sevcikova I, Stikarovska D, Pikulova Z, Pazdirkova A, Lokaj J. IgA deficiency in Czech healthy individuals and selected patient groups. Int Arch Allergy Immunol. 2000;123:177–80.

Lu P, Ling B, Wang N, Hammarstrom L. Study on immunoglobulin A Deficiency(IgAD) in Chinese Shanghai blood donors. Zhongguo Shi Yan Xue Ye Xue Za Zhi. 2016;24:1216–20. https://doi.org/10.7534/j.issn.1009-2137.2016.04.047.

Ludvigsson JF, Neovius M, Ye W, Hammarstrom L. IgA deficiency and risk of cancer: a population-based matched cohort study. J Clin Immunol. 2015;35:182–8. https://doi.org/10.1007/s10875-014-0124-2.

Ludvigsson JF, Neovius M, Hammarstrom L. Risk of infections among 2100 individuals with IgA deficiency: a nationwide cohort study. J Clin Immunol. 2016;36:134–40. https://doi.org/10.1007/s10875-015-0230-9.

Macpherson AJ, Koller Y, McCoy KD. The bilateral responsiveness between intestinal microbes and IgA. Trends Immunol. 2015;36:460–70. https://doi.org/10.1016/j.it.2015.06.006.

Ozkan H, Atlihan F, Genel F, Targan S, Gunvar T. IgA and/or IgG subclass deficiency in children with recurrent respiratory infections and its relationship with chronic pulmonary damage. J Investig Allergol Clin Immunol. 2005;15:69–74.

Rezaei N, Abolhassani H, Kasraian A, Mohammadinejad P, Sadeghi B, Aghamohammadi A. Family study of pediatric patients with primary antibody deficiencies. Iran J Allergy Asthma Immunol. 2013;12:377–82.

Roberton DM, Colgan T, Ferrante A, Jones C, Mermelstein N, Sennhauser F. IgG subclass concentrations in absolute, partial and transient IgA deficiency in childhood. Pediatr Infect Dis J. 1990;9:S41–5.

Wood P, et al. Recognition, clinical diagnosis and management of patients with primary antibody deficiencies: a systematic review. Clin Exp Immunol. 2007;149:410–23.

IgG Subclass Deficiency and Specific Polysaccharide Antibody Deficiency (SPAD)

Taco W. Kuijpers[1] and Joris M. van Montfrans[2]
[1]Department of Pediatric Immunology, Rheumatology and Infectious Diseases, Emma Children's Hospital, Amsterdam University Medical Center (Amsterdam UMC), Amsterdam, The Netherlands
[2]Department of Pediatric Immunology and Infectious Diseases, Wilhelmina Children's Hospital, University Medical Center Utrecht (UMCU), Utrecht, The Netherlands

Definition IgG Subclass Deficiency

An immunodeficiency defined by a deficiency in one or more IgG subclasses (>2 SD below age-matched reference values) with normal or near normal IgG concentration. It is important to emphasize that the low levels of IgG subclasses as such do not necessarily indicate an underlying pathology or the presence of clinical disease.

Definition Specific Polysaccharide Antibody Deficiency (SPAD)

An immunodeficiency diagnosed when there is profound decrease of the antibody response to polysaccharide antigens, either after documented invasive infection with, e.g., *S. pneumoniae*, or after test immunization with an unconjugated pneumococcal (or other) polysaccharide vaccine.

Four IgG subclasses have been recognized since the early 1960s (Terry and Fahey 1964). Approximately 65% of the total circulating IgG in normal persons is of the IgG1 subclass. IgG2 constitutes 20 to 25% of circulating IgG, and IgG3 and IgG4 each represent less than 10%. Assessment is readily available but cannot easily be compared between assays. IgG subclass deficiency and selective polysaccharide antibody deficiency (SPAD) present similarly and are part of an overlapping spectrum of antibody deficiencies.

The antibody response to polysaccharide antigens after test immunization with an unconjugated pneumococcal (or other) polysaccharide vaccine is required in both conditions to verify the correlate of the clinical finding with the immunological correlate of unresponsiveness (Oxelius 1974; Kuijpers et al. 1992).

Prevalence

Little is known about the exact prevalence of IgG subclass deficiencies. An inventory of IgG subclass deficiency among more than 8000 healthy adult blood donors demonstrated that there were more individuals with low IgG2 concentrations than predicted by the log-normal distribution and some had a combined IgA-IgG2-IgG4 subclass deficiency without any clinical symptoms (Nahm et al. 1990).

In a cohort of 575 healthy children, 2% showed IgG2 concentrations >2SD below the mean for age. These asymptomatic children with subnormal IgG2 levels showed normal antibody responses to immunization with *Haemophilus*

influenzae type b (Hib) polysaccharide antigens. These findings reinforce the fact that isolated IgG subclass deficiency does not tell us much and some may wonder whether we should determine IgG subclasses at all (Shackelford et al. 1990). Studies in *selected* populations mentioned a prevalence of about 20% for IgG subclass deficiency in symptomatic populations (screened for immunodeficiency) (Ochs et al. 2004; Meulenbroek and Zeijlemaker 2000). IgG3 subclass deficiency has been variably reported to be slightly more prevalent than IgG2 subclass deficiency and is especially found in patients with asthma or atopic disease. Isolated IgG4 subclass deficiency is considered to be innocent and without clinical relevance; its prevalence in the normal population is unknown.

As a note of caution – retesting IgG subclasses in different assays may give different results, and interpretation of specific antipneumococcal assays remains notoriously difficult and requires expert advice (Perez et al. 2017).

Clinical Presentation

IgG subclass deficiency may have no clinical consequences, while in other individuals, it can cause an increased susceptibility to (mainly) airway infections. Even patients with complete absence of multiple IgG subclasses may be asymptomatic. In symptomatic patients, infections are usually restricted to the upper airway infections (including otitis, sinusitis) and sometimes lower airway infections (bronchitis, pneumonia). Only rarely, individuals with IgG subclass deficiency have more serious (invasive) infections (such as osteomyelitis, meningitis, and septicemia). The presence of this type of infections should prompt a search for another cause of these infections. IgG3 deficiency may be associated with bronchial asthma.

When pulmonary bronchiectasis is present, other T- and B-cell defects ought to be excluded, such as common variable immunodeficiency in development (together with a low hypogammaglobulinemia and IgA or IgM deficiency), APDS (due to constitutively activated PI3K), ataxia-telangiectasia or other breakage syndromes, and NEMO deficiency (due to hypomorphous IKBKG mutations in male subjects).

In both abovementioned instances, an IgG subclass deficiency as the primary cause seems unlikely. Advice of a clinical immunologist can help to confirm the proper diagnosis.

Diagnosis

Diagnosis is made by IgG subclass measurement, and the clinical relevance of IgG subclass deficiency can be best underpinned by a polysaccharide vaccine response, using an unconjugated vaccine (such as 23-valent pneumococcal capsular polysaccharide vaccine).

Genetic analysis is not indicated unless progressive deterioration in clinical terms (fever, respiratory infections, bronchiectasis, weight loss, etc.), in lung function tests, or if suspected of a broader syndromic appearance.

Identifying children with clinically relevant IgG subclass deficiency and/or SPAD among the many children seen in everyday practice can be challenging. While in adults the IgG subclass levels and concomitant lack of polysaccharide reactivity reflect the inherent inability to mount an appropriate antibody response against encapsulated bacterial pathogens, in children these findings may change over time representing more of a developmental issue of the humoral immune response. Because of physiological maturation of the humoral immune system, it is probably not useful to measure IgG subclasses in patients under 2 years of age.

After 2 years of age, the antibody response to polysaccharide antigens after test immunization with an *unconjugated* pneumococcal (or other validated) polysaccharide vaccine is required to verify the humoral antibody reactivity. Different assays are available for testing specific antibody deficiency for pneumococcal antibodies. It is felt that the global assay may not be as sensitive as the serotype specific assay according to the WHO

protocol (PMID: 30682575, PMID: 28588580), which however is only offered by few centers.

The value of evaluation of lymphocyte and B-cell phenotyping in the context of IgG subclass deficiency has still not been fully evaluated.

Given potential changes in time follow-up, control of total IgG or subclasses may be required if clinically indicated in order to detect the transition into full-blown antibody deficiency or the transitory character of the antibody deficiency.

Pathophysiology

The exact pathophysiology of IgG subclass deficiency has not yet been elucidated.

In contrast to most adults, in children the findings of IgG subclass deficiency and/or SPAD may disappear before the age of 10–12, being a developmental maturation phenomenon. In very rare cases, mutations (deletions) in the gene encoding C-gamma-1, C-gamma-2, and C-gamma-3, underlying complete IgG subclass deficiency, have been reported, and these are without clinical symptoms (Kuijpers et al. 1992).

Routine genetic analysis is not indicated in patients with IgG subclass deficiency. IgG1 and IgG3 are the product of a T-cell-dependent B lymphocyte response; IgG1 and G3 subclass deficiency thus may also be caused by T-cell-related immune defects. IgG2 is more associated with antibody responses against the polysaccharides of encapsulated bacteria.

Apart from low IgG subclasses being the result of a primary immunodeficiency, they may also be caused secondarily to protein losing enteropathy, renal conditions, or the use of certain types of medication.

Therapy

As mentioned above, many individuals with IgG subclass deficiency are asymptomatic (expressing no increased frequency, duration, or severity of infections). These persons have no indication for treatment or prophylaxis, and it is commonly believed that they will have no long-term sequelae.

For patients who are symptomatic (preferably objectified by microbial cultures and/or imaging), the following treatments are commonly applied in a step-up manner:

1. Additional vaccinations. In patients who can mount an adequate response to conjugate vaccines, extra vaccinations against pneumococci and *Haemophilus influenzae* type b are often prescribed. There is no proof of efficacy of this type of protection.
2. Early treatment of (suspected) bacterial infections. By applying a watchful waiting strategy including treatment of bacterial infections early in their course, the burden of infections can be decreased.
3. Antibiotic prophylaxis for airway infections is offered for those with a considerable disease burden despite abovementioned measures. This type of prophylaxis is usually sufficient to significantly reduce the number of bacterial infections. Daily administration of low dose co-trimoxazole (trimethoprim-sulfamethoxazole) or an antibiotic with similar spectrum of activity is often used, usually prescribed during winter months and paused during spring and summer.
4. Immunoglobulin supplementation. Some patients with IgG subclass deficiency (especially those with recurrent pneumonia despite adequate antibiotic prophylaxis) have insufficient benefit of the abovementioned measures and benefit from immunoglobulin replacement therapy.

A limited period of 6–12 months of IgG substitution can be initiated under strict monitoring (infections, pulmonary symptoms, imaging). Monitoring and the comparison with historical findings prior to substitution therapy will help to determine the benefits of IgG substitution in a more objective manner. Also, if IgG substitution is considered beneficial and when substitution is continued in patients with IgG subclass deficiency or SPAD, it should be advised to stop substitution after 2 or 3 years – both in pediatric and adult

patients – and to retest the relevant immune parameters (including T- and B-cell counts) after (at least) 3–4 months washout period, together with polysaccharide vaccine responses to reconfirm the persistent and stable nature of the underlying immunodeficiency and continued need of IgG substitution.

No controlled trials have been published showing evidence of such an approach; however, a small number of non-controlled studies showed a benefit for IgG replacement in a subset of more severely affected IgG subclass deficiency patients (Hajjar et al. 2020).

A recent randomized-controlled crossover clinical trial was performed in 114 patients with IgG subclass deficiency and/or selective anti-polysaccharide antibody deficiency, who suffered from recurrent respiratory tract infections. This prospective trial showed that antibiotic prophylaxis or IgG substitution was equally effective in preventing infections. No differences could be found between the number and duration of infections and consequences of these infections. More adverse drug reactions occurred during IVIG treatment, but they were mostly mild and transient. The conclusion of this study can be that it is not useful to treat patients with IgG subclass deficiency upfront with IgG supplementation and to reserve this type of treatment for those who continue to have a severe burden of infections despite adequate alternative measures, including antibiotic prophylaxis [Dutch National Working Party on Immunodeficiencies, unpublished data].

Prognosis and Follow-Up

It is commonly believed that asymptomatic patients, and those that respond well on antibiotic prophylaxis, have a normal long-term prognosis. In a small fraction of patients, IgG subclass deficiency is the first finding of a later developing more severe primary antibody deficiency or other immunodeficiency. Therefore, serum immunoglobulin levels and if indicated other signs of immunodeficiency should be checked once every 1 to 2 years in patients during a watch-and-see approach.

References

Hajjar J, Nguyen AL, Constantine G, Kutac C, Syed MN, Orange JS, Sullivan KE. Prophylactic antibiotics versus immunoglobulin replacement in specific antibody deficiency. J Clin Immunol. 2020;40(1):158–64.

Kuijpers TW, Weening RS, Out TA. IgG subclass deficiencies and recurrent pyogenic infections, unresponsiveness against bacterial polysaccharide antigens. Allergol Immunopathol. 1992;20(1):28–34.

Meulenbroek AJ, Zeijlemaker WP. Human IgG subclasses: useful diagnostic markers for immunocompetence. 2nd ed. Amsterdam: CLB; 2000.

Nahm MH, Macke K, Kwon OH, Madassery JV, Sherman LA, Scott MG. Immunologic and clinical status of blood donors with subnormal levels of IgG2. J Allergy Clin Immunol. 1990;85(4):769–77.

Ochs HD, Stiehm ER, Winkelstein JA, et al. In: Ochs HD, Stiehm ER, Winkelstein JA, editors. Antibody deficiencies. In: Immunologic disorders in infants and children. 5th ed. Philadelphia: Elsevier; 2004.

Oxelius VA. Chronic infections in a family with hereditary deficiency of IgG2 and IgG4. Clin Exp Immunol. 1974;17(1):19–27.

Perez E, Bonilla FA, Orange JS, Ballow M. Specific antibody deficiency: controversies in diagnosis and management. Front Immunol. 2017;8:586.

Shackelford PG, Granoff DM, Madassery JV, Scott MG, Nahm MH. Clinical and immunologic characteristics of healthy children with subnormal serum concentrations of IgG2. Pediatr Res. 1990;27(1):16–21.

Terry WD, Fahey JL. Subclasses of human gamma-2-globulin based on differences in the heavy polypeptide chains. Science. 1964;146(3642):400–1.

Igα Deficiency

Vassilios Lougaris and Alessandro Plebani
Pediatrics Clinic and Institute for Molecular Medicine A. Nocivelli, Department of Clinical and Experimental Sciences, University of Brescia and ASST-Spedali Civili of Brescia, Brescia, Italy

Definition

Igα deficiency (OMIM #613501) is a rare primary immunodeficiency characterized by reduced serum levels of all immunoglobulin classes in the absence of peripheral B cells (peripheral B cells<2%). To date, a small number of patients have been described. Igα deficiency is caused by biallelic mutations in the gene encoding for CD79A, located in chromosome 19q13.2.

Pathogenesis

Early B cell development takes place in the bone marrow. An important maturational step is the progression from the pro-B to the pre-B stage (Espeli et al. 2006; Rudin and Thompson 1998; Bartholdy and Matthias 2004). This passage depends on the expression of a functional B-cell receptor composed of the μ heavy chain (*IGHM*; OMIM∗147020), Igα (CD79A; OMIM∗112205), Igβ (CD79B; OMIM∗147245), VpreB, and λ5 (*IGLL1*; OMIM∗146770) that initiates downstream signaling necessary for early B-cell differentiation through kinases such as BTK and *BLNK* (OMIM∗604615). Animal models and in vitro studies over the years have underlined the importance of each of the pre-BCR components and associated transcription factors for the transition from pro-B to pre-B stage of maturation (Conley and Cooper 1998).

Igα and Igβ form the signaling transducing elements that associate with the pre-BCR and allow the initiation of the downstream signaling cascade, rendering both valid candidates for this disease. In 1999, Minegishi et al. reported on the first patient with a mutation in the Igα gene, resulting in alternative exon 3 splicing of the gene product which abolishes the expression of the protein on the cell surface. The second male patient was reported in 2002 by Wang et al. and had a homozygous alteration at an invariant splice donor site of intron 2, which presumably resulted in the truncation of the protein. Khalili et al. reported in 2014 the third patient with a homozygous nonsense mutation in *CD79A*. Langereis et al. described a patient with compound heterozygous mutations, a previously splicing mutation and a frame shift (p.Cys119fs∗). Patient was diagnosed at age 2 and received immunoglobulin supplementation.

Clinical Presentation

Minegishi et al. reported the first patient affected with Igα deficiency: she was a female patient that presented chronic diarrhea with failure to thrive starting from her 1st month of life. At 1 year of age, she was admitted for bronchitis and neutropenia. Immunological work-up showed severely reduced levels of all immunoglobulin classes and absence of peripheral B cells. Bone marrow analysis evidenced a specific block at the transition from pro-B to pre-B cell. Interestingly, no lymph nodes were detectable during clinical examination. Wang et al. reported the second patient affected with Igα deficiency: he was a boy with a history of respiratory infections, diarrhea, and a dermatomyositis-like phenotype. Unfortunately, he died of a pulmonary infection. The female patient described by Khalili et al. in 2014 presented an unusual onset at the age of 6 months with a febrile convulsion that progressed in encephalitis; HHV8 and JC viruses were isolated from the CFS liquid. The patient progressively responded to broad-spectrum antibiotics, high-dose immunoglobulins, and antiviral treatment.

Diagnosis

Immunological work-up in affected patients shows almost undetectable levels of serum immunoglobulins and complete absence of peripheral B cells. T-cell number or functions are not affected. Once BTK mutations are excluded for male patients, genetic screening for mutations in components of the pre-BCR should be performed. Bone marrow studies show impaired maturation of B cells.

Management

As in other forms of primary humoral immunodeficiencies, immunoglobulin replacement treatment should be undertaken once the immunological diagnosis of agammaglobulinemia is established. Currently two options are available: intravenous or subcutaneous. Normally, a dose of 400 mg/kg/dose every 3–4 weeks is sufficient to maintain pre-infusion IgG levels >500 mg/dl that should be able to reduce the number of infectious episodes, especially that of invasive infections.

Antibiotic usage should be undertaken for every infectious episode, and in some case, prophylactic regimen may also be prescribed.

Considering the limited number of affected patients, long-term disease progression is not well- known. Respiratory function should be monitored because of the increased frequency of bronchiectasis and chronic lung disease in antibody deficiencies.

References

Bartholdy B, Matthias P. Transcriptional control of B cell development and function. Gene. 2004;327:1–23.

Conley ME, Cooper MD. Genetic basis of abnormal B cell development. Curr Opin Immunol. 1998;10(4): 339–406.

Espeli M, Rossi B, Mancini SJ, Roche P, Gauthier L, Schiff C. Initiation of pre-B cell receptor signaling: common and distinctive features in human and mouse. Semin Immunol. 2006;18:56–66.

Khalili A, Plebani A, Vitali M, Abolhassani H, Lougaris V, Mirminachi B, Rezaei N, Aghamohammadi A. Autosomal recessive agammaglobulinemia: a novel nonsense mutation in CD79a. J Clin Immunol. 2014;34(2):138–41.

Langereis JD, Henriet SS, Kuipers S, Weemaes CMR, van der Burg M, de Jonge MI, van der Flier M. IgM augments complement bactericidal activity with serum from a patient with a novel CD79a mutation. J Clin Immunol. 2018;38(2):185–92.

Minegishi Y, Coustan-Smith E, Rpalus L, Ersoy F, Campana D, Conley ME. Mutations in Igalpha (CD79a) result in a complete block in B cell development. J Clin Invest. 1999;104(8):1115–21.

Rudin CM, Thompson CB. B-cell development and maturation. Semin Oncol. 1998;25:435–46.

Wang Y, Kanegane H, Sanal O, Tezcan I, Ersoy F, Futatani T, Miyawaki T. Novel Igalpha (CD79a) gene mutation in a Turkish patient with B cell-deficient agammaglobulinemia. Am J Med Genet. 2002;108: 333–6.

Igβ Deficiency

Vassilios Lougaris and Alessandro Plebani
Pediatrics Clinic and Institute for Molecular
Medicine A. Nocivelli, Department of Clinical
and Experimental Sciences, University of Brescia
and ASST-Spedali Civili of Brescia, Brescia, Italy

Definition

Igβ deficiency (OMIM #612692) is a rare primary immunodeficiency characterized by reduced serum levels of all immunoglobulin classes in the absence of peripheral B cells (peripheral B cells <2%). To date, a small number of patients have been described. Igβ deficiency is caused by biallelic mutations in the gene encoding for CD79B.

Pathogenesis

Early B cell development takes place in the bone marrow. An important maturational step is the progression form the pro-B to the pre-B stage (Espeli et al. 2006; Rudin and Thompson 1998; Bartholdy and Matthias 2004). This passage depends on the expression of a functional B cell receptor composed of the μ heavy chain (*IGHM*; OMIM∗147020), Igα (CD79A; OMIM∗112205), Igβ (CD79B; OMIM∗147245), VpreB and λ5 (*IGLL1*; OMIM∗146770), that initiates downstream signalling necessary for early B cell differentiation through kinases such as BTK and *BLNK* (OMIM∗604615). Animal models and in vitro studies over the years have underlined the importance of each of the pre-BCR components and associated transcription factors for the transition from pro-B to pre-B stage of maturation (Conley and Cooper 1998).

Igα and Igβ form the signalling transducing elements that associate with the pre-BCR and allow the initiation of the downstream signalling cascade, rendering both essential for B cell differentiation and function.

In 2007, Dobbs et al. (2007) reported on a 15-year-old female patient with a hypomorphic, homozygous, mutation in Igβ (p.G137S), which impaired the binding with Igα and resulted in a leaky defect in B cell development. In the same year, Ferrari et al. (2007) reported on a 20-year-old male patient with a homozygous nonsense mutation in Igβ, resulting in a stop codon. Evaluation of the bone marrow revealed a complete block of B cell development at the pro-B to pre-B cell transition, closely resembling the one observed in the animal knockout model for this gene deficiency. Additional in vitro studies confirmed that the nonsense Igβ mutation abrogates the expression of the pre-BCR on the B cell surface. Lougaris et al. in 2014 reported on the third patient affected with Igβ deficiency due to a novel nonsense mutation in the CD79B gene.

Clinical Presentation

The patient described by Dobbs et al. carrying the hypomorphic mutation in Igβ presented recurrent lower respiratory tract infections from the age of 5 months. IVIG therapy was initiated at the age of 15 months with good clinical response. The patient reported by Ferrari et al. carrying the nonsense mutation in the Igβ gene was first admitted at the age of 8 months for pneumonia and Salmonella-caused enteritis; his immunological work-up showed a complete absence of peripheral B cells (CD19 <1%) and hypogammaglobulinemia. Intravenous immunoglobulin (IVIG) therapy was initiated immediately but the patient's clinical history was complicated by recurrent bronchitis, sinusitis, otitis media, and bacterial conjunctivitis. The third patient reported by Lougaris et al. harboring the novel nonsense mutation presented a history of mild respiratory infections. Her clinical history was complicated at the age of 14 months with the onset of fever, neutropenia, and ecthyma of the left gluteus caused by *Staphylococcus aureus*. Her immunological work-up showed panhypogammaglobulinemia with absence of peripheral B cells (CD19+ B cells: <1%). Antibiotic treatment and

IVIG were started with good clinical response. Her clinical conditions improved and neutropenia progressively resolved.

Diagnosis

Immunological work-up in patients with recurrent infections, most commonly respiratory, demonstrate undetectable levels of serum immunoglobulins and absence of peripheral B cells. T cell, NK cell number and function are not compromised. Once BTK mutations are excluded for male patients, genetic screening for mutations in components of the pre-BCR should be performed.

Management

As in other forms of primary humoral immunodeficiencies, immunoglobulin replacement treatment should be undertaken once the immunological diagnosis of agammaglobulinemia is established. Currently two options are available: intravenous or subcutaneous. Normally, a dose of 400 mg/kg/dose every 3–4 weeks is sufficient to maintain pre-infusion (trough) IgG levels >500 mg/dl that should be able to reduce the number and severity of infectious episodes, especially that of invasive infections.

Antibiotic usage should be undertaken for every infectious episode, and in some cases, when infections continue to occur, prophylactic regimen may be considered.

Considering the limited number of affected patients, long-term complications and prognosis are not well defined. Two of the three reported cases were diagnosed in adolescence. Nonetheless, antibody deficiencies are often associated with recurrent lung infections leading to low respiratory function (bronchiectasis, chronic lung disease).

References

Bartholdy B, Matthias P. Transcriptional control of B cell development and function. Gene. 2004;327:1–23.

Conley ME, Cooper MD. Genetic basis of abnormal B cell development. Curr Opin Immunol. 1998;10(4): 339–406.

Dobbs AK, Yang T, Farmer D, Kager L, Parolini O, Conley ME. Cutting edge: a hypomorphic mutation in Igbeta (CD79b) in a patient with immunodeficiency and a leaky defect in B cell development. J Immunol. 2007;179:2055–9.

Espeli M, Rossi B, Mancini SJ, Roche P, Gauthier L, Schiff C. Initiation of pre-B cell receptor signaling: common and distinctive features in human and mouse. Semin Immunol. 2006;18:56–66.

Ferrari S, Lougaris V, Caraffi S, Zuntini R, Yang J, Soresina A, Meini A, Cazzola G, Rossi C, Reth M, Plebani A. Mutations of the Igbeta gene cause agammaglobulinemia in man. J Exp Med. 2007;204: 2047–51.

Lougaris V, Vitali M, Baroniuo M, Moratto D, Tampella G, Biasini A, Badolato R, Plebani A. Autosomal recessive agammaglobulinemia: the third case of Igb deficiency due to a novel non-sense mutation. J Clin Immunol. 2014;34(4):425–7.

Rudin CM, Thompson CB. B-cell development and maturation. Semin Oncol. 1998;25:435–46.

IIAE1

▶ UNC93B1 Deficiency

IIAE2

▶ TLR3 Deficiency

IIAE3

▶ IRF3 Deficiency

IIAE5

▶ TRAF3 Deficiency

IKAROS (*IKZF1*) Deficiency

Attila Kumánovics
Department of Pathology, University of Utah,
Salt Lake City, UT, USA

Definitions

Dominant-negative variant: The heterozygous altered gene product inhibits the function of the wild-type one. One of the mechanisms that can cause dominant inheritance.

Hypomorphic variants cause an incomplete loss of gene function. The mechanism can be through reduced expression or reduced function.

Haploinsufficiency occurs when the loss of one of the two copies of a gene leads to disease or phenotype. One of the mechanisms that can cause dominant inheritance.

Germline sequence variants are present in the germ cells and inherited by the progeny. Somatic sequence variants are genetic alterations acquired by the non-germ cells; these can be passed on by mitotic cell division (as in a malignant cell growth), but are not inherited by the progeny.

De novo variants result from genetic alterations that occur in the germ cells of one of the parents or in the fertilized egg; therefore, the parents of the patient are unaffected.

Zinc finger is a protein structural motif stabilized by one or more zinc ions. The zinc fingers in IKAROS coordinate one zinc ion through two cysteine and two histidine residues (C_2H_2).

Next-generation sequencing (NGS) methods are various forms of high-throughput DNA sequencing technologies that were invented after Sanger sequencing ("next generation"). NGS is also known as massively parallel sequencing.

Introduction

IKAROS deficiency is a novel primary immunodeficiency disease, which affects the B-cell system most severely, but can present initially with either recurrent infections, cytopenias, autoimmunity, acute lymphoblastic leukemias or remain asymptomatic. Currently, there is no explanation for this variability, and routinely available laboratory tests provide no prognostic value. B-cell and antibody deficiency increases with age, but serum immunoglobulins and peripheral blood B-cell numbers only weakly correlate with the clinical course. No IKAROS-specific treatments are available, and management follows clinical presentation. Diagnosis requires the detection of pathogenic variants in the gene encoding IKAROS, called *IKZF1* (IKAROS family zinc finger 1).

Background

IKAROS deficiency was first described as an autosomal dominant primary immunodeficiency disease (PIDD) in 2016 (Kuehn et al. 2016), and within a year, additional cases have been reported all over the world (there are now over 50 cases identified), suggesting that it is not a rare cause of PIDDs and it occurs in many different ethnic backgrounds. The population frequency is unknown at this point.

IKZF1 is a novel gene to cause human disease, but the function of IKAROS has long been studied in various animal models (Heizmann et al. 2018). Mouse studies using complete loss-of-function, dominant-negative, and hypomorphic variants demonstrated that all hematopoietic lineages are affected by IKAROS expression, although the degree to which they are compromised by the loss of IKAROS varied greatly. Similar to human, B-cell development was found to be the most sensitive to decreased IKAROS function in mouse as well, but the development of all lymphoid, myeloid, megakaryocytic, and erythroid cells is affected in homozygous complete loss-of-function or dominant-negative mouse models. These studies demonstrated that IKAROS plays a role in many stages of B-cell development in the bone marrow and function in the periphery.

IKAROS was originally identified in mouse as a transcription factor that binds to the promoter of genes required for early lymphoid cell development (Heizmann et al. 2018). IKAROS can directly and indirectly activate or repress the expression of a large number of genes. It achieves this due to its direct DNA-binding activity and its interaction with large multimeric chromatin-remodeling complexes, which include acetylases, deacetylases, methylases, and others. IKAROS binds to DNA as a dimer; it can form homo- or heterodimers with other IKAROS family members (IKZF2–5). Structurally, the four N-terminal zinc fingers form the DNA-binding domain, whereas the two C-terminal zinc fingers form the dimerization domain.

All heterozygous missense variants described in PIDD patients thus far affect the DNA-binding zinc finger regions and were shown to be loss-of-function variants. In addition, whole-gene deletions and frameshift variants have been identified, strongly suggesting that the mechanism of IKAROS deficiency is haploinsufficiency (Bogaert et al. 2018; Hoshino et al. 2017; Kuehn et al. 2016; Yoshida et al. 2017). Since IKAROS works as part of a large complex or as a dimer, it is possible that some of the missense variants or in-frame deletions lead to dominant-negative effects (Heizmann et al. 2018): heterozygous pathogenic variants can lead to expression of a protein that can dimerize with the wild-type IKAROS expressed from the other allele but cannot bind to DNA, hence decreasing IKAROS function to less than 50%. Although no such effects have been published to date in germline IKAROS deficiency, dominant-negative variants are commonly seen as somatic variants in leukemias. Approximately 30% of pediatric B-cell ALL cases show somatic inactivation of *IKZF1*.

Clinical Presentation

IKAROS deficiency can present with (1) infections, (2) autoimmunity, (3) cytopenias, or (4) acute leukemias or (5) remain asymptomatic.

1. Recurrent infection is the most common clinical presentation in IKAROS deficiency (~50%), and the most common clinical diagnosis is common variable immunodeficiency (CVID). IKAROS-deficient CVID patients

do not have major distinguishing features. Patients can be diagnosed from early childhood to late in life. The infections seen in these patients are the same as in CVID, affecting mainly the respiratory tract, but diarrhea due to *Giardia lamblia*, *Blastocystis hominis*, and *Clostridium difficile* has also been reported. Mainly bacterial infections are seen, and *S. pneumoniae* is a common infectious organism in these patients. There is no evidence of increased susceptibility to viral or fungal infections, although *Pneumocystis jirovecii* pneumonia was reported. Similar to CVID in general, these patients can have autoimmune manifestations, mainly cytopenias, and have increased risk of hematological malignancies. The laboratory findings, however, often show a striking progressive decrease in B-cell numbers with age, which is only seen in a minority of CVID patients. The laboratory findings, such as serum immunoglobulins and B-cell counts, often appear more severe than the clinical course with mild infections in many of the cases. One possible explanation is the persistence of long-lived plasma cells in the bone marrow. As IKAROS-deficient patients often have normal B-cell counts during childhood, it is possible that plasma cells generated early in life provide lasting protection. This could be verified by additional bone marrow studies, but these are rarely done in CVID. Antibody response to vaccination is also variable, most patients reported had no response, but normal response was also seen. The fraction of patients with B-cell and antibody deficiency increases with age, but serum immunoglobulins and peripheral blood B-cell numbers only weakly correlate with the clinical course. Moreover, age cannot be the only risk factor, as antibody deficiency, leukemias, and autoimmunity often present very early in childhood, preceding B-cell deficiency. Overall, it is likely that the heterozygous loss of IKAROS leads to hematopoietic stem and progenitor cell defects that result in abnormal B-cell development.

Family history can indicate IKAROS deficiency. Majority of CVID patients have no known first-degree relatives with antibody deficiency, but a history consistent with an autosomal dominant inheritance increases the likelihood of IKZF1 deficiency, especially if B lymphopenia is present. It should be noted, however, that the absence of family history does not rule out IKAROS deficiency, as de novo mutations are the most common cause in most human dominant diseases, including *IKZF1* deficiency.

2. Autoimmunity is the second most common presentation in IKAROS deficiency (~20%). Autoimmunity can be either part of CVID or the primary clinical presentation. Autoimmune cytopenias, mainly immune thrombocytopenic purpura (ITP), are often seen in CVID and have been described in IKAROS-deficient CVID patients as well. Intriguingly, ITP with or without dysgammaglobulinemia can occur within the same family with *IKZF1* mutations. Moreover, familial ITP without recurrent infections can also occur. ITP is the most common, but not the only autoimmune, manifestation. In one IKAROS-deficient family, one sister was diagnosed with monocyclic systemic-onset juvenile idiopathic arthritis at the age of 6 and reactive arthritis at 9 years of age, whereas her younger sister was first seen for reactive arthritis at the ages of 3 and 5 and later diagnosed with myasthenia gravis confirmed by positive acetylcholine receptor auto-antibodies. IgA vasculitis was described in one IKAROS-deficient patient with bacterial pneumonias and agammaglobulinemia. SLE was diagnosed in one IKAROS-deficient 8-year-old boy, who at the time of diagnosis presented with elevated serum immunoglobulins but later developed hypogammaglobulinemia. The development of CVID or hypogammaglobulinemia in SLE is rare but has been reported before. Although SLE was only seen once with IKAROS mutation, genome-wide association studies (GWAS) identified genetic variants in *IKZF1* associated with SLE, supporting a connection between IKAROS and systemic autoimmunity.

3. Nonimmune cytopenias are a rare presentation of IKZF1 deficiency (<5%). Two patients have been reported with nonimmune pancytopenia at birth. Both patients required red blood cell and platelet transfusion after birth. One of the patients also required fetal red cell transfusion before delivered by emergency C-section due to fetal distress. Both patients had absence of B cells at birth with normal or increased T-cell counts. One patient was treated on day of life 47 with allogeneic bone marrow transplant following a reduced intensity myeloablative regimen but died at day 40 posttransplant due to multi-organ failure. The second patient was also planned for transplantation but started to recover from pancytopenia around 1 month of age and has survived without treatment. His B cells spontaneously recovered, although the hypogammaglobulinemia persisted. Red blood cell and platelet numbers also recovered. No somatic reversion in *IKZF1* was identified in the patients purified B cells (Hoshino et al. 2017).

Interestingly, the presentation of these two patients is very different from all the other published IKAROS-deficient patients. Both of them carried the heterozygous p.Tyr210Cys change, suggesting that there might be genotype-phenotype correlations in IKAROS deficiency. The exact effect of this Tyr-to-Cys change in the fourth DNA-binding zinc finger domain remains unknown at this point, as the experimental studies published by different groups disagree. Nonetheless, mouse studies clearly demonstrated that altering the different DNA-binding zinc finger domains (1 through 4) results in different phenotypes. Currently, p.Tyr210Cys is the only pathogenic variant in the fourth zinc finger to date. One patient was born in the USA to Caucasian parents, and the other is in Japan, suggesting that the effect is not specific to one ethnic group.

Mouse studies indicated that the development of all hematopoietic lineages requires IKAROS expression, including not only B and other lymphoid cells but also all myeloid cells, megakaryocytes, and red blood cells (Heizmann et al. 2018). It should be noted that most of these studies used complete loss-of-function mutant animals, whereas the IKAROS-deficient patients identified thus far are all heterozygous, perhaps explaining the difference. Although severe granulocyte defects were only seen in the two patients with the p.Tyr210Cys mutation, there are decreased numbers of nonclassical monocytes and plasmacytoid dendritic cells in the peripheral blood of most IKAROS-deficient patients. One study looked at red blood cells in patients with mutations other than the p.Tyr210Cys mutation and found no abnormalities.

4. Acute lymphoblastic leukemia (ALL). A minority (<5%) of IKAROS-deficient patients presented with ALL, suggesting smaller penetrance for ALL than for hypogammaglobulinemia. Still, this is a much higher risk than in the general population. Two of the patients presented with typical childhood B-cell ALL (positive for CD19, CD10, CD22, CD24, HLA-DR, CD34, and TdT). One of them died from relapse of ALL; the other was successfully transplanted after his ALL relapsed after chemotherapy. The third patient first presented with severe pulmonary infection and acute respiratory distress and was diagnosed with combined immunodeficiency due to nearly complete absence of B cells and low number of T cells with markedly reduced T-cell proliferation induced by mitogens. The patient was transplanted from her haploidentical mother at 10 months of age, but the graft was rejected. However, her T-cell numbers and mitogen-induced T-cell proliferation spontaneously recovered, although the B-cell numbers and hypogammaglobulinemia remained. Her infections continued, and she has developed a T-ALL (CD8[+]CD4[int]) at age 13. She had successful unrelated bone marrow transplantation after reduced intensity preconditioning (Yoshida et al. 2017).

   Although these three patients alone are not enough to draw solid conclusions about the risk of ALL in germline heterozygous IKAROS deficiency, it should be noted that somatic *IKZF1* variants are a hallmark of high-risk B-progenitor ALL, mainly in BCR-ABL1-positive (Philadelphia chromosome positive, Ph+) but also in Ph-like ALL. These somatic mutations occur as secondary events during clonal evolution. Germline variants in IKAROS are just now starting to be recognized as part of the childhood cancer predisposition syndromes. Germline disruptions of IKAROS are specifically associated with lymphoid malignancies in mouse models as well. Interestingly, in engineered mice, IKAROS deficiency leads to T-cell but not B-cell malignancies, and the penetrance is very high. These findings suggest that mutations in *IKZF1* are not the initiating events in leukemias, but loss of IKAROS activity leads to the acquisition of a hematopoietic stem cell-like phenotype with an altered gene expression profile (e.g., adhesion molecule expression and signaling), which can increase the risk of malignant transformation and stem cell exhaustion leading to progressive loss of B cells.

5. Based on family studies, about 25% of mutation carriers are clinically asymptomatic (Bogaert et al. 2018; Hoshino et al. 2017; Kuehn et al. 2016). It appears that some degree of antibody deficiency is present in almost all individuals carrying heterozygous loss-of-function mutations, but it may not always be severe enough to cause clinical disease. Based on the limited data currently available, the immunological penetrance (laboratory evidence of immunodeficiency) is close to complete (~95%), but the penetrance of clinical disease is estimated to be about 72–75% (Hoshino et al. 2017; Kuehn et al. 2016). The antibody deficiency in IKAROS deficiency is progressive and increases with age. This increasing risk strongly suggests that all germline IKZF1 mutation carriers may eventually develop clinical disease; therefore, regular follow-up is indicated.

As previously stated, the degree of B-cell and antibody deficiency only weekly correlates with clinical course, and mutation in carrier siblings with similar age and serum immunoglobulins may require immunoglobulin replacement therapy (IRT) for recurrent infections or report no significant infectious history and appear clinically unaffected. Moreover, age cannot be the primary risk factor, as ALL and autoimmunity often presents very early in childhood, preceding B-cell deficiency. This observation indicates that the clinical manifestations of IKAROS deficiency are not solely caused by loss of B cells and antibody production, but there is a functional defect in B cells, even early in life, when there is no numerical defect. This heterogeneity, including asymptomatic mutation carriers, is often seen in autosomal dominant PIDDs (e.g., GATA2, NFkB1).

Laboratory Findings/Diagnostic Testing

Diagnosis. There are no screening tests for IKAROS deficiency. IKZF1 should be in the differential diagnosis of CVID, autoimmunity and cytopenias, as well as ALLs, especially in familial cases. Due to the heterogeneous clinical presentation and lack of other specific tests, genetic testing is required for diagnosis. Gene panels and whole-exome (or genome) sequencing are the most prudent way to identify IKAROS deficiency. Gene panels for antibody deficiency diseases, combined immunodeficiencies, cytopenias, and ALL should now include *IKZF1*. If these are not available, exome (or genome) sequencing can be pursued. Genetic tests that include deletion/duplication testing are preferred, as partial- or whole-gene deletions are common causes of IKAROS deficiency both in inherited diseases and in leukemias and next-generation sequencing (massively parallel sequencing) often cannot identify large deletions and duplications. Whole- or partial-gene deletions, frameshift, and canonical splice site mutations lead to the loss of protein expression. In these cases, haploinsufficiency is the assumed mechanism. Missense mutations and some of the in-frame partial-gene deletions can have loss-of-function and/or dominant-negative effects. The pathogenicity of the missense mutations in the published studies was shown by the loss of characteristic pattern of DNA binding of the pathogenic IKAROS proteins, but these tests are not available clinically.

Heterozygous IKAROS deficiency in human subjects causes progressive B-cell and antibody deficiency (Kuehn et al. 2016). The workup for these patients should follow the general laboratory testing recommended for autoimmunity, cytopenias, or CVID. Flow cytometric examination of almost all IKAROS-deficient individuals, including those clinically asymptomatic, can identify abnormalities. Absolute B-cell deficiency is progressive and may not be present in pediatric patients. Declining fraction or count in class-switched B cells can be seen before the absolute B-cell deficiency manifests. Transitional B cells are often increased. Increase in CD8+ T cells and reversed CD4:CD8 ratios are usually seen. Both CD4+ and CD8+ cells appeared to be polyclonal, as detected by T-cell receptor Vβ flow cytometry. Nonclassical monocyte (CD16 positive) and plasmacytoid dendritic cell are usually decreased, and a subset of conventional dendritic cell (CD141 and CLEC9A positive) is increased. No consistent change in NK cell numbers or function has been noted.

Functional studies. Most patients tested had no antibody response to vaccination, but normal response was also seen. T-cell proliferation tests are usually normal, but in one patient with history of *Pneumocystis jirovecii* pneumonia, a poor response was seen to anti-CD3/CD28 antibody stimulation (Hoshino et al. 2017; Kuehn et al. 2016).

Among the autoimmune manifestations, thrombocytopenia is the most common. In one case, similar to ITP in general, antiplatelet antibodies were not detected, and bone marrow examination showed increased number of megakaryocytes without other significant abnormalities. The two cases of neonatal pancytopenia in p.Tyr210Cys mutation carriers suggests that cytopenia may be transient in these patients (Hoshino et al. 2017).

Although autoimmunity and hematological malignancies in general associated with PIDDs and CVID, but the risk for ALL is especially high in IKAROS deficiency. The risk cannot be estimated precisely currently, but thus far about 5% of IKAROS-deficient individuals presented with ALL. The role and frequency of leukemia monitoring are unknown at this point, especially in adults, as all the known ALL cases presented in the pediatric age range. Bone marrow biopsy was reported in six patients, demonstrating a highly variable defect in B-cell development, but its role of monitoring ALL is unknown.

Treatment/Prognosis

There is no specific treatment for IKAROS deficiency. Most of the IKAROS-deficient patients diagnosed with CVID are treated with immunoglobulin replacement therapy following standard regimens and have done well. Response to the treatment of ITP is reportedly highly variable. One patient did not respond to steroid therapy but anti-D immunoglobulin therapy controlled the disease for 2 years. The second episode of ITP in this patient was successfully treated with four doses of anti-CD20 therapy. Splenectomy was used successfully in one patient years before IKAROS deficiency was identified. Steroid treatment and high-dose intravenous immunoglobulin (IVIG) were needed in another patient to control thrombocytopenia.

Nonimmune neonatal pancytopenia due to IKAROS deficiency represents a special challenge, as these may improve spontaneously over a couple months; therefore, bone marrow transplantation may not be indicated. The acute treatment of these patients required frequent platelet and red blood cell transfusion. High doses of granulocyte colony-stimulating factor (G-CSF) did not increase the absolute neutrophil count in one patient with near zero absolute neutrophil count.

Somatic IKAROS inactivation is often seen in Ph + and Ph-like ALL cases and currently considered the best predictor of treatment failure in B-ALL even using chemotherapies incorporating tyrosine kinase inhibitors. These patients usually require bone marrow transplantation. Of the two patients with germline mutation in IKAROS who developed B-ALL, one died, and the other also relapsed following chemotherapy but had successful bone marrow transplantation. One patient with T-ALL was successfully treated with bone marrow transplantation. If relatives are considered as donors, they should be tested for the presence of the *IKZF1* mutation, as IKAROS deficiency is dominantly inherited and may be asymptomatic.

References

Bogaert DJ, Kuehn HS, Bonroy C, Calvo KR, Dehoorne J, Vanlander AV, Bruyne MD, Cytlak U, Bigley V, Baets FD, et al. A novel IKAROS haploinsufficiency kindred with unexpectedly late and variable B-cell maturation defects. J Allergy Clin Immunol. 2018;141:432–435.e7.

Heizmann B, Kastner P, Chan S. The Ikaros family in lymphocyte development. Curr Opin Immunol. 2018;51:14–23.

Hoshino A, Okada S, Yoshida K, Nishida N, Okuno Y, Ueno H, Yamashita M, Okano T, Tsumura M, Nishimura S, et al. Abnormal hematopoiesis and autoimmunity in human subjects with germline IKZF1 mutations. J Allergy Clin Immunol. 2017;140:223–31.

Kuehn HS, Boisson B, Cunningham-Rundles C, Reichenbach J, Stray-Pedersen A, Gelfand EW, Maffucci P, Pierce KR, Abbott JK, Voelkerding KV, et al. Loss of B cells in patients with heterozygous mutations in IKAROS. N Engl J Med. 2016;374: 1032–43.

Yoshida N, Sakaguchi H, Muramatsu H, Okuno Y, Song C, Dovat S, Shimada A, Ozeki M, Ohnishi H, Teramoto T, et al. Germline IKAROS mutation associated with primary immunodeficiency that progressed to T-cell acute lymphoblastic leukemia. Leukemia. 2017;31:1221–3.

IkB-Alpha Gain of Function

▶ Autosomal Dominant Anhidrotic Ectodermal Dysplasia with Immunodeficiency (AD-EDA-ID)

IKBKB Deficiency

Robert P. Nelson
Divisions of Hematology and Oncology, Stem
Cell Transplant Program, Indiana University (IU)
School of Medicine and the IU Bren and Simon
Cancer Center, Indianapolis, IN, USA
Pediatric Immunodeficiency Clinic, Riley
Hospital for Children at Indiana University
Health, Indianapolis, IN, USA
Medicine and Pediatrics, Indiana University
School of Medicine, Immunohematology and
Transplantation, Indianapolis, IN, USA

Synonyms

IκB kinase-beta; IKK2; IKKB; NF-κB IKB

Definition

IKBKB is the gene that encodes IκB kinase-beta
(IKK2), a key regulator of NF-κB activation. It is
located in chromosome 8p11.21.

Introduction

Transcription factors of the nuclear factor of
kappa B (NF-κB) family regulate immunological
function, cellular differentiation, proliferation,
and survival. NF-κB is maintained in an inactive
form in the cytoplasm by the inhibitory kappa B
kinase (IKK) complex, which consists of two
kinases IKBK-alpha (IKK1) and IKBK-beta
(IKK2) (Mercurio et al. 1997). Upon signaling,
IKK is phosphorylated, facilitating its degradation
that frees cytoplasmic NF-κB to translocate to the
nucleus. In the nucleus, NF-κB initiates transcription of a variety of inflammatory genes, including
interleukin-2 (IL-2) receptor alpha (Shirakawa
and Mizel 1989). IKK2, a key protein involved
with the canonical activation sequence of immune
cells, maps to chromosome 8p11.21. Several

signaling pathways converge at IKBKB, which
participates in the regulation of the innate host
defense, adaptive immunity, and epidermal
differentiation. Loss-of-function mutations in the
gene encoding IKBKB causes a combined human
T- and B-cell immunodeficiency (Delhase and
Karin 1999; Ambros et al. 1998).

Function

A diverse group of upstream stimuli advance
toward the IKK complex, including double
stranded RNA (virus infections), lipopolysaccharides (endotoxins), and inflammatory cytokines
(IL-1; TNF-α). IKBKB targets two adjacent serine
residues of IκB, rendering it susceptible to
ubiquitination and proteasome degradation,
enabling the release and translocation of cytoplasmic NF-κB to the nucleus. IKBKB function is
relevant to a number of common acute and
chronic inflammatory diseases, and dysregulated
constitutive activity of NF-κB inhibits apoptosis
and increases the frequency of transformative
neoplastic events.

Most clinical research concerning IKK2
predates its recognition as a cause of primary
immunodeficiencies. In this regard, IκB kinases
are constitutively expressed in fibroblasts from
patients with both rheumatoid and osteoarthritis,
and mutations in IKBKB, but not IKBKA, alter
TNF-α-mediated NF-κB nuclear translocation in
these diseases (Aupperle et al. 1999; Schmid and
Birbach 2008). Co-stimulation of TCR/CD3 and
CD28 receptors in T cells activates the Jun kinase
(JNK) cascade that plays a role in activating the
CD28 response element (CD28RE) in the IL-2
promoter. Kempiak provided evidence that the
activation of the CD28RE occurs in part by
"cross talk" with IKBKB, and Koshnan et al.
demonstrated that stimulation of primary human
CD4+ T cells by CD3/CD28 activates a hetero-
dimeric IKBKA/IKBKB and a homodimeric
IKBKB complex (Kempiak et al. 1999).

The widely used anti-inflammatory pharma-
ceuticals, aspirin and sodium salicylate, specifically inhibit IKK activity, and the binding of a

nonsteroidal to IKK2 impairs ATP binding (Yin et al. 1998). Sodium salicylate, an inhibitor of IKBKB, but not IKBKA, inhibits IL-2 promoter activation as well as IL-2 secretion. Recently, Homer3, an adaptor and signaling protein, was found to specifically associate with an ubiquitin-like domain of IKBKB in T cells. Although Homer3 is not required for NF-κB activation, the IKK complex appears to recruit Homer3 to the immune synapse, where it may play a role in the regulation of actin dynamics in T cells (Yatherajam et al. 2010).

Clinical Manifestations

Cuvelier et al. reported the largest and most recent cohort of IKBKB deficiency, describing 16 cases with early-onset bacterial, viral, fungal, and mycobacterial infections (Cuvelier et al. 2019). All patients carried a homozygous duplication–c.1292dupG in exon 13 of *IKBKB*, (R286X), associated with undetectable IKBKB. Pannicke et al. had analyzed four children from four Northern Cree families with the same *IKBKB* mutation (R286X), presenting with early-onset, severe viral, bacterial, and fungal infections consistent with severe combined immunodeficiency (SCID) (Pannicke et al. 2013). T- and B-cell numbers were normal, predominantly of the naïve phenotype. T-cell proliferation to mitogens and antigens were abnormal. Infections included oral candidiasis, parainfluenza virus type 1 and 3, pneumonias, and bloodstream infections with *Escherichia coli*, *Listeria monocytogenes* and *Serratia marcescens*. They presented with a homozygous, loss-of-function mutation in IKBKB.

Mousallem et al. reported four patients from two families who presented with early-onset fungal, viral, and bacterial infections and hypogammaglobulinemia (Mousallem et al. 2014). Nielsen et al. described an infant with a novel immunodeficiency related to homozygous nonsense (R272X) mutations in *IKBKB* (Nielsen et al. 2014). She presented early in life with respiratory insufficiency secondary to *Pneumocystis jirovecii*. At 9 months, she developed disseminated vaccination-associated *Mycobacterium bovis* infection that led to death at 14 months of age.

Cardinez et al. reported patients from two separate kindreds with a clinical presentation of recurrent upper respiratory infections, mild hypogammaglobulinemia, and features consistent with ectodermal dysplasia (Cardinez et al. 2018). Remarkably, they reported that the patients carried a heterozygous mutation in the *IKBKB* gene, appeared de novo in the probands and inherited in an autosomal dominant form, which changed the highly conserved valine at codon 203 for isoleucine (V203I). The mutant protein had kinase activity but was not stable. IkB-alpha phosphorylation was increased at resting state and after activation. Patients had T- and B-cell lymphopenia and impaired T-cell proliferation to mitogens and antigens. Thus, both loss-of-function and gain-of-function mutations in IKBKB result in different immunodeficiency syndromes.

Diagnostic and Laboratory Findings

Whereas B- and T-cell numbers may be normal by the standard immunophenotype screening tests, there may be decreases in the number of regulatory T cell and NK cells. T and B are mostly naïve (CD45RA+) cells and T-cell activation through the T-cell receptor is impaired. The patients might be hypo- or agammaglobulinemic. Functional analysis of T- and B-cell receptors, mitogens, toll-like receptors, and inflammatory cytokine receptors was abnormal. Gamma/delta T cells were absent. Laboratory findings in the Nielsen et al. report were similar to those observed with hyper-IgM syndrome. In the largest series, most had normal numbers of T and B cells, with naïve phenotype and severe hypo-gammaglobulinemia. T-cell receptor excision circles were normal (Cuvelier et al. 2019).

Analyses of lymphocyte function from affected patients suggest that human immunity may develop without functional IKBKB, but defects in IKBKB render mature lymphocytes unable to respond normally to a broad array of innate and antigen-based stimulation (Pannicke et al. 2013).

In cases presenting with IKBKB gain of function mutations, there was lymphopenia, mild hypogammaglobulinemia, and defective T-cell proliferation to mitogen and antigens of adult onset.

Treatment

To date, eight patients have received hematopoietic stem cell transplantation (HSCT), all reported by the Canadian group (Cuvelier et al. 2019). Graft sources were HLA matched parent or sibling ($n = 4$) or unrelated umbilical cord blood ($n = 4$). Methods varied with respect to conditioning and intensity; some of the patients had systemic infections at the time of transplant. Three patients receiving transplant were alive 6-month, 6-year, and 7-year post-HSCT. The spectrum of infections that patients with the IKBKB deficiency experience before and after transplant attests to the importance of IKBKB in mediating the innate and adaptive host defense. New viral, bacterial, fungal, and mycobacterial infections occur in patients at least 6 months after transplant and were still occurring years after transplant despite full and mixed lymphoid and myeloid donor chimerism and normal neutrophil and lymphocyte counts. One patient who developed tuberculous pneumonia at 1-year post-HSCT was successfully treated with antituberculosis medications and remains a long-term survivor.

All patients achieved normal numbers of CD3+, CD4+, CD8+, CD56+, and CD19+ cells post-HSCT. Immunoglobulin replacement was variable between patients and generally continued between 3- and 12-month post-HSCT. PHA responses were normal (above 50%) for all patients. Despite these findings, specific antibody production to post-transplant vaccinations once immunoglobulin was discontinued was deficient. Two patients did not make antipneumococcal antibodies, despite pneumococcal vaccinations or natural infection with *Streptococcus pneumoniae*. One patient received

six combined hepatitis A and B vaccinations and, despite this, did not make antibody against either. Detailed autopsy reports from 2 of the deceased exhibited severe thymic hypoplasia, minimal lymph tissue, and absence of germinal follicles in the spleen. One patient experienced secondary graft failure 3-year post-HSCT, developed disseminated mycobacterial infection, and died. At autopsy, the spleen was entirely replaced by atypical mycobacteria.

General precautions for immunodeficient patients should be considered. Inactivated childhood vaccines are indicated but live vaccines are not. BCG infection was reported in these patients. Other measures include the use of prophylactic antibiotics as indicated, with guidance informed by serial assessments of clinical and laboratory findings, including antibody production capacity.

Patients with a SCID phenotype can be treated with timely hematopoietic cell transplantation. An ideal outcome of allotransplantation for SCID is characterized as complete immunological reconstitution, minimal transplant-related toxicity, and achievement of full lymphohematopoietic donor chimerism without graft-versus-host disease (GVHD). Important hurdles that must be overcome for healthy survival include delays in diagnosis, identification of a suitable donor, delays in referral to a transplant center, lack of access, avoidance of severe conditioning toxicities, life-threatening infections, and long-term toxicities. The goal is the timely correction of immunological function (de la Morena and Nelson Jr. 2014).

Cross-References

▶ NF-Kappa-B Essential Modulator (NEMO) Deficiency

References

Ambros PF, Schmid J, Rumpler S, Binder BR, de Martin R. Localization of the human I-kappaB kinase-beta (IKBKB) to chromosome 8p11.2 by fluorescence in situ hybridization and radiation hybrid mapping. Genomics. 1998;54:575–6.

Aupperle KR, Bennett BL, Boyle DL, Tak PP, Manning AM, Firestein GS. NF-kappa B regulation by I kappa B kinase in primary fibroblast-like synoviocytes. J Immunol. 1999;163:427–33.

Cardinez C, Miraghazadeh B, Tanita K, et al. Gain-of-function IKBKB mutation causes human combined immune deficiency. J Exp Med. 2018;215:2715–24.

Cuvelier GDE, Rubin TS, Junker A, et al. Clinical presentation, immunologic features, and hematopoietic stem cell transplant outcomes for IKBKB immune deficiency. Clin Immunol. 2019;205:138–47.

de la Morena MT, Nelson RP Jr. Recent advances in transplantation for primary immune deficiency diseases: a comprehensive review. Clin Rev Allergy Immunol. 2014;46:131–44.

Delhase M, Karin M. The I kappa B kinase: a master regulator of NF-kappa B, innate immunity, and epidermal differentiation. Cold Spring Harb Symp Quant Biol. 1999;64:491–503.

Kempiak SJ, Hiura TS, Nel AE. The Jun kinase cascade is responsible for activating the CD28 response element of the IL-2 promoter: proof of cross-talk with the I kappa B kinase cascade. J Immunol. 1999;162:3176–87.

Mercurio F, Zhu H, Murray BW, et al. IKK-1 and IKK-2: cytokine-activated IkappaB kinases essential for NF-kappaB activation. Science. 1997;278:860–6.

Mousallem T, Yang J, Urban TJ, et al. A nonsense mutation in IKBKB causes combined immunodeficiency. Blood. 2014;124:2046–50.

Nielsen C, Jakobsen MA, Larsen MJ, et al. Immunodeficiency associated with a nonsense mutation of IKBKB. J Clin Immunol. 2014;34:916–21.

Pannicke U, Baumann B, Fuchs S, et al. Deficiency of innate and acquired immunity caused by an IKBKB mutation. N Engl J Med. 2013;369:2504–14.

Schmid JA, Birbach A. IkappaB kinase beta (IKKbeta/IKK2/IKBKB)–a key molecule in signaling to the transcription factor NF-kappaB. Cytokine Growth Factor Rev. 2008;19:157–65.

Shirakawa F, Mizel SB. In vitro activation and nuclear translocation of NF-kappa B catalyzed by cyclic AMP-dependent protein kinase and protein kinase C. Mol Cell Biol. 1989;9:2424–30.

Yatherajam G, Banerjee PP, McCorkell KA, et al. Cutting edge: association with I kappa B kinase beta regulates the subcellular localization of Homer3. J Immunol. 2010;185:2665–9.

Yin MJ, Yamamoto Y, Gaynor RB. The anti-inflammatory agents aspirin and salicylate inhibit the activity of I (kappa)B kinase-beta. Nature. 1998;396:77–80.

IKK-Gamma Deficiency

▶ Anhidrotic Ectodermal Dysplasia with Immunodeficiency (EDA-ID), X-linked

IL-1 Receptor Antagonist

▶ Deficiency of the IL-1 Receptor Antagonist (DIRA)

IL-17R Deficiency

▶ Chronic Mucocutaneous Candidiasis: IL-17RA Deficiency

IL-1Ra

▶ Deficiency of the IL-1 Receptor Antagonist (DIRA)

IL-21 Deficiency

▶ Interleukin-21 Deficiency

IL-21 Receptor (IL-21R) Deficiency

Robert P. Nelson
Divisions of Hematology and Oncology, Stem Cell Transplant Program, Indiana University (IU) School of Medicine and the IU Bren and Simon Cancer Center, Indianapolis, IN, USA
Pediatric Immunodeficiency Clinic, Riley Hospital for Children at Indiana University Health, Indianapolis, IN, USA
Medicine and Pediatrics, Indiana University School of Medicine, Immunohematology and Transplantation, Indianapolis, IN, USA

Synonyms

IL-21R deficiency

Definition

IL-21R deficiency results from deleterious mutations in the *IL21R* gene, located in chromosome 16p12. IL-21R-deficient patients present with cellular and humoral immunity defects, including variable NK cell dysfunction.

Introduction

Cytokines regulate the immune system by regulating lymphocyte development, survival, differentiation, and function. Cytokine binding to their specific receptors on immune cells results in intracellular signaling pathways that activate specific transcription factors and promote certain gene expression. IL-21 receptor is a type I cytokine receptor that shares homology with the beta subunit of the IL-2 receptor and associates with the IL-2R common gamma chain (γc) for function (Asao et al. 2001). Unlike γc-deficiency, IL-21R deficiency is not associated with severe combined immunodeficiency (SCID), but rather a life-threatening combined immunodeficiency that presents in late childhood.

The gene for the interleukin-21 receptor (IL-21R) had first been reported to be associated with the oncogene *BCL6* in t(3;16)(q27;p11) translocation found in patients with diffuse, large B cell lymphoma (Ueda et al. 2002). The IL-21R receptor system contains the common cytokine-receptor γ chain that is associated with IL-2, IL-4, and IL-15. Loss-of-function mutations in γ chain cause human X-linked severe combined immunodeficiency (SCID).

Function

Innate Host Defense

IL-21 affects dendritic cells and NK cells; NK cells express a low-affinity receptor for the Fc region of immunoglobulin G (FcγRIIIa). Following FcR stimulation in vitro, there is an increase in transcription of IL-21R that peaks at approximately 8 h. The increased expression of the IL-21R sensitizes NK cells to IL-21 stimulation,

leading to increased phosphorylation of STAT1 and STAT3 (Wendt et al. 2007).

IL21/IL-21R system is also involved in the pathogenesis of muscle inflammatory diseases. IL21R is upregulated in the endothelial cells from ischemic muscle in mice and humans. Patients with peripheral artery disease have 1.7-fold higher levels of circulating IL-21 than normal individuals (Wang et al. 2016).

Adaptive Immunity

IL-21 promotes proliferation of T and B cells and the cytolytic activity of NK cells (Parrish-Novak et al. 2002). This cytokine appears to be important for a durable, T cell response to viral infections (Frohlich et al. 2009). Interaction with the IL-21R on CD8+ T cells helps to maintain cell proliferation and cytokine production. Mice with mutated IL-21R can expand functional CD8+ T cells, regulate memory homeostasis, and execute recall responses to nonpersistent viruses; however, IL-21R signaling is required for the sustenance of T cell responsiveness during chronic viral infections (Yi et al. 2009). The binding of IL-21 to its receptor regulates the activation and proliferation of T cells, B cells, and NK cells through activating JAKs-STATs signaling pathways.

The IL-21/IL-21R signaling axis regulates cytokine production of T cells by enhancing the expression of T-bet and STAT4 in human T cells, resulting in an augmented production of IFN-gamma; mice deficient in IL-21 or IL-21R generate reduced inflammatory responses following parasitic infections, such as toxoplasmosis (Stumhofer et al. 2013). Borte et al. demonstrated that combination of IL-21, IL-4, and anti-CD40 stimulation induced class-switch recombination to IgG and IgA and differentiation to Ig-secreting cells in patients with common variable immunodeficiency and isolated IgA deficiency (Borte et al. 2009).Conversely, IL-21R-deficient mice present reduced numbers of germinal center and IgA+ B cells and decrease of intestine IgA+ plasmablasts and plasma cells, leading to higher bacterial burdens and subsequent expansion of Th17 and Treg cells (Cho et al. 2019).

Clinical Manifestations

The spectrum of microbial infections that may affect patients with IL-21R deficiency includes encapsulated bacteria, viruses, and fungi, and the most common sites of infection are the gastrointestinal tissues and lungs. In addition, patients might report opportunistic pathogens and develop cryptosporidiosis, norovirus, and atypical *Mycobacterium* infections.

IL-21 was first reported in two kindreds (Kotlarz et al. 2013). A 4-year-old boy born to consanguineous parents of Lebanese descent developed chronic upper respiratory infections and liver failure secondary to chronic cryptosporidiosis. His liver was found completely cirrhotic, and he received a liver transplant, after which examination of the resected liver revealed purulent cholangitis associated with marked epithelial and lymphoid hyperplasia. His 10-year-old sister experienced recurrent pneumonia, chronic diarrhea, failure to thrive, sinusitis, *Helicobacter pylori*-associated gastritis, and esophageal candidiasis. Her liver was also large, with dilated biliary tract system, lymphadenopathy, extensive fibrosis, and *Cryptosporidium* infection in the bile ducts and duodenum. Thus, the predominant clinical findings in both siblings were severe cholangitis and liver fibrosis associated with cryptosporidiosis. Two distinct homozygous loss-of-function mutations in the *IL-21R* were detected and found to cause aberrant trafficking of the IL-21R to the plasma membrane, abrogation of IL-21 ligand binding, and impaired phosphorylation of STAT1, STAT3, and STAT5.

The second kindred included two brothers from a consanguineous Colombian family who experienced recurrent otitis media, *P. jirovecii* pneumonia, recurrent *P. aeruginosa*, and *S. pneumoniae* pneumonias and bronchiectasis and liver disease secondary to *Cryptosporidium* sp. infection. Laboratory evaluation revealed low numbers and functional defects in lymphocytes. Gene sequencing demonstrated nonsynonymous variants that were both rare and homozygous in both patients; amino acid substitutions in the protein abrogated phosphorylation of downstream mediators. STAT proteins phosphorylation

via other γc-related cytokines (IL-2, IL-4, and IL-15) was not affected by the IL-21R mutation. Serum IgE was increased in all cases.

Stepensky and collaborators reported a 5-year-old girl with a deleterious homozygous mutation in IL-21R gene who presented with hypogammaglobulinemia and *P. jirovecii* pneumonia, but without gastrointestinal pathology (Stepensky et al. 2015). She required prolonged mechanical ventilation. Immunology testing revealed reduced IgG and IgA, while IgM was increased. Lymphocyte subset numbers, proliferative response to mitogens, T cell receptor Vβ repertoire, and T cell receptor excision circle (TREC) numbers) were normal. CD40L upregulation was impaired.

IL-21R deficiency might present with NK cell lymphopenia. Erman et al. reported a 7-year-old boy born to consanguineous parents with chronic diarrhea since infancy (Erman et al. 2015). He had failure to thrive, sclerosing cholangitis, tinea corporis, and recurrent otitis media, but no pneumonia. His sister had chronic diarrhea and died at the age of 5. Genetic testing revealed a homozygous frameshift mutation in the IL-*21R* gene, causing a premature stop codon (p.Asp179Thrfs∗51). Immunological testing showed normal B and T cell counts, and natural killer (NK) cells were almost absent. T cell proliferation to antigens and mitogens was impaired. There was increased transitional B cells with decreased switched memory B cells. Normal serum immunoglobulin levels in the patient suggested sufficiency of IL21R-independent pathways for plasma cell differentiation despite near absence of memory B cells. Serum IgE was elevated.

The above experiences suggest that IL-21R deficiency presents with a form of combined immunodeficiency, with variable presentation.

Laboratory Findings and Diagnosis

IL-21R-deficient patients may be initially diagnosed with common variable immunodeficiency before opportunistic infections occur. Antibody levels may be low or normal and IgE levels normal, increased, or quite elevated. Antibody responses may be intact to tetanus toxoid vaccine but not to the pneumococcal vaccine. Immunophenotyping reveals low or normal T and NK cells. B cells may be normal or high, but number of switched memory B cells are consistently low. T cell proliferation to mitogens and antigens may be normal or reduced. NK may show impaired NK cell lysis of 51^{Cr}-labeled K562 target cells, but normal antibody-dependent cellular cytotoxicity.

Treatment and Prognosis

An index of suspicion will enable early laboratory testing to expedite management. *Cryptosporidium*-associated cholangitis in a non-HIV-infected patient may prompt consideration of PIDs, in which case the differential diagnosis includes HLA class II deficiency, hyper-IgM syndrome, and IL-21 defects.

Referral to centers for the management of primary immunodeficiency diseases should be considered. Preventive measures for immunocompromised patients are recommended. Inactivated immunizations are indicated but live vaccines are not.

Extreme isolation or avoidance of normal schooling may not be necessary or recommended, but rather prompt medical evaluation for early unusual consequences of infection is paramount to the care of patients with combined immunodeficiencies.

Hematopoietic cell transplantation (HSCT) is a potentially curative procedure but one that can shorten the patient's life span as well. Presence of *Cryptosporidium* sp. infection, which is common in IL-21R deficiency, has been shown to increase mortality in HSCT for CD40L deficiency. The index patient underwent transplant, and the clinical course was complicated by abdominal abscesses, pneumonia, recurrent septicemia, systemic cytomegalovirus infection, and subsequent multiorgan failure leading to death on day +542. His sibling underwent HLA-identical HSCT, and the post-transplant was complicated by increased cholangitis, cytomegalovirus infection, and graft rejection that necessitated a second transplant that was complicated by multiorgan failure and death on day +84.

Although the targeting of the IL-21/IL-21R signaling axis may provide novel approaches to the prevention or treatment of certain infections, autoimmune illness, and cancer, medications that alter the IL-21/IL-21R circuit will likely generate iatrogenic risks that will require recognition, definition, and therapeutic strategies. It is also possible that rigorous inquiry into this cytokine signaling may provide an adjunct to transplant therapy (Tormo et al. 2017).

Cross-References

▶ HLA Class I Deficiency
▶ IL-21 Deficiency

References

Asao H, Okuyama C, Kumaki S, Ishii N, Tsuchiya S, Foster D, Sugamura K. Cutting edge: the common gamma-chain is an indispensable subunit of the IL-21 receptor complex. J Immunol. 2001;167:1–5.

Borte S, Pan-Hammarstrom Q, Liu C, et al. Interleukin-21 restores immunoglobulin production ex vivo in patients with common variable immunodeficiency and selective IgA deficiency. Blood. 2009;114:4089–98.

Cho H, Jaime H, de Oliveira RP, Kang B, Spolski R, Vaziri T, Myers TG, et al. Defective IgA response to atypical intestinal commensals in IL-21 receptor deficiency reshapes immune cell homeostasis and mucosal immunity. Mucosal Immunol. 2019;12:85–96.

Erman B, Bilic I, Hirschmugl T, Salzer E, Çagdas D, Esenboga S, et al. Combined immunodeficiency with CD4 lymphopenia and sclerosing cholangitis caused by a novel loss-of-function mutation affecting IL21R. Haematologica. 2015;100(6):e216–9.

Frohlich A, Kisielow J, Schmitz I, et al. IL-21R on T cells is critical for sustained functionality and control of chronic viral infection. Science. 2009;324:1576–80.

Kotlarz D, Zietara N, Uzel G, et al. Loss-of-function mutations in the IL-21 receptor gene cause a primary immunodeficiency syndrome. J Exp Med. 2013;210:433–43.

Parrish-Novak J, Foster DC, Holly RD, Clegg CH. Interleukin-21 and the IL-21 receptor: novel effectors of NK and T cell responses. J Leukoc Biol. 2002;72:856–63.

Stepensky P, Keller B, Abuzaitoun O, Shaag A, Yaacov B, Unger S, et al. Extending the clinical and immunological phenotype of human interleukin-21 receptor deficiency. Haematologica. 2015;100(2):e72–6.

Stumhofer JS, Silver JS, Hunter CA. IL-21 is required for optimal antibody production and T cell responses during chronic *Toxoplasma gondii* infection. PLoS One. 2013;8(5):e62889.

Tormo A, Khodayarian F, Cui Y, et al. Interleukin-21 promotes thymopoiesis recovery following hematopoietic stem cell transplantation. J Hematol Oncol. 2017;10:120.

Ueda C, Akasaka T, Kurata M, et al. The gene for interleukin-21 receptor is the partner of BCL6 in t (3;16)(q27;p11), which is recurrently observed in diffuse large B-cell lymphoma. Oncogene. 2002;21:368–76.

Wang T, Cunningham A, Houston K, Sharma AM, Chen L, Dokun AO, et al. Endothelial interleukin-21 receptor up-regulation in peripheral artery disease. Vasc Med. 2016;21(2):99–104.

Wendt K, Wilk E, Buyny S, Schmidt RE, Jacobs R. Interleukin-21 differentially affects human natural killer cell subsets. Immunology. 2007;122:486–95.

Yi JS, Du M, Zajac AJ. A vital role for interleukin-21 in the control of a chronic viral infection. Science. 2009;324:1572–6.

IL-21R Deficiency

▶ IL-21 Receptor (IL-21R) Deficiency

Immune-Osseous Dysplasia

▶ Schimke Immuno-osseous Dysplasia

Immunodeficiency 31C (IMD31C)

▶ Chronic Mucocutaneous Candidiasis, STAT1 Gain of Function

Immunodeficiency 51 (IMD51)

▶ Chronic Mucocutaneous Candidiasis: IL-17RA Deficiency

Immunodeficiency with Multiple Intestinal Atresias (TTC7A)

Silvia Giliani[1] and Gaetana Lanzi[2]
[1]Department of Molecular and Translational Medicine, University of Brescia, Brescia, Italy
[2]Department of Molecular and Translational Medicine, University of Brescia, Angelo Nocivelli Institute for Molecular Medicine, Brescia, Italy

Synonyms

KIAA1140; TTC7

Definition

Multiple intestinal atresia and combined immunodeficiency MIA-CID (MIM 243150) is an autosomal recessive disorder caused by mutations in the TTC7A gene (MIM 609332).

Introduction/Background

Tetratricopeptide repeat domain 7A (TTC7A) is a gene encoding for the TTC7A protein, characterized by the tetratricopeptide repeat (TPR) region. This domain is known to be involved in protein-protein interaction in the assembly of multiprotein complexes. Proteins containing TPR domains are involved in multiple crucial biological processes, such as cell cycle regulation and transcriptional control.

TTC7A has been shown to interact with EFR3 and phosphatidylinositol 4-kinase

(PI4KA-PI4KIIIα), which in turn catalyzes the conversion of phosphatidylinositol to phosphatidylinositol 4-phospate (PI4P), primary blocks of phosphoinositides involved in plasma membrane functions, polarity, and homeostasis (Avitzur et al. 2014; Lees et al. 2017; Chen et al. 2013). Lack of TTC7A diminished transport of the PI4KIIIα enzyme from the Golgi to the plasma membrane blocking phosphatidylinositol phosphorylation, which is crucial in cell polarity maintenance (Kammermeier et al. 2016).

TTC7A protein is mainly expressed in thymocytes and enterocytes, thus its crucial role in these cell types' homeostasis. Its lack is known to lead to a reduction in thymocytes and enterocytes, as TTC7A depletion affects actin cytoskeleton rearrangements enhancing RhoA signaling, being required in its regulated form for all the major cellular functions, such as polarization, proliferation, and migration (Lemoine et al. 2014).

Clinical Presentation

Lack of TTC7A leads to different degrees of intestinal epithelial disruption. In the most severe form, multiple intestinal atresias (MIA) are evident even in the antenatal period, requiring immediate surgical interventions soon after birth. These cases are usually associated with different forms of immunodeficiency, usually lacking T-lymphocytes (Samuels et al. 2013; Chen et al. 2013; Bigorgne et al. 2014; Notarangelo 2014). More recently TTC7A deficiency has been described in association with early-onset IBD (Avitzur et al. 2014), but also isolates MIA or isolated CID were described (Lien et al. 2017), extensive enteropathy or apoptotic enterocolitis, a clinical phenotype resembling CVID (Lawless et al. 2017), enteropathy-lymphocytopenia-alopecia (Lemoine et al. 2014), or tricho-hepato-enteric syndrome (SD/THE) (Neves et al. 2017). In this broad spectrum of clinical phenotypes involving at the moment less than 50 cases (Lien et al. 2017), some intermediate cases with mild immunological and intestinal involvement have also been published, such as one case resembling CVID (Lawless et al. 2017).

Autoimmune manifestations (hemolysis, thyroiditis, alopecia, diabetes, psoriasis, and onychomycosis) are frequently associated with the different forms of TTC7A deficiency (Lien et al. 2017) as well as different dermatological features, in particular ichthyosis (Leclerc-Mercier et al. 2016). The CID/SCID phenotype is mainly caused by the not-organized thymus in which lymphocytes could not develop properly. Early fatal outcome is usually related to sepsis or intestinal obstructions, underlying the impairment of both epithelial cells and lymphocytes, which cooperatively causes the disorder (Lemoine et al. 2014).

Laboratory Findings/Diagnosis

The high heterogeneity of the clinical presentations does not allow depicting a single laboratory protocol for the diagnosis of the disease, but in the most severe cases, MIA is evident soon after birth. In those cases usually, the immunological phenotype displays severe T cell lymphopenia in all the subsets, with variably reduced number of B and NK cells and low TRECs number consistent with thymopoiesis impairment leading to a CID phenotype (Fullerton et al. 2018); moreover proliferative T cell response to PHA and anti-CD3 is markedly reduced as is reduced immunoglobulin production. All these laboratory findings are consistent with high occurrence of severe bacterial and viral infections in the patients.

These CID-MIA patients are often hypogammaglobulinemic, requiring IVIG administration, and do not respond to vaccinations displaying lymphoid depletion.

Thymus biopsies in multiple observations showed different abnormalities: small size and depleted organization, with few and small Hassall's corpuscles and a not-defined cortico-medullary organization (Chen et al. 2013; Bigorgne et al. 2014).

The gut in MIA is characterized by severe villous atrophy, with evidences of apoptosis and abolition of epithelial organization probably due to the in vitro demonstrated inversion of the apicobasal polarity (Bigorgne et al. 2014; Avitzur et al. 2014).

A final diagnosis is achieved by gene sequencing of the TTC7A gene. Mutations have been described on all the length of the gene and include all the possible kind of mutations, with a possible founder effect for a 4nucleotide deletion in exon 7 found in multiple French-Canadian patients with MIA-CID (Samuels et al. 2013). There not seems to exist a genotype-phenotype correlation, as the same mutation could give the complete MIA-CID phenotype, or only the MIA one, but it seems clear that the more severe cases usually do not express TTC7A protein, while cases with a phenotype limited to bowel with no MIA usually express protein at low levels as a result of double missense mutations (Samuels et al. 2013). What is not yet clear is if a partial defect due to hypomorphic mutations could affect only the expression in the intestinal epithelium, while more severe mutations could affect also the thymus giving the more complex clinical phenotype.

Treatments

Due to the broad range of clinical presentation, no standardized protocol for TTC7A deficiency treatment is actually in use. The kind of treatment is usually dictated by the clinical phenotype. The soon after birth bowel resection is the needed intervention to remove atresias, and liver and small bowel transplantation could be an option (Gilroy et al. 2004; Lien et al. 2017). In the MIA cases with CID phenotype, hematopoietic stem cell transplantation has been attempted to correct the thymus defect. Treatment demonstrated efficacy and safeness from the immunological point of view, but the persistent lack of TTC7A in the enterocytes hesitates in HSCT as a non-definitive curative measure with refractory diarrhea and fatal outcome in the need for intestinal transplantation (Lien et al. 2017) Anyhow longer follow-up data on HSCT in TTC7A deficiency will help to understand whether the treatment will be at least partially efficient (Kammermeier et al. 2016).

In cases characterized by isolated enteropathy, usually total parenteral nutrition (TPN) is required for life, while in cases with mild immune involvement, IVIG and antibiotic prophylaxis will be added. Refractory diarrhea seen in apoptotic enteropathy usually does not respond to immunosuppression with steroids, azathioprine, methotrexate, cyclosporine, sirolimus, tacrolimus, and anti-TNF-α agonists (Lien et al. 2017).

Due to TTC7A involvement in modulation of Rho kinase activity and effective use in vitro of Rho kinase (ROCK) inhibitors to revert enterocytes apoptosis in patients' organoids, it has been suggested that the use of ROCK inhibitors could become a possible therapeutic option (Bigorgne et al. 2014).

References

Avitzur Y, Guo C, Mastropaolo LA, Bahrami E, Chen H, Zhao Z, Elkadri A, Dhillon S, Murchie R, Fattouh R, Huynh H, Walker JL, Wales PW, Cutz E, Kakuta Y, Dudley J, Kammermeier J, Powrie F, Shah N, Walz C, Nathrath M, Kotlarz D, Puchaka J, Krieger JR, Racek T, Kirchner T, Walters TD, Brumell JH, Griffiths AM, Rezaei N, Rashtian P, Najafi M, Monajemzadeh M, Pelsue S, McGovern DP, Uhlig HH, Schadt E, Klein C, Snapper SB, Muise AM. Mutations in tetratricopeptide repeat domain 7A result in a severe form of very early onset inflammatory bowel disease. Gastroenterology. 2014;146(4): 1028–39.

Bigorgne AE, Farin HF, Lemoine R, Mahlaoui N, Lambert N, Gil M, Schulz A, Philippet P, Schlesser P, Abrahamsen TG, Oymar K, Davies EG, Ellingsen CL, Leteurtre E, Moreau-Massart B, Berrebi D, Bole-Feysot C, Nischke P, Brousse N, Fischer A, Clevers H, de Saint Basile G. TTC7A mutations disrupt intestinal epithelial apicobasal polarity. J Clin Invest. 2014;124(1):328–37.

Chen R, Giliani S, Lanzi G, Mias GI, Lonardi S, Dobbs K, Manis J, Im H, Gallagher JE, Phanstiel DH, Euskirchen G, Lacroute P, Bettinger K, Moratto D, Weinacht K, Montin D, Gallo E, Mangili G, Porta F, Notarangelo LD, Pedretti S, Al-Herz W, Alfahdli W, Comeau AM, Traister RS, Pai SY, Carella G, Facchetti F, Nadeau KC, Snyder M, Notarangelo LD. Whole-exome sequencing identifies tetratricopeptide repeat domain 7A (TTC7A) mutations for combined immunodeficiency with intestinal atresias. J Allergy Clin Immunol. 2013;132(3):656–664.e17.

Fullerton BS, Velazco CS, Hong CR, Carey AN, Jaksic T. High Rates of Positive Severe Combined Immunodeficiency Screening Among Newborns with Severe

Intestinal Failure. JPEN J Parenter Enteral Nutr. 2018;42(1):239–46.

Gilroy RK, Coccia PF, Talmadge JE, et al. Donor immune reconstitution after liver-small bowel transplantation for multiple intestinal atresia with immunodeficiency. Blood. 2004;103:1171–4.

Kammermeier J, Lucchini G, Pai SY, Worth A, Rampling D, Amrolia P, Silva J, Chiesa R, Rao K, Noble-Jamieson G, Gasparetto M, Ellershaw D, Uhlig H, Sebire N, Elawad M, Notarangelo L, Shah N, Veys P. Stem cell transplantation for tetra-tricopeptide repeat domain 7A deficiency: long-term follow-up. Blood. 2016;128(9):1306–8.

Lawless D, Mistry A, Wood PM, Stahlschmidt J, Arumugakani G, Hull M, Parry D, Anwar R, Carter C, Savic S. Bialellic Mutations in Tetra-tricopeptide Repeat Domain 7A (TTC7A) Cause Common Variable Immunodeficiency-Like Phenotype with Enteropathy. J Clin Immunol. 2017;37(7):617–22.

Leclerc-Mercier S, Lemoine R, Bigorgne AE, Sepulveda F, Leveau C, Fischer A, Mahlaoui N, Hadj-Rabia S, de Saint Basile G. Ichthyosis as the dermatological phenotype associated with TTC7A mutations. Br J Dermatol. 2016;175(5):1061–4.

Lees JA, Zhang Y, Oh MS, Schauder CM, Yu X, Baskin JM, Dobbs K, Notarangelo LD, De Camilli P, Walz T, Reinisch KM. Architecture of the human PI4KIIIα lipid kinase complex. Proc Natl Acad Sci USA. 2017;114(52):13720–5.

Lemoine R, Pachlopnik-Schmid J, Farin HF, Bigorgne A, Debré M, Sepulveda F, Héritier S, Lemale J, Talbotec C, Rieux-Laucat F, Ruemmele F, Morali A, Cathebras P, Nitschke P, Bole-Feysot C, Blanche S, Brousse N, Picard C, Clevers H, Fischer A, de Saint Basile G. Immune deficiency-related enteropathy-lymphocytopenia-alopecia syndrome results from tetratricopeptide repeat domain 7A deficiency. J Allergy Clin Immunol. 2014;134(6):1354–1364.e6.

Lien R, Lin YF, Lai MW, Weng HY, Wu RC, Jaing TH, Huang JL, Tsai SF, Lee WI. Novel Mutations of the Tetratricopeptide Repeat Domain 7A Gene and Phenotype/Genotype Comparison. Front Immunol. 2017;8:1066.

Neves JF, Afonso I, Borrego L, Martins C, Cordeiro AI, Neves C, Lacoste C, Badens C, Fabre A. Missense mutation of TTC7A mimicking tricho-hepato-enteric (SD/THE) syndrome in a patient with very-early onset inflammatory bowel disease. Eur J Med Genet. 2017

Notarangelo LD. Multiple intestinal atresia with combined immune deficiency. Curr Opin Pediatr. 2014;26(6):690–6.

Samuels ME, Majewski J, Alirezaie N, Fernandez I, Casals F, Patey N, Decaluwe H, Gosselin I, Haddad E, Hodgkinson A, Idaghdour Y, Marchand V, Michaud JL, Rodrigue MA, Desjardins S, Dubois S, Le Deist F, Awadalla P, Raymond V, Maranda B. Exome sequencing identifies mutations in the gene TTC7A in French-Canadian cases with hereditary multiple intestinal atresia. J Med Genet. 2013;50(5):324–9.

Immunodeficiency, Centromeric Instability, and Facial Dysmorphism (ICF Syndrome) (ICF1-DNMT3B, ICF-2 ZBTB24)

Vera Goda
Pediatric Hematology and Stem Cell Transplantation Department, South-Pest Central Hospital, United Szent Istvan and Szent Laszlo Hospital Budapest, Budapest, Hungary

Definition

Immunodeficiency-centromeric instability-facial anomalies syndrome (ICF) is a rare autosomal recessive (AR) primary immunodeficiency (PID) characterized by a profound hypogammaglobulinemia with characteristic rearrangements in the proximity of the centromeres of chromosomes 1, 16, and occasionally 9 in mitogen-stimulated lymphocytes. Other variable symptoms include characteristic facial dysmorphism, growth retardation, failure to thrive, and mental retardation. The main immunological defect is the lack of CD19+CD27+ memory B cells while B cells are usually present. Serum immunoglobulins are variably low. There are limited data on T-cell function; however, in reported cases T cell function is severely impaired. These patients suffer mainly from recurrent or chronic bacterial respiratory infections as presenting symptoms. Bronchiectasis, gastrointestinal and skin infections are also common from early childhood. According to the severity of the concomitant T-cell defect, opportunistic and severe viral infections may be present. In several cases, autoimmune manifestations and malignancies can also be part of the clinical spectrum (Ehrlich et al. 2006; Sterlin et al. 2016).

Introduction/Background

Patients with immunodeficiency-centromeric instability-facial anomalies syndrome (ICF) are of diverse ethnicity, mainly European, Turkish, Japanese, and African American. Although consanguinity has been noted, most cases are not familial, and the prevalence is less than 1 in 1,000,000 (Ehrlich et al. 2006).

ICF is a rare AR disease, first described in 1978. There are three different forms (ICF1 to 4) recognized and linked to specific genetic defects with distinct clinical features. All forms are characterized by the branching of chromosomes 1, 9, and 16 after phytohemagglutinin (PHA) stimulation of lymphocytes. The underlying abnormality is linked to abnormal hypomethylation of juxtacentromeric heterochromatin repeats (Velasco et al. 2014). This is similar to what is observed after treatment of cells with demethylating agents. In recent years, the number of disease genes has expanded from 1 to 4, there are still cases left unexplained.

The most common type is ICF type 1 is the biallelic mutation of deoxyribonucleic acid (DNA) methyltransferase B (DNMT3B) on chromosome 20q11.2 found in approximately 50% of the patients. DNMT3B as a de novo DNA methyltransferase acts during early cell development with a preference for CpG dense regions, so *ICF1* mutations in the catalytic domain of DNMT3B result in a largely reduced methyltransferase activity and hypomethylation of regions that should be active during lymphocyte development. These cases most often carry missense partial loss of function mutations (Sterlin et al. 2016; Velasco et al. 2014).

Thirty percent of patients have ICF type 2 with biallelic deletion in the *ZBTB24* gene on chromosome 6q21, that belongs to a zinc finger and BTB domain family of transcription factors responsible in B cell differentiation. The biallelic missense mutation of *ZBTB24* strengthen the hypothesis that ICF2 patients suffer from a ZBTB24 loss of function mechanism and confirms that complete absence of ZBTB24 is compatible with human life. This is in contrast to the observed early embryonic lethality in mice lacking functional *zbtb24* gene (van den Boogaard et al. 2017; Velasco et al. 2014).

In the remaining 20% of ICF cases, two more genes are involved acting in converging pathways leading to the ICF phenotype. ICF3 has been described with mutation in cell division cycle associated 7 (*CDCA7*) genes, while ICF4 is a compound heterozygous or homozygous mutation of the helicase lymphoid-specific gene (*HELLS*) (Sterlin et al. 2016).

The diagnosis of ICF on the basis of cytogenetic hallmarks occurs at a median age of 5.2 years (range: 1 month to 11.4 years). Life expectancy is poor. In a study of 45 patients, 40.5% died. Cause of death were predominantly severe respiratory tract infections, sepsis and failure to thrive, with a median age at death at 8 years of age (range 6 months to 42 years) (Hagleitner et al. 2008).

Clinical Presentation

Based on a recent French national cohort study (Sterlin et al. 2016), the first clinical signs of ICF syndrome, mostly recurrent infections or a failure to thrive, occur at a median age of 4 months (range: 1–12 months). Hypogammaglobulinemia was diagnosed at a median age of 3.3 years (range: 2 months to 11 years). ICF syndrome is characterized by recurrent severe respiratory, gastrointestinal and skin infections. Gastrointestinal problems are commonly seen at initial presentation with history of several episodes of acute or chronic diarrhea. The combination of gastrointestinal complications and recurrent respiratory infections imply poor prognosis. Failure to thrive is often related to chronic diarrhea. In some cases, nodular gastritis or colon stenosis in association with CD3+ lymphocyte infiltration have been described. The spectrum of infections range from chronic bronchitis, pneumonia, otitis media (often caused by Streptococcus pneumoniae), and sepsis to meningitis/encephalitis with main causative organisms including *Staphylococcus aureus*, *Pseudomonas aeruginosa*, and *Klebsiella* species. Severe infections with *Candida albicans* and *Pneumocystis jirovecii* reflect a component of T cell defect. Infections are the leading cause of death occurring mainly before immunoglobulin replacement therapy is implemented (Sterlin et al. 2016).

The **facial anomalies** are typical: high forehead with frontal bossing, hypertelorism, epicanthus, broad flat nasal bridge, low-set ears, macroglossia with some other possible abnormalities, including hyperpigmented spots, microcrania, micrognathia, sparse hair, short limbs, and hypospadias. Delayed growth and mental retardation are typical and common for ICF type 2 wheres ICF type 1 patients present as slight cognitive and motor developmental delay in the first few years of life. In ICF type 2 cortical atrophy, generalized tonic-clonic seizures can develop within the first years of life (Ehrlich et al. 2006; Sterlin et al. 2016; Hagleitner et al. 2008).

Autoimmune and immune-mediated manifestations include autoimmune hepatitis, arthritis, synovitis, nephritis, thyreoiditis, and psoriasis (Sterlin et al. 2016; Hagleitner et al. 2008).

Malignancies: Hematologic malignancies (myelodysplastic syndrome, acute lymphoblastic leukemia, Hodgkin disease) are reported. Acquired cytopenias, including thrombocytopenia can be detected in several cases (Hagleitner et al. 2008).

Laboratory Findings/Diagnostic Testing

ICF is diagnosed by standard metaphase chromosome analysis of phytohemagglutinin-stimulated peripheral blood lymphocytes from patients (Maraschio et al. 1988) Fig. 1.

Classical findings include multibranched chromosomes with whole-arm deletions and pericentromeric breaks of chromosomes 1 and 16 and rarely 9; where three or more arms of chromosomes 1 and 16 joined in the proximity of the centromere (mostly at the 1qh or 16qh region). Occasional isochromosomes and translocations with breaks are in the vicinity of the centromere. In addition, prominent stretching in the 1qh and 16qh region is seen. Stimulation with pokeweed mitogen produces similar anomalies. In most, but not all patients, chromosome 1 is affected more frequently than chromosome 16 (Ehrlich et al. 2006; van den Boogaard et al. 2017).

B cell immunity is severely impaired in all patients. Serum levels of isotypes (IgG, IgM, IgE, IgA) are variable, low level of IgA is associated with gastrointestinal problems mostly diarrhea. While naive flow cytometry studies reveal the absence of CD27+ memory B cells against normal circulating B cell count and can explain severe hypogammaglobulinemia. In vitro B cells might show a weak or no response to CD40L activation and are more prone to undergo apoptosis. This B cell abnormality is more severe in ICF1 than in ICF2 patients. The absence of specific antibodies against recall antigens is typical in both type.

Immunodeficiency, Centromeric Instability, and Facial Dysmorphism (ICF Syndrome) (ICF1-DNMT3B, ICF-2 ZBTB24), Fig. 1 Associations of the centromeric regions of chromosomes 1/1 (**a, b**), 1/16 (**c, d**), 111116 (**e**), 119 (**f**), 16116 (**g**), and 1116p (**h**). (**a, c, e–h**) Q banding, (**b, d**) DA-DA PI. In the latter, the two centromeric regions appearfused in a single heterochromatic block. J Med Genetics 1988, 25, 173–180

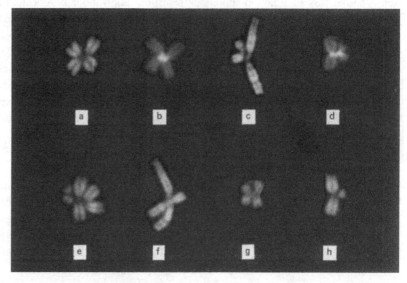

In some cases, there is a decrease in CD4+ and CD8+ T cell counts. CD45RA+CD31+ recent thymic immigrant cell count is always low, naive CD8+ T-cell count is usually preserved. Lymphocyte proliferation to PHA stimulation is normal by contrast low levels of T cell proliferation can be seen in response to antigens such as candida and tetanus toxoid (Sterlin et al. 2016).

In case of autoimmune hepatitis, histology of liver biopsy is notable for infiltration of the portal area by inflammatory cells, including a few macrophages and CD8+ T cells (Sterlin et al. 2016; Hagleitner et al. 2008).

Treatment/Prognosis

The long-term outcome can be improved by immunoglobulin replacement therapy and antibiotic prophylaxis, that control well infectious complications (Sterlin et al. 2016). In case of severe autoimmune complications, immune modulation is indicated that can negatively impact outcome (Sterlin et al. 2016). Alternative therapy for autoimmune cytopenias may include allogenic hematopoetic stem cell transplantation (HSCT) with an HLA identical sibling donor can be an experimental therapeutic option, conditioning regimen usually contains treosulfan, fludarabine, and thiotepa. (There are centers using alemtuzumab, fludarabine and melphalan containing regimens.) Long-term follow up data after HSCT are not available.

ICF1 patients usually need iron supplementation while ICF2 has not shown this feature. ICF2 patient often require anticonvulsive treatments and education at a specialized institution because of severe progressive mental defects, while almost 70% of ICF1 patients have normal intelligence or mild deficit (Hagleitner et al. 2008).

References

Ehrlich M, Jackson K, Weemaes C. Immunodeficiency, centromeric region instability, facial anomalies syndrome (ICF). Orphanet J Rare Dis. 2006;1:2. https://doi.org/10.1186/1750-1172-1-2.

Hagleitner MM, Lankester A, Maraschio P, Hultén M, Fryns JP, Schuetz C, Gimelli G, Davies EG, Gennery A, Belohradsky BH, de Groot R, Gerritsen EJA, Mattina T, Howard PJ, Fasth A, Reisli I, Furthner D, Slatter MA, Cant AJ, Cazzola G, van Dijken PJ, van Deuren M, de Greef JC, van der Maarel SM, Weemaes CMR. Clinical spectrum of immunodeficiency, centromeric instability and facial dysmorphism (ICF syndrome). J Med Genet. 2008; 45:93–9. https://doi.org/10.1136/jmg.2007.053397.

Maraschio P, Zuffardi O, Dalla Fior T, Tiepolo L. Immunodeficiency, centromeric heterochromatin instability of chromosomes 1, 9, and 16, and facial anomalies: the ICF syndrome. J Med Genet. 1988;25:173–80.

Sterlin D, Velasco G, Moshous D, Touzot F, Mahlaoui N, Fischer A, Suarez F, Francastel C, Picard C. Genetic, cellular and clinical features of ICF syndrome: a French national survey. J Clin Immunol. 2016;36:149–59. https://doi.org/10.1007/s10875-016-0240-2.

van den Boogaard ML, Thijssen PE, Aytekin C, Licciardi F, Kıykım AA, Spossito L, Dalm VASH, Driessen GJ, Kersseboom R, de Vries FE, van Ostaijenten Dam MM, Ikinciogullari A, Dogu F, Oleastro M, Bailardo E, Daxinger L, Nain E, Baris S, van Tol MJD, Weemaes C, van der Maarel SM. Expanding the mutation spectrum in ICF syndrome: evidence for a gender bias in ICF2. Clin Genet. 2017;92:380–7.

Velasco G, Walton EL, Sterlin D, Hédouin S, Nitta H, Ito Y, Fouyssac F, Mégarbané A, Sasaki H, Picard C, Francastel C. Germline genes hypomethylation and expression define a molecular signature in peripheral blood of ICF patients: implications for diagnosis and etiology. Orphanet J Rare Dis. 2014;9:56.

Immunoglobulin Class Switch Recombination Defects

A. Durandy and Sven Kracker
INSERM UMR 1163, Human Lymphohematopoiesis Laboratory, Paris, France
Imagine Institute, Université Paris Descartes, Sorbonne Paris Cité, Paris, France

Synonyms

This group of primary antibody deficiencies are also known as Hyper IgM syndromes (HIGMs)

Introduction

Immunoglobulin (Ig) class switch recombination (CSR) defects are rare inherited immune deficiencies, with a frequency estimated around 1/200,000 births. By definition, all CSR-deficient patients present with an absence or a strong decrease of switched immunoglobulin isotypes (IgG, IgA and IgE) in serum, although IgM levels are increased or normal (Cooper et al. 1973). As a consequence of the CSR defect and IgG deficiency, patients suffer from recurrent bacterial infections that predominantly affect the respiratory tract, including chronic sinusitis and bronchiectasis. Chronic infections of the digestive tract might also occur and result in malabsorption and failure to thrive. Molecular defects affecting both B and T cells are associated with additional defective cellular response leading to severe viral and opportunistic infections that strongly worsen the prognosis. Other complications, lymphadenopathies, autoimmunity, and susceptibility to cancers, can also be observed.

Two main causes lead to CSR deficiency, either a defect in the germinal center reaction (T-B cooperation) or a defect in the CSR machinery (B cell-intrinsic defect).

Pathophysiology

Antibody Maturation Process

Antibody maturation takes place within the secondary lymphoid organs (spleen, lymph nodes, and tonsils). When naive B cells (IgM+ IgD+) encounter a specific antigen, and with a close interaction with T follicular helper cells (T_{FH}), they proliferate, acquire the activation marker CD27, and undergo processes of antibody maturation. Interaction between T_{FH} and B cells involves CD40L, a molecule transiently expressed on $T_{FH,}$ and CD40 constitutively expressed on B cells. Antibody maturation is thus antigen and T cell dependent.

CSR is a DNA recombination process occurring into the Ig locus between two different switch (S) regions, leading to deletion of the intervening DNA as an excision circle (Iwasato et al. 1990; Matsuoka et al. 1990; von Schwedler et al. 1990) and ultimately to the expression of one of the different immunoglobulin isotypes with the same variable (V) region and thus the same antigen specificity and affinity. Each constant (C) region

is preceded by an S region, except Cδ region. The Cμ region is replaced by a downstream Cx (Cα, Cγ, or Cε) region (coding, respectively, for IgA, IgG, or IgE). Secondary CSR events have also been reported, in already IgM-switched B cells, using downstream S regions (Du et al. 2008). The first step of CSR is the transcription of the S region, which is induced by cytokines. Interestingly, each cytokine specifically targets specific S regions (e.g., IL4 for Sε, IL10 for Sα). The activation-induced cytidine deaminase (AID) gain access to the single-strand DNA or DNA in the transcription bubbles, and change cytosine (C) into uracil (U) residues (Petersen-Mahrt et al. 2002). This lesion (U:G mismatch) is further recognized and processed by the uracil N-glycosylase (UNG) that removes the uracil residues and produces an abase site, which is eventually cleaved by apurinic/apyrimidinic endonucleases (APEs) (Guikema et al. 2007); this ultimately leads to the formation of single-strand DNA breaks which, if present on both strands of DNA, result in the formation of the double-strand breaks (DSBs) required for recombination between the two targeted S regions. DSB can also occur through the endonuclease activity of postmeiotic segregation 2 (PMS2), an enzyme of the mismatch repair (MMR) machinery (Peron et al. 2008). The DSBs in the S regions are repaired mainly through the conventional non-homologous end-joining (c-NHEJ) pathway although alternative end joining (AEJ) can perform the repair (Yan et al. 2007).

Somatic hypermutation (SHM) introduces stochastically mutations into the Ig variable (V) regions (that recognize antigen) at a very high frequency (1×10^{-3} bases/generation). As in CSR, the first step of SHM is the DNA transcription of V regions and the introduction of uracil residues by AID. No DNA breaks are needed for SHM, and the U:G mismatch is repaired either during replication or through MMR (MSH2/MSH6 complex) repair and the error-prone polymerase η (Faili et al. 2004). Alternatively, as in CSR, UNG leads to an abasic site that is repaired by error-prone translesion synthesis polymerases. Altogether, these pathways introduce mutations in V regions, modifying their affinity for antigens, without changing the C region, thus the isotype of the Ig. This process is the basis for the selection and proliferation of B cells expressing a BCR with a high affinity for antigen in close interaction with the follicular dendritic cells within the germinal center.

CSR Deficiency Caused by a Defective Germinal Center Reaction

T cell defects can lead to a CSR deficiency since CSR is a T cell-dependent process. Some defects are directly linked to defective cooperation between T_{FH} and B cells within the follicles in lymphoid organs, such as CD40L (and its counterpart CD40) and ICOS deficiencies.

X-Linked CSR Deficiency, due to CD40L Deficiency

CD40L deficiency accounts for around 50% of all CSR deficiencies. It is characterized by the lack of T_{FH}-B interaction in lymphoid organs and an absence of germinal centres, with low numbers of CD27+ B cells in peripheral blood. Patients suffer from recurrent and severe bacterial infections but also from viral and opportunistic infections since CD40L interaction with CD40 also expressed on dendritic cells is required for efficient cellular immune responses. Liver disease is very common; sclerosing cholangitis (often associated with *Cryptosporidium* spp. infection) is particularly severe and may lead to terminal liver damage. Intermittent or chronic neutropenia is also a common feature (Levy et al. 1997). Some patients present with normal or even increased IgA serum levels, suggesting an alternative diversification pathway for IgA (upon CpG- or proliferating inducible ligand (APRIL)-induced activation of B cells in the gut lamina propria) (He et al. 2007). Some patients also exhibit residual SHM, suggesting an innate defence mechanism in the splenic marginal zone (Weller et al. 2001).

This X-linked condition is due to deleterious mutations in *CD40L* gene, most of them affecting exon 5, which contains most of the tissue necrosis factor (TNF) homology domain. Most mutations lead to a markedly low or no membrane CD40L expression.

Treatment of CD40L deficiency is based on intravenous or subcutaneous IgG infusion, antibiotic prophylaxis, and administration of G-CSF (in cases of severe neutropenia). Treatment by subcutaneous administration of rCD40L has been attempted, showing a partial restoration of T_{H1} cell function but no effect on B cell function (Jain et al. 2011). Therefore, hematopoietic stem cell transplantation (HSCT) appears as the best curative treatment, at least whenever a human leukocyte antigen (HLA)-identical donor is available (Gennery and Cant 2008). If required by severe liver damage, liver transplantation should be performed before HSCT. The prognosis of this CSR remains severe, and genetic counseling should be proposed.

Autosomal Recessive CSR Deficiency, Due to CD40 Deficiency

The autosomal recessive (AR) defect in CD40, the surface receptor for CD40L, is much less common than the CD40L deficiency but the phenotype is quite similar. Bi-allelic deleterious mutations in *CD40* gene are responsible for this condition (Ferrari et al. 2001). Diagnosis can be easily made when CD40 expression on B cells' membrane is absent, although expression can be found normal in a few cases (Karaca et al. 2012). HLA-identical HSCT, the only curative treatment, has been successfully used in a few cases (Al-Dhekri et al. 2012; Mazzolari et al. 2007).

X-Linked CSR Deficiency, Due to Defective NF-κB Activation

Crosslinking of CD40 results in activation of the canonical NF-κB signaling pathway which appears critical in CSR, as shown by the observation of patients affected with the X-linked ectodermal dysplasia associated with immunodeficiency (EDA-ID) (Smahi et al. 2000; Zonana et al. 2000). Besides ectodermal dysplasia, patients suffer from an immune deficiency characterized by normal-to-elevated serum IgM levels, low levels of serum IgG (especially IgG2 and IgG4) and IgA, and impaired antibody responses (to polysaccharide antigens in particular). Susceptibility to mycobacterial infections is also frequently associated. SHM is variably impaired in the decreased CD27+ B cell subset. X-linked EDA-ID is caused by hypomorphic mutations, most frequently found in the zinc-finger domain of the *NF-κB essential modulator* (NEMO, also known as IKKγ) gene. Treatment associates antibiotics and IgG replacement but HSCT is often required as a curative treatment in severe forms.

Of note, other defects in proteins involved in the NFκB pathway lead to a common variable immunodeficiency-like phenotype, rather than to CSR deficiency features (Fliegauf et al. 2013; Chen et al. 2013).

Autosomal Recessive CSR Deficiency, Due to ICOS Deficiency

Inducible co-stimulatory molecule (ICOS) deficiency leads to elevated or normal IgM levels and low IgG and IgA levels (Warnatz et al. 2006). ICOS is expressed on activated T cells (including the T_{FH}) and is involved in the generation and function (i.e., cytokine production, especially IL21) of T_{FH} in germinal centers (Bossaller et al. 2006). Furthermore, ICOS must interact with its cognate ligand (ICOS-L, which is constitutively expressed on B cells) for full antibody production. The SHM process is impaired in the CD27+ B cell subset. A cell-mediated immune defect has also been reported in some patients (Takahashi et al. 2009). This condition appears to be rare and only two different *ICOS* gene mutations have been reported to date (Takahashi et al. 2009; Grimbacher et al. 2003). IgG replacement is the usual treatment, although HLA-identical HSCT should be considered in case of severe associated T cell defect.

CSR Deficiency Caused by a Defect in the CSR Machinery

CSR deficiencies caused by an intrinsic B cell defect affecting the CSR machinery are less severe than those due to germinal center defects, because T cell function is generally conserved. However, autoimmunity and cancers can occur.

Autosomal Recessive CSR Deficiency, Due to AID Deficiency

This condition appears to be the second most frequent molecularly defined CSR deficiency. It is clinically characterized by recurrent bacterial infections mainly affecting the upper respiratory tract but no susceptibility to opportunistic or viral infections is reported. The hallmark of the disease is the presence of impressive lymphadenopathies (cervical, mesenteric, mediastinal) characterized histologically by the presence of giant germinal centers filled with IgM+IgD+ proliferating B cells.

Autoimmunity induced by IgM autoantibodies is a frequent complication, affecting 30% of patients, affecting mostly the blood cells (autoimmune anemia, thrombocytopenia), but also other organs (autoimmune hepatitis, sclerosing lupus erythroid). This frequent complication emphasizes the role of AID in central and peripheral tolerance (Durandy et al. 2012). In the absence of functional AID, the B cells cannot generate either IgG, IgA, or IgE via CSR (Revy et al. 2000). The proportion of peripheral blood B cells carrying the CD27 marker is normal (20–50%), although all of these are IgM+ and IgD+, thus unswitched "memory" B cells. Strikingly, this CD27+ B cell population is completely devoid of SHM. This observation linked, for the first time, CSR and SHM, the two events of antibody maturation, through AID activity (Revy et al. 2000; Muramatsu et al. 2000).

Deleterious mutations scattered throughout the *AICDA* gene are responsible for this disease. Some rare mutations located in the C terminal part of AID do not affect the cytidine deaminase activity nor the SHM process (although CSR is completely abolished), suggesting a further role of AID in CSR, either in AID stabilization or its subcellular localization (Ta et al. 2003). Moreover, deletions of the nuclear export signal lead to an autosomal dominant disease with a milder phenotype (Imai et al. 2005). AID-deficient patients do well under IgG replacement that reduces susceptibility to bacterial infections, unless autoimmunity complications develop.

Autosomal Recessive CSR Deficiency Due to UNG Deficiency

This is a very rare form of CSR-D since only five patients have been up to now reported in the literature (aan de Kerk et al. 2013; Imai et al. 2003; Cantaert et al. 2016). The clinical and immunological phenotype is very similar to that of AID deficiency except that SHM are not absent since U:G mismatches can be repaired during replication or through the MMR pathway in the absence of Uracil-N glycosylase. Nevertheless, the SHM pattern is abnormal with transition mutations predominant on G:C mismatches. Six different mutations in *UNG* gene have been described. Patients with UNG deficiency do well on IgG replacement therapy. However, UNG is part of the DNA base excision pathway involved in the repair of spontaneously occurring lesions and therefore constitutes an antimutagenic defence strategy. Indeed, UNG-deficient mice develop B cell lymphomas when elderly (Nilsen et al. 2003).

Autosomal Recessive CSR Deficiency Due to INO80 Deficiency

Recently a very rare form of CSR-D caused by an intrinsic B cell defect has been shown to be caused by hypomorphic mutations in *INO80* gene. This syndrome leads to a partial CSR defect without affecting SHM, although number of circulating CD27+ B cells is low. The exact role of INO80 during CSR is not completely elucidated. INO80 belongs to a complex that binds AID and plays a role in cohesin activity. It has been found to be located on S regions during CSR, suggesting that it could play a role in the Sμ-Sx synapsis during the CSR-induced DNA repair process. Three different bi-allelic hypomorphic mutations in *INO80* have been described. Both reported patients do well, one of them being treated by regular IgG replacement (Kracker et al. 2015).

Autosomal Recessive CSR-D Due to PMS2 Deficiency

Whereas heterozygous mutations in one of the genes coding for MMR lead to hereditary non-polyposis colic cancer (syndrome de Lynch), bi-allelic mutations lead to the early occurrence of a variety of cancers in the first few years of life. Among the MMR-deficient patients, those affected by a complete lack of PMS2 suffer also from a CSR deficiency that can be the prominent symptom or, indeed, the sole symptom for several years. Affected patients have a marked susceptibility to bacterial infections requiring Ig substitution and biologically by elevated serum IgM levels, with low IgG (especially IgG2 and IgG4) and IgA levels (Peron et al. 2008). The CSR defect is very likely linked to the lack of the endonuclease activity of PMS2 in patients, as shown by the defective generation of CSR-induced DSB (Peron et al. 2008).

In terms of SHM, the frequency and nucleotide substitution pattern is normal but the peripheral blood CD27+ B cell count is always low. Although infections are well controlled by Ig substitution, the prognosis is very poor and is linked to the occurrence of cancers, thus limiting life expectancy to less than 20 years of age.

CSR Deficiency Caused by a Defect in the DNA Repair Machinery

CSR-D can occur in patients with a DNA repair deficiency since a complex DNA repair machinery is required for CSR and/or SHM-induced DNA lesions. Among them, MMR deficiency can be associated to an immunodeficiency and susceptibility to infectious complications. Besides the CSR-D due to PMS2 deficiency reported above that is mostly linked to defective PMS2 endonuclease activity, deficiencies in MSH2/MSH6 lead to a partial CSR-D with abnormal pattern of SHM, pinpointing to the role of these enzymes in recognition and repair of AID-induced U:G mismatches on both S and V regions (Gardes et al. 2012).

CSR-D is also a complication of ataxia telangiectasia (AT), a devastating disease due to bi-allelic mutations in the *ATM* gene, which combines progressive neurodegeneration (ataxia), cutaneous abnormalities (telangiectasia), predisposition to malignancy, and immunodeficiency. Of note, the immunodeficiency may be the sole symptom for several years. It is characterized by susceptibility to bacterial infections (especially of the respiratory tract) requiring Ig replacement therapy. In addition to a progressive T-cell defect, some AT patients present with elevated IgM and very low IgG and IgA levels and B cells that are unable to undergo CSR in vitro, in accordance to the known role of ATM in CSR-induced DSB repair (Pan et al. 2002). In contrast, the presence of normal SHM in the CD27+ B cell subpopulation (which is normal in number) indicates that ATM is not essential for DNA repair in V regions.

As is the case for ATM, the MRE11/RAD50/NBS1 complex is involved in the repair of CSR-induced DSBs. Hence, a CSR deficiency can be observed in the "AT-like" disease due to *MRE11* mutations and Nijmegen breakage syndrome (due to *NBS1* mutations). A CSR deficiency associated with elevated radiosensitivity of fibroblasts has been reported in RIDDLE syndrome and is caused by mutations in the gene for ubiquitin ligase RNF168 (Stewart et al. 2009). A CSR deficiency phenotype has also been observed as part of a combined immunodeficiency related to leaky mutations in genes encoding NHEJ factors (such as Cernunnos, DNA ligase IV, and Artemis) (Du et al. 2008, 2012; Buck et al. 2006; Pan-Hammarstrom et al. 2005).

Conclusion

CSR deficiencies are phenotypically and genetically extremely heterogeneous: The most frequent are caused by defects in T cells or in T cell-B cell cooperation in germinal centers. They combine a humoral and a cellular immunodeficiency. The only curative treatment is HSCT. Other CSR deficiencies, caused by an intrinsic B cell defect that affects the CSR machinery itself, are treated with IgG replacement and have a good prognosis. Some of these conditions are caused by defects in the DNA repair pathway and consequently are prone to cancers. Molecular characterization of these diseases is essential for establishing a precise diagnosis, offering appropriate genetic counseling and accurate follow up and opening up the way to specific targeted therapies. Lastly, the detailed analysis of these conditions has been

essential for a better understanding of the two events of antibody maturation, the CSR and the SHM processes.

References

aan de Kerk DJ, Jansen MH, ten Berge IJ, van Leeuwen EM, Kuijpers TW. Identification of B cell defects using age-defined reference ranges for in vivo and in vitro B cell differentiation. J Immunol. 2013; 190(10):5012–9. Epub Apr 12.

Al-Dhekri H, Al-Sum Z, Al-Saud B, Al-Mousa H, Ayas M, Al-Muhsen S, et al. Successful outcome in two patients with CD40 deficiency treated with allogeneic HCST. Clin Immunol. 2012;143(1):96–8.

Bossaller L, Burger J, Draeger R, Grimbacher B, Knoth R, Plebani A, et al. ICOS deficiency is associated with a severe reduction of CXCR5+CD4 germinal center Th cells. J Immunol. 2006;177(7):4927–32.

Buck D, Malivert L, de Chasseval R, Barraud A, Fondaneche MC, Sanal O, et al. Cernunnos, a novel nonhomologous end-joining factor, is mutated in human immunodeficiency with microcephaly. Cell. 2006;124(2):287–99.

Cantaert T, Schickel JN, Bannock JM, Ng YS, Massad C, Delmotte FR, et al. Decreased somatic hypermutation induces an impaired peripheral B cell tolerance checkpoint. J Clin Invest. 2016;126:4289.

Chen K, Coonrod EM, Kumanovics A, Franks ZF, Durtschi JD, Margraf RL, et al. Germline mutations in NFKB2 implicate the noncanonical NF-kappaB pathway in the pathogenesis of common variable immunodeficiency. Am J Hum Genet. 2013;93(5): 812–24.

Cooper MD, Faulk WP, Fudenberg HH, Good RA, Hitzig W, Kunkel H, et al. Classification of primary immunodeficiencies. N Engl J Med. 1973;288(18): 966–7.

Du L, van der Burg M, Popov SW, Kotnis A, van Dongen JJ, Gennery AR, et al. Involvement of Artemis in nonhomologous end-joining during immunoglobulin class switch recombination. J Exp Med. 2008;205(13):3031–40.

Du L, Peng R, Bjorkman A, Filipe de Miranda N, Rosner C, Kotnis A, et al. Cernunnos influences human immunoglobulin class switch recombination and may be associated with B cell lymphomagenesis. J Exp Med. 2012;209(2):291–305. Epub 2012 Feb 6.

Durandy A, Cantaert T, Kracker S, Meffre E. Potential roles of activation-induced cytidine deaminase in promotion or prevention of autoimmunity in humans. Autoimmunity. 2012;46(2):148–56. Epub 2013 Jan 10.

Faili A, Aoufouchi S, Weller S, Vuillier F, Stary A, Sarasin A, et al. DNA polymerase {eta} is involved in hypermutation occurring during immunoglobulin class switch recombination. J Exp Med. 2004;199(2): 265–70.

Ferrari S, Giliani S, Insalaco A, Al-Ghonaium A, Soresina AR, Loubser M, et al. Mutations of CD40 gene cause an autosomal recessive form of immunodeficiency with hyper IgM. Proc Natl Acad Sci USA. 2001;98(22):12614–9.

Fliegauf M, Bryant VL, Frede N, Slade C, Woon ST, Lehnert K, et al. Haploinsufficiency of the NF-kappaB1 subunit p50 in common variable immunodeficiency. Am J Hum Genet. 2013;97(3):389–403.

Gardes P, Forveille M, Alyanakian MA, Aucouturier P, Ilencikova D, Leroux D, et al. Human MSH6 deficiency is associated with impaired antibody maturation. J Immunol. 2012;188(4):2023–9. Epub 2012 Jan 16.

Gennery AR, Cant AJ. Advances in hematopoietic stem cell transplantation for primary immunodeficiency. Immunol Allergy Clin North Am. 2008;28(2):439–56, x–xi.

Grimbacher B, Hutloff A, Schlesier M, Glocker E, Warnatz K, Drager R, et al. Homozygous loss of ICOS is associated with adult-onset common variable immunodeficiency. Nat Immunol. 2003;4(3):261–8.

Guikema JE, Linehan EK, Tsuchimoto D, Nakabeppu Y, Strauss PR, Stavnezer J, et al. APE1- and APE2-dependent DNA breaks in immunoglobulin class switch recombination. J Exp Med. 2007;204(12):3017–26.

He B, Xu W, Santini PA, Polydorides AD, Chiu A, Estrella J, et al. Intestinal bacteria trigger T cell-independent immunoglobulin A(2) class switching by inducing epithelial-cell secretion of the cytokine APRIL. Immunity. 2007;26(6):812–26.

Imai K, Slupphaug G, Lee WI, Revy P, Nonoyama S, Catalan N, et al. Human uracil-DNA glycosylase deficiency associated with profoundly impaired immunoglobulin class-switch recombination. Nat Immunol. 2003;4(10):1023–8.

Imai K, Zhu Y, Revy P, Morio T, Mizutani S, Fischer A, et al. Analysis of class switch recombination and somatic hypermutation in patients affected with autosomal dominant hyper-IgM syndrome type 2. Clin Immunol. 2005;115(3):277–85.

Iwasato T, Shimizu A, Honjo T, Yamagishi H. Circular DNA is excised by immunoglobulin class switch recombination. Cell. 1990;62(1):143–9.

Jain A, Kovacs JA, Nelson DL, Migueles SA, Pittaluga S, Fanslow W, et al. Partial immune reconstitution of X-linked hyper IgM syndrome with recombinant CD40 ligand. Blood. 2011;118(14):3811–7. Epub 2011 Aug 12.

Karaca NE, Forveille M, Aksu G, Durandy A, Kutukculer N. Hyper-immunoglobulin M syndrome type 3 with normal CD40 cell surface expression. Scand J Immunol. 2012;76(1):21–5.

Kracker S, Di Virgilio M, Schwartzentruber J, Cuenin C, Forveille M, Deau MC, et al. An inherited immunoglobulin class-switch recombination deficiency associated with a defect in the INO80 chromatin remodeling complex. J Allergy Clin Immunol. 2015;135(4):998–1007. Epub 2014 Oct 11.

Levy J, Espanol-Boren T, Thomas C, Fischer A, Tovo P, Bordigoni P, et al. Clinical spectrum of X-linked hyper-IgM syndrome. J Pediatr. 1997;131(1 Pt 1):47–54.

Matsuoka M, Yoshida K, Maeda T, Usuda S, Sakano H. Switch circular DNA formed in cytokine-treated mouse splenocytes: evidence for intramolecular DNA deletion in immunoglobulin class switching. Cell. 1990;62(1):135–42.

Mazzolari E, Lanzi G, Forino C, Lanfranchi A, Aksu G, Ozturk C, et al. First report of successful stem cell transplantation in a child with CD40 deficiency. Bone Marrow Transplant. 2007;40(3):279–81.

Muramatsu M, Kinoshita K, Fagarasan S, Yamada S, Shinkai Y, Honjo T. Class switch recombination and hypermutation require activation-induced cytidine deaminase (AID), a potential RNA editing enzyme. Cell. 2000;102(5):553–63.

Nilsen H, Stamp G, Andersen S, Hrivnak G, Krokan HE, Lindahl T, et al. Gene-targeted mice lacking the Ung uracil-DNA glycosylase develop B-cell lymphomas. Oncogene. 2003;22(35):5381–6.

Pan Q, Petit-Frere C, Lahdesmaki A, Gregorek H, Chrzanowska KH, Hammarstrom L. Alternative end joining during switch recombination in patients with ataxia-telangiectasia. Eur J Immunol. 2002;32(5):1300–8.

Pan-Hammarstrom Q, Jones AM, Lahdesmaki A, Zhou W, Gatti RA, Hammarstrom L, et al. Impact of DNA ligase IV on nonhomologous end joining pathways during class switch recombination in human cells. J Exp Med. 2005;201(2):189–94.

Peron S, Metin A, Gardes P, Alyanakian MA, Sheridan E, Kratz CP, et al. Human PMS2 deficiency is associated with impaired immunoglobulin class switch recombination. J Exp Med. 2008;205(11):2465–72.

Petersen-Mahrt SK, Harris RS, Neuberger MS. AID mutates *E. coli* suggesting a DNA deamination mechanism for antibody diversification. Nature. 2002;418(6893):99–104.

Revy P, Muto T, Levy Y, Geissmann F, Plebani A, Sanal O, et al. Activation-induced cytidine deaminase (AID) deficiency causes the autosomal recessive form of the hyper-IgM syndrome (HIGM2). Cell. 2000;102(5):565–75.

Smahi A, Courtois G, Vabres P, Yamaoka S, Heuertz S, Munnich A, et al. Genomic rearrangement in NEMO impairs NF-kappaB activation and is a cause of incontinentia pigmenti. The International Incontinentia Pigmenti (IP) Consortium. Nature. 2000;405(6785):466–72.

Stewart GS, Panier S, Townsend K, Al-Hakim AK, Kolas NK, Miller ES, et al. The RIDDLE syndrome protein mediates a ubiquitin-dependent signaling cascade at sites of DNA damage. Cell. 2009;136(3):420–34.

Ta VT, Nagaoka H, Catalan N, Durandy A, Fischer A, Imai K, et al. AID mutant analyses indicate requirement for class-switch-specific cofactors. Nat Immunol. 2003;4(9):843–8.

Takahashi N, Matsumoto K, Saito H, Nanki T, Miyasaka N, Kobata T, et al. Impaired CD4 and CD8 effector function and decreased memory T cell populations in ICOS-deficient patients. J Immunol. 2009;182(9):5515–27.

von Schwedler U, Jack HM, Wabl M. Circular DNA is a product of the immunoglobulin class switch rearrangement. Nature. 1990;345(6274):452–6.

Warnatz K, Bossaller L, Salzer U, Skrabl-Baumgartner A, Schwinger W, van der Burg M, et al. Human ICOS deficiency abrogates the germinal center reaction and provides a monogenic model for common variable immunodeficiency. Blood. 2006;107(8):3045–52.

Weller S, Faili A, Garcia C, Braun MC, Le Deist FF, de Saint Basile GG, et al. CD40-CD40L independent Ig gene hypermutation suggests a second B cell diversification pathway in humans. Proc Natl Acad Sci USA. 2001;98(3):1166–70.

Yan CT, Boboila C, Souza EK, Franco S, Hickernell TR, Murphy M, et al. IgH class switching and translocations use a robust non-classical end-joining pathway. Nature. 2007;449(7161):478–82.

Zonana J, Elder ME, Schneider LC, Orlow SJ, Moss C, Golabi M, et al. A novel X-linked disorder of immune deficiency and hypohidrotic ectodermal dysplasia is allelic to incontinentia pigmenti and due to mutations in IKK-gamma (NEMO). Am J Hum Genet. 2000;67:6.

Immunoglobulin Heavy Chain Deficiency

▶ Ig Heavy Chain Deletions

Innate Immune Defects, Clinical Presentation

Jennifer W. Leiding
Department of Pediatrics, Division of Allergy and Immunology, University of South Florida at Johns Hopkins – All Children's Hospital, St. Petersburg, FL, USA

The innate immune system includes several cell types: neutrophils, monocytes, and natural killer cells. Innate immune defects often present in childhood and cause patients to be susceptible to invasive bacteria, mycobacteria, fungi, and viral infections.

Phagocyte Defects

Granulocytes, a type of leukocyte are differentiated by other white blood cells based on the presence of cytoplasmic granules and a segmented nucleus. Because of the segmented nature of their nuclei, granulocytes are often also referred to as polymorphonuclear leukocytes (PML).

Neutrophils are the most abundant cell within the granulocyte population leading to the title of neutrophil and granulocyte becoming synonymous. Eosinophils, basophils, and mast cells are other types of granulocytes.

Neutrophils, also known as granulocytes, are important for host defense against bacteria and fungi. These are bone marrow derived and have a short life span in the peripheral blood (~7 h) and tissue (1–2 days). Disorders of neutrophils can be subdivided into disorders of neutrophil production, defects in neutrophil chemotaxis, defects in neutrophil degranulation, and disorders of neutrophil killing.

Chronic neutropenia refers to conditions that cause the peripheral neutrophil count to be <500 cells/uL for more than 6 weeks. There are five types of severe chronic neutropenia (SCN), SCN types 1–4 and X-linked neutropenia, detailed in Table 1. SCN is usually diagnosed in early infancy during or after recurrent or a severe infection with pyogenic bacteria. Various molecular defects cause SCN but all cause impairment of myeloid differentiation in the bone marrow. This defect in myeloid differentiation can aid in the diagnosis of affected patients (Boztug 2011).

The majority of SCN patients have mutations in *ELANE* which codes for the neutrophil elastase. Mutations in *ELANE* cause both chronic SCN and cyclic neutropenia. The cyclic form has oscillating neutrophil counts every 21 days. Diagnosis of SCN is established by determining the molecular defect. Chronic neutropenia, arrest of myeloid differentiation, and susceptibility to infections are hallmarks of these diseases.

For efficient neutrophil killing, the neutrophil must first leave the vasculature and migrate into peripheral tissues. This complex process of neutrophil migration includes neutrophil rolling along the endothelial surface, firm attachment of neutrophils to the endothelial surface, and migration through endothelial cells. Leukocyte adhesion deficiencies (LAD) occur when neutrophils are unable to migrate efficiently. Three types of LAD have been described. All three types are characterized by an elevated leukocyte count, specifically neutrophilia in the peripheral blood, delayed separation of the umbilical cord in neonates, and recurrent bacterial infections, skin ulcers, defective wound healing, gingivitis, and periodontitis. The three types of LAD are detailed in Table 2. A diagnosis of LADI, II, or III can be established by direct measurement of CD18, CD15s, and Kindlin3 in the serum by flow cytometry. Neutrophil chemotaxis assays performed in a research setting can also be performed and would be abnormal. Lastly, the disease can be diagnosed by identifying the specific molecular defect (Boztug 2011).

Once the neutrophil reaches the sight of infection, phagosomes within the neutrophil ingest the infectious pathogen, and killing of the infectious agent occur directly with neutrophil granules. Chediak-Higashi syndrome (CHS) is an autosomal recessive disorder characterized by defects in neutrophil granule development and granule release. Clinical manifestations include susceptibility to bacterial infections, oculocutaneous albinisim, and neurologic disease. A peripheral smear of an affected patient's blood shows classic giant peroxidase positive granules that coalesce azurophilic and specific granules which are hallmark of the disease. Determining the molecular defect is necessary to fully establish the diagnosis (Boztug 2011).

Production of reactive oxygen species by the NADPH oxidase system within phagosomes is another method employed by neutrophils for killing of infectious agents. Chronic granulomatous disease (CGD), first described in the 1950s, occurs due to mutations in any of the five components of the NADPH oxidase (Table 3). Patients

Innate Immune Defects, Clinical Presentation, Table 1 Severe congenital neutropenias

Disease	Genetic Defect	Inheritance	Other manifestations
SCN1	*ELANE*	AD	
SCN2	*GFI1*	AD	
SCN3	*HAX1*	AR	Neurologic impairment
SCN4	*G6PC3*	AR	Congenital heart defects Facial dysmorphism Increased visibility of superficial veins Urogenital malformations Endocrine abnormalities Hearing loss Skin hyperelasticity
XLN	*WAS*	XL	

SCN severe congenital neutropenia, *XLN* X-linked neutropenia, *GFI1* growth factor independent 1, *HAX1* HCLS1 Associated Protein X-1, *G6PC3* glucose-6-phosphatase catalytic subunit 3, *WAS* Wiskott Aldrich syndrome, *AD* autosomal dominant, *AR* autosomal recessive

Innate Immune Defects, Clinical Presentation, Table 2 Leukocyte adhesion deficiencies

Disease	Gene	Protein	Inheritance	Other manifestations
LAD-I	*ITGB2*	CD18	AR	
LAD-II	*SLC35C1*	CD15s	AR	Growth and mental retardation Hypotonia Seizures Dysmorphic features Bombay blood type
LAD-III	*Kindlin 3*	Kindlin3	AR	Bleeding diathesis

LAD leukocyte adhesion deficiency, *AR* autosomal recessive, *AD* autosomal dominant with CGD are susceptible to invasive bacterial and fungal infections that primarily affect the lungs, liver, lymph nodes, and skin. More rarely brain abscesses and bacteremia can occur. In addition to infections, patients with CGD are susceptible to the formation of granuloma. Pyloric outlet, bladder outlet, and ureteral obstruction are common due to the development of granulomata.

Innate Immune Defects, Clinical Presentation, Table 3 Genetic defects in chronic granulomatous disease

Gene	Protein	Inheritance pattern	Percentage
CYBA	p22^{phox}	AR	6%
NCF1	p47^{phox}	AR	20%
NCF2	p67^{phox}	AR	6%
NCF4	p40^{phox}	AR	1 individual
CYBB	gp91^{phox}	XL	70%

AR autosomal recessive, *XL* X-linked

Crohn's like colitis occurs in ~50% of patients and can lead to growth failure.

Diagnosis of CGD relies on direct measurement of superoxide production. The dihydrorhodamine assay uses flow cytometry to measure superoxide production (Fig. 1). Dihydrorhodamine123 is converted to rhodamine123 which fluoresces upon stimulation and superoxide production. In addition to diagnosing CGD, the DHR can also give some insight into the specific gene mutated and inheritance pattern (Fig. 2) (Leiding and Holland 2012).

Hyper IgE Syndromes

Loss of function mutations in signal transducer activator of transcription (STAT) 3 cause a multisystem disease known as hyper IgE syndrome or

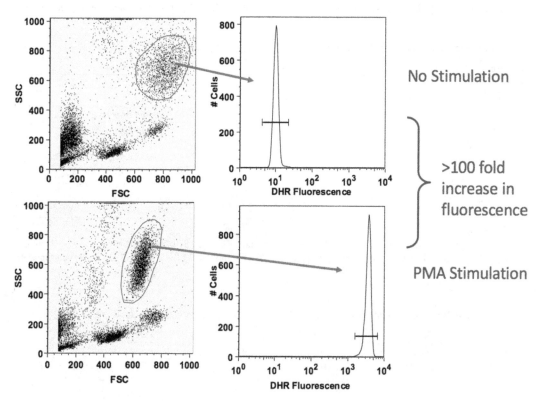

Innate Immune Defects, Clinical Presentation, Fig. 1 Gated neutrophils stimulated with phorbol myrisate acetate (Figure provided by Matt Morrow, MS, Johns Hopkins-All Children's Hospital)

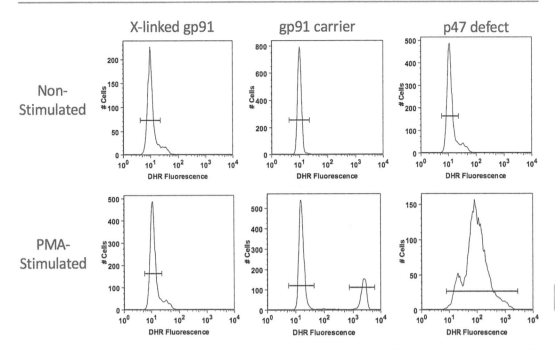

Innate Immune Defects, Clinical Presentation, Fig. 2 DHR Results. Characteristic histograms show absence of florescence indicating absent superoxide production in gp91phox deficient CGD, 2 populations of mutated and non-mutated cells in X-linked gp1phox carriers, and some residual florescence and superoxide production in autosomal recessive p47phox deficient CGD (Figure provided by Matt Morrow, MS, Johns Hopkins-All Children's Hospital)

Job's syndrome. Clinical characteristics include: eczema, high IgE (>2000 IU/ml), recurrent boils, pneumonia, mucocutaneous candidiasis, characteristic facies, lung pneumatoceles, scoliosis, hyperextensible joints, bone fractures, and delayed shedding of the primary teeth. Primary pulmonary infections occur with *S. aureus, S. pneumoniae,* and *H. influenzae.* Once pneumatoceles develop, superinfection with *Aspergillus sp.* and *Pseudomonas* are common. Mutations in STAT3 disrupt production of IL-17 producing T cells (Th17) (Sowerwine 2012).

DOCK8 deficiency also known as autosomal recessive hyper IgE syndrome has some similar characteristics as Job's syndrome: eczema, high IgE, eosinophilia. However, patients with DOCK8 deficiency also suffer from severe atopic diseases such as food allergies, asthma, and eosinophilic esophagitis. DOCK8 deficient patients are also susceptible to common cutaneous viruses including human papilloma virus, molluscum contagiosum virus, and herpes simplex virus.

Diagnosis of hyper IgE syndromes is based on clinical constellation of symptoms. Meausrement of Th17 cells in the peripheral blood of Job's syndrome patients will be low or absent. Determining the molecular defect is diagnostic (Sowerwine 2012).

Disorders of the IL-12-IFNγ Pathway

Over the last two decades, multiple defects affecting interferon (IFN) γ-mediated immunity have been described. Many of these disorders have been grouped into a class of diseases known as Mendelian susceptibility to Mycobacterial disease. Susceptibility to mycobacterial and viral infections are hallmark of these diseases (Bustamante 2014).

Innate Immune Defects, Clinical Presentation, Table 4 Defects in IL-12-IFNγ pathway

Gene	Protein Expression	Inheritance	Infectious susceptibility	Other Symptoms
IFNγR1	Complete	AR	Disseminated NTM or BCG Nontyphoid Salmonella *Listeria monocytogenes* HHV-8	Impaired granuloma formation
	Partial	AR	Disseminated NTM or BCG Salmonellosis, Shigella, *Haemophilus influenzae*, *Mycoplasma pneumoniae*, *Klebsiella* sp.	
	Partial	AD	NTM or BCG often affecting bone Disseminated NTM or BCG Salmonellosis *Histoplasma*	
IFNγR2	Complete	AR	Disseminated NTM or BCG CMV	Impaired granuloma formation
	Partial	AR	Disseminated NTM or BCG	
IL-12β	Complete	AR	NTM or M. tuberculosis Salmonellosis *Nocardia* sp.	
IL-12Rβ1	Complete	AR	NTM or M. tuberculosis Salmonellosis CMC	
STAT1	Partial LOF	AD	NTM	
	Partial GOF	AD	NTM CMC VZV, HSV, CMV *Coccidiomycosis, Histoplasma*	IPEX-like symptoms CID
	Complete LOF	AR	NTM HSV, EBV	
IRF8	Complete	AR	NTM	
	Partial	AD	NTM	

LOF loss of function, *GOF* gain of function, *AR* autosomal recessive, *AD* autosomal dominant, *NTM* non-tuberculous mycobacteria, *BCG* bacillus Calmette–Guérin, *HHV-8* human herpes virus-8, *CMC* chronic mucocutaneous candidiasis, *VZV* varicella zoster virus, *HSV* herpes simplex virus, *CMV* cytomegalovirus, *EBV* Epstein Barr virus

The genetic etiologies of the IL-12 - IFNγ pathway are described in Table 4. IFNγ is the key cytokine produced as a result of activation of the IFNγ pathway. Upon infection with intracellular bacteria, viruses, and other pathogens, phagocytes and dendritic cells secrete IL-12. IL-12 binds to its cognate receptor made of β1 and β2 subunits expressed on NK and T cells. IFNγ is produced and secreted by NK and T cells binding to its cognate receptor made of two subunits, IFNγR1 and IFNγR2. IFNγ leads to the phosphorylation of signal transducer and activator of transcription (STAT1) and translocates into the nucleus where it activates IFNγ responsive genes.

Table 4 describes the clinical manifestations of patients with defects in IL-12 -IFNγ axis (Bustamante 2014). Mutations in IFNγR1 or IFNγR2 can lead to complete or partial absence of protein expression. In those with absent protein expression, disease onset is earlier and more severe. Without HSCT, patients will die of overwhelming infection. In partial autosomal recessive IFNγR1 and IFNγR2 deficiency, disease manifestations are similar but less severe. Mutations leading to partial autosomal dominant IFNγR1 deficiency are downstream from segments encoding the transmembrane domain of the protein and impact downstream IFNγR1 signaling but not IFNγ binding. With large doses of exogenous IFNγ, the defect can be overcome and allow clinical improvement in those affected.

Diagnosis is established by determining the individual molecular defect. The clinical presentation of patients with severe or disseminated infections with non-tuberculous mycobacteria and herpes-related viruses may alert the clinician to think about this group of diseases. Functional testing can be obtained as well to investigate IFNγ production and STAT1 phosphorylation in response to cell activation.

Nuclear Factor κB (NFκB Defects)

Defects in the canonical and non-canonical pathways in NFκB signaling are detailed in Table 5 (Bustamante 2014). Upon cellular activation, both pathways lead to translocation of NFκB into the nucleus. NFκB along with IKBKα and IKBKβ comprise the IKK complex. At rest, NFκB is stored in the cytoplasm bound to an inhibitor of NFκB (IκB). Upon cell stimulation, IκB is phosphorylated freeing NFκB to translocate into the nucleus.

Patients with defects in the NFκB pathway are susceptible to opportunistic infections, specifically *Pneumocystis jiroveci* pneumonia, severe viral infections (HSV, CMV), mycobacterium, and encapsulated bacterial infections. The immune deficiency includes hypogammaglobulinemia, defects in specific antibody production in response to recall antigens, and variability in T cell quantities and function.

Diagnosis is established by determining the molecular defect. Presence of ectodermal dysplasia, specific infectious susceptibility, and immune abnormalities alert the clinician to think of NFκB-pathway-related diseases.

Toll Like Receptor Defects

This group of disorders lead to impaired Toll-like receptor (TLR) 3 signaling. TLRs are present on

Innate Immune Defects, Clinical Presentation, Table 5 NFκB-mediated defects

Gene	Inheritance	Infectious susceptibility	Other manifestations
IKBKG (NEMO)	XL	Mycobacteria PJP Encapsulated bacteria HSV, CMV, EBV	Ectodermal dysplasia Colitis
IKBA	AR	PJP CMC	Ectodermal dysplasia Colitis
NF κB1	AD	Recurrent sinopulmonary infections Superficial skin infections	Pyoderma gangrenosum Lymphoproliferation Cytopenia Autoimmunity Enteritis LIP Lung adenocarcinoma
NF-κB2	XL	Sinopulmonary viral and bacterial infections HSV *Giardia lamblia* Onychomycosis	Alopecia Trachyonychia Psoriaform dermatitis Thyroid dysfunction

NEMO nuclear factor κ B essential modulator, *XL* X-linked, *AR* autosomal recessive, *AD*, autosomal dominant, *PJP* Pneumocystis jiroveci, *CMC* chronic mucocutaneous candidiasis, *HSV* herpes simplex virus, *CNV* cytomegalovirus, *EBV* Epstein Barr virus, *LIP* lymphocytic interstitial pneumonitis the surface of most innate cells and when activated, upregulate NFκB pathways leading to the production of IFNγ. Patients have a characteristic susceptibility to herpes simplex encephalitis. Mutations in TLR3, UNC-93B, and TRAF3 have shown impaired TLR3 agonist stimulation and susceptibility to herpes simplex encephalitis.

Natural Killer Cell Deficiencies

Natural killer (NK) cells are critical in defense of virally infected cells and tumor surveillance. NK cell deficiency syndromes are divided into:

- Classical NK cell deficiency – Patients lack NK cells as well as have abnormal NK cell function.
- Functional NK cell deficiency – Patients have NK cells but have absent or very decreased NK cell function.

Patients with NK cell deficiency are characteristically susceptible to invasive viral infections, specifically herpes simplex virus. Diagnosis of NK cell deficiency is established by showing very low quantities of CD56+ NK cells, or very decreased NK cell function, or both. NK cell function is assessed with cytotoxicity testing by way of a chromium release assay (Orange 2013).

References

Boztug K, Klein C. Genetic etiologies of severe congenital neutropenia. Curr Opin Pediatr. 2011;23(1):21–6.

Bustamante J, Boisson-Dupuis S, Abel L, Casanova JL. Mendelian susceptibility to mycobacterial disease: genetic, immunological, and clinical features of inborn errors of IFN-γ immunity. Semin Immunol. 2014;26(6):454–70.

Leiding JW, Holland SM. Chronic granulomatous disease. In: Pagon RA, Adam MP, Ardinger HH, Wallace SE, Amemiya A, Bean LJH, Bird TD, Ledbetter N, Mefford HC, Smith RJH, Stephens K, editors. GeneReviews® [Internet]. Seattle: University of Washington; 1993–2017. 9 Aug 2012 [updated 11 Feb 2016].

Orange JS. Natural killer cell deficiency. J Allergy Clin Immunol. 2013;132(3):515–25.

Sowerwine KJ, Holland SM, Freeman AF. Hyper-IgE syndrome update. Ann N Y Acad Sci. 2012;1250:25–32.

Interleukin-21 Deficiency

Robert P. Nelson[1,2,3] and Javier Chinen[4]
[1]Divisions of Hematology and Oncology, Stem Cell Transplant Program, Indiana University (IU) School of Medicine and the IU Bren and Simon Cancer Center, Indianapolis, IN, USA
[2]Pediatric Immunodeficiency Clinic, Riley Hospital for Children at Indiana University Health, Indianapolis, IN, USA
[3]Medicine and Pediatrics, Indiana University School of Medicine, Immunohematology and Transplantation, Indianapolis, IN, USA
[4]Division of Allergy and Immunology, Department of Pediatrics, Baylor College of Medicine, Texas Children's Hospital, The Woodlands, TX, USA

Synonyms

IL-21 deficiency

Definition

IL-21 deficiency is caused by deleterious mutations in the *IL-21* gene, on chromosome 4q27, and is associated with a clinical presentation of very early onset inflammatory bowel disease (VEOIBD) and common variable immunodeficiency (CVID).

Introduction

Cytokines regulate hematopoiesis and immunity by influencing lymphocyte development, survival, differentiation, and function. The binding of cytokines to specific receptors on immune cells activates intracellular signaling pathways that induce specific transcription factors that trigger gene expression. The largest group of membrane receptors for cytokines is termed class I or hematopoietin receptors.

Parrish-Novak et al. discovered that conditioned media from activated human CD3+ T cells supported proliferation of a lymphoid cell line and functionally cloned a four-helix-bundle structure protein and designated it as interleukin-21 (IL-21) (Parrish-Novak et al. 2000). This cytokine was closely related to IL-2 and IL-15, and its signaling facilitated proliferation of T cells costimulated with anti-CD3, mature B cells costimulated with anti-CD40, and natural killer (NK) cells.

Function

Innate Host Defense
Within the innate host defense system, IL-21 promotes terminal differentiation of NK cells, enhances cytotoxic function, and decreases NK cell viability (Wendt et al. 2007). IL-21 also stimulates dendritic cells, as it is linked to and interacts synergistically with IL-2, in a process that may or may not augment the activity of the other cytokine, regulated by selective engagement of particular STAT pathways (Nutt et al. 2004). NK cells express a low-affinity receptor for the Fc constant region of immunoglobulin G (FcγRIIIa), and following FcR stimulation in vitro, there is an increase in transcription of IL-21R that peaks at approximately 8 h. The increased expression of the IL-21R sensitizes NK cells to IL-21 stimulation, leading to increased phosphorylation of STAT1 and STAT3 (Nutt et al. 2004). Paidipally et al. studied the effects of IL-21 on human NK cells and monocytes during *Mycobacterium tuberculosis* (Mtb) infection (Paidipally et al. 2018). CD4+ T and NK cells from latently infected healthy individuals produced more IL-21 compared to the CD4+ T cells from patients with active Mtb. These findings suggested that IL-21 production from activated T cells enhances NK cell killing of Mtb-infected monocytes. Furthermore, IL-21-activated NK cells augmented the production of IL-1b, IL-18, and macrophage inflammatory protein-1β (MIP-1β, CCL4) while reducing IL-10 production by monocytes in response to the intracellular pathogen.

Adaptive Immunity

IL-21 interactions are important for early and late stages of the development of T, B, and NK lymphocytes (Nutt et al. 2004). IL-21 is produced by activated T cells and is expressed preferentially by TH2 CD4+ cells. IL-21 influences proliferation of T and B cells and the cytolytic activity of NK cells (Parrish-Novak et al. 2002). This cytokine is important for a durable, initial T-cell response to viral infections and is critical in controlling chronic viral infections (Yi et al. 2009). One of several examples was reported by Tang et al. who investigated the effect of IL-21 on CD8+ T-cell responses to hepatitis B infections (HBV). Phenotypic and functional analyses of samples from patients with chronic HBV infection and a mouse model with HBV expression demonstrated IL-21 to promote proliferation of HBV-specific CD8+ T cells and downregulate the inhibitory receptors programmed death 1 and T-cell immunoglobulin domain and mucin domain 3 (TIM3). Also, IL-21 upregulated interferon-gamma, granzyme B, and CD107a in HBV-specific CD8+ T cells while enhancing the cytolytic activity of CD8+ T cells against HepG2.2.15 target cells. Recombinant murine IL-21 accelerated HBsAg clearance in a hepatitis mouse model. These findings show IL-21 enhances the antiviral effect of HBV-specific CD8+ T cells. IL-21 modulates antitumor immune responses mediated by NK and T lymphocytes.

Acting on B cells, IL-21 regulates differentiation to plasma cells, participates in immunoglobulin class switching, and downregulates IgE production by inhibiting germ line epsilon chain transcription from IL-4-stimulated B cells. TH2 cell-derived IL-21 also downregulates TH1 cells, further favoring the TH2 response (Wurster et al. 2002). Thus, IL-21 and its cognate receptor are highly expressed in parasitized organs of infected humans. The IL-21/IL-21R signaling axis regulates cytokine production of T cells by enhancing the expression of T-bet and STAT4 in human T cells, resulting in an augmented production of IFN-gamma. IL-21 has different roles in T-cell-dependent B-cell activation, germinal center reactions, and humoral immune regulation and effector function (Tangye and Ma 2020). Borte et al. demonstrated that combination of IL-21, IL-4, and anti-CD40 stimulation might induce class-switch recombination to IgG and IgA and differentiation to Ig-secreting cells in patients with common variable immunodeficiency and isolated IgA deficiency (Borte et al. 2009).

Clinical Manifestations

Salzer et al. reported a 4-year-old boy born to consanguineous parents, with recurrent respiratory infections, elevated IgE, and decreased IgG. He presented at 2 months of age with severe diarrhea, aphthous ulcers, and failure to thrive. Investigations of infections were negative. Colonoscopy and colon biopsy were suggestive of Crohn's disease, and he was diagnosed with inflammatory bowel disease. Two of his seven siblings had died in infancy because of dehydration and malnutrition secondary to diarrhea. Other immunology studies included normal neutrophil oxidative test, positive anti-hepatitis B antibodies, and absence of autoimmune antibodies. He had reduced naïve B cells and absent switched memory B cells. T-cell subsets were normal in number and function, and T-cell repertoire was polyclonal. Proliferation to mitogens and antigens was conserved, except when tetanus toxoid was used as stimulus. Exome sequencing analysis reported homozygous gene mutations in *IL21* (c.T147C, p.Leu49Pro), which segregated in the patient family with the occurrence of severe diarrhea (Salzer et al. 2014).

Laboratory Findings and Diagnosis

Diagnosis should be suspected in a patient with very early onset inflammatory bowel disease (VEOIBD) and humoral immunity deficiency. Antibody levels may be low or normal and IgE levels normal, slightly increased, or quite elevated. Immunoglobulin levels may be normal or low. Antibody responses may be intact or low. Immunophenotyping reveals normal T and NK cells. T-cell proliferation to mitogens and antigens may be normal or reduced.

Treatment and Prognosis

Because only one case has been reported and he presented with a missense mutation rather than a null mutation, it is unclear if the clinical presentation described above is representative of IL-21 deficiency. Additional cases might expand the disease phenotype.

Management of IBD, in addition to antibiotic prophylaxis and immunoglobulin supplementation, was helpful to support the reported patient. Hematopoietic cell transplantation is a potentially curative procedure.

Cross-References

▶ CVID
▶ HLA Class I Deficiency
▶ IL-21R Deficiency
▶ Neonatal-Onset Multisystem Inflammatory Disease (NOMID)

References

Borte S, Pan-Hammarstrom Q, Liu C, et al. Interleukin-21 restores immunoglobulin production ex vivo in patients with common variable immunodeficiency and selective IgA deficiency. Blood. 2009;114:4089–98.

Nutt SL, Brady J, Hayakawa Y, Smyth MJ. Interleukin 21: a key player in lymphocyte maturation. Crit Rev Immunol. 2004;24:239–50.

Paidipally P, Tripathi D, Van A, et al. Interleukin-21 regulates natural killer cell responses during *Mycobacterium tuberculosis* infection. J Infect Dis. 2018;217:1323–33.

Parrish-Novak J, Dillon SR, Nelson A, et al. Interleukin 21 and its receptor are involved in NK cell expansion and regulation of lymphocyte function. Nature. 2000;408:57–63.

Parrish-Novak J, Foster DC, Holly RD, Clegg CH. Interleukin-21 and the IL-21 receptor: novel effectors of NK and T cell responses. J Leukoc Biol. 2002;72:856–63.

Salzer E, Kansu A, Sic H, Májek P, Ikincioğullari A, Dogu FE, et al. Early-onset inflammatory bowel disease and common variable immunodeficiency-like disease caused by IL-21 deficiency. J Allergy Clin Immunol. 2014;133(6):1651–9.

Tangye SG, Ma CS. Regulation of the germinal center and humoral immunity by interleukin-21. J Exp Med. 2020;217:pii: e20191638.

Wendt K, Wilk E, Buyny S, Schmidt RE, Jacobs R. Interleukin-21 differentially affects human natural killer cell subsets. Immunology. 2007;122:486–95.

Wurster AL, Rodgers VL, Satoskar AR, et al. Interleukin 21 is a T helper (Th) cell 2 cytokine that specifically inhibits the differentiation of naive Th cells into interferon gamma-producing Th1 cells. J Exp Med. 2002;196:969–77.

Yi JS, Du M, Zajac AJ. A vital role for interleukin-21 in the control of a chronic viral infection. Science. 2009;324:1572–6.

Introduction to Autoinflammatory Diseases

Raphaela Goldbach-Mansky
Translational Autoinflammatory Diseases Section (TADS), National Institute of Allergy and Infectious Diseases (NIAID), National Institutes of Health (NIH), Bethesda, MD, USA

Abbreviations

AGS	Aicardi-Goutières syndrome
Blau syndrome	See also PGA
CAMPS	CARD14-mediated psoriasis
CANDLE	Chronic atypical neutrophilic dermatitis with lipodystrophy and elevated temperatures
CAPS	Cryopyrin-associated periodic syndrome
CINCA	Chronic infantile neurologic, cutaneous, and articular syndrome
DADA2	Deficiency of adenosine deaminase 2
DIRA	Deficiency of interleukin-1 receptor antagonist
DITRA	Deficiency of interleukin-36 receptor antagonist
FCAS	Familial cold autoinflammatory syndrome
FMF	Familial Mediterranean fever
HA20	Haploinsufficiency of A20
HIDS	Hyperimmunoglobulinemia D and periodic fever syndrome
MKD	Mevalonate kinase deficiency
MWS	Muckle-Wells syndrome
N4AID	NLRC4-mediated autoinflammatory diseases
NDAS	NEMO-deleted exon 5 autoinflammatory syndrome
NEMO	NF-κB essential modulator
NOMID	Neonatal-onset multisystem inflammatory disease
ORAS	OTULIN-related autoinflammatory syndrome/otulipenia
PAPA	Pyogenic arthritis, pyoderma gangrenosum, and acne (syndrome)
PGA	Pediatric granulomatous arthritis
PLAID	PLCG2-associated antibody deficiency and immune dysregulation
PRAAS	Proteasome-associated autoinflammatory syndrome
SAVI	STING-associated vasculopathy with onset in infancy
TRAPS	TNF receptor-associated periodic syndrome

Definition of Autoinflammatory Diseases

Autoinflammatory diseases are genetically defined immune-dysregulatory conditions that typically present in early childhood with systemic inflammation (i.e., fever, rashes) and with disease-specific sterile organ inflammation, with the recruitment of a predominantly innate immune cell infiltrate in affected tissues. Most mutations that cause autoinflammatory diseases affect key innate immune sensor pathways that lead to cytokine dysregulation including IL-1, type 1 IFN, IL-18, and IL-17 and, more generally, increased NFκB signaling.

Background

The term "autoinflammatory diseases" was introduced in 1999 in a seminal paper by Drs. Michael McDermott and Daniel Kastner et al. that reported the genetic cause for the tumor necrosis factor (TNF) receptor-associated periodic syndrome (TRAPS) (McDermott et al. 1999). This concept aimed to distinguish familial Mediterranean fever (FMF) and TRAPS, the then only genetically defined "periodic fever syndrome," from autoimmune diseases such as systemic lupus erythematosus and rheumatoid arthritis. The latter are both conditions that were thought to be caused by adaptive immune dysregulation, marked by high-titer autoantibodies and autoreactive lymphocytes. Over the last two decades, the genetic revolution and the technologic developments that reduced the cost of whole exome and genome sequencing allowed to sequence patients with rare immune-dysregulatory diseases which fueled the discovery of novel autoinflammatory diseases.

The monographs in this section describe the genetically defined autoinflammatory diseases and recapitulate the exiting journey of the discovery of the currently known autoinflammatory diseases and their treatment (de Jesus et al. 2015; Manthiram et al. 2017).

Autoinflammatory Diseases, Cytokine Dysregulation, Pathomechanisms, and Treatment

The diseases summarized in the monographs in this section are listed in Table 1 below and are grouped by their most prominent clinical manifestations and by their response to targeted cytokine-blocking therapies.

The genetic discovery and understanding of the disease pathogenesis combined with the often impressive responses to targeted treatments led to the discovery of shared innate immune pathways that drive the chronic systemic and the organ-specific inflammation in these patients. The diseases can be grouped by a combination of clinical phenotypes and response to cytokine-targeting agents (Table 1).

A. *Significant clinical and laboratory responses to IL-1 blocking therapies led to the discovery of the prominent role of IL-1 in autoinflammation.* These insights started with the genetic discovery of gain-of-function mutations in *NLRP3* as the cause of the cryopyrin-associated periodic syndromes (CAPS) including FCAS, MWS, and NOMID/CINCA and with the simultaneous deciphering of the molecular components of the NLRP1 and NLRP3 inflammasomes that link danger sensing to IL-1β activation and release (Broderick et al. 2015) (Table 1, Group 2). The significant clinical responses to IL-1 blocking treatment clinically confirmed the pivotal role of IL-1 in disease pathogenesis of CAPS and later also in the periodic fever syndromes (FMF, mevalonate kinase deficiency (MKD), and TRAPS) (Table 1, Group 1) (Jesus and Goldbach-Mansky 2014). While IL-1α and IL-1β activate signaling through the IL-1 receptor, IL-1 receptor antagonist competitively inhibits IL-1α and IL-1β binding and therefore downregulates and eventually stops IL-1 signaling. The discovery of loss-of-function (LOF) mutations in *IL1RN* that causes deficiency of the interleukin-1 receptor antagonist (DIRA) clinically demonstrated the potent role of uninhibited IL-1 signaling and amplification in causing a systemic inflammation, osteomyelitis, and pustulosis and if untreated can progress to organ failure and death and forged the concept of IL-1 in autoinflammation. More recently, mutations in *LPIN2* encoding the phospholipase Lipin-2 also cause IL-1-dependent osteomyelitis and underscore the concept of IL-1/cytokine amplification as contributing to the systemic and organ-specific disease manifestations in these conditions (5). However, the pathogenesis of pyogenic arthritis, pyoderma gangrenosum, and acne (PAPA) syndrome, an autoinflammatory syndrome presenting with pyoderma gangrenosum and pyogenic arthritis, is more complex and remains incompletely understood. Some PAPA syndrome patients only partially respond to IL-1 blockade and often

Introduction to Autoinflammatory Diseases, Table 1 Clinical classification of genetically defined autoinflammatory diseases

Clinical presentations	Sensor	Diseases	Cytokine dysregulation
Group 1. Recurrent/episodic fever and abdominal pain with absence or sporadic presence of maculopapular rashes (hereditary periodic fever syndrome)	Pyrin, Other	**FMF** **HIDS** **TRAPS**	*All IL-1:* *FMF*: Intrinsic inflammasome activation *HIDS*: Inactive rho GTPase due to prenylation defect increases pyrin inflammasome activation
Group 2. Neutrophilic urticaria (cryopyrin-associated periodic syndrome – CAPS)	NLRP3	**FCAS** **MWS** **NOMID/CINCA**	*All IL-1:* *FCAS, MWS, NOMID/CINCA:* Intrinsic NLRP3 inflammasome activation with increasing severity from FCAS to NOMID
Group 3. Pustular skin rashes and episodic fevers	NLRP3 and amplification of cytokine signals CARD14	*IL-1:* **DIRA** **Majeed synd.** **PAPA** *IL-17, IL-36:* **CAMPS** **DITRA** *NF-kB:* **HA20**	*IL-1:* *DIRA*: Unopposed IL-1 signaling *Majeed*: Impaired Lipin-2 activity reduces cholesterol deposition in monocyte cell membrane which sensitizes P2X7 receptor signaling and NLRP3 inflammasome activation *IL-17, IL-36:* *CAMPS, DITRA*: Increased keratinocyte activation with recruitment of IL-17 ad TNF-producing cells *NF-kB:* *HA20*: Reduced A20 deubiquitylation increases NF-kB activation
Group 4. Vasculopathy and panniculitis/lipodystrophy syndromes	Unknown	*Type 1 IFN:* **CANDLE/PRAAS** *NF-kB:* **ORAS/otulipenia** **NDAS/NEMO**	*Type 1 IFN:* *PRAAS*: Proteasome dysfunction and accumulation of ubiquitylated proteins drive mainly type 1 IFN; *NF-kB:* *NDAS*: Increased NF-kB/IRF3 activation drives type 1 IFN production
Group 5. Vasculopathy and/or vasculitis with livedo reticularis syndromes with and without neurological symptoms	Viral sensors, IFIH1, STING, other	*Type 1 IFN:* **SAVI** **AGS1–7** *TNF:* **DADA2**	*Type 1 IFN:* *SAVI*: Constitutive STING activation leads to IFNβ production *AGS*: Nucleic acid accumulation due to defective exonuclease, endonuclease function triggers viral sensors and IFN production, *Decreased adenosine deaminase activity*: *DADA2*: Leads to increased NF-kB and TNF and likely IFN production
Group 6. Autoinflammatory disorders with granulomatous skin diseases	NOD2, PLCG2	*Unknown:* **Blau synd**rome **PLAID and APLAID**	Unknown but NOD2 deficiency leads to granuloma formation and partial responses to IL-1, TNF, IL-6
Group 7. Autoinflammatory syndromes – Presenting with macrophage activation syndrome and hyperferritinemia	NLRC4	*IL-18 and IL-1:* **NLRC4-mediated autoinflammatory diseases (N4AID)**	*IL-18, IL-1, IL-6:* *N4AID*: Increased IL-1 leads to autoinflammatory disease and elevated IL-18 levels predispose to the development of MAS in the context of microbial triggers
Group 8. Other autoinflammatory syndromes	Unknown	*Unknown:* **Cherubism** **COPA**	

require combination treatment with TNF inhibitors (Table 1, Group 3, IL-1) (Cox and Ferguson 2018).

B. *Mutations that lead to activation of the IL-23/IL-17/IL-36 axis of cytokine amplification in the skin cause psoriasiform diseases and/or pustulosis.* The characterization of this group of conditions was spearheaded by the discovery that gain-of-function mutations in *CARD14* cause the autosomal dominant disease *CARD14*-mediated psoriasis (CAMPS) and loss-of function mutations in *IL36RN* which encodes the IL-36 receptor antagonist cause the homozygous or compound heterozygous disease, deficiency of the IL36 receptor antagonist (DITRA). The clinical responses to treatments with IL-23/IL-12 or IL-17 inhibiting treatments confirmed the clinical role of IL-17 in amplifying and perpetuating a spectrum of psoriasiform to pustular skin inflammation (Table 1, Group 3, IL-17).

C. *More recently, mutations affecting intracellular pathways that lead to chronic type 1 IFN signatures are referred to as autoinflammatory interferonopathies.* Chronic atypical neutrophilic dermatitis with lipodystrophy and elevated temperatures (CANDLE)/proteasome-associated autoinflammatory syndrome (PRAAS) syndromes present with panniculitis and progressive lipoatrophy and a high IFN signature during active disease flares (Table 1 Group 4, type 1 IFN), and STING-associated vasculopathy with onset in infancy (SAVI) presents with acral vasculitis/vasculopathy and interstitial lung disease and is caused by gain-of-function mutations in the double-stranded DNA sensor and adaptor molecule, STING. The clinical responses to IFN-blocking agents of several of these patients initially confirm a role of type 1 interferon in causing these diseases (Rodero and Crow 2016; Kim et al. 2016). Last but not least, the Aicardi-Goutières syndrome (AGS 1–7), with AGS 1 caused by loss-of-function mutation in the endonuclease,

TREX1, was the first monogenic interferonopathy described; patients present with demyelination, CNS vasculopathy, and variable degrees of autoimmunity, and due to the lack of systemic inflammation, they are only rarely seen by rheumatologists. A total of seven monogenic forms of AGS have been described caused by loss-of-function mutations in endo- and exonucleases that regulate nucleic acid metabolism and by gain-of-function mutations in the ds RNA sensor, *IFIH1*/MDA5 (Table 1, Group 5, type 1 IFN).

D. *Disorders that present with extremely elevated IL-18 serum levels predispose to the development of macrophage activation syndrome (MAS).* While macrophage activation syndrome (MAS) is not a common feature of the diseases caused by mutations regulating the NLRP3 and pyrin inflammasomes, gain-of-function mutations in the *NLRC4* (alias *IPAF, CARD12*) inflammasome are associated with the development of periodic fever syndromes and the development of MAS, with hallmark clinical features of MAS including hyperinflammation, hyperferritinemia, and hemophagocytosis in the context of high levels of unbound or free IL-18 (Table 1, Group 7).

E. **Mutations that prevent deubiquitination of molecules in the NF-kB signaling pathway and those that affect NEMO can cause a spectrum of autoinflammatory diseases with overlapping clinical phenotypes.** OTULIN-related autoinflammatory syndrome (ORAS)/otulipenia and NEMO-deleted exon 5 autoinflammatory syndrome (NDAS) can present with panniculitis and hypogammaglobulinemia in the latter. ORAS/otulipenia is caused by loss-of-function mutations in the deubiquitylase, OTULIN, and NDAS an X-linked disease is caused by splice-site mutations in *IKBKG* encoding NEMO that result in loss of exon 5, which both increase NF-kappa B and IRF3 signaling that affect innate and adaptive immune dysregulation and tissue differentiation (Table

1, Group 4, NFκB). Patients with HA20 have clinical symptoms of disrupted mucosal barriers that include Behcet's like oral ulcers and gastrointestinal inflammation (Table 1, Group 3, NFκB). Deficiency of adenosine deaminase 2 (DADA2) is caused by loss-of-function mutations in *ADA2* (alias *CECR1)* encoding the enzyme adenosine deaminase 2. Loss-of-function mutations in *ADA2* cause early-onset stroke, vasculopathy and periarteritis nodosa, and arterial hypertension (Table 1, Group 5, TNF).

F. *NOD2* and *LACC1* **mutations can cause granulomatous inflammation and point to mechanisms that may provide better insights into the cause of granulomatous diseases.** Noninfectious granulomas are seen in the context of autoinflammatory diseases caused by mutations in *NOD2* and *PLCG2* that cause Blau syndrome or pediatric granulomatous arthritis (PGA) and PLAID/APLAID *(PLCG2*-related antibody deficiency with immune dysregulation/autoinflammation PLCG2-related antibody deficiency with immune dysregulation), respectively (Table 1, Group 7). Granulomatous tissue responses in chronic inflammatory conditions indicate a form of macrophage dysfunction with no specific pathomechanism that can yet be therapeutically targeted.

While the characterization of intracellular sensor pathways that are linked to cytokine production is helpful in understanding the pathogenesis of some autoinflammatory diseases, others cannot currently be characterized based on pathogenic dominance of a single inflammatory pathway. These include the immune dysregulatory syndrome, COPA, and the autoinflammatory bone disease, cherubism (Table 1, Group 8).

These monographs of seminal autoinflammatory disease summarize their clinical manifestations, genetics, and currently known pathogenic mechanisms. These diseases taught us about key proinflammatory cytokines that contribute to the autoinflammatory phenotypes and provided insights into targets for effective therapies while confirming the pathogenic roles of IL-1, type 1 IFN, IL-23/IL-17, TNF, and IL-18 in the respective diseases.

Reference for genetic mutations causing autoinflammatory diseases: http://fmf.igh.cnrs.fr/ISSAID/infevers/

References

Broderick L, De Nardo D, Franklin BS, Hoffman HM, Latz E. The inflammasomes and autoinflammatory syndromes. Annu Rev Pathol. 2015;10:395–424.

Cox AJ, Ferguson PJ. Update on the genetics of non-bacterial osteomyelitis in humans. Curr Opin Rheumatol. 2018;30(5):521–5.

de Jesus AA, Canna SW, Liu Y, Goldbach-Mansky R. Molecular mechanisms in genetically defined autoinflammatory diseases: disorders of amplified danger signaling. Annu Rev Immunol. 2015;33:823–74.

Jesus AA, Goldbach-Mansky R. IL-1 blockade in autoinflammatory syndromes. Annu Rev Med. 2014;65:223–44.

Kim H, Sanchez GA, Goldbach-Mansky R. Insights from Mendelian Interferonopathies: comparison of CANDLE, SAVI with AGS monogenic lupus. J Mol Med (Berl). 2016;94(10):1111–27.

Manthiram K, Zhou Q, Aksentijevich I, Kastner DL. The monogenic autoinflammatory diseases define new pathways in human innate immunity and inflammation. Nat Immunol. 2017;18(8):832–42.

McDermott MF, Aksentijevich I, Galon J, McDermott EM, Ogunkolade BW, Centola M, et al. Germline mutations in the extracellular domains of the 55 kDa TNF receptor, TNFR1, define a family of dominantly inherited autoinflammatory syndromes. Cell. 1999; 97(1):133–44.

Rodero MP, Crow YJ. Type I interferon-mediated monogenic autoinflammation: the type I interferonopathies. A conceptual overview. J Exp Med. 2016;213(12):2527–38.

IPAF

▶ NLRC4-Associated   Autoinflammatory
Diseases

IRF3 Deficiency

Henry Y. Lu[1] and Stuart E. Turvey[2,3]
[1]Department of Pediatrics and Experimental
Medicine Program, British Columbia Children's
Hospital, The University of British Columbia,
Vancouver, BC, Canada
[2]Division of Allergy and Clinical Immunology,
Department of Pediatrics and Experimental
Medicine Program, British Columbia Children's
Hospital, The University of British Columbia,
Vancouver, BC, Canada
[3]Willem-Alexander Children's Hospital, Leiden
University Medical Center, Leiden, the
Netherlands

Synonyms

IIAE3

Definition

Interferon regulatory factor (IRF) 3 is a transcription factor that regulates the secretion of type I interferons and innate immunity. Patients with IRF3 deficiency can be more susceptible to developing herpes simplex encephalitis.

Introduction

Please refer to the introductory section listed for ▶ UNC93B1 deficiency.

Molecular Genetics and Pathogenesis

Inteferon (IFN) regulatory factor 3 (IRF3) belongs to a family of transcription factors, which collectively have diverse roles in regulating gene

OMIM: 616532

networks in immunity (Honda and Taniguchi 2006). IRF3 is activated by most pattern recognition receptors and is particularly important for its role in inducing type I IFNs to promote antibacterial and antiviral innate immunity (Honda and Taniguchi 2006; Ysebrant de Lendonck et al. 2014). It is therefore a crucial signaling intermediate in the TLR3 pathway.

The identification of IRF3 deficiency provided the first description of defects in an IRF transcription factor conferring susceptibility to HSE (Andersen et al. 2015). Thus far, there has been one form of IRF3 deficiency described (Table 1). This was identified in a young Danish girl who possessed an AD heterozygous mutation caused by a guanine to adenine substitution at nucleotide position 854 in exon 6 (c.854G>A), ultimately leading to an arginine to glutamine substitution at the highly conserved amino acid position 285 (R285Q) (Andersen et al. 2015). This mutation was also present in the father, but without history of HSE, suggesting incomplete clinical penetrance. Patient cells were unable to undergo phosphorylation and homodimerization, leading to an inability to activate IFN target genes in response to both stimulation and infection (Andersen et al. 2015).

Diagnosis

Please refer to the diagnosis section listed for ▶ UNC93B1 deficiency.

Prognostic Factors

Please refer to the prognosis section listed for ▶ UNC93B1 deficiency.

Treatment

Please refer to the treatment section listed for ▶ UNC93B1 deficiency.

IRF3 Deficiency, Table 1 Known IRF3 mutation implicated in HSE susceptibility

Mutation(s)	Inheritance	Gene expression	Protein expression	Functional impact	Molecular mechanism	No. of HSE episodes	Age of episodes	References
p. R285Q	AD	–	Unchanged	Partial	Haploinsufficiency	1	15 years	Andersen et al. (2015)

Cross-References

▶ TBK1 Deficiency
▶ TLR3 Deficiency
▶ TRAF3 Deficiency
▶ TRIF Deficiency
▶ UNC93B1 Deficiency

References

Andersen LL, Mork N, Reinert LS, Kofod-Olsen E, Narita R, Jorgensen SE, et al. Functional IRF3 deficiency in a patient with herpes simplex encephalitis. J Exp Med. 2015;212(9):1371–9.
Honda K, Taniguchi T. IRFs: master regulators of signalling by toll-like receptors and cytosolic pattern-recognition receptors. Nat Rev Immunol. 2006;6(9):644–58.
Ysebrant de Lendonck L, Martinet V, Goriely S. Interferon regulatory factor 3 in adaptive immune responses. Cell Mol Life Sci. 2014;71(20):3873–83.

Isolated Congenital Asplenia (ICA) and Mutations in RPSA

Luis Murguia-Favela
Pediatric Immunology and Allergy, Alberta Children's Hospital, Calgary, AB, Canada
The University of Calgary, Calgary, AB, Canada

Synonyms

ICA: Familial isolated congenital asplenia; RPSA: Ribosomal protein SA, Human 40S ribosomal protein SA, Laminin receptor 1 (LamR1)

Definition

Isolated congenital asplenia is defined as the absence of a spleen at birth in individuals who do not have other developmental defects. These patients are prone to life-threatening bacterial infections, mainly by encapsulated organisms (Myerson and Koelle 1956).

Mutations in ribosomal protein SA (RPSA), a component of the small subunit of the ribosome, have been found to cause autosomal dominant ICA (Bolze et al. 2013).

Isolated Congenital Asplenia

Isolated congenital asplenia (ICA) is a rare primary immunodeficiency disease that has been recognized since the late 1950s (Myerson and Koelle 1956). ICA should not be confused with asplenia/polysplenia syndrome, which can be characterized by absence of splenic tissue, hyposplenia, or in some cases polysplenia. Patients with asplenia/polysplenia syndrome also suffer from various anomalies of the heart and great vessels, which ICA patients do not have (Mahlaoui et al. 2011).

ICA is very rare. Less than 80 patients from almost 50 families have been reported to date (Imashuku et al. 2012; Uchida et al. 2012; Mahlaoui et al. 2011; Almoznino-Sarafian et al. 2007; Myerson and Koelle 1956). ICA is mostly diagnosed in early childhood, although a few rare cases have been diagnosed only in adulthood (Unic-Stojanovic et al. 2014).

The majority of cases with ICA have developed severe, invasive bacterial infections early in childhood, most often by *Streptococcus pneumoniae* in more than 60% of cases and with a mortality rate as high as 45%. Infections present early in life, with a median age of presentation of 12 months, and range from otitis to meningitis, septicemia, and purpura fulminans. Infections by *Haemophilus influenzae* have also been reported (Mahlaoui et al. 2011).

Up until 2013, the genetic etiology of ICA was unknown. Whole exome sequencing of ICA patients has revealed mutations in the ribosomal protein SA (RPSA) gene. Expression studies confirmed that these mutations are indeed the cause of ICA (Bolze et al. 2013).

Ribosomal Protein SA

The human 40S ribosomal protein SA (RPSA) is involved in preribosomal RNA processing (O'Donohue et al. 2010) and is part of the small subunit of the ribosome (Ben-Shem et al. 2011). It is also known as laminin receptor 1 (LamR1) (Ould-Abeih et al. 2012).

RPSA is also ubiquitously expressed in most cellular compartments. It is a multifunctional protein, which belongs to the ribosome but is also a membrane receptor for laminin, growth factors, prions, bacteria, toxins, and even anticarcinogens such as epigallocatechin gallate in green tea (Ould-Abeih et al. 2012). It also contributes to the crossing of the blood-brain barrier by neurotropic viruses and bacteria (Ould-Abeih et al. 2012).

RPSA Mutations and ICA

In 2013, Bolze et al. found seven mutations in RPSA in 18 out of 33 patients with ICA from 23 families studied. The patients with mutations were from eight different families. The heterozygous mutations included one nonsense mutation, one frameshift duplication, and five missense mutations. All ICA patients in these eight families carried a mutation in RPSA, and all individuals carrying an RPSA mutation had ICA. This complete penetrance, the high mortality of the disease,

and the finding that many cases are spontaneous within the families studied suggest an autosomal dominant inheritance pattern.

Prior to this study, RPSA was not known to be involved in spleen development, which is controlled by a cascade of transcription factors. Mutations in other ribosomal proteins are associated with Diamond-Blackfan anemia, which is characterized by bone marrow failure and developmental defects such as craniofacial and thumb abnormalities. However, patients with RPSA mutations do not express this phenotype and the opposite is also true, Diamond-Blackfan anemia patients do not display splenic abnormalities (Bolze et al. 2013).

To date, the exact role of RPSA in the pathogenesis of ICA is still not known.

Immunological Aspects of Patients with ICA

The absence of a spleen has consequences for the immune system. Splenic macrophages play an important role in removal of complement-opsonized pneumococci and other encapsulated organisms from the blood, a process that is enhanced by the presence of specific antibodies against the polysaccharide capsule of these organisms (Ahmed et al. 2010).

Immunological evaluation of a series of patients with ICA revealed normal levels of IgG, IgA, and IgM, normal lymphocyte subpopulations, and normal complements C3 and C4. ICA patients with documented *Streptococcus pneumoniae* infections were found to have protective antipneumococcal plasma antibodies, post-infection (Mahlaoui et al. 2011).

Conclusions

Heterozygous mutations in RPSA gene cause autosomal dominant ICA, a rare form of primary immunodeficiency. RPSA is involved, among other processes, in preribosomal processing. At this point in time, the role of RPSA in the development of the spleen or its exact participation in the pathogenesis of ICA is unknown.

Any child with invasive bacterial infection by an encapsulated organism should be evaluated for absence of a spleen by searching for Howell-Jolly bodies in peripheral blood smears and imaging studies such as abdominal ultrasound, computed tomography, or magnetic resonance imaging. The cardiovascular system should also be reviewed to rule out the more common asplenia/polysplenia syndrome. Given the autosomal dominant inheritance pattern of RPSA mutations causing ICA, family members of affected patients should also be evaluated.

If the diagnosis of ICA is made, proper steps should be taken to protect these patients from severe infections such as vaccinating for encapsulated microorganisms (*Streptococcus pneumoniae*, *Haemophilus influenzae* type b, and *Neisseria meningitidis*), daily antimicrobial prophylaxis, and aggressive parenteral antibiotic treatment in the event of acute febrile illness.

Cross-References

▶ Evaluation of Suspected Immunodeficiency, Overview

▶ Innate Immune Defects, Clinical Presentation

References

Ahmed SA, Zengeya S, Kini U, Pollard AJ. Familial isolated congenital asplenia: case report and literature review. Eur J Pediatr. 2010;169:315–8.

Almoznino-Sarafian D, Dotan E, Sandbank J, Gorelik O, Chachashvily S, Shteinshnaider M, Cohen N. Unusual manifestations of myelofibrosis in a patient with congenital asplenia. Acta Haematol. 2007;118(4):226–30.

Ben-Shem A, Garreau de Loubresse N, Melnikov S, Jenner L, Yusupova G, Yusupov M. The structure of the eukaryotic ribosome at 3.0 Å resolution. Science. 2011;334(6062):1524–9.

Bolze A, Mahlaoui N, Bruyn M, Turner B, Trede N, Elis S, Abhyankar A, Itan Y, Patin E, Brebner S, Sackstein P, Puel A, Picard C, Abel L, Quintana-Murci L, Faust SN, Williams AP, Baretto R, Duddridge M, Kini U, Pollard AJ, Gaud C, Frange P, Orbach D, Emile JF, Stephan JL, Sorensen R, Plebani A, Hammarstrom L, Conley ME, Selleri L, Casanova JL. Ribosomal protein SA haploinsufficiency in humans with isolated congenital Asplenia. Science. 2013;340:96–978.

Imashuku S, Kudo N, Kubo K, Takahashi N, Tohyama K. Persistent thrombocytosis in elderly patients with rare hyposplenias that mimic essential thrombocythemia. Int J Hematol. 2012;95(6):702–5.

Mahlaoui N, Minard-Colin V, Picard C, Bolze A, Kui CL, Toumilhac O, Gilbert-Dussadier B, Pautard B, Durard P, Devictor D, Lachassinne E, Guillois B, Morin M, Gouraud F, Valensi F, Fischer A, Puel A, Abel L, Bonnet D, Casanova JL. Isolated congenital Asplenia: a French nationwide retrospective survey of 20 cases. J Pediatr. 2011;158:142–148.e1.

Myerson RM, Koelle WA. Congenital absence of the spleen in an adult; report of a case associated with recurrent Waterhouse-Friderichsen syndrome. N Engl J Med. 1956;254(24):1131–2.

O'Donohue MF, Choesmel V, Faubladier M, Fichant G, Gleizes PE. Functional dichotomy of ribosomal proteins during the synthesis of mammalian 40S ribosomal subunits. J Cell Biol. 2010;190(5):853–66.

Ould-Abeih MB, Petit-Topin I, Zidane N, Baron B, Bedouelle H. Multiple folding states and disorder of ribosomal protein SA, a membrane receptor for laminin, anticarcinogens, and pathogens. Biochemistry. 2012;51:4807–21.

Uchida Y, Matsubara K, Wada T, Oishi K, Morio T, Takada H, Iwata A, Yura K, Kamimura K, Nigami H, Fukaya T. Recurrent bacterial meningitis by three different pathogens in an isolated asplenic child. J Infect Chemother. 2012;18(4):576–80.

Unic-Stojanovic D, Vukovic P, Miomir J. Cardiac surgery in an adult patient with congenital asplenia and thrombocytopenia. J Anesth Clin Res. 2014;5:1–2.

ITK Deficiency

Thomas G. Fox
Department of Pediatrics, Section of Pediatric Infectious Diseases, Indiana University School of Medicine, Riley Hospital for Children, Indianapolis, IN, USA
Department of Pediatrics, Division of Pediatric Infectious Disease, Emory University School of Medicine, Atlanta, GA, USA

Synonyms

EBV-associated autosomal lymphoproliferative syndrome; Lymphoproliferative syndrome 1 (LPFS1)

Introduction/Background

Interleukin 2-inducible T-cell kinase (ITK) deficiency is caused by a genetic defect of T cell signaling that results in an inadequate cytotoxic T-lymphocyte response to EBV infection, leading to the polyclonal proliferation of EBV-infected B cells that usually transforms into malignancies (Linka et al. 2012). ITK is an intracellular, non-receptor tyrosine kinase member of the TEC family kinases (which includes Bruton's tyrosine kinase) that is critical for proximal T cell receptor (TCR) signaling and T cell proliferation/differentiation (Cohen 2015). ITK phosphorylates phospho-inositide-specific phospholipase C gamma 1 (PLCγ1), a key enzyme that generates second messengers during T cell receptor signaling. Deficient ITK activity impairs downstream calcium flux and signaling through the extracellular receptor kinase (ERK) that deregulates actin (Kapnick et al. 2017). T cells begin to activate, but signals are abnormal that emanate through the TCR leading to impaired responses in TCR-dependent pathways that are indispensable for IL-2 transactivation and T cell responses (Teku and Vihinen 2017). In mice, the absence of ITK decreases TCR stimulation, T cell proliferation, and IL-2 production. ITK deficiency also alters thymic selection of CD4 and CD8 T cells and poor CD4 differentiation with functional deficits (Kapnick et al. 2017). Invariant natural killer T (iNKT) cells appear particularly affected by ITK deficiency, given the enzyme provides important signals for terminal maturation, survival, and cytokine production in these cells. The lack of iNKT cells in ITK deficiency explains certain aspects of the clinical phenotype (Huck et al. 2009).

The *ITK* gene is contained on 5q33.3. Autosomal recessive inheritance of mutant ITK alleles leads to the phenotype. Several different mutations have been implicated that span all the protein's domains and differ in their impact on protein function, but all ultimately confer a loss of function due to protein instability (Cipe et al. 2015). Mutations at analogous positions within the SH2 domain on BTK (Bruton's tyrosine kinase) and SAP (SLAM-associated protein) also destabilize the protein, causing X-linked agammaglobulinemia (XLA) and X-linked lymphoproliferative syndrome (XLP), respectively (Huck et al. 2009). To date, all patients with ITK deficiency are of Middle Eastern descent and parental consanguinity was common.

The clinical features are similar to X-linked lymphoproliferative syndrome (XLP) but with select differences. Epstein-Barr virus (EBV) infection appears a requisite for lymphoproliferation in patients with ITK deficiency; however, three patients were diagnosed prior to developing lymphoma (Cipe et al. 2015). T cell immune function is broadly compromised in ITK deficiency, as evidenced by reports of severe infections with *Pneumocystis jirovecii*, cytomegalovirus, varicella, and BK virus in these patients (Ghosh et al. 2014). The prognosis is poor but hematopoietic stem cell transplantation (HCT) can be curative (Stepensky et al. 2011).

Clinical Presentation

The initial manifestation of ITK deficiency is most often lymphoproliferative disease (LPD) due to unchecked EBV infection. Patients, thus far, presented between ages three and thirteen (Ghosh et al. 2014). All cases except one were diagnosed after EBV infection. The phenotype prior to EBV infection is not well-characterized. Huck et al. (2009) reported the first clinical description of ITK deficiency in two Turkish sisters born to consanguineous parents. The first child presented at age six with severe mucosal candidiasis, *Pneumocystis jirovecii* pneumonia, cytopenias, hepatosplenomegaly, and hypogammaglobulinemia. She had EBV viremia and an axillary lymph node biopsy revealed EBER (EBV-encoded small RNAs) positive polymorphic B cell proliferation. She received rituximab prior to the development of Hodgkin lymphoma of the nasal concha 16 months later. The cancer responded to standard therapy but T cell function declined and she succumbed to *P. jirovecii* pneumonia at ten years of age. Her sister presented at age five with similar clinical features but failed to achieve remission from EBV-associated Hodgkin lymphoma. She underwent haploidentical peripheral blood HCT but died prior to engrafting secondary to ischemic brain injury following airway obstruction and cardiac arrest.

Serwas et al. reported a unique case of ITK deficiency in an EBV-seronegative patient without LPD (Serwas et al. 2014). A 17-year-old Turkish male of consanguineous background developed bronchiectasis after recurrent pulmonary infections beginning at seven years of age. Persistent CD4 lymphopenia was detected at age 10. Functional T cell analysis revealed decreased proliferation to CD3/CD28 stimulation, but normal responses to phytohemagglutinin (PHA). iNKT cells by flow cytometry were undetectable. Homozygosity mapping and exome sequencing defined the ITK mutations and he remained EBV seronegative at the time of the report.

The LPD in ITK deficiency is caused by an ineffective T cell response to EBV-infected B cells. Hodgkin lymphoma and rarely non-Hodgkin lymphoma are the malignancies thus far reported in ITK- deficient patients. This contrasts with XLP, which is more commonly complicated by Burkitt's lymphoma (Cipe et al. 2015). Lymphoma is usually present at the time of diagnosis of ITK deficiency. Patients with XLP may occasionally develop LPD in the absence of EBV infection but it appears required in the context of ITK deficiency (Ghosh et al. 2014).

Autoimmune phenomena may also occur in ITK-deficient patients. Three patients in the case series by Ghosh et al. (2014) developed cytopenias, nephritis, and thyroiditis; two patients developed hemophagocytic lymphohistiocytosis (HLH). A Palestinian patient had diffuse mesangial and focal segmental glomerulonephritis (Stepensky et al. 2011). Interstitial pulmonary nodules were also observed.

Diagnosis and Laboratory Testing

Patients with ITK deficiency experience progressive declines in total immunoglobulins and CD4+ lymphocyte numbers. CD8 cells are usually normal in number. iNKT cells, which are critical components for the control of EBV infection, are substantially reduced in ITK deficiency, similar to other immunodeficiencies in which EBV drives LPD. Most patients diagnosed with ITK deficiency presented with EBV+ LPD, and all patients with LPD in ITK deficiency have been EBV IgG

seropositive with EBV viremia, suggesting that EBV infection is required for permitting the immune dysregulation that leads to LPD (Ghosh et al. 2014). The presence of CD4 lymphopenia and pulmonary conditions (recurrent infections, bronchiectasis, and interstitial pulmonary nodularity), particularly in a child born to consanguineous parents, should prompt the consideration of ITK deficiency, even in the EBV naïve patient. HLH occurred in a minority of patients. As with many combined immunodeficiencies, the diagnosis of ITK deficiency is confirmed with molecular genetic sequencing.

Treatment and Prognosis

Given the small number of cases reported to date, an optimal treatment strategy for ITK deficiency is not established; however, thus far, there appears to be a grim prognosis overall. The experience with HCT is insufficient to consider it standard, although the severity, early onset, and early mortality in the developing cohort suggest that it is the only current reasonable therapy with curative intent. Patients who did not receive HCT died 1–15 years after the onset of disease manifestations, but the transplanted patient died during pretransplant conditioning. Immune globulin intravenous should be administered regularly to those with documented deficits in antibody production capacity. As with all immunocompromised patients, systemic glucocorticosteroid therapy is not absolutely contraindicated, but the additional iatrogenic immunosuppression added to a combined natural deficit should prompt the clinician to consider appropriated antimicrobial prophylaxis and a multidisciplinary approach to treatment is warranted (Ghosh et al. 2014). The presence of autoimmune disease and lymphoma increase the mortality risk (Tanyildiz et al. 2016). One child achieved remission and was living following chemotherapy for Hodgkin lymphoma; the second child died from HLH; and the third underwent a successful matched sibling HCT (Stepensky et al. 2011). Future investigation of patients with this disease promises to help correlate individual mutations with the nature of the disease. At present, one would encourage a personalized approach, familial testing and genetic counseling, and close monitoring of patients with ITK deficiency who are naïve to EBV (Ghosh et al. 2014).

References

Cipe FE, Aydogmus C, Serwas NK, Tugcu D, Demirkaya M, Bicici FA, et al. ITK deficiency: how can EBV be treated before lymphoma? Pediatr Blood Cancer. 2015;62(12):2247–8.

Cohen JI. Primary immunodeficiencies associated with EBV disease. Curr Top Microbiol Immunol. 2015;390(Pt 1):241–65.

Ghosh S, Bienemann K, Boztug K, Borkhardt A. Interleukin-2-inducible T-cell kinase (ITK) deficiency - clinical and molecular aspects. J Clin Immunol. 2014;34(8):892–9.

Huck K, Feyen O, Niehues T, Ruschendorf F, Hubner N, Laws HJ, et al. Girls homozygous for an IL-2-inducible T cell kinase mutation that leads to protein deficiency develop fatal EBV-associated lymphoproliferation. J Clin Invest. 2009;119(5):1350–8.

Kapnick SM, Stinchcombe JC, Griffiths GM, Schwartzberg PL. Inducible T cell kinase regulates the acquisition of cytolytic capacity and degranulation in CD8(+) CTLs. J Immunol. 2017;198(7):2699–711.

Linka RM, Risse SL, Bienemann K, Werner M, Linka Y, Krux F, et al. Loss-of-function mutations within the IL-2 inducible kinase ITK in patients with EBV-associated lymphoproliferative diseases. Leukemia. 2012;26(5):963–71.

Serwas NK, Cagdas D, Ban SA, Bienemann K, Salzer E, Tezcan I, et al. Identification of ITK deficiency as a novel genetic cause of idiopathic CD4+ T-cell lymphopenia. Blood. 2014;124(4):655–7.

Stepensky P, Weintraub M, Yanir A, Revel-Vilk S, Krux F, Huck K, et al. IL-2-inducible T-cell kinase deficiency: clinical presentation and therapeutic approach. Haematologica. 2011;96(3):472–6.

Tanyildiz HG, Dincaslan H, Yavuz G, Unal E, Ikinciogullari A, Dogu F, et al. Lymphoma secondary to congenital and acquired immunodeficiency syndromes at a Turkish pediatric oncology center. J Clin Immunol. 2016;36(7):667–76.

Teku GN, Vihinen M. Simulation of the dynamics of primary immunodeficiencies in CD4+ T-cells. PLoS One. 2017;12(4):e0176500.

IVIG

► Management of Immunodeficiency, IgG Replacement (IV)

IκB Kinase-Beta

► IKBKB Deficiency

IKK2

► IKBKB Deficiency

IKKB

► IKBKB Deficiency

J

Jacobsen Syndrome

Virgil A. S. H. Dalm
Internal Medicine, Clinical Immunology,
Erasmus MC, Rotterdam, The Netherlands

Synonyms

Chromosome 11q deletion syndrome; Partial 11q monosomy syndrome

Introduction

Jacobsen syndrome (JBS) is a contiguous gene syndrome initially described in 1973 by the Danish physician Dr. Petra Jacobsen et al. (1973). JBS is a rare disorder with an estimated occurrence of about 1/100,000 births and a female to male ratio of 2:1 (Jacobsen et al. 1973; Grossfeld et al. 2004, #2). JBS is caused by partial deletion of the long arm of chromosome 11, del(12)(q23) (Jacobsen et al. 1973). The deletion size ranges from 5 to 20 Mb. Breakpoints typically arise within or distal to subband 11q23.3 and the deletion usually extends to the telomere. The 11q23 chromosomal region is gene rich with 342 functional genes and several possible breakpoints (Mattina et al. 2009). Partial JBS with a 5 Mb deletion has been described as well (Grossfeld et al. 2004).

The most common clinical features include pre- and postnatal physical growth retardation, psychomotor retardation, behavioural changes, characteristic facial dysmorphism, and thrombocytopenia/thrombocyte dysfunction (Paris-Trousseau thrombocytopenia with dysmegakaryopoiesis) or pancytopenia. A subset of patients has malformations of the heart, kidney, gastrointestinal tract, genitalia, central nervous system, and/or skeleton. Ocular, hearing, and endocrine problems may be present as well (Mattina et al. 2009; Grossfeld et al. 2004).

Over the past decades, several groups have described patients with JBS with a clinical and immunological phenotype compatible with an immunodeficiency state and it has been nowadays recognized that immunodeficiency is part of the clinical spectrum of JBS.

Clinical Presentation of Immunodeficiency in JBS

Antibody deficiency was the first reported immune defect in patients with JBS (Puglisi et al. 2009; Sirvent et al. 1998). One patient had a history of recurrent upper respiratory tract infections (Sirvent et al. 1998), while two other patients showed increased incidence of both upper and lower respiratory tract infections (Puglisi et al. 2009). In a prospective study of 110 JBS patients, recurrent episodes of otitis media and/or

© Springer Science+Business Media LLC, part of Springer Nature 2020
I. R. Mackay et al. (eds.), *Encyclopedia of Medical Immunology*,
https://doi.org/10.1007/978-1-4614-8678-7

sinusitis were described in 42 out of 78 subjects from which clinical data were available (54%). Only serum IgA levels were evaluated in a minority of subjects and were found to be normal or low normal for age, while no further thorough immunological analysis was performed at that time (Grossfeld et al. 2004). Over the past years, several case reports and case series have described the presence of an immunodeficiency state in patients with JBS. The most important findings in these published cases or case series are summarized in Tables 1 and 2 (Puglisi et al. 2009; Sirvent et al. 1998; Blazina et al. 2016; Dalm et al. 2015; Fernandez-San Jose et al. 2011; Seppanen et al. 2014; von Bubnoff et al. 2004).

Various patterns of immunodeficiency can be recognized in patients with JBS. It is clearly shown from Table 1 that antibody deficiency with disturbed response to immunization with a polysaccharide vaccine is a common feature in patients with JBS. These features are compatible with a predominant primary antibody deficiency, like common variable immunodeficiency (CVID), a primary humoral immunodeficiency defined by reduction in levels of serum IgG in combination with low levels of IgA and/or IgM, poor or absent response to immunizations and/or low number of switched memory B cells. These patients mainly present with recurrent infections of the upper and lower respiratory tract (otitis, sinusitis, pneumonia), predominantly caused by encapsulated bacteria including *S. pneumoniae* and *H. influenzae*. As summarized in Table 2, a significant number of patients may present with additional immunological findings, compatible with a combined immunodeficiency. In these patients, an increased propensity of viral or opportunistic infections can be found. Apart from the B lymphocyte dysfunction (low immunoglobulin levels, disturbed response to pneumococcal polysaccharide immunization and lower numbers of memory B lymphocytes), a decrease in the total number or function of T lymphocytes is described. Moreover, low numbers of natural killer (NK) cells have been described in a number of patients.

The genetic cause of the immunodeficiency in JBS remains unknown. In the common deleted region, six genes are related to immune system regulation and response, including TIRAP, ETS1, FLI-1, NFRKB, THYN1, and SNX19. In previous studies, particular interest has been on ETS-1, which is highly expressed in NK-cells, B- and T-lymphocytes in physiological conditions, is involved in NK cell development, B-cell differentiation and T-lymphocyte development (Garrett-Sinha 2013). In ETS-1 knockout mice, several aberrations in B lymphocyte differentiation have been described (Garrett-Sinha 2013). ETS-1 knockout mice also have a variety of defects in the T-cell lineage, including aberrant thymic differentiation, reduced peripheral T-cell numbers, reduced IL-2 production, and impairments in Th1 and Th2 cytokine production. Finally, in ETS-1 deficient mice, lower numbers of NK cells and lower NK progenitors in the bone marrow are found (Garrett-Sinha 2013). This could be explained by a deletion of ETS-1. Also, Friend Leukemia virus Integration-1 (FLI-1), which belongs to the ETS transcription factor family, is mainly expressed in haematopoietic cells. Loss of normal FLI-1 activation in mice resulted in significantly fewer splenic follicular B cells, an increased number of transitional and marginal zone B cells when compared to control mice (Zhang et al. 2008). There are no studies that have evaluated the role of FLI-1 on immune cell functions in human. Further studies are needed to reveal whether these or other genes are responsible for immunodeficiency in JBS.

Evaluation of Immunodeficiency in JBS

It is recommended that in all patients with JBS immunological evaluation is performed, as immunodeficiency is part of the clinical phenotype in these patients (Dalm et al. 2015). Thorough examination is warranted as infections may be severe, recurring and life threatening and a proper diagnosis may direct therapeutic strategies. Functional analysis should be considered in patients suspected for an immunodeficiency state as quantitative evaluation of lymphocytes could be insufficient in determining qualitative dysfunction of these cells.

Jacobsen Syndrome, Table 1 Described immune deficiencies in patients with Jacobsen syndrome

	Clinical phenotype	IgG	IgA	IgM	Specific antibody titers against S. pneumoniae	Specific antibody titers against H. influenzae	Antibody response upon vaccination with polysacharide vaccine against S. pneumoniae	Antibody response upon vaccination with polysacharide-protein conjugate vaccine against H. influenzae
Patient 1, ♀ 12 years (Sirvent et al. 1998)	Recurrent respiratory tract infections	540 mg/dL (normal)	28 mg/dL (low)	15 mg/dL (low)	N.A.	N.A.	N.A.	N.A.
Patient 2, ♂ 12 years (Fernandez-San Jose et al. 2011)	Chronic diarrhea, recurrent respiratory tract infections	226 mg/dL (low)	31 mg/dL (low)	17 mg/dL (low)	Low	Low	Decreased	Decreased
Patient 3, ♂ 4 years (Puglisi et al. 2009)	Recurrent respiratory tract infections, otitis media, sinusitis	281 mg/dL (low)	17 mg/dL (low)	15 mg/dL (low)	Low	Present	Decreased	N.A.
Patient 4, ♂ 5 years (Puglisi et al. 2009)	*Enterobacter Cloacae* mediastinitis, *Klebsiella* tracheitis, CNS bacteriemia	161 mg/dL (low)	19 mg/dL (low)	25 mg/dL (low)	Absent	N.A.	Vaccinated, but no response measured	N.A.
Patient 5, ♂ 34 years (von Bubnoff et al. 2004)	Increased incidence of viral and bacterial infections	N.A.	N.A.	35 mg/dL (low)	N.A.	N.A.	N.A.	N.A.
Patient 6, ♀ 45 years (Seppanen et al. 2014)	Recurrent pneumococcal pneumoniae, genital and cutaneous condylomata	340 mg/dL (low)	66 mg/dL (normal)	40 mg/dL (low)	Low	N.A.	Decreased	N.A.
Patient 7, ♂ 24 years (Dalm et al. 2015)	Recurrent otitis, sinusitis, upper and lower respiratory tract infections	580 mg/dL (low)	45 mg/dL (low)	<30 mg/dL (low)	Low	N.A.	Decreased	N.A.
Patient 8, ♀ 35 years (Dalm et al. 2015)	No recurrent infections	750 mg/dL (normal)	189 mg/dL (normal)	<30 mg/dL (low)	Normal	N.A.	N.A.	N.A.
Patient 9, ♀ 14 years (Dalm et al. 2015)	Recurrent otitis, upper and lower respiratory tract infections	520 mg/dL (low)	65 mg/dL (normal)	97 mg/dL (normal)	Low	N.A.	Decreased	N.A.
Patient 10, ♂ 14 years (Dalm et al. 2015)	Recurrent upper and lower respiratory tract infections	310 mg/dL (low)	30 mg/dL (low)	<30 mg/dL (low)	Low	N.A.	Decreased	N.A.
Patient 11, ♀ 6 years (Dalm et al. 2015)	Recurrent otitis, sinusitis, upper and lower respiratory tract infections	320 mg/dL (low)	88 mg/dL (normal)	17 mg/dL (low)	Low	N.A.	Decreased	N.A.
Patient 12, ♀ 10 years (Dalm et al. 2015)	Recurrent otitis, sinusitis, upper and lower respiratory tract infections	350 mg/dL (low)	61 mg/dL (normal)	<30 mg/dL (low)	Low	N.A.	Decreased	N.A.
Patient 13, ♀ 16 years (Blazina et al. 2016)	Recurrent viral and bacterial upper and lower respiratory tract infections	891 mg/dL (normal)	53 mg/dL (normal)	<17 mg/dL (low)	Normal	N.A.	Normal	N.A.

This table summarizes clinical and immunological laboratory findings in 13 patients with Jacobsen syndrome described in literature until now. Results depicted in red represent abnormal findings when compared to healthy controls. In between brackets interpretation of measured values when compared to healthy controls is described. *IgG* immunoglobulin G, *IgA* immunoglobulin A, *IgM* immunoglobulin M, *N.A.* not available

Jacobsen Syndrome, Table 2 Described immune cell defects in patients with Jacobsen syndrome

	B cells (total and specific findings)	T cells (total and specific findings)	NK cells (total)
Patient 1, ♀ 12 years (Sirvent et al. 1998)	Decreased	Decreased	Not specified
Patient 2, ♂ 12 years (Fernandez-San Jose et al. 2011)	Decreased	Decreased Decreased CD4+ and CD8+ T cells	Decreased
Patient 3, ♂ 4 years (Puglisi et al. 2009)	Normal	Normal	Not specified
Patient 4, ♂ 5 years (Puglisi et al. 2009)	Normal	Decreased Decreased CD4+ and CD8+ T cells	Not specified
Patient 5, ♂ 34 years (von Bubnoff et al. 2004)	Not specified	Decreased CD4+ T cells Decreased mitogen respons to PHA	Normal
Patient 6, ♀ 45 years (Seppanen et al. 2014)	Decreased Decreased numbers of memory B cells	Decreased Decreased CD4+ T cells	Decreased
Patient 7, ♂ 24 years (Dalm et al. 2015)	Normal Decreased numbers of memory B cells	Normal Decreased CD4+ T cells	Decreased
Patient 8, ♀ 35 years (Dalm et al. 2015)	Decreased Decreased numbers of memory B cells	Decreased Decreased CD8+ T cells	Decreased
Patient 9, ♀ 14 years (Dalm et al. 2015)	Normal	Normal	Normal
Patient 10, ♂ 14 years (Dalm et al. 2015)	Decreased Decreased numbers of memory B cells	Normal	Normal
Patient 11, ♀ 6 years (Dalm et al. 2015)	Decreased Decreased numbers of memory B cells	Normal	Decreased
Patient 12, ♀ 10 years (Dalm et al. 2015)	Decreased Decreased numbers of memory B cells	Decreased Decreased CD8+ T cells	Decreased
Patient 13, ♀ 16 years (Blazina et al. 2016)	Decreased	Decreased Decreased CD4+ and CD8+ T cells Decreased mitogen respons to PHA	Normal

This table summarizes the described immune cell defects in patients with Jacobsen syndrome. Abnormal total numbers of B, T, and NK cells are described as well as specific deficiencies in B and/or T cell subsets. In a small number of patients, specific functional defects have been described

Initial immunological analysis of patients with JBS should include measurement of total blood count, levels of immunoglobulins A, G, and M, total numbers of B and T lymphocytes, preferably including the number of memory B cells and NK cells. Additional functional analysis including response to immunizations using T cell independent- and T cell dependent-vaccines, and functional T cell testing (proliferation assays, response to viral antigens) should be considered in patients in which an underlying immunodeficiency is strongly suspected.

Nowadays, newborn screening for severe combined immunodeficiency (SCID) has been introduced in various countries. T cell receptor excision circle (TREC) assay is used to detect T cell lymphopenia. Using this approach, patients with JS were identified shortly after birth, based on abnormal findings of low TRECS in neonatal screening assays in these patients (Verbsky et al. 2012). However, those patients who develop T cell deficiency later in life and older patients may be missed in NBS screening for SCID.

Treatment of Immunodeficiency in JBS

In patients with recurrent upper and/or lower respiratory tract infections, due to antibody deficiency, antibiotic treatment on demand, prophylactic antibiotic treatment, or immunoglobulin supplementation therapy should be considered based on severity and/or frequency of infections. Treatment approaches are in accordance with those applied for other primary antibody deficiencies, including CVID (Jolles et al. 2017).

In patients with T cell dysfunction, specific prophylactic treatment can be considered, based on involved and isolated pathogens.

Follow-Up of Immunodeficiency in JBS

It is recommended that patients with JBS-associated immunodeficiency are regularly evaluated by an immunologist and follow-up for end organ damage (amongst others bronchiectasis) is required.

References

Blazina S, Ihan A, Lovrecic L, Hovnik T. 11q terminal deletion and combined immunodeficiency (Jacobsen syndrome): case report and literature review on immunodeficiency in Jacobsen syndrome. Am J Med Genet A. 2016;170(12):3237–40.

Dalm VA, Driessen GJ, Barendregt BH, van Hagen PM, van der Burg M. The 11q terminal deletion disorder Jacobsen syndrome is a syndromic primary immunodeficiency. J Clin Immunol. 2015;35(8):761–8.

Fernandez-San Jose C, Martin-Nalda A, Vendrell Bayona T, Soler-Palacin P. Hypogammaglobulinemia in a 12-year-old patient with Jacobsen syndrome. J Paediatr Child Health. 2011;47(7):485–6.

Garrett-Sinha LA. Review of Ets1 structure, function, and roles in immunity. Cell Mol Life Sci. 2013;70(18):3375–90.

Grossfeld PD, Mattina T, Lai Z, Favier R, Jones KL, Cotter F, et al. The 11q terminal deletion disorder: a

prospective study of 110 cases. Am J Med Genet A. 2004;129A(1):51–61.

Jacobsen P, Hauge M, Henningsen K, Hobolth N, Mikkelsen M, Philip J. An (11;21) translocation in four generations with chromosome 11 abnormalities in the offspring. A clinical, cytogenetical, and gene marker study. Hum Hered. 1973;23(6):568–85.

Jolles S, Chapel H, Litzman J. When to initiate immunoglobulin replacement therapy (IGRT) in antibody deficiency: a practical approach. Clin Exp Immunol. 2017;188(3):333–41.

Mattina T, Perrotta CS, Grossfeld P. Jacobsen syndrome. Orphanet J Rare Dis. 2009;4:9.

Puglisi G, Netravali MA, MacGinnitie AJ, Bonagura VR. 11q terminal deletion disorder and common variable immunodeficiency. Ann Allergy Asthma Immunol. 2009;103(3):267–8.

Seppanen M, Koillinen H, Mustjoki S, Tomi M, Sullivan KE. Terminal deletion of 11q with significant late-onset combined immune deficiency. J Clin Immunol. 2014;34(1):114–8.

Sirvent N, Monpoux F, Pedeutour F, Fraye M, Philip P, Ticchioni M, et al. [Jacobsen's syndrome, thrombopenia and humoral immunodeficiency]. Syndrome de Jacobsen, thrombopenie et deficit immunitaire humoral. Arch Pediatr. 1998;5(12):1338–40.

Verbsky JW, Baker MW, Grossman WJ, Hintermeyer M, Dasu T, Bonacci B, et al. Newborn screening for severe combined immunodeficiency; the Wisconsin experience (2008–2011). J Clin Immunol. 2012;32(1):82–8.

von Bubnoff D, Kreiss-Nachtsheim M, Novak N, Engels E, Engels H, Behrend C, et al. Primary immunodeficiency in combination with transverse upper limb defect and anal atresia in a 34-year-old patient with Jacobsen syndrome. Am J Med Genet A. 2004;126A(3):293–8.

Zhang XK, Moussa O, LaRue A, Bradshaw S, Molano I, Spyropoulos DD, et al. The transcription factor Fli-1 modulates marginal zone and follicular B cell development in mice. J Immunol. 2008;181(3):1644–54.

JAGN1 Deficiency

Gesmar Rodrigues Silva Segundo
Pediatrics Allergy and Immunology,
Universidade Federal de Uberlandia, Uberlandia,
Brazil

Introduction

Severe congenital neutropenia (SCN) caused by homozygous mutation in the gene encoding Jagunal homolog 1 (JAGN1) was described as a novel disease in 2014 by Bostug et al. (2014). JAGN1 is an endoplasmic reticulum transmembrane protein involved in vesicle-mediated transport, which is required for neutrophil function and acts as a regulator of neutrophil function, probably via its role in vesicle-mediated transport: required for defense against fungal pathogens and for granulocyte-macrophage colony-stimulating factor (GM-CSF) signaling pathway, possibly by regulating glycosylation and/or targeting of proteins contributing to the viability and migration of neutrophils (Boztug et al. 2014; Wirnsberger et al. 2014). Up to date, there are only 2 reports with 16 patients diagnosed as JAGN1 deficiency (OMIM 616012) (Boztug et al. 2014; Baris et al. 2015).

Clinical and Laboratory Findings

The first study in 2014 reported 14 patients from 9 families with severe congenital neutropenia that presented recurrent bacterial including respiratory tract infections, sepsis, skin abscesses, and pancolitis in association with neutropenia and sinopulmonary and skin infections. Additionally, extra-hematopoietic manifestations such as short stature, pyloric stenosis, scoliosis, convulsion, hip dysplasia, osteoporosis, bone abnormalities, pancreatic insufficiency, amelogenesis imperfecta, and coarctation of the aorta were also mentioned in this group of patients. Histological analysis of bone marrow smears revealed maturation arrest at the promyelocyte/myelocyte stage. Electron microscopy of patient neutrophils showed an abnormal and enlarged endoplasmic reticulum (ER) with almost complete absence of granules, as well as evidence of increased ER stress (Boztug et al. 2014).

Subsequently, Baris et al. published in 2015 two more patients, products of consanguineous parents, with SCN also presenting mutated JAGN1 gene and multisystemic involvement reported previously and other abnormalities, including mild facial dysmorphism, urogenital anomalies, and hypothyroidism (Baris et al. 2015).

JAGN1 is ubiquitously expressed; however, only congenital neutropenia phenotype was found in all JAGN1-deficient patients in their first report, and their hypothesis was that this cell specificity could happen because some other protein carries out the function of JAGN1 in other cell types (as G6PC1 can replace G6PC3 but not in hematopoietic cells) or because JAGN1 is essential for the secretion/membrane localization of proteins necessary for neutrophil function (Boztug et al. 2009, 2014). Otherwise, immunological assessment of the additional two patients described in the second report also revealed CD4 + T-cell lymphopenia, low recent thymic emigrants, and hypogammaglobulinemia. The hypogammaglobulinemia mechanism should be better investigated in patients with JAGN1 diagnosis, but the recent explanation of hypogammaglobulinemia observed in patients with congenital disorder of glycosylation type IIb by intrinsic defects in immunoglobulin glycosylation patients could be important; once JAGN1-deficient neutrophil has been shown to be defectively glycosylated (Sadat et al. 2014). *JAGN1*-mutant granulocytes are characterized by ultrastructural defects, paucity of granules, aberrant N-glycosylation of multiple proteins, and increased apoptosis. JAGN1 participates in the secretory pathway and is required for granulocyte colony-stimulating factor receptor-mediated signaling. JAGN1 emerges as a factor necessary in differentiation and survival of neutrophils (Boztug et al. 2014).

Recently, JAGN-1 mRNA also was detected in primary rodent islets and in insulinoma cell lines, and the levels were augmented in response to ER stress. The function of Jagn1 was to evaluate in insulinoma cells by both knockdown and overexpression approaches (Nosak et al. 2016). Knockdown of JAGN-1 caused an increase in glucose-stimulated insulin secretion resulting from an increase in proinsulin biosynthesis. On the other hand, overexpression of JAGN1 in insulinoma cells resulted in reduced cellular proinsulin and insulin levels. Our results identify a novel role for Jagn1 in regulating proinsulin biosynthesis in pancreatic β-cells. Under ER stress conditions, Jagn1 is induced which might contribute to reducing proinsulin biosynthesis, in part by helping to relieve the protein-folding load in the

ER in an effort to restore ER homeostasis (Nosak et al. 2016). Consequently, it is notable that these individuals presenting JAGN-1 AR disease often have other abnormalities in addition to neutropenia including some with abnormal pancreatic function, although it does not appear, these young individuals have major metabolic abnormalities.

Treatment and Prognosis

The treatment and prognosis of patients with JAGN1 deficiency remain under evaluation as only 16 patients have been described worldwide. From this cohort, one patient died at age 5 years; the others, aged 5–28 years, were alive and well (Boztug et al. 2014; Baris et al. 2015). Two patients underwent hematopoietic bone marrow transplantation.

The majority of JAGN1-deficient patients showed no or poor therapeutic response to G-CSF in both studies. Its cognate interaction partner GCSF-R is heavily glycosylated and relevant for development of neutrophils. Global assessment of glycosylation implicated a defect of N-glycosylation in patient neutrophils, and authors hypothesized that inadequate G-CSF receptor (G-CSF-R)-mediated signaling may offer an explanation for defective neutrophil differentiation. Recurrent respiratory tract infections led to bronchiectasis which responded favorably to IVIG and prophylactic antibiotic therapy in two patients with associated hypogammaglobulinemia (Baris et al. 2015).

As described previously, JAGN-1 plays a role in the secretory pathway and certain cell surface receptors such as the G-CSF receptor which are reduced in patient neutrophil cells, and this finding could explain the reduced response to G-CSF.

References

Baris S, Karakoc-Aydiner E, Ozen A, Delil K, Kiykim A, Ogulur I, et al. JAGN1 deficient severe congenital neutropenia: two cases from the same family. J Clin Immunol. 2015;35:339–43.

Boztug K, Appaswamy G, Ashikov A, Schäffer AA, Salzer U, Diestelhorst J, et al. A syndrome with congenital neutropenia and mutations in G6PC3. N Engl J Med. 2009;360:32–43.

Boztug K, Järvinen PM, Salzer E, Racek T, Mönch S, Garncarz W, et al. JAGN1 deficiency causes aberrant myeloid cell homeostasis and congenital neutropenia. Nat Genet. 2014;46:1021–7.

Nosak C, Silva PN, Sollazzo P, Moon KM, Odisho T, Foster LJ, et al. Jagn1 is induced in response to ER stress and regulates proinsulin biosynthesis. PLoS One. 2016;11:e0149177.

Sadat MA, Moir S, Chun TW, Lusso P, Kaplan G, Wolfe L, et al. Glycosylation, hypogammaglobulinemia, and resistance to viral infections. N Engl J Med. 2014;370:1615–25.

Wirnsberger G, Zwolanek F, Stadlmann J, Tortola L, Liu SW, Perlot T, et al. Jagunal homolog 1 is a critical regulator of neutrophil function in fungal host defense. Nat Genet. 2014;46:1028–33.

Job's Syndrome

▶ Autosomal Dominant Hyper IgE Syndrome

Joint Contractures, Muscle Atrophy, Microcytic Anemia, and Panniculitis-Induced Lipodystrophy (JMP)

▶ Chronic Atypical Neutrophilic Dermatosis with Lipodystrophy and Elevated Temperature Syndrome (CANDLE)/Proteasome-Associated Auto-inflammatory Syndromes (PRAAS)

K

Kabuki Syndrome

Soma Jyonouchi
Division of Allergy and Immunology, Department
of Pediatrics, The Children's Hospital of
Philadelphia, Philadelphia, PA, USA

Synonyms

KMT2D mutation; MLL2 mutation; Niikawa-Kuroki syndrome

Definition

Kabuki syndrome is a multisystem disease characterized by distinct facial features, short stature, congenital heart disease, skeletal abnormalities, humoral immunodeficiency, and autoimmunity.

Introduction/Background

Kabuki or Niikawa-Kuroki syndrome (KS) is an autosomal dominant congenital syndrome originally described in Japan in 1981 which derives its name from the resemblance of patients to the actors wearing highly stylized make-up in traditional Japanese kabuki theater. The incidence is 1 per 30,000–40,000 in the population and believed to occur in all ethnic groups (Adam and Hudgins 2005).

Approximately 70% of patients with disease carry a mutation in the *KMT2D* (*MLL2*) gene which encodes a histone methyltransferase (Lin et al. 2015). KMT2D functions to regulate the expression of numerous genes during embryogenesis through methylation of histone 3, lysine 4 (H3K4); as a result, mutations in KMT2D result in multisystem abnormalities including immunodeficiency. During activation of B cells, epigenetic modifications from H3K4 methylation are involved in the recruitment of activation-induced cytidine deaminase (AID) to the immunoglobulin switch regions which is required for subsequent class switch recombination. In somatic hypermutation, similar epigenetic modification through H3K4 methylation at the V(D)J coding sequence leads to recruitment of AID and affinity maturation of the antibody (Lindsley et al. 2016). A small number of KS patients with mutations in the *KDM6A* gene have also been described (the product of this gene is involved in histone demethylation). Causative gene mutations are not found in 30% of patients with a clinical diagnosis of KS (Lin et al. 2015).

Clinical Presentation (History/PE)

There are currently no consensus clinical diagnostic criteria for KS. The unique characteristic facial features of this syndrome include long palpebral fissures with eversion of the lateral portion of the lower eyelids, prominent eyelashes, arched

© Springer Science+Business Media LLC, part of Springer Nature 2020
I. R. Mackay et al. (eds.), *Encyclopedia of Medical Immunology*,
https://doi.org/10.1007/978-1-4614-8678-7

eyebrows with sparse lateral third, ptosis, large protuberant ears, and open mouth with tented upper lip.

Additional clinical features include short stature, mild intellectual disability, congenital heart disease (coarctation of the aorta, ventricular septal defect and atrial septal defect), musculoskeletal anomalies (short 5th digit, joint laxity, scoliosis, deformed vertebrae, and ribs), persistent fingertip pads, and cleft palate (Adam and Hudgins 2005).

A majority of patients suffer from recurrent infections, most commonly bacterial ear infections and pneumonia. Opportunistic infections such as pneumocystis pneumonia, mucocutaneous candidiasis, or recurrent viral infections do not appear to be a typical feature of this syndrome (Adam and Hudgins 2005).

KS patients can also develop autoimmune manifestations later in life including autoimmune hemolytic anemia (AIHA), idiopathic thrombocytopenic purpura (ITP), thyroiditis, and vitiligo (Ming et al. 2005).

Laboratory Findings/Diagnostic Testing

Any KS patient who suffers from recurrent infections warrants a formal evaluation by a clinical immunologist. The immunodeficiency reported in KS includes low IgG, IgA, and IgM levels. Some patients have a common variable immunodeficiency (CVID) phenotype with both low IgG and impaired responses to specific vaccine responses. Absolute major lymphocyte subset values (T, B, and NK cells) and lymphocyte function (as measured by response to mitogens) are typically normal. However, low memory (CD27+) and class-switched memory (CD27+IgM−) B cell populations and impaired somatic hypermutation have been reported. T cell receptor excision circles (TRECs), kappa deleting excision circles (KRECs), neutrophil superoxide formation, and complement activity were all normal in one cohort (Hoffman et al. 2005; Lin et al. 2015; Lindsley et al. 2016).

Initial testing to confirm the diagnosis of KS should include *KMT2D* (*MLL2*) and *KDM6A*

gene sequencing. Patients with mutations in the *KMT2D* gene are more likely to have classic facial features associated with KS as well as short stature, joint laxity, intellectual disability, and recurrent infections (Makrythanasis et al. 2013).

The immune evaluation of patients with KS should include measurement of IgG, IgM, IgA levels and testing of specific IgG vaccine responses such as tetanus, diphtheria, and *Streptococcus pneumoniae*. Enumeration of memory and class-switched memory B cells by flow cytometry is also useful.

Treatment/Prognosis

For patients with recurrent sinopulmonary infections due to hypogammaglobulinemia and impaired vaccine responses (CVID phenotype), treatment with immunoglobulin replacement therapy is indicated. Patients can receive intravenous immunoglobulin replacement therapy every 3–4 weeks (400–600 mg/kg/dose) or once weekly subcutaneous immunoglobulin therapy (100–150 mg/kg/dose).

KS patients with milder antibody immunodeficiency (e.g., IgA deficiency) and recurrent infections may benefit from prophylactic antibiotic therapy (e.g., Amoxicillin 20 mg/kg/day divided BID up to 250 mg BID).

It is presumed that with appropriate management of congenital defects such as heart abnormalities and immune abnormalities (antibody deficiency, autoimmune disease), patients have a high likelihood of survival into adulthood (Adam and Hudgins 2005).

References

Adam MP, Hudgins L. Kabuki syndrome: a review. Clin Genet. 2005;67(3):209–19.

Hoffman JD, Ciprero KL, Sullivan KE, Kaplan PB, McDonald-McGinn DM, Zackai EH, et al. Immune abnormalities are a frequent manifestation of Kabuki syndrome. Am J Med Genet A. 2005;135(3):278–81.

Lin JL, Lee WI, Huang JL, Chen PK, Chan KC, Lo LJ, et al. Immunologic assessment and KMT2D mutation detection in Kabuki syndrome. Clin Genet. 2015;88(3): 255–60.

Lindsley AW, Saal HM, Burrow TA, Hopkin RJ, Shchelochkov O, Khandelwal P, et al. Defects of B-cell terminal differentiation in patients with type-1 Kabuki syndrome. J Allergy Clin Immunol. 2016;137(1): 179–87.e10.

Makrythanasis P, van Bon BW, Steehouwer M, Rodríguez-Santiago B, Simpson M, Dias P, et al. MLL2 mutation detected in 86 patients with Kabuki syndrome; a genotype-phenotype study. Clin Genet. 2013;84:539–45.

Ming JE, Russell KL, McDonald-McGinn DM, Zackai EH. Autoimmune disorders in Kabuki syndrome. Am J Med Genet A. 2005;132A(3):260–2.

KIAA1140

▶ Immunodeficiency with Multiple Intestinal Atresias (TTC7A)

KMT2D Mutation

▶ Kabuki Syndrome

K

L

Lactoferrin Deficiency

▶ Specific Granule Deficiency

LAP1

▶ TRAF3 Deficiency

Laron Syndrome Due to Post-Receptor Defect

▶ STAT5b Deficiency, AR

Late Component Complement Deficiency

▶ C5b-C9 Deficiency

Leukocyte Adhesion Deficiency Syndromes

Amos Etzioni
Ruth Children Hospital, Faculty of Medicine, Technion, Haifa, Israel

Introduction

One of the crucial events during the inflammatory response is the adhesion of the leukocytes to the blood vessels endothelium. This process is very dynamic and involves several precise steps. Different types of adhesion molecules take part in each of the steps of the adhesion cascade. Once the endothelium is stimulated by various insults, the selectins, which are expressed only on activated endothelium, will bind to their ligands on the leukocytes. These saylated ligands, which contain fucose in their structure, are constitutively expressed on the leukocyte. This binding is a loose one and thus the leukocyte will start rolling on the endothelium. During this rolling, which is the first step of the cascade, the leukocyte will come in contact with various chemokines and thus will activate the integrin molecules on the

© Springer Science+Business Media LLC, part of Springer Nature 2020
I. R. Mackay et al. (eds.), *Encyclopedia of Medical Immunology*,
https://doi.org/10.1007/978-1-4614-8678-7

leukocyte surface. Once the activation occurs, integrins will bind to their ligand, intracellular adhesion molecules (ICAMs), which is normally expressed on the endothelium. This third phase of the cascade will lead to firm adhesion of the leukocytes to the endothelium which is followed by transmigration of the leukocyte to the inflamed tissue (Nourshargh and Alon 2014).

During the last 40 years genetic defects in several of these adhesion molecules were discovered. The leukocyte adhesion deficiencies (LAD) syndromes are a rare autosomal recessive group of disorders in which there is a specific defect in one of the steps of the adhesion cascade leading to the inability of leukocyte to migrate from the blood vessel to the inflamed tissue. Aside from the adhesion defect they all share the tendency to severe bacterial infections and a very high neutrophil count. The designated LAD I, II, and III was given respectively to the time each one was discovered, and not to the specific defective step in the adhesion cascade (Etzioni and Alon 2014).

Clinical Presentation

LAD I was first described in 1982 and up to now hundreds of patients were reported worldwide. Clinically it is characterized by delay separation of the umbilical cord, omphalitis, recurrent severe bacterial and fungal infections without pus formation, defective wound healing, and marked leukocytosis (up to 150,000 mm^3). Later in life they all also suffer from severe periodontitis. This recessive condition, which effects equally male and female, is due to mutations in the ITGB2 gene which encodes for the β2 subunit of the integrin (CD18), the main player in the leukocyte adhesion. Up to now more than 80 different mutations were described all along the gene without any hot spot. No genotype-phenotype correlation was found and patients can have the severe form (less than 3% CD18 expression) or the moderate type (3–25% expression). In the severe type infants will not survive the first years of life, if transplantation is not performed.

LAD II is the rarest of all LADs, described so far in less than 10 patients from various ethnic

groups. Although it shares with the other LADs syndromes increase tendency to infections and leukocytosis, this syndrome is also characterized by severe psychomotor retardation, growth retardation, and the very rare "Bombay" blood group. It should be noted that later in life, there is a marked decrease in the incidence of severe infections, but they still suffer from severe periodontitis. The primary defect here is in the fucosylation of macromolecules, which leads to the absence of the fucosylated carbohydrate ligand (Sialyle Lewis X- CD15), the H antigen on red blood cells (Bombay) among other glycoproteins. CD15 is essential for the binding to the selectins which thus will lead to defective rolling. As opposed to the other LADs syndromes, in LAD II there is no delay in cord separation and the severity of the infections is less. The genetic defect resides in the gene encoded for the guanosine diphosphate (GDP)-fucose transporter (SLC35C1) (Gazit et al. 2010). This is a specific transporter which delivers fucose from the cytoplasma to the Golgi apparatus, where it is incorporated into glycans, which can then be expressed at the cell membrane. Since this is a general defect in fucose metabolism, the syndrome was also designated as congenital disorder of glycosylation (CDG-IIc). Indeed, while the infection episodes decrease in time, the metabolic manifestations remain. Interestingly enough, recently, several children with short stature were found to have mutation in the gene, without any immunological abnormalities.

LAD III. While in LAD I and II only leukocytes are defective in their adhesion ability, in LAD III leukocytes and platelets are involved. Clinically, these patients have similar symptoms as LAD I but in addition they also have a severe tendency for bleeding which can be life threatening. Several dozen of patients were reported mainly from Turkish origin. As opposed to LAD I, the structure and expression of the integrins is normal, but they cannot be activated by physical stimuli. The defect is common to all integrins (β1, 2, and 3) leading to increase bleeding tendency (β3) and infections (β2) (Malinin et al. 2010). All the patients with LAD III have mutation in FERMT3, a gene which encoded for Kindlin 3. This protein is essential for the activation and the strong binding of all integrins to their ligand on the blood endothelial vessels. Transfecting the defective cells with normal FERMT3 restore their integrins activation completely. In some cases there is also a second mutation in Cal-DAG-GEF1 which can cause a bleeding tendency but has no effect on leukocyte adhesion.

Recently, another defect in the activation phase was found in monocytes from patients with cystic fibrosis (CF) and was designated LAD IV. Gene mutation in cystic fibrosis transmembrane conductance regulator (CFTR) can lead to adhesion deficiency in monocytes but not in lymphocytes or neutrophils in patients with CF (Fan and Lew 2016). Although integrin expression is normal, they are not activated (no binding to KIM127, a monoclonal antibody which recognize integrin activation confirmation). This is due to the fact that the small GTPase which are involved in integrin inside-outside activation is impaired in CF monocytes. This defect may play an important role in the severe inflammatory process in the lung. Interestingly, the CFTR-corrected drug VTR325 reconstituted monocyte adhesion.

Laboratory Findings/Diagnostic Testing

In all LADs syndromes the clinical picture is the most important factor in making the right diagnosis. In most cases the diagnosis can be made early in infancy. In a child with high leukocyte count, delay separation of the cord with omphalitis should raise the possibility of an adhesion molecule defect. Aside from a CBC (complete blood count) a flow cytometric test for CD18 (LAD I) and CD15 (LAD II) can confirm the diagnosis. In some cases the expression of the CD18 is normal but the mutation caused a nonfunctional β integrin2 (LAD I variant). Platelets aggregation test should be performed in cases suspected of LAD III. Leukocyte adhesion assays are not done routinely and are mainly for research purposes. While the clinical features and the laboratory tests mentioned above is sufficient to make the correct diagnosis, genetic analysis is recommended in all cases mainly for genetic counseling and for final confirmation.

Treatment/Prognosis

All patients with LADs should be treated with antibiotics and in many cases the intravenous route will be used due to the severity of the infections. In LAD I and III antibiotics should be given prophylactically until hematopoietic stem cell transplantation (HSCT) is performed. In the severe form of LAD I and in LAD III hematopoietic stem cell transplantation (HSCT) is the treatment of choice. In the moderate type of LAD I, antibiotic therapy alone is enough to keep the patient in good condition and no transplantation is needed. The overall success rate of HSCT in LAD I was above 75%, while the prognosis in LAD III is less favorable. In LAD III blood transfusion will be needed occasionally until the transplantation. While gene therapy gave promising results in a canine model of LAD, clinical trials in humans have thus far been unsuccessful. Recently, it was shown that the periodontitis is not due to persistent bacterial overgrowth in the gingiva area, but rather an inflammatory process and bone loss due to excessive local production of IL-17 and IL-23. Indeed, treatment with an anti-IL-23 monoclonal antibody improved dramatically refractory periodontitis in a patient with LAD I (Moutsopoulos et al. 2017).

In LAD II antibiotics should be given in infancy but later in life only when infections occur. In some cases fucose supplementation may be beneficial restoring the immune defect, but has no effect on the psychomotor retardation or growth retardation and thus is not generally recommended.

References

Etzioni A, Alon R. Cell adhesion and leukocyte adhesion defects. In: Ochs HD, Smith CIE, Puck JM, editors. Primary immunodeficiency diseases. 3rd ed; 2014. p. 723–41.

Fan Z, Lew K. Leukocyte adhesion deficiency IV- monocyte integrin activation deficiency in cystic fibrosis. Am J Respir Crit Care Med. 2016;193(5):1075–6.

Gazit Y, Mory A, Etzioni A, Frydman M, Scheuerman O, Baruch R, et al. Leukocyte adhesion deficiency type II; long term follow-up and review of the literature. J Clin Immunol. 2010;30(2):308–13.

Malinin NL, Plow EP, Byzova TV. Kindlins in FERM adhesion. Blood. 2010;115(20):4011–7.

Moutsopoulos NM, Zerbe CS, Wild T, Dutzan N, Brenchley L, DiPasquale G, et al. Interleukin 12 and interleukin 23 blockade in leukocyte adhesion deficiency type 1. N Engl J Med. 2017;376(2):1141–6.

Nourshargh S, Alon R. Leukocyte migration into inflamed tissue. Immunity. 2014;41(11):694–707.

Localized Juvenile Periodontitis

Raz Somech and Tali Stauber
Pediatric Department, Allergy and the Immunology Services, "Edmond and Lily Safra" Children's Hospital, Sackler School of Medicine, Tel Aviv University, Tel Aviv, Israel
Jeffrey Modell Foundation Center, Sackler School of Medicine, Tel Aviv University, Tel Aviv, Israel
[3]Sheba Medical Center, Tel Hashomer, Sackler School of Medicine, Tel Aviv University, Tel Aviv, Israel

Synonyms

CTSC deficiency

Definition

Localized aggressive periodontitis (LAP) is a clinical form of aggressive periodontal inflammation during childhood or adolescence. Although single monogenetic defect was not described so far for LAP, it was reported that LAP is linked to human chromosome 1q25 or chromosome 11q14. The latter overlaps a region containing the CTSC gene.

Introduction

Localized aggressive periodontitis (LAP) is one of the forms of aggressive periodontitis, characterized by early-onset periodontal inflammation during childhood or adolescence, with rapid alveolar bone loss, tooth mobility, and tooth loss. The process usually involves the first molars and incisors teeth of an otherwise healthy adolescent (Armitage and Cullinan 2010). Epidemiological evidence estimates that LAP affects 0.1–7.6% of children and adolescents worldwide; there is a familial tendency, and in the USA, the disease is more prevalent among African-Americans (Albandar and Tinoco 2002).

Clinical Presentation

The extent of the LAP disease is considered localized if less than 30% of the sites (or teeth) are affected and generalized if >30% of the sites (or teeth) are involved. Pathogenic clinical findings include bone loss pockets of ≥5 mm with bleeding on probing (BOP), with radiographically detected bone loss. In localized aggressive periodontitis, especially in its early stages, there are often only minimal signs of clinical inflammation (i.e., redness and swelling) associated with a thin and unimpressive biofilm on the affected tooth surfaces and little or no calculus. In few cases, the levels of inflammation and amounts of plaque are approximately the same as in generalized aggressive periodontitis, with the only difference being the number of affected teeth. The two forms of aggressive periodontitis appear to be associated with somewhat different bacterial profiles in the subgingival microbiota (Gunsolley et al. 1995) and immunological response (Saraiva et al. 2014) and have separate genetic risk factors (Shapira et al. 1994).

Laboratory Findings

LAP is thought to be the result of a combination of microbial infection (most notable pathogen is *Aggregatibacter actinomycetemcomitans*) together with a presumed genetic susceptibility. Although single monogenetic defect was not described so far for LAP, it was reported that LAP is linked to human chromosome 1q25. Interestingly, a consanguineous Jordanian family in which four members had pre-pubertal periodontitis were found to have abnormal genetic variant in the interval on chromosome 11q14 flanked by D11S916 and D11S1367. This interval overlapped the region containing the CTSC gene, mutations of which can cause Papillon-Lefevre and Haim-Munk syndromes. Few genetic changes were also putatively reported in association to LAP including in GPR126 and in GLT6D1 as well as in interleukin-1, interleukin-17, and tumor necrosis factor-alpha genes. Association between HLA alleles and susceptibility to periodontitis have been also reported.

Studies have shown that patients with LAP present a hyperinflammatory response to bacterial LPS, phagocyte abnormalities, and a hyper-responsive phenotype, and similar immune response defects are observed in families of dis-eased individuals (Shaddox et al. 2016). It is suggested that disease onset may be due to biofilm composition shifting to include more Gram-negative anaerobes capable of releasing various toxins, including lipopolysaccharides (LPS), which activate innate and adaptive immunity, per-petuating the cycle of disease. Another possible explanation for the hyperinflammatory state is an imbalance between the proinflammatory lipid metabolites to the proresolving (resolution of inflammation) ones, specifically maresin 1. Maresin 1 was found to be low in patients' blood and when supplemented in vitro restored patient's phagocytic activity (Wang et al. 2015).

Treatment/Prognosis

LAP is treated by combination therapy of mechanical debridement with systemic antibiotic therapy. The suggested regimen is amoxicillin/metronidazole combination for 7–14 days. For prognosis, the loss of alveolar bone may progress only to a certain point and then may remain sta-tionary for many years. In a few patients, the disease may be self-limiting or, on the other hand, become generalized (Miller et al. 2017).

References

Armitage GC, Cullinan MP. Comparison of the clinical features of chronic and aggressive periodontitis. Peri-odontol 2000. 2010;53:12–27.

Albandar JM, Tinoco EM. Global epidemiology of peri-odontal diseases in children and young persons. Peri-odontol 2000. 2002;29:153–76.

Gunsolley JC, Califano JV, Koertge TE, Burmeister JA, Cooper LC, Schenkein HA. Longitudinal assessment of early onset periodontitis. J Periodontol. 1995;66:321–8.

Miller KA, Branco-de-Almeida LS, Wolf S, Hovencamp N, Treloar T, Harrison P, Aukhil I, Gong Y, Shaddox LM. Long-term clinical response to treatment and maintenance of localized aggressive peri-odontitis: a cohort study. J Clin Periodontol. 2017;44(2):158–68.

Saraiva L, Rebeis ES, Martins Ede S, Sekiguchi RT, Ando-Suguimoto ES, Mafra CE, Holzhausen M, Romito GA, Mayer MP. IgG sera levels against a subset of peri-odontopathogens and severity of disease in aggressive periodontitis patients: a cross-sectional study of selected pocket sites. J Clin Periodontol. 2014;41(10):943–51.

Shapira L, Eizenberg S, Sela MN, Soskolne A, Brautbar H. HLA A9 and B15 are associated with the general-ized form, but not the localized form, of early-onset periodontal diseases. J Periodontol. 1994;65:219–23.

Shaddox LM, Spencer WP, Velsko IM, Al-Kassab H, Huang H, Calderon N, Aukhil I, Wallet SM. Localized aggressive periodontitis immune response to healthy and diseased subgingival plaque. J Clin Periodontol. 2016;43(9):746–53.

Wang CW, Colas RA, Dalli J, Arnardottir HH, Nguyen D, Hasturk H, Chiang N, Van Dyke TE, Serhan CN. Maresin 1 biosynthesis and proresolving anti-infective functions with human-localized aggressive periodontitis leukocytes. Infect Immun. 2015;84(3):658–65.

LPIN2: Gene Encoding the Phosphatidate Phosphatase Lipin 2

▶ Majeed Syndrome

LRBA (Lipopolysaccharide-Responsive and Beige-Like Anchor Protein) Deficiency (OMIM# 614700)

Lisa J. Kobrynski
Children's Healthcare of Atlanta, Department of Pediatrics, Emory University School of Medicine, Atlanta, GA, USA

Introduction/Background

Mutations in the LRBA gene cause an autosomal recessive form of combined immunodeficiency affecting both cellular and humoral immunity. The LRBA gene is located on chromosome 4q31.3 and encodes a multidomain protein, which contains a highly conserved domain called BEACH [beige and Chediak-Higashi (CH) syndrome 1] and multiple terminal tryptophan-aspartic acid (WD) repeats. Several of these domains have functions implicated in regulating endosomal trafficking. BEACH domains are conserved regions which appear to be important as regulators of lysosomal trafficking and may have roles in apoptosis and receptor signaling (Cullinane et al. 2013). The WD domain can play roles in transcription regulation, signal transduction, apoptosis, and vesicle trafficking (Li and Roberts 2001). LRBA is constitutively associated with protein kinase A. It colocalizes with lysosomes, the cytosolic endoplasmic reticulum (ER) and perinuclear ER, the trans-Golgi network, and in endocytic vacuoles.

LRBA Function

Upon LPS stimulation, LRBA binds to intracellular vesicles and is transported to the plasma membrane. LRBA upregulates cytotoxic T lymphocyte-associated protein 4 (CTLA4) expression and prevents degradation of CTLA4 by blocking its transport into lysosomes (Wang et al. 2001) (Fig. 1). LRBA deficiency results in increased CTLA4 turnover with a decreased level of CTLA4 and a subsequent loss of FOXP3+ T-cell regulation of conventional T cells. T-regulatory (Tregs) cells from patients with LRBA deficiency have decreased expression of FOXP3, CD25, CTLA4, and Helios (Charbonnier et al. 2015). Consequently, loss of LRBA impairs control of T-cell activation and regulation mediated by CTLA4.

Clinical Presentation

An initial report identified a group of patients from a large kindred in which five individuals were affected with early-onset inflammatory bowel disease. Four of the five had autoimmunity

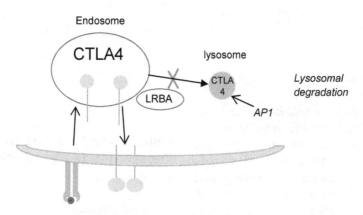

LRBA (Lipopolysaccharide-Responsive and Beige-Like Anchor Protein) Deficiency (OMIM# 614700), Fig. 1 Activation of T cell through TCR causes mobilization of endosomal intracellular CTLA4 to the cell membrane where it exerts an inhibitory effect. LRBA stabilizes intracellular CTLA4 stores by blocking trafficking of CTLA4 to lysosomes and preventing its degradation (thrombocytopenia, autoimmune hemolytic anemia, and arthritis). All patients had inflammatory bowel disease, and two-fifths of patients developed various autoimmune disorders with a combined immune deficiency. One patient had IBD with immune deficiency but no autoimmunity. Serum immunoglobulins, specific antibody production, lymphocyte subsets, and T cell proliferation to mitogens were normal in two patients and decreased in three patients. A homozygous two base pair deletion in exon 44 of the LRBA gene was subsequently identified. This deletion caused premature termination and production of a truncated protein. The truncated protein was rapidly degraded and was not detectable on immunoblotting. Thus, this mutation resulted in a complete loss of function (Alangari et al. 2012).

LRBA deficiency has been identified in other kindreds as a cause of early onset inflammatory bowel disease associated with immune dysregulation. One patient from a consanguineous family presented with inflammatory bowel disease in early childhood and then developed several autoimmune diseases (thyroiditis and type 1 insulin-dependent diabetes mellitus). However, this patient had elevated serum immunoglobulins with normal numbers of CD19+ B cells but increased CD21^{lo} B cells. T cell number and proliferation to mitogens was normal. The missense mutation did not result in a decreased expression of LRBA protein, however, its function was seen to be markedly impaired (Serwas et al. 2015). In another family, two children born to consanguineous parents had type 1 diabetes mellitus, growth hormone deficiency with a severe enteropathy due to a homozygous mutation in LRBA which resulted in an absence of LRBA protein (Schreiner et al. 2016).

Importantly, patients with LRBA deficiency may present with an "IPEX-like" phenotype that is characterized by enteropathy, early onset autoimmunity, and failure to thrive. This clinical phenotype mimics that of IPEX patients in whom a lack of expression of FOXP3 is characteristic. However, patients with LRBA do not have mutations in FOXP3. Alternatively, the clinical phenotype may resemble common variable immunodeficiency (CVID) associated with early-onset autoimmunity, known as CVID8 (Lo et al. 2015). In these cases, autoimmune diseases frequently affect multiple organs. Insulin-dependent diabetes mellitus, hypothyroidism, ITP, autoimmune hemolytic anemia, intrinsic factor deficiency, autoimmune enteropathy, and growth hormone production.

LRBA deficiency may also present with a phenotype similar to autoimmune lymphoproliferative syndrome (ALPS) but have normal numbers of double negative (DN) T cell subsets (Revel-Vilk et al. 2015).

The largest cohort of patients with LRBA deficiency published to date consisted of 22 patients either lacking LRBA expression or with homozygous or compound heterozygous deleterious mutations in LRBA (Gamez-Diaz et al. 2016). Immune dysregulation was seen in 95%, organomegaly in 86%, recurrent infections in 71%, decreased immunoglobulins in 57%, and lung disease in 52%. Autoimmunity included: autoimmune enteropathy (62%), autoimmune hemolytic anemia (57%), autoimmune ITP (52%), GLILD (38%), type 1 diabetes mellitus (24%), neutropenia (24%), autoimmune hepatitis (14%), uveitis (10%), and alopecia (5%) (Gamez-Diaz et al. 2016).

Diagnosis and Laboratory Testing

LRBA deficiency has a very heterogenous clinical and laboratory phenotype. Patients with CVID phenotype, especially if associated with autoimmunity and/or enteropathy or patients with early onset IBD with normal FOXP3 sequencing should be considered for genetic LRBA testing. Those patients with history of recurring infections are likely to have reduced serum IgG and IgA. IgM levels may be decreased, normal, or increased. Therefore, LRBA deficiency should also be considered in the differential diagnosis of X-linked hyper IgM syndrome if CD40Ligand genetic testing is reported as wild-type. Specific antibody responses, especially to polysaccharides, are frequently impaired. Lymphocyte proliferation to PHA may be decreased and B cell proliferation to PWM is reduced. Total CD3+ and

CD19+ cell numbers are usually normal. However, patients with LRBA deficiency show a decrease in the frequency of Treg cells in peripheral blood. These CD4+ regulatory T cells show decreases in FOXP3, IL-2RA, and CTLA4 expression. IL10 production may be normal or increased. Some patients have been shown to have a marked increase in T_{FH} cells in peripheral blood (Charbonnier et al. 2015). Patients with immune deficiency have decreased numbers of switched memory B cells (despite normal numbers of CD19+ B cells). In vitro B cells fail to differentiate into plasma cells and have an increased susceptibility to apoptosis (Lopez-Herrera et al. 2012). Regulatory T cells have an increase in staining for Annexin V, suggesting an increase in apoptosis and cell death (Charbonnier et al. 2015).

Patients in whom the phenotype is predominately IBD and autoimmunity without immune deficiency may have increased serum immunoglobulins (Lopez-Herrera et al. 2012). Autoantibodies directed against the thyroid, red blood cells, platelets, enterocytes, pancreatic islet cells, and intestinal parietal cells. GAD antibodies have been detected in patients with autoimmunity (Gamez-Diaz et al. 2016).

Immunoblotting can be used to show a reduction or absence of LRBA protein. Caution is necessary due to the few reported cases of affected patients with near normal levels of LRBA protein production.

Sequencing of LRBA is indicated to confirm the diagnosis. Many of the reported cases occur in patients from consanguineous families. These patients were more likely to have homozygous mutations. Since the heterozygous carriers were not affected this suggested autosomal recessive inheritance. Mutations described include missense mutations causing amino acid substitutions or premature stop codons and deletions occurring in multiple different exons. Compound heterozygous mutations have been reported in more than 50% of patients described (Schreiner et al. 2016; Lopez-Herrera et al. 2012; Charbonnier et al. 2015; Lo et al. 2015; Serwas et al. 2015; Gamez-Diaz et al. 2016).

Treatment

Replacement with gamma globulin to reduce the frequency of infection is indicated in patients with LRBA deficiency and recurrent infections. Gamma globulins have been used to treat autoimmune cytopenias with some benefit. Patients with autoimmunity may require additional immunomodulatory therapy. Agents used include systemic corticosteroids, mycophenolate mofetil, tacrolimus, cyclosporine, TNF inhibitors, hydroxychloroquine, azathioprine, and rapamycin (Gamez-Diaz et al. 2016).

Abatacept, a CTLA4-Ig fusion molecule, has been reported to treat severe IBD and interstitial lung disease in patients with LRBA deficiency. Clinical improvement was seen in their autoimmune disease associated with an increase in FOXP3 expression and CTLA4 expression on T cells (Lo et al. 2015).

Hematopoietic cell transplantation (HCT) has been reported in five patients to date. Of these, only three have survived. The authors suggested that although HCT should be considered as a treatment for LRBA deficiency, careful consideration regarding the pretransplant comorbidities of the patient may preclude transplant as a treatment option (Gamez-Diaz et al. 2016; Sari et al. 2016). The availability of CTLA4 agonists (such as abatacept) and newer immunomodulatory drugs may offer good therapeutic options with less morbidity and lower mortality than HCT (Lo et al. 2015).

References

Alangari A, Alsultan A, Adly N, et al. LPS-responsive beige-like anchor (LRBA) gene mutation in a family with inflammatory bowel disease and combined immunodeficiency. J Allergy Clin Immunol. 2012;130:481–8.

Charbonnier LM, Janssen E, Chou J, et al. Regulatory T-cell deficiency and immune dysregulation, polyendocrinopathy, enteropathy, X-linked-like disorder caused by loss-of-function mutations in LRBA. J Allergy Clin Immunol. 2015;135(1):217–27.

Cullilane AR, Schaeffer AA, Huizing M. The BEACH is hot: A LYST of emerging roles for BEACH-domain containing proteins in human disease. Traffic. 2013;14:749–66.

Gamez-Diaz L, August D, Stepensky P, et al. The extended phenotype of LPS-response beige-like anchor protein (LRBA) deficiency. J Allergy Clin Immunol. 2016;137:223–30.

Li D, Roberts R. WD-repeat proteins: structure characteristics, biological function and their involvement in human diseases. Cell Mol Life Sci. 2001;58:2085–97.

Lo B, Zhang K, Lu W, et al. Patients with LRBA deficiency show CTLA4 loss and immune dysregulation responsive to abatacept therapy. Science. 2015;2015(49):436–40.

Lopez-Herrera G, Tampella G, Pan-Hammarstrom Q, et al. Deleterious mutations in LRBA are associated with a syndrome of immune deficiency and autoimmunity. Am J Hum Genet. 2012;90:985–1001.

Revel-Vilk S, Fischer U, Keller B, et al. Autoimmune lymphoproliferative syndrome-like disease in patients with LRBA mutation. Clin Immunol. 2015;159(1): 84–92.

Sari S, Doqu F, Hwa V, et al. A successful HSCT in a girl with novel LRBA mutation with refractory celiac disease. J Clin Immunol. 2016;36:8–11.

Schreiner F, Plamper M, Dueker G, et al. Infancy-onset T1DM, short stature, and severe immunodysregulaton in two siblings with a homozygous LRBA mutation. J Clin Endocrinol Metab. 2016;101:989–04.

Serwas N, Kinus A, Schto-Valente E, et al. Atypical manifestations of LRBA deficiency with predominantly IBD-like phenotype. Inflamm Bowel Dis. 2015;21:40–7.

Wang JW, Howson J, Haller E, Kerr WG. Identification of a novel lipopolysaccharide-inducible gene with key features of both a kinase anchor protein and chs1/beige proteins. J Immunol. 2001;166:4586–95.

LUBAC Deficiencies

Julia Zinngrebe[1] and Catharina Schuetz[2]
[1]Department of Pediatrics and Adolescent Medicine, Ulm University Medical Center, Ulm, Germany
[2]Pediatric Immunology, Technical University Dresden, Dresden, Germany

Synonyms

Amylopectinosis; HOIL-1 deficiency; HOIP deficiency; Polyglucosan body myopathy 1 with or without immunodeficiency (PGBM1); Polyglucosan body myopathy, early-onset, with or without immunodeficiency (PBMEI); Systemic autoinflammation; Systemic lymphangiectasia

Definition

Linear ubiquitin chain assembly complex (LUBAC) deficiencies are caused by mutations in the *HOIL1* or *HOIP* genes. LUBAC is a tripartite protein complex consisting of heme-oxidized IRP2 ubiquitin ligase-1 (HOIL-1; also known as RBCK1), HOIL-1-interacting protein (HOIP; also known as RNF31), and SHANK-associated RH domain-interacting protein (SHARPIN), known to assemble linear ubiquitin linkages (M1-linked ubiquitin chains) to substrate proteins. Linear ubiquitin linkages assembled by LUBAC are important for the regulation of many different immune signaling pathways. Mutations in the *HOIL1* or *HOIP* genes can result in perturbation of linear ubiquitination which might then result in dysregulation of the host's immune response. Patients with mutations in the *HOIL1* gene suffer from polyglucosan storage myopathy of yet unknown etiology associated with early-onset progressive muscle weakness and progressive dilated cardiomyopathy (Boisson et al. 2012; Nilsson et al. 2013; Wang et al. 2013). In severe cases these patients may require a cardiac transplant (Nilsson et al. 2013). Some patients present with severe autoinflammation and immunodeficiency (Boisson et al. 2012). Only one patient has been published with a disease-causing mutation in the *HOIP* gene (Boisson et al. 2015). This patient suffered from multi-organ autoinflammation, combined immunodeficiency, polyglucosan storage myopathy with weakness of the lower extremities, and systemic lymphangiectasia but no cardiomyopathy (Boisson et al. 2015).

Whether the phenotype of the published patients is entirely caused by defective linear ubiquitination, or is partially due to LUBAC-independent functions of the respective proteins, is currently unknown.

Introduction

LUBAC deficiency was first described by Boisson et al. in 2012 who identified mutations in the *HOIL1* gene as causative for a fatal phenotype encompassing autoinflammation, immunodeficiency, and amylopectinosis (or polyglucosan storage myopathy) resulting in death of the patients during early childhood (Boisson et al. 2012). LUBAC is the only known complex in humans capable of forming linear ubiquitin linkages. Since its initial discovery in 2006, LUBAC was shown to play an important role in the regulation of a number of immune signaling pathways. One year after the initial description of LUBAC deficiency in humans, 13 additional patients with mutations in the *HOIL1* gene were described in two independent studies (Nilsson et al. 2013; Wang et al. 2013). These patients also suffered from polyglucosan storage myopathy. Their muscle weakness and cardiomyopathy, however, were more severe, but they failed to show signs of autoinflammation or immunodeficiency (Nilsson et al. 2013; Wang et al. 2013). Thus, mutations in the *HOIL1* gene can result in variable clinical manifestations. LUBAC deficiency can also occur when the central and catalytically active component HOIP is mutated as was shown in 2015 for a patient with a missense mutation in the *HOIP* gene (Boisson et al. 2015). This HOIP-deficient patient suffered from autoinflammation, immunodeficiency, and amylopectinosis (Boisson et al. 2015).

Background

Ubiquitination, like phosphorylation, is a posttranslational modification of proteins. Posttranslational modifications are required to regulate a protein's stability, enzymatic activity, or interaction with other proteins. Ubiquitination describes the biochemical process in which ubiquitin molecules are covalently attached to substrate proteins (Hershko 1983). Ubiquitin molecules can also be attached to one another resulting in the formation of ubiquitin chains. Eight different ubiquitin chain types exist in the human body. These different ubiquitin chain types were identified to fulfill different and very distinct functions ranging from protein degradation to activation of signaling pathways. Linear ubiquitin chains, also known as M1-linkages, were demonstrated to be required for NF-κB and MAPK signaling downstream of many different innate immune receptors, including tumor necrosis factor receptor (TNFR) 1, cluster of differentiation (CD) 40, interleukin (IL)-1β, nucleotide-binding oligomerization domain containing (NOD) 2, and toll-like receptors (TLRs) 1/2, 3, 4, and 9 (Damgaard et al. 2012; Gerlach et al. 2011; Tokunaga et al. 2009; Zinngrebe et al. 2016). LUBAC was also shown to prevent excessive cell death in different models in vitro and in vivo. NEMO and RIPK1 or RIPK2 were identified as LUBAC substrates upon ligation of TNFR1 with TNF or NOD2 with muramyl dipeptide (MDP), respectively (Damgaard et al. 2012; Gerlach et al. 2011). Additional substrates of LUBAC in these two and other signaling pathways remain to be identified.

Clinical Presentation

HOIL-1 Deficiency

In 2012, three patients from two independent families were identified with mutations in the *HOIL1* gene who suffered from a syndrome encompassing severe systemic autoinflammation, immunodeficiency, and polyglucosan storage myopathy (or muscular amylopectinosis). All three patients developed early-onset periodic fever syndrome with elevation of acute-phase markers accompanied by hepatosplenomegaly, lymphadenitis, and failure to thrive. Gastrointestinal symptoms like abdominal pain and blood and mucus in the stools were reported in all three patients. Furthermore, they showed signs of cardiomyopathy with amylopectin-like deposits in the muscles. The patients suffered from severe infections with, e.g., *S. pneumoniae*, *H. influenzae*, *E. coli*, *Enterococcus*, *Malassezia furfur*, and *Candida albicans* and viral infections such as roseola, chicken pox, or CMV. Two patients presented with episodes of skin inflammation. All three patients died in early childhood (Boisson et al. 2012).

In two independent studies, truncating mutations in the *HOIL1* gene were suggested to cause a phenotype consisting of myopathy and dilated cardiomyopathy due to accumulation of polyglucosan in the muscle. However, none of these patients suffered from severe immunodeficiency or overt hyperinflammation (Nilsson et al. 2013; Wang et al. 2013).

This phenotypic variability in HOIL-1-deficient patients may be due to different mutation sites in the HOIL1 gene. For instance, the three HOIL-1-deficient patients with immune dysfunction harbored homozygous or compound heterozygous mutations affecting the N-terminal region of HOIL-1, whereas most other patients have been homozygous or compound heterozygous for mutations in the central or C-terminal part of HOIL-1 (Boisson et al. 2012; Nilsson et al. 2013; Wang et al. 2013). The exact underlying mechanism, however, needs further clarification.

HOIP Deficiency

HOIP deficiency in humans has been described for a single case of a 19-year-old woman suffering from multi-organ autoinflammation and recurrent viral and bacterial infections (Boisson et al. 2015). During the neonatal period, the patient suffered from omphalitis requiring antibiotic treatment. During the first years of life, she repeatedly presented with fever episodes as well as splenohepatomegaly. Since early childhood, she had growth retardation, and, at the age of 7 years, she developed recurrent fatty diarrhea and oral ulcers. During adolescence, she developed arthralgia and muscular weakness, in particular of the lower extremities. Furthermore, intestinal lymphangiectasia was diagnosed at the age of 16 years. Immunization with BCG resulted in generalized lymphadenopathy. Immunization against *H. influenzae* and *S. pneumoniae* resulted in non-protective titers, whereas the vaccination response to tetanus toxoid was normal (Boisson et al. 2015).

An overview of the different symptoms associated with LUBAC deficiencies is given in Table 1 and Fig. 1.

Laboratory Findings/Diagnostic Testing

No validated functional test is available for diagnosis of LUBAC deficiencies.

Patients with LUBAC deficiencies can present with immune abnormalities including highly elevated IgA and impaired proliferation with anti-CD3. Additional laboratory findings include elevated white blood cells and thrombocyte count, anemia, hypoproteinemia, and cholestasis. So far, autoantibodies were not detected in patients.

Patients with LUBAC deficiencies should be monitored for development of cardiomyopathy and myopathy on a regular basis. In case of first clinical symptoms suggestive of disease, a muscle biopsy should be performed to check for the presence of amylopectin-like structures. Routine blood testing should also be performed regularly including blood counts and analysis of B- and T-cell populations, acute phase markers, electrolytes, albumin, gamma globulins, vitamins, and liver and kidney values.

Treatment/Prognosis

A targeted, causative treatment strategy for LUBAC-deficient patients directly modulating the level of M1-linked ubiquitin chains is not yet available. Patients with LUBAC deficiencies should receive antibiotic prophylaxis. Pyogenic bacterial infections should be treated with broad-spectrum antibiotics. In patients with impaired B-cell function, treatment with intravenous immunoglobulins may be indicated. Patients should receive vaccination against *S. pneumoniae*, *H. influenzae*, and *N. meningitidis*. An immunosuppressive therapy may be necessary for patients with signs of autoinflammation. Corticosteroids are effective in patients with HOIL-1 deficiency, whereas treatment with anti-TNF and anti-IL-1R shows minor or no effects in these patients (Boisson et al. 2012). One patient with HOIL-1 deficiency was treated with stem cell transplantation preventing further septic episodes; however,

LUBAC Deficiencies, Table 1 Overview of patient characteristics with mutations in *HOIL-1* or *HOIP* genes

	Function	Phenotype	ID	Laboratory findings	Age	Inheritance	n	References
HOIL-1	Component of LUBAC; E3 ligase; and assembles M1 linkages	Polyglucosan storage myopathy associated with early-onset progressive muscle weakness Progressive dilated cardiomyopathy (8/10) Heart transplantation (4/10) Myopathy	n	Serum CK elevated (4/10)	15–50	AR	10	Nilsson et al. (2013)
		Polyglucosan storage myopathy and cardiomyopathy		Not determined	>8		3	Wang et al. (2013)
		1. Infections: Severe bacterial infections such as *S. pneumoniae, H. influenzae, E. coli,* and *Enterococcus* Fungal infections such as *Malassezia furfur* and *Candida albicans* Viral infections such as roseola, chicken pox, or CMV 2. Chronic autoinflammation: Hepatosplenomegaly Lymphadenitis Gastrointestinal symptoms Failure to thrive Skin inflammation (2/3) 3. Other: Polyglucosan storage myopathy Cardiomyopathy	y	1. Immunological abnormalities: Low memory B cells (2/3), Highly elevated IgA (2/3), Impaired proliferative response to antiCD3 (1/3) No autoantibodies detected 2. Other: Hyperleukocytosis (2/3) Thrombocytosis (1/3) Anemia (1/3) CRP ↑ (3/3) Hypoproteinemia (1/3) Cholestasis (1/3)	0–4		3	Boisson et al. (2012)
HOIP	Central and main catalytic component of LUBAC; E3 ligase; and assembles M1 linkages	1. Combined immunodeficiency 2. Chronic autoinflammation: Multi-organ autoinflammation Hepatosplenomegaly Gastrointestinal symptoms Failure to thrive Arthralgia 3. Other: Polyglucosan storage myopathy and muscular weakness Systemic lymphangiectasia	y	1. Immunological abnormalities: T cell lymphopenia and impaired proliferative response to antiCD3 Hypogammaglobulinemia 2. Other: Anemia Hypoalbuminemia Hypocalcemia Iron deficiency Vitamin D deficiency ESR ↑ CRP ↑	19		1	Boisson et al. (2015)

ID immunodeficiency

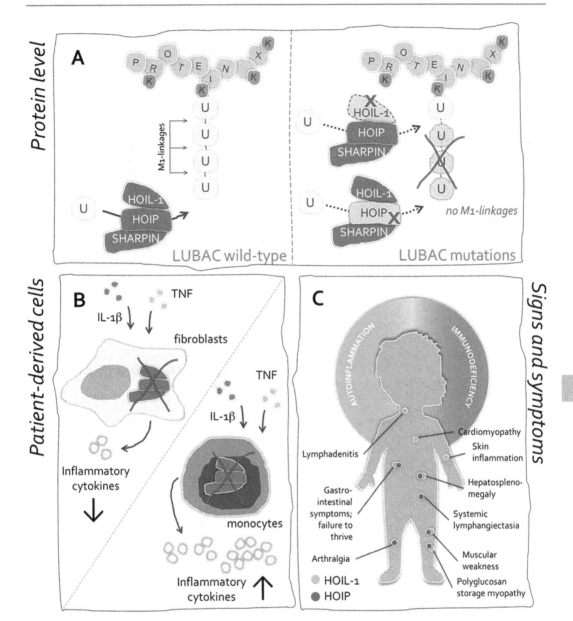

LUBAC Deficiencies, Fig. 1 (**a**) The linear ubiquitin chain assembly complex (LUBAC) consisting of SHARPIN, HOIL-1 and HOIP, is the only complex capable of assembling linear ubiquitin (also known as M1-) linkages in human cells. LUBAC attaches linear ubiquitin linkages to substrate proteins (Protein X). Mutations in the *HOIL-1* or *HOIP* genes result in perturbed linear ubiquitin linkage formation. (**b**) Absence of linear ubiquitin linkages can alter a cell's signaling output: patient-derived fibroblasts showed diminished gene activation upon stimulation with TNF or IL-1beta whereas the same innate immune stimuli resulted in an increased activation of patient-derived monocytes as compared to control cells. This differential response of different cell types was suggested to be causative, at least in part, for the paradoxical and pleiotropic effects observed in LUBAC-deficient patients. (**c**) The variable signs and symptoms of HOIL-1-deficient patients are indicated by blue circles, those of the only described HOIP-deficient patient by red circles growth retardation and amylopectinosis persisted (Boisson et al. 2012).

The prognosis of LUBAC deficiency is dependent on the severity of the symptoms which are variable between patients. All three HOIL-1-deficient patients who showed signs of immunodeficiency died during early childhood. The outcome of LUBAC-deficient patients without signs of immunodeficiency depends on severity of cardiomyopathy.

Cross-References

▶ Otulipenia/ORAS   Otulipenia/Otulin-Related Autoinflammatory Syndrome

References

Boisson B, Laplantine E, Prando C, Giliani S, Israelsson E, Xu Z, et al. Immunodeficiency, autoinflammation and amylopectinosis in humans with inherited HOIL-1 and LUBAC deficiency. Nat Immunol. 2012;13(12):1178–86.
Boisson B, Laplantine E, Dobbs K, Cobat A, Tarantino N, Hazen M, et al. Human HOIP and LUBAC deficiency underlies autoinflammation, immunodeficiency, amylopectinosis, and lymphangiectasia. J Exp Med. 2015;212(6):939–51.
Damgaard RB, Nachbur U, Yabal M, Wong WW, Fiil BK, Kastirr M, et al. The ubiquitin ligase XIAP recruits LUBAC for NOD2 signaling in inflammation and innate immunity. Mol Cell. 2012;46(6):746–58.
Damgaard RB, Walker JA, Marco-Casanova P, Morgan NV, Titheradge HL, Elliott PR, et al. The deubiquitinase OTULIN is an essential negative regulator of inflammation and autoimmunity. Cell. 2016;166(5):1215–30 e20.
Gerlach B, Cordier SM, Schmukle AC, Emmerich CH, Rieser E, Haas TL, et al. Linear ubiquitination prevents inflammation and regulates immune signalling. Nature. 2011;471(7340):591–6.
Hershko A. Ubiquitin: roles in protein modification and breakdown. Cell. 1983;34(1):11–2.
Nilsson J, Schoser B, Laforet P, Kalev O, Lindberg C, Romero NB, et al. Polyglucosan body myopathy caused by defective ubiquitin ligase RBCK1. Ann Neurol. 2013;74(6):914–9.
Tokunaga F, Sakata S, Saeki Y, Satomi Y, Kirisako T, Kamei K, et al. Involvement of linear polyubiquitylation of NEMO in NF-kappaB activation. Nat Cell Biol. 2009;11(2):123–32.
Wang K, Kim C, Bradfield J, Guo Y, Toskala E, Otieno FG, et al. Whole-genome DNA/RNA sequencing identifies truncating mutations in RBCK1 in a novel Mendelian disease with neuromuscular and cardiac involvement. Genome Med. 2013;5(7):67.
Zhou Q, Yu X, Demirkaya E, Deuitch N, Stone D, Tsai WL, et al. Biallelic hypomorphic mutations in a linear deubiquitinase define otulipenia, an early-onset autoinflammatory disease. Proc Natl Acad Sci U S A. 2016;113(36):10127–32.
Zinngrebe J, Rieser E, Taraborrelli L, Peltzer N, Hartwig T, Ren H, et al. –LUBAC deficiency perturbs TLR3 signaling to cause immunodeficiency and autoinflammation. J Exp Med 2016;213(12):2671–89.

LUBAC Deficiency

▶ TIR Signaling Pathway Deficiency, HOIL1 Deficiency

LUBAC Linear Ubiquitin Chain Assembly Complex

▶ OTULIN   Deficiency-Associated   Disease Spectrum

Lymphocyte-Specific Protein Tyrosine Kinase: LCK

Robert P. Nelson
Divisions of Hematology and Oncology, Stem Cell Transplant Program, Indiana University (IU) School of Medicine and the IU Bren and Simon Cancer Center, Indianapolis, IN, USA
Pediatric Immunodeficiency Clinic, Riley Hospital for Children at Indiana University Health, Indianapolis, IN, USA
Medicine and Pediatrics, Indiana University School of Medicine, Immunohematology and Transplantation, Indianapolis, IN, USA

Synonyms

p56LCK

Definition

Gene located on human chromosome 1 that encodes a cell membrane-associated protein that transduces signals through the T cell receptor.

Introduction/Background

The lymphocyte-specific protein tyrosine kinase (LCK) belongs to the Src family of proto-oncogene kinases that regulate cell proliferation, motility, activation, and survival. The LCK gene product, expressed in lymphoid cells, is required for normal signal transduction through the T cell receptor (TCR) and enables T cell development and maturation (Perlmutter et al. 1988). LCK also affects signaling through the B cell receptor (BCR) (Ulivieri et al. 2003). Located on murine chromosome 4 and human chromosome 1, LCK is a membrane-associated protein initially recognized as a Moloney murine leukemia virus proto-oncogene. Its position at p32-35 is near a site of frequent structural abnormalities observed in human lymphomas and neuroblastomas, which suggested its importance in preventing human malignant transformation (Marth et al. 1986). Loss-of-function (LOF) genetic lesions cause defective T cell receptor (TCR)-associated signaling and decreased CD4+ helper T cell activity leading to combined immunodeficiencies.

Members of the Src family each contain unique amino-terminal regions, followed by Src-homology domains SH3 and SH2, and a tyrosine kinase domain. LCK is regulated by phosphorylation of a tyrosine in the short C-terminal tail of its catalytic domain (Eck et al. 1994).

Function

Innate Defense

The cell surface receptor Fc gamma RIIIA (CD16) on human NK cells is essential for antibody-dependent cellular cytotoxicity (ADCC). Engagement of the CD16 receptor, cross-linking of CD16 and interleukin-12 stimulation all induce tyrosine phosphorylation of LCK, which regulates cytotoxicity. LCK overexpression enhances the association of ZAP-70 with the zeta chain of the Fc gamma R complex (Pignata et al. 1993, 1995).

Adaptive Immunity

LCK participates in T cell selection to the repertoire during development and maturation in the thymus and mediates cell fate decisions throughout the life of the cell. Human fetal thymocytes express LCK at 70 days of gestation, which coincides with the appearance of lymphoid cells (Van Laethem et al. 2013). The functional consequences of TCR engagement depend on whether the maturing T cell is committing to a CD4+ or CD8+ lineage. In CD4+ cells, antigen-stimulated TCR activation elicits the biochemical organization of a complex containing LCK and a CD4 cell surface glycoprotein (Shaw et al. 1989).

Antigen receptor signaling of naïve T cells requires the sequential activities of LCK and zeta chain of T cell receptor associated protein-70 (ZAP70). Upon TCR stimulation, LCK phosphorylates the TCR, which leads to the recruitment, phosphorylation, and activation of ZAP70. LCK binds and stabilizes phosho-ZAP70 with its SH2 domain. ZAP70 phosphorylates the critical adaptor linker of activated T cells (LAT) with its SH3 domain, thus connecting ZAP70 and LAT (Lo et al. 2018).

Clinical Presentation

The small number of patients documented with combined immunodeficiencies secondary to LCK deficiency speaks to its importance in immunophysiology and suggests that pathogenic variants are perhaps embryonically lethal. Loss-of-function (LOF) genetic lesions cause defective TCR-associated signaling and decreased CD4+ helper T cell activity leading to combined immunodeficiency. Clinical consequences include respiratory tract infections, early onset inflammation, and autoimmune manifestations; clinical findings may overlap with those of common variable immunodeficiency (CVID), severe combined immuno-deficiency (SCID), and idiopathic CD4 lymphopenia.

Human cases of defective LCK demonstrated infections, inflammation, and autoimmunity. Complete loss of kinase activity secondary to a missense mutation (L341P) in LCK caused SCID with selective CD4 lymphopenia (Hauck et al. 2012). Loss of LCK full length expression secondary to aberrantly splicing of the LCK transcript, with expression of a LCK protein lacking the entire exon 7 has been reported in a patient with CVID and a patient with CD4 T cell lymphopenia (Sawabe et al. 2001) (Goldman et al. 1998). Three siblings with T cell defects, HPV infection, and virus-induced malignancy were reported with a homozygous splicing mutation (c.188-2A > G) that caused an exon 3 deletion, frameshift mutation, and mRNA decay (Li et al. 2016).

Diagnoses and Laboratory Testing

History
Patients are diagnosed in childhood. There may be a history of autoimmune manifestations; current or previous cancers; enteritis; recurrent, persistent, and/or severe infections; failure to thrive; positive family history of PID; opportunistic infections; persistent or recurrent dermatological manifestations; and recurrent or severe infections with encapsulated bacterial pathogens.

Physical
Signs of failure to thrive.

Diagnostic Tests
Screening immunological evaluation may demonstrate a normal complete blood count (CBC) or signs of autoimmune cytopenias. Total lymphocytes percentages may be normal or decreases. Patients have low levels of CD4 and CD8 expression on T cells and a restricted repertoire (oligoclonality). B cell counts are normal. Functional assays demonstrate marked TCR signaling defects including weak tyrosine phosphorylation

signals and failure to mobilize calcium after TCR stimulation.

Clinical consequences include respiratory tract infections, early onset inflammation, and autoimmune manifestations. CD8 expression may be deficient and the T lymphocyte repertoire restricted.

Cross-References

▶ ZAP70 Deficiency (OMIM # 176947)

References

Eck MJ, Atwell SK, Shoelson SE, Harrison SC. Structure of the regulatory domains of the Src-family tyrosine kinase Lck. Nature. 1994;368(6473):764–9.

Goldman FD, Ballas ZK, Schutte BC, Kemp J, Hollenback C, Noraz N, Taylor N. Defective expression of p56lck in an infant with severe combined immunodeficiency. J Clin Invest. 1998;102:421–9.

Hauck F, Randriamampita C, Martin E, et al. Primary T-cell immunodeficiency with immunodysregulation caused by autosomal recessive LCK deficiency. J Allergy Clin Immunol. 2012;130:1144–52.e11.

Li SL, Duo LN, Wang HJ, Dai W, Zhou EH, Xu YN, et al. Identification of LCK mutation in a family with atypical epidermodysplasia verruciformis with T-cell defects and virus-induced squamous cell carcinoma. Br J Dermatol. 2016;175(6):1204–9.

Lo WL, Shah NH, Ahsan N, Horkova V, Stepanek O, Salomon AR, Kuriyan J, Weiss A. Lck promotes Zap70-dependent LAT phosphorylation by bridging Zap70 to LAT. Nat Immunol. 2018;19(7):733–41.

Marth JD, Disteche C, Pravtcheva D, Ruddle F, Krebs EG, Perlmutter RM. Localization of a lymphocyte-specific protein tyrosine kinase gene (lck) at a site of frequent chromosomal abnormalities in human lymphomas. Proc Natl Acad Sci U S A. 1986;83:7400–10.

Perlmutter RM, Marth JD, Lewis DB, Peet R, Ziegler SF, Wilson CB. Structure and expression of lck transcripts in human lymphoid cells. J Cell Biochem. 1988;38(2):117–26.

Pignata C, Prasad KV, Robertson MJ, Levine H, Rudd CE, Ritz J. Fc gamma RIIIA-mediated signaling involves src-family lck in human natural killer cells. J Immunol. 1993;151(12):6794–800.

Pignata C, Prasad KV, Hallek M, Druker B, Rudd CE, Robertson MJ, Ritz J. Phosphorylation of src family lck tyrosine kinase following interleukin-12 activation of human natural killer cells. Cell Immunol. 1995;165(2):211–6.

Sawabe T, Horiuchi T, Nakamura M, et al. Defect of lck in a patient with common variable immunodeficiency. Int J Mol Med. 2001;7:609–14.

Shaw AS, Amrein KE, Hammond C, Stern DF, Sefton BM, Rose JK. The lck tyrosine protein kinase interacts with the cytoplasmic tail of the CD4 glycoprotein through its unique amino-terminal domain. Cell. 1989;59(4): 627–36.

Ulivieri C, Valensin S, Majolini MB, Matthews RJ, Baldari CT. Normal B-1 cell development but defective BCR signaling in Lck−/− mice. Eur J Immunol. 2003;33(2):441–5.

Van Laethem F, Tikhonova AN, Pobezinsky LA, et al. Lck availability during thymic selection determines the recognition specificity of the T cell repertoire. Cell. 2013;154:1326–41.

Lymphoproliferative Syndrome 1 (LPFS1)

▶ ITK Deficiency

L

Magnesium Transporter 1 (MAGT1) Deficiency

▶ MAGT1 Deficiency

MAGT1 Deficiency

Thomas G. Fox
Department of Pediatrics, Section of Pediatric
Infectious Diseases, Indiana University School of
Medicine, Riley Hospital for Children,
Indianapolis, IN, USA
Department of Pediatrics, Division of Pediatric
Infectious Disease, Emory University School of
Medicine, Atlanta, GA, USA

Synonyms

Magnesium transporter 1 (MAGT1) deficiency;
X-linked immunodeficiency with magnesium
defect, Epstein-Barr virus infection, and neoplasia
(XMEN disease)

Introduction/Background

Magnesium transporter 1 (MAGT1) deficiency
causes X-linked magnesium defect, Epstein-Barr
virus infection, and neoplasia (XMEN) disease,
which is a genetic disorder of intracellular
magnesium ion (Mg^{2+}) regulation that results in
a combined immunodeficiency. Some consider it
a mild form of primary immunodeficiency disease
(PID). It is characterized by chronic Epstein-Barr
virus (EBV) infection, CD4+ T-cell lymphopenia,
impaired NK and CD8+ T-cell cytolytic function,
and increased susceptibility to EBV-associated
B-cell lymphomas (Ravell et al. 2014). The disorder was initially described in two brothers with
chronic EBV infection and CD4 lymphopenia
(Li et al. 2011). Genetic sequencing of the siblings
revealed a ten-base pair deletion on *MAGT1* that
resulted in nonsense-mediated decay and
decreased messenger RNA expression and
undetectable gene product (Li et al. 2011). This
research group subsequently screened a cohort of
patients with CD4 cell lymphopenia and identified
an additional five unrelated individuals with other
MAGT1 mutations and similar clinical phenotypes. Three additional patients with MAGT1
deficiency have been reported to date.

Magnesium ion (Mg^{2+}) is the most abundant
divalent cation in eukaryotic cells and participates
in fundamental physiologic biochemical processes. *MAGT1* consists of ten exons and is
located on Xq21.1. Expressed in all mammalian
cells, MAGT1 encodes a transmembrane ion
channel that specifically takes up Mg^{2+}. Although
the vast majority of intracellular Mg^{2+} is bound to
proteins, MAGT1 is a key regulator of the <5% of
free cation (Ravell et al. 2014).

The regulation of intracellular magnesium is
important in anti-EBV cellular immunity by two

© Springer Science+Business Media LLC, part of Springer Nature 2020
I. R. Mackay et al. (eds.), *Encyclopedia of Medical Immunology*,
https://doi.org/10.1007/978-1-4614-8678-7

distinct molecular mechanisms that rely on functional MAGT1, both of which are impaired in MAGT1 deficiency. In T cells, stimulation of the T-cell receptor (TCR) leads to a rapid but transient influx of Mg^{2+} through MAGT1. Mg^{2+} influx leads to phosphorylation of phospholipase $C\gamma 1$ ($PLC\gamma 1$) and subsequent calcium release that activates T cells (Ravell et al. 2014). Patients with MAGT1 deficiency have impaired Mg^{2+} influx, decreased downstream generation of calcium, and depressed T-cell activation. The defect in MAGT1 in NK and CD8 cells results in a chronically low basal level of Mg^{2+}, which reduces the expression of natural killer group 2, member D (NKG2D). NKG2D is an important stimulatory molecule in these cell types that is important in cytolytic control of EBV-infected cells as well as tumor surveillance (Ravell et al. 2014).

Clinical Presentation

The initial report of MAGT1 deficiency described two brothers with chronic EBV, CD4+ lymphopenia, and intermittently abnormal immunoglobulin levels and vaccine responses (Li et al. 2011). Skewed or unbalanced lyonization was discovered in the mother that led to X-linked inheritance of the affected gene as the functional gene was inactivated in her T cells. The mutation in the mother and her sons was detected by X-chromosome exon capture and single-end next-generation sequencing (Li et al. 2011). Li et al. subsequently screened a 61-patient cohort of individuals with CD4 lymphopenia, chronic EBV infection, and/or EBV B-cell lymphoma and discovered 5 additional unrelated XMEN cases. All seven patients with MAGT1 deficiency had persistent EBV viremia and splenomegaly. Age at diagnosis ranged from 3 to 45, and EBV lymphoma at diagnosis was common. All postpubertal patients developed EBV-related lymphoproliferative disease (LPD). Some patients seemed susceptible to pathogens other than EBV; the two index patients had experienced sinopulmonary infections, diarrhea, and viral pneumonias (Li et al. 2014). One patient had severe varicella zoster virus infection with recurrent zoster. One patient developed to CMV and severe autoimmune disease (Patiroglu et al. 2015). Other interesting conditions reported in XMEN cases include autoimmune phenomena, Kaposi sarcoma, and progressive multifocal leukoencephalopathy (Brigida et al. 2017; Dhalla et al. 2015).

Compared to other CID associated with EBV-driven LPD, patients with MAGT1 deficiency tend to experience an indolent course, perhaps as a function of a less severe T-cell defect (Ravell et al. 2014). In contrast, patients with interleukin-2-inducible T-cell kinase (ITK) deficiency present earlier in life with severe and rapidly progressive disease, and those with X-linked lymphoproliferative (XLP) syndrome often present with fulminant mononucleosis due to EBV. A lack of invariant NK T-cell (iNKT) numbers is observed in both ITK deficiency and XLP syndrome, but not in MAGT1 deficiency. Hemophagocytic lymphohistiocytosis (HLH) has not been reported in XMEN disease (Ravell et al. 2014).

Diagnosis and Laboratory Testing

The prevalence of MAGT1 deficiency is likely low but needs to be considered in the differential diagnosis of any male with unexplained chronic EBV viremia, splenomegaly, and a personal or family history of EBV B-cell LPD. Total serum magnesium is normal in MAGT1-deficient patients given that the Mg+ deficiency is subtle and intracellular. The most consistent finding in XMEN is persistent EBV viremia and EBV-associated LPD. Mild hepatitis associated with chronic EBV infection can be observed. Most patients are seropositive consistent with past EBV infection but have varying levels of EBV viremia. CD4 lymphopenia is common, and the clinician should consider percentages rather than solely absolute numbers as they may be normal. In this regard, a decreased CD4/CD8 ratio is universal. Abnormalities in humoral immunity, vaccine responses, and T-cell proliferation are not consistent among reported cases. Absolute B-cell lymphocyte numbers are often elevated due to chronic EBV infection.

Establishing the diagnosis of MAGT1 deficiency prior to EBV infection is a challenge, given that most clinical consequences occur as a function of unchecked EBV. However, male patients with a family history of EBV LPD, recurrent infections, and CD4 lymphopenia deserve an evaluation for this immune deficiency. It is noteworthy that patients with MAGT1 deficiency do not experience failure to thrive, mental retardation, or developmental delay.

Flow cytometry for NKG2D expression on CD8 and NK cells is commercially available and will be low in patients with MAGT1 deficiency; however, NKG2D is also low in certain malignancies. To date, sequencing of the *MAGT1* exon is available at a few genetics laboratories. It is also important to perform mRNA expression studies to rule out noncoding mutations that result in abnormal MAGT1 protein expression.

Treatment and Prognosis

Hematopoietic cell transplantation (HCT) is the only known cure for this disease; however, theoretically, oral magnesium supplementation may be helpful. Chaigne-Delalande et al. demonstrated that magnesium supplementation leads to a partial and significant recovery of NKG2D expression with improved cytolytic CD8/NK function (Chaigne-Delalande et al. 2013). It is unclear whether magnesium supplementation will prevent EBV LPD, however. The anti-CD20 monoclonal antibody rituximab may have some effect, but since it does not deplete all tissue CD20+ B cells, cure is unlikely (Li et al. 2014). Adjunctive specific antiviral T-cell therapy may be a consideration but there is no data.

The mortality in XMEN disease and much of the morbidity are usually due to uncontrolled EBV infection; however, whether EBV infection is a sine qua non for the development of LPD is unknown (Ravell et al. 2014). The natural history of the disease is also unclear since only a handful of cases are reported to date. Some patients survive into adulthood. The prognosis may depend in part on the timing of acquisition of EBV infection. If infected with EBV later in life, the lymphoproliferative sequelae would be expected to be delayed. On the other hand, CD4 lymphopenia may worsen with age such that the prognosis without EBV infection is unknown (Li et al. 2014).

HCT may be considered for patients with XMEN disease; two patients with MAGT1 deficiency underwent HCT to date. They were 23 and 45 at the time of transplant, and both died of complications shortly afterward (Li et al. 2014). From the transplanter's perspective, HCT attempted earlier would likely be associated with better outcomes, but this remains to be seen.

References

Brigida I, Chiriaco M, Di Cesare S, Cittaro D, Di Matteo G, Giannelli S, et al. Large Deletion of MAGT1 Gene in a Patient with Classic Kaposi Sarcoma, CD4 Lymphopenia, and EBV Infection. J Clin Immunol. 2017;37(1):32–35.

Chaigne-Delalande B, Li FY, O'Connor GM, Lukacs MJ, Jiang P, Zheng L, et al. Mg2+ regulates cytotoxic functions of NK and CD8 T cells in chronic EBV infection through NKG2D. Science. 2013;341(6142):186–91.

Dhalla F, Murray S, Sadler R, Chaigne-Delalande B, Sadaoka T, Soilleux E, et al. Identification of a novel mutation in MAGT1 and progressive multifocal leucoencephalopathy in a 58-year-old man with XMEN disease. J Clin Immunol. 2015;35(2):112–8.

Li FY, Chaigne-Delalande B, Kanellopoulou C, Davis JC, Matthews HF, Douek DC, et al. Second messenger role for Mg^{2+} revealed by human T-cell immunodeficiency. Nature. 2011;475(7357):471–6.

Li FY, Chaigne-Delalande B, Su H, Uzel G, Matthews H, Lenardo MJ. XMEN disease: a new primary immunodeficiency affecting Mg^{2+} regulation of immunity against Epstein-Barr virus. Blood. 2014;123(14):2148–52.

Patiroglu T, Haluk Akar H, Gilmour K, Unal E, Akif Ozdemir M, Bibi S, et al. A case of XMEN syndrome presented with severe auto-immune disorders mimicking autoimmune lymphoproliferative disease. Clin Immunol. 2015;159(1):58–62.

Ravell J, Chaigne-Delalande B, Lenardo M. X-linked immunodeficiency with magnesium defect, Epstein-Barr virus infection, and neoplasia disease: a combined immune deficiency with magnesium defect. Curr Opin Pediatr. 2014;26(6):713–9.

M

Majeed Syndrome

Polly J. Ferguson
Rheumatology, Allergy and Immunology,
Department of Pediatrics, University of Iowa
Carver College of Medicine, Iowa City, IA, USA

Synonyms

CNO: Chronic non-bacterial osteomyelitis; CRMO: Chronic recurrent multifocal osteomyelitis; *LPIN2*: gene encoding the phosphatidate phosphatase lipin 2

Definition

Majeed syndrome is an autosomal recessive autoinflammatory disorder characterized by an array of symptoms including early-onset chronic recurrent multifocal osteomyelitis, recurrent fever, and dyserythropoietic anemia that may be accompanied by a neutrophilic dermatosis. The disease is caused by mutations in *LPIN2* (MIM# 609628). *LPIN2* encodes the phosphatidate phosphatase, LIPIN2.

Introduction and Background

Majeed syndrome is an autosomal recessive syndrome recognized by Dr. Hasan Majeed in three children, from two consanguineous families, affected with multifocal sterile osteomyelitis and congenital dyserythropoietic anemia; two from one family also had neutrophilic dermatosis (Sweet syndrome) (Majeed et al. 1989). It is an exceedingly rare disorder with 20 cases from 9 families reported in the literature since its initial description in 1989 (Majeed et al. 1989, 2000, 2001; Al-Mosawi et al. 2007; Herlin et al. 2013; Rao et al. 2016; Pinto-Fernandez and Seoane-Reula 2017; Moussa et al. 2016; Liu et al. 2019; Roy et al. 2019).

Genetics

Majeed syndrome is a Mendelian genetic disorder caused by homozygous mutations in *LPIN2* which encodes the LIPIN2 protein (Al-Mosawi et al. 2007; Ferguson et al. 2005). Seven mutations have been reported in nine families. The initial reports were all Arabic families but have subsequently been reported in other races/ethnicities. Consanguinity was present in eight families all with homozygous mutations; one family in which the parents were not related had an affected child was a compound heterozygote (paternal allele c.2327 + 1 G > C affecting a donor splice site at exon 17 and a truncation mutation in the maternal allele c.1691_1694delGAGA; p.Arg564Lysfs*3) (Liu et al. 2019). One mutation which changes a highly conserved serine to a leucine at amino acid 734 (p.Ser734Leu) is present in two families, and another missense mutation (c.G2207A; pR736H) was recently reported to be homozygous in all six members of one family; this affects an amino acid in a highly conserved region which is two amino acids downstream from the previously reported p. Ser734Leu mutation. Both are in a highly conserved area of the gene. The other mutations are private mutations predicted to result in early truncation of the protein.

Pathogenesis

LIPIN2 is a phosphatidic acid phosphatase (PAP) important in lipid metabolism (Reue 2009; Zhang and Reue 2017). This p.Ser734Leu no longer maintains its PAP activity; however, the role of LIPIN2 PAP activity in the pathogenesis of Majeed syndrome remains to be determined (Donkor et al. 2009).

Interleukin-1 was identified as a key inflammatory cytokine in disease pathogenesis using various cytokine-blocking agents to treat children with Majeed syndrome. Blockade of either IL-1 receptor I and IL-1β in vivo, but not tumor necrosis factor-alpha (TNF-α), results in healing of the inflammatory skin lesions and improved hemoglobin levels in children with Majeed syndrome (Herlin et al. 2013; Pinto-Fernandez and Seoane-Reula 2017). Lorden et al. went on to demonstrate using two different in vitro models that under-expression of *LPIN2* resulted in enhanced secretion of IL-1β (human macrophages and mouse bone marrow-derived macrophages). They then went on to show that this was due to increased activation of the NLRP3 inflammasome at multiple levels including increased $P2X_7$ receptor sensitization. In these cellular models, the authors went on to demonstrate that the enhanced IL-1β production could be normalized by normalization of cholesterol levels in the in vitro system (Lorden et al. 2017).

Clinical Manifestations

Nearly all affected individuals developed sterile multifocal osteomyelitis consistent with chronic recurrent multifocal osteomyelitis (CRMO). The age of onset of CRMO was younger than in non-syndromic forms of the disease with nearly all presenting prior to the second birthday (reported ages range 0.75 to 96 months). Recent reports suggest that penetrance may be incomplete (Roy et al. 2019).

Systemic and Cutaneous Manifestations
Recurrent fever and/or failure to thrive was reported in nearly half the cases, and hepatosplenomegaly was reported in a third, systemic inflammation present in all tested as manifest by elevated acute-phase reactants. The neutrophilic dermatosis, Sweet syndrome, was reported in two of the initial patients reported by Dr. Majeed in 1989 but has not been reported in any other cases (Majeed et al. 1989).

Musculoskeletal Manifestations
More than 90% presented with joint or limb pain, and most of those had objective swelling in the joints near the bone lesions. However, two individuals did not have any bone or joint symptoms to prompt MRI imaging (Liu et al. 2019; Roy et al.

2019). The bone lesions were present in the long bones in all children in cases that had imaging performed. Involvement of the bones of the lower extremity was slightly more common, but many had upper extremity involvement as well. Other bones were less commonly involved. Roy et al. described a consanguineous Pakistani family in which all six individuals (both parents and four children) were homozygous for the p.R736H mutation in *LPIN2*. The father was asymptomatic except for non-specific knee pain. The mother and the oldest child (a female) had mild anemia and limb pains requiring NSAIDs. The proband had typical Majeed syndrome (see below). The two younger brothers subsequently developed CRMO, high inflammatory markers, and chronic microcytic anemia (Roy et al. 2019).

Radiographic Imaging

Sterile osteomyelitis has been described in all patients with Majeed syndrome. Plain films may show osteolytic lesions surrounded by sclerosis, located preferentially in the metaphyses of the long bones of the extremities but can occur in other bones (Ferguson and El-Shanti 2007). Bone scan showed increased uptake in the metaphyseal regions of the long bones (Al-Mosawi et al. 2007; Rao et al. 2016). Magnetic resonance imaging shows findings consistent with osteomyelitis with decreased signal intensity on T1-weighted images and increased signal intensity on T2 fat-saturated images and on short tau inversion recovery (STIR) images (Herlin et al. 2013; Rao et al. 2016; Pinto-Fernandez and Seoane-Reula 2017; Moussa et al. 2016).

Hematological Manifestations
Dyserythropoietic anemia is present in all patients tested. The anemia is of variable severity ranging from transfusion dependent to mild with minimal symptoms. All 15 of the patients who underwent bone marrow biopsy had dyserythropoiesis seen on pathologic evaluation of the marrow (Majeed et al. 1989; Al-Mosawi et al. 2007; Herlin et al.

2013; Rao et al. 2016; Moussa et al. 2016; Liu et al. 2019; Roy et al. 2019). All six of the children reported by Dr. Majeed et al. required one or more red blood cell transfusions with one patient reported to be transfusion dependent (Majeed et al. 1989). One patient reported by Roy et al. was reported to have severe microcytic anemia with hemoglobin as low as 6.9, but no information was given about transfusions in this report (Roy et al. 2019). The remaining patients were reported to have less severe anemia (Al-Mosawi et al. 2007; Herlin et al. 2013; Rao et al. 2016; Moussa et al. 2016).

Laboratory Testing

All patients who had inflammatory markers drawn had a moderately to highly elevated erythrocyte sedimentation rate (18 of 18 tested). Anemia is present in all patients tested but is variable in severity. The anemia was microcytic in >90% (13 of 14 in which the MCV was reported) (Majeed et al. 1989; Al-Mosawi et al. 2007; Rao et al. 2016; Moussa et al. 2016; Liu et al. 2019; Roy et al. 2019). Only one individual had a normocytic anemia with an MCV of 86.8 (Rao et al. 2016). Bone biopsies were performed in six patients with five showing osteomyelitis (Majeed et al. 1989; Herlin et al. 2013; Pinto-Fernandez and Seoane-Reula 2017) and one osteonecrosis (Moussa et al. 2016).

Diagnosis

The diagnosis is made by recognition of the typical clinical features of Majeed syndrome including CRMO and microcytic anemia with or without Sweet syndrome and confirmed by DNA sequencing demonstrating recessive, deleterious mutation (s) in LPIN2.

Treatment

There have been no controlled trials in the treatment of Majeed syndrome. Prior to the advent of biologic agents, treatment of Majeed syndrome was based on a combination of NSAIDs and corticosteroids. And for some with very mild disease, NSAIDs alone has been all that is needed. However, most have more severe disease requiring more aggressive therapy. Diseases modifying antirheumatic medications such as colchicine and methotrexate have also been used with variable success. Pamidronate has also been used with some improvement in bone pain (Roy et al. 2019). The use of IL-1, but not TNF, antagonists has been shown to dramatically improve bone outcomes and to improve the anemia in all five individuals in which it has been used (Herlin et al. 2013; Pinto-Fernandez and Seoane-Reula 2017; Roy et al. 2019). However, it remains to be seen if IL-1 blockade reverses the dyserythropoietic anemia as no child has had an indication for repeat bone marrow biopsy after the initiation of treatment with an IL-1 inhibitor.

Prognosis

Majeed syndrome presents with sterile bone inflammation, recurrent fever, and dyserythropoietic anemia in most, but we are learning that disease severity is not uniform. There is a range of phenotypes from severe with fevers, high inflammatory markers, failure to thrive, severe CRMO, and symptomatic anemia to those with no fevers and much milder disease, and one adult individual had minimal to no symptoms, requiring treatment with NSAIDs only or in one person no treatment. For the majority of affected individuals, treatment with NSAIDs alone is inadequate and can result in severe flexion contractures that cause disability. DMARDs such as methotrexate have been used with reported success in a few children with mild disease. Pamidronate can help bone pain but has not been used as monotherapy. Biologic therapy has changed the outcomes for these children. While TNF inhibitors have not been reported to be successful, treatment of severe cases with IL-1 inhibition (either IL-1 receptor blockade or inhibiting IL-1β) has been reported to control the fevers and bone inflammation. It remains unclear if this prevents dyserythropoiesis in the bone marrow as no child has required repeated bone marrow biopsies after treatment with an IL-1 inhibitor. Although there is limited long-term follow-up in these patients, it is presumed that lifelong therapy will be required for those with severe disease.

Conclusion

Majeed syndrome is an ultra-rare Mendelian disorder that is caused by recessive mutations in LPIN2. The disease presents with sterile bone inflammation, recurrent fever, and dyserythropoietic anemia. There is a range of phenotypes from severe with fevers, high inflammatory markers, failure to thrive, severe CRMO, and symptomatic anemia to those with no fevers and much milder disease, and one adult individual had minimal to no symptoms. In vitro and in vivo data implicates dysregulation of the NLRP3 inflammasome with subsequent IL-1β hypersecretion in the pathogenesis. Treatment with IL-1β inhibitors has markedly improved outcomes.

Cross-References

▶ Introduction to Autoinflammatory Diseases

Acknowledgment PJF is funded by NIH/NIAMS R01AR059703 and Marjorie K. Lamb Professorship.

References

Al-Mosawi ZS, Al-Saad KK, Ijadi-Maghsoodi R, El-Shanti HI, Ferguson PJ. A splice site mutation confirms the role of LPIN2 in Majeed syndrome. Arthritis Rheum. 2007;56(3):960–4.

Donkor J, Zhang P, Wong S, O'Loughlin L, Dewald J, Kok BP, et al. A conserved serine residue is required for the phosphatidate phosphatase activity but not the transcriptional coactivator functions of lipin-1 and lipin-2. J Biol Chem. 2009;284(43):29968–78. Pubmed Central PMCID: 2785625. Epub 2009/09/01. eng.

Ferguson PJ, El-Shanti HI. Autoinflammatory bone disorders. Curr Opin Rheumatol. 2007;19(5):492–8.

Ferguson PJ, Chen S, Tayeh MK, Ochoa L, Leal SM, Pelet A, et al. Homozygous mutations in LPIN2 are responsible for the syndrome of chronic recurrent multifocal osteomyelitis and congenital dyserythropoietic anaemia (Majeed syndrome). J Med Genet. 2005;42(7):551–7. Pubmed Central PMCID: 1736104. Epub 2005/07/05. eng.

Herlin T, Fiirgaard B, Bjerre M, Kerndrup G, Hasle H, Bing X, et al. Efficacy of anti-IL-1 treatment in Majeed syndrome. Ann Rheum Dis. 2013;72(3):410–3. Pubmed Central PMCID: 3660147.

Liu J, Hu XY, Zhao ZP, Guo RL, Guo J, Li W, et al. Compound heterozygous LPIN2 pathogenic variants in a patient with Majeed syndrome with recurrent fever and severe neutropenia: case report. BMC Med Genet. 2019; 20(1):182. Pubmed Central PMCID: 6857307.

Lorden G, Sanjuan-Garcia I, de Pablo N, Meana C, Alvarez-Miguel I, Perez-Garcia MT, et al. Lipin-2 regulates NLRP3 inflammasome by affecting P2X7 receptor activation. J Exp Med. 2017;214(2):511–28. Pubmed Central PMCID: 5294860.

Majeed HA, Kalaawi M, Mohanty D, Teebi AS, Tunjekar MF, al-Gharbawy F, et al. Congenital dyserythropoietic anemia and chronic recurrent multifocal osteomyelitis in three related children and the association with sweet syndrome in two siblings. J Pediatr. 1989;115(5 Pt 1):730–4.

Majeed HA, El-Shanti H, Al-Rimawi H, Al-Masri N. On mice and men: an autosomal recessive syndrome of chronic recurrent multifocal osteomyelitis and congenital dyserythropoietic anemia. J Pediatr. 2000;137(3): 441–2.

Majeed HA, Al-Tarawna M, El-Shanti H, Kamel B, Al-Khalaileh F. The syndrome of chronic recurrent multifocal osteomyelitis and congenital dyserythropoietic anaemia. Report of a new family and a review. Eur J Pediatr. 2001;160(12):705–10.

Moussa T, Bhat V, Kini V, Fathalla BM. Clinical and genetic association, radiological findings and response to biological therapy in seven children from Qatar with non-bacterial osteomyelitis. Int J Rheum Dis. 2016;43:1258–9.

Pinto-Fernandez C, Seoane-Reula ME. Efficacy of treatment with IL-1RA in Majeed syndrome. Allergol Immunopathol. 2017;45(1):99–101.

Rao AP, Gopalakrishna DB, Bing X, Ferguson PJ. Phenotypic Variability in Majeed Syndrome. J Rheumatol. 2016;43(6):1258–9. Pubmed Central PMCID: 4898189.

Reue K. The lipin family: mutations and metabolism. Curr Opin Lipidol. 2009;20(3):165–70. Pubmed Central PMCID: 2875192.

Roy NBA, Zaal AI, Hall G, Wilkinson N, Proven M, McGowan S, et al. Majeed syndrome: description of a novel mutation and therapeutic response to bisphosphonates and IL-1 blockade with anakinra. Oxford: Rheumatology; 2019.

Zhang P, Reue K. Lipin proteins and glycerolipid metabolism: Roles at the ER membrane and beyond. Biochimica et biophysica acta Biomembranes. 2017;1859(9 Pt B):1583–95. Pubmed Central PMCID: 5688847.

M

MALT1 Deficiency

Robert P. Nelson
Divisions of Hematology and Oncology, Stem
Cell Transplant Program, Indiana University (IU)
School of Medicine and the IU Bren and Simon
Cancer Center, Indianapolis, IN, USA
Pediatric Immunodeficiency Clinic, Riley
Hospital for Children at Indiana University
Health, Indianapolis, IN, USA
Medicine and Pediatrics, Indiana University
School of Medicine, Immunohematology and
Transplantation, Indianapolis, IN, USA

Synonyms

MALT1 protease; Paracaspase 1; PCASP1

Definition

A gene that encodes a protein that augments
BCL10-induced activation of NF-kappa B.

Background/Introduction

In the 1980s, Isaacson et al. suggested that histo-
chemical and genetic similarities exist between
Mediterranean lymphoma and primary gastrointestinal lymphoma of follicle center cell origin.
These include a dense, noninvasive monotypic
lamina propria plasma cell infiltrate, individual
gland invasion, clonality, and a common histogen-
esis from mucosa-associated lymphoid-tissue
(MALT) (Isaacson and Wright 1983; Diebold
1988; Horsman et al. 1992). The *MALT1* gene
product is a caspase-like (paracaspase) cysteine protease that participates in the signal transduction cascade triggered by the formation of immunoreceptor/
peptide-MHC complexes at T and B cell surfaces.
Caspase recruitment domain-containing membrane-
associated guanylate kinase protein-1 (CARMA1)
mediates T and B cell receptor-induced NF-kappa
B activation by recruiting B-cell lymphoma-10
(BCL10) and MALT1 adaptor proteins to lipid
rafts following stimulation (Lin and Wang 2004).
MALT1 provides scaffolding and proteolytic functions consequential to downstream signaling of a
variety of different receptors (Hachmann and
Salvesen 2016). In humans, pathogenic mutations
in MALT1 impair normal NF-kappa B activation
and paracaspase activity causing combined T and
B cell immunodeficiency.

Function

Host Defense: Innate and Adaptive Immune Responses

An important step of membrane-to-nucleus signaling includes BCL10, which recruits and activates MALT1. The CARMA1/BCL-10/MALT1
(CBM) complex converts monomers to macromolecular complexes by finite polymerization and
interacts with tumor necrosis factor receptor-
associated factor six (TRAF6), which activates
the IκB kinase (IKK) complex that phosphorylates the inhibitor IκBα, resulting in proteasome
ubiquitination and degradation (Wegener et al.
2006; Oeckinghaus et al. 2007). Multiple roles
in T cell activation were summarized comprehensively by Thome (2008) The p50 and p65/avian
reticuloendotheliosis viral oncogene homolog
A (RelA) subunits liberate NF-κB from IκBα,
enabling NF-κB to migrate to the nucleus and
initiate gene transcription that activates the cell.
Mice deficient in MALT1 fail to activate autoreactive T cells in the experimental autoimmune
encephalomyelitis (EAE) model (Mc Guire et al.
2013). MALT1 is also essential for dectin-1- and
dectin-2-driven production of the IL-1β,
IL-23p19, and IL-17 by dendritic cells
(DC) (Brustle et al. 2012).

MALT1 activates NF-κB in marginal zone
developing B cells via the B-cell activating factor
(BAFF) receptor (Tusche et al. 2009). MALT1-
deficient mice have no thymus-generated natural
Tregs and induced Tregs in the periphery are
diminished. Murine Malt1 (−/−) iTregs express
relatively high levels of Toll-like receptor
2 (TLR2). Treatment of WT and Malt1 (−/−) Th
cells in-vitro with a TLR-2 ligand induced
Malt1(−/−) iTregs to proliferate, which suggests

that MALT1 supports Treg development in the thymus but suppresses iTreg induction in the periphery. These findings implicate MALT1 as a facilitator of immune tolerance at ambiance and immune reactivity under stress (Rosenbaum et al. 2019). Thus, MALT1 deficiency results in unbalanced regulatory and effector T and B cell responses leading to multiorgan inflammation (Bornancin et al. 2015).

Hematological Malignancies

MALT1 is associated with and was discovered by recognition of its relatedness to MALT lymphoma, and it appears also active in chronic lymphocytic leukemia (CLL). CLL with antibody deficiency was one of the initial Food and Drug Agency (FDA)-indications for intravenous immunoglobulin (IVIG) replacement therapy in humans. Bruton's tyrosine kinase (BTK) loss-of-function mutations render the affected infant void of B cells, thus causing Bruton's or X-linked agammaglobulinemia, while gain-of-function mutations enhance malignant B cell production in CLL. Furthermore, inhibition of BTK developed into an approved therapy for CLL. Most patients resistant to BTK inhibition CLL clones carry mutations in BTK or phospholipase C Gamma 2 (PLCG2), a downstream effector target of BTK. Inhibition of MALT1 with the small molecule inhibitor MI-2 is effective in killing CLL clones resistant to ibrutinib in preclinical models. Clinical development of MALT1 inhibitors for the treatment of CLL will take into consideration the naturally occurring immunodeficiencies suggesting risk of iatrogenic induction of MALT-deficiency in patients with cancer (Saba et al. 2017).

Clinical Presentation

Jabbara et al. described the initial patients with MALT1 deficiency, who experienced a spectrum of infections that included recurrent pneumonia and bronchiectasis in early infancy. Bronchial lavage (BAL) cultures revealed a broad group of organisms, including *Pseudomonas*, *Streptococcus pneumoniae*, *Candida albicans*, *Haemophilus influenzae*, *Klebsiella pneumoniae*, and *Staphylococcus aureus*. Pneumococcal and *H. influenzae* meningitis occurred early in life. Other infections included mastoiditis, chronic aphthous ulcers, cheilitis, gingivitis, esophagitis, gastritis, and duodenitis. Small intestinal biopsies revealed villous atrophy in one child and increased numbers of intraepithelial lymphocytes in the second. Growth was delayed but neurological development was normal (Jabara et al. 2013). McKinnon et al. reported a 15-year-old girl born from consanguineous parents, who presented with skin viral and bacterial infections and eczema since infancy. She had chronic inflammatory bowel disease and recurrent pneumonias. Clinical immunology testing revealed very low B cell counts and abnormal T cell proliferation to mitogens. There was absent of IκBα degradation and NF-κB phosphorylation in the patient's T cells that was rescue with expression of wild-type MALT1 (McKinnon et al. 2014).

Weigmann et al. described a female infant with severe immune dysregulation leading to recurrent systemic infections, failure to thrive, and severe crises of ichthyosiform erythroderma associated with high levels of serum IgE. The differential diagnosis included Netherton and Omenn syndromes; however, serine protease inhibitor Kazal-type 5 (SPINK5) and recombinase activating gene 1 and 2 sequences were normal. The patient received intensive care but died in the hospital. Whole exome sequencing revealed two compound heterozygous mutations in MALT1 gene associated with a low MALT1 protein level and findings were confirmed by immunofluorescence staining of key proteins in the skin (Wiegmann et al. 2019).

Frizinsky et al. described two cousins with recurrent infections, failure to thrive, lymphadenopathy, dermatitis, and autoimmunity and novel autosomal recessive homozygous c.1799T>A; p. I600N missense mutation in *MALT1*. Immunological evaluation revealed lymphocytosis but low or normal total serum immunoglobulin levels and normal CD19+ B cells. Both patients had group A+ red blood cells but no detectable

M

anti-hemagglutinin B antibodies. Specific antibody to protein and polysaccharide antigens were also nonprotective. Peripheral blood immunophenotype revealed normal percentages of CD3+, CD4+, and CD8+ T cells that proliferated poorly to anti-CD3, tetanus toxoid (TT), diphtheria toxoid (DT), and Candida antigens, and the T cell repertoire was restricted. Regulatory T cells were absent. Delayed cutaneous hypersensitivity to Candida antigen was absent in both patients. CD56+ NK cells were normal in one and low in the other (Frizinsky et al. 2019).

Diagnostic Laboratory Testing

Patients may have lymphocytosis or normal numbers of circulating T and B cells, low or normal total immunoglobulins but poor functional antibody capacity. Although CD19+ B cells may be normal, anti-hemagglutinin may be undetectable and specific antibody to protein and other polysaccharide antigens nonprotective. Candida cutaneous sensitivity may be absent and T cells may proliferate poorly to anti-CD3 and antigens. Detailed T cell functional analysis may reveal impaired IκBα degradation and IL-2 expression following T cell stimulation with phorbol myristate acetate and ionomycin. Patients may have elevated serum IgE and CD56+ NK cells are normal or low. Gene sequencing analysis of *MALT1* should be performed to provide with molecular diagnosis.

Treatment

Pathogenic MALT1 variants impair normal NF-kappa B activation and paracaspase activity that leads to combined immunodeficiency. General treatment considerations for immunocompromised patients apply. Patients who are not receiving IVIG should be immunized per standard protocol with the exception of live viral vaccines. It may be prudent to mainstream a pediatric patient in school, while providing prompt evaluation for early unusual consequences of infection. Prolonged courses of antibiotics may be necessary

for infections, particularly sinus infections. Prophylactic antimicrobials and immunoglobulin replacement therapy are recommended for those with cellular immune impairment or demonstrably low functional antibody production capacity.

Early diagnosis is crucial, as curative treatment by hematopoietic cell transplantation may be warranted and the successful execution of the transplant is predicated on access to a suitable transplant protocol and center before debilitating clinical consequences ensue. Consider referral to a multidisciplinary clinical program that is engaged in research related to the disease. Input from the family is paramount with this process that affects their financial health and care of other children. Social workers play an important role in connecting with services and advocacy groups.

Punwani et al. and Rozmus et al. successfully corrected the clinical and immunological phenotype of MALT1 deficiency with hematopoietic stem cell transplantation following reduced intensity conditioning (Punwani et al. 2015; Rozmus et al. 2016).

There has been a novel approach reported in which MALT1 substrate cleavage was rescued, in part by incorporation of a molecular corrector known to be an allosteric inhibitor for MALT1. Using lymphocytes from a patient with the biallelic mutation W580S in MALT1, NFkB, and JNK signaling was restored with binding of the allosteric inhibitor. This approach provides another example of precise, targeted therapy made possible by understanding the molecular pathophysiological underpinnings of the defect (Quancard et al. 2019).

Cross-References

▶ IKBKB Deficiency

References

Bornancin F, Renner F, Touil R, et al. Deficiency of MALT1 paracaspase activity results in unbalanced regulatory and effector T and B cell responses leading to multiorgan inflammation. J Immunol. 2015;194: 3723–34.

Brustle A, Brenner D, Knobbe CB, et al. The NF-kappaB regulator MALT1 determines the encephalitogenic potential of Th17 cells. J Clin Invest. 2012;122:4698–709.

Diebold J. Malignant lymphoma of mucosa-associated lymphoid tissue. Ann Pathol. 1988;8:340.

Frizinsky S, Rechavi E, Barel O, et al. Novel MALT1 mutation linked to immunodeficiency, immune dysregulation, and an abnormal T cell receptor repertoire. J Clin Immunol. 2019;39:401–13.

Hachmann J, Salvesen GS. The paracaspase MALT1. Biochimie. 2016;122:324–38.

Horsman D, Gascoyne R, Klasa R, Coupland R. t(11;18) (q21;q21.1): a recurring translocation in lymphomas of mucosa-associated lymphoid tissue (MALT)? Genes Chromosomes Cancer. 1992;4:183–7.

Isaacson P, Wright DH. Malignant lymphoma of mucosa-associated lymphoid tissue. A distinctive type of B-cell lymphoma. Cancer. 1983;52:1410–6.

Jabara HH, Ohsumi T, Chou J, et al. A homozygous mucosa-associated lymphoid tissue 1 (MALT1) mutation in a family with combined immunodeficiency. J Allergy Clin Immunol. 2013;132:151–8.

Lin X, Wang D. The roles of CARMA1, Bcl10, and MALT1 in antigen receptor signaling. Semin Immunol. 2004;16:429–35.

Mc Guire C, Wieghofer P, Elton L, et al. Paracaspase MALT1 deficiency protects mice from autoimmune-mediated demyelination. J Immunol. 2013;190:2896–903.

McKinnon ML, Rozmus J, Fung SY, Hirschfeld AF, Del Bel KL, Thomas L, et al. Combined immunodeficiency associated with homozygous MALT1 mutations. J Allergy Clin Immunol. 2014;133(5):1458–62.

Oeckinghaus A, Wegener E, Welteke V, et al. Malt1 ubiquitination triggers NF-kappaB signaling upon T-cell activation. EMBO J. 2007;26:4634–45.

Punwani D, Wang H, Chan AY, Cowan MJ, Mallott J, Sunderam U, et al. Combined immunodeficiency due to MALT1 mutations, treated by hematopoietic cell transplantation. J Clin Immunol. 2015;35(2):135–46.

Quancard J, Klein T, Fung SY, et al. An allosteric MALT1 inhibitor is a molecular corrector rescuing function in an immunodeficient patient. Nat Chem Biol. 2019;15(3):304–13.

Rosenbaum M, Gewies A, Pechloff K, et al. Bcl10-controlled Malt1 paracaspase activity is key for the immune suppressive function of regulatory T cells. Nat Commun. 2019;10:2352.

Rozmus J, McDonald R, Fung SY, et al. Successful clinical treatment and functional immunological normalization of human MALT1 deficiency following hematopoietic stem cell transplantation. Clin Immunol. 2016;168:1–5.

Saba NS, Wong DH, Tanios G, et al. MALT1 inhibition is efficacious in both naive and ibrutinib-resistant chronic lymphocytic leukemia. Cancer Res. 2017;77:7038–48.

Thome M. Multifunctional roles for MALT1 in T-cell activation. Nat Rev Immunol. 2008;8:495–500.

Tusche MW, Ward LA, Vu F, et al. Differential requirement of MALT1 for BAFF-induced outcomes in B cell subsets. J Exp Med. 2009;206:2671–83.

Wegener E, Oeckinghaus A, Papadopoulou N, et al. Essential role for IkappaB kinase beta in remodeling Carma1-Bcl10-Malt1 complexes upon T cell activation. Mol Cell. 2006;23:13–23.

Wiegmann H, Reunert J, Metze D, et al. Refining the dermatological spectrum in primary immunodeficiency: MALT1 deficiency mimicking Netherton- and Omenn syndrome. Br J Dermatol. 2019; https://doi.org/10.1111/bjd.18091.

MALT1 Protease

▶ MALT1 Deficiency

Mammalian Sterile 20-Like 1 (MST1) Deficiency

Robert P. Nelson
Divisions of Hematology and Oncology, Stem Cell Transplant Program, Indiana University (IU) School of Medicine and the IU Bren and Simon Cancer Center, Indianapolis, IN, USA
Pediatric Immunodeficiency Clinic, Riley Hospital for Children at Indiana University Health, Indianapolis, IN, USA
Medicine and Pediatrics, Indiana University School of Medicine, Immunohematology and Transplantation, Indianapolis, IN, USA

MST1/STK4 (OMIM: #614868)

Synonyms

Serine/Threonine Kinase 4 (STK4)

Introduction/Background

Mammalian sterile 20-like 1 kinase (MST1, official gene name serine/threonine kinase 4, STK4), a member of the "sterile 20" family of proteins, is a cytosolic kinase that participates in a broad array of biological processes affecting immune function and hematopoiesis. It is activated upstream of other mitogen-activated kinases, in response to stress. The gene encoding MST1/STK4 is mapped to chromosome 20q13.12. As a major component of the Hippo pathway, MST1/STK4 regulates apoptosis and plays an important role in the cellular response to oxidative stress. Given that the Hippo pathway is key to the regulation of cell proliferation and survival, MST1/STK4 is a link in the signaling pathway that contributes to governing the self-renewal and differentiation of stem and progenitor cells (Torres-Bacete et al. 2015).

Consistent with the majority of T- and B-cell combined immunodeficiencies, MST1 is pleotropic also participates in the early phase of the immune response and immune regulation. It helps dendritic cells move quickly by mediating CCR7-dependent changes in cytoarchitecture and endocytosis. In a kindred of three siblings affected, homozygous nonsense mutation in MST1/*STK4* (c.442C > T, p.Arg148Stop) was found to eliminate MST1 protein expression and normal chemotaxis stimulated with CXCL11; therefore, abnormal chemotaxis is one of the defining features of the defect (Robertson et al. 2017). This trafficking defect among human MST1-deficient lymphocytes is predicted by the murine knockout mode, in which T-cell development, positive selection, thymic egress, and immune synapse formation are impaired (Dang et al. 2016). In addition, in T cells, MST1/STK4 enhances the transcriptional activity of Foxp3 and modulates the Foxp3 protein at the posttranslational level (Li et al. 2015). Defective MST1-FOXO1 signaling downregulates Treg cells, while Th2 and T follicular helper cells expand, which suggest MST1/STK4 participates in the maintenance of tolerance by regulating T-cell-mediated B-cell activation (Park et al. 2017). Defective MST1/STK4 is associated with prostate and breast cancer, as MST1/STK4 suppresses tumor growth by helping to maintain lymphoid cell chromosomal instability (Kim et al. 2012; Collak et al. 2012). Defects are strongly associated with poor overall survival for patients with

breast cancer, as demonstrated by findings collected from a 110-patient breast cancer cohort, where MST1/STK4 was expressed in over 70% in breast cancers. Multivariate analysis revealed MST1/STK4 expression independently impacted survival ($P = 0.030$). Plasma MST1/STK4 levels also predicted survival (Lin et al. 2013; Lin et al. 2017). Exemplifying the breadth of its activity, MST1/STK4 defects cause cardiomyocyte apoptosis and dilated cardiomyopathy (You et al. 2009; Anand et al. 2009). Taken together, these findings illustrate the rich connectivity between an inborn errors of immunity, autoimmunity, and cancer.

Clinical Presentation

The human MST1/STK4 defect may present as a combined immunodeficiency with recurrent cutaneous lesions caused by a specific group of related human papillomavirus genetic variants. Although autosomal recessive mutations in EVER1 (TMC6) and EVER2 account for the majority of epidermodysplasia verruciformis (EV), Crequer et al. described a 19-year-old patient with an MST1/STK4 defect that caused a T-cell deficiency associated with EV-HPV, bacterial, and fungal infections (Crequer et al. 2012). MST1/STK4 defects thus represent another genetically determined susceptibility to infection-driven cancer. MST1/STK4 mutations were responsible for combined immunodeficiencies described in seven cases from unrelated kindreds with T-cell deficiencies, viral and bacterial infections, EBV-induced lymphoproliferation, autoimmunity, inflammation, allergy, and malignancy. Halici et al. described a pair of siblings with autoimmune cytopenias, molluscum contagiosum, perioral herpetic infections, bacterial infections, mild onychomycosis, mild atopic and seborrheic dermatitis, lymphopenia (particularly CD4 lymphopenia), and intermittent mild neutropenia (Halacli et al. 2015). Thus, this clinical phenotype can be similar to those of DOCK-8 deficiency. Abdollapour et al. reported three affected members of a family with recurrent infections and heart anomalies. Studies revealed loss of mitochondrial membrane potential and increased susceptibility to apoptosis in lymphocytes and neutrophils, with significantly reduced numbers (Abdollahpour et al. 2012). Nehme reported four patients from two families with homozygous mutations in MST1/STK4, presenting with recurrent bacterial and viral infections, very low naive T cells, and very reduced T-cell survival in vitro (Nehme et al. 2012).

Diagnosis and Laboratory Testing

Patients with the MST1/STK4 defect present in childhood or young adulthood and may have a family history of PIDD. There may be recurrent persistent and/or severe infections or infections with nonvirulent organisms. Other findings may include autoimmune manifestations, current or previous cancer (especially EBV-lymphoproliferative disease), enteritis, failure to thrive, and persistent or recurrent dermatological manifestations (HPV-related papilloma/warts). Physical signs of failure to thrive are not always present; there is no facial dysmorphia and no particular distinguishing physical features related to MST1/STK4 deficiency. The thymus should be present unless another preceding intragestational event occurred. SCID screening T cell receptor excision circles (TRECs) will likely be normal, as will the absolute neutrophil count. A relative hypereosinophilia (i.e., over 10%) may be observed and IgA will be normal or less than 7 mg/d. IgE and IgM levels may be normal or elevated. CD4 cells may be normal or less than 20%, and complement levels likely normal. Patients with CD4 lymphopenia may demonstrate absence of naive T cells and poor pneumococcal antibody responses. The presentation can be consistent with a leaky form of autosomal recessive SCID; a negative screen for genes associated with SCID will prompt the obtainment of whole exome sequencing (WES) followed by Sanger sequencing and Western blot analysis of patient fibroblasts

and lymphoblastoid B cell lysates to confirm the loss of protein expression. Although CXCR3 expression is preserved, patient leukocytes exhibit deficient chemotaxis after stimulation with CXCL11, and lymphocytes will not bind effectively to immobilize ICAM-1 (Dang et al. 2016).

Treatment

It is important to define cases of EV-HPV molecularly, given that prognosis and treatment differ according to the genetic lesion. Patients with MST1/STK4 deficiency are treated with gamma globulin replacement therapy, either intravenous (IVIG) or subcutaneous, if there is a demonstrable antibody production defect. Bacterial infections are treated with appropriate antimicrobial therapy, a prolonged course may be necessary (Ballow et al. 2018). Antiviral therapy is recommended for viral infections. *Pneumocystis jirovecii* prophylaxis in the context of CD4+ lymphopenia is recommended; first line is trimethoprim-sulfamethoxazole, and alternatives include pentamidine, dapsone, or atovaquone. Hematopoietic cell transplantation has been successful in selected cases. It is important to define cases of EV-HPV molecularly, given that prognosis and treatment differ according to the genetic lesion.

Cross-References

▶ DOCK8 Deficiency

References

Abdollahpour H, Appaswamy G, Kotlarz D, Diestelhorst J, Beier R, Schäffer AA, et al. The phenotype of human STK4 deficiency. Blood. 2012;119(15):3450–7.

Anand R, Maksimoska J, Pagano N, et al. Toward the development of a potent and selective organoruthenium mammalian sterile 20 kinase inhibitor. J Med Chem. 2009;52:1602–11.

Ballow M, Paris K, de la Morena M. Should antibiotic prophylaxis be routinely used in patients with antibody-mediated primary immunodeficiency? J Allergy Clin Immunol Pract. 2018;6:421–6.

Collak FK, Yagiz K, Luthringer DJ, Erkaya B, Cinar B. Threonine-120 phosphorylation regulated by phosphoinositide-3-kinase/Akt and mammalian target of rapamycin pathway signaling limits the antitumor activity of mammalian sterile 20-like kinase 1. J Biol Chem. 2012;287:23698–709.

Crequer A, Picard C, Patin E, et al. Inherited MST1 deficiency underlies susceptibility to EV-HPV infections. PLoS One. 2012;7:e44010.

Dang TS, Willet JD, Griffin HR, et al. Defective leukocyte adhesion and chemotaxis contributes to combined immunodeficiency in humans with autosomal recessive MST1 deficiency. J Clin Immunol. 2016;36:117–22.

Halacli SO, Ayvaz DC, Sun-Tan C, et al. STK4 (MST1) deficiency in two siblings with autoimmune cytopenias: a novel mutation. Clin Immunol. 2015;161:316–23.

Kim TS, Lee DH, Kim SK, Shin SY, Seo EJ, Lim DS. Mammalian sterile 20-like kinase 1 suppresses lymphoma development by promoting faithful chromosome segregation. Cancer Res. 2012;72:5386–95.

Li J, Du X, Shi H, Deng K, Chi H, Tao W. Mammalian sterile 20-like kinase 1 (Mst1) enhances the stability of forkhead box P3 (Foxp3) and the function of regulatory T cells by modulating Foxp3 acetylation. J Biol Chem. 2015;290:30762–70.

Lin X, Cai F, Li X, et al. Prognostic significance of mammalian sterile 20-like kinase 1 in breast cancer. Tumour Biol. 2013;34:3239–43.

Lin XY, Cai FF, Wang MH, et al. Mammalian sterile 20-like kinase 1 expression and its prognostic significance in patients with breast cancer. Oncol Lett. 2017;14:5457–63.

Nehme NT, Schmid JP, Debeurme F, Andre-Schmutz I, Lim A, Nitschke P, Rieux-Laucat F, Lutz P, Picard C, Mahlaoui N, Fischer A, de Saint Basile G. MST1 mutations in autosomal recessive primary immunodeficiency characterized by defective naive T-cell survival. Blood. 2012;119:3458–68.

Park E, Kim MS, Song JH, Roh KH, Lee R, Kim TS. MST1 deficiency promotes B cell responses by CD4(+) T cell-derived IL-4, resulting in hypergammaglobulinemia. Biochem Biophys Res Commun. 2017;489:56–62.

Robertson A, Mohamed TM, El Maadawi Z, et al. Genetic ablation of the mammalian sterile-20 like kinase 1 (Mst1) improves cell reprogramming efficiency and increases induced pluripotent stem cell proliferation and survival. Stem Cell Res. 2017;20:42–9.

Torres-Bacete J, Delgado-Martin C, Gomez-Moreira C, Simizu S, Rodriguez-Fernandez JL. The mammalian sterile 20-like 1 kinase controls selective CCR7-dependent functions in human dendritic cells. J Immunol. 2015;195:973–81.

You B, Yan G, Zhang Z, et al. Phosphorylation of cardiac troponin I by mammalian sterile 20-like kinase 1. Biochem J. 2009;418:93–101.

Management of Immunodeficiency, Antibiotic Therapy

Panida Sriaroon
Department of Pediatrics, Division of Allergy and Immunology, University of South Florida/Johns Hopkins All Children's Hospital, Tampa, FL, USA

Most immunodeficient patients are susceptible to infections (See details in entry "► Management of Immunodeficiency, Overview"). Depending on the type of primary immunodeficiency diseases (PID), the infections can be severe, recurrent, or prolonged and can be due to usual or opportunistic pathogens. Risks and benefits must be considered thoroughly prior to administration of antimicrobial agents either for treatment or prophylactic use. Several factors influence antibiotic selection, dosage, and length of therapy, including type and location of infections, other comorbidities, and culture and susceptibility results. Body fluid or drainage cultures and tissue biopsy are helpful in identifying infectious organisms and should be obtained whenever possible, especially when evaluating unusual or invasive infections in immunocompromised hosts.

The choice and dosage of antibiotics used to treat mild to moderate infections are similar to those used in immunocompetent hosts. For example, streptococcal pharyngitis can be treated with penicillins. Amoxicillin/clavulanic acid is the first line therapy for sinopulmonary infections that are likely due to *Streptococcus pneumoniae* or *Haemophilus influenzae*. Macrolides should be prescribed if *Mycoplasma spp.* is suspected. In patients with PID, any suspected bacterial infection must be treated early with antibiotics and some may require a longer treatment course than would be normally prescribed (Cunningham-Rundles 2010). Treatment should be adjusted according to clinical responsiveness and laboratory results, including culture and sensitivity tests, PCR assays, or the presence of specific antibodies to the organism. However, antibody-based laboratory assays might not be helpful in patients who have antibody defects or are receiving IgG replacement therapy.

Patients with antibody deficiency usually suffer from sinopulmonary infections. Occasionally, short- or long-term antibiotic prophylaxis against upper and lower respiratory bacterial infections are used as a conservative therapy when there are no clear indications for IgG replacement therapy or other specific treatment measures (Bonilla et al. 2015). In some cases, antibiotic prophylaxis is used in addition to IgG replacement therapy although there are no published data that compare IgG therapy with or without prophylactic antibiotics.

Prophylactic antibiotics are not, however, routinely recommended for all patients with PID. The need for antibiotic prophylaxis depends on the type and severity of the underlying immunodeficiency and the history of previous infections. The decision to start prophylactic antibiotics should be made on a case-by-case basis due to possible risks associated with antibiotic therapy such as development of drug-resistant organisms, yeast overgrowth, or diarrhea due to *C. difficile* infection. Trimethoprim/sulfamethoxazole (TMP/SMX) and amoxicillin are commonly used to treat respiratory infections prophylactically because of their reasonably broad coverage against common gram-positive and gram-negative bacteria. A list of regimens for prophylaxis of bacterial respiratory tract infections is provided in Table 1.

Patients with cellular immune deficiency, particularly those with diagnosis of severe combined immunodeficiency (SCID), CD40, and CD40L deficiencies, and nuclear factor kB essential modulator (NEMO) deficiency, should receive antimicrobial prophylaxis for opportunistic infections (Bonilla et al. 2015). The prophylaxis should be considered in other combined immunodeficiencies when there is a reduction in T-cell numbers, function, or both. TMP/SMX is the first-line prophylaxis for *Pneumocystis jiroveci* pneumonia (PCP). Alternative drugs, such as pentamidine, dapsone, and atovaquone, can be used in patients with sulfa antibiotic hypersensitivity. Patients with profound lymphopenia should also receive prophylaxis for atypical mycobacterium infections and be considered for prophylaxis against some viral, such as varicella or respiratory syncytial virus (RSV), or fungal infections (Bonilla et al. 2015).

Patients with chronic granulomatous disease have defective phagocytic cell function. In addition to receiving interferon-γ injections, they should receive antifungal and antibiotic prophylaxis against catalase-positive organisms, such as *S. aureus, Nocardia spp., Burkholderia spp.,* and *Aspergillus spp.* The most commonly used regimen is a combination of TMP/SMX and an antifungal agent, such as itraconazole, voriconazole, or posaconazole. However, adherence might be an issue because of side effects, and breakthrough infections still occur.

Some PID diagnoses may have associated specific recommendations regarding antimicrobial prophylaxis. Patients with congenital asplenia are at risk of developing invasive infections due to encapsulated organisms (Schutze et al. 2002). They should receive antibiotic prophylaxis, such

Management of Immunodeficiency, Antibiotic Therapy, Table 1 Antibiotic prophylaxis regimens for bacterial respiratory tract infections (Adapted from Bonilla et al. (2015))

Antibiotic	Regimen for children	Regimen for adults
Amoxicillin (consider with clavulanate, if needed)	10–20 mg/kg daily or twice daily	500–1000 mg daily or twice daily
Trimethoprim (TMP)/sulfamethoxazole (dosing for TMP)	5 mg/kg daily or twice daily	160 mg daily or twice daily
Azithromycin	10 mg/kg weekly or 5 mg/kg every other day	500 mg weekly or 250 mg every other day
Clarithromycin	7.5 mg/kg daily or twice daily	500 mg daily or twice daily
Doxycycline	Age >8 years; 25–50 mg daily or twice daily	100 mg daily or twice daily

as penicillin or amoxicillin, and vaccination for encapsulated organisms especially *S. pneumoniae, H. influenzae type B*, and *N. meningitidis*. The optimal duration of antibiotic prophylaxis in individuals with asplenia is unknown and some experts recommend lifelong prophylaxis (Bonilla et al. 2015). Prophylaxis should be maintained at least until the age of 5 years in fully immunized children.

Infectious complications are uncommon in patients with autoimmune lymphoproliferative syndrome (ALPS). However, long-term antibiotic prophylaxis is strongly indicated in patients with ALPS after splenectomy due to a high risk of sepsis and mortality because of infectious complications (Rao and Oliveira 2011).

NEMO deficiency is associated with impaired humoral immunity, low NK cell function, and poor Toll-like receptor response. Patients usually suffer from recurrent sinopulmonary infections with encapsulated bacterial organisms. Some patients are also susceptible to mycobacterial and severe viral infections, particularly herpesviruses (Hanson et al. 2008). PCP has also been reported. Patients with NEMO deficiency should receive IgG replacement therapy. PCP, antibacterial, antimycobacterial, and antiviral prophylaxis should be considered for patients with NEMO deficiency.

Cross-References

▶ Management of Immunodeficiency, Overview

References

Bonilla FA, Khan DA, Ballas ZK, Chinen J, Frank MM, Hsu JT, et al. Practice parameter for the diagnosis and management of primary immunodeficiency. J Allergy Clin Immunol. 2015;136(5):1186–205.e1-78. PubMed PMID: 26371839. Epub 2015/09/16. eng

Cunningham-Rundles C. How I treat common variable immune deficiency. Blood. 2010;116(1):7–15. PubMed PMID: 20332369. Pubmed Central PMCID: PMC2904582. Epub 2010/03/25. eng

Hanson EP, Monaco-Shawver L, Solt LA, Madge LA, Banerjee PP, May MJ, et al. Hypomorphic nuclear factor-kappaB essential modulator mutation database and reconstitution system identifies phenotypic and immunologic diversity. J Allergy Clin Immunol. 2008;122(6):1169–77.e16. PubMed PMID: 18851874. Pubmed Central PMCID: PMC2710968. Epub 2008/10/15. eng

Rao VK, Oliveira JB. How I treat autoimmune lymphoproliferative syndrome. Blood. 2011;118(22):5741–51. PubMed PMID: 21885601. Pubmed Central PMCID: PMC3228494. Epub 2011/09/03. eng

Schutze GE, Mason EO Jr, Barson WJ, Kim KS, Wald ER, Givner LB, et al. Invasive pneumococcal infections in children with asplenia. Pediatr Infect Dis J. 2002;21(4):278–82. PubMed PMID: 12075756. Epub 2002/06/22. eng

Management of Immunodeficiency, Bone Marrow Transplantation

Jennifer W. Leiding
Department of Pediatrics, Division of Allergy and Immunology, University of South Florida at Johns Hopkins – All Children's Hospital, St. Petersburg, FL, USA

For many primary immunodeficiency diseases, hematopoietic stem cell transplantation (HSCT) otherwise known as bone marrow transplant is the only curative therapy available. Genetic mutations in hematopoietic stem cells or stem cell subsets give rise to many immunodeficiencies. Replacement of the defective hematopoietic system can allow for development of a functional immune system. Without HSCT, severe combined immunodeficiency (SCID) is lethal in the first few years of life. For other primary immunodeficiencies, HSCT can cure disease, increase life expectancy, and improve quality of life (Griffith et al. 2008).

Donor Matching

Successful HSCT requires a significant degree of matching of human leukocyte antigen (HLA) markers between the donor and the recipient in order to reduce complications such as graft-versus-host disease (GvHD). The first successful HSCT occurred in 1968 in a patient with severe combined immunodeficiency using marrow from an identical donor. An HLA-identical donor is usually a sibling (matched related donor, MRD) and is the most desirable donor. A MRD HSCT carries the most favorable prognosis with rapid immune reconstitution and lower risk of GvHD. Matched unrelated donors (MUD) are identified from individuals registered in the National Marrow Donor Program. Initially, MUD HSCT had lower survival than MRD HSCT; however, more recent studies suggest that outcomes are comparable. Mismatched related donors (MMRD) are often parents and are currently utilized as donors when there is not a more desirable bone marrow source. There is a much higher risk of GvHD with this type of transplant (Filipovich 2008; Hagin and Resner 2010).

Donor Sources

Sources of hematopoietic cells for transplantation include bone marrow, peripheral blood, or umbilical cord blood from neonates. Bone marrow is harvested typically from the pelvis and peripheral blood from apheresis. Umbilical cord blood is a rich source of stem cells and is collected when the newborn infant is born.

Preconditioning Regimens

In order for the newly transplanted immune system to be accepted by the host, the host often must be treated with pretransplant chemotherapy to ablate or reduce the function of their own immune system (Szabolcs 2010; Filipovich 2008). Preparative regimens are variable in intensity and toxicity. Generally accepted definitions of the different types of regimens include:

- Myeloablative regimen – A single agent or combination of therapies that are expected to destroy all hematopoietic cells in the bone marrow resulting in profound long-lasting or irreversible pancytopenia within 1 week of infusion.

- Non-myeloablative regimen – A regimen that will cause minimal reductions in cell counts with the exception of lymphocytes.

- Reduced intensity regimens – These regimens are an intermittent category of regimens that do not fit the definition of myeloablative or non-myeloablative. Such regimens may result in reduced cell counts that require cell support but that may be reversible.

The underlying condition being treated, patient clinical status and other comorbidities, and risk of rejection are all considerations when determining the type of preparative regimen for any given HSCT.

Common toxicities include mucositis, nausea and vomiting, alopecia, diarrhea, rash, peripheral neuropathies, and infertility. Pulmonary and liver toxicity are also common. Busulfan, a common agent in both myeloablative and reduced intensity regimens, can cause interstitial lung disease and hepatic sinusoidal obstructive syndrome.

Complications of HSCT (Szabolcs 2010)

- Chemotherapy-related toxicity – Chemotherapeutic agents can cause short-term or long-term sequelae. Damage of the liver endothelium by agents such as busulfan or cyclophosphamide can cause veno-occlusive disease (VOD). VOD consists of painful hepatomegaly, jaundice, ascites, and fluid retention and can progress into multi-organ failure. Busulfan can also cause lung damage and fibrosis. Cyclophosphamide can cause hemorrhagic cystitis, syndrome of inappropriate antidiuretic hormone secretion, and cardiac toxicity. Total body irradiation is associated with long-term hormonal imbalance causing delayed puberty, infertility, and thyroid dysfunction.

- Infection – Patients undergoing HSCT are at increased risk of invasive bacterial, fungal,

M

viral, and opportunistic infections depending on the degree of myeloablation. Patients are at the highest risk when cell (lymphocyte and neutrophil) counts are the lowest. Strict isolation of patients during and after HSCT and use of prophylactic antimicrobials help to prevent the development of infections.

- Blood product and growth factor support – Blood product support is often necessary before and after HSCT. Transfusion with red blood cells and platelets are often required frequently in the 14–21 days following transplant; transfusion need is reduced with non-myeloablative conditioning regimens. Cloned hematopoietic growth factors such as granulocyte colony-stimulating factor provide clear benefit in encouraging neutrophil recovery following transplant.
- Graft rejection – Graft rejection occurs when the host's immune system mounts a sufficient response against the donor cells. Pre-conditioning regimens are intended to prevent this complication by destroying or blunting the response of immunocompetent cells within the host.
- Acute graft versus host disease – GvHD occurs when T cells present within the graft are activated and react to the host's immune system. A variety of methods have been developed to deplete mature T cells from the graft and to prevent the development of autoreactive T cells within the graft especially if there is a strong degree of mismatching between donor and host. Clinical symptoms include rash, diarrhea, and liver abnormalities.
- Chronic GvHD – Chronic GvHD is traditionally defined as symptoms that persist or appear more than 100 days post HSCT. Symptoms include scleroderma-like skin changes, tissue fibrosis with limitation of joint mobility, fibrosis of the exocrine glands, fibrosis of the lungs and liver, autoimmunity, and increased susceptibility to infections.
- Posttransplant immune-mediated hemolysis – Autoimmune cytopenias occur more frequently following non-myeloablative rather than myeloablative transplant. The most

common cause occurs due to donor B cells producing antibodies against the donor's red blood cell antigens.

Immune Reconstitution

In order to assess immune reconstitution, chimerism studies are assessed periodically. Chimerism studies determine the genetic origin of hematopoietic cells – donor or host. With most primary immunodeficiencies, mixed donor chimerism, in which the recipient's immune system has not been fully replaced by that of the donor, is often acceptable.

Immune reconstitution of hematopoietic cells occurs in a stepwise and often predictable pattern after transplant (Szabolcs 2010):

- Neutrophils: 14–21 days.
- Natural killer cells: 30–100 days.
- T cells: 100 days.
- B cells: 1–2 years.

Prognosis

The overall prognosis for patients transplanted for primary immunodeficiency has increased significantly with improvement in advances of early recognition of disease, improved HLA typing, refined conditioning regimens, and improved treatment of infections.

References

Filipovich A. Hematopoietic cell transplantation for correction of primary immunodeficiencies. Bone Marrow Transplant. 2008;42(Suppl 1):S49.

Griffith LM, Cowan MJ, Kohn DB, et al. Allogeneic hematopoietic cell transplantation for primary immune deficiency diseases: current status and critical needs. J Allergy Clin Immunol. 2008;122:1087.

Hagin D, Reisner Y. Haploidentical bone marrow transplantation in primary immune deficiency: stem cell selection and manipulation. Immunol Allergy Clin N Am. 2010;30:45.

Szabolcs P, Cavazzana-Calvo M, Fischer A, Veys P. Bone marrow transplantation for primary immunodeficiency diseases. Pediatr Clin N Am. 2010;57:207.

Management of Immunodeficiency, IgG Replacement (IV)

Elena E. Perez
Allergy Associates of the Palm Beaches, North Palm Beach, FL, USA

Synonyms

Antibody replacement therapy; IVIG

Primary immunodeficiency was the first FDA-approved indication for immunoglobulin therapy. Immunoglobulin therapy is a life-saving treatment for primary immunodeficiencies characterized by absent or deficient antibody production. The goal of therapy with intravenous immunoglobulin is to decrease (or eliminate) the incidence and severity of infections in patients with antibody deficiency. Clinical phenotypes of primary immunodeficiency for which immunoglobulin replacement (by either intravenous or subcutaneous route) is or may be indicated include (1) agammaglobulinemia due to absence of B cells, (2) hypogammaglobulinemia with poor antibody function, (3) normal immunoglobulins with poor antibody function, (4) hypogammaglobulinemia with normal antibody function, (5) isolated IgG subclass deficiency with recurrent infections, and (6) recurrent infections due to a complex immune mechanism related to a genetically defined primary immunodeficiency disease (Perez et al. 2017). Immunoglobulin replacement is also indicated for certain conditions associated with secondary immunodeficiency such as chronic lymphocytic leukemia, pediatric HIV infection, and hypogammaglobulinemia following bone marrow transplantation (Perez et al. 2017). Immunoglobulin replacement also may be considered for secondary antibody deficiencies found in multiple myeloma, genetic syndromes associated with immunodeficiency, patients receiving solid organ transplantation, and patients treated with B-cell-depleting therapies (Perez et al. 2017). The accurate diagnosis of antibody deficiencies is crucial prior to initiation of gammaglobulin replacement therapy and generally requires evidence of hypogammaglobulinemia and poor antibody responses to vaccinations. In severe combined immunodeficiency or agammaglobulinemia, titers to vaccines are not necessary, due to absence of B-cell numbers or function.

Dosage and Administration

The usual replacement dose for intravenous gammaglobulin is between 400 mg/kg/month and 600 mg/kg/month. The frequency of infusions is every 3–4 weeks. Placement of peripheral IVs monthly is preferred over use of central ports due to the risk of infection. Intravenous gammaglobulin is usually infused over 4–6 h, depending on the patient's tolerance and adverse effects. The rate is gradually ramped up, to avoid rate-related side effects. Each product has specific parameters for infusion times in the prescribing information; however, slower rates tend to be associated with less side effects. Trough levels are monitored after the third dose and approximately every 6–12 months or after changes in dose or frequency. Higher trough levels are associated with less incidence of infection (Perez et al. 2017; Lucas et al. 2010), but every patient may have an individual "biologic trough" (Bonagura et al. 2008) below which they have recurrent infections.

Adverse Reactions

Intravenous immunoglobulin is generally well tolerated but can be associated with mild to severe adverse events, which range from common to rare (Table 1). Immunoglobulin therapy is considered a blood product as it is derived from the plasma of thousands of healthy donors who have been screened for infectious diseases. Adverse reactions can affect up to half of all individuals receiving intravenous immune globulin (IVIG). Reactions are most likely to occur during the

Management of Immunodeficiency, IgG Replacement (IV), Table 1 Adverse events with IVIG administration (table from Perez et al. 2017)

Common[a]	Headache, myalgia, back pain, arthralgia, chills, malaise, fatigue, anxiety, fever, rash, flushing, nausea, vomiting, tingling, infusion site pain/swelling, erythema, hypo- or hypertension, tachycardia, fluid overload
Uncommon (multiple reports)	Chest pain or tightness, dyspnea, severe headaches, aseptic meningitis, pruritis, urticarial, thromboembolic[b] (cerebral ischemia, strokes, myocardial infarction, deep vein thrombosis, pulmonary emboli, renal toxicity[c]), hemolytic reactions due to isoagglutinins to Rh or other blood groups, anaphylactic/anaphylactoid reactions
Rare (isolated reports)	Anaphylaxis due to IgE or IgG antibodies to IgA in the immunoglobulin product, progressive neurodegeneration, arthritis, cardiac rhythm abnormalities, transfusion-related acute lung injury (granulocyte antibody mediated), neutropenia, pseudohyponatremia, uveitis, noninfectious hepatitis, hypothermia, lymphocytic pleural effusion, skin (leukocytoclastic vasculitis of the skin, erythema multiforme, urticaria, dyshidrotic eczema, maculopapular or eczematoid rashes, alopecia)

[a]Infusion rate related and/or at higher doses (2 g/kg)
[b]Related to the procoagulant activity in the IVIG (Factor XIa and hyperosmolality)
[c]Majority due to sucrose containing IVIG products, osmotic nephrosis with injury to proximal renal tubules

first infusion or the first infusion of new product after changing brands. Most adverse reactions are mild and rate related and occur in 5–15% of infusions (Perez et al. 2017). The most common adverse reactions include back or abdominal pain, nausea, breathing difficulties, chills, flushing, rash, anxiety, low-grade fever, arthralgia, myalgias, and/or headache (Perez et al. 2017). Symptoms of common adverse reactions may be improved by slowing or temporarily stopping the infusion. Strategies including oral or IV hydration, pretreatment with NSAIDs, antihistamines, and steroids prior to infusion may help prevent adverse reactions, although data is lacking regarding the best regimen. A recent or ongoing bacterial infection or underlying chronic inflammation may be risk factors for adverse events (Perez and Silverglied 2017). Other factors contributing to adverse reactions include higher concentrations, lyophilized products, and rapid infusion rates. Caution is advised when switching IVIG products because significant adverse reactions occur during the process (Perez et al. 2017).

Serious adverse events include anaphylaxis, aseptic meningitis, thromboembolic events, acute kidney injury, and hemolysis. Anaphylaxis during IVIG administration is extremely rare, but it may be life-threatening. Thromboembolic event risk is increased in the presence of underlying cardiovascular risk factors or hyperviscosity. Strategies to minimize thromboembolic events include ensuring adequate hydration, avoiding prolonged immobilization, spacing large doses over several days, slowing infusions, and using low osmolarity products (Perez and Silverglied 2017). The prescribing information for all IVIG products includes a boxed warning about thromboembolic events (especially in patients with risk factors of advanced age, prolonged immobilization, hypercoagulable conditions, history of venous or arterial thrombosis, use of estrogens, indwelling vascular catheters, hyperviscosity, and cardiovascular risk factors), renal dysfunction, and acute renal failure (especially with sucrose-containing products). Hemolytic anemia ranging from mild to severe can occur from blood group reactive antibodies in the IVIG product (Perez and Silverglied 2017).

The use of intravenous gammaglobulin therapy for the treatment of patients with primary or secondary antibody deficiency is complex and requires the clinician to have a familiarity with the products available, prescribing guidelines, and possible adverse events. The American Academy of Allergy, Asthma, and Immunology has published the "Eight guiding principles for effective use of IVIG for patients with primary immunodeficiency" (Perez et al. 2017; AAAAI 2017) as a resource for clinicians who take care of these patients. These guiding principles include:

1. **Indication of immunoglobulin therapy**: Immunoglobulin is indicated as replacement therapy for patients with primary immunodeficiency characterized by absent or deficient antibody production. Primary immunodeficiency is an FDA-approved indication of immunoglobulin, for which all currently available products are licensed.
2. **Diagnoses**: A large number of primary immunodeficiency diagnoses exist for which IVIG is indicated and recommended. Many diagnoses have low total levels of IgG, but some have a normal level with documented specific antibody deficiency.
3. **Frequency of immunoglobulin treatment**: Treatment is indicated as ongoing replacement therapy for and should not be interrupted once a definitive diagnosis has been established.
4. **Dose**: IVIG is indicated for patients with PI at a starting dose of 400–600 mg/kg every 3–4 weeks (SCIG is generally used at a starting dose of 100–200 mg/kg/week; see "SCIG" chapter). Less frequent treatment, or use of lower doses, is not substantiated by clinical data.
5. **IgG trough levels**: IgG trough levels can be useful in some diagnoses to guide care but should Not be a consideration in access to immunoglobulin therapy.
6. **Site of care**: The decision to infuse IVIG in a hospital, hospital outpatient, community office, or home-based setting must be based on clinical characteristics of the patient.
7. **Route**: Route of immunoglobulin administration must be based on patient characteristics. Throughout life, certain patients may be more appropriate for IV or SC therapy depending on many factors, and patients should have access to either route as needed.
8. **Product**: IVIG and SCIG are not generic drugs and products are not interchangeable. A specific product needs to be matched to patient characteristics to ensure patient safety; a change of product should occur only with the active participation of the prescribing physician.

Cross-References

► Management of Immunodeficiency, IgG Replacement (SC)
► Management of Immunodeficiency, Overview

References

AAAAI. IVIG toolkit. 2017. https://www.aaaai.org/practice-resources/Practice-Tools/ivig-toolkit. Accessed 25 Nov 2017.

Bonagura VR, Marchlewski R, Cox A, Rosenthal DW. Biologic IgG level in primary immunodeficiency disease: the IgG level that protects against recurrent infection. J Allergy Clin Immunol. 2008;122:210–2.

Lucas M, Lee M, Lortan J, Lopez-Granados E, Misbah S, Chapel H. Infection outcomes in patients with common variable immunodeficiency disorders: relationship to immunoglobulin therapy over 22 years. J Allergy Clin Immunol. 2010;125:1354.e4–60.e4.

Perez EE, Silverglied AJ. Intravenous immune globulin: adverse effects. UptoDate. 2017. Last modified 3 Apr 2017.

Perez EE, Orange JS, Bonilla F, et al. Update on the use of immunoglobulin in human disease: a review of evidence by members of the Primary Immunodeficiency Committee of the American Academy of Allergy, Asthma & Immunology. J Allergy Clin Immunol. 2017;139(3 Suppl):S1–S46.

M

Management of Immunodeficiency, IgG Replacement (SC)

Elena E. Perez
Allergy Associates of the Palm Beaches, North Palm Beach, FL, USA

Definition

SCIG   Subcutaneous immunoglobulin
fSCIG   Facilitated subcutaneous immunoglobulin

The use of subcutaneous immunoglobulin (SCIG), to treat a patient with agammaglobulinemia, was first published in the USA by Dr. Ogden Bruton in 1952 (Bruton 1952). This route of therapy was replaced by IM and then IV over the years. However, over the past decade, the renewed availability of SCIG has expanded treatment options available for patients needing gammaglobulin therapy for primary antibody deficiencies (Perez et al. 2017). SCIG provides an option for patients with poor venous access and for patients who prefer not to have monthly infusions for a variety of reasons including busy lifestyles and a need for independence among others. The number of products available for SCIG is expanding as well. Smaller more frequent doses can be delivered daily, twice per week, once per week, every 2 weeks, or once per month depending on the SCIG product chosen and patient preferences.

SCIG Dosing and Administration

The use of SCIG is growing among patients with antibody deficiency. SCIG is given in smaller and more frequent doses compared to IVIG. As in IVIG, the typical starting dose is between 400 mg/kg/month and 600 mg/kg/month (Perez et al. 2017). The monthly dose is divided into infusions daily, weekly, or every 2 weeks. In general, SCIG is dosed at 100–200 mg/kg/week (or the monthly IV dose multiplied by a conversion factor and divided weekly) (Perez et al. 2017). With facilitated SCIG, the whole monthly dose is infused every 3–4 weeks. Doses are titrated to clinical effect, with the goal of minimizing the frequency and severity of recurrent infections. IgG levels are monitored over time, correlated with clinical outcomes, and the dose is adjusted as necessary. With SCIG, there is a steady level of IgG present in the bloodstream due to the more frequent dosing (Perez et al. 2017; Wasserman et al. 2010). With facilitated SCIG, peak levels are not as high, and trough levels are not as low, as with IVIG. SCIG offers a greater flexibility in dosing and a steady state plasma level of gammaglobulin (instead of high peaks and lower troughs as experienced with IVIG). See Fig. 1 for a representative comparison of IV and SC pharmacokinetics (Wasserman et al. 2010; Ponsford et al. 2015).

SCIG is infused under the skin at one or multiple sites, in the abdomen, thighs, or buttocks. The volume being infused determines the number of sites needed. The total monthly dose is calculated by the prescriber and then divided according to the interval between infusions. The number of needle sticks (sites) is also calculated for the patient depending on the volume to be infused. The greater the interval between infusions, the greater the volume of product will need to be infused to achieve the same total

Management of Immunodeficiency, IgG Replacement (SC),
Fig. 1 Graph representing serum levels of IgG over time when administered via IVIG (black), SCIG (dotted), or facilitated SCIG (purple). (Source: Ponsford et al. 2015)

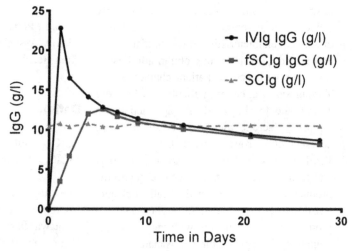

dose. SCIG can be given daily, weekly, every 2 weeks, or multiple times per week, as long as the total monthly dose is divided appropriately (Perez et al. 2017). Facilitated SCIG refers to the use of hyaluronidase, a naturally occurring enzyme that catalyzes the breakdown of hyaluronic acid and increases the permeability of tissue to fluids, administered SC prior to the gammaglobulin (Perez et al. 2017). Facilitated SCIG can be given every 3–4 weeks, to deliver the total monthly dose at once, into the subcutaneous space.

The length of SCIG infusions varies depending on the volume of product and the tubing and pump used. SCIG generally takes up to 1–2 h (or less). Preparations currently available for SC use include certain 10% products (suitable for IV or SC), 20% preparations (SC only), and facilitated SCIG (hyaluronidase plus a 10% preparation) (Table 1). In general, SCIG regimens require the patient or caregiver to learn how to self-administer at home. In the USA, facilitated SCIG allows for self-administration or nurse supervised in-office administration, depending on insurance and preference.

Several of the standard 10% IVIG preparations can be used via the SC route. Twenty percent preparations, allowing half the volume to deliver the same dose, are indicated for SC use only. With the 20% preparations, less needlesticks are needed, and allowable volume/site can range from 30 ml to 60 ml, depending on patient tolerance. With facilitated SCIG, about 300–600 ml can be delivered in one site or divided into two sites as tolerated. SCIG is delivered using a small needle attached to tubing and a syringe that is placed in a portable pump. The SCIG products come in a variety of vial sizes depending on the manufacturer. Several needle and tubing sizes are also available.

Adverse Events

SCIG is associated with fewer severe adverse events than IVIG (Perez et al. 2017). Side effects are usually mild, although systemic adverse reactions have been reported. Severe reactions rarely occur, and patients who have had severe reactions to IVIG might be at a higher risk. As with the 10% products, the prescribing information for the 20% SCIG products also contain a boxed warning for the risk of thrombosis, which may occur with immune globulin products. Risk factors for thrombosis may include advanced age, prolonged immobilization, hypercoagulable conditions, history of venous or arterial thrombosis, use of

Management of Immunodeficiency, IgG Replacement (SC), Table 1 Current immunoglobulin products available in the USA for subcutaneous administration

IV or SC	Formulation	Refrigeration?	Sodium	pH	IgA (ug/ml)	Stabilizer
Gammagard	10% liquid	Not required	None added	4.6–5.1	37	Glycine
Gammaked	10% liquid	Not required[a]	None added	4–4.5	46	Glycine
Gamunex-C	10% liquid	Not required[a]	None added	4–4.5	46	Glycine
SC	Formulation	Refrigeration?	Sodium	pH	IgA (ug/mL)	Stabilizer
Cuvitru	20% solution	Not required[b]	None added	4.6–5.1	80	Glycine
Hizentra	20% liquid	Not required	Trace[c]	4.6–5.2	≤50	Proline
HyQvia	10% liquid + hyaluronidase	Not required	None added	4.6–5.1	37	Glycine

[a]Storage is 2–8 °C for 36 months or 25 °C for 6 months
[b]Storage is 2–8 °C for 36 months or room temperature 25 °C for 12 months
[c]<10 mmol/l

estrogens, indwelling vascular catheters, hyperviscosity, and cardiovascular risk factors. Premedication is usually not required for SCIG. The most common adverse reaction reported is a redness and irritation at the injection site. These mild localized reactions improve with repeated infusions. In rare cases, the injection site reactions can be severe. To avoid the infusion site reactions, and decrease the chance of other problems, patients need to receive thorough training regarding proper technique. SCIG is an option for patients who do not tolerate IVIG, have poor venous access, or prefer SCIG due to lifestyle. Candidates for SCIG include children, adults, pregnant women, and patients with IgA deficiency or those who have had adverse reactions with IVIG. Needle phobia can be helped using topical anesthetics prior to the SC infusion.

Practical Considerations

SCIG requires more frequent administrations (daily, weekly, every 2 weeks), unless the facilitated SCIG route is chosen (every 3–4 weeks). SCIG provides the freedom to administer gammaglobulin at home at any time of day. This has been shown to enhance the quality of life for some patients (Perez et al. 2017). Medical supervision is not required for home infusion; therefore patient adherence is an important consideration. Manual dexterity is required to prepare the syringes and manage the pump for SCIG. Fear of needlesticks may be an important barrier to SCIG, but thorough training and use of topical anesthetics may help. The optimal route of infusion (SCIG vs. IVIG) may change over time for any given patient (Perez et al. 2017). Therefore, clinicians should discuss options with patients regarding changes in route as appropriate.

Monitoring

With SCIG, a steady state level of IgG is achieved in the circulation due to more frequent infusions

of smaller doses. Peak and trough levels are not as extreme, and the level is more consistent on a daily basis. Routine lab work including blood counts and markers of liver and kidney function should be performed at least once per year and more often depending on clinical circumstances or insurance requirements. None of the currently available products for SCIG are stabilized with sucrose, making renal complications less likely (Perez et al. 2017). Smaller doses given subcutaneously also minimize risks due to fluid overload (Perez et al. 2017).

Summary of Products Available

There are three 10% products (which can be used IV or SC), two 20% products (for SC use only), and one 10% product facilitated with hyaluronidase (Perez et al. 2017) (Table 1). Other products are being developed and will likely be available in the near future.

Cross-References

▶ IVIG

References

Bruton OC. Agammaglobulinemia. Pediatrics. 1952;9(6):722–8.

Perez EE, Orange JS, Bonilla F, et al. Update on the use of immunoglobulin in human disease: a review of evidence by members of the Primary Immunodeficiency Committee of the American Academy of Allergy, Asthma & Immunology. J Allergy Clin Immunol. 2017;139(3 Suppl):S1–S46.

Ponsford M, Carne E, Kingdon C, et al. Facilitated subcutaneous immunoglobulin (fSCIg) therapy – practical considerations. Clin Exp Immunol. 2015;182:302–13.

Wasserman RL, Irani AM, Tracy J, et al. Pharmacokinetics and safety of subcutaneous immune globulin (human), 10% caprylate/chromatography purified in patients with primary immunodeficiency disease. Clin Exp Immunol. 2010;161:518–26.

Management of Immunodeficiency, Overview

Panida Sriaroon
Department of Pediatrics, Division of Allergy and Immunology, University of South Florida/Johns Hopkins All Children's Hospital, Tampa, FL, USA

Immunodeficiency (or immune deficiency) is a state in which the immune system's ability to fight infectious diseases is compromised. Most immunodeficiency diseases are chronic and life-long conditions that require close clinical monitoring and aggressive interventions to optimize health and quality of life. The management of immunodeficiency depends on which component of the immune system is defective and whether function can be restored.

General Care

Depending on the degree of immune defect, most patients with immunodeficiency need to modify their lifestyle to minimize risks of acquiring new infections. They should avoid crowded areas and limit exposure to people who are ill or have signs of an obvious infection. Young children with immunodeficiency might benefit from smaller schools or daycare facilities.

Treatment of Infections and Underlying Conditions

It is crucial that infections be treated properly to avoid persistence or complications of infections or development of resistance to antimicrobial agents. Immunodeficient subjects might need longer treatment or higher dosages of antimicrobial agents, depending on the type of infections. Infections can be difficult to treat and surgical interventions such as abscess drainage, removal of infected tissues or organs might be required. When immune deficiency occurs as a result of other diseases, those underlying conditions should be evaluated and managed aggressively. For example, management of secondary hypogammaglobulinemia from protein losing enteropathy or nephrosis should aim at preventing further IgG loss by treating underlying gastrointestinal and renal conditions, respectively.

Immunization

Patients with immune deficiency and their family members should keep their immunizations up-to-date. Most patients can safely receive inactivated vaccinations unless there is a contraindication or history of hypersensitivity reactions to vaccine or its components. Nevertheless, patients with severe immune defects might not respond adequately to vaccinations.

Live vaccines, such as those for mumps, measles, and rubella (MMR); rotavirus; varicella; BCG; yellow fever; and oral polio vaccines, are contraindicated in patients with profound cellular, humoral, or combined immune defects due to increased risk of developing infections from the vaccine strains (Sobh and Bonilla 2016). Patients with milder immune defects must be evaluated individually, especially for their cellular function, to assess risk versus benefit ratio from receiving live vaccinations.

Patients who are receiving IgG replacement therapy can safely receive inactivated vaccines although the usefulness of vaccination during IgG treatment remains unclear. Most vaccine-preventable diseases are prevented by the administration of intravenous immunoglobulin (IVIG) or subcutaneous immunoglobulin (SCIG) since all IgG preparations are prepared from pooled donors (Sriaroon and Ballow 2015). However, antibodies to new strains of pathogens, such as seasonal influenza, may not be present in therapeutic IgG, thereby requiring the administration of the indicated vaccine to patients receiving IgG treatment.

M

IgG therapy has been shown to reduce MMR vaccine response (Siber et al. 1993). Therefore, it is recommended that the administration of MMR vaccine be delayed up to 11 months after receiving IgG therapy (McLean et al. 2013). IgG therapy does not appear to reduce immunogenicity of other live attenuated vaccines such as oral polio and yellow fever vaccines and they can be administered as scheduled, only if indicated in the context of a particular patient's immune deficiency (see above regarding live vaccines).

Antibiotic Prophylaxis

Sometimes prophylactic antibiotics are prescribed for patients with immunodeficiency as a conservative therapy for recurrent infections, especially when there are no indications for IgG replacement therapy or other specific treatment measures. However, prophylactic antibiotics should not be routinely prescribed for all patients with recurrent infections because of possible side effects associated with prolonged antibiotic therapy such as development of antibiotic-resistant organisms, *C. difficile* colitis, and candidiasis. See details in entry "▶ Management of Immunodeficiency, Antibiotic Therapy."

IgG Replacement Therapy

Therapeutic IgG, which is derived from pooled plasma of 10,000–60,000 healthy donors, is a standard replacement therapy in patients with PID (Sriaroon and Ballow 2015). IgG can be given via monthly intravenous or weekly subcutaneous infusions. The goal of therapy is to reduce the incidence of serious bacterial infections in individuals with antibody function defects. Although newer IgG products are safe and well-tolerated, approximately one-third of patients receiving the treatment experience adverse reactions. IgG replacement therapy should be reserved for patients who demonstrate clinical and laboratory evidence of a defect in antibody production or function and have failed conservative therapy

with antibiotics; economic costs should also be considered. See details in entries "▶ Management of Immunodeficiency, IgG Replacement (IV)" and "▶ Management of Immunodeficiency, IgG Replacement (IV)."

Hematopoietic Stem Cell Transplantation

In hematopoietic stem cell transplantations (HSCT), stem cells obtained from bone marrow, umbilical cord blood, or peripheral blood are infused to re-build the immune system of the recipient. This high risk procedure often requires pretransplant conditioning chemotherapy and immune suppression. Patients with severe defects in cellular or phagocytic immunity may require HSCT as the only curative therapy to reverse the condition. Patients with various primary immunodeficiency disease (PID) conditions have been successfully treated with HSCT, including severe combined immunodeficiency (SCID), chronic granulomatous disease (CGD), X-linked hyper-IgM syndrome, Immune dysregulation, polyendocrinopathy, enteropathy, X-linked syndrome (IPEX), and Wiskott-Aldrich syndrome (WAS). Ideally, HSCT should be performed as early as possible before infections and other complications occur. In the last decade, HSCT outcomes have improved as a result of early diagnosis, preemptive detection and treatment of infections, effective conditioning regimens, and the increased availability of alternative donors. Although the use of HSCT for the treatment of PID has increased significantly, significant complications can still occur including infections, venoocclusive disease (GVHD), graft-versus-host disease, and graft failure.

Gene Therapy

Gene therapy (GT) has been proposed as a life-saving alternative treatment to allogeneic HSCT, especially for patients with severe PID conditions caused by single gene mutation who do not have a matched sibling donor. GT has been used to treat patients with X-linked SCID, SCID secondary to adenosine deaminase (ADA) deficiency, CGD, and WAS. The key concept of GT for the treatment of PID has been to perform autologous HSCT using the patient's own hematopoietic stem cells that are genetically corrected (Kohn and Kuo 2017). The hematopoietic stem cells, typically derived from patients' bone marrow or mobilized peripheral mononuclear cells, are corrected ex vivo by addition of a normal copy of the gene into stem cells. Different forms and gene delivery systems have been examined. Approximately two thirds of GT clinical trials worldwide have used a virus as vector, with the most commonly used viral vectors being adenovirus and lentivirus class of retroviruses. Unlike in HSCT, graft rejection and GVHD are not seen in GT since the gene of interest is inserted into the patient's own hematopoietic stem cells. See details in entry "▶ Management of Immunodeficiency: Gene Therapy."

Cross-References

- ▶ Management of Immunodeficiency, Antibiotic Therapy
- ▶ Management of Immunodeficiency, IgG Replacement (IV)
- ▶ Management of Immunodeficiency: Gene Therapy

References

Kohn DB, Kuo CY. New frontiers in the therapy of primary immunodeficiency: from gene addition to gene editing. J Allergy Clin Immunol. 2017;139(3):726–32. PubMed PMID: 28270364. Epub 2017/03/09. eng

McLean HQ, Fiebelkorn AP, Temte JL, Wallace GS. Prevention of measles, rubella, congenital rubella syndrome, and mumps, 2013: summary recommendations of the Advisory Committee on Immunization Practices (ACIP). MMWR Recomm Rep. 2013;62(RR-04):1–34. PubMed PMID: 23760201. Epub 2013/06/14. eng

Siber GR, Werner BG, Halsey NA, Reid R, Almeido-Hill J, Garrett SC, et al. Interference of immune globulin with measles and rubella immunization. J Pediatr. 1993;122(2):204–11. PubMed PMID: 8429432. Epub 1993/02/01. eng

Sobh A, Bonilla FA. Vaccination in primary immunodeficiency disorders. J Allergy Clin Immunol Pract. 2016;4(6):1066–75. PubMed PMID: 27836056. Epub 2016/11/12. eng

Sriaroon P, Ballow M. Immunoglobulin replacement therapy for primary immunodeficiency. Immunol Allergy Clin N Am. 2015;35(4):713–30. PubMed PMID: 26454315. Epub 2015/10/12. eng

---

Management of Immunodeficiency, Quality of Life

Panida Sriaroon
Department of Pediatrics, Division of Allergy and Immunology, University of South Florida/Johns Hopkins All Children's Hospital, Tampa, FL, USA

Primary immunodeficiency diseases (PID) are a heterogeneous group of diseases characterized by recurrent infections and associated conditions such as autoimmune diseases, chronic lung or gastrointestinal diseases, cytopenia, lymphoproliferative disorders, and, in limited cases, malignancy. Prior to PID diagnosis, many patients suffer from several years of physical illness before being evaluated for an immunologic disorder. Once a PID diagnosis has been made, patients usually require close follow-up with healthcare professionals and lifelong treatment given the risk of infections and other associated complications. Fewer than 15% of adults with PID never experience severe or life-threatening conditions (Barlogis et al. 2017). Living with a chronic illness like PID can take a significant emotional toll, which in turn can affect the quality of life (QOL).

QOL is an intricate concept that involves physical, psychological, and social aspects of one's well-being. General health questionnaires, such as the Medical Outcomes Study in the Short

Form-36 (SF-36), Short Form-12 (SF-12), and General Health Questionnaire-12 Items (GHQ-12), are widely used to assess health status and QOL in the general population and have been used in patients with PID. Recently, specific PID-related QOL questionnaires have been created and validated for use in patients with antibody deficiency conditions who are on IgG replacement therapy (Ballow et al. 2017; Quinti et al. 2016). These tools were developed with the goal of having health-related QOL instruments that are PID-specific, easy to use, and useful in optimizing treatment and gauging PID disease burden. However, the utility of these questionnaires still needs to be evaluated in larger groups of PID patients with different ages, disease severity, comorbidities, and changes in disease status over time.

In the past decade, several studies demonstrated that patients with PID have lower QOL than healthy controls (Barlogis et al. 2017). Patients with common variable immunodeficiency (CVID) have much lower SF-12 scores than the general US population, and the scores are higher in those who have mild disease, lack physical impairments, are not disturbed by treatment, and receive IgG treatments at home. A survey conducted by the Immune Deficiency Foundation reported that 39% of patients with PID perceived their health status as fair or very poor (Seeborg et al. 2015). Children with PID had similar QOL scores to children with cancer (Sultan et al. 2017) and much lower emotional and social functioning than children with juvenile inflammatory arthritis (Kuburovic et al. 2014).

Due to their susceptibility to infections and other complications, patients with certain PIDs require lifelong immunoglobulin (Ig)G replacement therapy, which now is available in intravenous Ig (IVIG) and subcutaneous Ig (SCIG) forms. The effects of IgG replacement therapy on QOL have been well described. The therapy improves QOL by reducing the frequency of infections and, as a result, the fear of getting frequent infections.

The increased use of SCIG during the past decade, particularly in North America and Europe, correlates with higher satisfaction and QOL than the traditional IVIG treatment mainly due to convenience and sense of independence.

However, pain and discomfort remain important issues, with children more frequently raising them as issues than their parents. Sultan et al. reported that while 69% of children who were receiving SCIG treatment for PID considered the treatment convenient, 24% considered it to be associated with discomfort (Sultan et al. 2017).

Similar to other chronic illnesses, the management of PID frequently becomes a challenge for work, school, and personal life. Many aspects of PID condition and treatment can be difficult for patients and their families to understand due to its complex and heterogeneous nature. Children who miss school often have difficulty functioning at school and with peers. Some children develop mood disturbances or depression as a result of having serious chronic illness. Adult patients with PID also face challenges in keeping up with job and family needs while managing their health. Moreover, the illness may affect work or interpersonal relations as well as self-esteem.

In addition to receiving proper medical treatment, it is crucial that patients with PID and their caregivers be evaluated for mental health issues and be offered proper management as needed. Some patients feel isolated, sad, or hopeless and may resent that they have a PID condition. Mental health providers can help identify factors that are most related to the patient's distress.

The support from multidisciplinary healthcare teams, family, friends, and community can significantly improve the QOL of patients with PID. Today, individuals living with PID can be connected to other people who share similar experiences via several platforms including social media groups, online forums, local group meetings, or national conferences held specifically for patients with PID and their families. Most people find these relationships and resources supportive. More educational strategies should be created to address the QOL issue in this vulnerable population.

References

Ballow M, Conaway MR, Sriaroon P, Rachid RA, Seeborg FO, Duff CM, et al. Construction and validation of a novel disease-specific quality-of-life instrument for patients with primary antibody deficiency disease (PADQOL-16). J Allergy Clin Immunol. 2017;139(6):2007.e8–10.e8.

Barlogis V, Mahlaoui N, Auquier P, Pellier I, Fouyssac F, Vercasson C, et al. Physical health conditions and quality of life in adults with primary immunodeficiency diagnosed during childhood: a French Reference Center for PIDs (CEREDIH) study. J Allergy Clin Immunol. 2017;139(4):1275–81 e7.

Kuburovic NB, Pasic S, Susic G, Stevanovic D, Kuburovic V, Zdravkovic S, Janicijevic Petrovic M, Pekmezovic T. Health-related quality of life, anxiety, and depressive symptoms in children with primary immunodeficiencies. Patient Prefer Adherence 2014;8:323–30. https://doi.org/10.2147/PPA.S58040. eCollection 2014.

Quinti I, Pulvirenti F, Giannantoni P, Hajjar J, Canter DL, Milito C, et al. Development and initial validation of a questionnaire to measure health-related quality of life of adults with common variable immune deficiency: the CVID_QoL questionnaire. J Allergy Clin Immunol. 2016;4(6):1169.e4–79.e4.

Seeborg FO, Seay R, Boyle M, Boyle J, Scalchunes C, Orange JS. Perceived health in patients with primary immune deficiency. J Clin Immunol. 2015;35(7):638–50.

Sultan S, Rondeau E, Levasseur MC, Dicaire R, Decaluwe H, Haddad E. Quality of life, treatment beliefs, and treatment satisfaction in children treated for primary immunodeficiency with SCIg. J Clin Immunol. 2017;37(5):496–504.

Management of Immunodeficiency: Gene Therapy

Jennifer W. Leiding
Department of Pediatrics, Division of Allergy and Immunology, University of South Florida at Johns Hopkins – All Children's Hospital, St. Petersburg, FL, USA

The use of gene-modified cells as a source of hematopoietic stem cell transplantation (HSCT) has grown significantly in the last 10 years. Although advances in supportive care, prevention of infections, improved HLA typing, and improved conditioning regimens have improved survival, HSCT can be complicated in those who lack well-matched donors or who have pre-existing infections.

The ability to develop viral vectors that stably integrate modified genes into cells occurred in the 1980s and 1990s. The first gene therapy trial occurred with a 4-year-old girl with adenosine deaminase (ADA)-deficient severe combined immunodeficiency (SCID). The patient received several infusions of a gamma retroviral vector containing normal ADA cDNA which led to endogenous production of ADA.

The sequence of events for gene modification therapy is as follows:

1. Stem cells collected from affected patient.
2. Stem cells cultured in vitro with modified virus carrying the corrective gene sequence.
3. Preconditioning chemotherapy is given to create bone marrow space.
4. Genetically modified stem cells are infused into the patient.

Gene Therapy for ADA SCID

ADA deficiency is an autosomal recessive disorder that manifests as T, B, and NK cell deficiency and dysfunction. The ADA enzyme is ubiquitously expressed, and deficiency of ADA leads to the buildup of toxic metabolites in lymphocytes and other cells. Enzyme replacement with pegylated ADA provides detoxification and some immune reconstitution, and over time the effects of pegylated ADA become blunted. HSCT is the treatment of choice for ADA deficiency, but for those without optimal donors, gene therapy is becoming standard of care. The gene therapy trials for ADA SCID are described below:

- The first trial used a murine gamma retroviral vector with patients maintained on enzyme replacement therapy. Although ADA expression developed, it was not high enough to confer significant benefit.
- The next trials used Moloney murine leukemia-derived replication-deficient recombinant retroviruses. Non-myeloablative doses of busulfan or melphalan were also used to create space in the bone marrow compartment. Enzyme replacement was stopped either

shortly before or at time of infusion. The majority of patients treated were able to discontinue IVIG and/or enzyme replacement therapy.

Overall, more than 100 patients have been treated with gene modification therapy with ADA SCID with 100% survival (Aiuti et al. 2009).

Gene Therapy for X-Linked SCID

X-linked SCID is caused by mutations in the *IL2RG* gene found on the X chromosome. *IL2RG* encodes for the common gamma chain that is responsible for IL-2, IL-4, IL-7, IL-9, IL-15, and IL-21 signaling. Defects in IL2RG lead to defective T and NK cell production with present B cells.

The first clinical trial for gene therapy for X-SCID occurred in 1999 in Paris and was followed closely in 2001 in London. X-SCID patients without an HLA-identical donor were treated without chemotherapy; hematopoietic stem cells were treated with a murine gamma retroviral vector in which the common gamma chain was under control of U3 region enhancers. Stable immune reconstitution was obtained and all patients had control of infections and increased growth. However, 31–68 months after gene therapy, five patients developed T cell acute lymphoblastic leukemia. In four patients, the gamma retroviral vector was integrated near and activated the LIM domain-only 2 (LMO2) proto-oncogene. Four of the five survived after receiving chemotherapy and bone marrow transplantation (Hacein-Bey Abina et al. 2008).

Subsequently, modifications were made to the gamma retrovirus vector, removing the enhancer sequences. This new self-inactivating gamma retroviral expressing IL2RG has been used in nine boys. Eight of the nine are still alive, and there have been no leukemic events following gene therapy. This trial is still open and enrolling (Hacein-Bey-Abina et al. 2014).

A newer approach using lentiviral vectors combined with low-exposure targeted busulfan has resulted in multilineage engraftment of functional T cells and B cells in 8 infants (reference Mamcarz E et al. "Lentiviral Gene Therapy Combined with Low-Dose Busulfan in Infants with SCID-X1" NEJM. 2019.

Gene Therapy for X-Linked Chronic Granulomatous Disease

X-linked CGD is caused by mutations in *CYBB* which encodes for gp91phox, a major component of the NADPH oxidase in neutrophils. Defects in the NADPH oxidase results in immunodeficiency characterized by severe bacterial and fungal infections and autoinflammation.

The first clinical trials used gamma retroviral vectors to deliver normal *CYBB*, some with and some without preconditioning regimens. Despite the presence of gene-corrected cells, these numbers decreased significantly in the first year after gene therapy. During these times of low but present gene-corrected neutrophils, severe life-threatening infections were able to improve or were cured. In an additional subset of patients, there was insertional activation of growth-promoting genes that led to myelodysplasia and monosomy 7 in two patients (Kang et al. 2010). Because of these problems with gamma retroviral vectors, use of a lentivirus vector to deliver *CYBB* is now being investigated (Farinelli et al. 2016). Initial results show >20% genetically modified neutrophils with resolution of infections and inflammatory disease in participants (Kohn et al. 2018) (Table 1).

Gene Therapy for Wiskott–Aldrich Syndrome

Wiskott-Aldrich Syndrome (WAS) is an X-linked disorder characterized by eczema, thrombocytopenia, and susceptibility to infections. WAS protein is required for functional leukocyte migration. The first clinical trial for gene therapy for WAS started in 2006. Ten patients received non-myeloablative doses of busulfan and

Management of Immunodeficiency: Gene Therapy, Table 1 Gene therapy trials for primary immunodeficiency diseases

Disease	Center	Status	NCT	Vector
ADA SCID	UCLA	Recruiting	NCT03765632	LV
	London	Recruiting	NCT01380990	LV
	Los Angeles, Bethesda, London	Complete	NCT0127972071, NCT02022696	LV
	Milan, Jerusalem	Complete	NCT00599781; NCT00598481	γ-RV
	Bethesda	Complete	NCT00018018	γ-RV
	London	Complete	NCT01279720	γ-RV
X-linked SCID	London	Recruiting	NCT01175239	SIN-γ-RV
	Paris	Recruiting	NCT01410019	SIN- γ-RV
	Memphis, San Francisco, Seattle	Recruiting	NCT01512888	LV
	Boston, Los Angeles	Recruiting	NCT03311503	LV
	Beijing	Recruiting	NCT03217617	LV
	Bethesda	Recruiting	NCT03315078	LV
	Bethesda	Recruiting	NCT01306019	LV
	London	Recruiting	NCT03601286	LV
	Boston, Cincinnati, London, Los Angeles, Paris	Complete	NCT01175239	SIN- γ-RV
	Bethesda	Complete	NCT00028236	RV
	Bethesda, Cincinnati, Los Angeles	Complete	NCT01129544	γ-RV
X-CGD	Frankfurt	Recruiting	NCT01906541	γ-RV
	Frankfurt, London, Paris, Zurich	Recruiting	NCT01855685	LV
	Bethesda, Boston, Los Angeles	Recruiting	NCT02234934	LV
	Paris	Recruiting	NCT02757911	LV
	Zurich	Complete	NCT00927134	γ-RV
	Bethesda	Complete	NCT00001476	γ-RV
	Seoul	Complete	NCT00778882	γ-RV
	Bethesda	Complete	NCT00394316	γ-RV
WAS	London	Recruiting	NCT01347242	LV
	Milan	Recruiting	NCT03837483	LV
	Boston	Recruiting	NCT01410825	LV
	Milan	Complete	NCT01515462	LV
	Paris London	Complete	NCT01347346	LV
	Paris	Complete	NCT02333760	LV

RV retrovirus, *LV* lentivirus

hematopoietic stem cells corrected with a Wiskott-Aldrich Syndrome protein (WASP) expressing gamma retrovirus (Hacein-Bey Abina et al. 2015). Immune reconstitution occurred in nine patients, along with increases in platelet count (Farinelli et al. 2016). Unfortunately, vector site insertion analysis showed clustering at sites of proto-oncogenes. Between 14 months and 5 years post gene therapy, seven of nine developed hematologic malignancy. All were treated with chemotherapy and HSCT, but two died of leukemia (Boztug et al. 2010).

In response, gene therapy trials using a self-inactivated lentiviral vector was developed. A total of 21 patients have been treated with stable engraftment of gene-marked cells. Patients had clinical benefit with decreased bleeding episodes and decreased incidence of infections, autoimmunity, and eczema. Platelet recovery has been variable (Braun et al. 2014).

There have been tremendous advances in gene therapy for treatment of primary immunodeficiency in the last 30 years, providing a new standard for treatment of patients. Newer technology to improve gene therapy strategies using genome editing tools to cause site-specific gene editing is underway8.

References

Aiuti A, Cassani B, Callegaro L, et al. Gene therapy for immunodeficiency due to adenosine deaminase deficiency. N Engl J Med. 2009;360(5):447–58.

Boztug K, Schmidt M, Schwarzer A, et al. Stem-cell gene therapy for the Wiskott- Aldrich syndrome. N Engl J Med. 2010;363(20):1918–27.

Braun CJ, Boztug K, Paruzynski A, et al. Gene therapy for Wiskott-Aldrich syn- drome–long-term efficacy and genotoxicity. Sci Transl Med. 2014;6(227):227–33.

Farinelli G, Jofra Hernandez R, Rossi A, Ranucci S, Sanvito F, Migliavacca M, Brombin C, Pramov A, Di Serio C, Bovolenta C, Gentner B, Bragonzi A, Aiuti A. Lentiviral vector gene therapy protects XCGD Mice from Acute *Staphylococcus aureus* Pneumonia and Inflammatory Response. Mol Ther. 2016;24(10):1873–80.

Hacein-Bey Abina S, Garrigue A, Wang GP, et al. Insertional oncogenesis in 4 patients after retrovirus-mediated gene therapy of SCID-X1. J Clin Invest. 2008;118(9):3132–42.

Hacein-Bey Abina S, Gaspar HB, Blondeau J, et al. Outcomes following gene therapy in patients with severe Wiskott-Aldrich Syndrome. JAMA. 2015;313(15):1550.

Hacein-Bey-Abina S, Pai S-Y, Gaspar HB, et al. A Modified γ-Retrovirus Vector for X-Linked Severe Combined Immunodeficiency. N Engl J Med. 2014;371(15):1407–17.

Kang EM, Choi U, Theobald N, et al. Retrovirus gene therapy for X-linked chronic granulomatous disease can achieve stable long-term correction of oxidase activity in peripheral blood neutrophils. Blood. 2010;115(4):783–91.

Kohn DBB C, Kang EM, Pai SY, Shaw KL, Kuo CY, Terrazas DR, Wang LD, Armant M, Santilli G, Bucklandd K, Rico DL, Snell K, De Ravin S, Choi U, Mavilio F, Galy A, Newburger P, Bushman FD, Gaspar HB, Williams DA, Malech HL, Thrasher AJ. Gene therapy for X-linked chronic granulomatous disease. Molecular Therapy. 2018;26(5S1):157–8.

Kohn. Consensus approach for the management of secvere combined immunodeficiency caused by ADA deficiency. JACI. 2019;143(3):852–863.

Mannose-Binding Lectin-Associated Serine Protease-2 (MASP-2) Deficiency

María Isabel García-Laorden[1,2] and Carlos Rodríguez-Gallego[1]
[1]Department of Immunology, Gran Canaria Dr. Negrín University Hospital, Las Palmas de Gran Canaria, Spain
[2]CIBER de Enfermedades Respiratorias (CIBERES), Instituto de Salud Carlos III, Madrid, Spain

Definition

MASP-2 deficiency refers to the congenital deficiency of the protein mannose-binding lectin-associated serine protease-2 (MASP-2) of the lectin pathway of the complement system, due to autosomal recessive mutations in the *MASP2* gene.

Introduction

The lectin pathway (LP) is one of the three pathways of activation of the complement system. To date five pattern recognition molecules (PRMs) have been found to trigger the activation of the LP of the complement system: mannose-binding lectin (MBL), ficolin-1, -2, and, -3 (also called M-, L-, and H-ficolin), and collectin 11 (CL11 or CL-K1). The LP is activated when one of these PRMs binds a pattern of oligosaccharides or acetylated residues on the surface of microorganisms or damaged host cells (Degn and Thiel 2013; Ma et al. 2013).

The PRMs of the LP circulate in complexes with the proenzyme form of MBL-associated serine proteases (MASPs): MASP-1, -2, and -3, as well as with two nonenzymatic proteins named sMAP (or Map19) and MAP-1 (Map44). MASP-1 and MASP-2 are produced mainly in the liver, and MASP-3 is produced in several other tissues besides the liver. Upon binding to the targets, MASP-1 becomes activated and activates

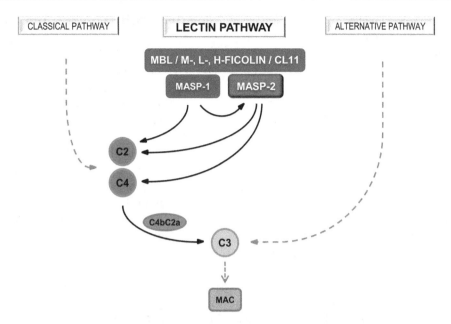

Mannose-Binding Lectin-Associated Serine Protease-2 (MASP-2) Deficiency, Fig. 1 Schematic representation of the lectin pathway of the complement system. The lectin pathway (*LP*) is triggered by five pattern recognition molecules (*PRM*): mannose-binding lectin (*MBL*), ficolin-1, -2, and -3, and collectin 11 (CL11 or CL-K1). The LP is initiated when these PRMs bind to pathogen-associated molecular patterns on the surface of pathogens or to apoptotic or necrotic cells. Circulating MBL, CL11, and ficolins form complexes with MASP-1 and MASP-2. After the binding of MBL, ficolins, and CL-11 to their targets, MASP-1 auto-activates and triggers MASP-2. Activated MASP-2 cleaves C4 and C2 allowing the assembly of the C3 (C4bC2a) and C5 (C4bC2a(C3)$_n$) convertases and the subsequent activation of the terminal pathway. Activated MASP-1 also cleaves C2. *MAC* membrane attack complex

MASP-2, which cleaves C2 and C4 to generate the C3 convertase, C4bC2a. Activated MASP-1 also cleaves C2. The LP, like the classic and alternative pathways, converges on C3, with the subsequent activation of the effector mechanisms of the complement system (Yongqing et al 2012; Degn and Thiel 2013; Frank and Sullivan 2014), (Fig. 1). The function of MASP-3, sMAP, and MAP-1 in humans remains unclear.

Polymorphisms in the gene for MBL (*MBL2*), conferring MBL deficiency, were first described in 1991. Since then, countless surveys have been conducted about the role of MBL in several pathologies. Nonetheless, there are many contradictory results, and hence there is still controversy about its role in susceptibility to infection and autoimmunity. It was suggested that MBL deficiency could play a role in susceptibility to infection under certain circumstances, such as in individuals with immunodeficiencies, toddlers, or cancer patients undergoing chemotherapy (Degn et al. 2011; Heitzeneder et al. 2012; Frank and Sullivan 2014).

Deficiency of MASP-2 was first reported in 2003 (Stengaard-Pedersen et al. 2003).

Clinical Phenotype

The first patient reported with MASP-2 deficiency was identified when MBL-dependent lectin pathway activity and MBL levels were measured in plasma from 125 patients with suspected immune deficiencies. The patient was completely deficient in LP activity despite having sufficient MBL, and he was later found to be MASP-2 deficient (Stengaard-Pedersen et al. 2003; Sørensen et al. 2005). He had been diagnosed with ulcerative colitis and systemic lupus erythematosus (SLE), and he had suffered from three episodes of severe

M

pneumococcal pneumonia, with one episode of sepsis requiring prolonged intensive care. The authors proposed that severe infections in this patient were due to MASP-2 deficiency. However, the patient also had anti-C1q antibodies, resulting in severely reduced serum C1q levels and a severe impairment of the classical pathway function. In addition he had low levels of C3 and C4, increased levels of C3dg, and a reduced alternative pathway function. These impairments of the classical and alternative pathways may have contributed to his susceptibility to severe pneumococcal infections.

In subsequent studies, nine MASP-2-deficient patients have been identified in genetic association studies on possible associations of MASP-2 genetic variants with a heterogeneous group of disorders: two children with recurrent respiratory infections (Cedzynski et al. 2004, 2009), one pediatric patient with cystic fibrosis (Olesen et al. 2006), two adult patients at lung clinics (Thiel et al. 2007), one hepatitis C virus-positive adult patient with hepatocellular carcinoma (Segat et al. 2008), one adult with colorectal cancer (Ytting et al. 2011), and two adults with pulmonary tuberculosis (Sokolowska et al. 2015) (Table 1).

However, deficiency of MASP-2 was also found by chance in seven adult healthy controls from genetic association studies (Stover et al. 2005; Garcia-Laorden et al. 2006, 2008; Segat et al. 2008; Olszowski et al. 2014; Sokolowska et al. 2015) (Table 1). In a study including 868 healthy Spaniard volunteers, 967 adult patients with community-acquired pneumonia, 43 children with recurrent respiratory infections, and 130 SLE patients, the only MASP-2-deficient individuals were a 37-year-old healthy control female from the hospital staff and a 39-year-old healthy female blood donor. Both healthy controls were further studied in order to confirm their health status; the 37-year-old female remains healthy 9 years after she was reported (Garcia-Laorden et al. 2006). Health status was also evaluated in at least another two healthy controls aged 19 and 29 years (Olszowski et al. 2014; Sokolowska et al. 2015).

Molecular Basis of MASP-2 Deficiency

MASP-1, -2, and -3 all exhibit domain structures identical with those of C1r and C1s, the C1 proteases of the classical pathway of the complement system. They consist of an N-terminal C1r/C1s, uEGF, and bone morphogenetic protein-1 (CUB1) domain, followed by an Ca^{2+}-binding epidermal growth factor (EGF)-like domain, a second CUB domain, two complement control protein (CCP) modules, an activation peptide, and a C-terminal serine protease domain. The CUB1 and EGF domains are responsible for binding to the collagenous regions of the PRMs of the LP, and the serine-protease domain is the catalytically active unit. The gene coding for MASP-2 (*MASP2*; 1p36.3-p36.2) comprises 12 exons. The mature polypeptide chain of human MASP-2 is composed of 686 residues, including a signal peptide of 15 amino acids (Thiel et al. 2009; Degn and Thiel 2013).

MASP-2 deficiency is caused in Caucasians by homozygosity for a *c.359A > G* (rs72550870, exon 3) mutation leading to a change of aspartic acid to glycine at amino acid position 120 (CUB1 domain) of the synthesized protein (p.D120G, p. D105G when excluding the signal peptide). The mutation results in very low serum levels of MASP-2. Since MASP-2 and sMAP are splice variants from the *MASP2* gene, the mutation also results in reduced serum levels of sMAP. In addition, the mutation affects the structure of the CUB1 domain which is directly involved in binding of calcium ions, a requisite for binding to PRM of the LP. As a consequence, the mutation D120G abolishes interaction with PRMs of the LP, and homozygotes for the mutation are unable to activate the LP. Heterozygotes for p.D120G had significantly lower MASP-2 levels (by 45%) than wild-type homozygous individuals (Stengaard-Pedersen K et al. 2003; García-Laorden et al. 2006; Thiel et al. 2009; Olszowski et al. 2014; Sokolowska et al. 2015).

The expected frequency of homozygosity for the p.D120G allele ranges between 6 and 10 cases in 10,000 individuals in populations of European ancestry, making this deficiency relatively

Mannose-Binding Lectin-Associated Serine Protease-2 (MASP-2) Deficiency, Table 1   Reported individuals with MASP-2 deficiency

Individuals with MASP-2 deficiency	Source	Reference
Adult Danish patient with SLE, UC, and severe pneumococcal infections	125 patients with suspected immune deficiencies	Stengaard-Pedersen et al. 2003
Pediatric Polish patient with recurrent pneumonias	335 Polish children with RRI, 78 healthy children	Cedzynski et al. 2004[a]
British healthy adult	314 based trios with offspring affected with psoriasis	Stover et al. 2005
Three healthy Spanish adults	967 adult patients with CAP, 43 children with RRI, 130 adult patients with SLE, 868 healthy adult controls, 514 patients without relevant infectious diseases	Garcia-Laorden et al. 2006, 2008[b]
Pediatric Danish patient with cystic fibrosis	109 patients with cystic fibrosis	Olesen et al. 2006
Two adult Danish patients at lung clinics	n.a.	Thiel et al. 2007
Italian HCV+ adult patient with hepatocellular carcinoma	215 adults with hepatocellular carcinoma, 164 controls	Segat et al. 2008
Italian healthy adult	215 adults with hepatocellular carcinoma, 164 controls	Segat et al. 2008
Pediatric Polish patient with recurrent upper respiratory infections and skin abscesses	331 children with allergy (N = 172) and/or RRI (N = 232), 91 healthy children	Cedzynski et al. 2009[a]
Danish adult patient with colorectal cancer	593 patients with colorectal cancer, 350 healthy controls	Ytting et al. 2011
Two adult Polish patients with TBC	440 patients with TBC, 276 healthy controls	Sokolowska et al. 2015
Polish healthy adult	440 patients with TBC, 276 healthy controls	Sokolowska et al. 2015
Polish healthy adult	179 Polish children with dental caries	Olszowski et al. 2014

MASP-2 levels and/or lectin pathway activity in MASP-2-deficient individuals were reported in Stengaard-Pedersen et al. 2003; Cedzynski et al. 2004; Garcia-Laorden et al. 2006, 2008; Olesen et al. 2006; Cedzynski et al. 2009; Sokolowska et al. 2015; and Olszowski et al. 2014

All the MASP-2-deficient individuals were homozygous for the p.D120G mutation in *MASP2*

SLE systemic lupus erythematosus, *UC* ulcerative colitis, *RRI* recurrent respiratory infections, *CAP* community-acquired pneumonia, *n.a.* not available, *HCV* hepatitis C virus, *TBC* pulmonary tuberculosis

[a]Data from this patient is detailed in Sokolowska et al. 2015

[b]Two individuals were described in Garcia-Laorden et al. 2006, and one additional MASP-2-deficient individual was identified in Garcia-Laorden et al. 2008

common (García-Laorden et al. 2006; Thiel et al. 2007). The mutation was not found in sub-Saharan African, Chinese, and Amerindian populations (Thiel et al. 2007).

Besides p.D120G, numerous genetic variants have been identified in *MASP2* among different populations (Thiel et al. 2007, 2009). Several of these variants are missense mutations. Most of them do not affect LP activation. However, the p.R439H variant (rs12085877, exon 12) displays

considerably reduced enzymatic activity despite binding to MBL (Thiel et al. 2009). When MASP-2 is activated, the polypeptide chain is cleaved at an arginine-isoleucine peptide bond (R444-I445) in the activation peptide. The mutation p.R439H is located in the activation peptide section, 5 aa N terminally from the R444 cleavage site. According to data from the National Center for Biotechnology Information SNP database (http://www.ncbi.nlm.nih.gov/snp) the variant is found at an allele frequency ranging from 0.056 to 0.146 in populations of sub-Saharan ancestry, but no clinical or LP activity data about homozygotes for the mutation have been reported. Another variant, a duplication of 12 bp, resulting in the insertion of four amino acids (156_159dupCHNH, EGF domain), was identified at very low frequency in Hong Kong Chinese (0.26%) (Thiel et al. 2007). The mutation severely impairs MBL binding and the ability to activate the LP (Thiel et al. 2009), but no homozygous individuals have been identified so far.

Concluding Remarks

The first description of a patient with MASP-2 deficiency led to suggest that this autosomal recessive deficiency would predispose to infection. MASP-2 deficiency might be more severe than MBL deficiency because complement activation via both ficolins and MBL are severely impaired in individuals homozygous for p. D120G. However, the finding of healthy adults homozygous for p.D120G, with demonstrated severely impaired LP activity, suggested that the clinical penetrance of MASP-2 deficiency could be low. At present, ten patients with a heterogeneous spectrum of clinical manifestations and seven healthy controls with MASP-2 deficiency have been reported; sixteen out of the seventeen individuals were identified in studies involving statistical analysis. Although a role of MASP-2 deficiency in susceptibility to infection in individuals with other underlying diseases impairing immune defence mechanisms cannot be excluded, MASP-2 deficiency is now considered a consequence of a common polymorphism with no clear clinical relevance.

Cross-References

▶ Complement System, C5, C6, C7, C8, C9, Component

▶ Ficolin-3

References

Cedzynski M, Szemraj J, Swierzko AS, Bak-Romaniszyn-L, Banasik M, Zeman K, et al. Mannan-binding lectin insufficiency in children with recurrent infections of the respiratory system. Clin Exp Immunol. 2004;136(2):304–11.

Cedzynski M, Atkinson AP, Swierzko AS, MacDonald SL, Szala A, Zeman K, et al. L ficolin (ficolin-2) insufficiency is associated with combined allergic and infectious respiratory disease in children. Mol Immunol. 2009;47(2–3):415–9.

Degn SE, Thiel S. Humoral pattern recognition and the complement system. Scand J Immunol. 2013;78(2):181–93.

Degn SE, Jensenius JC, Thiel S. Disease-causing mutations in genes of the complement system. Am J Hum Genet. 2011;88(6):689–705.

Frank MM, Sullivan KE. Deficiencies of the complement system. In: Sullivan KE, Stiehm ER, editors. Stiehm's immune deficiencies. San Diego: Academic; 2014. p. 731–63.

Garcia-Laorden MI, Garcia-Saavedra A, de Castro FR, Violan JS, Rajas O, Blanquer J, et al. Low clinical penetrance of mannose binding lectin-associated serine protease 2 deficiency. J Allergy Clin Immunol. 2006;118(6):1383–6.

Garcia-Laorden MI, Sole-Violan J, Rodriguez de Castro F, Aspa J, Briones ML, Garcia-Saavedra A, et al. Mannose binding lectin and mannose-binding lectin-associated serine protease 2 in susceptibility, severity, and outcome of pneumonia in adults. J Allergy Clin Immunol. 2008;122(2):368–74.

Heitzeneder S, Seidel M, Förster-Waldl E, Heitger A. Mannan-binding lectin deficiency – good news, bad news, doesn't matter? Clin Immunol. 2012;143(1):22–38.

Ma YJ, Skjoedt MO, Garred P. Collectin-11/MASP complex formation triggers activation of the lectin complement pathway – the fifth lectin pathway initiation complex. J Innate Immun. 2013;5(3):242–50.

Olesen HV, Jensenius JC, Steffensen R, Thiel S, Schiotz PO. The mannan-binding lectin pathway and lung disease in cystic fibrosis – disfunction of mannan-binding lectin-associated serine protease 2 (MASP-2) may be a major modifier. Clin Immunol. 2006;121(3):324–31.

Olszowski T, Poziomkowska-Gęsicka I, Jensenius JC, Adler G. Lectin pathway of complement activation in a Polish woman with MASP-2 deficiency. Immunobiology. 2014;219(4):261–2.

Segat L, Fabris A, Padovan L, Milanese M, Pirulli D, Lupo F, et al. MBL2 and MASP2 gene polymorphisms in patients with hepatocellular carcinoma. J Viral Hepat. 2008;15(5):387–91.

Sokolowska A, Szala A, St Swierzko A, Kozinska M, Niemiec T, Blachnio M, et al. Mannan-binding lectin-associated serine protease-2 (MASP-2) deficiency in two patients with pulmonary tuberculosis and one healthy control. Cell Mol Immunol. 2015;12(1):119–21.

Sørensen R, Thiel S, Jensenius JC. Mannan-binding-lectin-associated serine proteases, characteristics and disease associations. Springer Semin Immunopathol. 2005;27(3):299–319.

Stengaard-Pedersen K, Thiel S, Gadjeva M, Moller-Kristensen M, Sorensen R, Jensen LT, et al. Inherited deficiency of mannan-binding lectin associated serine protease 2. N Engl J Med. 2003;349(6):554–60.

Stover C, Barrett S, Lynch NJ, Barker JN, Burden D, Trembath R, et al. Functional MASP2 single nucleotide polymorphism plays no role in psoriasis. Br J Dermatol. 2005;152(6):1313–5.

Thiel S, Steffensen R, Christensen IJ, Ip WK, Lau YL, Reason IJ, et al. Deficiency of mannan-binding lectin associated serine protease-2 due to missense polymorphisms. Genes Immun. 2007;8(2):154–63.

Thiel S, Kolev M, Degn S, Steffensen R, Hansen AG, Ruseva M, Jensenius JC. Polymorphisms in mannan-binding lectin (MBL)-associated serine protease 2 affect stability, binding to MBL, and enzymatic activity. J Immunol. 2009;182(5):2939–47.

Yongqing T, Drentin N, Duncan RC, Wijeyewickrema LC, Pike RN. Mannose-binding lectin serine proteases and associated proteins of the lectin pathway of complement: two genes, five proteins and many functions? Biochim Biophys Acta. 2012;1824(1):253–62.

Ytting H, Christensen IJ, Steffensen R, Alsner J, Thiel S, Jensenius JC, et al. Mannan-binding lectin (MBL) and MBL associated serine protease 2 (MASP-2) genotypes in colorectal cancer. Scand J Immunol. 2011;73(2):122–7.

MCM4 Deficiency

Bhumika Patel
Asthma, Allergy and Immunology of Tampa Bay, Tampa, FL, USA

Definition

Minichromosome maintenance complex component 4 (MCM4) deficiency is an autosomal recessive disease affecting DNA replication and resulting in natural killer (NK) cell deficiency, increased chromosomal breakage, adrenal insufficiency, growth failure, and predisposition to viral infections.

Introduction/Background

NK cells are lymphocytes of the innate immune system that have a vital role in antiviral immunity and tumor surveillance. They lack antigen-specific T cell and B cell receptors and are classified as CD56$^+$CD3$^-$. NK cells are found primarily in the functionally distinct CD56^{dim} and CD56^{bright} subsets. The CD56^{dim} subset expresses low levels of CD56 and CD16 and accounts for most of the peripheral blood NK cell population. CD56^{bright} NK cells are believed to be the developmental precursor to CD56^{dim} mature NK cells. CD56^{dim} NK cells are primarily involved in contact-dependent toxicity, whereas the CD56^{bright} NK cells are potent producers of cytokines.

To date, there are only five identified primary immunodeficiencies that selectively affect the NK cell population. Classical NK cell deficiency (cNKD) is defined as an absent or profoundly decreased CD56$^+$CD3$^-$ NK cell population. In functional NKD (fNKD), there are normal levels of NK cells, but they have impaired function.

MCM4 deficiency (OMIM 609981) is a cNKD that involves disruption of cell replication. MCM4 is part of the hexameric MCM helicase complex MCM2-7. The complex, along with MCM10 and Go-Ichi-Ni-San complex subunit 1 (GINS1), is crucial in the initiation and elongation of eukaryotic DNA replication (Orange 2012).

MCM4 deficiency was first described in 2012 in a consanguineous Irish traveler population. The causative mutation in these individuals was identified as a homozygous substitution (adenine to guanine) in the acceptor splice site in the *MCM4* gene located on chromosome 8p11.23-q11.21 (Gineau et al. 2012). This mutation caused a frameshift, which resulted in a premature stop codon and a severely truncated protein (p.Pro24-ArgfsX4). The mutated protein is able to form the MCM complex but fails to promote normal DNA replication (Hughes et al. 2012). The prevention of re-replication is affected leading to genomic instability, which is characterized by an accumulation of chromosomal aberrations.

M

Clinical Presentation (History/PE)

In 2012, Gineau et al. and Hughes et al. first described MCM4 deficiency in a consanguineous Irish traveler community. Patients in this cohort had NK cell deficiency, increased chromosomal breakage, adrenal insufficiency, pre- and postnatal growth failure, and predisposition to viral infections. The eldest child from the first family died from cytomegalovirus (CMV) and others were felt to have complications from viral illnesses. Susceptibility to viral infections is felt to be secondary to low NK cell numbers, especially decreased $CD56^{dim}$ NK cell population. Growth failure could be seen ante- and postnatal and included microcephaly. Cortisol deficiency in this population is not as severe as seen in other forms of familial glucocorticoid deficiency (FGD) and onset is typically seen in childhood after a period of normal adrenal sufficiency (Hughes et al. 2012).

Laboratory Findings/Diagnostic Testing

MCM4 deficiency is extremely rare, and to date, it has only been reported in those of Irish descent thus obtaining ethnicity history is important. These affected individuals have a normal complete blood count and normal numbers of T and B cells. However, they have a decreased absolute NK cell population with decreased numbers of $CD56^{dim}$ NK cells but normal levels of $CD56^{bright}$ NK cells (Orange 2012). Patients have glucocorticoid deficiency, raised adrenocorticotropic hormone (ACTH), and normal renin and aldosterone levels. Patient fibroblasts from this Irish community contain excessive chromosomal breaks and cell-cycle abnormalities. If MCM4 deficiency is suspected, genetic testing may be used to confirm the diagnosis.

Treatment/Prognosis

Those affected with MCM4 have a predisposition to viral infections because of decreased NK cell populations; especially, a decrease in the $CD56^{dim}$ mature NK cells subset. Thus, prevention of viral infections is important, as well as aggressively treating suspected viral infections promptly. The increase in viral susceptibility and DNA instability results in an increased risk of malignancy. In the Hughes et al. cohort, one of the patients developed an Epstein-Barr virus (EBV) driven lymphoproliferative disorder and another developed osteosarcoma. Hematologic and tumor surveillance is therefore recommended. Patients should be followed by endocrinology and started on glucocorticoid replacement since adrenal insufficiency can be life threatening. Hughes et al. described seven children with adrenal failure from three families within the Irish traveler community who were maintained on replacement hydrocortisone, 10–14 $mg/m^2/day$. Growth and nutrition should also be followed closely. Hematologic stem cell transplantation may also be a potential treatment depending on the clinical status of the patient.

References

Gineau L, Cognet C, Kara N, et al. Partial MCM4 deficiency in patients with growth retardation, adrenal insufficiency, and natural killer cell deficiency. J Clin Invest. 2012;122:821–32.

Hughes CR, Guasti L, Meimaridou E, et al. MCM4 mutation causes adrenal failure, short stature, and natural killer cell deficiency in humans. J Clin Invest. 2012; 122:814–20.

Mace EM, Orange JS. Genetic causes of human NK cell deficiency and their effect on NK cell subsets. Front Immunol. 2016;7:545.

Orange JS. Unraveling human natural killer deficiency. J Clin Invest. 2012;122:798–801.

Mevalonate Kinase Deficiency (MKD)

Jerold Jeyaratnam and Joost Frenkel
Department of Pediatrics, University Medical Center Utrecht, Utrecht, The Netherlands

Introduction

Mevalonate kinase deficiency (MKD) is a rare autoinflammatory syndrome characterized by fever and generalized inflammation (van der

Burgh et al. 2013). The disease was first described in the 1980s as two different phenotypes, namely, the hyper-immunoglobulinemia D and periodic fever syndrome (HIDS, MIM#260920) and mevalonic aciduria (MA, MIM#610377). Initially, both phenotypes were considered to be unrelated, until two groups independently described that both phenotypes were caused by mutations in the same gene.

Nowadays, mevalonate kinase deficiency is considered to be a clinical continuum between the HIDS and the MA phenotype. All patients with MKD may experience fever, gastrointestinal complaints, lymphadenopathy, mucosal ulcers, myalgia, arthralgia, and skin rash. In addition, patients with the more severe MA phenotype can also present with dysmorphic features, pre- and postnatal growth retardation, and ocular and neurological manifestations (van der Burgh et al. 2013; ter Haar et al. 2016).

MKD is caused by mutations in the mevalonate kinase (*MVK*) gene. Mevalonate kinase is an essential enzyme in the mevalonate pathway, which produces cholesterol and non-sterol isoprenoids. In MKD patients, the mevalonate kinase activity is reduced. Most HIDS patients have a residual activity of 1.8–28%, while patients with a MA phenotype usually show a residual activity below 0.5%. Recently, this biochemical defect was associated with an uncontrolled activation of the *MEFV* gene product, pyrin, which in turn results in caspase-1-mediated IL-1β release, fever, and inflammation.

Currently, there are about 300 known cases of MKD, of whom the vast majority have the HIDS phenotype. This number of known MKD patients is certainly an underestimate, since many patients go undiagnosed or do not end up in registries. MKD is seen more frequently in people with Caucasian ethnicity; a founder mutation (p. V377I) in the Dutch population has led to a disproportionate number of Dutch HIDS patients (ter Haar et al. 2016).

Pathophysiology

The mevalonate pathway is essential for the production of cholesterol and non-sterol isoprenoids.

The pathophysiology of MKD has not been unraveled completely yet. Recently, an association between the pyrin inflammasome and MKD was made (Park et al. 2016). Inflammasomes are multi-protein complexes, which produce the interleukins (IL)-1β and IL-18, if stimulated by specific microbial or endogenous danger signals. Uncontrolled activation of inflammasomes is the cause of some autoinflammatory diseases, such as Familial Mediterranean Fever, which is the result of uncontrolled activation of pyrin.

In MKD patients, the deficient mevalonate kinase leads to a lower production of geranylgeranyl pyrophosphate, the substrate of protein geranylgeranyl transferases. Geranylgeranylation is a posttranslational modification, which is crucial for the normal activity of the proteins involved. Decreased geranylgeranylation is responsible for the inactivation of the GTPase RhoA. Inactivation of RhoA eventually leads to activation of the pyrin inflammasome, which produces IL-1β and IL-18 in turn. IL-1β, secreted by macrophages and monocytes, is a strong inducer of fever and inflammation (Park et al. 2016). Although this theory explains a part of the pathophysiology, there is still a lot unknown. Future (molecular) studies should yield more information about the pathophysiology of this rare disease.

Clinical Presentation

MKD patients typically present with febrile episodes within the first 6 months of life and only in rare cases later than 19 months. Most patients suffer from 11 to 15 episodes per year, with most episodes lasting 3–7 days. Febrile episodes are often unprovoked but can be triggered by specific events, such as vaccination, emotional stress, and infection. Especially vaccination is a well-known trigger of MKD (ter Haar et al. 2016).

Febrile episodes are often accompanied by symptoms that can involve many organ systems. Gastrointestinal complaints are common during febrile episodes and include mainly abdominal pain, diarrhea, and vomiting. Recurrent sterile serosal inflammation can lead to peritoneal adhesions, which might require surgical intervention (Fig. 1). Mucocutaneous manifestations

Mevalonate Kinase Deficiency (MKD),
Fig. 1 Acute intestinal obstructions due to peritoneal adhesions in MKD

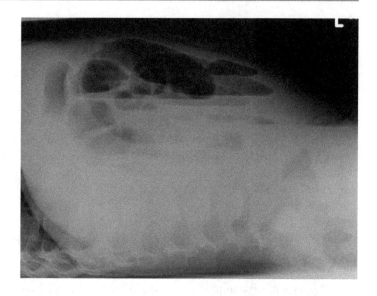

commonly include oral ulcers but can also affect the genital or rectal mucosa. Further, many patients experience a maculopapular rash (Fig. 2) or erythema nodosum (Fig. 3). Ninety-six percent of patients experience cervical lymphadenopathy during attacks. Arthralgia is seen in 70% of patients, while arthritis is seen in about one in three patients. Arthritis is usually non-erosive, but can be erosive in rare cases, leading to flexion contractures. Besides organ-specific symptoms, many patients experience constitutional symptoms, such as headache, fatigue, and malaise. These symptoms are typically present during febrile episodes but can also affect patients between episodes (ter Haar et al. 2016).

A complication of MKD that occurs in around 4% of patients is amyloid A amyloidosis. The amyloid A protein is produced in the liver under influence of interleukin-6. In case of continuous or recurrent inflammation, amyloid A accumulates in organs, especially in the kidneys. This can lead to kidney failure, which might require dialysis or kidney transplantation. Another rare complication of MKD is macrophage activation syndrome (MAS), which can initially present as a febrile episode. Macrophage activation syndrome is a life-threatening condition that presents with high fever, liver failure, and pancytopenia (ter Haar et al. 2016). MAS is

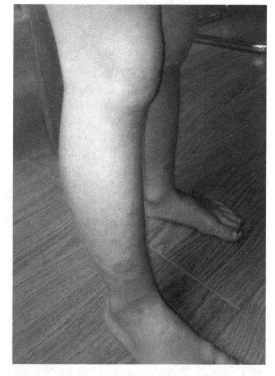

Mevalonate   Kinase   Deficiency   (MKD),
Fig. 2 Maculopapular rash in MKD

seen in about 1% of MKD patients. Whenever a patient has a "normal" ESR or platelet counts despite progressively severe inflammation, MAS should be suspected.

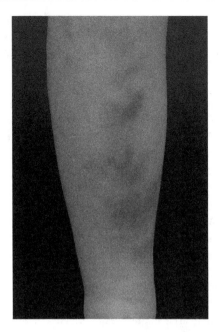

**Mevalonate Kinase Deficiency (MKD),
Fig. 3** Erythema nodosum in MKD

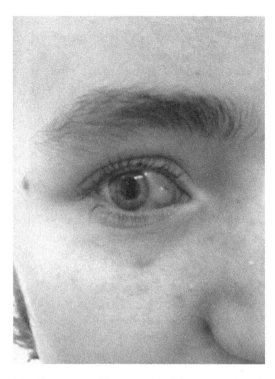

**Mevalonate Kinase Deficiency (MKD),
Fig. 4** Episcleritis in a patient with MKD

MKD patients appear to be unusually susceptible to bacterial infections like pneumonia and otitis media (van der Burgh et al. 2013).

Ocular symptoms mainly include conjunctivitis and episcleritis (Fig. 4). Tapetoretinal degeneration (retinitis pigmentosa) is a rare but debilitating complication, leading to night blindness, sometimes progressing to visual impairment (ter Haar et al. 2016).

A rare kidney tumor, angiomyolipoma, may be associated with MKD (Bader-Meunier et al. 2011).

In addition to physical complaints, MKD also affects patients in their educational and professional careers. MKD patients score significantly lower on social functioning, physical role functioning, general health perception, and vitality when compared to healthy controls. The disease delays education in 45% of patients and also leads to a sixfold increase in unemployment in comparison to the general population (van der Hilst et al. 2008).

MA patients are more severely affected than HIDS patients. Disease onset can be antenatal with some patients dying in utero. Patients often have congenital defects, ranging from dysmorphic features to cataracts. After birth children often suffer from failure to thrive and hypotonia. Many MA patients have severe neurological manifestations, mainly cerebellar ataxia and dysarthria and psychomotor retardation, which can vary from mild to very severe (van der Burgh et al. 2013).

Diagnostic Testing

MKD should be considered in patients with recurrent febrile episodes, especially when these started before the age of 6 months. The combination of abdominal pain, diarrhea, vomiting, lymphadenopathy, maculopapular rash, and aphthous ulcers might help to distinguish MKD from other autoinflammatory diseases. Febrile episodes are further characterized by a brisk acute phase response, which can be seen as an elevation of erythrocyte sedimentation rate (ESR),

C-reactive protein (CRP), serum amyloid A protein, and the presence of granulocytosis (ter Haar et al. 2016).

The name HIDS suggest an important role of IgD in the diagnostic process of MKD. However, IgD appears to be an unreliable marker for the disease. IgD can be normal in over 20% of patients, while healthy controls also show elevated IgD levels. Besides IgD, also, other immunoglobulins can be elevated, especially IgA (van der Burgh et al. 2013; ter Haar et al. 2016).

The diagnosis can be made by detection of two known pathogenic *MVK* mutations, either by targeted sequencing of the *MVK* gene or simultaneous analysis of multiple genes by next-generation sequencing. If genetic testing is inconclusive, the diagnosis may be confirmed by measurement of mevalonate kinase activity in leukocytes or fibroblasts. The residual activity varies from below undetectable to 28% in comparison to healthy controls. Measurement of urinary mevalonic acid is a sensitive marker to select patients for genetic testing. Mevalonic acid, the substrate of the enzyme mevalonate kinase, accumulates in MKD patients and is excreted in the urine. In MKD patients the mevalonic acid excretion can be 10,000-fold elevated in comparison to healthy controls. In order to collect a reliable sample, urine should be collected during a febrile episode. Between febrile episodes the mevalonic acid excretion might be entirely normal in patients with the HIDS phenotype (van der Burgh et al. 2013).

Treatment

A curative treatment for MKD is not available yet. Treatment is used to suppress symptoms and in order to prevent complications. Continuous inflammation might lead to continuously elevated amyloid A levels. Therefore, amyloid A levels should be measured regularly and should be within normal range in between episodes.

The only drug with proven efficacy in a prospective randomized placebo-controlled trial is the monoclonal anti-IL-1β antibody, canakinumab.

However, most patients can be managed with cheap and readily available drugs. Therefore, a stepped approach is used in the treatment of MKD (van der Hilst et al. 2008). Nonsteroidal anti-inflammatory drugs (NSAIDs) can provide symptom relief when used during febrile episodes. If NSAIDs are ineffective, high-dose corticosteroids (1–2 mg/kg) can be effective, especially when given at the start of an episode. If patients do not respond to corticosteroids or require continuous treatment with corticosteroids, treatment with biologicals might provide further improvement.

The biochemical pathway of mevalonate kinase suggests a role for statins in the treatment of MKD. Yet, statins are not effective in the treatment of MKD and may even worsen the disease in some patients. Colchicine, a drug that is often used to treat Familial Mediterranean Fever, is usually not effective in MKD (ter Haar et al. 2016).

Anakinra, an interleukin (IL)-1 antagonist, may be used during attacks only or as maintenance therapy, depending on the frequency of attacks. If anakinra is unavailable, is poorly tolerated, or fails to control disease, canakinumab is indicated. If IL-1 blockade is ineffective, the tumor necrosis factor (TNF) blocking agent etanercept or the IL-6 blocking agent tocilizumab may be considered (ter Haar et al. 2015, 2016).

A disadvantage of these biological treatments is the increased susceptibility of patients to infections. Therefore, it is recommended to vaccinate patients completely before starting such treatments. Further, tuberculosis should be ruled out, either by Mantoux testing or by interferon-gamma release assay.

In very severe, therapy-resistant MA patients allogeneic hematopoietic stem cell transplantation can be considered. This treatment has been used in a few patients with promising results. Stem cell transplantation led to complete remission and also improved neurological manifestations. However, hematopoietic stem cell transplantation carries many risks and should only be performed if all other therapies fail (van der Burgh et al. 2013).

Prognosis

Generally, the prognosis of HIDS is good. The frequency of attacks decreases and attacks become less severe with years passing by. Some HIDS patients may even achieve complete remission by the time they are adults. Although rare, AA amyloidosis may result in end-stage kidney failure (van der Burgh et al. 2013).

MA patients are affected more severely with many dying in utero or in early childhood. MA patients surviving childhood will often suffer from severe neurological manifestations, such as ataxia and psychomotor retardation.

References

Arostegui JI, Anton J, Calvo I, Robles A, Iglesias E, Lopez-Montesinos B, et al. Open-Label, Phase II Study to Assess the Efficacy and Safety of Canakinumab Treatment in Active Hyper-immunoglobulinemia D With Periodic Fever Syndrome. Arthritis Rheumatol. 2017;69(8):1679–1688.

Bader-Meunier B, Florkin B, Sibilia J, Acquaviva C, Hachulla E, Grateau G, et al. Mevalonate kinase deficiency: a survey of 50 patients. Pediatrics. 2011;128(1): e152–9.

Park YH, Wood G, Kastner DL, Chae JJ. Pyrin inflammasome activation and RhoA signaling in the autoinflammatory diseases FMF and HIDS. Nat Immunol. 2016;17(8):914–21.

ter Haar NM, Oswald M, Jeyaratnam J, Anton J, Barron KS, Brogan PA, et al. Recommendations for the management of autoinflammatory diseases. Ann Rheum Dis. 2015;74(9):1636–44.

ter Haar NM, Jeyaratnam J, Lachmann HJ, Simon A, Brogan PA, Doglio M, et al. The phenotype and genotype of mevalonate kinase deficiency: a series of 114 cases from the Eurofever registry. Arthritis Rheumatol. 2016;68(11):2795–805.

van der Burgh R, Ter Haar NM, Boes ML, Frenkel J. Mevalonate kinase deficiency, a metabolic

autoinflammatory disease. Clin Immunol. 2013; 147(3):197–206.

van der Hilst JC, Bodar EJ, Barron KS, Frenkel J, Drenth JP, van der Meer JW, et al. Long-term follow-up, clinical features, and quality of life in a series of 103 patients with hyperimmunoglobulinemia D syndrome. Medicine (Baltimore). 2008;87(6):301–10.

MHC Class I, A Deficiency of

Caroline Y. Kuo
Allergy and Immunology, David Geffen School of Medicine at the University of California, Los Angeles, Los Angeles, CA, USA

Synonyms

HLA class I deficiency

Introduction/Background

Major histocompatibility complex class I deficiency (HLA Class I Deficiency), also referred to as bare lymphocyte syndrome type I, is an extremely rare autosomal recessive primary immunodeficiency arising from defects in the transporter associated with antigen processing (*TAP*) 1, *TAP2*, or *TAPBP* genes (Hamosh 2012). MHC class I molecules are composed of a heavy chain encoded by HLA-A, HLA-B, and HLA-C genes on chromosome 6 associated with β2-microglobulin. MHC I molecules interact with CD8+ T cells and natural killer cells. The HLA genes themselves are unaffected in bare lymphocyte syndrome type I, but mutations in the transporter associated with antigen processing result in abnormal transfer of antigenic peptides that have been degraded from intracellular proteins in the cytoplasm to the endoplasmic reticulum lumen where they are loaded onto MHC class I molecules and then transported to the cell surface (Hanna and Etzioni 2014). In patients

M

affected by bare lymphocyte syndrome type I, unoccupied MHC I/β2-microglobulin molecules remain trapped between the endoplasmic reticulum and Golgi compartment, unable to be properly expressed on the cell surface (Yabe et al. 2016).

Clinical Presentation

There are only a handful of case reports and series describing HLA type I deficiency in the world, with the most known about TAP1- and TAP2-deficient patients (Hamosh 2012). Unlike patients with MHC class II deficiency who present with a SCID phenotype within the first year of life, those with defects in MHC class I expression are generally asymptomatic throughout infancy. A subset of patients remains asymptomatic, likely due to a less pronounced reduction in surface expression of HLA class I molecules. For others, recurrent bacterial pulmonary infections begin in the first decade of life and result in long-term sequelae such as bronchiectasis and chronic inflammatory lung disease. In addition, some patients have been reported to have necrotizing granulomatous lesions in the upper respiratory tract and skin similar to that found in granulomatosis with polyangiitis (Wegener's granulomatosis) but resistant to immunosuppression (Moins-teisserenc et al. 1999). There is one reported case of a patient with a mutation in TAPBP, which encodes tapasin needed to bridge the MHC I heavy chain and TAP (Yabe et al. 2016). Interestingly, the affected individual did not experience the typical infections associated with TAP1/2 deficiency and suffered primarily from chronic glomerulonephritis with an unknown mechanism.

Unlike the severe presentation of class II HLA deficiency, isolated class I defects are generally not life-threatening. Unexpectedly, individuals with MHC I defects do not exhibit a predisposition to viral infections or increased rates of cancer even though intracellular antigen presentation to CD8+ T cells through MHC class I molecules is important for protection against viral infections and immune surveillance against malignancy. This is likely due to overlapping protection from antibodies, HLA class I-independent cytotoxic T cells, and normal CD8+ T cell responses to antigens that do not require processing by TAP (Markel et al. 2004).

After a latency period of 5–10 years free of severe infections, affected individuals begin to develop recurrent bacterial infections of the upper respiratory tract manifesting as sinusitis and otitis media. This is thought to occur due to increased T- and NK-cell inflammatory responses leading to ciliary cell damage, poor bacterial clearance, and increased neutrophil influx (Yabe et al. 2016). Nasal polyposis and postnasal drip also common, and as upper respiratory infections become chronic and more complicated, pneumonias and bronchiectasis of the lower respiratory tracts occur. *Haemophilus influenza, Streptococcus pneumoniae, Klebsiella* spp., *Escherichia coli, Pseudomonas aeruginosa*, and *Staphylococcus aureus* are frequently identified.

In addition, necrotizing granulomatous lesions of the skin can begin in childhood or adulthood. Lesions begin as small pustules or subcutaneous nodules that progress and ulcerate. Skin findings are asymmetrically distributed with lymphocyte (particular NK cell) and macrophage infiltrates on biopsy. No specific organism has been identified in skin lesions, including mycobacteria, fungi, and other pathogens. Necrotizing, granulomatous lesions can also be found in upper airway biopsies but not in the lungs.

Diagnosis and Laboratory Testing

The differential diagnosis for patients who present with recurrent upper respiratory infections, resultant bronchiectasis, and granulomatous skin disease includes chronic granulomatous disease, granulomatosis with polyangiitis, sarcoidosis, mycobacterial infections, cystic fibrosis, and common variable immunodeficiency among many others (Gadola et al. 2000). Immunologic evaluation demonstrates normal absolute T cells numbers and a normal or increased CD4+/CD8+ ratio due to decreased CD8+ αβ T cell numbers. Despite decreased CD8+ αβ T cells, T-cell receptor repertoire is normal. T cells maintain appropriate proliferative responses to mitogens and antigens. Immunoglobulin levels and NK cells numbers are normal, although both T and NK cells exhibit increased cytotoxic reactivity towards autologous cells. This phenotype may explain the inflammatory features associated with MHC class I deficiency. Flow cytometry can be used to identify very large reductions of 30- to 100-fold of HLA class I on peripheral blood mononuclear cells in affected patients. Serological (not molecular) HLA typing is also diagnostic.

Treatment

Given the wide range of clinical presentations, there is no standardized treatment protocols for MHC Class I deficiency, and therapy should be guided by disease severity. Prevention and prompt attention to upper and lower respiratory infections is important in the prevention of progressive inflammation and irreversible bronchiectasis. This includes immunoglobulin replacement, prudent use of antibiotics, and chest physiotherapy. Topical steroids, saline/steroid washes, and antibiotics can be used to address chronic sinus disease. Surgical debridement should be avoided if possible since it is frequently ineffective in HLA I deficiency, and nasal pathology can be worsened by granulomatous lesions. Cutaneous lesions are generally treated with basic antiseptic care; immunomodulatory treatment with interferon-alpha and -gamma have led to worsening of skin lesions (Gadola et al. 2000), which are generally slow-healing and result in hyperpigmented scars. Gentle debridement can be performed for ulcerated lesions to decrease bacterial colonization. Psoralen and UV-A photochemotherapy has resulted in transient improvement in two patients (Gadola et al. 2000). There is currently no curative treatment option for those with symptomatic HLA Class I deficiency. Bone marrow transplant,

while curative in HLA Class II deficiency, has not been reported. Lung transplantation may be indicated with severe pulmonary fibrosis, although this also has not been reported.

References

Gadola SD, Moins-Teisserenc HT, Trowsdale J, Gross WL, Cerundolo V. TAP deficiency syndrome. Clin Exp Immunol. 2000;121(2):173–8. https://doi.org/10.1046/j.1365-2249.2000.01264.x.

Hamosh A. Bare lymphocyte syndrome, type I. 2012. http://www.omim.org/entry/604571.

Hanna S, Etzioni A. MHC class I and II deficiencies. J Allergy Clin Immunol. 2014;134(2):269–75. https://doi.org/10.1016/j.jaci.2014.06.001.

Markel G, Mussaffi H, Ling KL, Salio M, Gadola S, Steuer G, Blau H, et al. The mechanisms controlling NK cell autoreactivity in TAP2-deficient patients. Blood. 2004;103(5):1770–8. https://doi.org/10.1182/blood-2003-06-2114.

Moins-teisserenc T, Gadola SD, Cella M, Rod Dunbar P, Exley A, Blake N, Baycal C, et al. Association of a syndrome resembling Wegener's granulomatosis with low surface expression of HLA class-I molecules. Lancet. 1999;354:1598–603.

Yabe T, Kawamura S, Sato M, Kashiwase K, Tanaka H, Ishikawa Y, Asao Y, Oyama J. Brief report: A subject with a novel type I bare lymphocyte syndrome has tapasin deficiency due to deletion of 4 exons by Alu-mediated recombination. Blood. 2016;100(4):1496–9. https://doi.org/10.1182/blood-2001-12-0252.Partly.

MHC Class II, Deficiency of

Caroline Y. Kuo
Allergy and Immunology, David Geffen School of Medicine at the University of California, Los Angeles, Los Angeles, CA, USA

Introduction/Background

Major histocompatibility complex class II deficiency, also referred to as bare lymphocyte syndrome type II, is a rare autosomal recessive combined immunodeficiency arising from defective MHC class II gene expression (Touraine et al.

1978). Since it was first described in 1978, there have been only approximately 200 cases reported to date (Hanna and Etzioni 2014). MHC class II molecules, or Human leukocyte antigens (HLA), are transmembrane proteins required for the presentation of extracellular peptides to CD4+ T cell receptors (TCR) and exist as three isotypes in humans (HLA-DR, HLA-DQ, and HLA-DP) (Converse 2002). Whereas MHC class I molecules are ubiquitously expressed, MHC II expression is generally limited to professional antigen presenting cells, such as B lymphocytes, dendritic cells, and other cells of the monocyte-macrophage lineage (Mach et al. 1996).

The MHC locus itself on chromosome 6 is unaffected by the disease, but its transcription is aberrantly affected by homozygous mutations in one of four regulatory transacting genes encoding regulatory factor X, 5 (*RFX5*), regulatory factor X-associated protein (*RFXAP*), class II transactivator (*CIITA*), and ankyrin repeat-containing regulatory factor X (*RFXANK*) located on chromosomes 1, 13, 16, and 19 respectively (Steimle et al. 1993; Mach et al. 1996). Gene mutations causing MHC II deficiency were initially characterized using somatic cell fusion experiments with patient-derived cell lines that identified four distinct complementation groups A, B, C, and D that represent the four MHC class I regulatory genes listed above (Durand et al. 1997). Most disease-causing mutations occur in splice sites that result in truncated or absent MHC type II proteins.

Clinical Presentation

In spite of the genetic heterogeneity contributing to MHC Class II deficiency, the clinical presentation is rather homogenous and presents as a severe combined immune deficiency (SCID). MHC class II deficiency is not typically categorized as a classical form of SCID, but the disease follows a similar clinical course and can be considered a SCID-related disorder. Affected individuals are susceptible to recurrent infections due to various bacterial, viral, and fungal organisms

frequently affecting the respiratory system and gastrointestinal tract (Mach et al. 1996). Recurrent pneumonias and upper respiratory infections are common in patients with bare lymphocyte syndrome. Intracellular organisms are most frequently involved, such as *Pneumocystis jirovecii, Salmonella, Cryptosporidium* species, cytomegalovirus, candida, and herpes simplex virus. As with typical SCID, patients with MHC class II deficiency have prolonged diarrhea due to various bacterial organisms resulting in failure to thrive. In addition, affected patients have a relatively higher predisposition for intestinal and hepatic cryptosporidial infections compared to other combined immunodeficiencies correlated with poor prognosis (Aguirre et al. 1994; Klein et al. 1993). Autoimmunity is also observed in about 20% of patients, manifesting as autoimmune cytopenias, anemia, neutropenia, or thrombocytopenia (Klein et al. 1993).

Diagnosis and Laboratory Testing

The clinical manifestations of MHC class II deficiency are explained by the lack of interaction between the MHC-antigen complex and the T cell receptor, leading to the impairment of both cellular and humoral immunity. Although mature B cells are present and can differentiate appropriately to plasma cells, no antigen-specific IgG antibodies are produced. Lymphocyte proliferation responses to mitogens are unaffected since the pathway is not restricted by the MHC class II/TCR complex. However, immune responses to specific antigens as measured by delayed hypersensitivity skin tests and in vitro stimulation with antigens such as tetanus toxoid or candida are absent (Hanna and Etzioni 2014). Humoral immunodeficiency manifests as hypogammaglobulinemia, typically with decreases in 1–2 immunoglobulin isotypes in most patients and panhypogammaglobulinemia in some (Hanna and Etzioni 2014).

Lymphocyte subpopulations in affected individuals characteristically demonstrate absent MHC class II molecule expression and decreased absolute CD4+ T cell numbers due to aberrant thymic selection and maturation, resulting in an inverted CD4+/CD8+ ratio (Klein et al. 1993). However, overall total circulating CD3+ T cell and CD19+ B cell numbers are generally within normal limits for age. Some patients can display residual MHC class II expression on B cells, although it is not sufficient to fully rescue the phenotype and expression will usually be absent on monocytes (Ouederni et al. 2011). Reduced levels of MHC class I molecules have also been reported, although this finding does not correlate with clinical disease severity or the known complementation groups responsible for MHC class II deficiency. NK cells are not known to be affected by this disease. Despite the severity of the immune defect, newborn screening for SCID through the quantification of T cell receptor excision circles may miss MHC class II deficiency, since early T cell development is normal (Kuo et al. 2013). Hypogammaglobulinemia with poor vaccine antibody responses is detected in the majority of patients. When MHC class II deficiency is suspected, further characterization of the exact molecular defect can be determined through targeted gene sequencing.

Treatment

As with SCID, the life expectancy for patients with MHC class II deficiency is poor without definitive therapy. Allogeneic hematopoietic stem cell transplant (HSCT) is currently the only curative modality for bare lymphocyte syndrome and is considered the treatment of choice (Ouederni et al. 2011). In the absence of HSCT, outcomes are poor due to severe and prolonged infections, with patients unlikely surviving past the first decade of life despite supportive care with immunoglobulin supplementation and prophylactic antimicrobials. Those who survive into adolescence or older generally have missense single base pair mutations that allow some residual expression of surface MHC class II.

For those who undergo bone marrow transplant, some case series have reported relatively poor outcomes in comparison to other primary immune deficiencies. This may be related to the high incidence of preexisting viral infections in affected patients resulting in an increased risk of graft versus host disease (Renella et al. 2006). Similar to transplant candidates for other conditions, it is important to address ongoing infections and nutritional status prior to transplant with immunoglobulin replacement, antibiotics, and parenteral nutrition. As bare lymphocyte syndrome is a relatively rare disease, conditioning protocols are not yet standardized. Full-intensity conditioning regimens with busulfan and cyclophosphamide are reported to result in high levels of donor engraftment with overall disease-free survival ranging from 60% to 76% in small case series after HLA-identical donor (Renella et al. 2006; Al-Mousa et al. 2010). More recently, improved outcomes have been reported in those who have HLA-identical sibling donors or those who receive reduced-intensity conditioning, particularly when there are comorbid conditions (Al-Mousa et al. 2010).

In summary, MHC class II deficiency is a rare primary immunodeficiency due to defective antigen presentation to CD4+ T cells. Despite the genetic heterogeneity that can result in defective MHC II protein expression, the clinical presentation is consistently a severe combined immunodeficiency that requires immunoglobulin supplementation and prophylactic antibiotics until a definitive cure with hematopoietic stem cell transplant can be performed. It is expected that therapeutic outcomes will continue to improve with better conditioning regimens and earlier recognition of disease that can allow for treatment prior to the onset of chronic infections.

References

Aguirre SA, Mason PH, Perryman LE. Susceptibility of major histocompatibility complex (MHC) class I- and MHC class II-deficient mice to *Cryptosporidium parvum* infection. Infect Immun. 1994;62(2):697–9. Available at http://www.ncbi.nlm.nih.gov/entrez/query.fcgi?cmd=Retrieve&db=PubMed&dopt=Citation&list_uids=7905464

Al-Mousa H, et al. Allogeneic stem cell transplantation using myeloablative and reduced-intensity conditioning in patients with major histocompatibility complex class II deficiency. Biol Blood Marrow Transplant. 2010;16(6):818–23. Available at http://www.ncbi.nlm.nih.gov/pubmed/20079864

Converse PJ. Bare lymphocyte syndrome, type II. 2002. Available at http://omim.org/entry/209920

Durand B, et al. RFXAP, a novel subunit of the RFX DNA binding complex is mutated in MHC class II deficiency. EMBO J. 1997;16(5):1045–55.

Hanna S, Etzioni A. MHC class I and II deficiencies. J Allergy Clin Immunol. 2014;134(2):269–75. https://doi.org/10.1016/j.jaci.2014.06.001.

Klein C, et al. Major histocompatibility complex class II deficiency: clinical manifestations, immunologic features, and outcome. J Pediatr. 1993;123(6):921–8.

Kuo CY, et al. Newborn screening for severe combined immunodeficiency does not identify bare lymphocyte syndrome. J Allergy Clin Immunol. 2013;131(6):1693–5.

Mach B, et al. Regulation of MHC class II genes: lessons from a disease. Annu Rev Immunol. 1996;14:301–31.

Ouederni M, et al. Major histocompatibility complex class II expression deficiency caused by a RFXANK founder mutation: a survey of 35 patients. Blood. 2011;118(19):5108–18.

Renella R, et al. Human leukocyte antigen-identical haematopoietic stem cell transplantation in major histocompatibility complex class II immunodeficiency: reduced survival correlates with an increased incidence of acute graft-versus-host disease and pre-existing viral infections. Br J Haematol. 2006;134(5):510–6.

Steimle V, et al. Complementation cloning of an MHC class II transactivator mutated in hereditary MHC class II deficiency (or bare lymphocyte syndrome). Cell. 1993;75(1):135–46.

Touraine J, et al. Combined immunodeficiency disease associated with absence of cell-surface HLA-A and -B antigens. J Pediatr. 1978;93(1):47–51.

MLL2 Mutation

▶ Kabuki Syndrome

MTHFD1: Methylenetetrahydrofolate Dehydrogenase 1

▶ Defects in B12 and Folate Metabolism (TCN2, SLC46A1 (PCFT Deficiency), MTHFD1)

μ Heavy Chain Deficiency

Vassilios Lougaris and Alessandro Plebani Pediatrics Clinic and Institute for Molecular Medicine A. Nocivelli, Department of Clinical and Experimental Sciences, University of Brescia and ASST-Spedali Civili of Brescia, Brescia, Italy

Definition

μ heavy chain deficiency (OMIM #601495) is a rare primary immunodeficiency characterized by reduced serum levels of all immunoglobulin classes and absent or very low peripheral B-cell counts (peripheral B cells <2% total lymphocytes). Affected individuals might be both males and females. μ heavy chain deficiency is caused by biallelic pathogenic mutations in the gene encoding for the μ heavy chain, located in chromosome 14q32.33.

Pathogenesis

B-cell development starts in the bone marrow from lymphoid progenitors. An important maturational step is the progression from the pro-B to the pre-B stage (Espeli et al. 2006; Rudin and Thompson 1998; Bartholdy and Matthias 2004). This passage depends on the expression of a functional B-cell receptor composed of the μ heavy chain (*IGHM*; OMIM∗147020), Igα (CD79A; OMIM∗112205), Igβ (CD79B; OMIM∗147245), and VpreB and λ5 (*IGLL1*; OMIM∗146770), which initiates downstream signalling necessary for B-cell differentiation through kinases such as BTK and *BLNK*. Animal models and in vitro studies over the years have underlined the importance of each of the pre-BCR components and associated transcription factors for the transition from pro-B to pre-B stage of maturation, suggesting the essential role that these genes may play in the presentation of agammaglobulinemia in humans (Conley and Cooper 1998).

Kitamura et al. described in 1991 the knockout mouse model for the μ heavy chain gene, resulting in agammaglobulinemia and absent B cells. A few years later, in 1996, Yel et al. described the first patients affected with autosomal recessive agammaglobulinemia due to biallelic mutations in the gene encoding for μ heavy chain. Following the first description, further genetic analysis in US and Italian patient cohorts revealed that mutations in μ heavy chain represent the second most frequent cause of agammaglobulinemia in humans, after the X-linked form, or BTK deficiency (Conley and Cooper 1998; Ferrari et al. 2007). The distribution and relative proportion of genetic causes might change in communities with significant proportion of consanguinity, which decreases the relative incidence of X-linked diseases.

Clinical Presentation

Clinical symptoms in patients with μ heavy chain deficiency are representative of agammaglobulinemia, although particular characteristics have been reported (Conley and Cooper 1998; Yel et al. 1996). For example, age at diagnosis appears to be younger for this disorder when compared to X-linked agammaglobulinemia (XLA) (Lopez Granados et al. 2002). Onset of the disease was reported to be variable, and illnesses at presentation include chronic enteroviral encephalitis, recurrent bronchitis, pneumonia, *Pseudomonas aeruginosa* sepsis, and otitis media. The clinical history of affected patients was reported to significantly improve, with reduction of number of infections, after regular immunoglobulin replacement therapy was initiated. Bone marrow analysis from μ heavy chain-deficient patients evidenced an early arrest of B-cell development. Physical exam reveals absence of tonsillar tissue.

Diagnosis

Immunological testing in affected patients reveals very low or undetectable levels of all serum immunoglobulins types, IgM, IgA, IgG, and IgE. There are very low numbers or absent peripheral B cells. Peripheral T-cell number and function are normal. Once BTK mutations are excluded for male patients, genetic screening for mutations in autosomal recessive genes, including μ heavy chain, should be performed.

Management

As with other forms of primary humoral immunodeficiencies, immunoglobulin replacement treatment should be promptly administered once the immunological diagnosis of agammaglobulinemia is established. Currently two options for immunoglobulin administration are available: intravenous or subcutaneous. Commonly, a dose of 400 mg/kg/dose every 3–4 weeks is sufficient to maintain pre-infusion (trough) IgG levels >500 mg/dl. This level has been used as a minimum goal to reduce the number of infectious episodes, especially that of invasive infections. Frequent determinations of the trough IgG levels might be helpful to achieve the IgG level that is associated with reduction of frequency of infections for each patient.

Antibiotic usage should be considered for every infectious episode, and in some cases who continue to present with frequent infections while receiving intravenous immunoglobulins, prophylactic antibiotic regimen may also be prescribed. Live viral vaccines might be avoided.

References

Bartholdy B, Matthias P. Transcriptional control of B cell development. Gene. 2004;327:1–23.

Conley ME, Cooper MD. Genetic basis of abnormal B cell development. Curr Opin Immunol. 1998;10(4):339–406.

Espeli M, Rossi B, Mancini SJ, Roche P, Gauthier L, Schiff C. Initiation of pre-B cell receptor signaling: common and distinctive features in human and mouse. Semin Immunol. 2006;18:56–66.

Ferrari S, Zuntini R, Lougaris V, Soresina A, Sourková V, Fiorini M, Martino S, Rossi P, Pietrogrande MC, Martire B, Spadaro G, Cardinale F, Cossu F, Pierani P, Quinti I, Rossi C, Plebani A. Molecular analysis of the pre-BCR complex in a large cohort of patients affected by autosomal recessive agammaglobulinemia. Genes Immun. 2007;8(4):325–33.

Kitamura D, Roes J, Kuhn R, Rajewsky K. A B cell-deficient mouse by targeted disruption of the membrane exon of the immunoglobulin mu chain gene. Nature. 1991;350:423–42.

Lopez Granados E, Porpiglia AS, Hogan MB, Matamoros N, Krasovec S, Pignata C, Smith CI, Hammarstrom L, Bjorkander J, Belohradsky BH, Casariego GF, Garcia Rodriguez MC, Conley ME. Clinical and molecular analysis of patients with defects in micro heavy chain gene. J Clin Invest. 2002;110(7):1029–35.

Rudin CM, Thompson CB. B-cell development and maturation. Semin Oncol. 1998;25:435–46.

Yel L, Minegishi Y, Coustan-Smith E, Buckley RH, Trubel H, Pachman LM, Kitchingman GR, Campana D, Rohrer J, Conley ME. Mutations in the μ heavy-chain gene in patients with agammaglobulinemia. N Engl J Med. 1996;335:1486–93.

Muckle-Wells Syndrome (MWS)

▶ Familial Cold Autoinflammatory Syndrome (FCAS) and Muckle-Wells Syndrome (MWS)

N

N4AID

▶ NLRC4-Associated Autoinflammatory Diseases

NAK

▶ TBK1 Deficiency

Nakajo-Nishimura Syndrome (NNS)

▶ Chronic Atypical Neutrophilic Dermatosis with Lipodystrophy and Elevated Temperature Syndrome (CANDLE)/Proteasome-Associated Autoinflammatory Syndromes (PRAAS)

NEMO Delta C-Terminus (NEMO-DCT)

▶ NEMO Disease Spectrum Including NEMO-Deleted Exon 5 Autoinflammatory Syndrome (NDAS) and NEMO-Delta C-Terminus (NEMO-DCT)

NEMO Delta Exon5 Autoinflammatory Syndrome (NDAS)

▶ NEMO Disease Spectrum Including NEMO-Deleted Exon 5 Autoinflammatory Syndrome (NDAS) and NEMO-Delta C-Terminus (NEMO-DCT)

NEMO Disease Spectrum Including NEMO-Deleted Exon 5 Autoinflammatory Syndrome (NDAS) and NEMO-Delta C-Terminus (NEMO-DCT)

Eric P. Hanson
Division Chief, Pediatric Rheumatology
Department of Pediatrics, Medical and Molecular Genetics, Riley Hospital for Children and Indiana University School of Medicine Herman B. Wells Center for Pediatric Research, Indianapolis, IN, USA

Synonyms

NEMO Delta exon5 Autoinflammatory Syndrome (NDAS); NEMO Delta C-terminus (NEMO-DCT); NF-kB essential modulator (NEMO)

© Springer Science+Business Media LLC, part of Springer Nature 2020
I. R. Mackay et al. (eds.), *Encyclopedia of Medical Immunology*,
https://doi.org/10.1007/978-1-4614-8678-7

Definition

NEMO- deleted exon 5 autoinflammatory syndrome (NDAS) is a condition with autoinflammatory features within the X-linked NEMO related disease spectrum. It is most frequently caused by splice variants resulting in a deletion in the C-terminal domain of the NEMO protein or by increased expression of an isoform lacking the domain encoded by exon5, respectively.

Introduction and Background

NF-κB is a transcription factor that is an essential activator of innate and adaptive immunity, and a regulator of cell differentiation and organ development, including embryonic ectoderm-derived structures such as the nervous system, hair follicles, sweat glands and teeth (Doffinger et al. 2001). The activation of diverse cell surface receptors (i.e. the tumor necrosis factor receptor (TNFR) superfamily members, pattern recognition receptors, and antigen receptors) signals the canonical IκB kinase (IKK) complex leading to NF-κB activation through a series of phosphorylation events and post-translational modifications. The signal transduction pathways that lead to NF-κB activation are tightly regulated. While activation of E3 ubiquitin ligases catalyzes the addition of distinct polyubiquitin chains that enable proteasomal degradation or protein-protein interactions, deubiquitinating enzymes (DUBs), including A20 and OTULIN, are negative regulators of NF-κB signaling and are essential for shutting down NF-κB activation and restoring homeostasis. In agreement with these observations, genetic defects that prevent ubiquitylation (i.e. in E3 ubiquitin ligases) impair the activation of NF-kB activation and cause primary immunodeficiency with immune dysregulation; loss of function mutations in DUBs that prevent the termination of NF-κB signaling, cause autoinflammatory diseases (See chapter ▶ "OTULIN Deficiency-Associated Disease Spectrum").

Function of Nemo and Nemo-ΔCT Gain-of-Function Mutations

The NF-κB essential modulator (NEMO) is a scaffolding protein that recruits the catalytically active components of the IKK complex in addition to multiple other signaling effectors and negative regulators of the NF-κB pathway. The IKK complex phosphorylates the inhibitor of NF-κB, IκB, which targets IκB for K48-linked polyubiquitination and proteasomal degradation, thus enabling stimulation-induced nuclear translocation of NF-κB dimers. Null NEMO mutations are lethal to males, but hypomorphic mutations can result in ectodermal dysplasia and immunodeficiency (Doffinger et al. 2001). This disease spectrum was defined by familial susceptibility to mycobacterial infection, recurrent infection with pyogenic bacteria, and abnormal immunoglobulin production (Hanson et al. 2008a). The ectodermal dysplasia results from an inability of the Ectodysplasin A receptor (a TNF Receptor family member) to induce NF-κB activation following ligation.

The incidence of NEMO hypomorphism have been estimated at 1/100,000 newborns (Keller et al. 2011). Autoimmune and autoinflammatory disease have occurred in up to a third of individuals who have been described. The clinical and immunological phenotypes attributed to NEMO hypomorphic mutations have expanded to highlight its function in recruiting negative regulators, as mutant forms with a C-terminal deletion (NEMO-ΔCT gain-of-function) have been shown to be associated with increased NF-κB activation and inflammatory disease resembling Behcet's disease (Hanson et al. 2008b; Miot et al. 2017). Hematopoietically derived cells expressing NEMO-Dex5 exhibit increased NF-kB activation and IFN production, and blood cells from these patients express a strong interferon and NF-kB transcriptional signature.

Genetics

Immune dysregulatory phenotypes occur in a subset of individuals due to mutations in *IKBKG*, the gene that encodes NEMO, located in chromosome Xq28. These patients generally exhibit immunodeficiency with a wide phenotypic spectrum. Autoimmunity and inflammatory disease has been associated with various difmferuetantti ons. One class of mutations in whcih a stop codon is gained leads to the expression of the 97 NEMO-DCT form. Another class of mutations all lead to alternative mRNA splicing and enhanced protein expression of a NEMO isoform lacking the domain encoded by exon 5. Although this is an X-linked disorder, female carriers have been identified with inflammatory disease resembling Behcet's Disease (Takada et al. 2010).

Pathogenesis

NF-kB activation depends on NEMO expression, as absence of NEMO leads to impaired formation of the IKK signaling complex. Inflammatory skin and intestinal disease are well characterized in NEMO deficient murine models and is explained by TNF driven apoptotic cell death (Nenci et al. 2006, 2007). Autoinflammatory disease in humans has been associated with mutations affecting two domains of the NEMO protein: the first coiled coil-leucine zipper and the C terminal domain. Mutant NEMO forms with partial or complete truncation of their C-terminal zinc finger domain exhibit gain of function in patient-derived monocytes, T cells and cell lines. These mutant proteins also fail to stabilize A20 following stimulation (Zilberman-Rudenko et al. 2016).

Clinical Manifestations

NDAS might present with a variety of skin rashes ranging from those resembling chronic GVHD, as well as features similar to seborrheic keratitis (Mancini et al. 2008a). Gastrointestinal infections might trigger atypical colitis and a sustained inflammatory response (Cheng et al. 2009). Patients with the frequent NEMO mutation E390Xfs4 have been reported with early onset inflammatory disease triggered in the first few

months of life (Tono et al. 2007; Pachlopnik Schmid et al. 2006; Mancini et al. 2008b).

Human females carrying null mutations in one of their X chromosome alleles are often diagnosed with incontinentia pigmenti soon after birth, with characteristic linear inflammatory lesions alternating with normal skin and reflecting random X-chromosome inactivation. These lesions might scar with hyperpigmentation. Female mice heterozygous for null IKKg mutation have a similar self-limiting inflammatory disease but males with null mutations die in utero (Makris et al. 2000).

Diagnosis

The diagnosis of NEMO-associated Autoiflammatory Disease is made with the presence of autoinflammatory disease features with or without ectodermal dysplasia and immunodeficiency. For classical NEMO hypomorphic disease, impaired TLR induced cytokine production from PBMC or impaired IκBα degradation or nuclear NF-κB translocation assay might be carried out in several specialized centers.

Diagnosis is confirmed by genetic sequencing analysis of *IKBKG* gene or cDNA sequencing that reveals a mutation predicted to lead to the expression of an altered NEMO protein. On a research basis, gain of function NF-κB activation can be demonstrated (Zilberman-Rudenko et al. 2016). Due to the presence of a non-transcribed pseudogene, ψNEMO, sequencing cDNA might be most useful for to identification of rare variants (Yates et al. 2017).

Treatment and Prognosis

TNF inhibitors have been used effectively in NDAS to reduce inflammatory manifestations. Hematopoietic stem cell transplantation is also an option, and outcomes inversely correlate with the degree of ectodermal dysplasia present (Chandrakasan et al. 2017). Due to the small number of cases identified, prognosis is not yet well defined.

References

Chandrakasan S, et al. Outcome of patients with NEMO deficiency following allogeneic hematopoietic cell transplant. J Allergy Clin Immunol. 2017;139:1040–3.

Cheng LE, et al. Persistent systemic inflammation and atypical enterocolitis in patients with NEMO syndrome. Clin Immunol. 2009;132:124–31.

de Jesus A, et al. Distinct interferon signatures and cytokine patterns define additional systemic autoinflammatory diseases. J Clin Inv. 2019; in press.

Doffinger R, et al. X-linked anhidrotic ectodermal dysplasia with immunodeficiency is caused by impaired NF-kappaB signaling. Nat Genet. 2001;27:277–85.

Hanson EP, et al. Hypomorphic nuclear factor-kappaB essential modulator mutation database and reconstitution system identifies phenotypic and immunologic diversity. J Allergy Clin Immunol. 2008a;122:1169. e1116–77.e1116.

Hanson E, et al. Hypomorphic nuclear factor-kappaB essential modulator mutation database and reconstitution system identifies phenotypic and immunologic diversity. J Allergy Clin Immunol. 2008b;122:1169. e1116–77.e1116.

Keller MD, et al. Hypohidrotic ectodermal dysplasia and immunodeficiency with coincident NEMO and EDA mutations. Front Immunol. 2011;2:61.

Makris C, et al. Female mice heterozygous for IKK gamma/NEMO deficiencies develop a dermatopathy similar to the human X-linked disorder incontinentia pigmenti. Mol Cell. 2000;5:969–79.

Mancini A, Lawley L, Uzel G. X-linked ectodermal dysplasia with immunodeficiency caused by NEMO mutation: early recognition and diagnosis. Arch Dermatol. 2008a;144:342–6.

Mancini AJ, Lawley LP, Uzel G. X-linked ectodermal dysplasia with immunodeficiency caused by NEMO mutation: early recognition and diagnosis. Arch Dermatol. 2008b;144:342–6.

Miot C, et al. Hematopoietic stem cell transplantation in 29 patients hemizygous for hypomorphic IKBKG/NEMO mutations. Blood. 2017;130:1456.

Nenci A, et al. Skin lesion development in a mouse model of incontinentia pigmenti is triggered by NEMO deficiency in epidermal keratinocytes and requires TNF signaling. Hum Mol Genet. 2006;15:531–42.

Nenci A, et al. Epithelial NEMO links innate immunity to chronic intestinal inflammation. Nature. 2007;446: 557–61.

Pachlopnik Schmid JM, et al. Transient hemophagocytosis with deficient cellular cytotoxicity, monoclonal immunoglobulin M gammapathy, increased T-cell numbers, and hypomorphic NEMO mutation. Pediatrics. 2006;117:e1049–56.

Takada H, Nomura A, Ishimura M, Ichiyama M, Ohga S, Hara T. NEMO mutation as a cause of familial occurrence of Behçet's disease in female patients. Clin Genet. 2010;78:575–9.

Tono C, et al. Correction of immunodeficiency associated with NEMO mutation by umbilical cord blood transplantation using a reduced-intensity conditioning regimen. Bone Marrow Transpl. 2007;39:801–4.

Yates TR, Wright BL, Bauer CS, Difficulty Finding NEMO. Functional pathways to sequencing. J Allergy Clin Immunol. 2017;139:Ab113-Ab113.

Zilberman-Rudenko J, et al. Recruitment of A20 by the C-terminal domain of NEMO suppresses NF-kappaB activation and autoinflammatory disease. Proc Natl Acad Sci U S A. 2016;113:1612–7.

Neonatal-Onset Multisystem Inflammatory Disease (NOMID)

Megha Garg and Raphaela Goldbach-Mansky
Translational Autoinflammatory Diseases Section (TADS), National Institute of Allergy and Infectious Diseases (NIAID), National Institutes of Health (NIH), Bethesda, MD, USA

Synonyms

CINCA: Chronic infantile neurological cutaneous and articular syndrome; NOMID: Neonatal-onset multisystem inflammatory disease

Definition

NOMID is a monogenic IL-1-mediated autoinflammatory disease caused by germline or gonosomal (somatic germline) gain-of-function mutations in the NACHT domain of the *NLRP3* gene. NOMID patients develop perinatal-onset systemic inflammation, neutrophilic urticaria, neutrophilic aseptic meningitis, cochlear inflammation with progressive neurosensory hearing loss, and patellar and/or epiphyseal overgrowth.

Introduction and Background

In 1981, Prieur and Griscelli identified a subgroup of patients, distinct from Still's disease, and termed their disease, chronic inflammatory neurologic cutaneous and arthritis (CINCA) syndrome (Prieur and Griscelli 1981), which is also called neonatal-onset multisystem inflammatory disease (NOMID) in the USA. NOMID is a rare, mostly sporadic autoinflammatory disease and is at the severe end of the spectrum of the cryopyrin-associated autoinflammatory syndromes (CAPS). The two mostly autosomal dominantly inherited conditions on the less severe end of the spectrum of CAPS include familial cold autoinflammatory syndromes (FCAS), at the mild, and Muckle-Wells syndrome (MWS), at the intermediate end of the spectrum. CAPS has an estimated prevalence of 1 case in every 1–3 million people based on reports from clinics in the USA and in Europe (Finetti et al. 2016). NOMID has no gender or ethnic predilection. The prevalence of NOMID is low; historically, patients with NOMID were unable to reproduce due to early mortality and morbidity thus limiting disease transmission (Prieur et al. 1987).

Genetics

In 1999 "Muckle-Wells syndrome" was linked to chromosome 1q44 (Cuisset et al. 1999), and in 2000, Hal Hoffman identified missense mutations in the NACHT domain of *NLRP3* (also previously called *CIAS1*, *PYPAF7*, and *NALP3*) in three families with autosomal dominant familial cold autoinflammatory syndrome (FCAS) and a family with Muckle-Wells syndrome (MWS) (Hoffman et al. 2001). Clinical similarities between MWS and NOMID prompted targeted candidate sequencing of *NLRP3* and led to the identification of spontaneous de novo mutations in about 50% of NOMID/CINCA (Feldmann et al. 2002; Aksentijevich et al. 2002). Later, the majority (~70%) of the "Sanger sequencing negative" NOMID/CINCA patients were found to have germline or gonosomal somaticism in *NLRP3*, with transcript levels of less than 10% in peripheral blood. The low transcript levels make mutation detection challenging for even standard next-generation sequencing protocols and may require

subcloning for detection (Saito et al. 2005; Tanaka et al. 2011). *NLRP3* encodes the protein cryopyrin which is expressed in monocytes, granulocytes, T cells, and in nonhematopoietic cells including chondrocytes, keratinocytes, microglial and reactive astrocytes in the CNS.

Pathogenesis

NLRP3/cryopyrin is a member of the NOD-like receptor (NLR) family and assembles a multi-molecular complex, the NLRP3 inflammasome. Upon stimulation, the NLRP3 inflammasome oligomerizes filaments of ASC/PYCARD adapter proteins and active caspase-1 molecules that enzymatically cleave pro-IL-1β and to a lesser extent pro-IL-18 into their active forms. CAPS mutations confer gain-of-function, and leukocytes isolated from CAPS patients have a lower threshold for NLPR3 inflammasome activation following LPS stimulation even in the absence of second signals such as ATP, nigericin, or crystals that are needed to activate wildtype inflammasomes in monocytes (Tassi et al. 2010). The NLRP3 inflammasome can be triggered by exogenous danger signals including conserved microbial components such as lipopolysaccharide (LPS), and large inorganic crystalline structures, such as asbestos and silica that lead to lysosomal lysis. Endogenous "danger signals" that can trigger the inflammasome include uric acid crystals, cholesterol crystals, ATP, and DNA and RNA fragments. In contrast to strong contribution of non-IL-1 activating pathways is murine CAPS, the clinical responses of human disease to IL-1 blocking agents points to the pivotal role of IL-1 in human disease (McGeough et al. 2017).

Clinical Manifestations

NOMID symptoms start in the perinatal period to early infancy. Patients present with urticaria-like rashes, fevers, malaise, fatigue, and myalgias with high granulocyte counts and elevation of ESR and CRP. Daily low-grade fevers or intermittent fevers usually accompany flares, but some patients report no fevers. Inflammatory organ manifestations include the skin, eye, ear, bone, and brain.

Cutaneous Manifestations

An urticaria-like rash occurs typically within 24 h of birth and begins with erythematous, maculopapular lesions that transition to wheals/hives within a few hours. The rash can be diffuse or limited to extremities or trunk (Fig. 1). In contrast to allergic reactions, the CAPS rash is nonpruritic and may be burning or stinging. Skin biopsies show a neutrophilic infiltrate in the dermis and the periadnexal area.

Ocular Manifestations

Conjunctivitis is the most common ophthalmologic presentation of all CAPS, but papilledema is only seen in severe MWS and NOMID patients; subepithelial corneal infiltrates can lead to corneal opacities requiring corneal transplants; posterior retinitis is a rare complication early in life. The inflammatory lesions in the anterior segment can lead to development of band keratopathies and corneal clouding. Optic nerve atrophy is the result of chronic increased intracranial pressures that leads to progressive loss of the visual field and/if severe also loss of visual acuity and blindness. Optical coherence tomography (OCT) which measures nerve fiber thickness and the Humphrey visual field test are used to monitor preservation of optic nerve thickness and function on treatment.

Audiologic Manifestations

High frequency sensorineural hearing loss with progression to the lower frequencies over time is the most common pattern of hearing loss in NOMID patients and a consequence of cochlear inflammation that leads to destruction of the neuroepithelial Corti cells. NOMID patients develop hearing loss that requires the use of hearing aids, in the first decade of life. Cochlear inflammation can be seen on FLAIR-MRIs of the inner ear and is used to monitor inner ear inflammation on treatment (Fig. 2). As chronic long-standing and severe hearing loss is irreversible, it is important to initiate IL-1 blocking treatment early in life.

Central Nervous System Manifestations

CNS manifestations can be most devastating. Chronic aseptic/neutrophilic meningitis is a common feature in NOMID and severe MWS patients and is diagnosed by leukocytosis on lumbar puncture and increased opening pressures. Chronic meningitis leads to swelling and occlusion of the arachnoid villi, resulting in decreased spinal fluid absorption and increased intracranial pressures

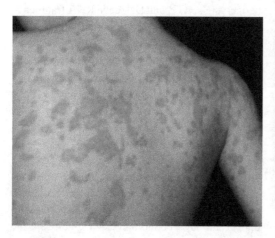

Neonatal-Onset Multisystem Inflammatory Disease (NOMID), Fig. 1 Urticaria-like rash in NOMID

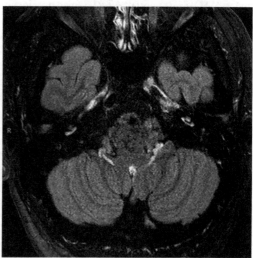

Neonatal-Onset Multisystem Inflammatory Disease (NOMID), Fig. 2 Inner ear enhancement in a patient with NOMID

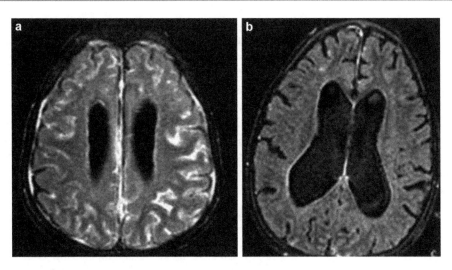

Neonatal-Onset Multisystem Inflammatory Disease (NOMID), Fig. 3 (**a**, **b**) Leptomeningeal enhancement in a patient with NOMID and presence of hydrocephalus and brain atrophy

(ICP). Clinical signs of increased ICP include early morning headaches that in younger children is associated with vomiting. Chronically increased ICPs lead to ventriculomegaly and brain atrophy and to cognitive impairment. Untreated, NOMID patients may require ventriculo-peritoneal shunt placements to alleviate ICP-related symptoms. Leptomeningeal and cochlear enhancement can be seen on contrast-enhanced MRIs; however, the MRI is less sensitive than the lumbar puncture in detecting CNS inflammation (Fig. 3a, b). Arachnoid adhesions, ventriculomegaly, and brain atrophy are sequelae of longstanding inflammation and increased ICPs and are visualized on MRI. Other CNS manifestations include seizures, stroke, spasticity, and vaso-occlusive events. Untreated, NOMID patients with hydrocephalus develop megalocephaly and what appears to be a "saddleback nose" with frontal bossing. Serial lumbar punctures and contrast-enhanced MRIs are used to monitor CNS inflammation on IL-1 blocking treatment in NOMID patients.

Musculoskeletal Manifestations

Arthralgias and arthritis are typically seen with flares, the arthritis is transient and nonerosive. NOMID patients develop chondroma-like lesion in the growth plates of the long bones that are

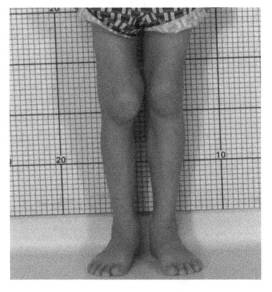

Neonatal-Onset Multisystem Inflammatory Disease (NOMID), Fig. 4 Limb length discrepancy and knee cap enlargement in a patient with NOMID

most common around the knee. The lesions are noninflammatory and represent immature chondrocytes that fail to differentiate and form palisading structures. The lesions develop into what clinically appears as "bony overgrowths," which can be misdiagnosed as "juvenile idiopathic arthritis" (Fig. 4). Many NOMID patients have large patellae for age due to premature ossification. The chondroma-like lesions reduce longitudinal growth at the affected site that results in the bone deformities and in premature closure of the growth plate of the long bones. Limb length discrepancy, bowing of long bones, and short statures as adults, below the third percentile, are common features. Osteopenia and osteoporosis are other common findings in untreated patients. Treatment with IL-1 blockade early in the course of the disease results in catch up of growth and normalization of the bone mineral density. Clubbing of fingers is seen in all CAPS including FCAS.

Diagnosis

The diagnosis of CAPS can be delayed due to poor awareness of the disease and due to non-specific features in the milder conditions particularly FCAS early in the disease. Diagnosis is made based on clinical presentation, and a mutation in *NLRP3* confirms the diagnosis. The presence of somatic mutations that are not seen on Sanger sequencing can make a genetic diagnosis challenging and require next-generation sequencing. New proposed CAPS diagnostic criteria are clinical and include the presence of raised inflammatory markers (CRP or SAA) plus at least two of six CAPS-typical signs or symptoms including: (1) urticaria-like rash, (2) cold-triggered episodes, (3) sensorineural hearing loss, (4) musculoskeletal symptoms of arthralgia/arthritis/myalgia, (5) chronic aseptic meningitis, and (6) skeletal abnormalities of epiphyseal overgrowth/frontal bossing is highly likely to confirm the diagnosis of CAPS (Kuemmerle-Deschner et al. 2017).

Laboratory Testing

Elevated inflammatory markers including ESR, CRP, and SAA (serum amyloid) correlate with clinical features. Leukocytosis with neutrophilic predominance and thrombocytosis are common. Mild hypochromic microcytic anemia resistant to iron supplementation can be present. CSF pleocytosis with neutrophilic predominance and elevated proteins >40 mg/dl are indicative of CNS inflammation. Increased intracranial pressure results in elevated CSF opening pressure, usually >20 cm of H_2O. Hypergammaglobulinemia is often present. Autoantibodies are negative except for lupus anticoagulant which is positive in untreated patients and becomes negative with treatment. Renal amyloidosis appears to be rare in NOMID patients, although case reports have been described. Disease activity is assessed through diary scores where patients record fever, rash, arthralgia, vomiting, and fatigue. Inflammatory markers help in gauging clinical disease activity and normalize with treatment.

Treatment

Treatment with IL-1 blocking agents has become standard of care for CAPS including NOMID. Three IL-1 blocking drugs are FDA approved for CAPS, anakinra, rilonacept, and canakinumab. Anakinra has been used as initial treatment for CAPS, the dose of anakinra that is needed to suppress inflammation in CAPS patients depends on disease severity and clinical phenotype and is lowest in patients with FCAS (0.5–1.5 mg/kg/d in most patients). Effective doses to achieve and maintain inflammatory remission in MWS and NOMID are around 3.5–5 mg/kg/d. Dose escalation as high as 10 mg/kg/d may be needed to optimally suppress CNS inflammation in severely affected NOMID patients. A recent study in NOMID with severe CNS disease indicated that anakinra is more efficacious than canakinumab in suppressing CNS inflammation (Rodriguez-Smith et al. 2017), which may be due to better blood-brain barrier penetration of anakinra. Of the three approved drugs, canakinumab is a monoclonal antibody against IL β approved in Europe for all subtypes of CAPS and for FCAS and MWS in USA. Rilonacept is a fusion protein derived from human sequence (IL-1 R, ACP, IgG Fc) and is injected weekly. It has been approved for milder forms of CAPS, including FCAS and MWS in children older than 12 years of age. Anakinra is approved for CAPS in Europe and for NOMID in the USA.

Prognosis

Before IL-1 blocking therapies were used to treat NOMID, the estimated mortality was greater than ~20%, and amyloidosis was reported in up to 30% of MWS patients. Hearing loss in the second to third decade was common but is not well documented. However, treatment with IL-1 blocking treatments has changed disease outcome. Early treatment can halt progression of organ damage including hearing loss (Sibley et al. 2012).

Reproductive Health

With improved disease outcomes, reproductive health issues become important. Patients with germline heterozygous mutation have a 50% chance to transmit the disease to each offspring. In case of somatic mosaicism, this risk of transmission depends on the possible presence of somatic mutations in the parental reproductive cells but is significantly lower than in patients with germline mutations. Prenatal diagnosis can be made through diagnostic techniques like chorionic villous sampling or amniocentesis. In a study of nine patients with CAPS, who received anakinra, "a category B drug" during pregnancy, miscarriage rates were lower compared to untreated patients and comparable to those in the general population. Anakinra treatment prevented disease flares during pregnancy and none of the women delivered preterm (Chang et al. 2014). Of nine men with MWS, oligospermia was the cause for infertility in two thirds of patients. It remains unclear whether treatment with anakinra will change this outcome (Tran et al. 2012).

Cross-References

▶ Familial Cold Autoinflammatory Syndrome (FCAS) and Muckle-Wells Syndrome (MWS)

References

Aksentijevich I, Nowak M, Mallah M, Chae JJ, Watford WT, Hofmann SR, et al. De novo CIAS1 mutations, cytokine activation, and evidence for genetic heterogeneity in patients with neonatal-onset multisystem inflammatory disease (NOMID): a new member of the expanding family of pyrin-associated autoinflammatory diseases. Arthritis Rheum. 2002;46(12):3340–8.

Chang Z, Spong CY, Jesus AA, Davis MA, Plass N, Stone DL, et al. Anakinra use during pregnancy in patients with cryopyrin-associated periodic syndromes (CAPS). Arthritis Rheumatol. 2014;66(11):3227–32.

Cuisset L, Drenth JP, Berthelot JM, Meyrier A, Vaudour G, Watts RA, et al. Genetic linkage of the Muckle-Wells syndrome to chromosome 1q44. Am J Hum Genet. 1999;65(4):1054–9.

Feldmann J, Prieur AM, Quartier P, Berquin P, Certain S, Cortis E, et al. Chronic infantile neurological cutaneous and articular syndrome is caused by mutations in CIAS1, a gene highly expressed in polymorphonuclear cells and chondrocytes. Am J Hum Genet. 2002;71(1):198–203.

Finetti M, Omenetti A, Federici S, Caorsi R, Gattorno M. Chronic infantile neurological cutaneous and articular (CINCA) syndrome: a review. Orphanet J Rare Dis. 2016;11(1):167.

Hoffman HM, Mueller JL, Broide DH, Wanderer AA, Kolodner RD. Mutation of a new gene encoding a putative pyrin-like protein causes familial cold autoinflammatory syndrome and Muckle-Wells syndrome. Nat Genet. 2001;29(3):301–5.

Kuemmerle-Deschner JB, Ozen S, Tyrrell PN, Kone-Paut I, Goldbach-Mansky R, Lachmann H, et al. Diagnostic criteria for cryopyrin-associated periodic syndrome (CAPS). Ann Rheum Dis. 2017;76(6):942–7.

McGeough MD, Wree A, Inzaugarat ME, Haimovich A, Johnson CD, Pena CA, et al. TNF regulates transcription of NLRP3 inflammasome components and inflammatory molecules in cryopyrinopathies. J Clin Invest. 2017;127:4488.

Prieur AM, Griscelli C. Arthropathy with rash, chronic meningitis, eye lesions, and mental retardation. J Pediatr. 1981;99(1):79–83.

Prieur AM, Griscelli C, Lampert F, Truckenbrodt H, Guggenheim MA, Lovell DJ, et al. A chronic, infantile, neurological, cutaneous and articular (CINCA) syndrome. A specific entity analysed in 30 patients. Scand J Rheumatol Suppl. 1987;66:57–68.

Rodriguez-Smith J, Lin YC, Li Tsai W, Kim H, Montealegre-Sanchez G, Chapelle D, et al. CSF cytokines correlate with aseptic meningitis and blood brain barrier function in Neonatal-Onset Multisystem Inflammatory Disease (NOMID). Arthritis Rheumatol. 2017;69(6):1325–1336.

Saito M, Fujisawa A, Nishikomori R, Kambe N, Nakata-Hizume M, Yoshimoto M, et al. Somatic mosaicism of

CIAS1 in a patient with chronic infantile neurologic, cutaneous, articular syndrome. Arthritis Rheum. 2005;52(11):3579–85.

Sibley CH, Plass N, Snow J, Wiggs EA, Brewer CC, King KA, et al. Sustained response and prevention of damage progression in patients with neonatal-onset multisystem inflammatory disease treated with anakinra: a cohort study to determine three- and five-year outcomes. Arthritis Rheum. 2012;64(7):2375–86.

Tanaka N, Izawa K, Saito MK, Sakuma M, Oshima K, Ohara O, et al. High incidence of NLRP3 somatic mosaicism in patients with chronic infantile neurologic, cutaneous, articular syndrome: results of an International Multicenter Collaborative Study. Arthritis Rheum. 2011;63(11):3625–32.

Tassi S, Carta S, Delfino L, Caorsi R, Martini A, Gattorno M, et al. Altered redox state of monocytes from cryopyrin-associated periodic syndromes causes accelerated IL-1beta secretion. Proc Natl Acad Sci U S A. 2010;107(21):9789–94.

Tran TA, Kone-Paut I, Marie I, Ninet J, Cuisset L, Meinzer U. Muckle-wells syndrome and male hypofertility: a case series. Semin Arthritis Rheum. 2012;42(3): 327–31.

Netherton Syndrome

▶ Comel-Netherton Syndrome (*SPINK5*)

Neutropenia with Myelodysplasia

▶ X-Linked Neutropenia/Myelodysplasia

Neutrophil Immunodeficiency Syndrome

▶ Rac2 Deficiency

Neutrophil-Specific Granule Deficiency

▶ Specific Granule Deficiency

NF-Kappa B-Inducing Kinase (NIK)

Robert P. Nelson
Divisions of Hematology and Oncology, Stem Cell Transplant Program, Indiana University (IU) School of Medicine and the IU Bren and Simon Cancer Center, Indianapolis, IN, USA
Pediatric Immunodeficiency Clinic, Riley Hospital for Children at Indiana University Health, Indianapolis, IN, USA
Medicine and Pediatrics, Indiana University School of Medicine, Immunohematology and Transplantation, Indianapolis, IN, USA

Definition

One of the many kinases which transduce signals from the cell membrane to the nucleus in select cells and processes.

Introduction/Background

Using TRAF2 to study proteins involved in NFKB pathways, Malinin et al. cloned NK-kappa B inducing kinase (NIK) (Malinin et al. 1997). NIK, which is a multifunctional, is officially known as mitogen-activated protein-kinase-kinase-kinase 14 (MAP 3K14) participates in the activation of NF-kB by TNF, CD95, IL1, but not TGF beta, which uses an NIK-independent mechanisms. (Sakurai et al. 1998) The "canonical" NF-kB pathway drives many inflammatory processes; however, the "noncanonical" pathway is also a crucial activation cascade (Zarnegar et al. 2008). The NIK-dependent pathway is "noncanonical," in that it does not require the NF-kappa essential modulator (NEMO, inhibitor of nuclear factor kappa-B kinase subunit gamma) (Gray et al. 2014). Effects are diverse, as NIK functions in epithelial and hematopoietic cells and interacts with developmental and activation programs important for innate defense, adaptive immune responses and hematopoiesis.

Function

Innate Host Defense

Inflammatory responses occur as an expanding matrix of simultaneous events that perturb multiple interacting cell activation pathways. Our capacity for understanding functional mechanisms of inflammation begins with the study of isolated events in-vitro, as if they occur sequentially. Activation of NF-kappa B by the inflammatory cytokines tumor necrosis factor (TNF) and interleukin-1 (IL-1) requires the successive action of NIK, IkappaB kinase-alpha (IKK-α), and IkappaB kinase-beta (IKK-β); IKK-α and IKK-β form heterodimers that interact with NIK (Woronicz et al. 1997). Interleukin-1 (IL-1), binding to its cell-surface receptor, starts a signaling cascade relayed through TNF receptor-associated factor 6 (TRAF6) via transforming growth factor-beta activated kinase 1, which phosphorylates NIK, permitting IKKα activation. NIK reaches the cellular-inhibitor of apoptosis (c-IAP) through a TRAF2-TRAF3 bridge whereby TRAF2 recruits c-IAP1/2 and TRAF3 binds to NIK, while constitutive proteasome-mediated degradation suppresses NIK. NIK is crucial for the generation of inflammation in multiple tissues. Dominant negative NIK mutants inhibit expression of the gene for pro-inflammatory IL-8, and structural interactions between NIK and Toll-like receptor-2 upregulate IL-1 beta, IL-8, and TNF-α. Autoimmune encephalomyelitis in mice, a model for human multiple sclerosis, requires NIK to induce Th17 cells and NIK participates with nucleotide-binding oligomerization domain-containing protein 2 (NOD2) signaling in intestinal epithelium (Pan et al. 2006; Awane et al. 1999).

Adaptive Immunity

The NIK protein transduces membrane-to-nucleus signals in many different cells that participate in the development, maintenance, and activation of immune function and hematopoiesis. Balanced NF-kappa B signaling is essential for maintaining normal hematopoiesis and the loss of noncanonical NF-kappa B signaling impairs the self renewal capacity of hematopoietic stem/progenitor cells (Yamada et al. 2000). A point mutation in NIK renders mice absent of lymph nodes/Peyer's patches, disrupting splenic and thymus development; mice with loss-of-function (LOF) NIK mutations fail to express peripheral tissue-restricted antigens normally, which implies that NIK is important for the establishment of central tolerance (Shinkura et al. 1999). Thymic dendritic cells (DCs) require NIK to form most α/β CD4 (+) T effector lineages. In this regard, NIK delivers costimulatory signals to CD4 (+) T cells and without DC NIK, they are anergic; reintroduction of NIK permits CD4 (+) T cells to become functional effectors (Kajiura et al. 2004). NIK also cooperates with protein kinase C (PKC) to set the threshold for T cell activation and deleterious NIK mutations impair T cell proliferation and IL-2 production in response to anti-CD3 stimulation (Matsumoto et al. 2002). B cells NIK interacts with B-cell activating factor (BAFF-R), which regulates activation of the alternative NF-kappa B pathway essential for mature B cell survival. Overexpression of NIK in mouse B-lymphocytes amplifies alternative NF-kappa B activation and peripheral B cell numbers in a BAFF-R-dependent manner, whereas uncoupling NIK from TNF receptor associated factors (TRAFs) and TRAF3-mediated control causes hyperplasia of BAFF-R-independent B cells. NIK also regulates naïve B cells homing to lymph nodes via production of B-cell homing chemokines (Yang et al. 2019).

Lymphoproliferative Disease and Cancer

The Akt/protein kinase B signaling inhibitor-2 (API2) mucosa-associated lymphoid tissue 1 (MALT1) fusion oncoprotein created by chromosomal t(11;18)(q21;q21) in MALT lymphoma induces proteolytic cleavage of NIK that renders it resistant to proteasomal degradation, resulting in constitutive noncanonical NF-kappa B signaling that enhances B cell adhesion and reduces apoptotic activity. Stable NIK protein is also prevalent in Hodgkin lymphoma cell lines and studies of biopsied tissue suggest

N

NIK and the noncanonical pathway are active. NIK is also expressed in primary human peripheral T cell lymphoma. These finding may offer an opportunity to target NIK for the treatment of these malignancies in the future, in which case the effects of iatrogenic NIK deficiency will require consideration. NIK in Nonhematopoietic Tissues Epidermal growth factor receptor (EGFR) also associates with NIK, creating a multiprotein signalosome between the EGFR, TNFR-interacting protein (RIP), and NIK (Habib et al. 2001). NIK dysfunction impairs osteoclastogenesis associated with inflammatory arthritis (Aya et al. 2005). Overactivation of liver NIK in obesity promotes hyperglycemia and glucose intolerance by increasing the hyperglycemic response to glucagon. Complement membrane attack complexes promote inflammatory functions in endothelial cells (ECs) by stabilizing NIK and activating noncanonical NF-kappa B signaling. An inhibitor of apoptosis binding motif at the amino terminus of NIK specifically recognizes and ubiquitylates hepatic NIK in response to exposure to damage-associated molecular patterns (DAMPs) that promotes liver inflammation, injury, and fibrosis.

Clinical Presentation

History

There is a paucity of human examples of defective NIK expression, which likely attests to its importance in human developmental immunophysiology. Three cases have been described. Willmann et al. reported a biallelic mutation producing (p.Pro565Arg) a NIK protein without kinase activity, in two cousins with recurrent bacterial, viral, and Cryptosporidium infections. They demonstrated defective activation of both canonical and noncanonical NF-kappaB signaling (Willmann et al. 2014). Another patient reported with an abscess at the BCG site at 2 years of age and received antituberculosis treatment. At age 4, she had brain granulomas and disease continue to progress despite treatment. She was found to have hypogammaglobulinemia, normal B cell numbers, and increased number of total lymphocytes. Exome sequencing revealed a homozygous mutation in exon 5 of the NIK gene (p.Val345Met). This mutation results in a protein with decreased kinase activity of NIK (Schlechter et al. 2017).

Based on the limited number of cases, there may be other characteristics expected, given the combined nature of the defect. Patients with the NIK defect will likely be 18 years of age or younger, may have a positive family history, and TRECs may be predicted to be normal or low newborn screening. A patient with this phenotype may have a history of recurrent or severe infections, particularly with mycobacteria, including BCG, other opportunistic organisms, and recurrent viral or Cryptosporidium infections.

Physical Exam

Signs of failure to thrive may be present, but facial features are normal. There are no specific, unusual, or unique pathognomonic signs that distinguish this phenotype from other combined T and B cell defects.

Laboratory Findings/Diagnostic Testing

Patients reported to date who suffer from homozygous loss-of function (LOF) have had total IgG, IgA, and/or IgM levels low or normal but not polyclonal gammopathies. Although overall T-cell numbers are normal, numbers of follicular helper and memory T cells were unbalanced. There were decreased numbers of switched memory B cells and impaired inducible co-stimulator ligand expression. Natural killer (NK) cells were decreased or normal in number and exhibited defective activation, leading to impaired formation of NK-cell immunological synapses (Willmann et al. 2014).

Treatment/Prognosis

The first clinical decision to make is whether to take care of the patent locally or consider referral to a multidisciplinary clinical program that is engaged in research related to the disease. It is paramount to consider input from the family with this process that impacts the family finances and care of other children. Social workers play an important role in connecting with services and advocacy groups for PIDD. General treatment considerations of immunocompromised patients apply, as is covered in this volume. Immunizations can be given with the exception of live viral vaccines. It may be prudent to mainstream the child in schools while providing prompt evaluation for early unusual consequences of infection. Prolonged courses of antibiotics may be necessary for infections, particularly sinus infections. Prophylactic antimicrobials and immunoglobulin replacement therapy is recommended for those with cellular immune deficiencies or functional antibody production is demonstrably low, respectively. Application of hematopoietic cell transplantation and gene therapy trials are investigational at present and may be forthcoming with advances in those areas. The two patients reported by Willman et al. received HCT, with only one patient survived (Willmann et al. 2014).

Cross-References

▶ Evaluation of Suspected Immunodeficiency, Overview

References

Awane M, Andres PG, Li DJ, Reinecker HC. NF-kappa B-inducing kinase is a common mediator of IL-17-, TNF-alpha-, and IL-1 beta-induced chemokine promoter activation in intestinal epithelial cells. J Immunol. 1999;162:5337–44.

Aya K, Alhawagri M, Hagen-Stapleton A, Kitaura H, Kanagawa O, Novack DV. NF-(kappa)B-inducing kinase controls lymphocyte and osteoclast activities in inflammatory arthritis. J Clin Invest. 2005;115:1848–54.

Gray CM, Remouchamps C, McCorkell KA, et al. Noncanonical NF-kappaB signaling is limited by classical NF-kappaB activity. Sci Signal. 2014;7:ra13.

Habib AA, Chatterjee S, Park SK, Ratan RR, Lefebvre S, Vartanian T. The epidermal growth factor receptor engages receptor interacting protein and nuclear factor-kappa B (NF-kappa B)-inducing kinase to activate NF-kappa B. Identification of a novel receptor-tyrosine kinase signalosome. J Biol Chem. 2001;276:8865–74.

Kajiura F, Sun S, Nomura T, et al. NF-kappa B-inducing kinase establishes self-tolerance in a thymic stroma-dependent manner. J Immunol. 2004;172:2067–75.

Malinin NL, Boldin MP, Kovalenko AV, Wallach D. MAP3K-related kinase involved in NF-kappaB induction by TNF, CD95 and IL-1. Nature. 1997;385(6616):540–4.

Matsumoto M, Yamada T, Yoshinaga SK, et al. Essential role of NF-kappa B-inducing kinase in T cell activation through the TCR/CD3 pathway. J Immunol. 2002;169:1151–8.

Pan Q, Kravchenko V, Katz A, et al. NF-kappa B-inducing kinase regulates selected gene expression in the Nod2 signaling pathway. Infect Immun. 2006;74:2121–7.

Sakurai H, Shigemori N, Hasegawa K, Sugita T. TGF-beta-activated kinase 1 stimulates NF-kappa B activation by an NF-kappa B-inducing kinase-independent mechanism. Biochem Biophys Res Commun. 1998;243:545–9.

Schlechter N, Glanzmann B, Hoal EG, Schoeman M, Petersen BS, Franke A, Lau YL, et al. Exome sequencing identifies a novel MAP3K14 mutation in recessive atypical combined immunodeficiency. Front Immunol. 2017;8:1624.

Shinkura R, Kitada K, Matsuda F, et al. Alymphoplasia is caused by a point mutation in the mouse gene encoding Nf-kappa b-inducing kinase. Nat Genet. 1999;22:74–7.

Willmann KL, Klaver S, Dogu F, et al. Biallelic loss-of-function mutation in NIK causes a primary immunodeficiency with multifaceted aberrant lymphoid immunity. Nat Commun. 2014;5:5360.

Woronicz JD, Gao X, Cao Z, Rothe M, Goeddel DV. IkappaB kinase-beta: NF-kappaB activation and complex formation with IkappaB kinase-alpha and NIK. Science. 1997;278:866–9.

Yamada T, Mitani T, Yorita K, et al. Abnormal immune function of hemopoietic cells from alymphoplasia (aly) mice, a natural strain with mutant NF-kappa B-inducing kinase. J Immunol. 2000;165:804–12.

Yang J, Zhang S, Zhang L, et al. Lymphatic endothelial cells regulate B-cell homing to lymph nodes via a NIK-dependent mechanism. Cell Mol Immunol. 2019;16:165–77.

Zarnegar BJ, Wang Y, Mahoney DJ, et al. Noncanonical NF-kappaB activation requires coordinated assembly of a regulatory complex of the adaptors cIAP1, cIAP2, TRAF2 and TRAF3 and the kinase NIK. Nat Immunol. 2008;9:1371–8.

NF-Kappa-B Essential Modulator (NEMO) Deficiency

▶ Anhidrotic Ectodermal Dysplasia with Immunodeficiency (EDA-ID), X-linked

NF-kB Essential Modulator (NEMO)

▶ NEMO Disease Spectrum Including NEMO-Deleted Exon 5 Autoinflammatory Syndrome (NDAS) and NEMO-Delta C-Terminus (NEMO-DCT)

NF-κB IKB

▶ IKBKB Deficiency

Niikawa-Kuroki Syndrome

▶ Kabuki Syndrome

Nijmegen Breakage Syndrome (*NBS1*)

Svetlana O. Sharapova[1] and
Larysa V. Kostyuchenko[2]
[1]Research Department, Belarusian Research Center for Pediatric Oncology, Hematology and Immunology, Minsk, Belarus
[2]Department of Clinical Immunology and Allergology, Danylo Halytsky Lviv National Medical University, West-Ukrainian Specialized Children's Medical Center, Lviv, Ukraine

Synonyms

Ataxia-telangiectasia variant 1 (AT-V1); Berlin breakage syndrome; Seemanova syndrome

Definition

Nijmegen breakage syndrome (NBS) is an autosomal-recessive chromosome instability disorder characterized by growth and developmental defects (growth retardation, severe and progressive microcephaly, a distinct facial appearance, lack of secondary sex characteristics in females, and frequent cryptorchism in males), immunodeficiency, high susceptibility to lymphoid malignancies, hypersensitivity to ionizing radiation, and aberrant cell-cycle checkpoint control (Varon et al. 2017; Seemanova et al. 2016). The disease is caused by mutations in the *NBN* gene (also abbreviated *NBS*, *NBS1*) and is located on chromosome 8q21 (GRCh38.p2: 89,933,336–89,984,733).

Introduction/Background

In 1981, Weemaes et al. from the University Hospital of Nijmegen, the Netherlands, first described the syndrome in two Dutch brothers with microcephaly, short stature, skin pigmentation abnormalities, mental retardation, immunologic defects, and a high prevalence of chromosome 7 and/or chromosome 14 rearrangements in cultured lymphocytes (Weemaes et al. 1981). It is assumed that the Dutch patients may have had Bohemian ancestors who immigrated to the Netherlands in the first half of the seventeenth century (Varon et al. 2000). In 1985, Eva Seemanova described a group of patients with an apparently new genetic disorder characterized by microcephaly with normal intelligence, cellular and humoral immune defects, and a striking predisposition to lymphoreticular malignancies. These cases were subsequently studied and found to fit into the category of Nijmegen breakage syndrome (Seemanova et al. 1985).

The disease is most common in people of Central and Eastern European with Slavic background, specifically those from Poland, Southeast Germany, the Czech Republic, and Ukraine (Varon et al. 2017; Seemanova et al. 2016). The frequency of the common *NBS1* heterozygous mutation c.657del5 is relatively high (0.5–1%) in the Slavic populations, and in homozygous form, it leads to the classical manifestation of NBS (Seemanova et al. 2016).

Pathogenesis

NBN gene product, nibrin protein, forms a tri-heteromeric complex with MRE11 (meiotic recombination 11 homolog) and RAD50 (repair of double-strand breaks protein 50) (the MRN complex – Mre11.Rad50.Nbs1). The complex is a primary sensor of DNA double-strand breaks (DSB) and is required for the effective mono-merization and autophosphorylation of ATM (ataxia-telangiectasia-mutated protein) after DNA DSB damage. This is an initial process in two major pathways of DNA DSB repair, e.g., homologous recombination and nonhomologous end joining. Thus, all patients with biallelic hypomorphic mutation in *NBN* gene have defective DSB repair machinery and their processing in immune gene rearrangements, telomere maintenance, and meiotic recombination, which lead to clinical features of the syndrome and are prone to develop malignancies (Seemanova et al. 2016; Pastorczak et al. 2016).

Clinical Presentation

Facial dysmorphism: All patients have a typical "bird-like" face, characterized by a receding forehead, a prominent midface with a long nose and a long philtrum, and a receding mandible. Most patients also show epicanthal folds, large ears, and sparse hair. Severe and progressive microcephaly has been detected intrauterine, from the birth, after the first month of life. Early closure of the fontanel (6 months) is observed in some NBS patients with a normal head circumference at birth (Fig. 1).

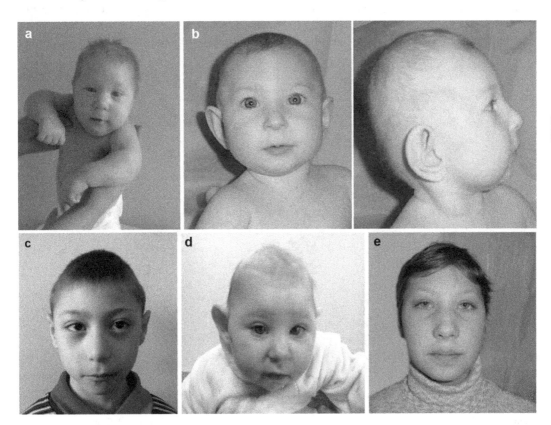

Nijmegen Breakage Syndrome (*NBS1*), Fig. 1 Facial presentation in children with NBS in different ages (**a**) Male patient at the age of 6 months. (**b**). Female patient at the age of 10 months. (**c**). Male patient at the age of 6 years. (**d**). Female patient at the age of 10 months. (**e**). Female patient at the age of 14 years. Written informed consent for photo was obtained from parents of patients

Growth retardation is more pronounced from birth until the age of 3 years, with mild improvement thereafter (Varon et al. 2017).

Recurrent infections include pneumonia, bronchitis, sinusitis, otitis media, and mastoiditis. Recurrent bronchopneumonia may result in bronchiectasis. Urinary and/or gastrointestinal tract infections are also relatively common. Opportunistic infections are rare and observed only in patients with severe T-cell deficiency (Wolska-Kuśnierz et al. 2015).

Autoimmunity. 10–30% of NBS patients with median onset age of 10.5 years (range 4–14 years) develop autoimmune complications comprising the following: skin changes (vitiligo, alopecia, granulomas, skin sarcoidosis, lupus-like skin changes); arthritis; thyroiditis and Graves disease; interstitial lymphocytic lung disease (ILLD); immune thrombocytopenic purpura, autoimmune hemolytic anemia, and neutropenia; uveitis and inflammatory tumor of the orbit; and coeliac

disease (Wolska-Kuśnierz et al. 2015; Deripapa et al. 2017) (Fig. 2).

In some patients with skin sarcoid-like granulomatous lesions, the RA27/3 vaccine strain of rubella virus has been found in homogenized granuloma tissue samples (Deripapa et al. 2017).

Malignancies: As commonly seen in patients with DNA repair, NBS prones patients for malignancy. By the age of 20 years, over 40% of NBS patients develop cancer, predominantly of lymphoid origin (Wolska-Kuśnierz et al. 2015; Deripapa et al. 2017). Recent large studies show the first episode of malignancy occurring at a median age of 10.25 years (range, 2–26 years) in a Polish cohort (n = 149) and 6.0 years (2–18 years) in a Russian cohort (n = 35) (Wolska-Kuśnierz et al. 2015; Deripapa et al. 2017). There is a strong predominance of diffuse large B-cell lymphoma (DLBCL) and T-cell lymphoblastic lymphoma (T-LBL/ALL). Regarding

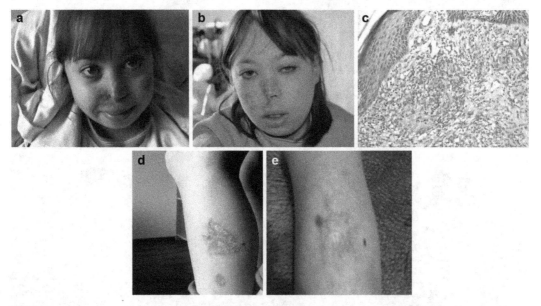

Nijmegen Breakage Syndrome (*NBS1*), Fig. 2 Macroscopic and microscopic images of granulomatous lesion in a girl with Nijmegen breakage syndrome (**a**). Chronic granulomatous skin lesions of the face with nose destruction in NBS patient at the age of 10 years. (**b**). The same patient at the age of 15 years. (**c**). Epithelioid granulomas with foci of necrosis, skin histology

demonstrating inflammatory infiltrates consisting of histiocytes, lymphocytes, and neutrophils, associated with basophilic alterations of collagen. H&E stain. (**d**). Chronic granulomatous skin lesions of the leg in NBS patient. (**e**). Regression of chronic granulomatous skin lesions of the leg in the same patient 6 months after HSCT. (Photographs are reproduced with parents' permission) other lymphoma subtypes, a few cases of ALCL, Hodgkin's lymphoma, and AILT-like B-cell and Burkitt-like lymphomas in NBS patients have also been documented. The common feature of lymphomas in NBS patients is the advanced stage of disease and multiorgan involvement resulting from a delayed diagnosis. Another characteristic feature of NBS lymphoma is the high incidence of disease recurrence and a high risk of secondary malignancies, again mainly lymphomas, but ALL and AML have been also described (Pastorczak et al. 2016). Other malignancies in NBS patients include medulloblastoma, neuroblastoma, dysgerminoma, lymphomatoid granulomatosis, ganglioglioma, and thyroid cancer (Wolska-Kuśnierz et al. 2015; Deripapa et al. 2017). Rarely, some patients develop more than once, and one patient from Poland had five episodes of cancer (Wolska-Kuśnierz et al. 2015).

Decline in intellectual ability occurs from normal or borderline-normal during early childhood to moderate intellectual disability in adolescence (Varon et al. 2017).

Laboratory Findings/Diagnostic Testing

Immunological studies reveal mild-to-moderate lymphopenia in nearly half of the patients with an evident decrease of T cells, CD4+ and CD45RA+ naïve subsets, and TREC levels. This may allow patients to be identified by newborn screening for SCID. With age, most patients develop profound immunodeficiency both of humoral and cellular type. This is frequently associated with recurrent sinopulmonary infections. The spectrum of humoral immunodeficiency is variable ranging from agammaglobulinemia to a moderate reduction in the immune response and subclasses of immunoglobulins (Varon et al. 2017; Seemanova et al. 2016; Wolska-Kuśnierz et al. 2015; Deripapa et al. 2017; Pastorczak et al. 2016).

Chromosome instability. Inversions and translocations involving chromosomes 7 and 14 are observed in phytohemagglutinin (PHA)-stimulated lymphocytes in 10%–50% of metaphases. The breakpoints most commonly

involved are 7p13, 7q35, 14q11, and 14q32, which are the loci for immunoglobulin and T-cell receptor genes (Varon et al. 2017).

Radiation sensitivity. Cells from individuals with NBS have a decrease in colony-forming ability following exposure to ionizing radiation and radiomimetics in vitro (Varon et al. 2017).

Genetics. The majority of NBS patients identified to date had homozygous five-base pair deletion in the *NBN* gene (c.657_661del5, pK219fsX19) with a founder effect observed in Caucasian European populations, especially of Slavic origin (Pastorczak et al. 2016). Similar founder phenomena were described among eight Pakistani patients from four consanguineous families with NBS features who were homozygous for c.C1089A (p.Y363X) mutation in *NBN* gene (Nakanishi et al. 2002; Gennery et al. 2004; New et al. 2005). Nine additional mutations have been identified among patients of different ethnicities (c.643C > T, p.R215W, Czech; c.681delT, Russian; c.698del4, English; c.742insGG and c.835del4, Italian; c.842insT, Mexican; c.900del25, African; c.976C > T (Q326X), Dutch; c.1142delC, Canadian) (Varon et al. 2006; 1998; Seemanová et al. 2006; Resnick et al. 2002).

Treatment

Infections. In individuals with hypogammaglobulinemia and frequent infections, immunoglobulin (Ig) replacement therapy should be considered. Ig replacement is typically administered either intravenously (IVIg) or subcutaneously (SCIg). According to the ESID registry database, IVIg was administered to 68% of NBS patients. The median onset age for Ig therapy was 6.5 years (ranging from 4 months to 18 years) (Wolska-Kusnierz et al. 2015). In most NBS patients, the spectrum of recurrent infections does not include opportunistic agents; therefore, prophylaxis against fungi, viruses, and *Pneumocystis jiroveci* is not routinely recommended, and the antibiotic selection should be appropriate for the microorganism being treated.

Malignancy. Standard treatment chemotherapy protocols for lymphoid malignancies in NBS need to be modified based on the individual's ability to tolerate radiosensitivity (Varon et al. 2017). Treatment of affected individuals with solid tumors is also challenging. Radiotherapy of central nervous system (CNS) tumors (medulloblastoma) has caused severe complications and death in some individuals with NBS (Varon et al. 2017).

For individuals who achieved first remission, hematopoietic stem cell transplantation (HSCT) may be considered:

HSCT. The first successful bone marrow transplantation was performed in a patient with NBS who was initially misdiagnosed with Fanconi anemia (FA) (Gennery et al. 2005; Slack et al. 2018). Latest updated results of HSCT in 26 patients with NBS, nineteen of whom were alive (73%), demonstarated broad spectrum of indication for transplantation. Four patients were transplanted for immunodeficiency, one for autoimmunity, 17 for malignancy treatment and two received preemptive therapy. A wide range of different donors, conditioning regimens, graft-versus-host disease prophylaxis, and stem cell sources were used. Median length of follow-up among living patients was 35 months (range, 2–150 months); 1 patient rejected the graft and is alive with disease. Overall mortality was 17%. Infections and relapse of malignancy were main factors in increased mortality among the post-HSCT patients. Reduced intensity conditioning (RIC) was best tolerated. Thus, HSCT can correct the hematopoietic defect and underlying immunodeficiency, particularly with RIC regimens (Slack et al. 2018). Long-term follow-up is yet to be done to determine the risk of remission of lymphoid malignancy; however, it is encouraging that HSCT might offer a viable treatment option.

Puberty and fertility. Females with NBS who are of pubertal age should be referred for evaluation by a gynecologist and/or endocrinologist to evaluate for hypergonadotropic hypogonadism. Hormonal replacement therapy should be considered with careful monitoring of secondary sexual characteristics and uterus development. Females are infertile; similarly, no male paternity has been reported.

Prognosis

According to the ESID database analysis, 60% of NBS patients died due to malignancies and/or complications of their treatment. In cases of severe immunodeficiency, infections before and after HSCT were the primary cause of death (Wolska-Kusnierz et al. 2015). Overall survival probabilities at 5, 10, 20, and 30 years of age are 95, 85, 50, and 35%, respectively (Wolska-Kusnierz et al. 2015).

References

Deripapa E, Balashov D, Rodina Y, et al. Prospective study of a cohort of Russian Nijmegen breakage syndrome patients demonstrating predictive value of low kappa deleting recombination excision circle (KREC) numbers and beneficial effect of hematopoietic stem cell transplantation (HSCT). Front Immunol. 2017;8:807.

Gennery AR, Slatter MA, Bhattacharya A, et al. The clinical and biological overlap between Nijmegen breakage syndrome and Fanconi anemia. Clin Immunol. 2004;113(2):214–9.

Gennery AR, Slatter MA, Bhattacharya A, et al. Bone marrow transplantation for Nijmegan breakage syndrome. J Pediatr Hematol Oncol. 2005;27(4):239.

Nakanishi K, Taniguchi T, Ranganathan V, et al. Interaction of FANCD2 and NBS1 in the DNA damage response. Nat Cell Biol. 2002;4(12):913–20.

New HV, Cale CM, Tischkowitz M, et al. Nijmegen breakage syndrome diagnosed as Fanconi anaemia. Pediatr Blood Cancer. 2005;44(5):494–9.

Pastorczak A, Szczepanski T, Mlynarski W. Clinical course and therapeutic implications for lymphoid malignancies in Nijmegen breakage syndrome. Eur J Med Genet. 2016;59(3):126–32.

Resnick IB, Kondratenko I, Togoev O, et al. Nijmegen breakage syndrome: clinical characteristics and mutation analysis in eight unrelated Russian families. J Pediatr. 2002;140(3):355–61.

Seemanova E, Passarge D, Beneskova J, et al. Familial microcephaly with normal intelligence, immunodeficiency, and risk for lymphoreticular malignancies: a new autosomal recessive disorder. Am J Med Genet. 1985;20(4):639–48.

Seemanová E, Sperling K, Neitzel H, et al. Nijmegen breakage syndrome (NBS) with neurological abnormalities and without chromosomal instability. J Med Genet. 2006;43(3):218–24.

Seemanova E, Varon R, Vejvalka J, et al. The Slavic NBN founder mutation: a role for reproductive fitness? PLoS One. 2016;11(12):e0167984.

Slack J, Albert MH, Balashov D, et al. Outcome of hematopoietic cell transplantation for DNA double-strand break repair disorders. J Allergy Clin Immunol. 2018;141(1):322–328.e10.

Varon R, Vissinga C, Platzer M, et al. Nibrin, a novel DNA double-strand break repair protein, is mutated in Nijmegen breakage syndrome. Cell. 1998;93(3): 467–76.

Varon R, Seemanova E, Chrzanowska K, et al. Clinical ascertainment of Nijmegen breakage syndrome (NBS) and prevalence of the major mutation, 657del5, in three Slav populations. Eur J Hum Genet. 2000;8:900–2.

Varon R, Dutrannoy V, Weikert G, et al. Mild Nijmegen breakage syndrome phenotype due to alternative splicing. Hum Mol Genet. 2006;15(5):679–89.

Varon R, Demuth I, Chrzanowska KH. In: Adam MP, Ardinger HH, Pagon RA, Wallace SE, Bean LJH, Stephens K, Amemiya A, editors. GeneReviews® [Internet]. Seattle (WA): University of Washington, Seattle; 1993–2018. 999 May 17 [updated 2017 Feb 2].

Weemaes CM, Hustinx TW, Scheres JM, et al. A new chromosomal instability disorder: the Nijmegen breakage syndrome. Acta Paediatr Scand. 1981; 70(4):557–64.

Wolska-Kuśnierz B, Gregorek H, Chrzanowska K, et al. Nijmegen breakage syndrome: clinical and immunological features, long-term outcome and treatment options – a retrospective analysis. J Clin Immunol. 2015;35(6):538–49.

NLRC4

▶ NLRC4-Associated Autoinflammatory Diseases

NLRC4-Associated Autoinflammatory Diseases

Scott W. Canna
University of Pittsburgh and UPMC Children's Hospital of Pittsburgh, Pittsburgh, PA, USA

Synonyms

AIFEC; Autoinflammation with infantile enterocolitis; CARD12; ICE-protease converting factor; IPAF; N4AID; NLRC4; NLRC4-mediated autoinflammatory diseases; Nucleotide-binding domain, Leucine-Rich Repeat, CARD domain 4

Definition

N4AID- or NLRC4-mediated autoinflammatory disease is a monogenic autoinflammatory disease with variable, but sometimes fatal, autoinflammatory presentation and is caused by gain-of-function mutations in the gene, NLRC4. (MIM#616050).

Introduction and Background

The association of gain-of-function NLRC4 mutations with autoinflammatory disease (AID) was first made in 2014 (Romberg et al. 2014; Canna et al. 2014), and the ongoing characterization of NLRC4-associated autoinflammatory diseases (N4AIDs) has evolved in the context of what we know about other AIDs, especially the NLRP3 and MEFV inflammasomopathies. Inflammasomopathies are AIDs caused by gain-of-function mutations in genes encoding inflammasome-nucleating proteins. The inflammasome is a massive innate immune complex that links cytosolic danger or pathogen sensing with an exponential increase in the ability to cleave (and thereby activate) the pro-inflammatory cytokines IL-1β and IL-18, and the mediator of inflammatory/pyroptotic cell death Gasdermin D (GSDMD). The proteins mutated in inflammasomopathies encode proteins at the early stages of this inflammatory cascade that themselves "nucleate" the aggregation of thousands of other inflammasome proteins, including the adaptor ASC and the enzymatic protease caspase-1. Thus, incremental increases in the activation state of these disease-associated nucleator proteins can have dramatic downstream effects both within the cells where they are expressed, and within neighboring phagocytes where the engulfed inflammasomes may retain their ability to perpetuate inflammation (Baroja-Mazo et al. 2014).

Genetics

Since 2014, ten distinct disease-associated NLRC4 mutations have been identified

(Romberg et al. 2014; Canna et al. 2014, 2016; Kitamura et al. 2014; Volker-Touw et al. 2016; Kawasaki et al. 2017; Liang et al. 2017; Moghaddas et al. 2018; Bracaglia et al. 2018) (Table 1). The mutations described to date have all been detected by whole exome sequencing with Sanger confirmation. The mutations have either occurred de novo or were inherited dominantly. In two patients who were born preterm, the NLRC4 mutations were somatic, meaning not every cell carried an NLRC4 mutation, although in both cases the majority of cells sequenced carried a mutation (Kawasaki et al. 2017; Liang et al. 2017). Currently, too few NLRC4 mutations have been reported to make solid genotype/phenotype correlations. Unlike NLRP3, however, the existence of crystal and cryo-EM structures for NLRC4 (Hu et al. 2013; Zhang et al. 2015; Diebolder et al. 2015) has suggested several "hot spots" associated with pathogenic mutations near amino acid positions 175, 340, and 445. Each of these positions maps in close proximity to NLRC4's ADP-binding site in the proposed tertiary structure.

Pathogenesis

As in Familial Mediterranean Fever (FMF) and the Cryopyrin-Associated Periodic Syndromes (CAPS), functional studies of N4AID patients/mutations confirm spontaneous or increased inflammasome activation. Unlike the other inflammasomopathies, N4AID patients (particularly those with features of macrophage activation syndrome, MAS, see below) have extremely high peripheral blood IL-18 levels. These may be used to distinguish N4AIDs both from other AIDs and from non-MAS causes of cytokine storm syndromes, like familial hemophagocytic lymphohistiocytosis (fHLH). IL-18 remains chronically and highly elevated in patients with NLRC4-MAS even during prolonged periods of disease quiescence (Romberg et al. 2014; Canna et al. 2014, 2016). IL-18 is an inflammasome-activated cytokine best known for its synergy with IL-12 in driving lymphocytes to secrete interferon (IFN)-γ. IL-18's effects in the absence of other cytokines (like IL-12) are quite modest in vitro, correlating with N4AID patients' lack of systemic inflammation between flares. IL-18 is naturally antagonized by a soluble inhibitor called

NLRC4-Associated Autoinflammatory Diseases, Table 1 Clinical and Genetic features of N4AID's

Mutation	Proposed mechanism	Phenotype	Long-term defect	Ref.
Ser171Phe[a]	Abnl nucleotide binding	Pre- and perinatal MAS, coagulopathy, enterocolitis	Death	Liang et al. (2017)
Thr177Ala[a]	Abnl nucleotide binding	NOMID[*]	Hearing loss	Kawasaki et al. (2017)
Thr337Ser/Asn	Abnl nucleotide binding	MAS, mild enterocolitis	N/A	Canna et al. (2014) and Bracaglia et al. (2018)
Val341Ala/Leu	Abnl nucleotide binding	MAS, severe enterocolitis	Death (1 of 5)	Romberg et al. (2014), Canna et al. (2016), and Barsalou et al. (2018)
Ile343Asn	Abnl nucleotide binding	MAS, vasculitis	N/A	Bracaglia et al. (2018)
His443Pro	Abnl nucleotide binding	Cold-urticaria	N/A	Kitamura et al. (2014)
Ser445Pro	Abnl nucleotide binding	Variable autoinflammatory	N/A	Volker-Touw et al. (2016)
Trp655Cys	Abnl oligomerization	MAS	Death (2 of 2)	Moghaddas et al. (2018)

[a]High-frequency somatic mutation
[*]Neonatal-Onset Multi-System Inflammatory Disease

IL-18 binding protein (IL-18BP), and measurement of IL-18 relative to, or unbound by, IL-18BP (so-called free IL-18) may be a surrogate for IL-18's targetability (Canna et al. 2016; Girard et al. 2016).

Clinical Manifestations

The clinical manifestations of the N4AIDs are quite variable but all consistent with auto-inflammatory origins. Disease severity can range from perinatal lethality to relatively benign, life-long, cold-induced urticaria. One severe pheno-type, combining the features of cytokine storm and intestinal inflammation, may be more uniquely associated with *NLRC4* mutations.

This section will address the published pheno-types from most mild to most severe.

Familial Cold-Induced Urticaria (FCU)
An extended Japanese kindred was noted to have recurrent cold-induced urticarial episodes that tracked with inheritance of a dominant NLRC4 mutation (Kitamura et al. 2014). There appeared to be minimal systemic inflammation in this kin-dred, but little clinical information was available.

Urticaria, Erythema Nodosum, and Arthralgia
A large Dutch kindred included family members with a rash that appeared more urticarial in youn-ger patients, but included erythematous nodules in older patients (Volker-Touw et al. 2016). Other organ manifestations that occurred in this kindred included conjunctivitis, lymphedema, erosive polyarthritis, and inflammatory bowel disease.

Neonatal Onset Multisystem Inflammatory Disease (NOMID)
Disease in a patient followed for many years with clinical features of NOMID, including fevers, urticarial rash, aseptic meningitis, sensorineural hearing loss, and response to IL-1 inhibition, was eventually attributed to a somatic gain-of-function NLRC4 mutation (Kawasaki et al. 2017).

Macrophage Activation Syndrome (MAS) with Infantile Enterocolitis
Best known as a potentially lethal complication of systemic juvenile idiopathic arthritis (SJIA), MAS consists of unremitting fever, pancytopenia, extremely high ferritin, coagulopathy, hepatosple-nomegaly, hepatobiliary dysfunction, and often bone marrow or tissue hemophagocytosis. It can progress to organ failure and death. Two groups independently and simultaneously published reports of life-threatening MAS concomitant with vomiting, infantile secretory diarrhea, and failure to thrive (Romberg et al. 2014; Canna et al. 2014). Several subsequent reports have cor-roborated this phenotype, although the presence and severity of enterocolitis was variable (Canna et al. 2016; Liang et al. 2017; Moghaddas et al. 2018; Bracaglia et al. 2018; Barsalou et al. 2018). One notable feature of the patients described with MAS and enterocolitis is that, if patients survive through infancy, their enterocolitis appears to resolve and does not recur.

Even within this severe phenotype, the spec-trum of severity can vary. One patient suffered from recurrent MAS episodes but otherwise grew and developed with relative normality (Canna et al. 2014). In another cohort, the index patient had infantile enterocolitis and recurrent MAS, but into adulthood had prolonged periods of complete dis-ease quiescence punctuated by (often stress-induced) severe MAS episodes (Romberg et al. 2014). This patient had two offspring: one whose course included resolving enterocolitis and smol-dering MAS-like inflammation, and another who died at 23 days of age due to complications of MAS. Notably, preterm delivery preceded neonatal disease in two patients (Kawasaki et al. 2017; Liang et al. 2017). One such patient was found to have severe fetal thrombotic vasculopathy involv-ing the placenta (Liang et al. 2017).

Laboratory Findings

As noted, the spectrum of phenotypes and severity in N4AIDs complicates specific laboratory testing.

In general, routine laboratory testing is commensurate with both the clinical features and severity of disease. Some patients with FCU had no baseline inflammatory abnormalities on routine testing (Kitamura et al. 2014). One potential source of differentiation from other AIDs is the character of the skin biopsy. Erythematous nodes were biopsied and found to have a lymphohistiocytic infiltrate (Volker-Touw et al. 2016). This is more consistent with the rash of SJIA than the mature neutrophilic infiltrate predominantly observed in *NLRP3* and *MEFV* inflammasomopathies, however the timing of the biopsy may have influenced the histology.

Patients with MAS had pancytopenia, hyperferritinemia, transaminitis, and coagulopathy consistent with active MAS. Severe enterocolitis was also accompanied by the hypoalbuminemia and hypogammaglobulinemia of a protein-losing enteropathy (Canna et al. 2016). Gut pathology in NLRC4-associated enterocolitis may focus on the duodenum; two patients had pathology reminiscent of celiac disease (Romberg et al. 2014; Canna et al. 2014), although profound inflammation can extend from the stomach to colon in severe disease (Canna et al. 2016). As stated above, N4AID patients, particularly those who have had MAS, exhibit chronically and strikingly elevated total IL-18 and detectable "free IL-18." Levels of total IL-18 in serum or plasma rarely fall below 40,000 pg/mL in such patients (Romberg et al. 2014; Canna et al. 2014, 2016; Weiss et al. 2018). Total IL-18 is quite elevated even in N4AID patients without MAS (Volker-Touw et al. 2016; Kawasaki et al. 2017), although not to the same degree as those with MAS.

Diagnosis

Diagnosis is made based on clinical suspicion followed by genetic confirmation. Rapid diagnosis may have profound therapeutic and prognostic consequences as detailed below. Deep sequencing may be required to identify N4AID patients with lower frequency somatic mutations.

Treatment

Treatments have largely been directed at the symptoms present in individual N4AID patients. The FCU kindred was managed with nothing more than NSAIDs (Kitamura et al. 2014). The NOMID-like patient and one recurrent MAS patient showed complete response to IL-1 inhibition (Canna et al. 2014; Kawasaki et al. 2017), whereas at best a partial response to IL-1 inhibition was observed in the complex Dutch cohort, and most other MAS/enterocolitis patients (Volker-Touw et al. 2016; Canna et al. 2016; Moghaddas et al. 2018; Barsalou et al. 2018). Infants with MAS/enterocolitis may have disease impressively refractory to conventional therapies including steroids, cyclosporine, TNF-inhibition, IL-1 inhibition, and integrin-inhibition (Canna et al. 2016; Moghaddas et al. 2018; Bracaglia et al. 2018; Barsalou et al. 2018). In these situations, investigational use of recombinant IL-18BP or inhibitors of the IL-18 induced cytokine Interferon-γ (IFNγ) have shown dramatic results in individual patients (Canna et al. 2016; Bracaglia et al. 2018). These patients were often able to achieve complete disease remission on therapy. However, given severe MAS episodes may occur after long periods of inactivity (Romberg et al. 2014) and no therapy appears to diminish IL-18 elevation (Romberg et al. 2014; Canna et al. 2016), patients will likely require at least close lifelong observation if not lifelong treatment. The efficacy of myeloablation and bone marrow transplant has not been reported. However, the case reports of effective management of severe MAS with IL-18- or IFNγ-targeted therapy, coupled with the potential for nonhematopoietic/transplant-resistant expression of IL-18 (Weiss et al. 2018), may tilt the balance against such interventions.

Prognosis

Those N4AID patients with more classic autoinflammatory features, like episodic fever or urticaria, appear to follow a course similar to these features in other AIDs (Kitamura et al. 2014; Canna et al. 2016; Kawasaki et al. 2017). The chronic features of other inflammasomopathies, like amyloidosis and bony overgrowth, have not been reported in N4AIDs with the notable exception of hearing loss in one NOMID-like patient (Kawasaki et al. 2017). Importantly, about half of the reported NLRC4-MAS patients have died in the perinatal period of coagulopathy and/or organ failure related to MAS (Romberg et al. 2014; Canna et al. 2014, 2016; Liang et al. 2017; Moghaddas et al. 2018; Bracaglia et al. 2018; Barsalou et al. 2018). Patients surviving infancy may have resolution of their enterocolitis, whereas MAS recurrences continue and can be severe (Romberg et al. 2014; Canna et al. 2014, 2016; Barsalou et al. 2018; Weiss et al. 2018). Thus, there is hope that efficient diagnosis and aggressive treatment, particularly with IL-18 or IFNγ targeting agents on the horizon, can prevent poor outcomes even in patients with life-threatening disease.

Cross-References

▶ Familial Cold Autoinflammatory Syndrome (FCAS) and Muckle-Wells Syndrome (MWS)
▶ *PRF1* Deficiency
▶ *STX11* Deficiency
▶ *STXBP2* Deficiency
▶ *UNC13D* Deficiency
▶ XIAP Deficiency

References

Baroja-Mazo A, Martin-Sanchez F, Gomez AI, Martinez CM, Amores-Iniesta J, Compan V, et al. The NLRP3 inflammasome is released as a particulate danger signal that amplifies the inflammatory response. Nat Immunol. 2014;15(8):738–48.

Barsalou J, Blincoe A, Fernandez I, Dal-Soglio D, Marchitto L, Selleri S, et al. Rapamycin as an adjunctive therapy for NLRC4 associated macrophage activation syndrome. Front Immunol. 2018;9:2162.

Bracaglia C, Prencipe G, Insalaco A, Caiello I, Marucci G, Ballabio M, et al. Abstract: Emapalumab, an anti-interferon gamma monoclonal antibody in two patients with NLRC4-related disease and severe hemophagocytic Lymphohistiocytosis. American College of Rheumatology Annual Meeting. 2018.

Canna SW, de Jesus AA, Gouni S, Brooks SR, Marrero B, Liu Y, et al. An activating NLRC4 inflammasome mutation causes autoinflammation with recurrent macrophage activation syndrome. Nat Genet. 2014;46(10):1140–6.

Canna SW, Girard C, Malle L, de Jesus A, Romberg N, Kelsen J, et al. Life-threatening NLRC4-associated hyperinflammation successfully treated with Interleukin-18 inhibition. J Allergy Clin Immunol. 2016;139(5):1698–701.

Diebolder CA, Halff EF, Koster AJ, Huizinga EG, Koning RI. Cryoelectron tomography of the NAIP5/NLRC4 inflammasome: implications for NLR activation. Structure. 2015;23(12):2349–57.

Girard C, Rech J, Brown M, Allali D, Roux-Lombard P, Spertini F, et al. Elevated serum levels of free interleukin-18 in adult-onset Still's disease. Rheumatology (Oxford). 2016;55(12):2237–47.

Hu Z, Yan C, Liu P, Huang Z, Ma R, Zhang C, et al. Crystal structure of NLRC4 reveals its autoinhibition mechanism. Science. 2013;341(6142):172–5.

Kawasaki Y, Oda H, Ito J, Niwa A, Tanaka T, Hijikata A, et al. Identification of a high-frequency somatic NLRC4 mutation as a cause of autoinflammation by pluripotent cell-based phenotype dissection. Arthritis Rheumatol. 2017;69(2):447–59.

Kitamura A, Sasaki Y, Abe T, Kano H, Yasutomo K. An inherited mutation in NLRC4 causes autoinflammation in human and mice. J Exp Med. 2014;211(12):2385–96.

Liang J, Alfano DN, Squires JE, Riley MM, Parks WT, Kofler J, et al. Novel NLRC4 mutation causes a syndrome of perinatal autoinflammation with hemophagocytic lymphohistiocytosis, hepatosplenomegaly, fetal thrombotic vasculopathy, and congenital anemia and ascites. Pediatr Dev Pathol. 2017;20(6):498–505.

Moghaddas F, Zeng P, Zhang Y, Schutzle H, Brenner S, Hofmann SR, et al. Autoinflammatory mutation in NLRC4 reveals an LRR-LRR oligomerization interface. J Allergy Clin Immunol. 2018;142(6):1956–1967.

Romberg N, Al Moussawi K, Nelson-Williams C, Stiegler AL, Loring E, Choi M, et al. Mutation of NLRC4 causes a syndrome of enterocolitis and autoinflammation. Nat Genet. 2014;46(10):1135–9.

Volker-Touw CM, de Koning HD, Giltay J, de Kovel C, van Kempen TS, Oberndorff K, et al. Erythematous nodes, urticarial rash and arthralgias in a large pedigree with NLRC4-related autoinflammatory disease, expansion of the phenotype. Br J Dermatol. 2016;176(1):244–8.

Weiss ES, Girard-Guyonvarc'h C, Holzinger D, de Jesus AA, Tariq Z, Picarsic J, et al. Interleukin-18 diagnostically distinguishes and pathogenically promotes human and murine macrophage activation syndrome. Blood. 2018;131(13):1442–55.

Zhang L, Chen S, Ruan J, Wu J, Tong AB, Yin Q, et al. Cryo-EM structure of the activated NAIP2-NLRC4 inflammasome reveals nucleated polymerization. Science. 2015;350(6259):404–9.

NLRC4-Mediated Autoinflammatory Diseases

▶ NLRC4-Associated Autoinflammatory Diseases

Nod, Leucine-Rich Repeat, Pyrin 3 (NLRP3)

▶ Familial Cold Autoinflammatory Syndrome (FCAS) and Muckle-Wells Syndrome (MWS)

NOMID: Neonatal-Onset Multisystem Inflammatory Disease

▶ Neonatal-Onset Multisystem Inflammatory Disease (NOMID)

Nucleotide-Binding Domain, Leucine-Rich Repeat, CARD Domain 4

▶ NLRC4-Associated Autoinflammatory Diseases

Nude SCID

▶ Winged Helix Deficiency (FOXN1)

O

OKT8 T Cell Antigen

▶ CD8 Alpha (CD8A) Deficiency

Omenn Syndrome (OS)

Robert P. Nelson
Divisions of Hematology and Oncology, Stem
Cell Transplant Program, Indiana University (IU)
School of Medicine and the IU Bren and Simon
Cancer Center, Indianapolis, IN, USA
Pediatric Immunodeficiency Clinic, Riley
Hospital for Children at Indiana University
Health, Indianapolis, IN, USA
Medicine and Pediatrics, Indiana University
School of Medicine, Immunohematology and
Transplantation, Indianapolis, IN, USA

Synonyms

Reticuloendotheliosis with eosinophilia

Definition

Omenn syndrome is a form of combined immunodeficiency characterized by severe rash, diarrhea, lymphadenopathy, hepatomegaly,
eosinophilia, and elevated IgE. It was initially
reported to be associated with some defects in
genes *RAG1* and *RAG2*, leading to ineffective
genetic recombination and an abnormal adaptive
lymphocyte repertoire.

Introduction

The Omenn syndrome (OS) represents a spectrum
of combined immunodeficiency disorders characterized by signs and symptoms secondary to
defects in genes essential for the adaptive immune
response. T and B lymphocytes express unique
immunoreceptors, the diversity of which depends
on the variable, diversity, and joining (VDJ) exon
recombination events. Genetic recombination
of these exons allows to expand the breadth of
adaptive immune T- and B-cell "repertoires"
needed for humans to survive in a divergent
microbial environment (Bernstein et al. 1994;
Wayne et al. 1994).

Function

VDJ exon recombination events are initiated
predominately by the proteins coded by
recombinase-activating genes 1 and 2 (*RAG1,
RAG2*). The nucleotide sequences of RAG genes
are highly conserved in animals, dating back to
their emergence in shark species millions of years
ago (Bernstein et al. 1994). RAG proteins create
double-stranded DNA breaks that initiate VDJ
recombination, participate in the joining phase,

and interact with post-cleavage complexes that prevent degradation of broken ends prior to joining. Some RAG mutants are proficient in cleaving DNA but defective in their ability to interact with coding ends following cleavage or to capture the target DNA for transposition. Such mutant proteins exhibit severe defects in their capacity to facilitate hybrid joint formation, hairpin coding end opening, and VDJ recombination. Patients with a loss-of-function (LOF) mutation in RAG genes display restricted, oligoclonal lymphocyte repertoires. Some self-reactive T-cell clones may survive negative thymic selection and cause autoimmune tissue injury, targeting most frequently the skin and GI tract (Harville et al. 1997).

Villa et al. described a cohort of children with immunodeficiencies characterized by the presence of activated, anergic, oligoclonal T cells, hypereosinophilia, and high serum IgE levels. Missense mutations within the RAG-1 homeodomain caused amino acid substitutions in the protein that reduced binding activity and lowered the efficiency of RAG-1/RAG-2 interactions (Villa et al. 1998; Notarangelo et al. 2001). These findings provided evidence that inefficiencies of VDJ recombination were pathologically implicated in OS. Homozygous mutations that completely abrogate RAG protein function cause T-B-severe combined immunodeficiency (SCID), whereas mutations that render partial VDJ recombination activity of RAG1 or RAG2 proteins cause "leaky" combined immunodeficiencies and OS. Pathogenic mutations in other genes including *Artemis*, *interleukin-7 receptor* (*IL-7R*), and *adenosine deaminase* (*ADA*) have been reported in sporadic OS cases. The *Artemis* gene interacts with DNA-dependent protein kinase catalytic subunits to open hairpin coding ends in the later stages of DNA VDJ recombination and repair. Artemis deficiency was discovered in a human with SCID and sensitivity to radiation and is characterized by absent B and T lymphocytes and increased sensitivity of fibroblasts and bone marrow to ionizing radiation. This phenotype is accompanied by a profound defect in VDJ recombination with normal signal joints but a lack of coding joint formation (Nicolas et al. 1998). Poliani et al. analyzed thymic maturation and

organization in several patients with combined immunodeficiencies. Those with OS had absent Foxp3 (+) T cells. In contrast, an IL2RG-R222C hypomorphic mutation permissive for T-cell development permitted thymic epithelial maturation, AIRE expression, and Foxp3 (+) T cells (Poliani et al. 2009).

Clinical Manifestations

Omenn's original report concerned 12 infants in 6 kindreds, with clinical findings of fevers, severe dermatitis, hepatosplenomegaly, generalized lymphadenopathy, and eosinophilia in the first weeks of life. The inheritance pattern was autosomal recessive, and the children experienced progressive failure to thrive and death within 2–6 months (Omenn 1965). The OS presents early in life and is characterized by diffuse erythroderma, elevated serum IgE, and dysfunctional oligoclonal T cells. The phenotype varies from the original description of SCID and non-SCID combined immunodeficiencies (Villa et al. 1998). In a large, registry retrospective study of 285 eligible SCID patients, 84% were classified as having typical SCID; 13% were classified as having leaky SCID, OS, or reticular dysgenesis; and 3% had a history of enzyme replacement or gene therapy (Shearer et al. 2014).

The clinical severity of partial deficiencies depends on the degree of impairment of the VDJ recombination process (Villa et al. 1999). Typically, a pruritic erythematous skin rash develops within weeks after birth may mimic seborrheic or atopic dermatitis. The rash may demonstrate purplish nodularity or reveal pustules or boils. The erythroderma progressively worsens, and the patient may develop crusts or scale, violaceous subcutaneous nodules, or exfoliation. There may be sparse scalp hair and morphologically normal eyebrow hair, and hair shaft analysis reveals no trichorrhexis. Generation of a few T cells that expand in the periphery can lead to autoimmune inflammatory injury, with some predilection for the gastrointestinal tract and skin.

Cassani et al. used next-generation sequencing to investigate the phenotypic heterogeneity of

RAG deficiency, analyzing the lymphocyte reper-toires in 12 patients with RAG mutations pre-senting with OS (n = 5), leaky SCID (n = 3), or combined immunodeficiency with granulomas and autoimmunity (CID-G/AI) (n = 4) (Cassani et al. 2010). Restriction of repertoire diversity and abnormalities of CDR3 length distribution were progressively more prominent in patients with a more severe phenotype. Patients with OS had a high proportion of class-switched immunoglobu-lin heavy chain transcripts and increased somatic hypermutation rate, suggesting in vivo activation of these B cells.

A patient with OS may come to the attention of the care team by the newborn screen that counts T-cell receptor excision circles (TRECs) on Guth-rie cards. A low TREC number equates with fail-ure to produce adequate naïve T cells. Thus a positive NBS and new rash in infancy suggests OS and requires immediate attention and consul-tation with an immunologist. Vaccine strain-related, life-threatening varicella infections and meningoencephalitis due to mumps virus might occur. Signs of failure to thrive may be present and lymph nodes likely palpable. Facial features are normal. Cutaneous granulomas without detectable infectious etiology may be a presenting sign (Van Horn et al. 2018). There may be history of autoimmune manifestations or enteritis, and the child may lack a thymus shadow. Cognitive impairment in the absence of an infectious cause or cardiovascular structural defects would not be expected (Aleman et al. 2001).

The differential diagnosis includes maternal T-cell transfer with GvHD-like disease in a SCID patient and DOCK8 deficiency, which is an autosomal recessive immunodeficiency char-acterized by elevated IgE, atopy, cutaneous viral infections, and increased susceptibility to cancer.

Diagnosis

OS infants might be identified by newborn screen-ing for SCID due to low number of TRECs. Com-plete blood count may be normal or demonstrate leukocytosis, anemia, and thrombocytopenia, and increased eosinophil percentage. Patients with OS

might present with normal or low numbers of T cells due to clonal expansion. T-cell repertoire is reported as oligoclonal. Serum levels of IgA, IgM, and IgG are low or undetectable.

Immunological Evaluation and Histology

In OS, the T-cell repertoire is oligoclonal and lacks capacity to respond to mitogens and anti-gens. Some residual abnormal T-cell clones in OS escaping negative selection expand in the periph-ery and react to the skin and gastrointestinal tis-sues. The dermatitis may mimic GvHD occurring in an infant with SCID; however, compared to GvHD, the OS spectrum of pathological skin changes is broad. There may be acanthosis, para-keratosis, with a dense psoriasiform hyperplasia, and spongiosis. Most inflammatory cells in an OS rash are T lymphocytes (Wiegmann et al. 2019).

Treatment and Prognosis

OS patients should be managed in a center that has a multidisciplinary team assembled for the man-agement of immunodeficiency diseases. Rapid initiation of adequate supportive treatment and timely referral for hematopoietic stem cell trans-plantation (HSCT) are essential. Generalized erythroderma, alopecia, and evidence of TH2 inflammation (eosinophilia and elevated serum IgE) are clinical elements that support initiation of immunosuppressive therapy, which serves as bridge to transplant. The calcineurin inhibitor cyclosporine A (CsA) may be useful for the treat-ment of erythroderma and lymphocytosis (Marrella et al. 2011). Under these circumstances, with abnormal T-cell function and immunosup-pression and anti-inflammatory therapy may increase susceptibility to opportunistic infections, therefore prophylactic antimicrobial therapy is indicated, preferably with pediatric infectious dis-ease consultation. OS patients require immuno-globulin supplementation. These supportive measures before HCST help with reducing risk of infections and mortality. Early prenatal diagnosis is another factor that reduces mortality and should be considered in those born in families with history of severe immunodeficiency (Santagata et al. 2000).

An occasional patient may spontaneously undergo corrective somatic mutations that restore some function, altering the clinical presentation from the severe to less severe immune deficiency (Wada et al. 2005).

Mazzolari et al. reported a series of 11 unselected patients with OS who underwent allogeneic HSCT at a median age of 8.4 months (Mazzolari et al. 2005). Two patients received two and one patient three transplant procedures. Donors included seven HLA-haploidentical parental, four with matched unrelated donors, and three from an HLA phenotypically identical-related donor and in one case from an HLA genotypically identical family donor. Nine out of 11 patients were alive at 30–146 months posttransplant. Nine survivors had normal T-cell function and eight normal antibody production. Overall mortality was 18.2%. Gene therapy may present another therapeutic option, particularly for those who lack a suitable donor for HSCT (Capo et al. 2018).

Cross-References

▶ DOCK8 Deficiency

References

Aleman K, Noordzij JG, de Groot R, van Dongen JJ, Hartwig NG. Reviewing Omenn syndrome. Eur J Pediatr. 2001;160:718–25.

Bernstein RM, Schluter SF, Lake DF, Marchalonis JJ. Evolutionary conservation and molecular cloning of the recombinase activating gene 1. Biochem Biophys Res Commun. 1994;205:687–92.

Capo V, Castiello MC, Fontana E, et al. Efficacy of lentivirus-mediated gene therapy in an Omenn syndrome recombination-activating gene 2 mouse model is not hindered by inflammation and immune dysregulation. J Allergy Clin Immunol. 2018;142: 928–41.e8

Cassani B, Poliani PL, Moratto D, et al. Defect of regulatory T cells in patients with Omenn syndrome. J Allergy Clin Immunol. 2010;125:209–16.

Harville TO, Adams DM, Howard TA, Ware RE. Oligoclonal expansion of CD45RO+ T lymphocytes in Omenn syndrome. J Clin Immunol. 1997;17:322–32.

Marrella V, Maina V, Villa A. Omenn syndrome does not live by V(D)J recombination alone. Curr Opin Allergy Clin Immunol. 2011;11:525–31.

Mazzolari E, Moshous D, Forino C, De Martiis D, Offer C, Lanfranchi A, Giliani S, Imberti L, Pasic S, Ugazio AG, Porta F, Notarangelo LD. Hematopoietic stem cell transplantation in Omenn syndrome: a single-center experience. Bone Marrow Transplant. 2005;36(2):107–14.

Nicolas N, Moshous D, Cavazzana-Calvo M, et al. A human severe combined immunodeficiency (SCID) condition with increased sensitivity to ionizing radiations and impaired V(D)J rearrangements defines a new DNA recombination/repair deficiency. J Exp Med. 1998;188:627–34.

Notarangelo LD, Santagata S, Villa A. Recombinase activating gene enzymes of lymphocytes. Curr Opin Hematol. 2001;8:41–6.

Omenn GS. Familial Reticuloendotheliosis with eosinophilia. N Engl J Med. 1965;273:427–32.

Poliani PL, Facchetti F, Ravanini M, et al. Early defects in human T-cell development severely affect distribution and maturation of thymic stromal cells: possible implications for the pathophysiology of Omenn syndrome. Blood. 2009;114:105–8.

Santagata S, Villa A, Sobacchi C, Cortes P, Vezzoni P. The genetic and biochemical basis of Omenn syndrome. Immunol Rev. 2000;178:64–74.

Shearer WT, Dunn E, Notarangelo LD, et al. Establishing diagnostic criteria for severe combined immunodeficiency disease (SCID), leaky SCID, and Omenn syndrome: the primary immune deficiency treatment consortium experience. J Allergy Clin Immunol. 2014;133:1092–8.

Van Horn SA, Johnson KM, Childs JM. Rheumatoid-nodule-like cutaneous granuloma associated with recombinase activating gene 1-deficient severe combined immunodeficiency: a rare case. J Cutan Pathol. 2018;45:940–3.

Villa A, Santagata S, Bozzi F, et al. Partial V(D)J recombination activity leads to Omenn syndrome. Cell. 1998;93:885–96.

Villa A, Santagata S, Bozzi F, Imberti L, Notarangelo LD. Omenn syndrome: a disorder of Rag1 and Rag2 genes. J Clin Immunol. 1999;19:87–97.

Wada T, Toma T, Okamoto H, et al. Oligoclonal expansion of T lymphocytes with multiple second-site mutations leads to Omenn syndrome in a patient with RAG1-deficient severe combined immunodeficiency. Blood. 2005;106:2099–101.

Wayne J, Suh H, Misulovin Z, Sokol KA, Inaba K, Nussenzweig MC. A regulatory role for recombinase activating genes, RAG-1 and RAG-2, in T cell development. Immunity. 1994;1:95–107.

Wiegmann H, Reunert J, Metze D, et al. Refining the dermatological spectrum in primary immunodeficiency: mucosa-associated lymphoid tissue lymphoma translocation protein 1 deficiency mimicking Netherton/Omenn syndromes. Br J Dermatol. 2019;

ORAI1 Deficiency

▶ Calcium Channel Defects (STIM1 and ORAI1)

OTULIN Deficiency-Associated Disease Spectrum

Ivona Aksentijevich
Inflammatory Disease Section, National Human Genome Research Institute (NHGRI), Bethesda, MD, USA

Synonyms

AIPDS Autoinflammation, panniculitis, and dermatosis syndrome; HOIL-1 Heme-oxidized IRP2 ubiquitin ligase 1; HOIP HOIL1 interacting protein; LUBAC Linear ubiquitin chain assembly complex; OTULIN OTU deubiquitinase with linear linkage specificity; Otulipenia/ORAS Otulipenia/Otulin-related autoinflammatory syndrome; SHARPIN SHANK-interacting protein like 1

Definition

Otulipenia or otulin-related autoinflammatory syndrome/ORAS is a rare autosomal recessive disease caused by loss-of-function mutations in *FAM105B*, which encodes the OTULIN (OTU deubiquitinase with linear linkage specificity) (MIM#617099).

Introduction and Background

Post-translational protein modification by ubiquitination (also known as ubiquitylation) has a pivotal role in the regulation of many biological processes and preservation of cellular homeostasis. As deregulation of these processes can result in pathological conditions, including immune disease, tight regulation of ubiquitination is of utmost importance. Ubiquitination is a highly dynamic process that can be reversed by the action of specific enzymes known as deubiqutylases or deubiquitinases (DUBs). Dysregulation of deubiquitination has been recently linked to autoinflammatory diseases (Aksentijevich and Zhou 2017).

Ubiquitination involves the attachment of evolutionarily conserved ubiquitin (Ub) molecules to target proteins in the form of a monomer or polymers (ubiquitin chains; Ub chains). The type of conjugated Ub polymer determines the function and fate of the modified protein by regulating protein activity, interactions, and degradation. Linear (Met1) Ub chains regulate a wide range of immune signaling pathways (Shimizu et al. 2015). Linear (Met1) ubiquitination is carried on by the function of E3 ligase known as the *L*inear *U*biquitin *C*hain *A*ssembly *C*omplex (LUBAC). LUBAC has a pivotal role in the regulation of innate and adaptive immune responses and regulation of cell death. Upon stimulation with proinflammatory stimuli, LUBAC is recruited to activate NF-kB and other signaling pathways. LUBAC depletion leads to attenuation of NF-kB and increases cell death.

LUBAC complex consists of the catalytic subunit HOIP and two accessory proteins: HOIL-1 and SHARPIN. LUBAC activity is counter-regulated by a highly specific DUB named OTULIN. OTULIN is an evolutionarily conserved protein that consists of an N-terminal

O

LUBAC-binding (PIM) domain and a C-terminal ovarian tumor (OTU) domain. Loss of HOIP-OTULIN interaction reduces the capacity of OTULIN capacity to restrict LUBAC-induced NF-kB activation.

Patients with deficiency in LUBAC have severe phenotype and die in early childhood. Their symptoms include features of auto-inflammation and immunodeficiency manifesting with invasive bacterial infections due to compromised NF-kB signaling. In addition, they present with amylopectinosis, which suggest a metabolic function of LUBAC. LUBAC-deficient cells display a variable and cell-dependent pheno-type. Patients' non-myeloid cells (B lymphocytes and fibroblasts) are unresponsive to immune stim-ulations, whereas their monocytes are highly responsive to IL-1 stimulation and produce high levels of proinflammatory cytokines. These obser-vations may explain features of systemic inflam-mation in conjunction with primary immunodeficiency in these patients (Boisson et al. 2012; Boisson et al. 2015).

Genetic loss of the catalytic subunit of LUBAC *Hoip* or the DUB *Otulin* (*gumby/gumby*) in mice results in embryonic lethality due to abnormalities in angiogenesis (Rivkin et al. 2013; Peltzer et al. 2014). Tamoxifen-induced deletion of *Otulin* in immune cells is viable, but mice present with spontaneous and severe neutrophil-mediated multiorgan systemic inflammation. Targeted abla-tion of *Otulin* in myeloid cells leads to chronic inflammation with features of autoimmunity, while loss of *Otulin* in T and B cells produces healthy mice with no overt inflammatory pheno-type. Together, the murine data demonstrate that OTULIN is an essential negative regulator of inflammation in myeloid cells (Damgaard et al. 2016).

Recently, patients with a severe early-onset autoinflammatory phenotype caused by a defect in OTULIN function have been reported. The disease is denoted by various names and acro-nyms: Otulipenia or ORAS or AIPDS (Damgaard et al. 2016; Zhou et al. 2016).

Genetics

Otulipenia/ORAS is caused by loss-of-function (LOF) biallelic mutations in the *FAM105B* gene, which encodes OTULIN. The first four patients with confirmed homozygous mutations in the *FAM105B* gene were identified in founder populations of the Pakistani and Turkish ancestry. Their parents and siblings, who are heterozygote carriers for a disease-causing mutation, are clini-cally asymptomatic. The disease-associated muta-tions have a deleterious effect on protein function since they affect the binding of OTULIN to linear Ub chains on various target molecules. The two missense pathogenic variants, p.Leu272Pro and p.Tyr244Cys, affect highly conserved residues in the OTU domain. The third mutation, p. Gly174Aspfs2*, creates a premature stop codon and results in a truncated mutant protein.

To date, there are only three living patients described in the literature and two siblings who died in early childhood. OTULIN deficiency was confirmed in one of the two postmortem DNA samples. Based on the severity of phenotype, disease-associated mutations are expected to be either novel (unreported in any population data-bases) or present at a very low frequency in the general population. Patients with Otulipenia/ORAS are more likely to be identified in consan-guineous families and in founder populations. More patients are needed to understand the genotype-phenotype correlations associated with the OTULIN deficiency.

Pathogenesis

Mutant OTULIN proteins have defective deubiquitinase function, and they fail to restrict the linear ubiquitination in the NF-κB immune signaling pathway (Fig. 1). As result, primary patients' cells accumulate excessive linear Ub chains upon stimulation with pro-inflammatory stimuli. The affected molecules include the inhibi-tor of nuclear factor kappa-B kinase subunit

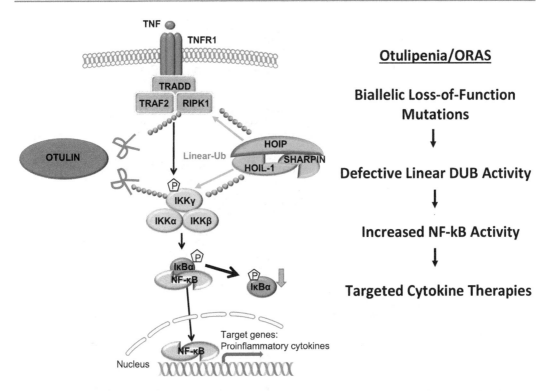

OTULIN Deficiency-Associated Disease Spectrum, Fig. 1 Proposed mechanisms of pathogenesis in otulipenia/ORAS. The canonical NF-κB pathway is regulated by reversible ubiquitination with K63 (Lys63)-linked and linear (Met1)-linked ubiquitin chains. RIPK1 is the central adaptor for assembly of the TNFR1 receptor-signaling complex and is a predominant target for ubiquitination by K63 and linear ubiquitin chains. Poly-ubiquitylated RIPK1 mediates recruitment of IKK complex that is also target for ubiquitination. The activated IKK complex phosphorylates inhibitor of kappa B (IκBα) and targets IκBα for proteasome-mediated degradation. Linear Ub chains are added to RIPK1 and IKKγ by linear ubiquitin chain assembly complex (LUBAC). OTULIN negatively regulates the NF-κB pathway by cleaving linear Ub chains from target molecules, RIPK1 and IKKγ. Decreased expression of OTULIN in patients with otulipenia/ORAS will lead to activation of the NF-κB pathway, increased expression of proinflammatory transcripts in immune cells, and systemic inflammation. TNF receptor 1 (TNFR1); TNFR1-associated death domain protein (TRADD); the death domain-containing protein kinase receptor-interacting protein1 (RIPK1); Inhibitor of nuclear factor kappa-B kinase subunit gamma (IKKγ/NEMO)

gamma (IKK/NEMO), tumor necrosis factor receptor 1 (TNFR1), the death domain-containing protein kinase receptor-interacting protein1 (RIPK1), and the apoptosis-associated speck-like protein with a caspase activation and recruitment domain (ASC/PYCARD). Consequently, patients' mononuclear leukocytes and fibroblasts display enhanced signaling of NF-κB as evidenced by increased phosphorylation of IKKα/IKKβ and IkBα, the hallmarks of the activated NF-kB pathway. Mitogen-activated protein kinases (MAPK) and inflammasome-mediated signaling pathways are also upregulated.

Clinical Manifestations

Patients with Otulipenia/ORAS present with early-onset severe autoinflammatory disease and failure to thrive (Fig. 2). Inflammatory

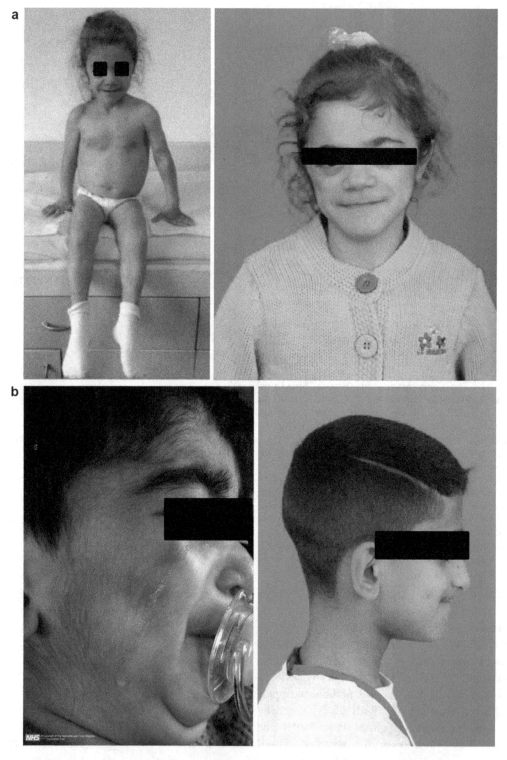

OTULIN Deficiency-Associated Disease Spectrum, Fig. 2 Clinical presentation of otulipenia/ORAS. (Photos were taken before and after the treatment with cytokine inhibitors. Patients had severe growth failure, prominent erythematous skin rash (**a**, **b**) or may have a cushingoid appearance due to treatment with high dose of corticosteroids (**b**))

manifestations include long and recurrent episodes of fever often accompanied with a prominent skin rash, arthralgia/arthritis, myalgia, lymphadenopathy, hepatosplenomegaly, and gastrointestinal inflammation. Acute phase reactants and blood counts, including neutrophils, are highly elevated during episodes of systemic inflammation. Although OTULIN has a critical role in the regulation of immune responses, OTULIN-deficient patients have no obvious immunodeficiency. Two patients suffered from iatrogenic infections coinciding with the use of immunosuppressive therapies.

Cutaneous Manifestations

The cutaneous phenotype is described as erythematous rash with painful skin nodules and may include a progressive fat loss (lipodystrophy). Pustular rash is noted in one patient. Skin biopsies showed evidence for neutrophilic dermatitis and mixed-type panniculitis, which are findings that might resemble patients with CANDLE (*C*hronic *A*typical *N*eutrophilic *D*ermatosis with *L*ipodystrophy and *E*levated Temperature).

Vascular Manifestations

One patient was diagnosed with vasculitis of small and medium-sized blood vessels.

Diagnosis

Diagnosis could be clinical or molecular. Patients may have a positive family history for a severe inflammatory disease. Other clinical features are nonspecific and may resemble patients with CANDLE. Molecular diagnostic testing involves targeted sequencing of the *FAM105B* (NM_138348. 5) gene. This gene has now been included in many targeted sequencing gene panels for immunodeficiency in private and research diagnostic laboratories. Protein diagnostic test is not available.

Laboratory Testing

Immunophenotyping is not diagnostic; preliminary investigations of the three affected patients revealed normal levels of immunoglobulins, normal to high T and B cell counts, and lower NK cell counts. The patients had adequate specific antibody responses to vaccines and adequate T and B cell proliferative responses to TCR and BCR stimulation. Cytokine profiling of patients' serum samples and supernatants of stimulated peripheral blood leucocytes showed highly increased levels of many proinflammatory cytokines and chemokines. Gene expression profiling of patients' whole blood RNA samples and RNA from stimulated fibroblasts demonstrated strong inflammatory signatures enriched for NF-κB, Jak-STAT, and TNF signaling (Zhou et al. 2016). Although the gene expression and cytokine inflammatory signatures are very significant, they are nonspecific for Otulipenia/ORAS and can be found in other diseases caused by upregulated NF-κB.

Treatment

Patients with OTULIN deficiency have excellent response to treatment with cytokine inhibitors. In particular, anti-TNF therapy is very effective in normalizing acute phase reactants and in controlling disease activity. One patient has been empirically treated with a TNF inhibitor (infliximab) for about 10 years prior to his molecular diagnosis. Within 1 month of starting infliximab, his fevers and rash subsided and 8 years after initiation of the treatment he is fully functional. IL-1 inhibitors may also be used for suppressing inflammation, although they appear less efficacious than TNF inhibitors. An interferon signature (IFN) was identified in two patients with active disease, but treatments targeting IFN signaling have not been used to treat patients.

Prognosis

The phenotype is very severe and potentially lethal if left untreated.

Cross-References

▶ Management of Immunodeficiency, Overview

References

Aksentijevich I, Zhou Q. NF-kappaB pathway in auto-inflammatory diseases: dysregulation of protein modifications by ubiquitin defines a new category of autoinflammatory diseases. Front Immunol. 2017;8: 399.

Boisson B, Laplantine E, Prando C, Giliani S, Israelsson E, Xu Z, et al. Immunodeficiency, autoinflammation and amylopectinosis in humans with inherited HOIL-1 and LUBAC deficiency. Nat Immunol. 2012;13(12): 1178–86.

Boisson B, Laplantine E, Dobbs K, Cobat A, Tarantino N, Hazen M, et al. Human HOIP and LUBAC deficiency underlies autoinflammation, immunodeficiency, amylopectinosis, and lymphangiectasia. J Exp Med. 2015;212(6):939–51.

Damgaard RB, Walker JA, Marco-Casanova P, Morgan NV, Titheradge HL, Elliott PR, et al. The Deubiquitinase OTULIN is an essential negative regulator of inflammation and autoimmunity. Cell. 2016;166(5):1215–30.e20.

Peltzer N, Rieser E, Taraborrelli L, Draber P, Darding M, Pernaute B, et al. HOIP deficiency causes embryonic lethality by aberrant TNFR1-mediated endothelial cell death. Cell Rep. 2014;9(1):153–65.

Rivkin E, Almeida SM, Ceccarelli DF, Juang YC, MacLean TA, Srikumar T, et al. The linear ubiquitin-specific deubiquitinase gumby regulates angiogenesis. Nature. 2013;498(7454):318–24.

Shimizu Y, Taraborrelli L, Walczak H. Linear ubiquitination in immunity. Immunol Rev. 2015; 266(1):190–207.

Zhou Q, Yu X, Demirkaya E, Deuitch N, Stone D, Tsai WL, et al. Biallelic hypomorphic mutations in a linear deubiquitinase define otulipenia, an early-onset autoinflammatory disease. Proc Natl Acad Sci U S A. 2016;113(36):10127–32.

OTULIN OTU Deubiquitinase with Linear Linkage Specificity

▶ OTULIN Deficiency-Associated Disease Spectrum

Otulipenia/ORAS Otulipenia/ Otulin-Related Autoinflammatory Syndrome

▶ OTULIN Deficiency-Associated Disease Spectrum

P

P14/LAMTOR2 Deficiency

Persio Roxo-Junior and Isabela Mina
Division of Immunology and Allergy, Department
of Pediatrics, Ribeirão Preto Medical School,
University of São Paulo, Ribeirão Preto, Brazil

Definition

P14/LAMTOR2 deficiency is a very rare primary
immunodeficiency syndrome due to a homozygous single point mutation in *p14* (also known
as *LAMTOR2*) gene that causes reduction in the
p14 protein expression, which is associated with
severe congenital neutropenia and abnormal function of specialized lysosomes in cells of innate and
adaptive immune system (Taub et al. 2012).

Introduction

The endosomal adaptor protein p14, also known
as the late endosomal/lysosomal adaptor and
mitogen-activated protein kinase (MAPK) and
mammalian target of rapamycin (mTOR) activa-
tor/regulator complex 2 (LAMTOR2) (Sparber
et al. 2015), is specifically required to regulate
endosomal traffic and cellular proliferation
(Rezaei et al. 2009). If there are biallelic mutations within its 3′-untranslated region (UTR),
proper processing of p14 mRNA is suppressed
(Speckmann et al. 2017).

The p14/LAMTOR2 deficiency is transmitted
through an autosomal recessive pattern (Rezaei
et al. 2009) and causes reduced p14 protein
expression (Taub et al. 2012).

This deficiency is characterized by severe neutropenia and leads to disorder at lysosomes in
neutrophils, cytotoxic T cells, and melanocytes,
besides reduced numbers of B cell subsets (Rezaei
et al. 2009).

Clinical Presentation

Patients with p14/LAMTOR2 deficiency present
early-onset recurrent respiratory infections (Taub
et al. 2012; Rezaei et al. 2009), oculocutaneous
hypopigmentation, short stature, and coarse facial
features (Rezaei et al. 2009; Klein and Welte
2010).

The infections usually occur by the age of
1 year. The most common present features are
cutaneous infections, superficial abscesses, oral
ulcers, otitis media, and recurrent pneumonia.
Frequent aphthous stomatitis and gingival hyperplasia lead to loss of permanent teeth in
childhood.

These patients have high susceptibility to
extracellular pathogens, such as *Pseudomonas
aeruginosa*, *Escherichia coli*, and *Streptococcus
pneumoniae*, which occurs on a secondary basis
because of deficient intracellular organelle fusion
in neutrophils and B and T cells. Furthermore, it
was demonstrated that the endosomal adaptor

© Springer Science+Business Media LLC, part of Springer Nature 2020
I. R. Mackay et al. (eds.), *Encyclopedia of Medical Immunology*,
https://doi.org/10.1007/978-1-4614-8678-7

protein p14 is an essential component of the defense against intracellular pathogens as well, such as *Salmonella* (Taub et al. 2012).

Laboratory Findings and Diagnostic Testing

Presence of severe neutropenia associated with early-onset severe and recurrent infections should raise suspicion of p14/LAMTOR2 deficiency, especially in the presence of short stature, oculocutaneous hypopigmentation, and coarse facial features.

Patients typically have persistent severe neutropenia with absolute neutrophil count of less than 500/mm³. In relation to complete blood cell count, patients usually present an increased number of platelets, monocytes, and eosinophils, while mild anemia is frequently seen. The p14/LAMTOR2 deficiency is associated with disorders in other elements of the immune system, such as reduced numbers of B cell subgroups and deficient function of cytotoxic T cells (Rezaei et al. 2009). Memory B cells can be reduced in these patients as well as low serum IgM levels. There are some reports of patients who presented low levels of IgG during adolescence. However, neutrophil maturation in the bone marrow seems to be normal (Rezaei et al. 2009; Klein and Welte 2010).

The diagnosis of this immunodeficiency is made through genetic evaluation that identifies homozygous point mutation in the 3'-untranslated region (3'-UTR) of the gene that encodes the endosomal adaptor molecule p14 (Rezaei et al. 2009; Klein and Welte 2010). This mutation causes a reduction at p14 protein levels that, consequently, leads to neutrophils with a modified ultrastructure of azurophilic granules and diminished microbicidal activity in phagosomes (Klein and Welte 2010). Besides that, the cells with p14 deficiency present a marked delocalization of late endosomes and show a deficiency in cytokine receptor-mediated ERK (extracellular signaling-regulated kinase) phosphorylation (Klein and Welte 2010; Klein 2009).

Treatment and Prognosis

Timely referral to a clinical immunologist and/or a hematologist remains key to the successful management of patients with p14/LAMTOR2 deficiency, as delay in starting the appropriate treatment reflects in high mortality.

The main goal of therapeutic for patients with severe congenital neutropenia is to reestablish the adequate antibacterial host defense. The first option of therapy is the use of recombinant human granulocyte colony-stimulating factor (GCSF) (Klein 2009). Before the emergence of this therapy, morbidity and mortality among patients with severe neutropenia in childhood were elevated due to severe and recurrent bacterial infections. Today, the improvement of quality of life and survival into adulthood is possible due to GCSF (Rezaei et al. 2009; Klein and Welte 2010). Approximately 90% or more of the patients have a good response to GCSF and experience an increase of neutrophil number and a consequently reduced number of infections and days of hospitalization.

Patients who do not respond to the therapy with GCSF are candidates to be submitted to allogeneic hematopoietic stem cell transplantation as a curative therapeutic strategy (Klein 2009).

Gammaglobulin replacement therapy can be indicated for the group of patients with low IgG levels, especially if these patients present recurrent infections (Speckmann et al. 2017).

It is strongly recommended that all patients should be followed up at least twice a year and complete blood cell counts should be performed at least every 3 months (Welte et al. 2006).

References

Klein C. Congenital neutropenia. Hematology Am Soc Hematol Educ Program. 2009;1:344–50.

Klein C, Welte K. Genetic insights into congenital neutropenia. Clin Rev Allergy Immunol. 2010;38(1):68–74.

Rezaei N, Moazzami K, Aghamohammadi A, Klein C. Neutropenia and primary immunodeficiency diseases. Int Rev Immunol. 2009;28(5):335–66.

Sparber F, Tripp CH, Komenda K, Scheffler JM, Clausen BE, Huber LA, et al. The late endosomal adaptor molecule p14 (LAMTOR2) regulates TGFβ1-mediated homeostasis of Langerhans cells. J Invest Dermatol. 2015;135(1):119–29.

Speckmann C, Borkhardt A, Gaspar B, Gambineri E, Ehl S. Genetic disorders of immune regulation. In: Rezaei N, Aghamohammadi A, Notarangelo LD, editors. Primary immunodeficiency diseases: definition, diagnosis, and management. 2nd ed. Berlin: Springer; 2017. p. 310–1.

Taub N, Nairz M, Hilber D, Hess MW, Weiss G, Huber LA. The late endosomal adaptor p14 is a macrophage host defense factor against *Salmonella* infection. J Cell Sci. 2012;125(Pt 11):2698–708.

Welte K, Zeidler C, Dale DC. Severe congenital neutropenia. Semin Hematol. 2006;43(3):189–95.

p56LCK

▶ Lymphocyte-Specific Protein Tyrosine Kinase: LCK

PAPA

▶ Pyogenic Arthritis, Pyoderma Gangrenosum, and Acne (PAPA) Syndrome

Papillon-Lefèvre Syndrome

Herberto Jose Chong-Neto
Division of Allergy and Immunology, Department of Pediatrics, Federal University of Parana Medical School, Curitiba, Brazil

Definition

Papillon-Lefèvre syndrome is an autosomal recessive disease classified as a type IV palmoplantar ectodermal dysplasia, caused by a cathepsin C mutation.

Introduction

Cathepsins are digestive enzymes with proteolytic activity in acidic environments. They were described by Willstatter and Bamnn in 1929, derived from the Greek words *kata* and *hepsein*, meaning boil down.

These lysosomal proteases have an essential role to maintain intracellular homeostasis, especially in the immunity, infection, cancers, and autoimmunity.

Papillon-Lefèvre syndrome was first described in 1924. It is a rare autosomal recessive disease, with no racial or sexual gender preference and prevalence estimated to 1–4 per million.

Humans have about 15 cathepsins, and some gene mutations are associated to severe inherited diseases, as the cathepsin C (*CTSC*) mutation that cause Papillon-Lefèvre syndrome.

The *CTSC* gene is localized on chromosome 11q14.1-q14.3 with seven exons. It is expressed in several tissues, especially in the lungs, kidneys, placenta, and liver as well as in areas commonly affected in Papillon-Lefèvre syndrome. Additionally *CTSC* is highly expressed in immune cells, including polymorphonuclear leukocytes and macrophages.

It has been shown to be required for the activation of neutrophil elastase, lymphocytes, and natural killer cells with a potential role in the immune system (Ketterer et al. 2017).

Clinical Presentation

The Papillon-Lefèvre syndrome is hallmarked by severe periodontal disease, and dysfunction of serine proteases and neutrophils can lead to the growth of periodontal pathogenic bacteria, associated to erythematous diffuse palmoplantar hyperkeratosis with thickening of the epidermis and slight increased susceptibility to infections. Parental consanguinity is reported in one third of cases. (Entry Figs. 1 and 2: **Hyperkeratosis palmoplantar. Collection of Division of Pediatric Dermatology, Federal University of Paraná**).

**Papillon-Lefèvre
Syndrome,
Fig. 1** Hyperkeratosis
palmar

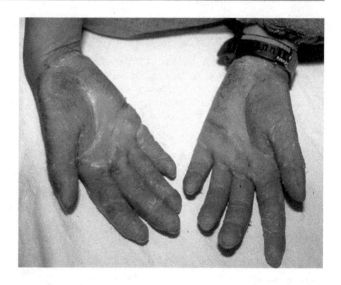

**Papillon-Lefèvre
Syndrome,
Fig. 2** Hyperkeratosis
plantar

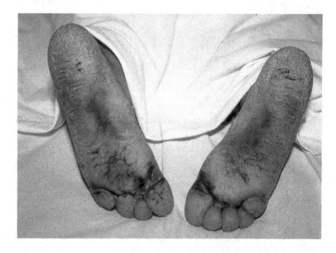

The diagnosis of the disorder may not be confirmed until inflammation and degeneration of the tissues surrounding and supporting the teeth (periodontium) become apparent. This usually occurs between the third and fifth year of life, when the infant teeth (deciduous) begin to erupt. In many people, abnormalities of the skin occur simultaneously with the loss of teeth.

Hyperhidrosis are reported with bromhidrosis and may appear in the elbows and knees. Besides the aggressive periodontal inflammation, the eruption of teeth starts at a normal age. The patient shows that gingivae harbor *Aggregatibacter actinomycetemcomitans* preferentially.

Differential diagnoses are Haim-Munk syndrome, also known as keratosis palmoplantaris with periodontopathia, Schopf-Schulz-Passarge syndrome, pachyonychia congenita, Meleda disease, Sjogren-Larsson syndrome, and Fitzsimmons syndrome (AlBarrak et al. 2016).

Laboratory Findings/Diagnostic Testing

The diagnosis of Papillon-Lefèvre syndrome may be confirmed by a thorough clinical evaluation that includes a detailed patient history and identification of characteristic physical findings.

A diagnosis can be made by a simple analysis of an infant's or child's urine (urinary analysis). The urine of a child suspected of having Papillon-Lefèvre syndrome is tested to see whether there is any activity of the enzyme cathepsin C. Little or no activity of this enzyme is diagnostic of the disorder. This is extremely important because early diagnosis and prompt treatment can potentially prevent aggressive periodontitis and tooth loss and improve overall quality of life of people with Papillon-Lefèvre syndrome (Hamon et al. 2016).

Molecular genetic testing can confirm a diagnosis and detect alterations in the *CTSC* gene known to cause Papillon-Lefèvre syndrome but is available only as a diagnostic service at specialized laboratories (Alkhiary et al. 2016).

Treatment/Prognosis

The treatment of Papillon-Lefèvre syndrome is focused in the hyperkeratosis and periodontitis. Combined periodontic and orthodontic treatments have been successfully applied in children.

Topical lubricants and moisturizers (emollients) have limited success in treating associated skin abnormalities.

Keratolic agents and topical steroids, which reduce inflammation of the skin, have been used to treat the palmoplantar hyperkeratosis. Acitretin treatment was used in cycles, for each 2 months, given 1 month apart. After 4 months, the extent relapse was observed, and improvement remained stable at the end of 1-year follow-up.

Etretinate, isotretinoin, and acitretin have been used reducing inflammation and decreasing the loss of teeth. Vitamin A may alleviate skin abnormalities and help to minimize recurrent pus producing. More research must be conducted before the long-term safety and effectiveness of using retinoids to treat Papillon-Lefèvre syndrome can be determined (Sarma et al. 2015).

References

AlBarrak ZM, Alqarni AS, Chalisserry EP, Anil S. Papillon-Lefèvre syndrome: a series of five cases among siblings. J Med Case Rep. 2016;10:260.

Alkhiary YM, Jelani M, Almramhi MM, et al. Whole-exome sequencing reveals a recurrent mutation in the cathepsin C gene that causes Papillon-Lefèvre syndrome in a Saudi family. Saudi J Biol Sci. 2016;23:571–6.

Hamon Y, Legowska M, Fergelot P, et al. Analysis of urinary cathepsin C for diagnosing Papillon-Lefèvre syndrome. FEBS J. 2016;283:498–509.

Ketterer S, Gomez-Auli A, Hillebrand LE, et al. Inherited diseases caused by miutations in cathepsin protease genes. FEBS J. 2017;284:1437–54.

Sarma N, Ghosh C, Kar S, Bazmi BA. Low-dose acitretin in Papillon-Lefèvre syndrome: treatment and 1-year follow-up. Dermatol Ther. 2015;28:28–31.

Paracaspase 1

▶ MALT1 Deficiency

Partial 11q Monosomy Syndrome

▶ Jacobsen Syndrome

PCASP1

▶ MALT1 Deficiency

PCFT: Proton-Coupled Folate Transporter

▶ Defects in B12 and Folate Metabolism (TCN2, SLC46A1 (PCFT Deficiency), MTHFD1)

Pediatric Granulomatous Arthritis

▶ Blau Syndrome

Periodic Neutropenia

▶ Cyclic Neutropenia

PGM3-Deficiency

Aniko Malik
Department of Pediatrics, Semmelweis
University, Budapest, Hungary
Pediatric Immunology, IWK Health Centre,
Halifax, NS, Canada

Introduction/Background

Initially, mutations in **phosphoglucomutase 3** (which is involved in protein glycosylation pathways) have been identified in autosomal recessive forms of Hyper IgE (HIES) syndrome, characterized by eczema, recurrent skin and sinopulmonary infections, and elevated serum IgE (**OMIM# 172100**) (Zhang et al. 2014; Sassi et al. 2014; Ben-Khemis et al. 2017; Yang et al. 2014). Later, whole exome sequencing (WES) led to the identification of diverse phenotypes associated with PGM3 mutations. Beyond HIES phenotype, SCID-like presentations with neutropenia were also described with homozygous or compound heterozygous *PGM3* mutations (Stray-Pedersen et al. 2014; Bernth-Jensen et al. 2015; Pacheco-Cuellar et al. 2017).

Glycosylation is a posttranslational modification, which essentially influences the function or fate of many proteins, including those related to immune mechanisms. Glycosylation has a pivotal role in altering interactions between cells and their environment (e.g., extra-cellular matrix and serum molecules). Since the immune response is based on uncountable contacts between cells and molecules, glycans play an essential role in immune interactions such as pathogen and other antigen recognition, inflammation, immune responses, and cancer (Monticelli et al. 2016).

Congenital disorders of glycosylation (CDG) lead to aberrant modification of serum glycoproteins such as immune receptors, immunoglobulins, proteins of complement cascade, and cytokines, which are essential for the integrity of immune functions. CDGs are typically multiorgan diseases since glycans play important roles in all organs and tissues. In the majority of CDGs, the skeletal and the nervous systems are involved, which leads to developmental delay, hypotonia, hyporeflexia, and ataxia (Monticelli et al. 2016).

PGM3 Function

Phosphoglucomutase 3 (PGM3) protein catalyzes the reversible conversion of N-acetyl-D-glucosamine-6-phosphate (GlcNAc-6-P) to N-acetyl-D-glucosamine-1-phosphate (GlcNAc-1-P), which is required for the synthesis of uridine diphosphate N-acetylglucosamine (UDP-GlcNAc), an important precursor for posttranslational protein glycosylation (Fig. 1).

Indeed, UDP-GlcNAc is an essential building block for N-glycans, O-glycans, proteoglycans, and glycolipids. Glycosylated proteins are found in various intracellular compartments, on the cell surface, in the cytoplasm, and in the extracellular matrix. In addition, UDP-GlcNAc is also a substrate for O-linked N-acetylglucosamine transferases in the cytosol or the nucleus, and thus participates in cell signaling.

Clinical Presentation

In humans, whole-exome sequencing (WES) led to the identification of diverse phenotypes and clinical heterogeneity associated with *PGM3* mutations in 26 AR-HIES patients from highly consanguineous families. The clinical presentation includes features of Hyper-IgE syndrome such as atopic disease (such as eczema, allergy, asthma), recurrent skin and pulmonary infections, skeletal, renal, and intestinal abnormalities, autoimmunity, as well as neurologic (developmental delay or severe mental retardation) and in some cases hematologic involvement (neutropenia, lymphopenia, anemia, Hodgkin lymphoma) (Zhang et al. 2014; Sassi et al. 2014; Ben-Khemis et al. 2017; Yang et al. 2014).

Furthermore, an early onset $T^-B^-NK^+$ SCID phenotype and skeletal dysplasia has been reported in six patients so far. Four cases had neutropenia (Stray-Pedersen et al. 2014; Bernth-Jensen 2015), two cases had bone marrow failure, renal malformations, and intestinal involvement (Pacheco-Cuellar et al.

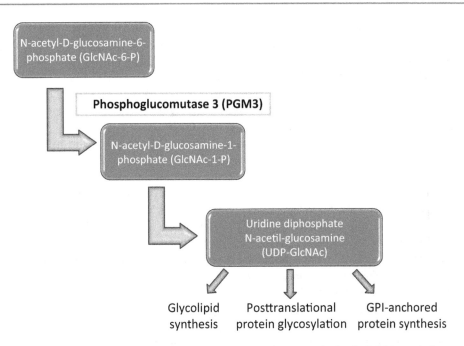

PGM3-Deficiency, Fig. 1 Role of phophoglucomutase 3 (PGM3) in the synthesis of UDP-N-acetyl-glucosamine, a critical building substrate for glycoproteins and glycolipids

2017). In one of the mentioned patients, the NK cell counts decreased by 9 weeks and the phenotype was then consistent with a T⁻B⁻NK⁻ phenotype (Bernth-Jensen et al. 2015).

An atypical presentation of normal IgE level and lack of the developmental defects in the nervous and skeletal systems was described in four siblings with immunodeficiency. The features of immunodeficiency were recurrent skin abscesses, otitis media, bronchitis, pneumonia, severe varicella infection, neutropenia, and eosinophilia (Lundin et al. 2015).

Thus, a total of 36 patients from 14 families have been reported to have pathogenic PGM3 mutations.

Infectious complications: Recurrent infections were highly frequent in patients with *PGM3* mutations. Majority of the patients had a history of skin infections (mostly secondary to eczema; subcutaneous abscesses), and most of them suffered from recurrent respiratory tract infections (otitis media, pneumonias). Pneumatoceles often developed as a complication of pneumonia, which was previously presumed to be pathognomonic for STAT3 HIES. Moderate-to-severe bronchiectasis developed among older patients, leading to chronic respiratory failure. Gastrointestinal infections (acute or chronic diarrhea) and encephalitis were also reported. Recurrent *Staphylococcus aureus* infection was highly prevalent. Other bacteria, like Enterococcus cloacae, group A Streptococcus, and Klebsiella pneumonia were also cultured from skin ulcers. Chronic candidiasis and severe viral infections were also prominent, including influenza virus, Epstein-Barr virus, respiratory syncytial virus, herpes simplex virus, and varicella zoster virus.

Allergic complications: Atopy was a characteristic clinical finding in patients with *PGM3* mutations and occurred in majority of the patients. Allergic manifestations included asthma, allergic rhinitis, food and drug allergy, and atopic dermatitis.

Autoimmunity: Autoimmune manifestations in a few patients were like polyarticular arthritis, cutaneous leukocytoclastic vasculitis, or membranoproliferative glomerulonephritis.

Musculoskeletal manifestations: Dysmorphic facial features, musculoskeletal, and connective tissue manifestations are frequently present, similarly as in patients with HIES due to *STAT3* mutations. Characteristic face with wide nostrils and prominent lips, downturned corners of the mouth, midface hypoplasia, and micrognathia, inverted epicanthal folds, short nose, low-set ears, hypertelorism were reported. Four patients had radiographic features of Debuquois-like dysplasia (extra ossification centers) associated with shortened tubular bones, brachydactyly, anomalies in metacarpals, metatarsal, and phalanges bones, clefting of vertebrae, exaggerated lesser trochanter (Stray-Pedersen et al. 2014; Pacheco-Cuellar et al. 2017).

Neurologic complications: Neurologic impairment is commonly seen in patients with CDGs and most likely due to defective glycosylation in the central nervous system. Similarly, among the published PGM3 deficient cases, the majority was reported to have a developmental delay and mental retardation, followed by psychomotor retardation, hypotonia, ataxia, dysarthria, sensorineural hearing loss, myoclonus, seizures, decreased myelinization, and periventricular lesions. But it should be noted, not all mutations in the PGM3 gene necessarily cause developmental or neurological disturbances (Lundin et al. 2015).

Other rare manifestations: One patient had unilateral renal agenesis, while three patients had horseshoe kidney. Intestinal manifestations were also described (esophageal stricture, intestinal malrotation, or obstruction). Two patients, identical twin boys, developed Hodgkin lymphoma and were successfully treated with chemotherapy (Zhang et al. 2014).

Laboratory Findings/Diagnostic Testing

According to the initial reports, high serum IgE was mentioned as a characteristic finding in PGM3 mutations, but later it turned out that not all mutation in this gene lead to HIES phenotype. Early onset with a severe combined immunodeficiency-like phenotype also has been described with or without increased serum IgE.

The immunologic phenotype of the HIES patients is not consistent, but in most cases, they presented with low CD4 and in some cases low CD8 numbers. Lymphocyte mitogen proliferation was also impaired, in those cases where it was measured. IgA levels were elevated in this group. Neutropenia and eosinophilia also frequently accompanied, but granulocytes showed normal chemotaxis and surface expression of glycosylphosphatidylinositol (GPI)-anchored proteins, which regulate leukocyte adhesion, polarization, and motility.

Four of those cases who had SCID phenotype (6/36) presented as $T^-B^-NK^+$ SCID. Interestingly, in one case, the NK cell counts decreased by 9 weeks, and the phenotype was then consistent with a $T^-B^-NK^-$ phenotype (Bernth-Jensen et al. 2015). In another family, two siblings had $T^-B^-NK^-$ SCID, developed bone marrow failure, and other organ involvement. Pacheco-Cuellar et al. (2017) IgE was high in one case, but normal in the others, while IgA was low in most of the cases. All of these patients had congenital neutropenia.

Eventually, in one family, four siblings had normal to low values of lymphopenia and neutropenia, eosinophilia, increased IgA, but normal IgE levels, and there was also a lack of the developmental defects in the nervous and skeletal systems (Lundin et al. 2015).

Clinical screening tests for CDG (e.g., serum transferrin and apolipoprotein CIII isoform analysis test) did not show abnormalities (Stray-Pedersen et al. 2014).

Reported Mutations

The mutations in *PGM3* reported in previous studies comprise four homozygous mutations predicting amino acid changes (p.Glu340del, p. Leu83Ser, p.Asp502Tyr, p.Ile322Thr) identified in seven affected HIES families (Sassi et al. 2014; Lundin et al. 2015; Ben-Khemis et al. 2017), a homozygous missense mutation (p. Asp325Glu) in two patients and compound heterozygous mutations (p.Glu529Gln and p. Leu480Serfs10) in four sequenced patients in another family (Zhang et al. 2014). The six SCID patients had either homozygous mutations (p.Asn246Ser; p.Asp239His; p.Phe379Leu) (Stray-Pedersen et al. 2014; Bernth-Jensen et al. 2015; Pacheco-Cuellar et al. 2017) or a compound heterozygous mutation (p.Asn246Lysfs*7 and p. Gln451Arg) (Stray-Pedersen et al. 2014).

In addition, enzymatic assays confirmed the diminished PGM3 enzyme activity with consequential reduction in UDP-GlcNAc in cells carrying some of the mentioned mutations with different degrees of residual activity, which possibly can be related with the severity of the clinical features.

Treatment/Prognosis

The management of patients with PGM3 deficiency is still being defined. The described treatments have generally been supportive, including antibiotic prophylaxis, eczema management, treatment of infections, and auto-inflammatory conditions as they arise. Antimicrobial prophylaxis proved moderately beneficial, but immunoglobulin replacement trials did not reduce these infections in a clinically significant way.

Nevertheless, several children have been described with severe combined immunodeficiency-like presentations and pancytopenia, and two of those received early and successful hematopoietic stem cell transplantation (HSCT) (Stray-Pedersen et al. 2014). However, treatment with HSCT is lifesaving; it remains unclear if HSCT will correct the neurologic and other somatic features. In other cases, HSCT was not performed due to the other respiratory, intestinal, and renal complications that rendered HSCT a high-risk procedure.

Other congenital disorders of glycosylation have been treated with dietary supplementation to bypass the pathway abnormalities. As to treatment, the administration of GlcNAc would be a logical approach. Indeed, GlcNAc supplementation restored intracellular UDP-GlcNAc levels in PGM3-deficient cells (Zhang et al. 2014), but its therapeutic value in patients remains unknown.

Cross-References

▶ Autosomal Dominant Hyper IgE Syndrome

References

Ben-Khemis L, et al. A founder mutation underlies a severe form of phosphoglucomutase 3 (PGM3) deficiency in Tunisian patients. Mol Immunol. 2017;90:57–63.

Bernth-Jensen JM, et al. Neonatal-onset T-B-NK+ severe combined immunodeficiency and neutropenia caused by mutated phosphoglucomutase 3. J Allergy Clin Immunol. 2015;137:321–4.

Lundin KE, et al. Susceptibility to infections, without concomitant hyper-IgE, reported in 1976, is caused by hypomorphic mutation in the phosphoglucomutase 3 (PGM3) gene. Clin Immunol. 2015;161:366–72.

Monticelli M, et al. Immunological aspects of congenital disorders of glycosylation (CDG): a review. J Inherit Metab Dis. 2016;39:765–80.

Pacheco-Cuellar G, et al. A novel PGM3 mutation is associated with severe phenotype of bone marrow failure, severe combined immunodeficiency, skeletal dysplasia, and congenital malformations. J Bone Miner Res. 2017;32:1853–9.

Sassi A, et al. Hypomorphic homozygous mutations in phosphoglucomutase 3 (PGM3) impair immunity and increase serum IgE levels. J Allergy Clin Immunol. 2014;133:1411–9.

Stray-Pedersen A, et al. PGM3 mutations cause a congenital disorder of glycosylation with severe immunodeficiency and skeletal dysplasia. Am J Hum Genet. 2014;95:96–107.

Yang L, et al. Hyper IgE syndromes: reviewing PGM3 deficiency. Curr Opin Pediatr. 2014;26:697–703.

Zhang Y, et al. Autosomal recessive phosphoglucomutase 3 (PGM3) mutations link glycosylation defects to atopy, immune deficiency, autoimmunity, and neurocognitive impairment. J Allergy Clin Immunol. 2014;133:1400–9.

P

PIK3R1 Deficiency-Associated Agammaglobulinemia

Vassilios Lougaris and Alessandro Plebani
Pediatrics Clinic and Institute for Molecular
Medicine A. Nocivelli, Department of Clinical
and Experimental Sciences, University of Brescia
and ASST-Spedali Civili of Brescia, Brescia, Italy

Definition

Phosphatidylinositol 3-kinase, regulatory subunit 1 (PIK3R1) deficiency (OMIM #615214) is a rare primary immunodeficiency characterized by reduced serum levels of all immunoglobulin classes, with absent or very low number of peripheral B cells (peripheral B cells <2%). To date, three patients have been described. PIK3R1 deficiency is caused by biallelic deleterious mutations (W298∗ in one patient and R301∗ in two patients) in the gene *PIK3R1* encoding for p85α, located in chromosome 5q13.1.

p85α is a regulatory protein that together with catalytic p110δ or PIK3CD form the lipid kinase phosphatidylinositol 3-kinase (PI3K).

The heterozygous mutation R649W and others in the c-SH2 domain of the PIK3R1 have been associated with SHORT syndrome (short stature, hyperextensibility, ocular depression, Rieger anomaly and teething delay, lipodystrophy, and insulin resistance) in several probands from at least 14 unrelated families (Nunes-Santos et al. 2019). Counterintuitively, monoallelic missense loss of function mutations in the intermediate SH2 domain of the *PIK3R1* gene disrupts the regulatory function of PIK3R1 and results in increased PI3K activity, which leads to a combined immunodeficiency of more clinical severity than the agammaglobulinemia resulting from absent PIK3R1.

Pathogenesis

Early B cell development takes place in the bone marrow. An important maturational step is the progression from the pro-B to the pre-B stage (Espeli et al. 2006; Rudin and Thompson 1998; Bartholdy and Matthias 2004). This passage depends on the expression of a functional B cell receptor composed of the μ heavy chain (*IGHM*; OMIM∗147020), Igα (CD79A; OMIM∗112205), Igβ (CD79B; OMIM∗147245), VpreB, and λ5 (*IGLL1*; OMIM∗146770) that initiates downstream signaling necessary for early B cell differentiation through kinases such as BTK and BLNK (OMIM∗604615). Animal models and in vitro studies over the years have underlined the importance of each of the pre-BCR components and associated transcription factors for the transition from pro-B to pre-B stage of maturation, suggesting that these genes may be

responsible for agammaglobulinemia in humans (Conley and Cooper 1998).

Engagement of the pre-BCR and BCR leads to activation of the PI3K pathway. Deficiency of the PI3K regulatory subunit, p85α, was identified as causative of agammaglobulinemia. The first patient was described by Conley et al. in 2012 and harbored a homozygous truncating mutation in PIK3R1. The second patient was described by Tang et al. in 2018, also with a homozygous truncating mutation. B cells were absent in the periphery. Bone marrow evaluation revealed an earlier block in B cell development than what was observed in patients with defects in components of the pre-BCR. Tang et al. also reported an affected sibling with autosomal recessive agammaglobulinemia due to PIK3R1 deficiency caused by a homozygous mutation in PIK3R1 leading to a premature stop codon.

Clinical Presentation

Conley et al. reported on a female patient born to consanguineous parents. The first evaluation was made at the age of 3.5 months for neutropenia, interstitial pneumonia, and gastroenteritis (de la Morena et al. 1995). Her immunological work-up showed lack of peripheral B cells (<1%) and agammaglobulinemia. She received immunoglobulin replacement therapy with progressive resolution of the neutropenia and the clinical manifestations. However, her clinical history worsened during follow-up with development of arthritis at the age of 12 years. At the age of 17 years, the patient was diagnosed with inflammatory bowel disease and Campylobacter bacteremia. The second patient reported by Tang et al. is a female born to consanguineous parents that was admitted at the age of 10 months for tongue ulcers and mucosal bleeding. She was found to have thrombocytopenia, neutropenia, and absence of B cells. Previous clinical history included diarrhea, recurrent respiratory infections, and oral thrush with progressive development of lung nodules. She is currently stable under weekly SCIG treatment. When she was almost 3 years old, a brother was born, and neonatal immunological evaluation showed absence of peripheral B cells allowing a diagnosis of autosomal recessive agammaglobulinemia. Initially, neutropenia and oral thrush were present that progressively resolved upon initiation of IVIG.

Diagnosis

Immunological work-up in affected patients shows almost undetectable levels of serum immunoglobulins and the absence of peripheral B cells. Genetic screening for mutations in components of the pre-BCR and downstream signaling molecules such as BLNK and p85α should be performed. If patient is male, BTK might be screened first due to its X-linked inheritance manner, otherwise, search for gene defects inherited in a recessive manner, especially if there is evidence of consanguinity.

Management

As in other forms of primary humoral immunodeficiencies, immunoglobulin replacement treatment should be undertaken once the immunological diagnosis of agammaglobulinemia is established. Currently two options are available: intravenous or subcutaneous. Normally, a dose of 400 mg/kg/dose every 3–4 weeks is sufficient to maintain pre-infusion IgG levels >500 mg/dl that should be able to reduce the number of infectious episodes, especially that of invasive infections.

Antibiotic usage should be considered for every infectious episode, and in some cases, prophylactic regimen may also be prescribed.

Considering that only three affected patients have been reported, long-term progress of disease is not well known.

References

Bartholdy B, Matthias P. Transcriptional control of B cell development and function. Gene. 2004;327:1–23.

Conley ME, Cooper MD. Genetic basis of abnormal B cell development. Curr Opin Immunol. 1998; 10(4):339–406.

Conley ME, Dobbs AK, Quintana AM, Bosompem A, Wang YD, Coustan-Smith E, Smith AM, Perez EE, Murray PJ. Agammaglobulinemia and absent B lineage cells in a patient lacking the p85alpha subunit of PI3K. J Exp Med. 2012;209:463–70.

de la Morena M, Haire RN, Ohta Y, Nelson RP, Litman RT, Day NK, Good RA, Litman GW. Predominance of sterile immunoglobulin transcripts in a female phenotypically resembling Bruton's agammaglobulinemia. Eur J Immunol. 1995;25:809–15.

Espeli M, Rossi B, Mancini SJ, Roche P, Gauthier L, Schiff C. Initiation of pre-B cell receptor signaling: common and distinctive features in human and mouse. Semin Immunol. 2006;18:56–66.

Nunes-Santos CJ, Uzel G, Rosenzweig SD. PI3K pathway defects leading to immunodeficiency and immune dysregulation. J Allergy Clin Immunol. 2019 May;143(5):1676–87.

Rudin CM, Thompson CB. B-cell development and maturation. Semin Oncol. 1998;25:435–46.

Tang P, Upton JEM, Barton-forbes MA, Salvadori MI, Clynick MP, Price AK, Goobie SL. Autosomal recessive agammaglobulinemia due to a homozygous mutation in PIK3R1. J Clin Immunol. 2018; 38(1):88–95.

PLAID – PLCγ2-Associated Antibody Deficiency and Immune Dysregulation

▶ PLAID and APLAID

PLAID and APLAID

Joshua D. Milner
Laboratory of Allergic Diseases, NIAID, NIH, Bethesda, MD, USA
Department of Pediatrics, Columbia University Irving Medical Center, New York, NY, USA

Synonyms

APLAID – autoinflammatory PLCG2-associated antibody deficiency and immune dysregulation; FCAS – familial cold autoinflammatory syndrome; PLAID – PLCγ2-associated antibody deficiency and immune dysregulation

Definition

Mutations in the gene encoding phospholipase C gamma 2 (PLCγ2) can lead to two distinct dominant disorders, PLAID (PLCG2-associated antibody deficiency and immune dysregulation) and APLAID (Autoinflammatory PLAID). PLAID, associated with deletions in *PLCG2*, presents with cold urticaria, along with variably penetrant skin granulomas, recurrent bacterial infection, and autoimmunity. APLAID, due to a gain-of-function missense mutation in *PLCG2*, leads to multiorgan autoinflammation. Both syndromes are enlightening on the complex pathways involved in cellular signaling via PLCγ2 (MIM PLAID #614468/MIM APLAID #614878).

Introduction and Background

Distinction Between Familial Cold Autoinflammatory Syndrome, Typical Cold Urticaria, and PLAID

The term "familial cold urticaria" was used to describe a dominant disorder now called familial cold autoinflammatory syndrome (FCAS). FCAS, due to *NLRP3* mutations, leads to excessive IL-1 production when patients are exposed to low temperatures, triggering the inflammatory phenotypes after several hours, one of which is a neutrophilic rash that might be mistaken for classical mast-cell degranulation-associated urticaria (Mathur and Mathes 2013). Classic cold urticarial is characterized by rapid onset to local or systemic cooling, and resolution with warming. The lesions are usually local to the contact with cold, or in the case of systemic cooling, can even be associated with anaphylaxis. The diagnosis of classic cold urticaria is made with the application of an ice cube and the appearance of a hive after exposure. The etiology is not clear – serum transfer from some, but not all, affected individuals leads to cold-induced hives in unaffected recipients, and importantly, the onset of responsiveness to cold tends to happen in the second or third decade of life and can be self-resolved after years (Abajian et al.

2012). Delayed cold urticaria, which appears clinically similar to typical cold urticaria except that symptom-onset is not immediately after cold exposure, had also been described to be inherited in a dominant fashion (Soter et al. 1977). PLAID was initially described by Ghandi et al., who reported families with dominantly inherited, immediate-onset classic cold urticaria which was present from birth and did not resolve (Gandhi et al. 2009). In another contrast to typical cold urticaria, patients reacted more often to evaporative cooling than contact with cold objects.

Genetics

The genetic basis for PLAID has been explained by large exonic deletions in a regulatory domain of PLCγ2. They were found in two of the families described by Ghandi et al., and in an additional family whose index patient was referred for diffuse granulomatous dermatitis, which had gradually worsened since birth (Ombrello et al. 2012). The mutations that lead to PLAID are quite unique. In the three families initially identified, each had a large, 4-8 kb in-frame, heterozygous genomic deletions in *PLCG2*. These deletions were not detected via whole-genome sequencing, but rather cDNA sequencing of the *PLCG2* transcript from peripheral blood. Several other families have been identified with clinical presentations identical to PLAID, but without *PLCG2* gene mutations (Ombrello et al. 2012).

Pathogenesis

Phospholipase C gamma 2 (PLCγ2) catalyzes the hydrolysis of phosphatidylinositol-4, 5-bisphosphate (PIP2) to inositol 1,4,5-trisphosphate (IP3) and diacylglycerol (DAG) in response to cell surface receptor ligation, which leads to a typical cellular activation cascade (Bunney et al. 2012). The disease-causing deletions disrupt a domain responsible for auto-inhibition, leaving the protein "on"/constitutively activated. The activating effect has been evaluated in a number of hematopoeitic lineage cells, including B, NK, and mast cells but is interestingly not observed in T cells. Despite the constitutive activation, the net cellular result at physiologic temperature is a loss of signaling function mediated by IP3 and DAG (Wang et al. 2014). The reduced B-cell receptor signaling and activation is the likely cause for the hypogammaglobulinemia leading to humoral immune deficiency. At the same time, a slight drop in the temperature leads to ligand-independent activation and degranulation of mast cells and explains the skin symptoms upon cooling (Ombrello et al. 2012) (Schade et al. 2016).

Clinical Manifestations

Cutaneous Manifestations

The granulomatous rash appeared in some – but not all patients – at birth, predominantly on their acral surfaces, presumably because these are the coldest body parts. The initial newborn rash appears almost like a burn. In many patients, the rash resolves as they get older, but in others, it progresses or reappears in adulthood. Despite histological findings of chronic granulomas that have similarity to sarcoidosis, angiotensin-converting enzyme (ACE) levels have been normal in all PLAID patients (Aderibigbe et al. 2015). To date, every PLAID patient has demonstrated an immediate skin hypersensitivity to cold, which is lifelong, beginning in infancy. Symptoms are elicited by cold water, but not by contact with cold objects. Evaporative cooling from air flow to wet surfaces – such as fans or air vents over perspiring skin – are the most common triggers. Patients have negative ice cube challenge but a positive challenge to forced air past a drop of water placed on the skin over several minutes.

Immune Manifestations

Additional features identified in PLAID include antibody deficiency and respiratory infections, which led to a diagnosis of common variable immune deficiency in some patients. Features of autoimmunity include the development of autoimmune hypothyroidism, vitiligo, and ANA-positivity (Ombrello et al. 2012; Aderibigbe et al. 2015). Syncope has been reported in situations of prolonged systemic cold exposure such as in insufficiently warm swimming pools. The rash elicited is erythematous, pruritic, and localized but not usually raised, unlike typical hives. Ingestion of cold items is a frequent trigger of burning sensations in the throat or retrosternal regions, but not of systemic symptoms (Gandhi et al. 2009). Aside from the urticaria, presence of other symptoms are quite variable and multiple affected patients reported that cold-induced urticaria was their only symptom.

APLAID (Autoinflammatory PLCG2-Associated Antibody Deficiency and Immune Dysregulation)

APLAID is a disorder caused by unique *PLCG2* mutations. This syndrome is differentiated because of the presence of autoinflammatory features. APLAID was initially described in a single family consisting of a father and daughter. They presented with early-onset multi-organ inflammation including sterile abscess, uveitis, colitis, interstitial pneumonitis with respiratory bronchiolitis, and recurrent bacterial and viral sinopulmonary infections (Zhou et al. 2012). They had a novel missense mutation in *PLCG2* in a domain similar to where the PLAID-associated mutations were found. The patients did not have cold urticaria, and in vitro studies suggested gain-of-function pattern when compared to PLAID mutations. The APLAID patients also had low or low-normal serum IgA and IgM levels, poor responses to pneumococcal vaccine, and nearly absent class-switched B cells. They did not have substantial autoantibody formation. Inflammatory markers were normal. Another APLAID patient was described with a vesiculopustular rash as a newborn, followed by inflammatory bowel disease, posterior uveitis, recurrent chest infections, interstitial pneumonitis, and

P

sensorineural deafness and cutis laxa (Neves et al. 2018). Immunological studies showed low serum IgM and IgA, absent antibody responses to protein antigens, and almost absent class-switched memory B cells. A de novo heterozygous missense L848P mutation was reported in the *PLCG2* gene, which demonstrated a gain-of-function feature.

Laboratory Findings

Despite the heterogeneity of symptoms, several laboratory measures are more consistent than the clinical findings. In addition to positive antinuclear antibodies, two thirds of the patients demonstrate humoral deficiency with low serum IgM levels and absence of circulating switched memory B cells (IgM-, IgD-CD27+). Many patients had low serum IgA levels, and have poor responses to anti-pneumococcal vaccines. NK cells number are low and with impaired function. In addition, cold agglutinins and cryoglobulins, which are seen in autoimmune-/antibody-mediated cold-induced inflammation, are absent. Most patients have normal acute phase reactants (ESR and CRP) even during periods of active cold-induced rashes. Serum immunoglobulin levels and specific antibody responses were impaired in relatives who had the mutation but were otherwise clinically asymptomatic.

Treatment

Treatment of patients with PLAID is largely symptomatic and includes avoidance of evaporative or systemic cooling. Specific instructions include, warming rapidly after showers, toweling off sweat during and after exercise, avoiding drafts whenever possible and avoiding cold pools. Short- and long-acting antihistamines can be effective as well. Patients typically do not describe massive changes in the urticarial symptoms over time, but become more aware of how to avoid situations which cause symptoms. The

antibody deficiency and CVID presentation can develop later in life, patients should be counselled, and infections should be carefully managed. If CVID develops, antibiotic prophylaxis and/or immunoglobulin supplementation should be considered as clinically indicated in the treatment plan. Immunosuppressive agents might be required in patients with APLAID.

References

Abajian M, Mlynek A, Maurer M. Physical urticaria. Curr Allergy Asthma Rep. 2012;12(4):281–7.

Aderibigbe OM, Priel DAL, Lee C-CR, Ombrello MJ, Prajapati VH, Liang MG, et al. Distinct cutaneous manifestations, autonomous and cold-induced leukocyte activation associated with PLCG2 mutations. JAMA Dermatol. 2015;151(6):627–34

Bunney TD, Esposito D, Mas-Droux C, Lamber E, Baxendale RW, Martins M, et al. Structural and functional integration of the PLCgamma interaction domains critical for regulatory mechanisms and signaling deregulation. Structure. 2012;20(12):2062–75.

Gandhi C, Healy C, Wanderer AA, Hoffman HM. Familial atypical cold urticaria: description of a new hereditary disease. J Allergy Clin Immunol. 2009;124(6):1245–50.

Mathur AN, Mathes EF. Urticaria mimickers in children. Dermatol Ther. 2013;26(6):467–75.

Neves JF, Doffinger R, Barcena-Morales G, Martins C, Papapietro O, Plagnol V, et al. Novel PLCG2 mutation in a patient with APLAID and cutis laxa. Front Immunol. 2018;9:2863.

Ombrello MJ, Remmers EF, Sun G, Freeman AF, Datta S, Torabi-Parizi P, et al. Cold urticaria, immunodeficiency, and autoimmunity related to PLCG2 deletions. N Engl J Med. 2012;366(4):330–8.

Schade A, Walliser C, Wist M, Haas J, Vatter P, Kraus JM, et al. Cool-temperature-mediated activation of phospholipase C-gamma2 in the human hereditary disease PLAID. Cell Signal. 2016;28(9):1237–51.

Soter NA, Joshi NP, Twarog FJ, Zeiger RS, Rothman PM, Colten HR. Delayed cold-induced urticaria: a dominantly inherited disorder. J Allergy Clin Immunol. 1977;59(4):294–7.

Wang J, Sohn H, Sun G, Milner JD, Pierce SK. The auto-inhibitory C-terminal SH2 domain of phospholipase C-gamma2 stabilizes B cell receptor signalosome assembly. Sci Signal. 2014;7(343):ra89.

Zhou Q, Lee GS, Brady J, Datta S, Katan M, Sheikh A, et al. A Hypermorphic missense mutation in PLCG2, encoding phospholipase Cgamma2, causes a dominantly inherited autoinflammatory disease with immunodeficiency. Am J Hum Genet. 2012;91(4):713–20.

PMS2 Deficiency

Bhumika Patel
Asthma, Allergy and Immunology of Tampa Bay, Tampa, FL, USA

Synonyms

Postmeiotic segregation increased 2: PMS2

Definition

Postmeiotic segregation increased 2 (PMS2) is a key component of the mismatch repair (MMR) pathway. Pathogenic variants in the *PMS2* gene have been associated with Lynch syndrome (formally known as hereditary nonpolyposis colorectal cancer or HPNCC), Turcot syndrome, and impaired immunoglobulin class-switch recombination (CSR) with somatic hypermutation (SHM). Pathogenic variants can be inherited in both autosomal dominant (Lynch and Turcot syndrome) and recessive patterns (CSR with SHM).

Introduction/Background

The DNA mismatch repair (MMR) system, a highly conserved pathway from bacteria to humans, involves many proteins that aid in the identifying and correcting of mismatched bases that may occur during DNA replication, recombination, and repair. The MMR proteins also stimulate DNA damage-induced apoptosis as part of the cytotoxic response to physical and chemical agents. The four key genes involved in the MMR pathway include *mutL homolog 1* (*MLH1*), *mutS homolog 2* (*MSH2*), *mutS homolog 6* (*MSH6*), and postmeiotic segregation increased 2 (PMS2). The MSH2-MSH6 heterodimer (mutSα) is involved in the initial identification of mismatched pairs. After binding to the mismatched pairs, mutSα undergoes a conformational change and recruits the PMS2 and MLH1 heterodimer (MutLα), which has endonuclease activity. The MutLα heterodimer introduces single-strand breaks near the mismatch and generates new entry points for the exonuclease EXO1 to degrade the strand containing the mismatch.

The MMR system is also involved in immunoglobulin class-switch recombination (CSR) and somatic hypermutation (SHM).

Pathogenic variants in a MMR system result in a condition called *constitutional mismatch repair deficiency syndrome* (CMMRD; OMIM 276300). CMMRD is characterized by the insertion or deletion of short, repetitive sequences of DNA termed microsatellites, thereby producing a mutator phenotype known as microsatellite instability (MSI). Individuals with CMMRD have an increased predisposition to cancer at an earlier age.

Clinical Presentation (History/PE)

Lynch Syndrome (OMIM 120435)

Lynch syndrome (formally known as hereditary nonpolyposis colorectal cancer; HPNCC) is an autosomal dominant disease that is associated with a high risk of colorectal cancer and also extra-colonic tumors, particularly endometrial cancer. Patients have an earlier age of onset of colorectal cancer with the average age being 45 years. The most common heterozygous pathogenic variants seen in Lynch syndrome are in *MLH1* (42%), followed by *MSH2* (33%), *MSH6* (18%), and *PMS2* (7%) (Richman 2015).

Turcot Syndrome (OMIM 276300)

Turcot syndrome (also known as brain tumor polyposis and mismatch repair cancer syndrome) may follow either an autosomal dominant or recessive pattern and is characterized by multiple adenomatous colon polyps and increased risk of colorectal and brain cancers. It may be associated with familial adenomatous polyposis (FAP) or Lynch syndrome. Turcot syndrome typically develops when the patient is in his or her teens. The genetic defect is typically seen in the APC

P

gene (for "adenomatous polyposis coli") when associated with FAP or in MLH1 and PMS2 when associated with Lynch syndrome. Individuals with the APC pathogenic variant typically have medulloblastoma, while those with pathogenic variants in the mismatch repair genes usually have glioblastoma multiforme (Dipro et al. 2012).

Impaired Immunoglobulin Class-Switch Recombination

Class-switch recombination deficiencies are rare primary immunodeficiencies that are characterized by normal or increased serum IgM levels and decreased or absent IgA, IgE, and IgG levels. Individuals with CSR deficiency may also have defects in the generation of somatic hypermutation (SHM) in the immunoglobulin variable region. Peron et al. in 2008 described impaired immunoglobulin CSR in three patients with homozygous or compound heterozygous pathogenic variants in the *PMS2* gene. Patient 1 had recurrent infections and café au lait skin spots and was found to have high serum IgM levels, profoundly low IgG levels, and an absence of IgA at 9 years of age. Patients 2 and 3 were found to have low levels of IgG2 and lack of IgG4. Tesch et al. in 2018 reviewed the clinical and laboratory data of a cohort of 15 patients with pathogenic variants in an MMR gene, 8 of which had homozygous or compound heterozygous pathogenic variants *PMS2*. Their review of patient-filled questionnaire or physician-reported history did not show any clinical signs of primary immunodeficiency in patients with pathogenic variants in *PMS2*. Most of the patients had variable combination of malignancies but no history of severe infections, autoimmunity, granulomas, autoinflammation, or lymphoproliferation. Patient did develop viral and fungal infections, especially after chemotherapy. Furthermore, immunoglobulin levels were highly variable, and analysis of B- and T-cell subsets in these patients revealed a reduction in the number of class-switched plasma blasts (in most patients) and B memory cells (in some individuals), but no abnormality of the cellular immune system was consistently found among these patients.

This is in contrast to other chromosomal instability syndromes, such as polymerase E1 deficiency (POLE1), ligase 4 (LIG4), Bloom and Nijmegen breakage syndrome, and Fanconi anemia which are often associated with immunodeficiency, growth retardation, and increased risk of malignancy.

Laboratory Findings/Diagnostic Testing

Family history of Lynch-associated tumors, relatives diagnosed with cancer at younger than average age, or multiple generations affected by a type of cancer warrant further evaluation of Lynch syndrome or Turcot syndrome. Tumor surveillance may include immunohistochemistry staining and microsatellite instability testing. Genetic testing may be used for confirmation. Immune evaluation includes immunoglobulin levels and B-cell subsets, with specific focus on class-switched compartments.

Treatment/Prognosis

Patients with genetic pathogenic variants associated with Lynch syndrome and Turcot syndrome require an aggressive screening protocol given the increased risk of developing malignancies. Surgical incision of the tumor and often the affected organ is a mainstay in treatment. Individuals may require immunoglobulin replacement if there is evidence of decreased IgG and clinical evidence of primary immunodeficiency.

References

Dipro S, Al-Otaibi F, Alzahrani A, et al. Turcot syndrome: a synchronous clinical presentation of glioblastoma multiforme and adenocarcinoma of the colon. Case Rep Oncol Med. 2012;2012:12.

Peron S, Metin A, Gardes P, Alyanakian MA, et al. Human PMS2 deficiency is associated with impaired immunoglobulin class switch recombination. J Exp Med. 2008;205:2465–72.

Richman S. Deficient mismatch repair: read all about it (Review). Int J Oncol. 2015;47:1189–202.

Tesch VK, Ijspeert H, Riach A, et al. No overt clinical immunodeficiency despite immune biological abnormalities in patients with constitutional mismatch repair deficiency. Front Immunol. 2018;9:1506.

POLE1

▶ Clinical Presentation of Polymerase E1 (POLE1) and Polymerase E2 (POLE2) Deficiencies

POLE2

▶ Clinical Presentation of Polymerase E1 (POLE1) and Polymerase E2 (POLE2) Deficiencies

Polyglucosan Body Myopathy 1 With or Without Immunodeficiency (PGBM1)

▶ LUBAC Deficiencies

Polyglucosan Body Myopathy, Early-Onset, With or Without Immunodeficiency (PBMEI)

▶ LUBAC Deficiencies

Postmeiotic Segregation Increased 2: PMS2

▶ PMS2 Deficiency

Predisposition to Severe Viral Infection, MCM4 Deficiency

Hannah Roberts[1] and Stuart E. Turvey[2,3]
[1]Division of Allergy and Clinical Immunology, Department of Pediatrics, BC Children's Hospital, University of British Columbia, Vancouver, BC, Canada
[2]Division of Allergy and Clinical Immunology, Department of Pediatrics and Experimental Medicine Program, British Columbia Children's Hospital, The University of British Columbia, Vancouver, BC, Canada
[3]Willem-Alexander Children's Hospital, Leiden University Medical Center, Leiden, the Netherlands

Definition

Minichromosome maintenance complex component 4 (MCM4) deficiency is a novel autosomal recessive condition that impairs DNA repair and is characterized by natural killer cell and glucocorticoid deficiency, growth failure, and viral infections.

Introduction

Natural killer (NK) cells are known for their role in innate immunity. They provide malignant cell surveillance and host defense against viral infections. NK cells develop from $CD34^+$ hematopoietic stem cells in the bone marrow and mature in lymphoid tissues. NK cells lack the T cell receptor complex and are identified by the neural cell adhesion molecule (CD56). Most peripheral blood NK cells express low levels of CD56 and CD16 and are considered mature. These are referred to as $CD56^{dim}$ NK cells. A minor subset of NK cells express high levels of CD56, without CD16, and are considered immature ($CD56^{bright}$). Selective NK cell deficiency is very rare but, when present, increases host susceptibility to viral illness. The *MCM4* gene encodes DNA helicase and is essential for cell proliferation and DNA replication. Minichromosome maintenance complex component 4 (*MCM4*) deficiency (OMIM 609981) is a novel autosomal recessive primary immunodeficiency that has been identified in a small cohort of consanguineous individuals of Irish descent. This rare condition impairs DNA repair and is characterized by NK cell and glucocorticoid deficiency, growth failure, and recurrent viral infections. Patient fibroblasts from this Irish community contain excessive chromosomal breaks and cell-cycle abnormalities. These individuals possess immature NK cells but lack mature NK cells and NK cell function. It remains to be determined mechanistically why a mutation in the *MCM4* would result in selective NK cell deficiency (Casey et al. 2012; Eidenschenk et al. 2006; Gineau et al. 2012; Hughes et al. 2012; Musahl et al. 1995; Orange 2013).

Genetics

In 1997, Satoh et al. mapped *MCM4* to chromosome 8q11.2. *MCM4* consists of 864 amino acids and has a molecular mass of 96 kDa (Musahl et al. 1995). The protein encoded by this gene is one of the minichromosome maintenance proteins that play an essential role in DNA replication. *MCM4*, in combination with *MCM2*, *MCM3*, *MCM4*, *MCM6*, and *MCM7*, forms a helicase complex known as the minichromosome maintenance (MCM2–7) complex which is involved in the initiation and elongation phases of DNA replication.

MCM4 deficiency is a novel autosomal recessive disorder caused by homozygous mutations in the *MCM4*. Affected individuals identified to date all share the same splice-site mutation causing early termination of the reading frame. In 2012, Gineau et al. first identified the splice defect in *MCM4* responsible for the condition; a homozygous adenine to guanine transition in intron 1 of *MCM4* shifts the splice site by one nucleotide, resulting in the insertion of a single guanine, causing a frameshift and premature termination at codon 27 (Phe24ArgfsTer4). Hughes et al. confirmed this splice-site shift with RT-PCR.

Immunoblotting of patient lymphocytes with *MCM4* deficiency has shown a loss of the typical 96-kDa *MCM4* protein and evidence of a truncated 85-kDa isoform. Considering the role of *MCM4*, it is evident why mutant cells demonstrate genomic instability and cause cell-cycle defects.

Disease

MCM4 deficiency has been recognized solely in a small number of consanguineous Irish families possessing the same autosomal recessive genetic mutation, presumably arising from a common founder. The condition, characterized by selective NK cell deficiency, adrenal insufficiency, growth failure, and recurrent viral infections, was first reported in 2006 in four patients of a consanguineous Irish kindred. Reported phenotypes to date are somewhat variable, specifically in terms of severity of viral infections. All patients had <1% NK cells in peripheral blood. In terms of growth, these individuals all had antenatal and postnatal growth retardation and, specifically, microcephaly (Eidenschenk et al. 2006). Two individuals sustained severe respiratory illnesses that were suspected to be of viral etiology. Interestingly, despite having evidence of adaptive immunity against Epstein-Barr virus (EBV), one individual developed EBV lymphoproliferative disorder. Eidenschenk et al. first mapped, by microsatellite homozygosity mapping, this novel primary immunodeficiency to chromosome 8. Via exome sequencing in 2012, Casey et al. found homozygosity for the *MCM4* mutation in ten affected members from three Irish families manifesting impaired DNA repair, NK cell deficiency, and adrenal insufficiency.

In 2012, Gineau et al. first identified the splice defect in *MCM4* which is responsible for the condition. A homozygous adenine to guanine transition in intron 1 of *MCM4* that shifts the splice site by one nucleotide results in the insertion of a single guanine, causing a frameshift and premature termination at codon 27 (Phe24ArgfsTer4). Gineau et al. identified six related individuals, from a consanguineous Irish family, with the same mutation and phenotype characterized by Eidenschenk et al. in 2006. In this group, patients' fibroblasts were studied and found to demonstrate genomic instability which was rescued by wild-type *MCM4* in vitro. Looking at *MCM4* in this cohort's cells, it was determined that mutant *MCM4* lacked the N terminus of wild-type *MCM4* and these truncated isoforms showed a lower proportion of cells in the G1 and S phases of the cell cycle and a higher proportion of cells in the G2/M phase, compared to controls. This was evidence that mutant *MCM4* has an impact on the mitotic phase. Along with this, these mutant cells showed increased chromosomal breakage. Like the first identified family, this group also had decreased mature NK cells, and immature or CD56[bright] NK cells showed impaired proliferation.

In 2012, Hughes et al. identified the same mutation as Gineau's team initially discovered, in eight children from three consanguineous Irish families with similar phenotypes as previously reported. This homozygous mutation was not identified in several exome databases and 300 control chromosomes. Seven of the children had adrenal failure and all were maintained on steroid replacement. To note, it appears that in this patient population, cortisol deficiency is often not as severe as other forms of familial glucocorticoid deficiency and onset is typically in childhood, following a period of adequate adrenal function. Patients had low birth weights and displayed growth failure, despite normal growth hormone. Four children had evidence of elevated DNA breakage on screening with diepoxybutane. Three children had levels of chromosomal breakage consistent with Fanconi anemia. All individuals had a normal complete blood count, and immunological investigations were evasive apart from selective NK cell deficiency. Seven had low NK cells; however, only one had a notable infectious history with recurrent pneumonitis and bronchiectasis on chest CT. Similar to human studies, studies with *mcm4*-deficient mice have shown markedly abnormal adrenal morphology, elevated chromosomal fragility, growth failure, and increased predisposition to mammary tumors, lymphomas, and sarcomas.

Diagnosis

MCM4 deficiency is extremely rare; however, based on literature to date, it should be considered as a differential diagnosis in those who display growth failure, adrenal insufficiency, and an exclusive predisposition to viral infections. To date, it has only been reported in those of Irish descent, and therefore ethnicity should also be discussed on history. Immunological investigations of patients to date demonstrate normal complete blood count and T and B cell enumeration. Individuals with *MCM4* deficiency have preservation of a small number of peripheral immature (CD56[bright]) NK cells but lack mature NK cells and NK cell cytotoxic function. If suspected based on clinical and immunological investigations, the condition can be confirmed by targeted genetic analysis.

Treatment

In the vast and rapidly expanding array of primary immunodeficiency disorders, selective NK cell deficiency and isolated predisposition to viral infections is a rare finding. Directed therapy to prevent viral infections is important, along with aggressively treating any suspected viral infection promptly. Adrenal insufficiency can be life-threatening, and therefore replacement with glucocorticoid and endocrinology assessment is essential. Patients demonstrate a phenotype similar to other DNA repair disorders, including chromosomal fragility and growth retardation. Growth and nutrition should be monitored. The combination of DNA instability and predisposition to viral infection increase the risk of malignancy. EBV lymphoproliferative disorder was present in one individual with *MCM4* deficiency, and predisposition to malignancy was found in *mcm4*-deficient mice; therefore, hematological and cancer surveillance is prudent. To date, the severity and frequency of viral illness is variable. Depending on clinical status of the individual patient, hematopoietic stem cell transplantation could be a potential treatment consideration.

P

Conclusion

MCM4 deficiency is a novel autosomal recessive primary immunodeficiency that has been identified in a small cohort of consanguineous individuals of Irish ancestry. This rare condition is characterized by selective NK cell deficiency, adrenal insufficiency, growth failure, and increased chromosomal breaks. Individuals reported to date all share the same homozygous splice-site mutation in the *MCM4* gene. From the available literature, affected individuals have increased susceptibility to viral infections, although frequency and severity is variable. Based on phenotypic features, it can be hypothesized that *MCM4* mutations have deleterious consequences on NK cells, the endocrine system, and development in general. The specific pathophysiology of these downstream effects remains unclear. Selective NK cell deficiency itself is extremely rare, and in *MCM4* deficiency, individuals exhibit variability in disease and infectious susceptibility, which suggests immunological management strategies may be best developed on an individual basis. Further research is needed to fully understand the impact of defective *MCM4* and its disease trajectory.

References

Casey JP, Nobbs M, McGettigan P, et al. Recessive mutations in MCM4/PRKDC cause a novel syndrome involving a primary immunodeficiency and a disorder of DNA repair. J Med Genet. 2012;49:242–5.

Eidenschenk C, Dunne J, Jouanguy E, et al. A novel primary immunodeficiency with specific natural-killer cell deficiency maps to the centromeric region of chromosome 8. Am J Hum Genet. 2006;78:721–7.

Gineau L, Cognet C, Kara N, et al. Partial MCM4 deficiency in patients with growth retardation, adrenal insufficiency, and natural killer cell deficiency. J Clin Invest. 2012;122(821–832):2012.

Hughes CR, Guasti L, Meimaridou E, et al. MCM4 mutation causes adrenal failure, short stature, and natural killer cell deficiency in humans. J Clin Invest. 2012;122:814–20.

Musahl C, Schulte D, Burkhart R, Knippers R. A human homologue of the yeast replication protein Cdc21: interactions with other Mcm proteins. Eur J Biochem. 1995;230:1096–101.

Orange JS. Natural killer cell deficiency. J Allergy Clin Immunol. 2013;132(3):515–26.

Satoh T, Tsuruga H, Yabuta N, et al. Assignment of the human CDC21 (MCM4) gene to chromosome 8q11.2. Genomics. 1997;46:525–6.

Predisposition to Severe Viral Infection, STAT2 Deficiency

Hannah Roberts[1] and Stuart E. Turvey[2,3]
[1]Division of Allergy and Clinical Immunology, Department of Pediatrics, BC Children's Hospital, University of British Columbia, Vancouver, BC, Canada
[2]Division of Allergy and Clinical Immunology, Department of Pediatrics and Experimental Medicine Program, British Columbia Children's Hospital, The University of British Columbia, Vancouver, BC, Canada
[3]Willem-Alexander Children's Hospital, Leiden University Medical Center, Leiden, the Netherlands

Definition

Signal transducer and activator of transcription (STAT2) deficiency is a novel autosomal recessive condition that impairs interferon (IFN) alpha/beta responses, leading to severe viral infections and mitochondrial defects.

Introduction

Cytokine signaling is mediated by seven STAT proteins that form homo- or heterodimers and translocate to the cell nucleus to drive signal transduction and transcription activation. STAT2 dimerizes with STAT1, and together with interferon regulatory factor (IRF) 9 encodes a transcription factor complex called interferon-stimulated gene factor 3 (ISGF3) (Fink and Grandvaux 2013). ISGF3 is involved in activating Type I and Type III interferons. Interferons elicit a multitude of effects in innate and adaptive immunity. Type 1 IFNs (IFN-alpha/beta) are necessary for inducing transcription genes which are crucial in host resistance to viral infections (Takaoka and Yanai 2006). STAT2 provides the transcriptional activation domain of the ISFG3 complex and is key for target gene transcription (Fink and Grandvaux 2013). STAT2 deficiency, also known as Immunodeficiency 44, is a novel autosomal recessive primary immunodeficiency first described in 2013 and has been shown to result in impaired antiviral responses specifically in interferon-alpha and interferon-beta signaling, leading to elevated susceptibility to viral infections, along with mitochondrial fission defects (Hambleton et al. 2013; Shahni et al. 2015).

Genetics and Function

The *STAT2* gene maps to chromosome 12q13.3 and is 24 exons in length. STAT2 consists of 851 amino acids and northern blot analysis has found it to be 4.8 kb in size (Fu et al. 1992). STAT2 has three helices in its N-terminal region: an SHs-like domain, heptad leucine repeats, and a C-terminal domain. IFNs are a group of cytokines secreted in response to pathogen exposure. Binding of IFN-alpha/beta to the type 1 IFN receptor (IFNAR) activates JAK kinases (TYK2 and JAK1), which in turn leads to tyrosine phosphorylation of STAT1 and STAT2 and signal transduction. Together with IRF9, phosphorylated STAT1 and STAT2 form the ISGF3. ISGF3 is 113 kD transcription factor that enters the nucleus and binds to IFN-stimulated response elements to activate the transcription of IFN-alpha/beta-stimulated genes, which invokes a protective antiviral state within the cell (Platanias 2005). STAT2 provides the transcriptional activation domain of the ISFG3 complex, for target gene transcription (Fink and Grandvaux 2013). STAT2 also appears to be a novel regulator of DRP1, a mitochondrial fission protein, implying that there are still not well-understood interactions between innate immunity and mitochondria (Shahni et al. 2015).

STAT2 deficiency is an autosomal recessive inherited disorder, caused by biallelic mutations in *STAT2*. The seven affected patients identified to date, from two unrelated families, carry homozygous mutations. Five patients of the same family were homozygous for a single variant within the donor splice site of introns 4 and 5 (c.381+5 G>C) in *STAT2*, while the two siblings in the second family were homozygous for a nonsense mutation (c.1836 C>A, p.C612X) (Hambleton et al. 2013; Shahni et al. 2015).

Disease

Innate immunity plays a crucial role in controlling infections and fundamental among innate antiviral defenses is the IFN response. Previously, increased susceptibility to viral infections has been observed in mice with genetic defects in the IFN signaling cascade. In mice, disabling mutations in *Stat2* have been associated with viral susceptibility both in vivo and in vitro. *Stat2*-null mice have been reported to be susceptible to vesicular stomatitis viral infection (Hambleton et al. 2013). STAT2 deficiency was first described in 2013 and is a novel primary immunodeficiency that to date has been reported in only two unrelated families, affecting a total of seven individuals. Phenotypic features of these seven individuals are variable. Overall, there appears to be an increased predisposition to viral infection, with severity ranging from quite benign to encephalopathy and infection-driven multisystem, neurologic decompensation. Of the seven patients described, there has been no evidence of predilection to bacterial infections.

The first case of STAT2 deficiency was reported in a 5-year-old male in 2013. At 18 months, he developed disseminated vaccine-strain measles 6 days after a standard measles/mumps/rubella (MMR) immunization. The severe infection was complicated by pneumonitis and hepatitis. Vaccine-strain measles was identified in his blood 14 days after immunization. His infant sibling died after an acute febrile illness with postmortem findings consistent with an overwhelming viral infection. These siblings were born to consanguineous parents. Further assessment of the sibling's extended family revealed three individuals with the same homozygous pathogenic variant. Two children had histories of severe viral illnesses, one being a 6-year-old who developed encephalitis post-MMR vaccination. The mother of these set of siblings, who was also homozygous for the mutation, had a benign infectious history, suggesting this condition may have incomplete penetrance or may only manifest if infection is encountered during a specific developmental window. Three of the five patients in this family were found to have nonthreatening cases of varicella. One individual had a herpes simplex infection complicated by gingivostomatitis. Surviving *STAT2*-deficient individuals in this family have remained healthy, suggesting type I IFN signaling is not essential for defense against various common viruses (Hambleton et al. 2013).

The other family, described in 2015, included two siblings born to nonconsanguineous Albanian parents who at about 1 year of age developed febrile illnesses post-MMR vaccinations. On immunological investigation, the two siblings had appropriate vaccine antibody titers. After immunization, the female sibling had recurrent fevers and septic shock ensued. The other child developed opsoclonus/myoclonus 1 month post-MMR vaccine and was managed with steroids and intravenous acyclovir. At age 2 he presented with disseminated infection and seizures, consistent with meningoencephalitis. He eventually developed multisystem deterioration including visual impairment, chorea, spasticity, and refractory seizures (Shahni et al. 2015).

Diagnosis

STAT2 deficiency is extremely rare; however, based on literature to date, it should be considered as a differential diagnosis in those who appear to have an exclusive predisposition to viral infections, particularly in any patient with a disseminated infection following live viral vaccination. Routine immunological investigations are typically inconclusive, emphasizing the importance of a high index of clinical suspicion. Immunological evaluations of patients to date demonstrate normal lymphocyte subset enumeration. More

directed investigations in a research laboratory in this patient population have identified impairment in interferon signaling. In vitro investigations via immunoblotting of interferon-stimulated genes in dermal fibroblasts demonstrated no expression of STAT2 protein, along with a block in ISGF3 signaling, increased predisposition to viral infection and failure of type I interferon signaling (Hambleton et al. 2013). Five out of seven patients with STAT2 deficiency have shown evidence of normal adaptive immunity with positive specific antibody titers to live and inactivated vaccinations, including MMR and common viruses (Hambleton et al. 2013; Shahni et al. 2015). In the two siblings who developed severe infection and neurologic sequelae post-MMR vaccination, laboratory investigations did not reveal evidence of mitochondrial dysfunction; however, skeletal muscle biopsy showed elongated mitochondria, rescued with wild-type *STAT2*. Three of the seven patients with STAT2 deficiency have been identified, by western blot analysis, to have inactive DRP1, a mitochondrial fission protein. This mitochondrial fission defect in patient fibroblasts was successfully rescued following transduction with wild-type *STAT2* (Shahni et al. 2015). If clinical suspicion is high, direct sequencing of *STAT2* may be the most effective strategy to reach a definitive diagnosis, since functional assays to assess STAT2 function are not typically available in standard clinical laboratories.

Treatment

In the broad array of primary immunodeficiency disorders, isolated predisposition to viral infections is rare. Autosomal-recessive STAT1 deficiency, less rare than STAT2 deficiency, is characterized by predisposition to lethal mycobacterial and viral infection. In those with STAT1 deficiency, hematopoietic stem cell transplant should be considered, as antimycobacterial and antiviral therapy has proven poor outcomes. Although those with STAT2 deficiency display a significant defect in IFN response with some showing predisposition to severe viral infection, others are healthy and can endure common viral pathogens. As there are an extremely small number of patients known to have this novel immunodeficiency, there is no established standard-of-care in terms of treatment. Based on case reports, it would be necessary to aggressively treat any suspected viral infection promptly with antiviral medication. Based on responses to MMR vaccination in some patients, it should also be a strong consideration to withhold live viral vaccines in patients with known STAT2 deficiency. With three of the seven patients having inactive DRP1, this could be an area of investigation for potential therapy options.

References

Fink K, Grandvaux N. STAT2 and IRF9: beyond ISGF3. JAK–STAT. 2013;2(4):e27521. https://doi.org/10.4161/jkst.27521.

Fu XY, Schindler C, Improta T, et al. The proteins of ISGF-3, the interferon alpha-induced transcriptional activator, define a gene family involved in signal transduction. Proc Natl Acad Sci. 1992;89:7840–3.

Hambleton S, Goodbourn S, Young D, et al. STAT2 deficiency and susceptibility to viral illness in humans. Proc Natl Acad Sci. 2013;110(8):3053–8.

Platanias L. Mechanisms of type-I-and type-II-interferon-mediated signaling. Nat Rev Immunol. 2005;5:375–86.

Shahni R, Cale C, Anderson G, et al. Signal transducer and activator of transcription 2 deficiency is a novel disorder of mitochondrial fission. Brain. 2015;138:2834–46.

Takaoka K, Yanai H. Interferon signaling network in innate defence. Cell Microbiol. 2006;8(6):907–22.

PRF1 Deficiency

Ivan K. Chinn
Section of Immunology, Allergy, and Retrovirology, Texas Children's Hospital, Houston, TX, USA
William T. Shearer Center for Human Immunobiology, Texas Children's Hospital, Houston, TX, USA
Department of Pediatrics, Baylor College of Medicine, Houston, TX, USA

Introduction

PRF1 is a three-exon gene located at 10q22.1 and encodes perforin, a 555 amino acid, 67 kDa glycoprotein that shares homology with complement factor 9 and which is nearly exclusively expressed in cytotoxic T cells and NK cells (Lichtenheld et al. 1988; Shinkai et al. 1988). The gene product is translated as a peptide precursor that must be processed into a mature form (Risma et al. 2006). Key domains include a membrane attack complex perforin-like/cholesterol-dependent cytolysin (MACPF/CDC) domain, an epidermal growth factor domain, and a C2 domain (Brennan et al. 2010; Willenbring et al. 2018).

Molecular Function

Activation of perforin requires binding of calcium to the C2 domain, which is inhibited by the acidic environment of the lytic granule (Brennan et al. 2010; Trapani and Voskoboinik 2007). During degranulation, perforin is released by cytotoxic T cells and NK cells into the intercellular space of immune synapses with target cells. This event allows for activation of perforin, which then inserts into the membrane of the target cell and multimerizes by means of the MACPF/CDC domain, forming a pore that allows granzyme serine proteases to transit and induce cell death (Blink et al. 1999).

Presentation

Familial hemophagocytic lymphohistiocytosis (HLH) type 2 represents the most well-recognized clinical consequence of *PRF1* deficiency (Stepp et al. 1999; Trapani and Voskoboinik 2013). HLH is defined by fulfillment of at least five of the following eight criteria: fever; splenomegaly; cytopenia; hypertriglyceridemia and/or hypofibrinogenemia; hemophagocytosis in the bone marrow, spleen, or lymph nodes; deficient NK cell function; hyperferritinemia; and elevated levels of serum soluble CD25 (Henter et al. 2007). In perforin deficiency, the most common presenting features include thrombocytopenia (100%), splenomegaly (98%), fever (96%), anemia (93%), and hyperferritinemia (90%) (Trizzino et al. 2008). This presentation typically appears in early infancy (median age of 3 months) (Trizzino et al. 2008). *PRF1* deficiency accounts for 20–40% of familial HLH cases (Gholam et al. 2011; Cetica et al. 2016; Göransdotter Ericson et al. 2001). Complete loss of perforin expression correlates with very early presentation of HLH and absent NK cell function, while the presence of a hypomorphic genetic change, such as a variant that permits translation of the precursor peptide but then impairs the maturation process, in at least one allele conveys later onset of disease (or an atypical presentation) and more variable NK cell cytotoxicity (Risma et al. 2006; Trapani and Voskoboinik 2013; Trizzino et al. 2008; Molleran Lee et al. 2004).

Loss of perforin can produce other clinical phenotypes. *PRF1* deficiency has been strongly linked to lymphomagenesis, which is postulated to be due to impaired eradication of malignant by CD8[+] T cells and NK cells (Clementi et al. 2002, 2005; Tesi et al. 2015; Mhatre et al. 2014). Monoallelic variants, particularly p.A91V or other variants that produce a misfolded product, have been proposed to increase the risk for lymphoma or leukemia development, but these potential associations require further investigations (Brennan et al. 2010; Trapani and Voskoboinik 2007, 2013). Perforin-deficient patients have been reported with isolated aplastic anemia and no other features of HLH (other than bone marrow hemophagocytosis) (Solomou et al. 2007). Other atypical presentations include systemic lupus erythematosus, colitis, and neuroinflammation (Tesi et al. 2015). Partial perforin deficiency has been associated with increased risk for multiple sclerosis (Brennan et al. 2010).

Conversely, perforin deficiency may offer protection against certain diseases. One intriguing study has observed that specific *PRF1* pathogenic variants are enriched in certain populations in a manner that correlates with geographic distance from the equator and proposes the hypothesis that decreased perforin activity may help to maintain blood-brain barrier integrity in the setting of endemic infections, such as malaria (Brennan et al. 2010; Willenbring et al. 2018). Partial perforin deficiency may also protect against the development of type 1 diabetes (Brennan et al. 2010).

Diagnosis

A number of tests are required to establish the diagnosis. Perforin deficiency is characterized by markedly decreased CD8[+] T cell and NK cell lysis of target cells in the presence of CD107a surface upregulation (Stepp et al. 1999; Marcenaro et al. 2006). Cytotoxicity testing alone is known to carry low specificity, however, for this condition (Rubin et al. 2017). The diagnosis can be strongly suspected if perforin expression in cytotoxic T cells and NK cells is decreased or absent by flow cytometry, although normal expression cannot fully exclude the condition (Rubin et al. 2017). A combination of cytotoxicity testing, perforin expression analysis, and CD107a screening is therefore recommended (Rubin et al. 2017). Genetic testing remains necessary to confirm the presence of biallelic pathogenic variants in *PRF1*.

Treatment

Protocols have not been developed specifically for treatment of HLH due to *PRF1* deficiency but instead apply to HLH in general. The initial HLH-94 protocol employed a combination of intravenous etoposide, oral or intravenous dexamethasone, and (if neurologic disease is present) intrathecal methotrexate (Henter et al. 1997). Subsequently, the HLH-2004 protocol was developed, which combines HLH-94 with the use of oral cyclosporine (Henter et al. 2007). Providers should be cognizant that cyclosporine use can be associated with the appearance of posterior reversible encephalopathy syndrome (Jordan et al. 2011). Adjunctive use of serotherapy has been reported to enhance outcomes (Ishii 2016; Tang and Xu 2011; Filipovich and Chandrakasan 2015). Supportive care with antibiotics and antifungal medications to minimize infections is necessary during treatment for HLH (Jordan et al. 2011; Ishii 2016). Patients may require additional support if bleeding or cardiac dysfunction is present (Jordan et al. 2011).

HSCT represents the only definitive therapy for this disease at this time. Optimal strategies continue to be developed, as overall 5-year survival after HSCT in the HLH-94 study was only 54% (Henter et al. 1997; Nikiforow 2015). For all forms of HLH taken as a whole, survival is superior with use of reduced intensity conditioning after successful induction of HLH remission (Jordan et al. 2011; Nikiforow 2015; Seo 2015). Primary graft loss is common, and donor chimerism must be monitored closely (Jordan et al. 2011). Successful transplantation using umbilical cord blood stem cells has also been reported (Nikiforow 2015). For *PRF1* deficiency, gene therapy may provide an excellent alternative definitive treatment option in the future (Ghosh et al. 2018).

Cross-References

▶ *STX11* Deficiency
▶ *STXBP2* Deficiency
▶ *UNC13D* Deficiency

References

Blink EJ, Trapani JA, Jans DA. Perforin-dependent nuclear targeting of granzymes: a central role in the nuclear events of granule-exocytosis-mediated apoptosis? Immunol Cell Biol. 1999;77:206–15.

Brennan AJ, Chia J, Trapani JA, Voskoboinik I. Perforin deficiency and susceptibility to cancer. Cell Death Differ. 2010;17:607–15.

Cetica V, Sieni E, Pende D, et al. Genetic predisposition to hemophagocytic lymphohistiocytosis: report on 500 patients from the Italian registry. J Allergy Clin Immunol. 2016;137:188–96.e4.

Clementi R, Emmi L, Maccario R, et al. Adult onset and atypical presentation of hemophagocytic lymphohistiocytosis in siblings carrying PRF1 mutations. Blood. 2002;100:2266.

Clementi R, Locatelli F, Lc D, et al. A proportion of patients with lymphoma may harbor mutations of the perforin gene. Blood. 2005;105:4424–8.

Filipovich AH, Chandrakasan S. Pathogenesis of hemophagocytic lymphohistiocytosis. Hematol Oncol Clin North Am. 2015;29:895–902.

Gholam C, Grigoriadou S, Gilmour KC, Gaspar HB. Familial haemophagocytic lymphohistiocytosis: advances in the genetic basis, diagnosis and management. Clin Exp Immunol. 2011;163:271–83.

Ghosh S, Carmo M, Calero-Garcia M, et al. T-cell gene therapy for perforin deficiency corrects cytotoxicity defects and prevents hemophagocytic lymphohistiocytosis manifestations. J Allergy Clin Immunol. 2018;142:904–13.e3.

Göransdotter Ericson K, Fadeel B, Nilsson-Ardnor S, et al. Spectrum of perforin gene mutations in familial hemophagocytic lymphohistiocytosis. Am J Hum Genet. 2001;68:590–7.

Henter J-I, Aricò M, Egeler RM, et al. HLH-94: a treatment protocol for hemophagocytic lymphohistiocytosis. Med Pediatr Oncol. 1997;28:342–7.

Henter J-I, Horne A, Aricó M, et al. HLH-2004: diagnostic and therapeutic guidelines for hemophagocytic lymphohistiocytosis. Pediatr Blood Cancer. 2007;48:124–31.

Ishii E. Hemophagocytic lymphohistiocytosis in children: pathogenesis and treatment. Front Pediatr. 2016;4:47.

Jordan MB, Allen CE, Weitzman S, Filipovich AH, McClain KL. How I treat hemophagocytic lymphohistiocytosis. Blood. 2011;118:4041–52.

Lichtenheld MG, Olsen KJ, Lu P, et al. Structure and function of human perforin. Nature. 1988;335:448–51.

Marcenaro S, Gallo F, Martini S, et al. Analysis of natural killer-cell function in familial hemophagocytic lymphohistiocytosis (FHL): defective CD107a surface expression heralds Munc13-4 defect and discriminates between genetic subtypes of the disease. Blood. 2006;108:2316–23.

Mhatre S, Madkaikar M, Jijina F, Ghosh K. Unusual clinical presentations of familial hemophagocytic lymphohistiocytosis type-2. J Pediatr Hematol Oncol. 2014;36:e524–7.

Molleran Lee S, Villanueva J, Sumegi J, et al. Characterisation of diverse PRF1 mutations leading to decreased natural killer cell activity in North American families with haemophagocytic lymphohistiocytosis. J Med Genet. 2004;41:137.

Nikiforow S. The role of hematopoietic stem cell transplantation in treatment of hemophagocytic lymphohistiocytosis. Hematol Oncol Clin North Am. 2015;29:943–59.

Risma KA, Frayer RW, Filipovich AH, Sumegi J. Aberrant maturation of mutant perforin underlies the clinical diversity of hemophagocytic lymphohistiocytosis. J Clin Invest. 2006;116:182–92.

Rubin TS, Zhang K, Gifford C, et al. Perforin and CD107a testing is superior to NK cell function testing for screening patients for genetic HLH. Blood. 2017;129:2993–9.

Seo JJ. Hematopoietic cell transplantation for hemophagocytic lymphohistiocytosis: recent advances and controversies. Blood Res. 2015;50:131–9.

Shinkai Y, Takio K, Okumura K. Homology of perforin to the ninth component of complement (C9). Nature. 1988;334:525–7.

Solomou EE, Gibellini F, Stewart B, et al. Perforin gene mutations in patients with acquired aplastic anemia. Blood. 2007;109:5234–7.

Stepp SE, Dufourcq-Lagelouse R, Deist FL, et al. Perforin gene defects in familial hemophagocytic lymphohistiocytosis. Science. 1999;286:1957.

P

Tang Y-M, Xu X-J. Advances in hemophagocytic lymphohistiocytosis: pathogenesis, early diagnosis/differential diagnosis, and treatment. Sci World J. 2011;11:697–708.

Tesi B, Chiang SCC, El-Ghoneimy D, et al. Spectrum of atypical clinical presentations in patients with biallelic PRF1 missense mutations. Pediatr Blood Cancer. 2015;62:2094–100.

Trapani JA, Voskoboinik I. Infective, neoplastic, and homeostatic sequelae of the loss of perforin function in humans. In: Shurin MR, Smolkin YS, editors. Immune-mediated diseases. New York: Springer; 2007. p. 235–42.

Trapani J, Voskoboinik I. Perforinopathy: a spectrum of human immune disease caused by defective perforin delivery or function. Front Immunol. 2013;4:441.

Trizzino A, zur Stadt U, Ueda I, et al. Genotype–phenotype study of familial haemophagocytic lymphohistiocytosis due to perforin mutations. J Med Genet. 2008;45:15.

Willenbring RC, Ikeda Y, Pease LR, Johnson AJ. Human perforin gene variation is geographically distributed. Mol Genet Genomic Med. 2018;6:44–55.

Primary and Secondary CD59 Deficiency

Dror Mevorach
Rheumatology Research Center, Department of Medicine, Hadassah-Hebrew University, Jerusalem, Israel

Definition

CD59 encodes a 77-amino acid glycosylphosphatidylinositol (GPI)-anchored cell surface glycoprotein, synthesized as a 128-amino acid protein that includes a signal sequence and the sequence for a GPI anchor replacement. The CD59 protein, formerly known as a membrane inhibitor of reactive lysis (MIRL) and HRF20, inhibits the final and most important step of membrane attack complex (MAC) formation. Erythrocytes that are deficient in GPI-anchored membrane proteins, including CD59, undergo complement-mediated hemolysis.

Introduction

Secondary CD59 deficiency is a common finding in adult patients with paroxysmal nocturnal hemoglobinuria (PNH). In this condition, there is clonal expansion of hematopoietic stem cells that have acquired a mutation in the PIGA gene (phosphatidylinositol glycan anchor biosynthesis, class A). PIGA encodes a GPI biosynthesis protein, phosphatidylinositol N-acetylglucosaminyltransferase subunit A (Takeda et al. 1993).

CD59 was identified by several groups (Sugita et al. 1988), and its relationship to the erythrocyte phenotypes of PNH was soon established. Later, in a murine model, Holt, Boto, and Morgan performed a targeted deletion of the CD59 gene that resulted in spontaneous intravascular hemolysis and hemoglobinuria (Holt et al. 2001).

Primary CD59 Deficiency

Primary CD59 deficiency in humans (Table 1) was first reported in a patient who suffered from hemolytic anemia and recurrent cerebral infarction (Yamashina et al. 1990; Motoyama et al. 1992). Disease onset was in adolescence, and peripheral nervous system involvement was not reported at 22 years of age. The primary molecular defect in the patient was reported to be homozygosity for two separate single-nucleotide deletions in the gene, resulting in a frameshift, which was initiated at codon 34 (Motoyama et al. 1992).

A novel primary homozygous Cys89Tyr CD59 deficiency (Table 1) was recently reported in humans (Nevo et al. 2013). The mutation resulted in the amino acid substitution p.Cys89Tyr and thus in failure of the proper localization of CD59 protein to the cell surface. Cys89Tyr mutation in CD59 is a founder mutation in Jewish subjects of North African ancestry. Sequence determination of CD59 in exon 3 in 197 anonymous Jewish subjects of North African origin identified three carriers, indicating a carrier rate of 1:66 in this community. The mutation was not found in 5379

Primary and Secondary CD59 Deficiency, Table 1 Homozygous mutations in primary CD59 deficiency

Authors	Homozygous mutation	Origin	Age at clinical manifestation	Clinical manifestations
Yamashina et al. (1990), Motoyama et al. (1992)	1 patient with a single-nucleotide deletion in codon 16 (GCC to GC) and codon 96 (GCA to CA). Homozygous deletion in codon 16 resulted in a frameshift and introduced a stop codon at position 54	Japanese	Adolescence	Stroke, hemolytic anemia
Nevo et al. (2013)	5 patients from 4 unrelated families. Homozygous c.266G-A transition in exon 3 of the CD59 gene, resulting in a cys89tyr (C89Y) substitution at a highly conserved residue that participates in the formation of a disulfide bond	North African Sephardic Jews	Infancy (3–4 months)	Recurrent polyneuropathy, hemolytic anemia
Ben-Zeev et al. (2015)	2 siblings from one family. Homozygous c.266G-A transition in exon 3 of the CD59 gene, resulting in a cys89tyr (C89Y) substitution at a highly conserved residue that participates in the formation of a disulfide bond	North African Sephardic Jews	Infancy (3–4 months)	Recurrent strokes Retinal and optic nerve disease
Hochsmann et al. (2014)	1 female. Homozygous 1-bp deletion (c.146delA) in exon 5 of the CD59 gene, resulting in a frameshift and premature termination (Asp49Valfs*)	Turkish	Infancy	Progressive peripheral and bulbar neurologic dysfunction, hemolytic anemia
Haliloglu et al. (2015)	3 patients. Homozygous missense mutation in the CD59 gene (c.A146T:p. Asp49Val)	Turkish	Infancy	Axonal peripheral neuropathy, strokes, hemolytic anemia

exomes from healthy subjects available through the Exome Variant Server of the National Heart, Lung, and Blood Institute Exome Sequencing Project. The Cys89Tyr mutation in CD59 was clinically manifested in infancy by chronic hemolysis, recurrent strokes, and relapsing peripheral demyelinating disease resembling recurrent Guillain-Barre syndrome (GBS) or chronic inflammatory demyelinating polyneuropathy (CIDP).

Two additional primary CD59 mutations were reported more recently. The third mutation to be described was identified in a German girl of Turkish origin with progressive neurologic dysfunction and hemolytic anemia (Hochsmann et al. 2014). The authors identified a homozygous 1-bp deletion (c.146delA) in exon 5 of the CD59 gene, resulting in a frameshift and premature termination (Asp49ValfsTer31). Her unaffected parents were heterozygous for the mutation. The patient first presented at age 7 months with generalized hypotonia, bulbar symptoms, and areflexia. During later febrile episodes, she developed hemolytic anemia with progressive neurologic deterioration, including T2-weighted hyperintense lesions on brain MRI, seizures, and visual impairment. Flow cytometric analysis of the patient's peripheral blood cells showed isolated CD59 deficiency. Treatment with eculizumab, an inhibitor of the complement membrane-attack complex, resulted in neurologic improvement about 6 months later. At age 5.5 years, the patient could eat and swallow normally, could walk short distances with support, and had improved cognition and speech production.

The fourth mutation to be described was identified in three children with early-onset immune-mediated axonal neuropathy, cerebrovascular events in both the anterior and posterior circulation, and chronic Coombs-negative hemolysis. Linkage analysis and homozygosity mapping allowed identification of a homozygous missense mutation in the CD59 gene (c.A146T:p. Asp49Val) (Haliloglu et al. 2015).

Unlike the first case, the three mutations identified later were characterized by early symptom onset starting from 3 to 4 months with recurrent peripheral neuropathy and/or strokes. Hemolytic anemia was often missed at presentation due to the predominantly neurological nature of symptoms.

Similarities and Differences in Primary and Secondary CD59 Deficiency

Primary and secondary Cys89Tyr mutations in CD59 have differences and similarities in their clinical presentation, which are summarized in Table 2.

Intravascular Hemolysis PNH, a disease of hematopoietic stem cells, arises as a consequence of a clonal expansion of one or more hematopoietic stem cells that have acquired a somatic mutation of the X chromosome gene PIGA. The protein encoded by PIGA is essential for synthesis of the GPI moiety that serves as the membrane anchor for a functionally diverse group of cellular proteins. As a consequence of mutant PIGA, all GPI-anchored proteins (several dozen) are deficient on progeny of the affected stem cells

(Hillmen et al. 1995). The complement regulatory proteins are CD55, also known as decay-accelerating factor (DAF), which inhibits complement activation, and CD59, which inhibits MAC formation. CD55 and CD59 are among the proteins that are not expressed on the membrane due to this mutation.

The clinical hallmarks of PNH, intravascular hemolysis and the resulting hemoglobinuria, were thought to be a direct consequence of deficiencies in CD55 and CD59, since peripheral blood erythrocytes derived from the mutant clone lack the capacity to restrict cell surface activation of the alternative complement pathway due to CD55 deficiency, and to block formation of the cytolytic MAC due to CD59 deficiency. Under conditions of acidification, activation of the alternative complement pathway does occur, but the amount of CD55 and CD59 on normal erythrocytes is sufficient to inhibit activity of the alternative complement pathway under these conditions. Indeed, studies have shown that susceptibility of PNH erythrocytes to acidified serum lysis is due to CD55 (DAF) and CD59 (MIRL) deficiency (Wilcox et al. 1991). Accordingly, following incubation in acidified serum, normal erythrocytes bear only small amounts of C3 activation products, and hemolysis is not observed. However, when CD55 (DAF) and CD59 are deficient, the capacity of PNH erythrocytes to inhibit activity of the alternative complement pathway is limited, alternative pathway complement activity proceeds on the cell surface, and PNH erythrocytes are hemolyzed.

Two questions are posed by these relationships: What is the relative contribution of each of the regulatory complement proteins CD55 and

Primary and Secondary CD59 Deficiency, Table 2 Clinical and laboratory manifestations in PNH and primary CD59 deficiency

	CD59 expression	CD55 expression	Intravascular hemolysis	Thrombophilia	Bone marrow dysfunction	Recurrent peripheral neurological symptoms
PNH	Variable	Variable	+	+	+	−
Primary CD59 deficiency	100% missing	100% present	+	+	−	+ (8/9)

CD59 to hemolysis and are additional GPI proteins involved in PNH manifestations?

It has been predicted based on laboratory investigations that, although CD55 and CD59 act in concert to control susceptibility to acidified serum lysis, CD59 is the main complement regulatory protein responsible for intravascular hemolysis. However, mice with targeted deletion of the CD59 gene that had spontaneous intravascular hemolysis and hemoglobinuria in these studies were not anemic (Holt et al. 2001), and in order to support the critical role of CD59, a "natural" human knockout was lacking. This was provided with the recognition of primary homozygous Cys89Tyr CD59 deficiency, where all patients exhibit intravascular hemolysis manifested by Coombs-negative hemolytic anemia with reticulocytosis, low haptoglobin, and high LDH and MAC deposition on red blood cell (RBC) membranes. The marked intravascular hemolysis observed in primary CD59 deficiency suggests that the previous observations were indeed correct and CD59 is the main complement-regulating GPI membrane protein responsible for intravascular hemolysis.

CD55-deficient erythrocytes were needed to finally verify this premise. Indeed, it was shown that antigens of the Cromer blood group complex are located on CD55, and rare cases of a null phenotype called Inab have been reported. Apparently, Inab erythrocytes are completely deficient in CD55, but, unlike PNH erythrocytes, other GPI-linked proteins that have been studied are expressed normally on Inab. Interestingly, Inab cells are resistant to reactive lysis, suggesting that CD59 or additional unknown GPI-linked proteins are needed for lysis in PNH. Inab cell susceptibility to acidified serum lysis has been examined by two groups. Telen and Green (1989) reported that Inab cells were resistant to acidified serum lysis, whereas Merry et al. (1989) reported that approximately 5% of Inab cells were hemolyzed in acidified serum. Although it has been reported that CD55 renders RBCs more susceptible to acidified serum lysis, we could conclude that the contribution of CD55 to hemolysis in the null CD55 phenotype Inab is very low and perhaps negligible.

What about other GPI-linked proteins? Additional GPI-linked proteins may contribute to this susceptibility to hemolysis; however, no other specific protein has been seriously suggested to be critical to the disease.

In conclusion, CD59 is the membrane complement regulatory protein that is the main and perhaps the only protein responsible for the massive intravascular hemolysis observed in PNH and primary CD59 deficiency.

Thrombophilia Thrombosis is the prognostic factor with the greatest effect on survival in PNH patients (Poulou et al. 2007). Data from several retrospective studies in the pre-eculizumab era showed that the cause of death was related to thrombosis in 22.2–37.2% of PNH patients. The extremely high incidence of thrombosis in PNH and its major effects on morbidity and mortality underline its clinical importance. The cumulative 10-year incidence of thrombosis in a retrospective study of 460 PNH patients with larger clones was 31–39% (Van Bijnen et al. 2012). The risk of venous thrombosis correlates with PNH granulocyte clone size and was 44% in patients with a PNH granulocyte clone of >50%.

In the PNH population with a classic presentation, such as the patients who participated in the various eculizumab trials, 15% of pretreatment thrombotic events were arterial, located in either the cerebral vasculature (13.6%) or coronary arteries (1.4%) (Hillmen et al. 2007); thus, risk of arterial thrombosis is probably also increased in this group in comparison with age-matched healthy controls. Ziakas et al. described 38 reports of arterial thrombosis, mainly in the central nervous system or coronary arteries. Thrombosis occurred in relatively young patients, with a median age of 35 years (range 22–47) for acute coronary syndromes and 39 years (range 11–76) for stroke (Ziakas et al. 2007). In primary Cys89Tyr CD59 deficiency, thrombophilia was only the second most important factor in the pre-eculizumab era (see below); however, we have recently reported recurrent strokes leading to premature death in young children in this population (Ben-Zeev et al. 2015).

Hemostasis is achieved via a balance of pro- and antithrombotic forces, maintained by coagulation and fibrinolysis, and is influenced by blood physiology and serum factors, as well as factors derived from vessel walls and blood cells. In PNH, prothrombotic mechanisms involving all components have been proposed to explain thrombophilia; however, it is not clear whether these mechanisms fully explain the extremely high risk of thrombosis. Deficiency of GPI-anchored fibrinolytic factors such as urokinase plasminogen activator receptor (u-PAR) as well as anticoagulant factors such as tissue factor pathway inhibitor (TFPI) and, potentially, proteinase 3 (PR3) was identified as a potential factor leading to a prothrombotic state in patients with PNH (Van Bijnen et al. 2012); however, the exact contribution of missing fibrinolytic and anticoagulant GPI-linked factors to PNH-related thrombosis remains unclear. Furthermore, the fact that primary CD59 deficiency presents a severe risk factor for stroke, and probably any arterial or venous thrombosis, does not support a major role for GPI-linked fibrinolytic or anticoagulant factors in the thrombophilic state in PNH, unless the fibrinolytic system is activated by another mechanism such as intravascular hemolysis.

In contrast to GPI-linked fibrinolytic or anticoagulant factors, intravascular hemolysis is seen in both PNH and primary CD59 deficiency, increasing the level of free hemoglobin. Normally, free hemoglobin is rapidly cleared from the circulation by several scavenging mechanisms. Excessive intravascular hemolysis saturates these scavengers, resulting in free hemoglobin in plasma that irreversibly reacts with nitric oxide (NO) to form nitrate and methemoglobin. Lysed erythrocytes release arginase, which catalyzes the conversion of arginine, the substrate for NO synthesis, to ornithine. Both processes decrease the availability of NO, which normally maintains smooth muscle cell relaxation, inhibits platelet activation and aggregation, and has anti-inflammatory effects on the endothelium. Through these mechanisms, decreased NO levels may increase the thrombotic tendency in both PNH and primary CD59 deficiency.

An additional shared mechanism may be related to free heme, which mediates direct pro-inflammatory, proliferative, and prooxidant effects on endothelial cells (Wagener et al. 2001). Endothelial cell damage, an additional possible contributor to thrombosis, may occur due to the free hemoglobin released from lysed PNH erythrocytes as well as cellular-derived microparticles (Simak et al. 2004). PNH patients probably do not harbor the PIGA mutation in endothelial cells and express CD59; however, endothelial cells of patients with primary CD59 deficiency definitely do not express CD59 and thus may have heightened susceptibility to complement damage and increased risk of thrombosis. An additional component that may be important in both PNH and primary CD59 deficiency is platelet function and activation.

The assumption is that platelets are not lysed in a manner similar to that discussed above for erythrocytes in PNH or CD59 deficiency. Normal platelets express CD55 and CD59. Both are absent on PNH platelets, whereas only CD59 is absent in patients with primary CD59 deficiency. While complement destroys PNH erythrocytes, it probably does not severely destroy PNH platelets, perhaps due to their ability to shed the MAC (Sims and Wiedmer 1991), and the lifespan of the platelet population is more or less normal in the majority of patients (Louwes et al. 2001). Thrombocytopenia in PNH is thus attributed to concomitant bone marrow failure rather than to complement-mediated damage, and the fact that patients with primary CD59 deficiency tend to have a normal or even a mildly elevated platelet count supports this hypothesis (Nevo et al. 2013).

In contrast, platelet activation has been shown to be present in PNH (Sims et al. 1989; Grunewald et al. 2004). Furthermore, microparticles that may be released by erythrocytes, white blood cells, or platelets have been suggested as an additional prothrombotic factor in PNH. Microparticles are small membrane-derived vesicles that are shed upon activation, inflammation, or cell death/damage. Under normal conditions, plasma membrane anionic phospholipid phosphatidylserine is restricted to the inner leaflet. Membrane asymmetry is lost upon cell stimulation or cell death, leading to phosphatidylserine exposure on the outer leaflet of the cell membrane, followed by microparticle release, providing a surface for the assembly of procoagulant enzyme complexes (Hugel et al. 1999; Owens and Mackman 2011). Complement activation at the cell surface of GPI-deficient cells may stimulate the release of pro-coagulant microparticles, increasing the risk of thrombosis. There are currently no data regarding platelet activation or microparticles in primary CD59 deficiency, although it seems plausible to suspect their existence.

In summary, thrombosis is an extremely important prognostic factor in PNH and a serious prognostic factor in primary CD59 deficiency. Common patterns of prothrombotic factors are most probably shared by both conditions although some differences apply, such as GPI-linked fibrinolytic or anticoagulant factors that exist only in PNH but not in primary CD59 deficiency.

Neurological Manifestations As indicated above, the risk of arterial thrombosis is increased in patients with PNH, and in the 38 patients described by Ziakas et al., arterial thrombosis occurred most often in the central nervous system (Ziakas et al. 2007). In three out of four groups of patients with different mutations leading to primary CD59 deficiency, strokes were documented (not reported in Hochsmann et al. (2014)). However, in contrast to PNH, additional neurological manifestations are common in primary CD59 deficiency and are the presenting symptom in most infants.

Relapsing peripheral neuropathy resembling recurrent Guillain-Barre syndrome (GBS) or chronic inflammatory demyelinating poly-neuropathy (CIDP) was first reported by Nevo et al., and later by others, with peripheral axonal with bulbar symptoms as well as strokes (Nevo et al. 2013; Hochsmann et al. 2014; Haliloglu et al. 2015). Only the earliest report of a homozygous mutation included no observation of peripheral neuropathy in infancy (Yamashina et al. 1990).

Renal Involvement An episode of renal crisis resembling hemolytic-uremic syndrome was reported by Nevo et al. (2013), but was eventually resolved.

Additional Clinical Manifestations Clinical manifestations in PNH that are distinct from those seen in primary CD59 deficiency include acquired aplastic anemia and evidence of bone marrow dysfunction (Inoue et al. 2006; Scheinberg et al. 2010; Pu et al. 2011). Understanding the relationship between PNH and aplastic anemia was suggested to be a key to unlocking the complex pathophysiology of this eccentric disease. The close association of PNH with aplastic anemia was suggested to be directly related to the acquired mutation, given that hematopoietic stem cells with mutant PIGA have a conditional growth or survival advantage in the setting of a specific type of bone marrow injury, with subsequent independent, nonmalignant expansion of the PIGA mutant clone in some cases. However, PIGA mutant stem cells appear to have no intrinsic growth or survival advantage, suggesting that clonal expansion is driven by factors that are distinct from, but work in concert with, mutant PIGA.

The peripheral blood of patients with PNH is a mosaic of normal and abnormal cells. The percentage of abnormal cells varies widely among patients, with the degree of mosaicism among different patients determined by the extent to which the PIGA mutant clone expands. In contrast, in primary CD59 deficiency, 100% of cells are CD59 deficient.

Another distinguishing feature is that in PNH, the PIGA mutation exists only in a hematopoietic clone, whereas in CD59 deficiency, the CD59 mutation appears in all cells of the body. As a result of the systemic presence of the mutation, patients suffer from recurring GBS- or CIDP-like disease, suggesting demyelination in the peripheral nervous system via MAC activation, which is not seen in PNH. MAC activation may cause nodal block and demyelination. An additional pathophysiological explanation could be the accumulation of unprocessed CD59 in neural or Schwann cells, causing endoplasmic reticulum stress. Although it was at first surprising, activation of MAC has been suggested to mediate demyelination in both the central and peripheral nervous systems, and deposits of MAC were observed in areas of demyelination in multiple sclerosis, GBS, and CIDP (Dalakas and Engel 1980; Lucchinetti et al. 2000; Wanschitz et al. 2003). CD59 deficiency in mice rendered all mutant animals susceptible to experimental autoimmune encephalomyelitis, which is seen in only 12–42% of wild-type animals. Inflammatory disease and axonal loss were more severe in the mutant animals, and demyelination was present only in the mutants, leaving the animals severely paralyzed. MAC deposits, which are abundant in C9, were found on perivascular tissue elements in the areas of demyelination (Mead et al. 2004).

Response to Eculizumab and Additional Therapies The MAC consists of complement components C5b, C6, C7, C8, and 16 C9 molecules. Eculizumab, a humanized monoclonal antibody, has a high binding affinity for human complement protein C5, preventing its cleavage to C5a and C5b and thus inhibiting formation of the MAC. In the last 10 years, therapeutic trials with eculizumab have been conducted in PNH patients. The results of the phase III multicenter, double-blind, placebo-controlled TRIUMPH trial demonstrated that the drug reduced intravascular hemolysis and the need for transfusions and improved fatigue in PNH patients (Hillmen et al. 2006). The conclusion of the SHEPHERD study, an open-label phase III safety and efficacy trial, substantiated the positive effect of the drug and its safety (Brodsky et al. 2008). Based on this evidence of efficacy, eculizumab was approved for the treatment of PNH in the United States and Europe in 2007. These observations also led to initiation of a clinical trial using eculizumab in primary Cys89Tyr CD59 deficiency (ClinicalTrials.gov number, NCT01579838). *Recent observations of additional novel therapies including early and terminal complement pathway inhibitors may be relevant to treatment of primary CD59 deficiency.*

Conclusion

Systematic investigation of the molecular basis of PNH provided a framework for management based on an understanding of disease pathophysiology, which led to the development of targeted therapy that has improved the lives of patients and changed the natural history of the disease. Much of our understanding of primary CD59 deficiency relies on previous knowledge of PNH pathophysiology, including the beneficial effect of eculizumab. Until now, four homozygous mutations affecting nine patients have been described, with eight of the nine cases manifesting in infancy. Insights derived from primary CD59 deficiency could deepen our understanding on the major, if not exclusive role of CD59 in the pathophysiology of PNH. Distinguishing features of both diseases, notably peripheral neuropathy in primary CD59 deficiency, expand our understanding of the role of MAC in pathophysiology of the nervous system.

Acknowledgments This chapter was supported by the Legacy Heritage BioMedical Program of the Israel Science Foundation (grant No. 1070/15 TO DM).

References

Ben-Zeev B, Tabib A, Nissenkorn A, Garti BZ, Gomori JM, Nass D, Goldshmidt H, Fellig Y, Anikster Y, Nevo Y, Elpeleg O, Mevorach D. Devastating recurrent brain ischemic infarctions and retinal disease in pediatric patients with CD59 deficiency. Eur J Paediatr Neurol. 2015;19:688–93.

Brodsky RA, Young NS, Antonioli E, Risitano AM, Schrezenmeier H, Schubert J, Gaya A, Coyle L, de Castro C, Fu CL, Maciejewski JP, Bessler M, Kroon HA, Rother RP, Hillmen P. Multicenter phase 3 study of the complement inhibitor eculizumab for the treatment of patients with paroxysmal nocturnal hemoglobinuria. Blood. 2008;111:1840–7.

Dalakas MC, Engel WK. Immunoglobulin and complement deposits in nerves of patients with chronic relapsing polyneuropathy. Arch Neurol. 1980;37:637–40.

Grunewald M, Grunewald A, Schmid A, Schopflin C, Schauer S, Griesshammer M, Koksch M. The platelet function defect of paroxysmal nocturnal haemoglobinuria. Platelets. 2004;15:145–54.

Haliloglu G, Maluenda J, Sayinbatur B, Aumont C, Temucin C, Tavil B, Cetin M, Oguz KK, Gut I, Picard V, Melki J, Topaloglu H. Early-onset chronic axonal neuropathy, strokes, and hemolysis: inherited CD59 deficiency. Neurology. 2015;84:1220–4.

Hillmen P, Lewis SM, Bessler M, Luzzatto L, Dacie JV. Natural history of paroxysmal nocturnal hemoglobinuria. N Engl J Med. 1995;333:1253–8.

Hillmen P, Young NS, Schubert J, Brodsky RA, Socie G, Muus P, Roth A, Szer J, Elebute MO, Nakamura R, Browne P, Risitano AM, Hill A, Schrezenmeier H, Fu CL, Maciejewski J, Rollins SA, Mojcik CF, Rother RP, Luzzatto L. The complement inhibitor eculizumab in paroxysmal nocturnal hemoglobinuria. N Engl J Med. 2006;355:1233–43.

Hillmen P, Muus P, Duhrsen U, Risitano AM, Schubert J, Luzzatto L, Schrezenmeier H, Szer J, Brodsky RA, Hill A, Socie G, Bessler M, Rollins SA, Bell L, Rother RP, Young NS. Effect of the complement inhibitor eculizumab on thromboembolism in patients with paroxysmal nocturnal hemoglobinuria. Blood. 2007;110:4123–8.

Hochsmann B, Dohna-Schwake C, Kyrieleis HA, Pannicke U, Schrezenmeier H. Targeted therapy with eculizumab for inherited CD59 deficiency. N Engl J Med. 2014;370:90–2.

Holt DS, Botto M, Bygrave AE, Hanna SM, Walport MJ, Morgan BP. Targeted deletion of the CD59 gene causes spontaneous intravascular hemolysis and hemoglobinuria. Blood. 2001;98:442–9.

Hugel B, Socie G, Vu T, Toti F, Gluckman E, Freyssinet JM, Scrobohaci ML. Elevated levels of circulating procoagulant microparticles in patients with paroxysmal nocturnal hemoglobinuria and aplastic anemia. Blood. 1999;93:3451–6.

Inoue N, Izui-Sarumaru T, Murakami Y, Endo Y, Nishimura J, Kurokawa K, Kuwayama M, Shime H, Machii T, Kanakura Y, Meyers G, Wittwer C, Chen Z, Babcock W, Frei-Lahr D, Parker CJ, Kinoshita T. Molecular basis of clonal expansion of hematopoiesis in 2 patients with paroxysmal nocturnal hemoglobinuria (PNH). Blood. 2006;108:4232–6.

Louwes H, Vellenga E, de Wolf JT. Abnormal platelet adhesion on abdominal vessels in asymptomatic patients with paroxysmal nocturnal hemoglobinuria. Ann Hematol. 2001;80:573–6.

Lucchinetti C, Bruck W, Parisi J, Scheithauer B, Rodriguez M, Lassmann H. Heterogeneity of multiple sclerosis lesions: implications for the pathogenesis of demyelination. Ann Neurol. 2000;47:707–17.

Mead RJ, Neal JW, Griffiths MR, Linington C, Botto M, Lassmann H, Morgan BP. Deficiency of the complement regulator CD59a enhances disease severity, demyelination and axonal injury in murine acute experimental allergic encephalomyelitis. Lab Investig. 2004;84:21–8.

Merry AH, Rawlinson VI, Uchikawa M, Daha MR, Sim RB. Studies on the sensitivity to complement-mediated lysis of erythrocytes (Inab phenotype) with a deficiency of DAF (decay accelerating factor). Br J Haematol. 1989;73:248–53.

Motoyama N, Okada N, Yamashina M, Okada H. Paroxysmal nocturnal hemoglobinuria due to hereditary nucleotide deletion in the HRF20 (CD59) gene. Eur J Immunol. 1992;22:2669–73.

Nevo Y, Ben-Zeev B, Tabib A, Straussberg R, Anikster Y, Shorer Z, Fattal-Valevski A, Ta-Shma A, Aharoni S, Rabie M, Zenvirt S, Goldshmidt H, Fellig Y, Shaag A, Mevorach D, Elpeleg O. CD59 deficiency is associated with chronic hemolysis and childhood relapsing immune-mediated polyneuropathy. Blood. 2013;121:129–35.

Owens 3rd AP, Mackman N. Microparticles in hemostasis and thrombosis. Circ Res. 2011;108:1284–97.

Poulou LS, Vakrinos G, Pomoni A, Michalakis K, Karianakis G, Voulgarelis M, Ziakas PD. Stroke in paroxysmal nocturnal haemoglobinuria: patterns of disease and outcome. Thromb Haemost. 2007;98:699–701.

Pu JJ, Mukhina G, Wang H, Savage WJ, Brodsky RA. Natural history of paroxysmal nocturnal hemoglobinuria clones in patients presenting as aplastic anemia. Eur J Haematol. 2011;87:37–45.

Scheinberg P, Marte M, Nunez O, Young NS. Paroxysmal nocturnal hemoglobinuria clones in severe aplastic anemia patients treated with horse anti-thymocyte globulin plus cyclosporine. Haematologica. 2010;95:1075–80.

Simak J, Holada K, Risitano AM, Zivny JH, Young NS, Vostal JG. Elevated circulating endothelial membrane microparticles in paroxysmal nocturnal haemoglobinuria. Br J Haematol. 2004;125:804–13.

Sims PJ, Wiedmer T. The response of human platelets to activated components of the complement system. Immunol Today. 1991;12:338–42.

Sims PJ, Rollins SA, Wiedmer T. Regulatory control of complement on blood platelets. Modulation of platelet procoagulant responses by a membrane inhibitor of the C5b-9 complex. J Biol Chem. 1989;264:19228–35.

Sugita Y, Nakano Y, Tomita M. Isolation from human erythrocytes of a new membrane protein which inhibits the formation of complement transmembrane channels. J Biochem. 1988;104:633–7.

Takeda J, Miyata T, Kawagoe K, Iida Y, Endo Y, Fujita T, Takahashi M, Kitani T, Kinoshita T. Deficiency of the GPI anchor caused by a somatic mutation of the PIG-A gene in paroxysmal nocturnal hemoglobinuria. Cell. 1993;73:703–11.

Telen MJ, Green AM. The Inab phenotype: characterization of the membrane protein and complement regulatory defect. Blood. 1989;74:437–41.

Van Bijnen ST, Van Heerde WL, Muus P. Mechanisms and clinical implications of thrombosis in paroxysmal nocturnal hemoglobinuria. J Thromb Haemost. 2012;10:1–10.

Wagener FA, Eggert A, Boerman OC, Oyen WJ, Verhofstad A, Abraham NG, Adema G, van Kooyk Y, de Witte T, Figdor CG. Heme is a potent inducer of inflammation in mice and is counteracted by heme oxygenase. Blood. 2001;98:1802–11.

Wanschitz J, Maier H, Lassmann H, Budka H, Berger T. Distinct time pattern of complement activation and cytotoxic T cell response in Guillain-Barre syndrome. Brain. 2003;126:2034–42.

Wilcox LA, Ezzell JL, Bernshaw NJ, Parker CJ. Molecular basis of the enhanced susceptibility of the erythrocytes of paroxysmal nocturnal hemoglobinuria to hemolysis in acidified serum. Blood. 1991;78:820–9.

Yamashina M, Ueda E, Kinoshita T, Takami T, Ojima A, Ono H, Tanaka H, Kondo N, Orii T, Okada N, et al. Inherited complete deficiency of 20-kilodalton homologous restriction factor (CD59) as a cause of paroxysmal nocturnal hemoglobinuria. N Engl J Med. 1990;323:1184–9.

Ziakas PD, Poulou LS, Rokas GI, Bartzoudis D, Voulgarelis M. Thrombosis in paroxysmal nocturnal hemoglobinuria: sites, risks, outcome. An overview. J Thromb Haemost. 2007;5:642–5.

Primary Immune Deficiency

▶ Clinical Presentation of Immunodeficiency, Overview
▶ Clinical Presentation of Immunodeficiency, Primary Immunodeficiency

Proline-Serine-Threonine Phosphatase-Interacting Protein 1

▶ Pyogenic Arthritis, Pyoderma Gangrenosum, and Acne (PAPA) Syndrome

Properdin Deficiency

Merja Helminen
Tampere Center for Child Health Research, Tampere University Hospital, Tampere, Finland

Synonyms

Complement factor P (CFP) deficiency; Properdin P factor (complement) (PFC) deficiency

Definition

Properdin deficiency is an X-chromosomally inherited disease with deficiency or dysfunction of the plasma protein properdin, which is the only known positive regulator of the complement activation cascade.

Introduction

Properdin is the only known positive regulator of the complement cascade and is essential for efficient complement activation via the alternative pathway (AP). It is synthesized, unlike other complement proteins, by leukocytes including monocyte/macrophages, T cells, and neutrophils and is present in serum at low levels of 11–30 mg/l (Späth et al. 1999). The regulation of its homeostasis in vivo is unknown. It is a glycoprotein that consists of identical 53 kDa subunits, monomers that form cyclic dimers, trimers, and tetramers in plasma (Kemper et al. 2010). Properdin functions as a positive regulator of AP by its ability to stabilize C3 convertase (C3bBb) and prolong its half-life. This allows increased C3 deposition on bacterial surfaces, more efficient opsonization and formation of the membrane attack complex (Kemper et al. 2010). Recent studies have suggested additional and more active roles for properdin. When properdin was initially discovered more than 50 years ago, it was considered as an initiator of AP activation. This concept was later abandoned, but some studies have recently shown that properdin may function as a pattern recognition molecule and when bound to selected surfaces initiate AP complement activation (Kemper et al. 2010).

Genetics

The *CFP* gene is located on the X chromosome at Xp11.23-p11.3. It consists of ten exons and has a length of 6 kb (Fijen et al. 1999b). Properdin deficiency is inherited as X chromosomal recessive trait: if the mother carries the mutation, she herself is asymptomatic, but her sons have 50%

risk to inherit the mutation and be symptomatic, and the daughters of a carrier mother have 50% risk to be carrier, whereas all daughters of a male patient have the mutation.

The molecular basis of properdin deficiency seems to be heterogeneous even in geographically limited areas (Table 1). Although most of the reported patients are of European origin, properdin deficiency has been diagnosed in patients of Pakistani and South American origin (Schejbel et al. 2009; Truedsson et al. 1997).

Three phenotypes on the basis of immunochemical and functional analysis have been described. Type I, which is the most common phenotype, is associated with undetectable properdin levels, type II has protein levels that are measurable but less than 10% of normal values, and type III has normal levels of properdin but the protein is not functional. Type II deficiency has been described in a Danish and Swedish family with mutations causing substitution of amino acids (Nordin Fredrikson et al. 1998; Westberg et al. 1995). Further analysis showed that the protein is synthesized and secreted in normal amounts but that oligomerization of the protein is abnormal. The low serum levels were suggested to result from increased catabolism of the abnormal protein (Nordin Fredrikson et al. 1998). Type III deficiency has been shown in one Dutch family in 1988 (Sjöholm et al. 1988). The mutation was caused by a missense mutation, which affected the binding of properdin to C3b (Nordin Fredrikson et al. 1996).

The serum properdin level of female carriers varies from normal values to values that are markedly reduced (Späth et al. 1999; van den Bogaard et al. 2000). This variation can be partly explained by uneven lyonization of the normal and mutated X chromosomes. No meningococcal infections have been reported in female carriers suggesting that even low levels of properdin are enough for efficient AP function in carriers.

Disease

Properdin deficiency was first described 1982 in a Swedish family in association with meningococcal infection (Sjöholm et al. 1982). Since then nearly all patients have been diagnosed because

Properdin Deficiency, Table 1 The properdin mutations published in literature 1987–2014 and listed in Human Gene Mutation Database (HGMD; http://www.hgmd.org; Stenson et al. 2014)

Mutation HGVS nucleotide(protein)	Exon	Phenotype	Origin	References
c.235C > T(p.R79*)	4	I	Swiss, Dutch	Truedsson et al. (1997), van den Bogaard et al. (2000)
c. 671_672delGT	6	I	Swedish	Truedsson et al. (1997)
c.617C > G(p.S206*)	6	I	Dutch	Van den Bogaard et al. (2000)
c.786_793delTTGGGGCC	7	I	Dutch	Van den Bogaard et al. (2000)
c.893G > T(p.G298V)	7	I	Dutch	Van den Bogaard et al. (2000)
c.961 T > G (p.W321G)	8	I	South American, Dutch	Truedsson et al. (1997), Van den Bogaard et al. (2000)
c.962G > C(p.W321S)	8	I	Dutch	Van den Bogaard et al. (2000)
c.1240 T > G(p.Y414D)	9	III	Dutch	Nordin Fredrikson et al. (1996)
c.481C > T(p.R161*)	5	I	Swedish	Westberg et al. (1995)
c.298C > T(p.R100W)	4	II	Swedish	Westberg et al. (1995)
c.1028A > G(p.Q343R)	8	II	Danish	Truedsson et al. (1997)
c.564_565delGGinsCCC	5	II	Pakistani	Schejbel et al. (2009)
c.1164G > A(p.W388*)	9	I	Finnish	Helminen et al. (2012)
c.559C > T(p.Q187*)	5	I	Israel (Moroccan), Israel (Tunisian)	Fijen et al. (1999b)
c. 1036C > T(p.R346C)	8	I	Israel (Tunisian)	Fijen et al. (1999b)

* Mutation giving rise to stop codon

of infection caused by *Neisseria meningitides*. In a Dutch study, the risk of contracting meningococcal infection was 250 times higher for the properdin deficient individuals, and the mortality was increased several fold (Fijen et al. 1999a). On the other hand, most patients with meningococcal infection do not have complement abnormalities, and not all patients with properdin deficiency seem to contract meningococcal infection (Fijen et al. 1999a). Additional factors may be needed or may increase the risk for meningococcal infection in properdin deficient individuals. Low activity of the lectin pathway and lack of immunoglobulin G2 m(n), which weakens antibody response against polysaccharide antigens, have been connected to increased risk of infection (Späth et al. 1999; Bathum et al. 2006).

The mechanism that underlies the clinically observed narrow susceptibility to meningococcal infections is unclear. In experimental mouse studies, it has been shown that the outer membrane complex of meningococci is a poor activator of classical and lectin pathways, whereas other gram-negative bacteria activate complement efficiently through both properdin-dependent and properdin-independent pathways (Kimura et al. 2008). The insufficient C3 deposition on the meningococcal surface in properdin deficiency that results in insufficient phagocytosis of the bacteria may also be a promoting factor for invasive infection (Fijen et al. 2000).

Properdin deficiency should be suspected in atypical cases and if the family has a history of meningococcal infection in males. In normal population, the peak incidence of meningococcal infection is at age of less than 2 years, and the lack of protective antibodies is an important risk factor. Patients with properdin deficiency usually contract the infection when they are older and should already have naturally acquired or cross-reactive antibodies. Properdin-deficient patients also have increased susceptibility to diseases caused by atypical *N. meningitides* strains (W-135, X, Y, Z) that seldom cause infections in healthy individuals (Fijen et al. 1999a). However, in an individual patient with properdin deficiency,

the infection can manifest at less than 2 years of age and be caused by a typical *N. meningitides* strain (A, B, C). Because properdin deficiency is extremely rare, all the data that is available on the clinical picture or prognosis of meningococcal infection in these patients is based on case reports and family studies and should be analyzed with scrutiny. Recurrent meningococcal infections seem to be nonexistent or extremely rare. In two recent reports, properdin deficiency was associated with history of recurrent pneumonia and otitis media (Schejbel et al. 2009; Lee et al. 2014). However, further studies are needed to clarify the association suggested by these reports. No association to autoimmune manifestations such as in early complement component deficiencies or more recently in other AP abnormalities has been described in properdin deficiency.

Diagnosis

Properdin deficiency should be suspected in patients with meningococcal disease especially if the infection is caused by an atypical strain or if the family has a history of meningococcal infections in male members. Properdin-deficient individuals can be identified by the LPS-based ELISA AP assay but not by the traditional AP-based hemolytic assay (Mollnes et al. 2007). When abnormal AP activity is detected, properdin levels should be measured in male patients. In type I properdin deficiency, the properdin level is below detection limit, in type II deficiency is <10% of normal values, and in type III deficiency, which has only been described in one family, the properdin level is normal, but the protein does not function. When properdin deficiency is diagnosed in a family, it is of utmost importance that all male members are screened for properdin deficiency because of risk for meningococcal disease. In asymptomatic female carriers, properdin level varies from normal to surprisingly low, and therefore carrier status should be determined by genetic methods. Properdin deficiency is confirmed by detecting the causative mutation.

Treatment

When properdin deficiency is identified, all male members of the family with a mutation should be vaccinated with meningococcal vaccine. Vaccination induces bactericidal antibodies and provides protection against the infection. Recommendations vary according to country and depend on the availability of the vaccine and age of the patient to be vaccinated. The Advisory Committee on Immunization Practices (ACIP) recommends that quadrivalent (ACWY) meningococcal conjugate vaccine should be used to immunize adults and children >2 months of age. First booster is recommended in children <7 years of age after 3 years and thereafter every 5 years and in adults and children >7 years every 5 years after the initial vaccination series (CDC 2013; MacNeil et al. 2014). Meningococcal group B vaccine is licensed from 2 months of age in several countries and is indicated for individuals with properdin deficiency. Antibiotic prophylaxis with penicillin at a dose of 50,000 IU/kg (one million units twice daily for adults) should be administered at least before protective antibodies have accumulated after vaccination.

References

Bathum L, Hansen H, Teisner B, Koch C, Garred P, Rasmussen K, Wang P. Association between combined properdin and mannose-binding lectin deficiency and infection with Neisseria meningitides. Mol Immunol. 2006;43:473–9.

CDC. Prevention and control of meningococcal disease: recommendation of the Advisory Committee on Immunization Practices (ACIP). MMWR. 2013;62(RR-02): 1–28.

Fijen CAP, Kuijper EJ, de Bulte MT, Daha MR, Dankert J. Assessment of complement deficiency in patients with meningococcal disease in the Netherlands. Clin Infect Dis. 1999a;28:98–105.

Fijen CAP, van den Bogaard R, Schipper M, Mannens M, Schlesinger M, Nordin FG, Dankert J, Daha MR, Sjöholm AG, Truedsson L, Kuijper EJ. Properdin deficiency: molecular basis and disease association. Mol Immunol. 1999b;36:863–7.

Fijen CAP, Bredius RGM, Kuijper EJ, Out TA, de Haas M, de Wit APM, Daha MR, van de Winkel JGJ. The role of Fcγ receptor polymorphisms and C3 in the immune defense against Neisseria meningitides in complement-deficient individuals. Clin Exp Immunol. 2000;120:338–45.

Helminen M, Seitsonen S, Jarvas H, Meri S, Järvelä IE. A novel mutation W388X underlying properdin deficiency in a Finnish family. Scand J Immunol. 2012;75:445–8.

Kemper C, Atkinson JP, Hourcade DE. Properdin: emerging roles of a pattern-recognition molecule. Annu Rev Immunol. 2010;28:131–55.

Kimura Y, Miwa T, Zhou L, Song W-C. Activator-specific requirement of properdin in the initiation and amplification of the alternative pathway complement. Blood. 2008;111:732–40.

Lee JXW, Yusin JS, Randhawa I. Properdin deficiency-associated bronchiectasis. Ann Allergy Asthma Immunol. 2014;112:551–62.

MacNeil JR, Rubin L, McNamara L, Briere EC, Clark TA, Cohn AC. Use of MenACWY-CRM vaccine in children aged 2 through 23 months at increased risk for meningococcal disease: recommendations of the advisory committee on immunization practices, 2013. MMWR. 2014;63:527–30.

Mollnes TE, Jokiranta TS, Truedsson L, Nilsson B, de Cordoba SR, Kirschfink M. Complement analysis in the 21st century. Mol Immunol. 2007;44:3838–49.

Nordin-Fredrikson G, Westberg J, Kuijper EJ, Tijssen CC, Sjöholm AG, Uhlen M, Truedsson L. Molecular characterization of properdin deficiency type III. J Immunol. 1996;157:3666–71.

Nordin-Fredrikson G, Gullstrand B, Westberg J, Sjöholm AG, Uhlen M, Truedsson L. Expression of properdin in complete and incomplete deficiency: normal in vitro synthesis by monocytes in two cases with properdin deficiency type II due to distinct mutations. J Clin Immunol. 1998;18:272–82.

Schejbel L, Rosenfeldt V, Marquart H, Valerius NH, Garred P. Properdin deficiency associated with recurrent otitis media and pneumonia, and identification of male carrier with Klinefelter syndrome. Clin Immunol. 2009;131:456–62.

Sjöholm AG, Braconier J-H, Söderström C. Properdin deficiency in a family with fulminant meningococcal infections. Clin Exp Immunol. 1982;50:291–7.

Sjöholm AG, Kuijper EJ, Tijssen CC, Jansz A, Bol P, Spanjaard L, Zanen HC. Dysfunctional properdin in a Dutch family with meningococcal disease. N Engl J Med. 1988;319:33–7.

Späth PJ, Sjöholm AG, Nordin Fredrikson G, et al. Properdin deficiency in a large Swiss family: identification of a stop codon in the properdin gene, and association of meningococcal disease with lack of the IgG2 allotype marker (G2 m(n)). Clin Exp Immunol. 1999;118:278–84.

Stenson PD, Mort M, Ball EV, Howells K, Phillips AD, Thomas NS, Cooper DN. The human Gene mutation

P

database: building a comprehensive mutation repository for clinical and molecular genetics, diagnostic testing and personalized genomic medicine. Hum Genet. 2014;133:1–9.

Truedsson L, Westberg J, Nordin Fredrikson G, Sjöholm AG, Kuijper EJ, Fijen CAP, Uhlen M. Human properdin deficiency has a heterogeneous genetic background. Immunopharmacology. 1997;38:203–6.

Van den Bogaard R, Fijen CAP, Schipper MGJ, de Galan L, Kuijper EJ, Mannens M. Molecular characterization of 10 Dutch properdin type I deficient families: mutation analysis and X-inactivation studies. Eur J Hum Genet. 2000;8:513–8.

Westberg J, Nordin Fredrikson G, Truedsson L, Sjöholm AG, Uhlen M. Sequence-based analysis of properdin deficiency: identification of point mutations in two phenotypic forms of an x-linked immunodeficiency. Genomics. 1995;29:1–8.

Properdin P Factor (Complement) (PFC) Deficiency

▶ Properdin Deficiency

Proteasome-Associated Autoinflammatory Syndrome (PRAAS)

▶ Chronic Atypical Neutrophilic Dermatosis with Lipodystrophy and Elevated Temperature Syndrome (CANDLE)/Proteasome-Associated Autoinflammatory Syndromes (PRAAS)

PRP

▶ CARD14-Mediated Psoriasis and Pityriasis Rubra Piliaris (PRP)

Pseudotoxoplasmosis Syndrome

▶ Aicardi-Goutières Syndrome (AGS1–AGS7)

PSTPIP1

▶ Pyogenic Arthritis, Pyoderma Gangrenosum, and Acne (PAPA) Syndrome

Pyogenic Arthritis, Pyoderma Gangrenosum, and Acne

▶ Pyogenic Arthritis, Pyoderma Gangrenosum, and Acne (PAPA) Syndrome

Pyogenic Arthritis, Pyoderma Gangrenosum, and Acne (PAPA) Syndrome

Deborah L. Stone and Daniel L. Kastner
National Human Genome Research Institute,
National Institutes of Health, Bethesda, MD, USA

Synonyms

CD2-binding protein 1; PAPA; Proline-serine-threonine phosphatase-interacting protein 1; PSTPIP1; Pyogenic arthritis, pyoderma gangrenosum, and acne

Definition

Pyogenic arthritis, pyoderma gangrenosum, and acne (PAPA) syndrome is a rare autoinflammatory condition presenting with inflammatory joint and skin disease that is caused by autosomal dominant, gain-of-function mutations in *PSTPIP1* (MIM #604416).

Introduction

PAPA syndrome was first described in a large family in 1997 (Lindor et al. 1997). The "streaky leukocyte syndrome" described in a teenage boy in 1975 was later confirmed by genetic testing to be a case of PAPA syndrome (Jacobs and Goetzl 1975).

Genetics

Familial PAPA syndrome is inherited in an autosomal dominant manner with phenotypic variability. De novo mutations are the cause of PAPA syndrome in other individuals. PAPA syndrome results from mutations in PSTPIP1 (proline-serine-threonine phosphatase-interacting protein 1), also known as CD2-binding protein 1 (CD2BP1), a tyrosine-phosphorylated protein involved in cytoskeletal organization.

Pathogenesis

Endogenous PSTPIP1/CD2BP1 interacts with pyrin, the protein mutated in the clinically distinct autoinflammatory syndrome familial Mediterranean fever (FMF). Both PSTPIP1/CD2BP1 and pyrin are expressed in monocytes and granulocytes. The most common PSTPIP1

mutations seen in patients with PAPA syndrome, p.A230T and p.E250Q, markedly increase pyrin-PSTPIP1 binding, as assayed by immunoprecipitation (Shoham et al. 2003).

Clinical Manifestations

Musculoskeletal Manifestations
Individuals affected by PAPA syndrome frequently have recurrent episodes of sterile pyogenic arthritis that can result in joint destruction (Fig. 1). Seemingly trivial injury may trigger episodes of arthritis, and the same joint may be involved repeatedly. Osteolytic lesions may also cause bone pain in people with PAPA syndrome (Fig. 2).

Cutaneous Manifestations
Pathergy in patients with PAPA syndrome may lead to the development of sterile skin abscesses at the sites of immunizations. Pyoderma gangrenosum (PG) lesions may develop spontaneously or after a minor skin injury or surgical procedure. PG lesions are painful and scarring,

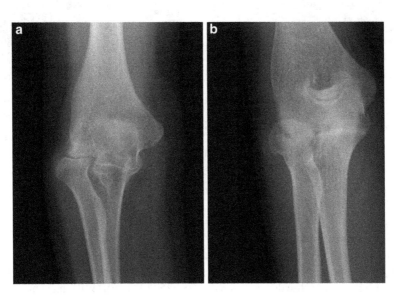

Pyogenic Arthritis, Pyoderma Gangrenosum, and Acne (PAPA) Syndrome, Fig. 1 Elbow x-rays from two patients with PAPA syndrome who have had recurrent sterile arthritis resulting in limitation of elbow movement: X-ray (**a**) shows loss of articular cartilage of the right elbow joint with subchondral changes noted in the distal elbow joint with subchondral changes noted in the distal right humerus with mild deformity of the radial head. X-ray (**b**) shows osteoarthritic degenerative changes greatest at the radiocapitellar joint, which are atypical for age, with apparent ventral bone excrescence off the distal humerus suggestive of a sessile osteochondroma or prior post-traumatic change

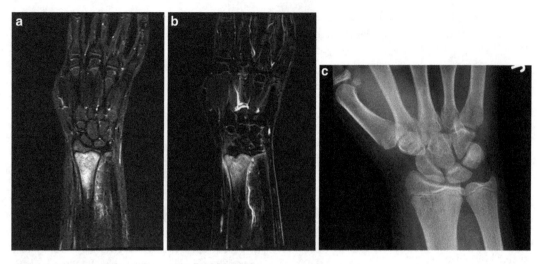

Pyogenic Arthritis, Pyoderma Gangrenosum, and Acne (PAPA) Syndrome, Fig. 2 MRI performed to evaluate wrist pain in the same patient seen in Fig. 3: coronal STIR (**a**) and 3D T1 post-contrast (**b**) images of distal right radius demonstrate increased STIR signal and enhancement of distal radial bone marrow. Plain anteroposterior radiograph (**c**) demonstrates a subtle lucency in the distal radius

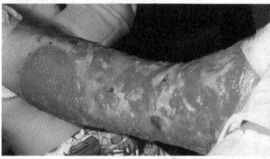

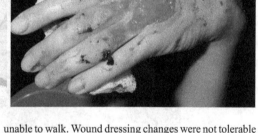

Pyogenic Arthritis, Pyoderma Gangrenosum, and Acne (PAPA) Syndrome, Fig. 3 These photos demonstrate the severe pyoderma gangrenosum lesions which were present on lower legs, arms, and hands of a 7-year-old child with the E250Q mutation in PSTPIP1. This child also had joint contractures from pyogenic arthritis and was unable to walk. Wound dressing changes were not tolerable without sedation. This child was treated with daily anakinra which appeared to prevent recurrence of pyogenic arthritis. These wounds did not respond to high doses (2 mg/kg) of etanercept but eventually healed after golimumab was prescribed

and the involved areas are vulnerable to recurrence with expansion into the nearby skin (Figs. 3 and 4). Eventually large areas, such as the lower extremities or buttocks, may be involved. Large PG lesions and joint destruction from recurrent arthritis may cause difficulties with walking and the activities of daily living.

After puberty begins, many people with PAPA syndrome develop severe, nodulocystic acne that is painful and scarring. PG lesions may also affect the face (Fig. 5). PG lesions may be misdiagnosed as cellulitis, with the resultant overuse of antibiotics.

Other Findings

Individuals with certain mutations (p.E250K and p.E257K) in PSTPIP1 may have splenomegaly and pancytopenia in addition to the usual findings of PAPA. This syndrome has sometimes been denoted as PSTPIP1-associated myeloid-related proteinemia inflammatory (PAMI) syndrome (Holzinger and Roth 2016).

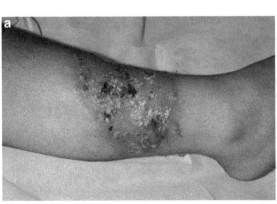
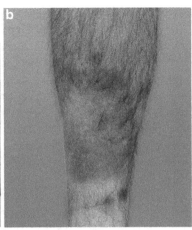

Pyogenic Arthritis, Pyoderma Gangrenosum, and Acne (PAPA) Syndrome, Fig. 4 Pyoderma gangrenosum (PG) lesion with pustules and crusting on the lower leg of a teenager with the E250Q mutation in PSTPIP1. The second photo shows the same area of the leg several years later after healing with an atrophic scar. This same area has become inflamed multiple times and expanded in size

Laboratory Findings

At the time of disease flare, inflammatory markers (CRP and ESR) are elevated, sometimes markedly so. A complete blood count (CBC) may show a microcytic anemia because of poor iron absorption associated with chronic disease and inflammation. Sequencing of *PSTPIP1* in patients with PAPA syndrome most frequently reveals mutations causing p.E250Q or p.A230T (Holzinger and Roth 2016). Sequencing has been found to be negative for *PSTPIP1* mutations in some individuals with overlapping clinical findings, such as PG lesions and osteolytic lesions, indicating genetic heterogeneity. Autoantibody testing is usually negative.

Treatment

Treatment of PAPA syndrome can be challenging, as there is variability in clinical presentation and response to treatment (Omenetti et al. 2016). High doses of corticosteroids can suppress inflammation and help heal the lesions of PAPA syndrome. However, corticosteroids work only partially and temporarily and cause many side effects. Good wound care is critical to promote the healing of the skin lesions associated with PAPA syndrome.

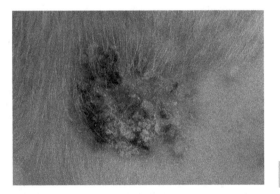

Pyogenic Arthritis, Pyoderma Gangrenosum, and Acne (PAPA) Syndrome, Fig. 5 Pyoderma gangrenosum lesion affecting the right temple of a teenage boy with PAPA syndrome and the A230T mutation in PSTPIP1

Inhibition of IL-1 with anakinra (a recombinant human IL-1 receptor antagonist) or canakinumab (a human anti-IL-1 beta monoclonal antibody) has prevented or ameliorated the arthritis associated with PAPA syndrome in some patients.

Treating the skin manifestations of PAPA syndrome is often more difficult. Both IL-1 inhibitors and TNF inhibitors have helped heal the skin lesions of PAPA syndrome in some individuals, but neither works consistently. Canakinumab appears to have greater efficacy than anakinra, whether owing to better patient compliance or to a more consistent steady-state level of drug in the body. Some patients have benefited from concurrent treatment with inhibitors of IL-1 and TNF; however, individuals treated with more than one cytokine inhibitor, especially long-acting ones, should be monitored closely and treated promptly for concerns of infection. Anti-TNF monoclonal antibodies, particularly infliximab and golimumab, have shown greater efficacy than etanercept in promoting the healing of severe PG lesions. Severely affected patients may continue to require daily corticosteroids, and intravenous corticosteroids may be given to calm a flare of disease. Isotretinoin has improved the severe acne of PAPA syndrome when given with cytokine inhibitors and corticosteroids. Bone marrow transplant has helped at least one patient.

Prognosis

Preventing the establishment of extensive areas of skin involvement and joint destruction with early diagnosis and aggressive treatment may prevent disability in individuals affected with PAPA syndrome. The diagnosis of PAPA should be considered in any patient with recurrent, sterile arthritis or PG lesions. Genetic testing for *PSTPIP1* mutations is commercially available. While treatment remains challenging in some patients with severe disease, all have shown some improvement when treated with a combination of TNF inhibitors, IL-1 inhibitors, and corticosteroids.

Cross-References

▶ Familial Mediterranean Fever and Pyrin-Associated Autoinflammatory Syndromes

References

Holzinger D Roth J. Alarming consequences – autoinflammatory disease spectrum due to mutations in proline-serine-threonine phosphatase-interacting protein 1. Curr Opin Rheumatol. 2016;28(5):550–559. PubMed: 27464597.

Jacobs JC, Goetzl EJ. 'Streaking leukocyte factor,' arthritis and pyoderma gangrenosum, Pediatrics. 1975;56:570–578. PubMed: 1165961.

Lindor NM, Arsenault TM, Solomon H, Seidman CE, McEvoy MT. A new autosomal dominant disorder of pyogenic sterile arthritis, pyoderma gangrenosum and acne: PAPA syndrome. Mayo Clin Proc. 1997; 72:611–615. PubMed: 9212761.

Omenetti A, Carta S, Caorsi R, Finetti M, Marotto D, Lattanzi B et al. Disease activity accounts for long-term efficacy of IL-1 blockers in pyogenic sterile arthritis pyoderma gangrenosum and severe acne syndrome Rheumatology (Oxford). 2016; 55(7):1325–1335. PubMed: 26989109.

Shoham NG, Centola M, Mansfield E, Hull KM, Wood G, Wise CA, et al. Pyrin binds the PSTPIP1/CD2BP1 protein, defining familial Mediterranean fever and PAPA syndrome as disorders in the same pathway. Proc Natl Acad Sci U S A. 2003;100:13501–13506. PubMed: 14595024.

R

Rac2 Deficiency

Raz Somech and Tali Stauber
Pediatric Department, Allergy and the
Immunology Services, "Edmond and Lily Safra"
Children's Hospital, Sackler School of Medicine,
Tel Aviv University, Tel Aviv, Israel
Jeffrey Modell Foundation Center, Sackler School
of Medicine, Tel Aviv University, Tel Aviv, Israel
Sheba Medical Center, Tel Hashomer, Sackler
School of Medicine, Tel Aviv University, Tel
Aviv, Israel

Synonyms

Neutrophil immunodeficiency syndrome

Definition

Rac2 which is expressed in cells of hematopoietic origin is a regulatory element that constitutes the predominant NADPH oxidase complex in leukocytes. Thus, it regulates superoxide production, direct migration in neutrophils and play distinct roles in actin organization, cell survival, and proliferation. Its deficiency leads to an immunodeficiency clinically similar to Chronic Granulomatous Diseases. Interestingly, it was shown that RAC2 is involved also in T and B cell immunity.

Introduction

Rho GTPases, members of the Ras superfamily of GTPases, regulate a wide variety of cellular activities including actin cytoskeleton reorganization, chemotaxis, gene transcription, cell growth, and development. These proteins are divided into six families based on sequence homology, protein domains, and function. Of them, Rac (Ras-related C3 botulinum toxin) proteins composed of three different isoforms, namely, Rac1, Rac2, and Rac3. Rac1 and Rac2 share over 90% identity. Rac2 expression is restricted to cells of hematopoietic origin, while Rac1 and Rac3 proteins are expressed in different tissues. The Rac2 gene is mapped to 22q13.1 and contained eight exoms spanning over 18 kb of DNA. Rac2 (with or without Rac1) has critical functions in neutrophil adhesion, migration, and killing. Importantly, Rac2 is one of four regulatory cytosolic subunits (the other three being p40phox, p47phox, p67phox) that together with two transmembrane components gp91phox (Nox2) and p22phox constitute the predominant nicotinamide adenine dinucleotide phosphate (NADPH) oxidase (Nox) complex in leukocytes (Pai et al. 2010). In mice models, Rac2 was shown to regulate superoxide production, direct migration in neutrophils, and play distinct roles in actin organization, cell survival, and proliferation. In many aspects, Rac2-deficient mice were found to have a phenotype similar to the human diseases of leukocyte

© Springer Science+Business Media LLC, part of Springer Nature 2020
I. R. Mackay et al. (eds.), *Encyclopedia of Medical Immunology*,
https://doi.org/10.1007/978-1-4614-8678-7

adhesion deficiency and chronic granulomatous disease, including increased susceptibility to Aspergillus infection. Interestingly, studies with Rac2 knockout mice have also shown defects in T- and B-cells.

Clinical Presentations

Rac2 fundamental value for the host immune defense has been confirmed as patients harboring mutations in Rac2 were found to have different types of immunodeficiencies.

Ambruso et al. (2000) identified a dominant negative inhibitory RAC2 mutation in a 5-week-old male infant with immunodeficiency syndrome suggestive of a neutrophil defect. The patient had delayed umbilical cord separation, perirectal abscesses, a failure to heal surgical wounds, and an absence of pus in infected areas. His blood tests revealed leukocytosis and neutrophilia. In addition, chemotaxis and phagocytosis were impaired, defective granule release was observed, and superoxide production was significantly reduced. An asp57-to-asn (D57N) amino acid substitution due to a G-to-A transition at nucleotide 169 in the RAC2 gene was identified. The site of the mutation is involved in nucleotide binding and is conserved in all mammalian Rho GTPases. Further, this mutant was found to have a dominant-negative fashion at the cellular level (Williams et al. 2000). The patient received successful marrow transplantation from his HLA-identical older brother. It was speculated that the Mutant D57N RAC2 in this patient bound GDP but not GTP and inhibited oxidase activation and superoxide anion production thus resulting in severe neutrophil defect. Chemotaxis was impaired due to abnormal Rac interaction with the actin cytoskeleton.

Another homozygous RAC2 mutation abolishing protein expression was identified (Alkhairy et al. 2015) in two siblings born from consanguineous parents that displayed symptoms suggestive of a humoral immunodeficiency. Both siblings presented with IgA deficiency that gradually evolved into CVID. Although severe clinical abnormalities in the associated with neutrophil

dysfunction were not documented, reduced chemotaxis activity and reduced numbers of neutrophil granules were observed. In both patients, a novel homozygous nonsense mutation in codon 56 (W56X) was identified in the RAC2 gene. The antibody deficiency observed in these patients supports an important role of RAC2 in T- and B-cell development.

Evidence of the role of RAC2 in T-cell development came from the identification of an apparently healthy 2-week-old infant, who exhibited reduced numbers of T-cell receptor excision circles (TRECs) in the Wisconsin statewide newborn screening for T-cell lymphopenia (Accetta et al. 2011). Further testing revealed leukocytosis, neutrophilia, CD4+ T-cell lymphopenia, and reduced serum IgA and IgM levels. He later had fever, omphalitis, and a paratracheal abscess, and neutrophil chemotaxis was severely reduced. This patient underwent successful matched unrelated umbilical cord blood transplantation at 3.5 months of life. Sequence analysis of patient's PBMCs demonstrated a guanine to adenine substitution at codon 57 (GAC → AAC) that resulted in the substitution of asparagine for aspartic acid.

Taken together, these cases together with the Rac2 targeted animal models, confirmed the important and nonredundant role of Rac2 in several blood cell lineages, particularly neutrophils (Pai et al. 2010).

Cross-References

▶ CYBB X-Linked Chronic Granulomatous Disease (CGD)

References

Accetta D, Syverson G, Bonacci B, Reddy S, Bengtson C, Surfus J, Harbeck R, Huttenlocher A, Grossman W, Routes J, Verbsky J. Human phagocyte defect caused by a Rac2 mutation detected by means of neonatal screening for T-cell lymphopenia. J Allergy Clin Immunol. 2011;127(2):535–8.
Alkhairy OK, Rezaei N, Graham RR, Abolhassani H, Borte S, Hultenby K, Wu C, Aghamohammadi A,

Williams DA, Behrens TW, Hammarström L, Pan-Hammarström Q. RAC2 loss-of-function mutation in 2 siblings with characteristics of common variable immunodeficiency. J Allergy Clin Immunol. 2015;135(5):1380–4.

Ambruso DR, Knall C, Abell AN, Panepinto J, Kurkchubasche A, Thurman G, Gonzalez-Aller C, Hiester A, deBoer M, Harbeck RJ, Oyer R, Johnson GL, Roos D. Human neutrophil immunodeficiency syndrome is associated with an inhibitory Rac2 mutation. Proc Natl Acad Sci U S A. 2000;97(9):4654–9.

Pai SY, Kim C, Williams DA. Rac GTPases in human diseases. Dis Markers. 2010;29(3–4):177–87.

Williams DA, Tao W, Yang F, Kim C, Gu Y, Mansfield P, Levine JE, Petryniak B, Derrow CW, Harris C, Jia B, Zheng Y, Ambruso DR, Lowe JB, Atkinson SJ, Dinauer MC, Boxer L. Dominant negative mutation of the hematopoietic-specific Rho GTPase, Rac2, is associated with a human phagocyte immunodeficiency. Blood. 2000;96(5):1646–54.

Ras Homolog Family Member H (RHOH) Deficiency

Robert P. Nelson
Divisions of Hematology and Oncology, Stem Cell Transplant Program, Indiana University (IU) School of Medicine and the IU Bren and Simon Cancer Center, Indianapolis, IN, USA
Pediatric Immunodeficiency Clinic, Riley Hospital for Children at Indiana University Health, Indianapolis, IN, USA
Medicine and Pediatrics, Indiana University School of Medicine, Immunohematology and Transplantation, Indianapolis, IN, USA

Synonyms

Translocation three four (TTF)

Definition

The RHOH is one membrane-bound adaptor protein related to a superfamily of small guanine triphosphate hydrolases (GTPases) that participate in signal transduction.

Introduction/Background

The Ras homolog gene H (RHOH) comprises one component of a family of small GTPases that includes Rho, Rac, and Cdc42, which participates in signaling from the plasma membrane downstream to the nucleus. RHOH is expressed only in hematopoietic cells (HPCs) and was initially recognized fused to the LAZ3/BCL6 gene in a non-Hodgkin's lymphoma (NHL) cell line that bore a (3; 4) (q27; p11-13) translocation (Galiegue-Zouitina et al. 1999).

Chromosomal mapping experiments located the gene on the chromosome 4p13, where it spans 35 kb and contains two exons (Dallery-Prudhomme et al. 1997). It had been previously named translocation three four (*TTF*), which was discovered as one of the genes activated in neutrophils induced by granulocyte-monocyte colony stimulating factor (GM-CSF) (Yousefi et al. 2000). Unlike most members of the Rho GTPase family, RHOH is GTPase-deficient and does not cycle between guanosine triphosphate and guanosine diphosphate-bound forms. It is noteworthy that RhoH is the first GTP-binding protein-encoding gene to be implicated as a cause of a human hematological malignancy (Preudhomme et al. 2000).

Function

Hematopoiesis
RHOH is expressed in hematopoietic progenitor cells (HPCs) and fully differentiated myeloid and lymphoid lineages. Knockdown of RHOH expression via RNA interference stimulates proliferation, survival, and stromal cell-derived factor-1 alpha-induced migration. RHOH overexpression in these cells impairs activation of Rac GTPases, alters actin polymerization and chemotaxis, reduces proliferation, and increases apoptosis. Therefore, RHOH overexpression in HPCs impairs hematopoietic reconstitution that suggests that RHOH serves as a negative regulator of both growth and actin-based function of HPCs (Gu et al. 2005).

RHOH is induced during human eosinophil differentiation is highly expressed in mature blood eosinophils and is upregulated in some patients with hypereosinophilic syndrome. The number of eosinophils in the blood is regulated by factors controlling their production in the bone marrow, such as extrinsic interleukin-5 that promotes eosinophil differentiation. Eosinophil-intrinsic factors may also play a role in the regulation of their own generation. Overexpression of RHOH increases the expression of GATA-2, a transcription factor involved in regulating eosinophil differentiation, and RhoH ($-/-$) mice have impaired GATA-2 expression as well as accelerated eosinophil differentiation both in vitro and in vivo. Taken together, Stoeckle concludes that RHOH is a negative regulator of eosinophilopoiesis (Stoeckle et al. 2016).

Adaptive Immunity

RHOH is active in thymic T cell production, in which it recruits Zap70 during double negative transitions and positive selection and favors T cell functional differentiation to the Th1 subset (Dorn et al. 2007). Consequential RHOH activity in T lymphocytes occurs early in the T cell receptor (TCR) activation sequence. At rest, lymphocyte-specific protein tyrosine kinase (LCK) is recruited to the plasma membrane by RHOH, which also binds C-terminal Src kinase (CSK), resulting in LCK inactivation. Upon ligand-mediated TCR activation, LCK is dephosphorylated, resulting in LCK auto-activation and release from RHOH. Low RHOH levels permit LCK autoactivation and constitutive activation of the TCR pathway (Wang et al. 2011; Li et al. 2002).

Rhoh$-/-$ mice have impaired CD3zeta phosphorylation, impaired translocation of zeta-chain-associated protein kinase 70 (Zap70) to the immunological synapse, and reduced activation of Zap70-mediated signaling in thymic and peripheral T cells, resulting in T cell immunodeficiency (Gu et al. 2006). In contrast, activation of the B cell receptor (BCR) in peripheral blood B cells is not associated with changes in RhoH levels, which suggests that RhoH function is regulated by lysosomal degradation of the RhoH protein

following TCR complex activation, but not BCR activation (Schmidt-Mende et al. 2010).

In a murine model, defective Rhoh signaling caused a 75% decrease in acute and chronic transplant rejection, reduced alloantigen-specific antibody levels, and improved graft function. Although dendritic cell antigen uptake was normal, mixed lymphocytes generated weaker alloreactivity secondary to lower cytotoxicity and cytokine release (Porubsky et al. 2011). Tamehiro et al. demonstrated that Rhoh deficiency induced Th17 polarization, resulting in chronic dermatitis similar to psoriasis. Rhoh deficiency impaired ubiquitin protein ligase E3 component N-recognin 5 (Ubr5) and reduced nuclear receptor subfamily 2 group F member 6 (Nr2f6) expression levels, resulting in increased IL-17 and IL-22 that resulted expansion of Th17 cells; treatment with IL-22 binding protein/Fc chimeric protein reduced psoriatic inflammation in Rhoh-deficient mice. Expression of RHOH in T cells was lower in patients with psoriasis with very severe symptoms and suggests that RHOH inhibits Th17 differentiation and plays a role in the pathogenesis of psoriasis.

RhoH expression enables T cells to switch between sensing chemokine-mediated "go" signals and TCR-dependent "stop" signals, and RhoH is required for maintenance of lymphocyte LFA-1 in a nonadhesive state (Troeger et al. 2012; Cherry et al. 2004). Mino et al. discovered new RhoH-interacting proteins by in-vivo biotinylating and mass spectrometry analyses. Kaiso is a 95 kDa zinc-finger transcription factor that regulates gene expression and p120 catenin-associated cell-cell adhesions. Kaiso and p120 catenin co-localize with RhoH at chemokine-induced actin-containing cell protrusion sites. These studies suggest that during T cell migration, actin-cytoskeleton structure and transcriptional activity is modulated by extracellular microenvironment signals that regulate RhoH and Kaiso (Dee et al. 2019).

Clinical Presentation: Susceptibility to Epidermodysplasia Verruciformis

Epidermodysplasia verruciformis (EV) is a rare genetic disorder characterized by increased susceptibility to specific human papillomaviruses (HPV), the beta papillomaviruses. Susceptibility to EV is caused by inactivating mutations in EVER-1, EVER-2 in most, but not all patients with autosomal recessive EV. In general, skin findings are characterized by disseminated hypo- or hyperpigmented macules and wart-like papules that can coalesce and scale. Flat warts persist, and there may be pityriasis versicolor-like lesions resembling generalized verrucosis. There is a high rate of transformation to squamous cell carcinoma (SCC). Homozygous inactivating mutations in transmembrane channel-like protein 6 (TMC6, EVER1) and TMC8 (EVER2) determine susceptibility to this disorder in 75% of cases; however, mutations in RHOH can augment human beta-papillomavirus replication and manifest as a EV-like phenotype (Przybyszewska et al. 2017).

Crequer et al. reported two young adult siblings who presented with various infectious diseases, including persistent EV-HPV infections and who were discovered to have homozygous mutations (p.Y38X) that created a stop codon in *RHOH*. The patients' circulating T cells contained predominantly effector memory T cells, which displayed impaired TCR signaling. Additionally, very few circulating T cells expressed the beta7 integrin subunit, a protein critical for T cell homing. Recapitulation of the defect in Rhoh-null mice rendered them T cell deficient. Expression of the wild type allele in Rhoh−/− hematopoietic stem cells corrected the T cell lymphopenia in mice after bone marrow transplantation, and the authors concluded that RHOH deficiency leads to T cell defects and persistent EV-HPV infections. This is consistent with T cells role in the pathogenesis of chronic EV-HPV infections (Crequer et al. 2012).

Treatment and Prognosis

The first clinical decision to make generally for patients with T and B combined immunodeficiency is whether to take care of the patent locally or consider referral to a center that has a multidisciplinary center for the management of these conditions, as exist for several of the classical immunodeficiency diseases. The patient and family may need input from social services regarding health care options and avenues to care that are either available or not. General treatment considerations of immunocompromised patients apply. Inactivated immunizations are indicated but live vaccines are not. Extreme isolation or avoidance of normal schooling may not be necessary or recommended, but rather prompt medical evaluation for early unusual consequences of infection is paramount to the care of patients with combined immunodeficiencies. The usual course of treatment for individual infectious episodes may require extension. Other measures include the use of prophylactic antibiotics as indicated, with guidance informed by serial assessments of clinical and laboratory findings, including antibody production capacity.

If the patient presents with EV, the current treatment modalities may be helpful but not curative. The skin lesions may respond to topical imiquimod and 5-fluorouracil, cryotherapy, systemic retinoids, and/or 5-aminolevulinic acid photodynamic therapy. Surgical excision is the treatment of choice for skin carcinoma secondary to EV. Sun exposure avoidance and photoprotection are recommended preventive measures that are crucial. Particular attention is given to the management of comorbid inflammatory or autoimmune conditions that require iatrogenic immunosuppression and anti-inflammatory therapy, as unintentional exacerbation of the condition may result from synergistic immunosuppressive influences. Early high-complexity care requires considerable effort by the clinical team, ideally before morbid complications ensue, as a bridge to potentially curative therapeutic approaches, such as hematopoietic cell transplantation. In a murine bone marrow transplantation model, expression of the wild type Rhoh corrected the T cell lymphopenia, an experiment that may facilitate development of corrective transplant therapy for patients with the defect in the future (Crequer et al. 2012).

Cross-References

▶ p56LCK

References

Cherry LK, Li X, Schwab P, Lim B, Klickstein LB. RhoH is required to maintain the integrin LFA-1 in a non-adhesive state on lymphocytes. Nat Immunol. 2004;5:961–7.

Crequer A, Troeger A, Patin E, et al. Human RHOH deficiency causes T cell defects and susceptibility to EV-HPV infections. J Clin Invest. 2012;122:3239–47.

Dallery-Prudhomme E, Roumier C, Denis C, Preudhomme C, Kerckaert JP, Galiegue-Zouitina S. Genomic structure and assignment of the RhoH/ TTF small GTPase gene (ARHH) to 4p13 by in situ hybridization. Genomics. 1997;43:89–94.

Dee RA, Mangum KD, Bai X, Mack CP, Taylor JM. Druggable targets in the Rho pathway and their promise for therapeutic control of blood pressure. Pharmacol Ther. 2019;193:121–34.

Dorn T, Kuhn U, Bungartz G, et al. RhoH is important for positive thymocyte selection and T-cell receptor signaling. Blood. 2007;109:2346–55.

Galiegue-Zouitina S, Quief S, Hildebrand MP, et al. Non-random fusion of L-plastin(LCP1) and LAZ3(BCL6) genes by t(3;13)(q27;q14) chromosome translocation in two cases of B-cell non-Hodgkin lymphoma. Genes Chromosomes Cancer. 1999;26:97–105.

Gu Y, Jasti AC, Jansen M, Siefring JE. RhoH, a hematopoietic-specific Rho GTPase, regulates proliferation, survival, migration, and engraftment of hematopoietic progenitor cells. Blood. 2005;105:1467–75.

Gu Y, Chae HD, Siefring JE, Jasti AC, Hildeman DA, Williams DA. RhoH GTPase recruits and activates Zap70 required for T cell receptor signaling and thymocyte development. Nat Immunol. 2006;7:1182–90.

Li X, Bu X, Lu B, Avraham H, Flavell RA, Lim B. The hematopoiesis-specific GTP-binding protein RhoH is GTPase deficient and modulates activities of other Rho GTPases by an inhibitory function. Mol Cell Biol. 2002;22:1158–71.

Porubsky S, Wang S, Kiss E, et al. Rhoh deficiency reduces peripheral T-cell function and attenuates allogenic transplant rejection. Eur J Immunol. 2011;41:76–88.

Preudhomme C, Roumier C, Hildebrand MP, et al. Non-random 4p13 rearrangements of the RhoH/TTF gene, encoding a GTP-binding protein, in non-Hodgkin's lymphoma and multiple myeloma. Oncogene. 2000;19:2023–32.

Przybyszewska J, Zlotogorski A, Ramot Y. Re-evaluation of epidermodysplasia verruciformis: reconciling more than 90 years of debate. J Am Acad Dermatol. 2017;76:1161–75.

Schmidt-Mende J, Geering B, Yousefi S, Simon HU. Lysosomal degradation of RhoH protein upon antigen receptor activation in T but not B cells. Eur J Immunol. 2010;40:525–9.

Stoeckle C, Geering B, Yousefi S, et al. RhoH is a negative regulator of eosinophilopoiesis. Cell Death Differ. 2016;23:1961–72.

Troeger A, Johnson AJ, Wood J, et al. RhoH is critical for cell-microenvironment interactions in chronic lymphocytic leukemia in mice and humans. Blood. 2012;119:4708–18.

Wang H, Zeng X, Fan Z, Lim B. RhoH modulates pre-TCR and TCR signalling by regulating LCK. Cell Signal. 2011;23:249–58.

Yousefi S, Cooper PR, Mueck B, Potter SL, Jarai G. cDNA representational difference analysis of human neutrophils stimulated by GM-CSF. Biochem Biophys Res Commun. 2000;277:401–9.

Recurrent Isolated Invasive Pneumococcal Disease 1 (IPD1)

▶ TIR Signaling Pathway Deficiency, IRAK-4 Deficiency

Reticuloendotheliosis with Eosinophilia

▶ Omenn Syndrome (OS)

RIDDLE Syndrome (RNF168)

Svetlana O. Sharapova
Research Department, Belarusian Research Center for Pediatric Oncology, Hematology and Immunology, Minsk, Belarus

Synonyms

RNF168 deficiency

Definition

RIDDLE is an acronym for **r**adiosensitivity, **immunod**eficiency **d**ysmorphic features, and **le**arning difficulties syndrome, due to mutations in the *RNF168* gene. Other clinical signs of

RIDDLE syndrome may include mild ataxia, microcephaly, normal intelligence, conjunctival telangiectasia, recurrent sinus infections, decreased serum IgG and IgA, increased alpha-fetoprotein (AFP), and late onset of pulmonary fibrosis.

Introduction/Background

Stewart et al. (2007) first described RIDDLE syndrome in a patient with increased radiosensitivity, immunodeficiency, mild motor control and learning difficulties, facial dysmorphism, and short stature. Mutations in the *RNF168* gene cause an autosomal recessive form of combined immunodeficiency with syndromic features and associated with immunoglobulin deficiency and cellular radiosensitivity (Stewart et al. 2009; Devgan et al. 2011; Chinn et al. 2017; Picard et al. 2018; Pietrucha et al. 2017). The *RNF168* gene is located on chromosome 3q29 and encodes a 571 amino acid protein that is a member of the "ring-finger nuclear factor" (RNF) family of ubiquitin ligases (Stewart et al. 2009). RNF168 is an E3 ubiquitin ligase that functions as a component of the ubiquitin-dependent DNA damage response to facilitate the relaxation of chromatin surrounding a double-strand breakage (DSB) to allow the subsequent recruitment of repair proteins. The RNF168-deficient cells fail to recruit the repair proteins 53BP1 and BRCA1 to sites of DSBs; they showed a defect in the G2M and mild impairment in intra-S-phase cell cycle checkpoints. The RNF168-deficient cells exhibit a hypersensitivity to ionizing radiation, cell cycle checkpoint abnormalities, impaired class switch, and V(D)J recombinations (Stewart et al. 2007; Pietrucha et al. 2017).

Clinical Presentation

Five patients have so far been described with biallelic mutations in the *RNF168* gene; one of them had additionally two mutations in *ZAP70* gene (Stewart et al. 2007, 2009; Devgan et al. 2011; Chinn et al. 2017; Pietrucha et al. 2017). The first case, an individual with absence of IgG since infancy and requiring immunoglobulin replacement, was described with slight ataxic gait, learning difficulty, mild facial dysmorphism, and short stature (Stewart et al. 2007).

A second patient has been diagnosed in a non-consanguineous Turkish family with no learning difficulties but with growth retardation, conjunctival and bronchial telangiectasias, and a wide-based gait and who died from respiratory failure at 30 years of age. He had reduced serum IgA and an elevated level of serum AFP (Devgan et al. 2011).

An adult patient with susceptibility to bacterial, herpesviral, and fungal infections was diagnosed by whole-exome sequencing. WES revealed missense variant in *RNF168* and compound heterozygous variants in *ZAP70*. Immunologic defects included CD8+ T-cell lymphopenia, decreased T-cell proliferative responses to mitogens, and hypogammaglobulinemia, and radiation sensitivity was reported (Chinn et al. 2017).

In a Polish family, two children born to consanguineous parents had immunoglobulin deficiency, telangiectasia, cellular radiosensitivity, and increased AFP levels due to a homozygous mutation in *RNF168* gene, which resulted in an absence of RNF168 protein. The younger sibling had a more pronounced neurological and morphological phenotype, and she also carried an *ATM* gene mutation in the heterozygous state (Pietrucha et al. 2017).

Detailed description of reported patients with RNF168 deficiency collected in Table 1.

Importantly, patients with RNF168 deficiency can survive to adulthood. Four out of five patients are alive, and in spite of radiosensitivity of patient's cells, malignancy was observed only in P3 with second genetic abnormalities in ZAP70 (Table 1).

RNF168 deficiency is consistently associated with immunoglobulin deficiency and cellular radiosensitivity, whereas ataxia, microcephaly, short stature, or learning difficulties are more variable phenotypes among the five patients.

RIDDLE Syndrome (RNF168), Table 1 Demographic, clinical, laboratory, and genetic characteristics of all reported *RNF168*-deficient patients

Patient № gender_country or ethnicity	Age of onset/ diagnosis	Mutation	Clinical data		Laboratory data		Follow-up
			Clinical features	Appearance	Ig and AFP	Lymphocytes	
P1_male_UK	1 y/21 y	*RNF168* p.A133Gfs*10 p. N441Rfs*16	Mild motor control and learning difficulties	Mild facial dysmorphism Short stature	IgG ↓↓ IgA ↓ IgM ↑	Radiosensitivity T and B – N T prolif – N B cell Ig prod in vitro -↓	Alive 22 y (SCIG)
P2_male_Turkish	16 y/29 y	*RNF168* p.R131X p.R131X	Normal intelligence Bronchial Telangiectasia Respiratory failure Dry skin with fine scaling (xerosis)	Mild gait ataxia Conjunctival telangiectasia Short stature Microcephaly	IgA ↓ AFP ↑	Radiosensitivity	Died 30 y (respiratory failure, pneumofibrosis)
P3_female_ Mexican-American	3 m/28 y	*RNF168* p.D103N p.D103N *ZAP70* p.G245R p.P502L	Otitis, URTI, warts, ChLD, bronchiectasis, chickenpox, repeated meningitis, HPV-lesions, squamous cell carcinomas	Normal	IgG ↓↓	Radiosensitivity T↓ CD8+ ↑ NK degranulation ↓ ZAP70 ↓	Alive 30 y (IVIg+fluconazol prophylaxis)
P4*_male_Polish	1 m/20 y	*RNF168* p.E99KfsX17 p.E99KfsX17	URTI, LRTI, nocturnal enuresis, generalized chronic lymphadenopathy, gait disturbances, mild arthritis, erythematous, scaly skin lesions on lower limbs	Conjunctival telangiectasia	IgG ↓↓ IgA ↓ AFP ↑	Radiosensitivity T and B – N B memory ↓	Alive 21 y (IVIG, *Helicobacter pylori* colon disease)
P5*_female_Polish	6 m/12 y	*RNF168* p.E99KfsX17 p.E99KfsX17 *ATM* c.1402_1403delAA	Psychomotor developmental delay, herpes infections, URTI	Mild facial dysmorphism	IgG2 ↓ IgA ↓ AFP ↑	Radiosensitivity T and B – N B memory ↓	Alive 13 y

UK United Kingdom

IgG/A/M immunoglobulin G/A/M, AFP alpha-fetoprotein

N normal, ↓ decreased, ↓↓ severely decreased, ↑ increased, y years

SCIG subcutaneous IgG replacement therapy, IVIg intravenous Ig therapy

URTI, upper respiratory tract infections, LRTI, lower respiratory tract infections, ChLD, chronic lung disease, HPV, human papillomavirus

*- Ter or X, stop codon

Laboratory Findings/Diagnostic Testing

Patients with ataxia and elevated serum AFP but without mutations in *ATM* gene should be considered for genetic testing of *RNF168* gene. Patients with RIDDLE syndrome may have history of recurring infections and are likely to have reduced serum IgG and IgA levels. IgM levels may be increased or normal. Total T (CD3+) and B (CD19+) cell numbers are usually normal. However, some patients with RNF168 deficiency have reduced numbers of switched memory B cells (Pietrucha et al. 2017) and reduced Ig production after in vivo stimulation of B cells (Stewart et al. 2007).

All described patients have abnormalities in cellular radiosensitivity as can be measured by means of colony survival assays and/or 53BP1 recruitment to DNA double-strand breaks (DSBs) and/or γH2AX foci accumulation in lymphoblasts or primary fibroblasts after irradiation.

Detection of pathogenic bi-allelic mutations of *RNF168* gene can confirm the diagnosis. Immunoblotting can be used to show a reduction or absence of RNF168 protein.

Treatment

Immunoglobulin replacement therapy can reduce the frequency of infection and is indicated in patients with RIDDLE syndrome and low IgG level. Hematopoietic cell transplantation (HCT) has not been reported in five described patients to date.

References

Chinn IK, Sanders RP, Stray-Pedersen A, et al. Novel combined immune deficiency and radiation sensitivity blended phenotype in an adult with biallelic variations in ZAP70 and RNF168. Front Immunol. 2017;8:576.

Devgan SS, Sanal O, Doil C, et al. Homozygous deficiency of ubiquitin-ligase ring-finger protein RNF168 mimics the radiosensitivity syndrome of ataxia-telangiectasia. Cell Death Differ. 2011;18(9):1500–6.

Picard C, Gaspar BH, Al-Herz W, et al. International Union of Immunological Societies: 2017 Primary immunodeficiency diseases committee report on inborn errors of immunity. J Clin Immunol. 2018;38(1):96–128.

Pietrucha B, Heropolitańska-Pliszka E, Geffers R, et al. Clinical and biological manifestation of RNF168 deficiency in two polish siblings. Front Immunol. 2017;4(8):1683.

Stewart GS, Stankovic T, Byrd PJ, et al. RIDDLE immunodeficiency syndrome is linked to defects in 53BP1-mediated DNA damage signaling. Proc Natl Acad Sci U S A. 2007;104(43):16910–5.

Stewart GS, Panier S, Townsend K, et al. The RIDDLE syndrome protein mediates a ubiquitin-dependent signaling cascade at sites of DNA damage. Cell. 2009;136(3):420–34.

RMRP

▶ Cartilage Hair Hypoplasia (RMRP)

RNase MRP

▶ Cartilage Hair Hypoplasia (RMRP)

RNF168 Deficiency

▶ RIDDLE Syndrome (RNF168)

RPSA

▶ Isolated Congenital Asplenia (ICA) and Mutations in RPSA

RTI Respiratory Tract Infections

▶ Wiskott-Aldrich Syndrome Protein-Interacting Protein (WIP) Deficiency

S

SAVI: STING-Associated Vasculopathy with Onset in Infancy

▶ STING-Associated Vasculopathy with Onset in Infancy (SAVI)

Schimke Immuno-osseous Dysplasia

Ilona DuBuske
Division of Allergy and Immunology, University of Cincinnati, Cincinnati, OH, USA

Synonyms

Immune-osseous dysplasia; Schimke immuno-osseous dysplasia; Schimke syndrome

Definition

Schimke immune-osseous dysplasia (SIOD, OMIM 242900) is a rare and fatal autosomal recessive disorder which includes T-cell deficiency, facial dysmorphism, spondyloepiphyseal dysplasia, nephropathy, and hyperpigmented macules.

Introduction

Initially was described by Schimke in 1971 as an immuno-osseous dysplasia due to chondroitin-6-sulfate mucopoly-saccharidosis in conjunction with lymphopenia, along with defective cellular immunity and nephrotic syndrome (Schimke et al. 1974). Spondyloepiphyseal dysplasia, nephrotic syndrome with progressive renal failure, recurrent lymphopenia, T-cell immunodeficiency typically occurs in SIOD in addition to, at times, hypothyroidism, bone marrow aplasia, autoimmune diseases, and malignancy.

Epidemiology

The incidence of SIOD is about 1:1,000,000 to 1:3,000,000 live births in North America (Santangelo et al. 2014). Prevalence of SIOD is unknown, as only 60 patients have been reported in North America.

Genetics and Pathophysiology

Approximately 50% of cases are associated with biallelic mutation in SMARCAL1 gene. Mutations in the *SMARCAL1 (SWI/SNF Related, Matrix Associated, Actin Dependent Regulator of Chromatin, Subfamily A Like 1)* gene which play an essential role in DNA stabilization, telomere

© Springer Science+Business Media LLC, part of Springer Nature 2020
I. R. Mackay et al. (eds.), *Encyclopedia of Medical Immunology*,
https://doi.org/10.1007/978-1-4614-8678-7

maintenance, and ataxia telangiectasia mutated (ATM) signaling, lead to disorders of intracellular signaling and DNA damage. SIOD disease severity is related to decreases in SMARCAL1 gene activity, suggesting that the SMARCAL1 protein is involved in the development of multiple organs.

T-cell immunodeficiency in SIOD appears to be related to lack of IL7Rα expression in T cells (Sanyal et al. 2015) believed to be associated with hypermethylation of the IL7R promoter in T cells and T cell progenitors. IL-7 is essential for T cell survival and early development. Therefore, SIOD patients lack CD4+CD45+CD31+ recent thymic emigrant cells, overall decrease of naïve T cells (CD45RA+-CD45RO−) including both CD4 and CD8 cells from an early life, indicative of defective thymic output and resultant developmental T-cell defect (Sanyal et al. 2015). However, peripheral T cells show normal proliferation with stimulation with mitogen (PHA) or anti-CD3/CD28 antibodies with IL-2 suggesting ability of T cells to proliferate, activate, and signal through the T cell receptor in SIOD patients (Sanyal et al. 2015). Focal segmental glomerulosclerosis development has been linked to increased Wnt and Notch activity consequent to SMARCAL1 deficiency (Morimoto et al. 2016).

Clinical Presentation

SIOD is a multisystem disease with prominent features of skeletal dysplasia, T cell deficiency, and renal failure.

The hallmark presentation of spondylo-epiphyseal dysplasia leads to short stature and intrauterine growth retardation. Among the most common musculoskeletal system disorders are abnormal femoral heads, short neck and trunk, lumbar lordosis, and hypoplastic pelvis. Renal involvement includes focal segmental glomerulosclerosis with severe proteinuria and renal failure. Development of recurrent infections is commonly seen following renal transplantation, including herpes zoster and Epstein-Barr virus infections. Immunologic abnormalities include lymphopenia and T-cell deficiency. Autoimmune complications

include hypothyroidism and immune cytopenias (anemia, thrombocytopenia, neutropenia). Non-Hodgkin's lymphoma has been reported in association with SIOD. Undifferentiated carcinoma of the sinus occurs due to a S859P missense mutation in SMARCAL1 gene.

Approximately, one-half of SIOD patients have atherosclerosis, migraine-like headaches and transient neurologic symptoms. Enteropathy with *Helicobacter pylori* has been reported in about 30% of SIOD patients. Tracheobronchial anomalies can occur due to decreased elasticity resulting in emphysema, pulmonary hypertension, and bronchiectasis. Oral abnormalities include microdontia and hypodontia.

Diagnostic Testing

Diagnosis of SIOD requires the combination of clinical features of spondylo-epiphyseal dysplasia, renal failure, and T-cell deficiency. If SIOD is suspected, genetic assessment should be performed for the sequence and deletion/duplication analysis of SMARCAL1 gene. Evaluation of growth, osteopenia, renal function including creatinine, urea, and urine protein, immune system or memory and naïve CD4 and CD8 T cells and B cells and immunoglobulin levels, hematologic assessments, neurologic assessment, thyroid hormone level assessment, and careful examination of the oral cavity and eyes are all necessary in assessment for SIOD.

Differential Diagnosis

Some other syndromes may appear in the differential diagnosis of SIOD including Braegger syndrome with B-cell defects, ischiadic hypoplasia, renal failure, and polydactyly; Cono-renal syndrome which is autosomal recessive disorder with skeletal dysplasia, chronic renal disease, retinal pigmentary dystrophy, and cerebellar ataxia; nail patella syndrome with autosomal dominant pattern, poorly developed nails, arthrodysplasia, and exostoses; short-limb skeletal dysplasia with severe combined immunodeficiency; short-limb skeletal dysplasia with humoral immunodeficiency; Sanjad-Sakati syndrome which is autosomal recessive disorder with hypoparathyroidism, growth hormone deficiency, dysmorphism, and intellectual disability; Kenny-Caffey syndrome with congenital hypoparathyroidism, calvarial osteosclerosis, and shortened stature. These syndromes, however, have some unique characteristics which distinguish them from SIOD.

Treatment

SIOD treatment includes appropriate therapy of scoliosis and/or kyphosis including orthopedic management. Hip replacement may be required in some older patients. Regarding infections, antiviral treatment such as acyclovir may be required for recurrent herpetic infections. Any immunization of SIOD patients should be done according to established T-cell immune deficiency protocols.

As for autoimmunity, levothyroxine is utilized if hypothyroidism occurs. For treatment of neutropenia, therapy may include granulocyte colony-stimulating factor or granulocyte-macrophage colony-stimulating factor. Systemic corticosteroids, cyclophosphamide, or intravenous immunoglobulin may be required for associated autoimmune disease. Autoimmune cytopenias can be multilinear and may be resistant to and-CD20 therapy (Zieg et al. 2011).

SIOD patient often have nephrotic syndrome which is resistant to systemic corticosteroid treatment but may respond partially to ACE inhibitors, renin-angiotensin channel blockers, and cyclosporine. Severe chronic renal failure may need renal transplantation.

For transient ischemic attacks or cerebral vascular insufficiency occurs, use of acetylsalicylic acid, dipyridamole, warfarin, or heparin is to be considered. Surgical revascularization may be needed for high-grade focal stenosis of the internal carotid artery.

Prognosis

SIOD patient most often succumb to their disease in the first two decades consequent to infections (23%), to cerebral vascular accidents (17%), to renal failure (15%), to pulmonary hypertension and congestive heart failure (15%), to organ transplant complications (9%), to complications of lymphoproliferative diseases (9%), to gastrointestinal hemorrhage (6%), to bone marrow aplasia (3%), and to acute restrictive lung disease (3%) (Baradaran-Heravi et al. 2013).

References

Baradaran-Heravi A, Lange J, Asakura Y, Cochat P, Massella L, Boerkoel CF. Bone marrow transplantation in Schimke immuno-osseous dysplasia. Am J Med Genet A. 2013;161A:2609–13.

Morimoto M, Myung C, Beirnes K, Choi K, Asakura Y, Bokenkamp A, et al. Increased Wnt and Notch signaling: a clue to the renal disease in Schimke immuno-osseous dysplasia? Orphanet J Rare Dis. 2016;11(1):149.

Santangelo L, Gigante M, Netti GS, Diella S, Puteo F, Carbone V, et al. A novel SMARCAL1 mutation associated with a mild phenotype of Schimke immuno-osseous dysplasia (SIOD). BMC Nephrol. 2014;15:41.

Sanyal M, Morimoto M, Baradaran-Heravi A, Choi K, Kambham N, Jensen K, et al. Lack of IL7Rα expression in T cells is a hallmark of T-cell immunodeficiency in Schimke immuno-osseous dysplasia (SIOD). Clin Immunol. 2015;161(2):355–65.

Schimke RN, Horton WA, King CR, Martin NL. Chondroitin-6-sulfate mucopoly-saccharidosis in conjunction with lymphopenia, defective cellular immunity and the nephrotic syndrome. Birth Defects Orig Artic Ser. 1974;10(12):258–66.

Zieg J, Krepelova A, Baradaran-Heravi A, Levtchenko E, Guillén-Navarro E, Balascakova M, Sukova M, Seeman T, Dusek J, Simankova N, Rosik T, Skalova S, Lebl J, Boerkoel CF. Rituximab resistant evans syndrome and autoimmunity in Schimke immuno-osseous dysplasia. Pediatr Rheumatol Online J. 2011;9(1):27. https://doi.org/10.1186/1546-0096-9-27.

Schimke Syndrome

▶ Schimke Immuno-osseous Dysplasia

SCN2 (GFI 1 Deficiency)

Anders Fasth
Department of Pediatrics, Institute of Clinical
Sciences, Sahlgrenska Academy at University of
Gothenburg, Gothenburg, Sweden

Synonyms

Severe congenital neutropenia 2 (SCN 2); Severe
congenital neutropenia with defect in transcription
factor Gfi1

Definition

Severe congenital neutropenia (SCN) is by the
European Society for Immunodeficiencies
(ESID) defined as neutropenia $<0.5 \times 10^9$/L
(500/μL) measured on at least three occasions *or*
neutropenia $<1.0 \times 10^9$/L (1000/μL) measured
on at least three occasions with at least one of the
following: deep-seated infection due to bacteria
and/or fungi, recurrent pneumonia, buccal and/or
genital aphthous lesions, omphalitis and affected
family members, *and* exclusion of secondary
causes of neutropenia (ESID Registry 2017).

In GFI1 deficiency, mutations are found in the
gene *GFI1* at1p22. Inheritance is autosomal dominant (Person et al. 2003).

Introduction/Background

Mutation in *GFI1* as etiology of SCN was
described in 2003. GFI1 is a transcription factor
with a SNAG and six zinc-finger domains. GFI1
acts as a transcriptional repressor that interacts
with myeloid-specific transcription factors
C/EBPα, C/EBPβ, and PU.1 to regulate among
others the expression of *ELANE*. GFI1 is essential
for full myeloid differentiation and also for full
T- and B-cell development (Person et al. 2003).

GFI1 deficiency is a very rare etiology of SCN.

Clinical Presentation

- First manifestation is often omphalitis and/or
  delayed detachment of the umbilical stump,
  later recurrent bacterial infections of the skin
  and the respiratory tract, and also severe infections such as septicemia, meningitis, and osteomyelitis (Skokowa et al. 2017).
- Typical is painful recurrent non-herpetic oral
  cavity aphthae and inflamed gingiva and periodontitis leading to premature tooth loss.

Laboratory Findings/Diagnostic Testing

- Severe neutropenia, usually $<0.2 \times 10^9$/L, but
  persons with less severe neutropenia are
  described.
- Moderate low numbers of B and T cells
  (= lymphopenia) in peripheral blood, but
  with normal isoagglutinins, specific antibodies, and normal T-cell function.
- Bone marrow does not always show typical
  maturation arrest at the level of promyelocytes
  seen in many forms of SCN.
- Diagnostic testing should verify severe neutropenia at least three occasions followed
  by DNA analysis to diagnose mutation in
  GFI1.

Treatment/Prognosis

- Vigorous treatment of any infection. Consider
  treatment/prophylaxis until normalization of
  neutrophils upon G-CSF treatment.
- Firm conclusions on response to recombinant
  G-CSF therapy cannot be drawn because of
  few patients described.
- Marked monocytosis in response to G-CSF
  was described. Without G-CSF treatment or
  response to G-CSF, mortality is very high,
  80–90%.
- Periodontitis and aphthae usually do not
  respond to G-CSF, which makes professional
  dental care important.

- The disorder carries at least a 15–20% lifetime risk for MDS/AML, and yearly bone marrow aspirations including cytogenetics and analysis of somatic mutations in *GCSFR* and *RUNX1* are mandatory.

References

ESID Registry. Clinical criteria. https://esid.org/content/download/15478/424246/file/ESIDRegistry_Clinical Criteria.pdf. Retrieved in October 2017.

Person RE, Li FQ, Duan Z, Benson KF, Wechsler J, Papadaki HA, Eliopoulos G, Kaufman C, Bertolone SJ, Nakamoto B, Papayannopoulou T, Grimes HL, Horwitz M. Mutations in proto-oncogene GFI1 cause human neutropenia and target ELA2. Nat Genet. 2003;34:308–12.

Skokowa J, Dale DC, Touw IP, Zeidler C, Welte K. Severe congenital neutropenias. Nat Rev Dis Prim. 2017;3:17032.

SCN3 (Kostmann Disease)

Anders Fasth
Department of Pediatrics, Institute of Clinical Sciences, Sahlgrenska Academy at University of Gothenburg, Gothenburg, Sweden

Synonyms

Severe congenital neutropenia 3 (SCN3)

Definition

Severe congenital neutropenia (SCN) is by the European Society of Immunodeficiency (ESID, www.esid.org) defined as neutropenia $<0.5 \times 10^9$/L (500/μL) measured on at least three occasions *or* neutropenia $<1.0 \times 10^9$/L (1000/μL) measured on at least three occasions with at least one of the following: deep-seated infection due to bacteria and/or fungi, recurrent pneumonia, buccal and/or genital aphthous lesions, omphalitis and affected family members, *and* exclusion of secondary causes of neutropenia (ESID Registry, esid.org/content/download/15478/424246/file/ESIDRegistry_ClinicalCriteria.pdf).

In Kostmann disease, mutations are found in the *HAX1* gene at 1q21.3. Inheritance is autosomal recessive (Klein et al. 2007).

Introduction/Background

Kostmann disease was the first inherited congenital neutropenia described. Rolf Kostmann investigated a large kindred in an isolated part of Northern Sweden in the 1940s and published his finding in a Swedish journal in 1950. Only in 2007 the gene, *HAX1*, behind Kostmann disease was found. *HAX1* codes for HS-1-associated protein XA, a mitochondria targeted protein with Bcl-2 homology domains. HAX1 is an apoptosis-regulating protein. Mutation in *HAX1* leads to reduced mitochondrial membrane potential, increased apoptosis, and abrogated G-CSFR signaling that induces mitochondrial endoplasmatic reticulum stress reaction (Klein et al. 2007).

Clinical Presentation

- First manifestation is often omphalitis/neonatal septicemia and/or delayed detachment of the umbilical stump, later recurrent bacterial infections of the skin and the respiratory tract, and also serious infections such as septicemia, meningitis, and osteomyelitis.
- Typical is painful recurrent non-herpetic oral cavity aphthae and inflamed gingiva and periodontitis leading to premature tooth loss.
- A neurological phenotype with moderate development delay and epilepsy is found in patients with mutations affecting both isoforms of HAX1.

- Also, gonadal insufficiency with delayed puberty, especially in females, is described (Skokowa et al. 2017).

Laboratory Findings/Diagnostic Testing

- Severe neutropenia, usually $<0.2 \times 10^9/L$.
- Bone marrow with typical maturation arrest at the level of promyelocytes.
- Diagnostic testing should verify severe neutropenia at least three occasions followed by DNA analysis to diagnose mutation in *HAX1*.

Treatment/Prognosis

- Vigorous treatment of any infection. Consider treatment/prophylaxis until normalization of neutrophils upon G-CSF treatment.
- Recombinant human G-CSF in doses 3–10 (60) μg/Kg restores neutrophil count and normalizes infection rate. Without G-CSF treatment, mortality is very high, 80–90%.
- Periodontitis and aphthae usually do not respond to G-CSF, which makes professional dental care important.
- The disorder carries a 15–20% lifetime risk for MDS/AML, and yearly bone marrow aspirations including cytogenetics and analysis of somatic mutations in *GCSFR* and *RUNX1* are mandatory.
- In case of resistance to G-CSF and/or development of MDS/AML hematopoietic stem cell transplantation.

References

ESID Registry. Clinical criteria. esid.org/content/download/15478/424246/file/ESIDRegistry_ClinicalCriteria.pdf. Retrieved in October, 2017.

Klein C, Grudzien M, Appaswamy G, Germeshausen M, Sandrock I, Schäffer AA, Rathinam C, Boztug K, Schwinzer B, Rezaei N, Bohn G, Melin M, Carlsson G, Fadeel B, Dahl N, Palmblad J, Henter JI, Zeidler C, Grimbacher B, Welte K. HAX1 deficiency causes autosomal recessive severe congenital neutropenia (Kostmann disease). Nat Genet. 2007;39:86–92.

Skokowa J, Dale DC, Touw IP, Zeidler C, Welte K. Severe congenital neutropenias. Nat Rev Dis Prim. 2017;3:17032.

SCN4 (G6PC3 Deficiency)

Anders Fasth
Department of Pediatrics, Institute of Clinical Sciences, Sahlgrenska Academy at University of Gothenburg, Gothenburg, Sweden

Synonyms

Severe congenital neutropenia 4 (SCN4)

Definition

Severe congenital neutropenia (SCN) is by the European Society of Immunodeficiency (ESID, www.esid.org) defined as neutropenia $<0.5 \times 10^9/L$ (500/μL) measured on at least three occasions *or* neutropenia $<1.0 \times 10^9/L$ (1000/μL) measured on at least three occasions with at least one of the following: deep-seated infection due to bacteria and/or fungi, recurrent pneumonia, buccal and/or genital aphthous lesions, omphalitis and affected family members, *and* exclusion of secondary causes of neutropenia (ESID Registry).

In glucose-6 phosphatase catalytic subunit 3 (G6PC3), deficiency mutations are found in the *G6PC3* gene at 17q21. Inheritance is autosomal recessive.

Introduction/Background

Normal glucose-6-phosphatase hydrolyzes glucose-6-phosphate to glucose and phosphate in the endoplasmatic reticulum (ER). The abnormal glycosylation of neutrophil proteins such as NOX2 in G6PC3 deficiency is reported to lead to increased ER stress with an unfolded protein response and apoptosis.

G6PC3 deficiency was first described in 2009 in five patients of Armenian descent, who besides severe neutropenia also had congenital heart defects and prominent superficial veins visible. Later a more extended phenotype was described including also a combined T and B cell deficiency (Boztug et al. 2009).

Clinical Presentation (History/PE)

- First manifestation is often omphalitis/neonatal septicemia and/or delayed detachment of the umbilical stump, later recurrent bacterial infections of the skin and the respiratory tract, and also serious infections such as septicemia, meningitis, and osteomyelitis.
- Cardiac defects, increased superficial veins visibility, urogenital malformations, endocrine abnormalities, and skin hyper-elasticity are other findings.
- Patients with inflammatory bowel disease-like symptoms have been described.
- Marked osteopenia is often found (Kiykim et al. 2015).

Laboratory Findings/Diagnostic Testing

- Common to all patients is severe neutropenia $<0.5 \times 109$/L.
- Intermittent thrombocytopenia and anemia are common.
- Some patients are also reported to have lymphopenia with low T cells and/or B cells. Other findings were low number of recent thymic emigrants and low proliferation upon stimulation with PHA.
- Typically, bone marrow aspirate shows maturation arrest at promyelocyte level, but this finding is not obligate as some patients did show only diminished myelopoiesis with slight left shift.
- Slight dysplastic bone marrow findings are common, but transformation to MDS/AML is only described in one single patient (Skokowa et al. 2017).

Treatment/Prognosis

- Vigorous treatment of any infection. Consider treatment/prophylaxis until normalization of neutrophils upon G-CSF treatment.

- Recombinant human G-CSF in doses 3–10 μg/Kg restores neutrophil count and normalizes infection rate. Without G-CSF treatment, mortality is high.
- Although the risk for development of MDS/AML is reported low, regular bone marrow aspirates about every 2–3 years with cytogenetics and DNA analysis of somatic mutations in *GCSFR* and *RUNX1* are recommended.

References

Boztug K, Appaswamy G, Ashikov A, Schaffer AA, Salzer U, Diestelhorst J, Germeshausen M, Brandes G, Lee-Gossler J, Noyan F, Gatzke A-K, Minkov M, 14 others. A syndrome with congenital neutropenia and mutations in G6PC3. New Engl J Med. 2009;360:32–43.

ESID Registry. Clinical criteria. esid.org/content/download/15478/424246/file/ESIDRegistry_ClinicalCriteria.pdf. Retrieved in October 2017.

Kiykim A, Baris S, Karakoc-Aydiner E, Ozen AO, Ogulur I, Bozkurt S, Ataizi CC, Boztug K, Barlan IB. G6PC3 deficiency: primary immune deficiency beyond just neutropenia. J Pediatr Hematol Oncol. 2015;37:616–22.

Skokowa J, Dale DC, Touw IP, Zeidler C, Welte K. Severe congenital neutropenias. Nat Rev Dis Prim. 2017;3:17032.

SCN5 (VPS45 Deficiency)

Anders Fasth
Department of Pediatrics, Institute of Clinical Sciences, Sahlgrenska Academy at University of Gothenburg, Gothenburg, Sweden

Synonyms

Severe congenital neutropenia 5 (SCN 5)

Definition

Severe congenital neutropenia (SNC) is by the European Society of Immunodeficiency (ESID, www.esid.org) defined as neutropenia $<0.5 \times 10^9$/L (500/μL) measured on at least three occasions *or* neutropenia $<1.0 \times 10^9$/L (1000/μL) measured on at least three occasions with at least one of the following: deep-seated infection due to bacteria and/or fungi, recurrent pneumonia, buccal and/or genital aphthous lesions, omphalitis and affected family members, *and* exclusion of secondary causes of neutropenia (ESID Registry).

In VPS45 deficiency, mutations are found in the *VPS45* gene at1q21.2. Inheritance is autosomal recessive.

Introduction/Background

Vacuolar protein sorting-associated protein 45 (VPS45) deficiency is a very rare cause of SCN and was first described in 2013. VPS45 regulates the assembly of the SNARE complex that plays an essential part in the vesicle trafficking and recycling of proteins through lysosomes, other endosomes, and the *trans*-Golgi complex. Defective VPS45 leads to defective transport of proteins from the *trans*-Golgi network to endosomes, impaired cell motility, increased apoptosis, dysfunction of NOXs with diminished superoxide production, and lack of surface expression of β1 integrin.

VPS45 deficiency was first reported in 2013 by two independent groups. In the same year, one of the groups reported the success of hematopoietic stem cell transplantation (Stepensky et al. 2013; Vilboux et al. 2013).

Clinical Presentation

- First manifestation is often omphalitis/neonatal septicemia and/or delayed detachment of the umbilical stump, later recurrent bacterial infections of the skin and the respiratory tract, and also severe infections such as septicemia, meningitis, and osteomyelitis.
- In addition to infections, the children present with poor growth, hepatosplenomegaly, and

development delay in addition to signs of pancytopenia developing to bone marrow failure without malignant transformation. The children might also show blindness and hearing loss (Skokowa et al. 2017).

Laboratory Findings/Diagnostic Testing

- Severe neutropenia with marked fluctuation over time.
- Anemia and thrombocytopenia develop over time.
- Already early during the course, bone marrow aspiration is difficult to perform, and biopsy is usually necessary. The bone marrow shows *no* maturation arrest but myeloid hyperplasia and myelofibrosis.
- Extramedullary hematopoiesis.
- Imaging will reveal thin corpus callosum, nephromegaly, and osteosclerosis.
- DNA analysis to find the mutation in *VPS45*.

Treatment/Prognosis

- Vigorous treatment of any infection. Consider prophylaxis, as there is poor or no response to G-CSF.
- As for other bone marrow failure syndromes, erythrocyte and thrombocyte transfusions are necessary and eventually hematopoietic stem cell transplantation.
- Prognosis is poor because diagnosis is difficult, and the children usually already have advanced myelofibrosis at time of diagnosis.
- Hematopoietic stem cell transplantation rescues the children. Only a handful of children have undergone transplantation and long-term prognosis for these are unknown.

References

ESID Registry. Clinical criteria. esid.org/content/download/ 15478/424246/file/ESIDRegistry_ClinicalCriteria.pdf.

Skokowa J, Dale DC, Touw IP, Zeidler C, Welte K. Severe congenital neutropenias. Nat Rev Dis Prim. 2017;3:17032.

Stepensky P, Simanovsky N, Averbuch D, Gross M, Yanir A, Mevorach D, Elpeleg O, Weintraub M. VPS 45-associated primary infantile myelofibrosis– successful treatment with hematopoietic stem cell transplantation. Pediatr Transplant. 2013;17:820–5.

Vilboux T, Lev A, Malicdan MC, Simon AJ, Järvinen P, Racek T, Puchalka J, Sood R, Carrington B, Bishop K, Mullikin J, Huizing M, Garty BZ, Eyal E, Wolach B, Gavrieli R, Toren A, Soudack M, Atawneh OM, Babushkin T, Schiby G, Cullinane A, Avivi C, Polak-Charcon S, Barshack I, Amariglio N, Rechavi G, van der Werff ten Bosch J, Anikster Y, Klein C, Gahl WA, Somech R. A congenital neutrophil defect syndrome associated with mutations in VPS45. N Engl J Med. 2013;369:54–65.

SDF-1 – Stromal Cell-Derived Factor 1

► Warts, Hypogammaglobulinemia, Infections, Myelokathexis (WHIM) Syndrome

Secondary Immune Deficiency

► Clinical Presentation of Immunodeficiency, Secondary Immunodeficiency

Seemanova Syndrome

► Nijmegen Breakage Syndrome (*NBS1*)

Serine/Threonine Kinase 4 (STK4)

► Mammalian Sterile 20-Like 1 (MST1) Deficiency

Serum Immunoglobulin Isotypes with Decreased or Absent B Cells, Reduction of

Vassilios Lougaris and Alessandro Plebani
Pediatrics Clinic and Institute for Molecular Medicine A. Nocivelli, Department of Clinical and Experimental Sciences, University of Brescia and ASST-Spedali Civili of Brescia, Brescia, Italy

Definition

Reduction of all serum immunoglobulin isotypes (IgM, IgG, and IgA) with decreased or absent B cells is an immunodeficiency syndrome that may result from several genetic defects, which might be inherited either X-linked (Bruton's agammaglobulinemia) or autosomal recessive (i.e., absent mu heavy chain, Ig-alpha deficiency, Ig-beta deficiency).

Pathogenesis

Immunoglobulins are produced by B lymphocytes and are divided in the following isotypes: IgG, IgA, IgM, and IgE. The first steps in B cell maturation take place in the bone marrow and are characterized by the sequential activation of diverse genes and the expression of diverse proteins involved in cell differentiation (Espeli et al. 2006; Rudin and Thompson 1998; Bartholdy and Matthias 2004). These events lead to the expression of the pre-B-cell receptor, which defines the passage from the pro-B to the pre-B step of early B-cell development. B-cell development in the bone marrow produces antigen-naive B cells that express IgM and are released to peripheral circulation, eventually leading to the formation of memory B cells and plasma cells.

Serum immunoglobulins are reduced in diverse forms of primary immunodeficiency that include impaired antibody production. When all immunoglobulin isotype production is deficient, with minimal or undetectable serum immunoglobulin levels, the immunological condition is defined as agammaglobulinemia and will be the subject of the following chapters. In some cases, absent immunoglobulin production is secondary to a reduction of peripheral B cells due to an early developmental block in the bone marrow. This may be due to defective expression of components of the pre-BCR or to defects in downstream signaling molecules that do not allow proper early B- cell maturation and thus lead to the lack of peripheral B cells (Gaspar and Conley 2000). When B cells are present in significant numbers, the clinical syndrome is called common variable immunodeficiency (CVID).

Clinical Presentation

Clinical presentation of low serum immunoglobulins may be variable, characteristically presenting with recurrent infections, often caused by encapsulated pyogenic bacteria and enteroviruses, and associated with impaired antibody production in affected patients (Plebani et al. 2002). The onset of recurrent and severe infections is common in infancy, approximately 6th–9th month of age, and coincides with the reduction of maternal IgG that had been transferred in utero. Infections involve mostly the respiratory and gastrointestinal tract, although joint infections may also be present. Invasive infections of the central nervous system may also occur in a limited number of patients. More details on the clinical presentation will be offered in the following chapters.

Diagnosis

Immunological work-up in affected patients shows very low or undetectable levels of all serum immunoglobulins, as well as low numbers of peripheral B cells. It is important to use normal ranges obtained from age-matched controls. Molecular diagnostics will be discussed in detail in the following chapters.

Management

As in other forms of primary humoral immunodeficiencies, immunoglobulin replacement treatment should be undertaken once the immunological diagnosis of agammaglobulinemia is established (Shillitoe and Gennery 2017). Currently two options are available: endovenous or subcutaneous. Normally, a dose of 400 mg/kg/dose every 3–4 weeks is sufficient to maintain pre-infusion IgG levels >500 mg/dl, which should be able to reduce the frequency and severity of infectious episodes, especially that of invasive infections. Subcutaneous immunoglobulins are used at a dosage of 100 mg/kg/dose and are administered once a week. Recently, a facilitated preparation of subcutaneous immunoglobulins (that includes the infusion of recombinant hyaluronidase) has been introduced and is used at the same dosage as the intravenous forms, every 3–4 weeks.

Infectious episodes still occur even though patients receive appropriate immunoglobulin replacement. Antibiotic usage should be considered for every infection, and in some cases when frequent infections occur, prophylactic antibiotic regimen may also be prescribed. Most commonly, the infectious episodes compromise the respiratory tract, upper and lower. However, they may also involve the gastrointestinal tract, the skin, and the musculoskeletal system. These latter infections may have a subtle, not clear clinical presentation and may be misdiagnosed for long periods, thus affecting the prognosis. In addition, the responsible infectious agent(s) are not easily detectable which renders the treatment decision difficult and not always efficient.

One of the major clinical problems during long-term follow-up is the development of bronchiectasis leading to chronic lung disease, affecting both quality of life and prognosis of affected patients (Stubbs et al. 2018). Considering the life expectancy of affected patients, respiratory physiotherapy use of bronchodilators and inhaled steroids is valid considerations in order to maintain acceptable lung function. In some cases, lung surgery is necessary in order to eliminate severely damaged lung areas favoring recurrent infections. Furthermore, in a small number of cases, lung transplantation has been undertaken due to the severity of the lung damage and the lack of response to classical medical treatment. Tumors have been reported in a small number of patients, mainly gastric cancer and leukemias (Abolhassani et al. 2015).

References

Abolhassani H, Hirbod-Mobarakeh A, Shahinpour S, Panahi M, Mohammadinejad P, Mirminachi B, Shakari MS, Samavat B, Aghamohammadi A. Mortality and morbidity in patients with X-linked agammaglobulinaemia. Allergol Immunopathol (Madr). 2015;43(1):62–6. https://doi.org/10.1016/j.aller.2013.09.013.

Bartholdy B, Matthias P. Transcriptional control of B cell development and function. Gene. 2004;327:1–23.

Espeli M, Rossi B, Mancini SJ, Roche P, Gauthier L, Schiff C. Initiation of pre-B cell receptor signaling: common and distinctive features in human and mouse. Semin Immunol. 2006;18:56–66.

Gaspar HB, Conley ME. Early B cell defects. Clin Exp Immunol. 2000;119(3):383–9. Review

Plebani A, Soresina A, Rondelli R, Amato GM, Azzari C, Cardinale F, Cazzola G, Consolini R, De Mattia D, Dell'Erba G, Duse M, Fiorini M, Martino S, Martire B, Masi M, Monafo V, Moschese V, Notarangelo LD, Orlandi P, Panei P, Pession A, Pietrogrande MC, Pignata C, Quinti I, Ragno V, Rossi P, Sciotto A. Stabile a; Italian pediatric group for XLA-AIEOP. Clinical, immunological, and molecular analysis in a large cohort of patients with X-linked agammaglobulinemia: an Italian multicenter study. Clin Immunol. 2002;104(3):221–30.

Rudin CM, Thompson CB. B-cell development and maturation. Semin Oncol. 1998;25:435–46.

Shillitoe B, Gennery A. X-linked Agammaglobulinaemia: outcomes in the modern era. Clin Immunol. 2017;183:54–62. https://doi.org/10.1016/j.clim.2017.07.008.

Stubbs A, Bangs C, Shillitoe B, Edgar JD, Burns SO, Thomas M, Alachkar H, Buckland M, McDermott E, Arumugakani G, Jolles MS, Herriot R, Arkwright PD. Bronchiectasis and deteriorating lung function in agammaglobulinaemia despite immunoglobulin replacement therapy. Clin Exp Immunol. 2018; 191(2):212–9. https://doi.org/10.1111/cei.13068.

Severe Congenital Neutropenia 1(SCN1)

▶ Elastase Deficiency, Severe Congenital Neutropenia (SCN) 1

Severe Congenital Neutropenia 2 (SCN 2)

▶ SCN2 (GFI 1 Deficiency)

Severe Congenital Neutropenia 3 (SCN3)

▶ SCN3 (Kostmann Disease)

Severe Congenital Neutropenia 4 (SCN4)

▶ SCN4 (G6PC3 Deficiency)

Severe Congenital Neutropenia 5 (SCN 5)

▶ SCN5 (VPS45 Deficiency)

S

Severe Congenital Neutropenia with Defect in Transcription Factor Gfi1

▶ SCN2 (GFI 1 Deficiency)

Severe T Cell Immunodeficiency, Congenital Alopecia, Nail Dystrophy Syndrome

▶ Winged Helix Deficiency (FOXN1)

SH3 Domain-Binding Protein 2

▶ Cranial Developmental Disorder Cherubism

SH3 Src Homology Domain 3

▶ Wiskott-Aldrich Syndrome Deficiency

SH3BP2

▶ Cranial Developmental Disorder Cherubism

SHARPIN SHANK-Interacting Protein Like 1

▶ OTULIN Deficiency-Associated Disease Spectrum

Short Telomere Syndromes

Mary Armanios[1] and Jolan Walter[2]
[1]Johns Hopkins University School of Medicine, Baltimore, MD, USA
[2]University of South Florida, St. Petersburg, FL, USA

Introduction

Short telomere syndromes (STS) represent a disease spectrum of variable severity that is caused by short telomere length (Armanios and Blackburn 2012). Their infant-onset manifestations are most severe but also most rare; they generally manifest as a primary immunodeficiency (PID) with enterocolitis (Jonassaint et al. 2013). Adult-onset disease is most common and manifests as pulmonary fibrosis (Armanios and Blackburn 2012). Liver disease is also a complication, and STS patients are cancer prone with an overall estimated lifetime risk of cancer around 10% (Armanios and Blackburn 2012). In general, the extent of telomere shortening predicts the age of onset and type of first disease to manifest (Alder et al. 2018). The telomere-mediated PID has variable severity and often manifests with other degenerative phenotypes (Jonassaint et al. 2013; Jyonouchi et al. 2011; Wagner et al. 2018). Because STS have attenuated phenotypes in adulthood, they are thought to be the most common of premature aging syndromes (Armanios and Blackburn 2012).

Clinical Presentations of Telomere-Mediated PID

Infancy. In infants, STS may present as severe lymphocyte deficiencies in B and NK lymphocytes (Jonassaint et al. 2013). IgA levels are often low or undetectable (Jonassaint et al. 2013). Newborn T cell receptor excision circle (TREC)-based screening may identify a subset of these infants who may also show variably low T cell numbers (Wagner et al. 2018). In a subset, severe cases may be recognized in the constellation of microcephaly, intrauterine growth restriction, cerebellar hypoplasia, and immunodeficiency, known as Hoyeraal-Hreidarsson syndrome (HHS) (Knight et al. 1999). It should be noted that PID may be the first and only manifestation of infant-onset STS even in the absence of classic HHS (Jonassaint et al. 2013). The natural history of disease in these infants is progressive marked by complications of colitis, and patients eventually develop bone marrow failure and other STS complications (Jonassaint et al. 2013).

Pediatric. Children with STS may also have PID as a first manifestation. In contrast to infants, they are more prone to developing common variable immunodeficiency (CVID) with a prominent T cell lymphopenia (Wagner et al. 2018). Childhood-onset STS was initially identified in the disease dyskeratosis congenita (DC) marked by classic features of oral leukoplakia, skin hyperpigmentation, and nail dystrophy. However, recent insights into the underlying genetic basis and availability of clinical telomere length testing have established that more than 95% of STS patients do not have these classic DC features (Alder et al. 2018). The T cell PID in STS patients can be severe with both quantitative and qualitative defects including a propensity to apoptosis, a depletion of naïve T cells, and a restriction of the T cell repertoire (Wagner et al. 2018). The severity of the defect is often variable across patients. STS patients may be prone to *P. jirovecii* pneumonia as well as herpes zoster and cytomegalovirus (CMV) infections (Wagner et al. 2018). It is important to note that the telomere-mediated PID may occur in the absence of bone marrow failure, and the STS diagnosis should be considered in the differential diagnosis of PIDs even when blood counts are normal (Wagner et al. 2018). Children often have quantitative immunoglobulin deficiency with IgM being most commonly affected (Wagner et al. 2018). Immunosuppression that is given without the diagnosis of STS can exacerbate an underlying subclinical PID and may provoke opportunistic infections such as with CMV (Wagner et al. 2018).

Adult-onset disease. Adults with STS usually manifest with liver and lung disease (Armanios and Blackburn 2012). In some cases these pathologies may be accompanied by bone marrow failure and subclinical PID (Parry et al. 2011). The most common liver pathologies are cryptogenic cirrhosis, but older children and young adults develop non-cirrhotic portal hypertension with hepatopulmonary syndrome (Gorgy et al. 2015; Calado et al. 2009). Adult-onset pulmonary fibrosis is the most common of the STS presentations and it represents >90% of all cases (Armanios and Blackburn 2012). Emphysema may also be a manifestation of telomere-related lung disease, alone or combined with pulmonary fibrosis (Stanley et al. 2015). Various lung histopathologies have been seen in patients with germline defects in telomere maintenance, but the most common is idiopathic pulmonary fibrosis (IPF) (70%) (Merck and Armanios 2016). The biology of telomere-mediated lung disease is thought to be driven at least in part by alveolar stem cell failure (Alder et al. 2015). Patients with telomere-mediated IPF are prone to complications of immunosuppressive therapy especially in the lung transplant setting (Silhan et al. 2014). Short telomere IPF patients have impaired CMV immunity and are more likely to suffer higher rates of CMV relapse and CMV morbidity and mortality after lung transplant (Popescu et al. 2019).

The Genetic Causes of STS

Thirteen genes have been linked to the STS phenotype (McNally et al. n.d.). The most common are mutation in *TERT*, the reverse transcriptase component of telomerase, followed by mutation in *TR* (also known as *TERC*), the telomerase RNA gene and *RTEL1*. Other causes include genes involved in telomerase RNA biogenesis: *DKC1*, *PARN*, *NAF1*, *NHP2*, and *NOP10*. Mutations in *ACD/TPP1* and *TINF2* affect telomerase recruitment and/or processivity, and mutant *CTC1* and *STN1* affect telomere length likely by interfering in lagging strand synthesis. Mutations in these genes explain 50–70% of STS cases, and the discovery of new genes is an active area of research. Autosomal dominant, autosomal recessive, de novo, and X-linked presentations have all been described. The infant-onset presentations are often caused by de novo *DKC1* mutations (X-linked), bi-allelic mutations in *TERT* or *RTEL1,* or de novo mutations in *TINF2*. Adult-onset disease is usually caused by mutations in *TERT* or *RTEL1*. Autosomal dominant is the most common mode of inheritance; it is associated with genetic anticipation, an earlier, more severe phenotype in later generations that is caused by the successive telomere shortening.

Telomere length, as measured by flow cytometry and fluorescence in situ hybridization

S

(flowFISH), is the gold standard for clinical testing (Alder et al. 2018). It can help make the diagnosis of telomere-mediated PID and aplastic anemia in patients with no identifiable mutation. In addition, it can inform the functional relevance of DNA sequence changes. It also has predictive potential in some clinical settings (Alder et al. 2018).

Evaluation and Treatment of PID in STS

Children and young adults with known STS should undergo a basic evaluation to assess their risk of PID-related complications. This should include enumeration of lymphocyte subsets and immunoglobulin quantification. Because the telomere-mediated PID is progressive, patients with severe T cell defects or a history of infection should be referred for evaluation for definitive hematopoietic stem cell transplantation if they are eligible. Attenuated, non-myeloablative protocols are required for STS patients, and hematopoietic stem cell transplantation should be performed in an experienced center (Dietz et al. 2010). Antibiotic prophylaxis, in bridge to transplant or in the cases where transplant options are not available, should be considered. Patients with STS have been reported to have adverse effects with dapsone (methemoglobinemia) and may be prone to excessive myelosuppressive and gastrointestinal toxicities with mycophenolate (Silhan et al. 2014). There are no studies evaluating the role of immunoglobulin replacement in STS.

References

Alder JK, Barkauskas CE, Limjunyawong N, Stanley SE, Kembou F, Tuder RM, et al. Telomere dysfunction causes alveolar stem cell failure. Proc Natl Acad Sci U S A. 2015;112(16):5099–104.
Alder JK, Hanumanthu VS, Strong MA, DeZern AE, Stanley SE, Takemoto CM, et al. Diagnostic utility of telomere length testing in a hospital-based setting. Proc Natl Acad Sci U S A. 2018;115(10):E2358–E65.
Armanios M, Blackburn EH. The telomere syndromes. Nat Rev Genet. 2012;13(10):693–704.
Calado RTRJ, Kleiner DE, Schrump DS, et al. A spectrum of severe familial liver disorders associate with telomerase mutations. PLoS One. 2009;4(11):e7926.
Dietz AC, Orchard PJ, Baker KS, Giller RH, Savage SA, Alter BP, et al. Disease-specific hematopoietic cell transplantation: nonmyeloablative conditioning regimen for dyskeratosis congenita. Bone Marrow Transplant. 2010;98–104.
Gorgy AI, Jonassaint NL, Stanley SE, Koteish A, DeZern AE, Walter JE, et al. Hepatopulmonary syndrome is a frequent cause of dyspnea in the short telomere disorders. Chest. 2015;148(4):1019–26.
Jonassaint NL, Guo N, Califano JA, Montgomery EA, Armanios M. The gastrointestinal manifestations of telomere-mediated disease. Aging Cell. 2013;12(2):319–23.
Jyonouchi S, Forbes L, Ruchelli E, Sullivan KE. Dyskeratosis congenita: a combined immunodeficiency with broad clinical spectrum – a single-center pediatric experience. Pediatr Allergy Immunol. 2011;22(3):313–9.
Knight SW, Heiss NS, Vulliamy TJ, Aalfs CM, McMahon C, Richmond P, et al. Unexplained aplastic anaemia, immunodeficiency, and cerebellar hypoplasia (Hoyeraal-Hreidarsson syndrome) due to mutations in the dyskeratosis congenita gene, DKC1. Br J Haematol. 1999;107(2):335–9.
McNally EJ, Luncsford PJ, Armanios M. Long telomeres and cancer risk: the price of cellular immortality. J Clin Invest. 2019; PMID: 31380804.
Merck SJ, Armanios M. Shall we call them "telomere-mediated"? Renaming the idiopathic after the cause is found. Eur Respir J. 2016;48(6):1556–8.
Parry EM, Alder JK, Qi X, Chen JJ, Armanios M. Syndrome complex of bone marrow failure and pulmonary fibrosis predicts germline defects in telomerase. Blood. 2011;117(21):5607–11.
Popescu I, Mannem H, Winters SA, Hoji A, Silveira F, McNally E, et al. Impaired cytomegalovirus immunity in idiopathic pulmonary fibrosis lung transplant recipients with short telomeres. Am J Respir Crit Care Med. 2019;199(3):362–76.
Silhan LL, Shah PD, Chambers DC, Snyder LD, Riise GC, Wagner CL, et al. Lung transplantation in telomerase mutation carriers with pulmonary fibrosis. Eur Respir J. 2014;44(1):178–87.
Stanley SE, Chen JJ, Podlevsky JD, Alder JK, Hansel NN, Mathias RA, et al. Telomerase mutations in smokers with severe emphysema. J Clin Invest. 2015;125(2):563–70.
Wagner CL, Hanumanthu VS, Talbot CC Jr, Abraham RS, Hamm D, Gable DL, et al. Short telomere syndromes cause a primary T cell immunodeficiency. J Clin Invest. 2018;128(12):5222–34.

Shwachman-Diamond Syndrome

Herberto Jose Chong-Neto[1] and
Debora Carla Chong-Silva[2]
[1]Division of Allergy and Immunology,
Department of Pediatrics, Federal University of
Parana Medical School, Curitiba, Brazil
[2]Division of Allergy and Immunology,
Department of Pediatrics, Federal University of
Paraná, Curitiba, Brazil

Definition

Shwachman-Diamond syndrome (SDS) is an autosomal recessive disorder associated with bone marrow failure and an increased risk of developing myelodysplastic syndrome (MDS) and acute myeloid leukemia (AML).

SDS is characterized by multiple developmental anomalies including poor growth, exocrine pancreatic insufficiency, skeletal abnormalities (metaphyseal chondrodysplasia, rib cage dysplasia and osteopenia), and cognitive impairment.

Introduction

It is first described as "congenital lipomatosis of the pancreas" in 1961 in two children with exocrine pancreatic insufficiency and leukopenia. SDS was named after the US physician Harry Shwachman, the British ophthalmologist Martin Bodian, and the American pediatrician Louis Diamond reported the syndrome in 1964 (Warren 2017).

SDS is a rare disease with estimated prevalence of 1 in 77,000 births; registry data indicate that the phenotypic spectrum is broad. Since the recognition of SDS as a distinct clinical entity in 1961, there have been several key advances in the characterization of the disease (Warren 2017; Isaev 2017).

First and a major advance was the identification of biallelic mutations in the SBDS gene (SBDS, ribosome maturation factor [*Homo sapiens* (human)]) in 90% of individuals with SDS. A second advance was the discovery that SBDS functions as a cofactor for elongation factor-like GTPase 1 (EFL1) in removing the anti-association factor eIF6 from the subunit joining face of the large (60S) ribosomal subunit in the final step of late cytoplasmic maturation. A third major advance was visualizing the human SBDS and EFL1 proteins bound to 60S ribosomal subunits carrying endogenous eIF6 using single-particle cryo-electron microscopy (cryo-EM) (Warren 2017).

Finally, the discovery of mutations in the 60S ribosome assembly factor DNAJC21 (yeast Jjj1) in SDS reveals genetic heterogeneity in this disorder but supports the original hypothesis that the primary defect in SDS is impaired maturation of the large ribosomal subunit (Warren 2017).

Clinical Presentation

The classical clinical presentation describing SDS includes exocrine pancreatic dysfunction and bone marrow failure. Skeletal abnormalities may include metaphyseal dysplasia, flared ribs, thoracic dystrophies, and osteopenia. Neurocognitive deficits have been described. A distinctive abnormal hepatic phenotype has also been reported. Progression and evolution of bone marrow disease occurs and remains a major source of morbidity and mortality in these patients (Isaev 2017; Myers 2013).

Gastrointestinal Manifestations

Exocrine pancreatic dysfunction is a classic feature of SDS resulting from severe depletion of pancreatic acinar cells. The majority (>90%) of patients with SDS are diagnosed with pancreatic dysfunction in the first year of life, often in the first 6 months. Clinical manifestations range widely from severe dysfunction with significant nutrient malabsorption, steatorrhea, and resultant failure to thrive to completely asymptomatic (Venet 2017; Myers 2013).

In many patients with SDS, clinical symptoms spontaneously improve with age. In as many as 50% of patients, pancreatic enzyme supplementation can be stopped by the age 4 years based on evidence of normal fat absorption, although enzyme secretion deficits remain. Both serum pancreatic and parotid isoamylase levels were lower in patients with SDS than in healthy controls, whereas pancreatic isoamylase levels were lower in other disease controls (like cystic fibrosis) than in normal controls. Secreted parotid amylase levels were also lower in patients with SDS than in healthy controls. These findings suggest a more generalized defect in acinar cell function in patients with SDS. Although the pancreatic manifestations of SDS are well known, patients with SDS often have other gastrointestinal involvement, most notably in the liver. Elevated levels of transaminases and hepatomegaly in younger patients with SDS were described and resolve with age. Elevated levels of bile acids (persistent cholestasis) and hepatic microcysts apparent on imaging studies were described in patients with SDS (Venet 2017; Myers 2013).

Hematologic Manifestations

Patients with SDS are at risk for cytopenias secondary to marrow failure. Neutropenia is reported in 88% to 100% of patients and can be either intermittent or persistent, with variable severity. Anemia and thrombocytopenia have also been reported in most patients, although both are often intermittent or asymptomatic. Elevated hemoglobin F levels can also be seen in a subset of patients. Severe aplastic anemia with trilineage cytopenias may also develop in a subset of patients. Prognostic factors reported with severe cytopenias in the cohort followed by the French Severe Chronic Neutropenia Registry included early age at diagnosis and hematologic parameters. Reports of progression to MDS or AML in patients with SDS have varied. The French Registry reported a rate of transformation to MDS or AML of 18.8% at 20 years and 36.1% at 30 years in a cohort of 55 patients with SDS. In contrast, data of NIH registry (17 patients) and the Israeli registry (3 patients) in which no patient developed MDS or AML are shown. Some of this

discrepancy arises from differences in the definition of MDS and may be partly due to the age of these cohorts. The median age of transformation for patients with SDS was 19.1 years in the French group, whereas the NIH and Israeli cohorts had median ages of 14 and 4 years, respectively, at the time of report. Transformation rates reported by the Severe Chronic Neutropenia International Registry (SCNIR) for patients with severe congenital neutropenia (SCN) are 11.8% at 10 years, whereas the rates for Fanconi's anemia (FA) and dyskeratosis congenita (DC) by the age of 50 years as reported by the NIH are 40% and 30%, respectively, for myelodysplasia (MDS), and 10% for both for AML. Together, these data suggest that the risk of malignant transformation in patients with SDS is significant but occurs with less frequency and longer latency than in patients with Fanconi's anemia. Published reports of solid tumors in patients with SDS are rare thus far (Myers 2013).

Reports suggest that a common cytogenetic abnormality, seen in patients with SDS, del(20) (q11), is not associated with a high risk of malignant transformation, and the cytogenetic anomaly, the isochromosome i(7)(q10), can come and go over years of time without progression to MDS/AML (Valli 2017).

Clinical observations have also demonstrated an increased frequency of infection beyond that attributable to simple neutropenia in patients with SDS, and sepsis is one of the most common fatal infections in SDS. However, patients with SDS also have susceptibility to recurrent bacterial, viral, and fungal infections. B-cell defects (less number of circulating B cell, low levels of IgG and IgG subclasses, and deficient antibody production) and T-cell defects (low CD3/CD4 cell subpopulations and decreased T-lymphocyte proliferation) were described in most patients with SDS studied. Abnormal neutrophil chemotaxis was also reported as described previously (Myers 2013).

Skeletal Manifestations

Skeletal dysplasias are also a frequent manifestation of SDS. The characteristic findings in SDS include short stature as well as delayed appearance of normally shaped epiphyses and progressive metaphyseal thickening/dysplasia in the long bones and costochondral junctions (Myers 2013).

The skeletal abnormalities were described in all individuals, although they were variable in severity and location, often evolving with age (Myers 2013).

In a recent study, demonstrated that SDS is also associated with low turnover osteoporosis, including markedly reduced bone mineral density, mild vitamin D deficiency, secondary hyperparathyroidism deficiency, and vitamin K deficiency, important situations are known to play an important role in skeletal health (Myers 2013).

Neurocognitive Manifestations

Patients with SDS have been shown to have neurocognitive impairment as well as structural brain alterations. Compared with sibling controls as well as patients with cystic fibrosis matched for age and gender patients with SDS, it ranged widely in their abilities from severely impaired to superior in some areas measured. Patients with SDS may have significant impairments in perceptual skills including reasoning and visual-motor skills, higher-order language, intellectual reasoning, and academic achievement.

About 20% of patients with SDS were found to have an intellectual disability, with perceptual reasoning being particularly difficult. Furthermore, children with SDS were 10 times more likely to be diagnosed with pervasive developmental disorder (6%) than the general population (0.6%). In addition, patients with SDS were more likely to have attention deficits than patients with cystic fibrosis (Myers 2013).

These findings were postulated that *SBDS* may have a role in neurodevelopment, especially because many patients with SDS have abnormalities on neuroimaging (Myers 2013).

Laboratory Findings/Diagnostic Testing

SDS patients with the classic presentation including failure to thrive, associated feeding difficulties, and variable recurrent or excessive infections, the diagnosis is often made in the first few years of life (Myers 2013).

Many patients may be diagnosed later in childhood or even adulthood, especially those with more mild pancreatic phenotype (Myers 2013).

The diagnosis is currently made clinically based on evidence of pancreatic dysfunction and hematologic abnormalities.

Regular complete blood cell counts and bone marrow evaluations should be emphasized to monitor for the evolution of marrow dysfunction or malignant transformation. To diagnose regular nutritional and growth assessments, laboratorial screening includes iron (Fe), folate, and B12 levels. To diagnose immunodeficiency, laboratorial screening includes IGA, IgG, and IgM levels. To diagnose pancreatic insufficiency, laboratorial screening including pancreatic enzymes (trypsinogen, pancreatic isoamylase), 72-h fat excretion, fecal elastase, fat-soluble vitamins (A, D, E) levels, and prothrombin time (surrogate for vitamin K) must be requested. To diagnose hepatic impairment, request a liver panel (Myers 2013).

Image exams such as pancreatic ultrasonography and radiological images of the skeleton should be requested for the diagnosis and during the follow-up of these patients (Myers 2013).

Molecular Findings

The majority of individuals with SDS have identified biallelic mutations in the highly conserved SBDS gene. Pathogenic mutations arise as a consequence of gene conversion due to recombination between SBDS and an unprocessed pseudogene located in a distal paralogous duplicon. More than 90% of affected individuals carry one of the three common pathogenic SBDS variants on one allele in exon 2: $183\_184TA > CT$, $258 þ2T > C$ or the combination of $183\_184TA > CT þ 258 þ2T > C$. The mutation $258 þ2T > C$ disrupts the donor splice site of intron 2, while the dinucleotide alteration, $183e184TA/CT$, introduces an in-frame stop codon (K62X) (Warren 2017; Myers 2013).

Although most parents of children with SDS are carriers, about 10% of SBDS mutations arise again. In addition, more than 40 novel sequence variants have been described in individuals who are compound heterozygotes with one of the three common gene conversion alleles (Warren 2017; Myers 2013).

As 5–10% of patients clinically diagnosed with SDS are negative for SBDS mutations, it was suspected that one or more additional genes might be linked to this disorder. The molecular pathology of SDS has indeed now been expanded to include biallelic mutations in DNAC21, the human homologue of the yeast Jjj1 protein that functions in cytoplasmic maturation of the 60S ribosomal subunit (Warren 2017; Myers 2013).

In summary, SDS is a genetically heterogeneous disorder caused by mutations that target a common pathway involved in maturation of the large ribosomal subunit. It is likely that additional gene variants may be identified in SDS in the near future by exome sequencing (Myers 2013).

Treatment/Prognosis

Supportive care for the complications of Shwachman-Diamond syndrome is critical for the medical management of these patients. Evidence of pancreatic insufficiency should be treated with pancreatic enzyme supplementation. Regarding of different degrees of cytopenias, regular transfusion requirements are uncommon outside the setting of severe aplastic anemia. Neutropenia is common, intermittent, and frequently mild to moderate, and patients do not require to use granulocyte colony-stimulating factor (GCSF). Patients with recurrent invasive bacterial/fungal infections and severe neutropenia should receive regular GCSF therapy (Venet 2017; Myers 2013).

Patients with progression to acute myeloid leukemia or myelodysplasia should be considered for the treatment using hematopoietic stem cell transplantation (HSCT). In acute myeloid leukemia, chemotherapy can be used to prepare patient to HSCT. However HSCT with donors other than HLA-identical siblings is associated with high mortality and unfavorable prognosis (Isaev 2017).

Recently was reported the first experience of HSCT treatment of Shwachman-Diamond using an unaffected HLA-identical sibling produced through preimplantation genetic diagnosis (PGD). The patient was a 6-year-old blood transfusion-dependent SDS baby girl with secondary myelodysplastic syndrome, for whom no HLA-identical donor was available. As a result of PGD, two unaffected HLA-matched embryos were identified; one of them was randomly selected for transfer, resulting in a clinical pregnancy and birth of an apparently healthy child. The patient underwent allogeneic transplantation of cord blood hematopoietic stem cells, together with bone marrow from this sibling, resulting in complete hematopoietic recovery. The patient was no longer transfusion-dependent and had normal blood values 160 days after transplantation (Isaev 2017).

References

Isaev AA, Deev RV, Kuliev A, et al. First experience of hematopoietic stem cell transplantation treatment of Shwachman-Diamond syndrome using unaffected HLA-matched sibling donor produced through preimplantation HLA typing. Bone Marrow Transplant. 2017;52:1249–52.

Myers K, Davies SM, Shimamura A. Clinical and molecular pathophysiology of Shwachman-Diamond syndrome: an update. Hematol Oncol Clin N Am. 2013;27:117–28.

Valli R, De Paoli E, Nacci L, et al. Novel recurrent chromosome anomalies in Shwachman-Diamond syndrome. Pediatr Blood Câncer. 2017;64(8):e26454.

Venet T, Masson E, Talbotec C, et al. Severe infantile isolated exocrine pancreatic insufficiency caused by the complete functional loss of the SPINK1 gene. Hum Mutat. 2017;38:1660. [Epub ahead of print]

Warren AJ. Molecular basis of the human ribosomopathy Shwachman-Diamond syndrome. Adv Biol Regul. 2017;67:109–27. [Epub ahead of print]

SIN Self-Inactivating

▶ Wiskott-Aldrich Syndrome Deficiency

SLC46A1: Solute Carrier Family 46, Member 1

▶ Defects in B12 and Folate Metabolism (TCN2, SLC46A1 (PCFT Deficiency), MTHFD1)

Sleeping Sickness

▶ APOL-1 Variants, Susceptibility and Resistance to Trypanosomiasis

Sp110 Deficiency

▶ Hepatic Veno-occlusive Disease with Immunodeficiency (VODI)

Specific Granule Deficiency

Herberto Jose Chong-Neto[1], Cristine Secco Rosario[2] and Nelson Augusto Rosario[3]
[1]Division of Allergy and Immunology, Department of Pediatrics, Federal University of Parana Medical School, Curitiba, Brazil
[2]Department of Pediatrics, Federal University of Paraná, Curitiba, Brazil
[3]Federal University of Paraná, Curitiba, Brazil

Synonyms

Lactoferrin deficiency; Neutrophil-specific granule deficiency

Definition

Neutrophil-specific granule deficiency (SGD) is an autosomal recessive congenital disorder in which the function and structure of neutrophils are altered, resulting in severe and recurrent bacterial infections, mainly by *Staphylococcus aureus*. SGD patients' neutrophils lack primary and secondary granule proteins, have abnormal migration and aggregation atypical bilobed nuclei and inadequate bactericidal activity. CEBPE, also known as CCAAT/enhancer binding protein (C/EBP) epsilon, which is a member of the C/EBP family of transcription factors, has been implicated in SGD. Those patients have normal neutrophil count in blood count.

Introduction/Background

Specific granule deficiency (SGD) is a rare congenital disorder provoked by an abnormal formation of peroxidase negative neutrophil granules. SGD patients suffer from recurrent infections, often in the form of abscesses. Their number of neutrophils is usually within the normal range, but these are structurally characterized by the pseudo-Pelger-Huet nuclear abnormality and by lack or minimal levels of proteins localized to the matrix of peroxidase negative granules such as lactoferrin and vitamin-B12-binding protein.

Since SGD individuals express normal levels of lactoferrin and transcobalamin in their saliva but not in either their plasma or neutrophils, the molecular basis for SGD was hypothesized to involve a mutation in a myeloid-specific transcription factor.

CEBPE, which is associated with SGD, is expressed primarily during granulocytic differentiation. CEBPE-deficient mice lack secondary granule proteins, including neutrophil gelatinase-associated lipocalin (NGAL), and germ-line mutations of CEBPE have been detected in several SGD patients (Glenthøj et al. 2014). Abnormalities in eosinophilic granule proteins and functional alterations of monocytes in SGD have been reported as well. These cells from SGD patients lacked eosinophil-specific granule contents, including eosinophil cationic protein, eosinophil-derived neurotoxin, and major basic protein.

A precise estimate of the incidence or prevalence of neutrophil-SGD is difficult to obtain because the disease is so rare. Only a few cases in a handful of families have been reported worldwide since 1980, when the disorder was first described.

Clinical Presentation (History/PE)

Clinical manifestations include susceptibility to severe invasive pyogenic infections with

Staphylococcus aureus, *Pseudomonas aeruginosa*, and *Candida albicans*. Most patients present in the first few years of life with severe infection. Patients with SGD usually present with severe, chronic cutaneous infections, often with ulcers and abscesses. Chronic and recurrent lung infections, including pneumonia and abscesses, are also common. Patients may also develop septicemia and recurrent mastoiditis, otitis media, and lymphadenitis with draining lymph nodes. One infant presented with vomiting, intractable watery diarrhea, and failure to thrive (Wynn et al. 2006).

Recurrent pulmonary infections can lead to chronic lung disease. The patient may be clinically stable if infections are controlled and there is no permanent damage to the lungs or other vital organs. Clinical characteristics of SGD in adults are unclear since only a few families have been reported (Shigemura et al. 2014).

Laboratory Findings/Diagnostic Testing

The diagnosis of SGD typically involves investigation of neutrophil granule components by Western Blot analysis or electron microscopy. Detection of neutrophil granules by flow cytometry is useful for a rapid diagnosis and a screening of SGD.

The expression of the primary granules and BPI (bactericidal/permeability-increasing protein) are nearly absent, but MPO (myeloperoxidase) and lysozyme expression are unaffected. Although the neutrophils of SGD patients produce normal levels of ROS (reactive oxygen species), the frequency and severity of infections are similar to those in chronic granulomatous disease, which exhibit defective ROS production. This indicates that both granule proteins and ROS play critical roles in neutrophils in neutrophil-mediated bactericidal activities. Neutrophils may also present abnormal nuclear segmentation, nuclear clefts, abnormally weak cytochemical reaction for alkaline phosphatase, and an increased number of mitochondria and ribosomes.

Lactoferrin is absent in neutrophils of patients with neutrophil-SGD, but normal levels of lactoferrin are secreted by nasal epithelial cells in these patients. Levels of RNA for neutrophil-specific granule products, including lactoferrin, transcobalamin F, neutrophil collagenase, neutrophil gelatinase, and defensins, are greatly reduced in SGD bone marrow compared with normal bone marrow. Lactoferrin deficiency in SGD neutrophils is tissue specific and is secondary to an abnormality of RNA production (Lomax et al. 1989).

Recent studies suggest that individual subunits of chromatin-remodeling complexes produce biologically specific meaning in different cells. Granulocyte development requires SMARCD2 (SWI/SNF related, matrix associated, actin-dependent regulator of chromatin, subfamily d, member 2 [*Homo sapiens* (human)], a subunit of ATP-dependent SWI/SNF (SWI/SNF protein [*Ciona intestinalis* (vase tunicate)] (BAF) chromatin-remodeling complexes. Mice with SMARCD2 deficiency do not produce functional neutrophils and eosinophils, a phenotype of SGD in humans.

SMARCD2-containing SWI/SNF complexes are necessary for CEBPε transcription factor recruitment to the promoter of neutrophilic secondary granule genes and for granulocyte differentiation (Priam et al. 2017).

Both CEBPE and SMARCD2 loss-of-function mutations identified in patients with SGD abolish the interaction with SWI/SNF and thereby secondary granule gene expression, thus providing a molecular basis for this disease (Witzel et al. 2017).

Deletion of the gene encoding growth factor independence-1 (GFI1) causes neutropenia and the neutrophils do not form specific granules and gelatinase granules, or their granule proteins. Gfi-1 works as a transcriptional repressor and as an activator of transcription. Genes encoding MPO, elastase, C/EBP-α, and PU.1 are repressed by Gfi-1, while lactoferrin and gelatinase need Gfi-1 for expression. C/EBP-ε and Gfi-1 are believed to form a complex that upturns transcription of genes encoding secondary and gelatinase granule proteins. A patient has been described with SGD and both a markedly reduced level of Gfi-1 expression as well as a mutated form of C/EBP-ε factor with an amino acid substitution.

Although, the mutated C/EBP-ε was able to induce transcription in a transient transfection assay, it could not induce transcription from genes encoding specific granule proteins as it could not form a functional complex with Gfi-1 (Wada et al. 2015). Gfi-1 has also been associated with severe congenital neutropenia as some GFI1 mutants are unable to repress transcription of the elastase gene (ELA2). This results in an increased level of synthesized elastase that produces the same phenotype as SGD patients with defects in the ELA2 gene.

The defect is not restricted to granule proteins of neutrophils but also includes eosinophil and monocyte granule proteins.

Treatment/Prognosis

Infections are often more severe than suggested by the clinical examination, because of defective inflammatory responses. Early diagnosis of infections, antimicrobial prophylaxis, and aggressive management of infectious complications are critical management components.

Treatment consists mainly of intensive intravenous antibiotics for active infections. Prophylactic antibiotics, such as trimethoprim-sulfamethoxazole, are recommended to prevent infection, such as in other primary phagocytic disorders. Growth factors such as granulocyte-colony stimulating factor might be considered. Surgical excision and debridement of the larger cutaneous and soft tissue abscesses are often required (Häger et al. 2010).

There has been one successful report of bone marrow transplantation as a treatment of SGD in a British child and further investigation is needed.

References

Glenthøj A, Dahl S, Larsen MT, Cowland JB, Borregaard N. Human a-defensin expression is not dependent on CCAAT/enhancer binding protein-e in a murine model. PLoS One. 2014;9(3):e92471.

Häger M, Cowland JB, Borregaard N. Neutrophil granules in health and disease (review). J Intern Med. 2010;268:25–34.

Lomax KJ, Gallin JI, Rotrosen D, Raphael GD, Kaliner MA, Benz EJ Jr, Boxer LA, Malech HL. Selective defect in myeloid cell lactoferrin gene expression in neutrophil specific granule deficiency. J Clin Invest. 1989;83(2):514.

Priam P, Krasteva V, Rousseau P, et al. SMARCD2 subunit of SWI/SNF chromatin-remodeling complexes mediates granulopoiesis through a CEBPε dependent mechanism. Nat Genet. 2017;49:753–64.

Shigemura T, Yamazaki T, Shiohara M, et al. Clinical course in a patient with neutrophil-specific granule deficiency and rapid detection of neutrophil granules as a screening test. J Clin Immunol. 2014;34:780–3.

Wada T, Akagi T, Muraoka M, et al. A novel in-frame deletion in the leucine zipper domain of C/EBPε leads to neutrophil-specific granule deficiency. J Immunol. 2015;195:80–6.

Witzel M, Petersheim D, Fan Y, et al. Chromatin-remodeling factor SMARCD2 regulates transcriptional networks controlling differentiation of neutrophil granulocytes. Nat Genet. 2017;49:742–52.

Wynn RF, Sood M, Theilgaard-Mönch K, Jones CJ, Gombart AF, Gharib M, et al. Intractable diarrhoea of infancy caused by neutrophil specific granule deficiency and cured by stem cell transplantation. Gut. 2006;55:292–6.

STAT3 Loss of Function

▶ Autosomal Dominant Hyper IgE Syndrome

STAT5b Deficiency, AR

David Hagin
Allergy and Clinical Immunology Unit, Department of Medicine, Tel-Aviv Sourasky Medical Center, Tel Aviv, Israel
Sackler Faculty of Medicine, University of Tel Aviv, Tel Aviv, Israel

Synonyms

Growth hormone insensitivity due to post-receptor defect; Growth hormone insensitivity with immunodeficiency (MIM #245590); Laron syndrome due to post-receptor defect

Definition

Autosomal recessive STAT5b deficiency is a combined disorder of growth failure due to growth hormone insensitivity and immune deficiency/immune dysregulation secondary to abnormal cytokine signaling.

Background

Deficiency in signal transducer and activator of transcription 5b (STAT5b) secondary to biallelic mutations was first described by Kofoed et al. as a cause for growth hormone insensitivity in the presence of normal growth hormone receptor (GHR) (Kofoed et al. 2003). In addition to growth failure, the affected patient suffered lymphoid interstitial pneumonia, recurrent viral infections and *Pneumocystis jirovecii* infection, suggesting that STATb plays an important role in immune function and regulation. To date, 8 pathogenic homozygous *STAT5B* variants in 11 patients with growth failure have been described, most suffering from significant symptoms of immune dysregulation.

STAT5b is one of seven STAT family proteins which induce gene transcription in multiple cell types in response to different cytokines, hormones, and growth factors. As their name suggests, STATs transduce an external signal and translate it into an effector function by inducing expression of target genes. This signaling pathway, known as the JAK-STAT pathway, is initiated by binding of an activating ligand to its target receptor, thereby inducing multimerization of the receptor subunits. This multimerization step brings the receptor cytoplasmic domains into close proximity. As a result, two receptor-associated tyrosine kinases of the Janus kinase (JAK) family can interact with each other and become activated by transphosphorylation. The activated JAKs in turn phosphorylate other targets, including the receptor's intracellular domain, creating docking sites for STAT proteins through their SH2 domain. In the next step, a conserved tyrosine residue at the carboxy terminus of the recruited STAT is being phosphorylated by the activated JAKs, which leads to rearrangement and dimerization of STATs through interaction of the phosphorylated tyrosine of each STAT with the SH2 domain of the other STAT. These STAT dimers can then translocate to the nucleus where they bind the DNA and regulate gene transcription.

Although this order of events is shared by all JAKs and STATs, the cell type involved, the activating ligand, receptor type, as well as the specific JAKs and STATs used in a specific pathway, will all determine the induced gene expression and will lead to a diverse effector function. It is therefore reasonable to assume that the clinical phenotype of an abnormal STAT function would be a reflection of its effect on the integrity of the pathways in which it is used. The case of STAT5b is more complicated as STAT5b shares more than 90% similarity with its highly related protein, STAT5a, differing by only 6 amino acids in their DNA binding domain, 20 amino acids in their carboxy terminus, and 18 amino acids in their amino terminus. Therefore, some genetic redundancy is expected, and the clinical phenotype of STAT5b deficiency depends on the pathways in which STAT5b plays a dominant role.

The mechanism underlying the abnormalities observed in STAT5b deficiency is the impaired STAT5b function in two major signaling pathways, namely, growth hormone receptor signaling and cytokine receptor signaling.

1. Mechanism of growth failure (Hwa 2016). Postnatal growth depends on insulin-like growth factor 1 expression (IGF1) and is regulated by pituitary-derived growth hormone (GH). Binding of GH to the GHR leads to JAK2 activation, which in turn activates three downstream pathways including STAT, mitogen-activated protein kinase (MAPK), and phosphoinositide-3 kinase (PI3K) pathways. These pathways mediate the metabolic effect and growth-driving effect of GH. Of these three pathways, the STAT pathway and

specifically STAT5b plays a crucial role in IGF1 production by stimulating *IGF1* gene transcription. Therefore, mutations in *STAT5b* are associated with severe growth failure and low to undetectable IGF1 levels. Although STAT5b deficiency leads to low IGF1 expression, the DNA elements within the human *IGF1* locus recognized by STAT5b are not well characterized, and evidence for remote upstream transcriptional enhancer elements, as well as intronic elements, suggests tightly regulated GH-activated STAT5b-mediated *IGF1* gene transcription.

2. Mechanism of immune deficiency and immune dysregulation. STAT5b plays an important role in downstream signaling of different cytokine and growth factor receptors. A common beta subunit (βc), shared by the receptors for GM-CSF, IL-3, and IL-5, induces STAT5b phosphorylation through its associated Janus kinase, JAK2. Perhaps more important for the observed immune dysfunction is the common gamma chain (γc) receptor subunit, shared by six immune-related cytokine receptors (IL-2, IL-4, IL-7, IL-9, IL-15, and IL-21). Since the γc activates STAT5b through its dedicated JAK3 and since γc cytokines are central for lymphocyte development and function, abnormal γc-STAT5b signaling is expected to have a significant impact on normal immune function. This is further supported by the identification of target genes induced specifically and non-redundantly by activated STAT5b. These genes include *DOCK8*, *SNX2*, *SKAP1*, *IL2R*, and *FOXP3*, all play a role in T cell development and function (Kanai et al. 2014). While abnormal IL-7 and IL-15 signaling could result in abnormal T cell and NK cell development, the most well-established effect of STAT5b deficiency is abnormal regulatory T cell (Treg) compartment as shown by reduced CD25 (IL2Rα subunit) expression, reduced numbers of CD4$^+$CD25^{high} FOXP3$^+$ Treg and reduced Treg suppression activity (Cohen et al. 2006). The combination of an abnormal immune cell development together with impaired regulatory

function results in a mixed clinical picture of immune deficiency and immune dysregulation.

Clinical Presentation

STAT5b plays an important role in signal transduction downstream of the growth hormone receptor and cytokine receptors. The clinical presentation of STAT5b deficiency is the result of abnormal STAT5b-dependent pathways. Most characterized are the GH-IGF1 pathway and the interleukin 2 (IL-2)-induced responses in T cells (see Table 1 for details).

1. GH-IGF1 axis. Postnatal growth retardation with resistance to growth hormone therapy is the most prominent clinical phenotype of STAT5b deficiency and was the presenting symptom leading to the investigation and the identification of STAT5b deficiency. Birth size was reported to be normal for gestational age but severe postnatal growth failure developed in all patients and was accompanied by delayed bone age when tested. Other dysmorphic features were described in 6 of the 11 patients and include prominent forehead, saddle nose, and high-pitched voice.

2. Immune dysregulation. Clinical symptoms of immune dysregulation could be expected given the central role of IL2 signaling in Treg development and function and the observed STAT5b-induced gene expression described above. Similar to other syndromes of immune dysregulation, several typical organ systems are involved in STAT5b deficiency.

   (a) Skin – Most patients described showed some degree of skin involvement ranging from pruritic skin lesions, through generalized eczema and atopic dermatitis to dyshidrotic ectodermal dysplasia, psoriasis, and alopecia.

   (b) Gastrointestinal – Early-onset chronic diarrhea was described in three patients, one of them was later diagnosed with celiac disease at the age of 20 years.

STAT5b Deficiency, AR, Table 1 Clinical features and laboratory evaluation of 11 patients described

Patient number	1	2	3	4	5	6	7	8	9	10	11
Reference	Kofoed EM et al. NEJM Sep 2003	Hwa V et al. J Clin Endocrinol Metab, Jul 2005	Vidarsdottir S et al. J Clin Endocrinol Metab, Sep 2006	Bernasconi A et al. Pediatrics Nov 2006	Cavallo MC et al. CIMEL, Dec 2006 (Spanish)	Hwa V et al. Horm Res, Mar 2007	Hwa V et al. Horm Res, Mar 2007	Pugliese-Pires PN et al. Eur J Endocrinol, Jun 2010	Pugliese-Pires PN et al. Eur J Endocrinol, Jun 2010	Scaglia PA et al. J Clin Endocrinol Metab May 2012	Acres MJ et al. J Allergy Clin Immunol, Sep 2018
Homozygous mutation	p.A630P	c.1191insG; p. N398EfsX15	c.1102-3insC; p. Q368PfsX8	p.R152X	p.R152X	c.1680delG (splice site) p. E561RfsX16	c.1680delG (splice site) p. E561RfsX16	c.424-427delCTCC, p. L142fsX19	c.424-427del CTCC, p. L142fsX19	c.1937T>C, p.F646S	c.452T>C, p. L151P
Origin	Argentine	Turkish	Dutch	Argentine	Argentine	Kuwaiti	Kuwaiti	Brazilian	Brazilian	Argentine	
Gender	Female	Female	Male	Female	Female	Female	Female	Male	Male	Female	Male
Physical features — Growth	Growth failure	Growth failure	Growth failure and delayed puberty	Growth failure and delayed puberty	Growth failure	Growth failure	Growth failure	Growth failure and delayed puberty	Growth failure	Growth failure, mildly delayed psychomotor and neurologic development	Growth failure, lethargy, delayed bone age. Delayed puberty
Physical features — Other	Prominent forehead, saddle nose, high pitched voice		Low testicular volume at age 16. Central obesity and pseudogynecomastia at age 30	Prominent forehead, saddle nose, high pitched voice	Prominent forehead, high palate, abnormal dentition			Mild facial dysmorphic features	Prominent forehead, depressed nasal bridge, centripetal fat distribution	Micro-cephaly, bird-like facies with micrognathia, frontal bossing, and synophrys	
Immune dysregulation — Lung	Respiratory difficulties; increased oxygen requirement; lymphoid interstitial pneumonia. Respiratory failure despite immunosuppressive treatment (prednisone and azathioprine)	Ground glass and generalized micronodular appearance. Suspected pulmonary fibrosis	Normal	Chronic lung disease with chronic hypoxemia and clubbing. Ground glass appearance on chest CT with generalized micronodules and bronchiectasis	Chronic respiratory failure with lymphoid interstitial pneumonitis per biopsy. Secondary cor-pulmonale	Bronchiectasis and interstitial pneumonitis		Interstitial lung disease since the first year of life. Severe lymphocytic interstitial pneumonitis on lung biopsy. Chronic steroid treatment and oxygen supplementation	Interstitial lung disease and impaired pulmonary function. On chronic steroid treatment	Normal	Normal

	P1	P2	P3	P4	P5	P6	P7	P8	P9	P10	P11
Skin	Generelized eczema with mild presentation until adulthood	Pruritic skin lesions	Congenital Ichthyosis	Generalized eczema since infancy	Periorbital desquamative dermatitis. Dyshidrotic ectodermal dysplasia per skin biopsy. Episodes of sporadic complete alopecia			Atopic eczema	Atopic eczema	Severe generalized seborrheic dermatitis at 1 year and psoriasis +alopecia at 4 years	Ichthyosis from infancy, severe eczema at 7 years and alopecia totalis at 9 years
GI	Chronic diarrhea and steatorrhea with normal gut biopsy			Chronic diarrhea since the age of 2 months						FTT. Celiac disease at 20 years	Constipation with antigliadin antibodies. No improvement on gluten free diet
Arthritis							Juvenile Idiopathic Arthritis				
Endocrine					Autoimmune thyroiditis					Autoimmune thyroiditis	Autoimmune thyroiditis
Hematologic		Epistaxis							Thrombocytopenic purpura requiring chronic steroid treatment		Iron-deficiency anemia
Infections Bacterial		Recurrent pulmonary infections		Recurrent severe skin and pulmonary infections	Recurrent bronchitis and Mycoplasma pneumonia (age 11)	Recurrent pulmonary infections				Recurrent infections (otitis media, cellulitis, pneumonia) since infancy	No severe infections
Viral	Severe hemorrhagic varicella; Recurrent herpes zoster		Hemorrhagic herpes zoster	Prolonged VZV infection (age 4 years). Recurrent herpes zoster keratitis and uveitis of the left eye + progressive visual loss	Severe life threatening VZV infection (age 4+age 10)					Severe varicella with secondary Strep pyogenas sepsis	No severe infections
Opportunisitc infections	Pneumocystis to jirovecii infection										No severe infections

(continued)

STAT5b Deficiency, AR, Table 1 (continued)

Patient number		1	2	3	4	5	6	7	8	9	10	11
Prognosis		Died of respiratory failure at age 30	Died of progressive pulmonary fibrosis and respiratory failure		Lost to follow up	Died of respiratory failure (age 12)			Underwent successful lung transplant at the age of 17.5. Surgical pathology report showed fibrosis, bronchiectasis and emphysema			No response to GH treatment. Eczema improved with cyclosporine
GH axis evaluation	Spontaneous GH (ng/mL) (N 0.06–5.0)	9.4 (N)	14.2 (N)	0.33 mU/L (N)	6.6 (N)	Normal	17 mU/L (N)	53mU/L (N)	1.7ng/mL (N)	1.0ng/mL (N)	1.7ng/mL (N)	Normal
	GHBP (pmol/L) (N 431–1892)	1236 (N)	1232 (N)	1542 (N)	NA	NA	1311	569	NA	NA	1200 (N)	
	IGF-I (ng/mL) (N 119–483)	38 (L)	7 (L)	3.8 (L)	Undetected	Low	<5	<5	34(L)	<25	16 (L)	62.5 (L)
	IGFBP-3 (ng/mL) (N 2100–7400)	874 (L)	543 (L)	180 (L)	Undetected	NA	700 (L)	800 (L)	520 (L)	754	840 (L)	
	ALS (ug/mL)	2.9 (L)	1.2 (L)	0.7 (L)	NA	NA	0.8 (L)	0.4 (L)	NA	NA	NA	
	Prolactin (ng/mL) (N 0–22)	NA	NA	110 (H)	168 (H)	NA	NA	NA	61 (H)	77 (H)	83 (H)	95.4 µIU/mL (N)
Immune-evaluation	Lymphocyte Subsets	Slightly reduced CD4 and CD8 numbers with skewed memory phenotype of CD4 T cells. Normal proliferation in response to	Normal T, B and NK cell numbers		Mild CD3 lymphopenia and CD8 lymphopenia. CD56 NK lymphopenia. Skewed mature T cell phenotyping. Impaired proliferation	Normal numbers of CD4, CD8 T cells with normal CD4/CD8 ratio			Significant CD3, CD4, and CD8 lymphopenia. Mild B cell and CD56 NK cell lymphopenia	Significant CD3, CD4, and CD8 lymphopenia. Mild B cell and CD56 NK cell lymphopenia	Significant CD3 lymphopenia, mild CD4 lymphopenia and significant CD8 lymphopenia. Mild CD16CD56	Normal lymphocyte counts. Slight reduction in naive CD4+ T cells and abundant activated HLA-DR+ T cells. Reduced naive CD27-IgM

	mitogens. Abnormal B cell phenotyping with reduced IgM memory B cells and increased CD27neg IgDneg class-switched memory B cells	in response to mitogens and antigens				NK cell lymphopenia. Skewed mature T cell phenotyping. Low TCRγδ CD3 T cells. B cell phenotyping showed low levels of IgM memory B cells and increased level of switched memory B cells	+IgD+ and increased class switched memory CD27 +IgMtl: 30 IgD- B cells
Regulatory T cells	Low level and reduced Treg function	Low percent of CD25high CD4 T cells				Low percent of CD4+ CD 25high FOXP3+ Treg (1%)	Low percent of CD4+ CD 25high CD127low Tregs
NK cell Function	Normal absolute number	Reduced NK cytolytic activity rescued by exogenous IL2				Low-normal NK activity	Normal absolute number
Antibody levels	Elevated IgG and IgA, normal IgM, and IgE	Elevated IgG, IgA, and IgE levels	Normal levels	Elevated IgG and IgA levels	Normal levels	Elevated IgG and IgA levels. Protective titers against tetanus and pneumococcus	Normal IgG, low IgA and IgM, increased IgE (491IU/mL).

(continued)

STAT5b Deficiency, AR, Table 1 (continued)

Patient number	1	2	3	4	5	6	7	8	9	10	11
Other	Enhanced GH induced STAT1 and STAT3 phosphorylation. Absent luciferase reporter assay activity. Positive AMA			Reduced IL2 induced STAT5 phosphorylation. Positive FANA	Normal CH50 and normal complement C3 level					Reduced T cell proliferation in response to PHA or CD3, corrected by IL2 supplementation. Absent luciferase reporter assay activity despite reduced residual STAT5 phosphorylation	Normal T cell proliferation in response to mitogens other than lower response to IL-2

GH growth hormone, *GHBP* growth hormone binding protein, *IGF-I* insulin-like growth factor 1, *IGFBP-3* IGF binding protein 3, *ALS* acid-labile subunit, *AMA* anti mitochondrial antibody, *FTT* failure to thrive

(c) Lung disease – Severe lung disease developed in 8 of the 11 patients during the first few years of life and in at least 2 patients, during the first year of life. Imaging studies showed evidence for interstitial lung disease with or without bronchiectasis and generalized micronodules. When obtained, lung biopsies demonstrated lymphoid interstitial pneumonitis (LIP). In some patients, diffuse lung disease was severe enough to justify immunosuppressive treatment and required oxygen supplementation. Three patients died of progressive respiratory failure and a fourth patient underwent lung transplant at the age of 17.5 years. Of all the complication described, pulmonary involvement seemed to be most severe and had a deleterious effect on overall prognosis.

(d) Other – Three patients were diagnosed with autoimmune thyroiditis and one with juvenile idiopathic arthritis. Finally, two patients had hematologic complications, one with idiopathic thrombocytopenic purpura and the other had epistaxis of unknown cause.

3. Immunodeficiency. Impaired signaling downstream of the γc cytokine receptors is expected to result in abnormal immune function and susceptibility to infections. Most patients suffered two types of infections:

(a) Bacterial infections – Recurrent pulmonary infections were described in 5 of 11 patients, 2 of them also had recurrent skin infections.

(b) Viral infections – Five of 11 patients suffered severe varicella-zoster virus (VZV) infection with recurrent zoster. Two developed severe hemorrhagic disease, one developed recurrent herpes zoster keratitis and uveitis with progressive visual loss, and one had two episodes of life-threatening VZV infection. This susceptibility to VZV infection might be explained by abnormal NK cell function as a result of impaired cytokine signaling (IL-2, IL-7, and, most important for NK cells, IL-15).

Laboratory Findings (See Table 1 for Detailed Available Laboratory Data)

1. Evaluation of the GH-IGF1 axis. In all patients, basal growth hormone levels were normal and were frequently elevated following stimulation. Similarly, the downstream effector IGF1, induced by STAT5b, was uniformly reduced and did not respond to GH treatment. Levels of IGF-binding protein-3 (IGFBP-3) and acid-labile subunit (ALS), which together with IGF1 form the major circulating IGF1 complex, were also significantly reduced.

   Interestingly, serum prolactin levels were elevated in five of six patients tested. since the prolactin receptor signals through JAK2-STAT5b activation, abnormal prolactin signaling could potentially disrupt a negative feedback singal and result in elevated serum prolactin levels.

2. Immunodeficiency and immune dysregulation. The clinical presentation of STAT5b deficiency clearly suggests inborn error of immunity with both immunodeficiency in the form of susceptibility to bacterial and viral infections and immune dysregulation in the form of autoimmunity and lymphocytic infiltration of target organs. Despite that, detailed immune evaluation was performed in only small number of the described patients (Bezrodnik et al. 2015). The more common findings include the following:

(a) T cell numbers and immunophenotyping – Three patients had normal lymphocyte numbers, two had mild lymphopenia, and three had significant T cell lymphopenia. An abnormal T cell phenotype was described in four patients; all had a skewed mature phenotype.

(b) Regulatory T cells – Low percent of CD25^{high} CD4$^+$ T cells was described in four patients tested with abnormal Treg function in one of the four.

(c) NK cell number and function – Other than mild CD56$^+$ NK cell lymphopenia in several patients, low NK function was described in two patients and was corrected by exogenous IL2 in one.

(d) B cell number and phenotyping – Mild B cell lymphopenia was described in some of the patients. When performed in two patients, B cell immunophenotyping showed increased levels of class-switched memory B cells.

(e) Antibody levels – Elevated IgG and IgA levels were observed in four out of seven patients tested.

All in all, a tendency for lymphopenia, skewed mature T cell and B cell immune-phenotyping, low Treg levels, and elevated IgG and IgA levels were the more common findings. An abnormal immune cytokine signaling could explain lymphopenia and low Treg numbers, while recurrent infections and abnormal Treg function could explain the skewed phenotype and elevated antibody levels.

Treatment/Prognosis

1. Growth failure – STAT5b is required for signaling downstream of the growth hormone receptor. Therefore, growth failure in STAT5b deficiency cannot be corrected by exogenous growth hormone treatment. However, since the STAT5b-induced IGF1 is the key component required for normal postnatal growth, treatment with recombinant IGF1 (rIGF1) could bypass STAT5b deficiency and should theoretically improve the observed growth failure. Despite that, evidence for the efficacy of rIGF1 is lacking, and a single patient treated with rIGF1 for 1.5 years did not show an increase in growth velocity. It is not clear whether this treatment failure suggests resistance to rIGF1 or was due to chronic illness.

2. Immunodeficiency – Descriptions of recurrent bacterial infections should support an active approach with early and aggressive treatment of infections, in an attempt to achieve better control and prevent end organ damage with emphasize on preventing further lung damage. In addition, since recurrent severe VZV infections were reported in five out of eleven patients, prophylactic treatment should be considered. Finally, although there are no clear guidelines regarding vaccines in STAT5b deficiency patients, recurrent VZV infections combined with tendency for lymphopenia and evidence for abnormal NK function should argue against live vaccine immunization in general and live varicella vaccine in particular.

3. Immune dysregulation – In the small number of patients reported, lung involvement with LIP leading to severe and progressive lung disease was the major reason for immunosuppressive treatment. The limited available data suggests ongoing disease progression despite suppressive treatment, although only steroids and azathioprine were used. Other immunosuppressive treatments and more recent combination protocols (such as rituximab and azathioprine) could result in better outcome. However, no data is available to support it, and more aggressive treatment would increase the risk of severe infections.

4. Prognosis – Out of the 11 patients described, 3 died of respiratory failure and another patient underwent a successful lung transplantation at the age of 17.5. Therefore, STAT5b deficiency should be considered as a severe disease with significant morbidity and mortality and might require a more active treatment approach.

5. Hematopoietic stem cell transplantation (HSCT) – HSCT should potentially correct the immunodeficiency and immune dysregulation aspects of the disease and prevent ongoing end organ damage. Although HSCT is not expected to improve growth failure, combining early stem cell transplantation with rIGF1 treatment could address the two major issues of STAT5b deficiency and improve overall survival and outcome. To date, no description of HSCT was published.

References

Bezrodnik L, Di Giovanni D, Caldirola MS, Azcoiti ME, Torgerson T, Gaillard MI. Long-term follow-up of STAT5B deficiency in three argentinian patients:

clinical and immunological features. J Clin Immunol. 2015;35(3):264–72.

Cohen AC, Nadeau KC, Tu W, Hwa V, Dionis K, Bezrodnik L, et al. Cutting edge: decreased accumulation and regulatory function of CD4+ CD25(high) T cells in human STAT5b deficiency. J Immunol. 2006;177(5):2770–4.

Hwa V. STAT5B deficiency: impacts on human growth and immunity. Growth Hormon IGF Res. 2016;28:16–20.

Kanai T, Seki S, Jenks JA, Kohli A, Kawli T, Martin DP, et al. Identification of STAT5A and STAT5B target genes in human T cells. PLoS One. 2014;9(1):e86790.

Kofoed EM, Hwa V, Little B, Woods KA, Buckway CK, Tsubaki J, et al. Growth hormone insensitivity associated with a STAT5b mutation. N Engl J Med. 2003;349(12):1139–47.

STIM1 Deficiency

▶ Calcium Channel Defects (STIM1 and ORAI1)

STING: Stimulator of Interferon Genes

▶ STING-Associated Vasculopathy with Onset in Infancy (SAVI)

STING-Associated Vasculopathy with Onset in Infancy (SAVI)

Adriana A. de Jesus
Translational Autoinflammatory Diseases Section (TADS), National Institute of Allergy and Infectious Diseases (NIAID), National Institutes of Health (NIH), Bethesda, MD, USA

Synonyms

SAVI: STING-associated vasculopathy with onset in Infancy; STING: Stimulator of interferon genes

Definition

SAVI is an autoinflammatory interferonopathy that presents with early-onset systemic inflammation, vasculitis, and vasculopathy in cold-exposed areas and interstitial lung disease (ILD) of variable severity. SAVI is caused by dominant gain-of-function (GOF) mutations in *TMEM173*, which encodes the protein, *STimulator of INterferon* (IFN) genes, STING (MIM#615934).

Introduction and Background

In 2014, Liu et al. described six patients from six families with de novo variants in *TMEM173* who presented with early-onset skin vasculopathy, failure to thrive, and variable degrees of ILD (Liu et al. 2014). Subsequently, Jeremiah et al. reported a family with four mutation positive members in three generations with variable clinical phenotype and onset, ranging from onset at 1 year of age with fevers, rash, and lung disease in one individual to adult-onset arthralgia and systemic inflammation (Jeremiah et al. 2014).

Genetics

SAVI is an ultra-rare autoinflammatory disease caused by de novo variants in *TMEM173/STING*. So far 11 disease-causing variants in *TMEM173* have been reported (Infevers). The mutations initially reported were located in exon 5, at or near the dimerization interface of the protein (V147L, V147M, N154S, V155M) (Liu et al. 2014; Jeremiah et al. 2014; Munoz et al. 2015). Later, patients with mutations in a second cluster in STING exon 6 (G206Y) and exon 7 (F279L, R281Q, R284G, R284S), have been reported (Melki et al. 2017; Seo et al. 2017; Saldanha et al. 2018). An additional variant close to the STING dimerization domain (G166E) was identified in five members from a four-generation family with a SAVI-like phenotype including peripheral vasculitis, but none of the affected members had lung disease (Konig et al. 2017). Recently, a new variant in exon 5 (F153L) has been detected in a Spanish patient with SAVI (Infevers). Of 32 patients with SAVI reported so far, 65% are sporadic cases.

Pathogenesis

SAVI is caused by de novo GOF mutations in *TMEM173*, which encodes the protein STING, an adaptor protein in the cytosolic DNA-sensing pathway (Liu et al. 2014). STING is a dimeric, endoplasmic reticulum (ER) transmembrane adaptor molecule, that coordinates viral immunity (Ahn et al. 2012; Wu et al. 2013). Upon activation, it recruits and activates TANK-binding kinase 1 (TBK1) and causes IRF3 phosphorylation/activation. Phosphorylated IRF3 is a transcription factor and leads to the transcription of *IFNB1* (Fig. 1) (Wu et al. 2013).

The disease-causing STING mutations cause constitutive transcription of *IFNB1* (Liu et al. 2014; Jeremiah et al. 2014) and the presence of a

Gain-of-function Mutations in STING

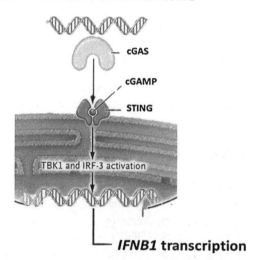

STING-Associated Vasculopathy with Onset in Infancy (SAVI), Fig. 1 Pathogenesis of SAVI. STING is an endoplasmic reticulum (ER) adaptor protein in the cytosolic DNA-sensing pathway that upon activation recruits and activates TANK-binding kinase 1 (TBK1) and causes transcription factor IRF3 phosphorylation/activation, which leads to the transcription of *IFNB1*

strong IFN response-gene-signature (IRS) in whole-blood RNA of SAVI patients (Liu et al. 2014), thus suggesting a critical role of chronic IFN stimulation in the disease pathogenesis. The STING/IFNβ pathway can be directly activated in endothelial cells indicating that the development of vasculitis may be triggered directly by dermal endothelial cell activation (Liu et al. 2014; Jeremiah et al. 2014).

In lesional skin biopsy endothelial cells, there is upregulation of endothelial inflammation (inducible nitric oxide synthase), coagulation (tissue factor), and endothelial cell adhesion and activation (E-selectin) (Liu et al. 2014).

A mouse model of SAVI (N153S knock-in) is characterized by lung disease, skin ulcerations, premature death, and T cell lymphopenia. SAVI mice have milder IRS than SAVI patients, and the mouse phenotype has been proven to be independent of IRF3 (Warner et al. 2017).

Because STING coordinates signals from multiple upstream dsDNA sensors, it may be a target for therapeutic interventions not only in SAVI but also in a wider phenotypic spectrum of IFN-mediated diseases (Liu et al. 2014; Jeremiah et al. 2014; Omoyinmi et al. 2015).

Clinical Manifestations

Onset of clinical manifestations in SAVI ranges from the first days of life to adulthood, but most patients develop disease in the first 3 years of life. Rash and fever typically develop in the first months of life (Liu et al. 2014; Jeremiah et al. 2014; Omoyinmi et al. 2015). Vasculopathic lesions are most prominent in cold-sensitive acral areas and present as telangiectasia, violaceous plaques, nodules on face, nose, ears, and distal ulcerations (Fig. 2a–e). Features of vascular and/or tissue damage include nail dystrophy, gangrene/infarcts of fingers/toes with tissues loss (Fig. 2d, f), and nasal septum perforation (Fig. 2g, h). Nailfold and gingival capillary changes are also observed. Other cutaneous

STING-Associated Vasculopathy with Onset in Infancy (SAVI), Fig. 2 Cutaneous manifestations and nasal septum perforation in SAVI. (**a**) Typical facial distribution of telangiectatic lesions on the nose and cheeks. (**b**) Violaceous, scaling, atrophic plaques on the right hand. (**c**) Telangiectasia, atrophy, and scarring of the skin with loss of deep tissue of the nose. (**d**) Violaceous and atrophic plaques with edema on feet. (**e**) Ulcerated lesions on the pinna of the ear with scales and crusts. (**f**) Erythematous, scaling plaques with atrophy, and scarring of the dorsal aspect of the foot and toes with digital swelling and extensive acral tissue loss. (**g**) Septal perforation at 3 o'clock (indicated by black stars). (**h**) Computed tomography (CT) of the sinuses revealing a septal defect (white star)

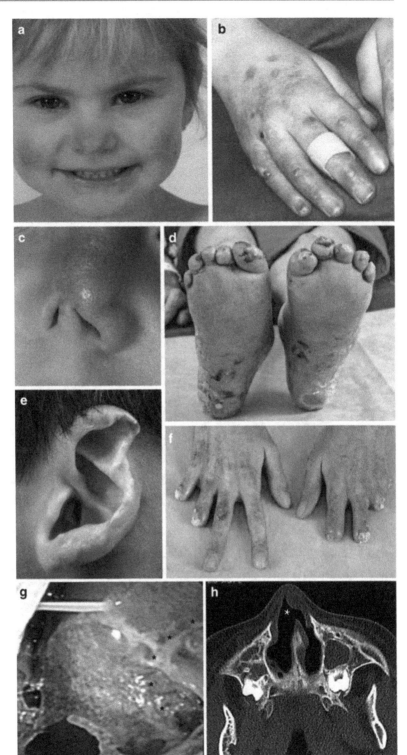

manifestations of SAVI include pustular and ulcerative rashes and eschars overlying non-healing wounds (Liu et al. 2014; Jeremiah et al. 2014; Munoz et al. 2015). All SAVI patients reported in the literature at the time of this review, presented with skin vasculopathy.

Lung disease is of variable severity. Some patients present with tachypnea in the first weeks of life and develop severe ILD and lung fibrosis (Liu et al. 2014; Jeremiah et al. 2014; Konig et al. 2017), other patients have no evidence of pulmonary disease (Liu et al. 2014; Jeremiah et al. 2014; Konig et al. 2017). Paratracheal adenopathy, abnormal pulmonary function tests, and variable interstitial lung disease on CT (Fig. 3c) are seen

with or without symptoms; the extent of lung fibrosis varies between patients (Liu et al. 2014; Jeremiah et al. 2014; Chia et al. 2016). ILD was described in 23 of the 32 cases and early mortality due to severe lung disease often in the context of infections is seen (Liu et al. 2014; Jeremiah et al. 2014; Munoz et al. 2015; Melki et al. 2017; Seo et al. 2017; Saldanha et al. 2018; Konig et al. 2017; Omoyinmi et al. 2015; Chia et al. 2016; Picard et al. 2016; Fremond et al. 2017).

Musculoskeletal manifestations in SAVI patients include myositis, arthritis, and arthralgia but are not consistently seen and may be influenced by additional genetic variants (Liu et al. 2014; Jeremiah et al. 2014; Chia et al. 2016). Basal ganglia

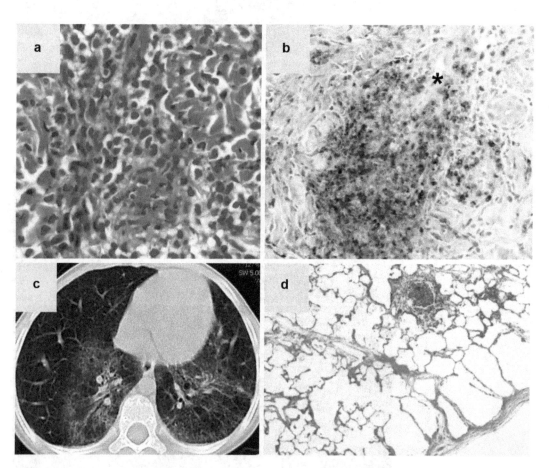

STING-Associated Vasculopathy with Onset in Infancy (SAVI), Fig. 3 Histopathology of skin biopsy and pulmonary findings in SAVI. (**a**) Dense inflammatory infiltrate surrounding a severely damaged vessel. (**b**) Myeloperoxidase immunohistochemical staining showing a dense neutrophilic inflammatory infiltrate surrounding a small blood vessel. (**c**) Interstitial lung disease and (**d**) lymphoid aggregate within the lung parenchyma and emphysematous changes in some alveolar spaces

calcification and systemic and pulmonary hypertension have also been observed (Kim et al. 2016).

Laboratory Findings

Systemic inflammation with increased acute phase reactants (erythrocyte sedimentation rate, ESR, and C-reactive protein, CRP) is seen in 80% of SAVI patients. Other frequent findings include normocytic and normochromic anemia, thrombocytosis, mild leukopenia, and T cell lymphopenia. Immunological abnormalities also detected in SAVI patients include hypergammaglobulinemia (increased IgG and IgA) and positive autoantibodies (ANA, antiphospholipid antibodies, c-ANCA).

Lesional skin biopsies show vasculitis with dense inflammatory infiltrates with predominance of neutrophils and leukocytoclasia surrounding dermal vessels (Fig. 3a, b), which are frequently damaged and show signs of fibrinoid necrosis. Although immune complexes (ICs) can be deposited in partially destroyed vessels, many vessels were void of immune complexes (IC) (Liu et al. 2014).

In SAVI lung biopsies, the number of alveolar macrophages is increased, type 2 pneumocytes appear activated, B cell follicles are found throughout the lung, and emphysematous changes and prominent fibrosis are signs of lung damage (Fig. 3d). Interestingly, vasculitis is not a feature of the SAVI lung disease (Liu et al. 2014).

Diagnosis

The diagnosis of SAVI can be suggested by typical clinical features, such as cold-induced vasculopathy and ILD. However, detection of a likely pathogenic variant in *TMEM173/STING* is mandatory for a definitive diagnosis.

Treatment

Immunosuppressive agents including high-dose steroids, azathioprine, colchicine, methotrexate, mycopheonlate mofetil, cyclophosphamide, tumor necrosis factor antagonist, IL-1 blockade, IL-6 blockade, anti-CD 20 therapy have not resulted in sustained responses (Liu et al. 2014; Jeremiah et al. 2014; Munoz et al. 2015; Omoyinmi et al. 2015; Chia et al. 2016). The discovery of STING mutations as the cause of SAVI led to the use of IFN blocking therapies, such as Janus kinase inhibitors, in patients with SAVI. Konig et al. reported the use of tofacitinib in two of five family members with SAVI. The patients had an improvement of skin manifestations and suppression of the IRS after treatment (Konig et al. 2017). Seo et al. described the use of tofacitinib in a 9-year-old patient with SAVI. The JAK inhibitor led to improvement of patient's skin manifestations, but the pulmonary findings remained unchanged with treatment (Seo et al. 2017). Fremond et al. reported the efficacy of treatment with the JAK1/2 inhibitor ruxolitinib in three children with SAVI. The three patients had a reduction of fever episodes and of CRP levels, significant improvement of skin lesions and of pulmonary function (Fremond et al. 2016). More recently, patients with SAVI were treated with the JAK1/2 inhibitor baricitinib in a study that included 18 patients with interferonopathies, 10 of those with CANDLE and 4 with SAVI. Although the clinical responses were most pronounced in patients with CANDLE, patients with SAVI presented with a reduced duration and severity of the cutaneous vasculitis flares and stabilization of their lung disease (Sanchez et al. 2018).

Prognosis

The mortality of SAVI is strongly associated with the severity of the lung involvement. Six out of the 32 (19%) patients with SAVI published thus far deceased between the ages of 5 and 29 years old (Kim et al. 2016). Since patients with heterozygous mutations have a 50% chance to transmit the disease to each offspring, genetic counseling is recommended.

Cross-References

▶ Chronic Atypical Neutrophilic Dermatosis with Lipodystrophy and Elevated Temperatures (CANDLE)

References

Ahn J, Gutman D, Saijo S, Barber GN. STING manifests self DNA-dependent inflammatory disease. Proc Natl Acad Sci U S A. 2012;109(47):19386–91.

Chia J, Eroglu FK, Ozen S, Orhan D, Montealegre-Sanchez G, de Jesus AA, et al. Failure to thrive, interstitial lung disease, and progressive digital necrosis with onset in infancy. J Am Acad Dermatol. 2016;74(1):186–9.

Fremond ML, Rodero MP, Jeremiah N, Belot A, Jeziorski E, Duffy D, et al. Efficacy of the Janus kinase 1/2 inhibitor ruxolitinib in the treatment of vasculopathy associated with TMEM173-activating mutations in 3 children. J Allergy Clin Immunol. 2016;138(6):1752–5.

Fremond ML, Uggenti C, Van Eyck L, Melki I, Bondet V, Kitabayashi N, et al. Brief report: blockade of TANK-binding kinase 1/IKKvarepsilon inhibits mutant stimulator of interferon genes (STING)-mediated inflammatory responses in human peripheral blood mononuclear cells. Arthritis Rheumatol. 2017;69(7):1495–501.

Infevers: an online database for autoinflammatory mutations. Copyright. Available at http://fmf.igh.cnrs.fr/ISSAID/infevers/. Accessed 25 Mar 2018. [Internet].

Jeremiah N, Neven B, Gentili M, Callebaut I, Maschalidi S, Stolzenberg MC, et al. Inherited STING-activating mutation underlies a familial inflammatory syndrome with lupus-like manifestations. J Clin Invest. 2014;124(12):5516–20.

Kim H, Sanchez GA, Goldbach-Mansky R. Insights from Mendelian Interferonopathies: comparison of CANDLE, SAVI with AGS, monogenic lupus. J Mol Med (Berl). 2016;94(10):1111–27.

Konig N, Fiehn C, Wolf C, Schuster M, Cura Costa E, Tungler V, et al. Familial chilblain lupus due to a gain-of-function mutation in STING. Ann Rheum Dis. 2017;76(2):468–72.

Liu Y, Jesus AA, Marrero B, Yang D, Ramsey SE, Montealegre Sanchez GA, et al. Activated STING in a vascular and pulmonary syndrome. N Engl J Med. 2014;371(6):507–18.

Melki I, Rose Y, Uggenti C, Van Eyck L, Fremond ML, Kitabayashi N, et al. Disease-associated mutations identify a novel region in human STING necessary for the control of type I interferon signaling. J Allergy Clin Immunol. 2017;140(2):543–52.e5.

Munoz J, Rodiere M, Jeremiah N, Rieux-Laucat F, Oojageer A, Rice GI, et al. Stimulator of interferon genes-associated vasculopathy with onset in infancy: a mimic of childhood granulomatosis with polyangiitis. JAMA Dermatol. 2015;151(8):872–7.

Omoyinmi E, Melo Gomes S, Nanthapisal S, Woo P, Standing A, Eleftheriou D, et al. Stimulator of interferon genes-associated vasculitis of infancy. Arthritis Rheumatol. 2015;67(3):808.

Picard C, Thouvenin G, Kannengiesser C, Dubus JC, Jeremiah N, Rieux-Laucat F, et al. Severe pulmonary fibrosis as the first manifestation of Interferonopathy (TMEM173 mutation). Chest. 2016;150(3):e65–71.

Saldanha RG, Balka KR, Davidson S, Wainstein BK, Wong M, Macintosh R, et al. A mutation outside the dimerization domain causing atypical STING-associated vasculopathy with onset in infancy. Front Immunol. 2018;9:1535.

Sanchez GAM, Reinhardt A, Ramsey S, Wittkowski H, Hashkes PJ, Berkun Y, et al. JAK1/2 inhibition with baricitinib in the treatment of autoinflammatory interferonopathies. J Clin Invest. 2018;128:3041.

Seo J, Kang JA, Suh DI, Park EB, Lee CR, Choi SA, et al. Tofacitinib relieves symptoms of stimulator of interferon genes (STING)-associated vasculopathy with onset in infancy caused by 2 de novo variants in TMEM173. J Allergy Clin Immunol. 2017;139(4):1396–9.e12.

Warner JD, Irizarry-Caro RA, Bennion BG, Ai TL, Smith AM, Miner CA, et al. STING-associated vasculopathy develops independently of IRF3 in mice. J Exp Med. 2017;214(11):3279–92.

Wu J, Sun L, Chen X, Du F, Shi H, Chen C, et al. Cyclic GMP-AMP is an endogenous second messenger in innate immune signaling by cytosolic DNA. Science. 2013;339(6121):826–30.

STX11 Deficiency

Ivan K. Chinn

Section of Immunology, Allergy, and Retrovirology, Texas Children's Hospital, Houston, TX, USA

William T. Shearer Center for Human Immunobiology, Texas Children's Hospital, Houston, TX, USA

Department of Pediatrics, Baylor College of Medicine, Houston, TX, USA

Introduction

STX11 is located at 6q24 and encodes syntaxin-11, a 287 amino acid protein that is predominantly expressed in immunologic cells and platelets (zur Stadt et al. 2005). Syntaxin-11 is considered an atypical member of the syntaxin family of proteins because it lacks a transmembrane domain (zur Stadt et al. 2005; Spessott et al. 2017). Instead, it is held to the membrane by prenyl- and palmitoyl-lipid modifications (Spessott et al.

2017). Syntaxin-11 serves as a Qa-Soluble NSF Attachment Protein Receptor (SNARE) protein (Dieckmann et al. 2015; Halimani et al. 2014). SNARE proteins are key molecules that interact with each other to mediate fusion of cellular membranes.

Molecular Function

Cytotoxic T cells and NK cells kill target cells by mobilizing secretory granules containing perforin and other agents, such as granzyme, to the cellular membrane and releasing the contents into the intercellular space at the immunologic synapse. Toward the final steps of the degranulation pathway, lytic granules are tethered to the plasma membrane through interactions between Rab27a and Munc13-4. Syntaxin-11 and Munc18-2 then work cooperatively to enable lytic granule secretion. Syntaxin-11 expression requires proteasome activity, and the protein is typically sequestered within cation-dependent-mannose-6-phosphate receptor-expressing vesicles (Dabrazhynetskaya et al. 2012). During degranulation, the molecule localizes to the plasma membrane at immunologic synapses to promote docking of lytic granules (Halimani et al. 2014). This initial syntaxin-11 plasma membrane localization requires Munc18-2 (Dieckmann et al. 2015). In human cytotoxic T cells, syntaxin-11 acting as a Qa-SNARE then complexes with the Qbc-SNARE, SNAP23, and binds to the R-SNARE, VAMP8 (Spessott et al. 2017). This complex yields incomplete membrane fusion in the absence of Munc18-2 (Spessott et al. 2017). Munc18-2 serves further as a catalyst for assembly of syntaxin-11/SNAP23/VAMP8 complexes to permit complete membrane fusion (Spessott et al. 2017). In this manner, Munc18-2 overcomes the inherent lack of a transmembrane domain within the syntaxin-11 molecule (Spessott et al. 2017).

In macrophages, endosomal syntaxin-11 regulates late endosome to lysosome fusion by sequestering the Qb-SNARE, Vti1b, from binding to syntaxin-6 and syntaxin-8 (Spessott et al. 2017; Offenhäuser et al. 2011). Syntaxin-11 is also required for upregulation of TLR4 on the surface of macrophages in response to IFN-γ or lipopolysaccharide (Kinoshita et al. 2019). Appropriate endosomal trafficking of TLR4 in these conditions is mediated by SNAP23 and involves a syntaxin-11-associated change to the conformation of SNAP23. Phagocytosis and cytokine secretion by macrophages do not appear to be impaired by syntaxin-11 deficiency (D'Orlando et al. 2013). Nonetheless, these examples underscore the ability of syntaxin-11 to regulate other SNARE molecules.

Syntaxin-11 has roles in other hematopoietic cells. Loss of syntaxin-11 in neutrophils results in defective degranulation (D'Orlando et al. 2013). In platelets, syntaxin-11 interacts with SNAP23, VAMP8, and Munc18-2 to promote fusion and granule secretion (Spessott et al. 2017).

Presentation

STX11 deficiency causes familial hemophagocytic lymphohistiocytosis (HLH) type 4 (zur Stadt et al. 2005). HLH is defined by fulfillment of at least five of the following eight criteria: fever; splenomegaly; cytopenia; hypertriglyceridemia and/or hypofibrinogenemia; hemophagocytosis in the bone marrow, spleen, or lymph nodes; deficient NK cell function; hyperferritinemia; and elevated levels of serum soluble CD25 (Henter et al. 2007). In a European cohort of 28 HLH families in whom perforin deficiency had been excluded, 4 families (14%) had *STX11* deficiency (Rudd et al. 2006). All four families were from Turkey and consanguineous. In a German familial HLH cohort of 63 patients, 6 (9.5%) had *STX11* deficiency (Stadt et al. 2006). All were Kurdish. Meanwhile, among 243 North American cases of familial HLH, *STX11* deficiency accounted for less than 1% (Marsh et al. 2010). Similarly, in an Italian cohort, only 1 case of *STX11* deficiency was identified among 171 patients who had genetically diagnosed familial HLH (Cetica et al. 2016). HLH due to *STX11* deficiency therefore occurs infrequently in outbred populations.

S

STX11 deficiency is known to produce a later and milder course of disease than other forms of familial HLH (Kram et al. 2019). In mouse models, the less severe presentation is due to exhaustion of IFN-γ producing CD8$^+$ T cells, although a mechanistic explanation for the exhaustion remains absent (Kögl et al. 2013).

Diagnosis

Establishment of a diagnosis remains difficult without genetic testing. In general, *STX11* deficiency results in reduced cytotoxic T cell and NK cell cytotoxicity and degranulation, which are partially restored by IL-2 (Bryceson et al. 2007). Notable exceptions have been reported, however. In one family, NK cell degranulation was not impaired, and NK cell cytotoxicity was only slightly decreased (Macartney et al. 2011). In another patient who had biallelic missense variants in *STX11*, normal NK cell degranulation and cytotoxicity were observed (Marsh et al. 2010). Even if cytotoxicity and degranulation defects are identified, *STX11* deficiency cannot be easily distinguished from familial HLH types 3 and 5. Genetic testing therefore remains essential to confirm the presence of biallelic pathogenic variants in *STX11*.

Treatment

Protocols have not been developed specifically for treatment of HLH due to *STX11* deficiency but instead apply to HLH in general. The initial HLH-94 protocol employed a combination of intravenous etoposide, oral or intravenous dexamethasone, and (if neurologic disease is present) intrathecal methotrexate (Henter et al. 1997). Subsequently, the HLH-2004 protocol was developed, which combines HLH-94 with the use of oral cyclosporine (Henter et al. 2007). Providers should be cognizant that cyclosporine use can be associated with the appearance of posterior reversible encephalopathy syndrome (Jordan et al. 2011). Adjunctive use of serotherapy has been reported to enhance outcomes (Ishii 2016; Tang and Xu 2011; Filipovich and Chandrakasan 2015). Supportive care with antibiotics and antifungal medications to minimize infections is necessary during treatment for HLH (Jordan et al. 2011; Ishii 2016). Patients may require additional support if bleeding or cardiac dysfunction is present (Jordan et al. 2011).

HSCT represents the only definitive therapy for this disease at this time. Optimal strategies continue to be developed, as overall 5-year survival after HSCT in the HLH-94 study was only 54% (Henter et al. 1997; Nikiforow 2015). For all forms of HLH taken as a whole, survival is superior with use of reduced intensity conditioning after successful induction of HLH remission (Jordan et al. 2011; Nikiforow 2015; Seo 2015). Primary graft loss is common, and donor chimerism must be monitored closely (Jordan et al. 2011).

Cross-References

▶ *PRF1* Deficiency
▶ *STXBP2* Deficiency
▶ *UNC13D* Deficiency

References

Bryceson YT, Rudd E, Zheng C, et al. Defective cytotoxic lymphocyte degranulation in syntaxin-11–deficient familial hemophagocytic lymphohistiocytosis 4 (FHL4) patients. Blood. 2007;110:1906–15.

Cetica V, Sieni E, Pende D, et al. Genetic predisposition to hemophagocytic lymphohistiocytosis: report on 500 patients from the Italian registry. J Allergy Clin Immunol. 2016;137:188–96.e4.

D'Orlando O, Zhao F, Kasper B, et al. Syntaxin 11 is required for NK and CD8+ T-cell cytotoxicity and neutrophil degranulation. Eur J Immunol. 2013;43:194–208.

Dabrazhynetskaya A, Ma J, Guerreiro-Cacais AO, et al. Syntaxin 11 marks a distinct intracellular compartment recruited to the immunological synapse of NK cells to colocalize with cytotoxic granules. J Cell Mol Med. 2012;16:129–41.

Dieckmann NMG, Hackmann Y, Aricò M, Griffiths GM. Munc18-2 is required for syntaxin 11 localization on the plasma membrane in cytotoxic T-lymphocytes. Traffic. 2015;16:1330–41.

Filipovich AH, Chandrakasan S. Pathogenesis of hemophagocytic lymphohistiocytosis. Hematol Oncol Clin North Am. 2015;29:895–902.

Halimani M, Pattu V, Marshall MR, et al. Syntaxin 11 serves as a t-SNARE for the fusion of lytic granules in human cytotoxic T lymphocytes. Eur J Immunol. 2014;44:573–84.

Henter J-I, Aricò M, Egeler RM, et al. HLH-94: a treatment protocol for hemophagocytic lymphohistiocytosis. Med Pediatr Oncol. 1997;28:342–7.

Henter J-I, Horne A, Aricó M, et al. HLH-2004: diagnostic and therapeutic guidelines for hemophagocytic lymphohistiocytosis. Pediatr Blood Cancer. 2007;48:124–31.

Ishii E. Hemophagocytic lymphohistiocytosis in children: pathogenesis and treatment. Front Pediatr. 2016;4:47.

Jordan MB, Allen CE, Weitzman S, Filipovich AH, McClain KL. How I treat hemophagocytic lymphohistiocytosis. Blood. 2011;118:4041–52.

Kinoshita D, Sakurai C, Morita M, Tsunematsu M, Hori N, Hatsuzawa K. Syntaxin 11 regulates the stimulus-dependent transport of Toll-like receptor 4 to the plasma membrane by cooperating with SNAP-23 in macrophages. Mol Biol Cell. 2019;30:1085–97.

Kögl T, Müller J, Jessen B, et al. Hemophagocytic lymphohistiocytosis in syntaxin-11–deficient mice: T-cell exhaustion limits fatal disease. Blood. 2013;121:604–13.

Kram DE, Santarelli MD, Russell TB, Pearsall KB, Saldaña BD. STX11-deficient familial hemophagocytic lymphohistiocytosis type 4 is associated with self-resolving flares and a milder clinical course. Pediatr Blood Cancer. 2019;66:e27890.

Macartney CA, Weitzman S, Wood SM, et al. Unusual functional manifestations of a novel STX11 frameshift mutation in two infants with familial hemophagocytic lymphohistiocytosis type 4 (FHL4). Pediatr Blood Cancer. 2011;56:654–7.

Marsh RA, Satake N, Biroschak J, et al. STX11 mutations and clinical phenotypes of familial hemophagocytic lymphohistiocytosis in North America. Pediatr Blood Cancer. 2010;55:134–40.

Nikiforow S. The role of hematopoietic stem cell transplantation in treatment of hemophagocytic lymphohistiocytosis. Hematol Oncol Clin North Am. 2015;29:943–59.

Offenhäuser C, Lei N, Roy S, Collins BM, Stow JL, Murray RZ. Syntaxin 11 binds Vti1b and regulates late endosome to lysosome fusion in macrophages. Traffic. 2011;12:762–73.

Rudd E, Göransdotter Ericson K, Zheng C, et al. Spectrum and clinical implications of syntaxin 11 gene mutations in familial haemophagocytic lymphohistiocytosis: association with disease-free remissions and haematopoietic malignancies. J Med Genet. 2006;43:e14.

Seo JJ. Hematopoietic cell transplantation for hemophagocytic lymphohistiocytosis: recent advances and controversies. Blood Res. 2015;50:131–9.

Spessott WA, Sanmillan ML, McCormick ME, Kulkarni VV, Giraudo CG. SM protein Munc18-2 facilitates transition of syntaxin 11-mediated lipid mixing to complete fusion for T-lymphocyte cytotoxicity. Proc Natl Acad Sci. 2017;114:E2176.

Stadt UZ, Beutel K, Kolberg S, et al. Mutation spectrum in children with primary hemophagocytic lymphohistiocytosis: molecular and functional analyses of PRF1, UNC13D, STX11, and RAB27A. Hum Mutat. 2006;27:62–8.

Tang Y-M, Xu X-J. Advances in hemophagocytic lymphohistiocytosis: pathogenesis, early diagnosis/differential diagnosis, and treatment. TheScientificWorldJOURNAL. 2011;11

zur Stadt U, Schmidt S, Kasper B, et al. Linkage of familial hemophagocytic lymphohistiocytosis (FHL) type-4 to chromosome 6q24 and identification of mutations in syntaxin 11. Hum Mol Genet. 2005;14:827–34.

STXBP2 Deficiency

Ivan K. Chinn

Section of Immunology, Allergy, and Retrovirology, Texas Children's Hospital, Houston, TX, USA

William T. Shearer Center for Human Immunobiology, Texas Children's Hospital, Houston, TX, USA

Department of Pediatrics, Baylor College of Medicine, Houston, TX, USA

Introduction

STXBP2 is located at 19p13 and encodes Munc18-2, a 19-exon, 593 amino acid, 66 kDa protein that is highly expressed in hematopoietic cells (Côte et al. 2009; zur Stadt et al. 2009).

Molecular Function

Cytotoxic T cells and NK cells kill target cells by mobilizing secretory granules containing perforin and other agents, such as granzyme, to the cellular membrane and releasing the contents into the intercellular space at the immunologic synapse. Toward the final steps of the degranulation pathway, lytic granules are tethered to the plasma membrane through interactions between Rab27a and Munc13-4. Syntaxin-11 and Munc18-2 then work cooperatively to enable lytic granule secretion. During degranulation, syntaxin-11 localizes to the plasma membrane at immunologic synapses to promote docking of lytic granules. This initial syntaxin-11 plasma membrane localization requires Munc18-2 (Dieckmann et al. 2015). In human cytotoxic T cells, syntaxin-11 then complexes with SNAP23 and binds to VAMP8 (Spessott et al. 2017). This complex yields incomplete membrane fusion in the absence of Munc18-2 (Spessott et al. 2017). Munc18-2 serves further as a catalyst for assembly of syntaxin-11/SNAP23/VAMP8 complexes to permit complete membrane fusion (Spessott et al. 2017). In this process, direct binding of Munc18-2 to the N-peptide and H_{ABC} domain of syntaxin-11 is required (Hackmann et al. 2013). In NK cells, interleukin-2 (IL-2) can upregulate expression of syntaxin-3, which may provide limited functional redundancy with syntaxin-11 (Hackmann et al. 2013).

Munc18-2 is required for mobilization and exocytosis of neutrophil granules (Zhao et al. 2013). In these cells, Munc18-2 colocalizes with primary granules and mediates membrane fusion through interactions with syntaxin-3 (Brochetta et al. 2008). Neutrophils from patients with STXBP2 deficiency demonstrate impaired granule exocytosis of proteolytic enzymes despite normal NADPH oxidase activity.

Munc18-2 plays distinct, essential roles in mast cell degranulation, as well, although the clinical relevance of this observation remains unclear (Brochetta et al. 2014; Gutierrez et al. 2018). In mast cells, IgE-induced degranulation becomes impaired with loss of Munc18-2. This defect is amplified by suppression of syntaxin-3, indicating the importance of interactions between the two molecules (Brochetta et al. 2014). Munc-18-2 also interacts with tubulin to effect granule mobilization (Brochetta et al. 2014; Martin-Verdeaux et al. 2003). In STXBP2-deficient mast cells, granule translocation to and fusion with the plasma membrane are therefore impaired (Brochetta et al. 2014).

In enterocytes, Munc18-2 serves as a catalyst for syntaxin-3:synaptotagmin-like protein 4a binding, which is necessary for exocytosis of vesicles from the apical membrane (Vogel et al. 2018). In Munc18-2 deficient intestinal organoid cells, syntaxin-3-positive vesicles mislocalize intracellularly, and microvillus inclusions form upon differentiation (Vogel et al. 2018; Mosa et al. 2018).

Presentation

STXBP2 deficiency causes familial hemophagocytosis (HLH) type 5 (Côte et al. 2009; zur Stadt et al. 2009). HLH is defined by fulfillment of at least five of the following eight criteria: fever; splenomegaly; cytopenia; hypertriglyceridemia and/or hypofibrinogenemia; hemophagocytosis in bone marrow, spleen, or lymph nodes; deficient NK cell function; hyperferritinemia; and elevated levels of serum soluble CD25 (Henter et al. 2007). STXBP2 deficiency may account for 5–20% of familial HLH (Côte et al. 2009; Cetica et al. 2016; Sieni et al. 2012; Degar 2015). Age of onset is below 1 year for patients with biallelic pathogenic missense, deletion (either in-frame or frameshift), and non-exon 15 splice site variants and above 1 year for patients with one or two pathogenic exon 15 canonical splicing site variants (Pagel et al. 2012; Usmani et al. 2013). Patients in the early-onset group tend to have a more rapidly progressive course, while patients in the latter group exhibit milder, more atypical presentations (Pagel et al. 2012).

STXBP2 deficiency can present with manifestations aside from HLH. Gastrointestinal symptoms, most notably enteropathy resembling microvillus inclusion disease, occur frequently (approximately 38% of cases) and are associated with the presence of highly damaging variants (zur Stadt et al. 2009; Vogel et al. 2018; Pagel et al. 2012; Stepensky et al. 2013). Hypogammaglobulinemia has been reported in as many as 59% of cases and is associated with exon 15 splicing variants (zur Stadt et al. 2009; Pagel et al. 2012; Esmaeilzadeh et al. 2015). Hearing impairment remains underappreciated but has been found in 35% of patients tested (Pagel et al. 2012; Bezdjian et al. 2018). Bleeding tendencies have also been identified in 22% of patients (zur Stadt et al. 2009; Pagel et al. 2012). Rarer features include the following: central nervous system disease (zur Stadt et al. 2009; Esmaeilzadeh et al. 2015; Meeths et al. 2010); renal Fanconi syndrome (one case) (Stepensky et al. 2013); and Hodgkin disease (linked to the presence of at least one hypomorphic variant) (Pagel et al. 2012; Machaczka et al. 2013).

Diagnosis

Munc-18-2 deficient NK and $CD8^+$ T cells generally demonstrate impaired cytotoxicity and degranulation, as measured by CD107a upregulation at the cellular membrane (Côte et al. 2009; zur Stadt et al. 2009; Usmani et al. 2013; Cetica et al. 2010). These defects have been reported to be partially restored with exogenous IL-2, although this characteristic may be constrained to the presence of one or more variants that do not completely abolish protein function, such as hypomorphic exon 15 splicing variants (Côte et al. 2009; zur Stadt et al. 2009; Pagel et al. 2012). In fact, the imprecise diagnostic sensitivity and specificity of these tests have been well-noted, and genetic testing for biallelic pathogenic variants in *STXBP2* is therefore ultimately required to establish the diagnosis (Côte et al. 2009; Pagel et al. 2012). (Providers should be aware that a pathogenic intronic variant [c.902+5G>A] has been reported, which may require targeted evaluation) (Vogel et al. 2018).

Monoallelic variants in two patients have been shown to impair lytic granule fusion in a dominant negative manner and have been proposed to result in HLH (Spessott et al. 2015). These missense variants were highly specific for the arginine at position 65 (c.194G>A:p.R65Q and c.193C>T:

p.R65W). Although genetic testing did not find any deletions in *STXBP2*, the potential presence of a pathogenic noncoding variant on the opposite allele cannot be excluded in these cases. Furthermore, healthy family members carrying these variants in monoallelic state did not develop HLH, and three of the four relatives tested had normal NK cell cytotoxicity or CD107a mobilization. Monoallelic pathogenicity of these variants therefore warrants deeper scrutiny.

Treatment

Protocols have not been developed specifically for treatment of HLH due to *STXBP2* deficiency but instead apply to HLH in general. The initial HLH-94 protocol employed a combination of intravenous etoposide, oral or intravenous dexamethasone, and (if neurologic disease is present) intrathecal methotrexate (Henter et al. 1997). Subsequently, the HLH-2004 protocol was developed, which combines HLH-94 with the use of oral cyclosporine (Henter et al. 2007). Providers should be cognizant that cyclosporine use can be associated with the appearance of posterior reversible encephalopathy syndrome (Jordan et al. 2011). Adjunctive use of serotherapy has been reported to enhance outcomes (Ishii 2016; Tang and Xu 2011; Filipovich and Chandrakasan 2015). Supportive care with antibiotics and antifungal medications to minimize infections is necessary during treatment for HLH (Jordan et al. 2011; Ishii 2016). Patients may require additional support if bleeding or cardiac dysfunction is present (Jordan et al. 2011).

Hematopoietic stem cell transplantation (HSCT) represents the only definitive therapy for this disease at this time. Optimal strategies continue to be developed, as overall 5-year survival after HSCT in the HLH-94 study was only 54% (Henter et al. 1997; Nikiforow 2015). In one cohort of 26 patients with *STXBP2* deficiency who received HSCT, disease-free survival was 69% at a median of 4 years of follow-up (Pagel et al. 2012). For all forms of HLH taken as a

S

whole, survival is superior with use of reduced intensity conditioning after successful induction of HLH remission (Jordan et al. 2011; Nikiforow 2015; Seo 2015). Primary graft loss is common, and donor chimerism must be monitored closely (Jordan et al. 2011).

Cross-References

▶ *PRF1* Deficiency
▶ *STX11* Deficiency
▶ *UNC13D* Deficiency

References

Bezdjian A, Bruijnzeel H, Pagel J, Daniel SJ, Thomeer HGXM. Low-frequency sensorineural hearing loss in familial hemophagocytic lymphohistiocytosis type 5. Ann Otol Rhinol Laryngol. 2018;127:409–13.

Brochetta C, Vita F, Tiwari N, et al. Involvement of Munc18 isoforms in the regulation of granule exocytosis in neutrophils. Biochim Biophys Acta (BBA) Mol Cell Res. 2008;1783:1781–91.

Brochetta C, Suzuki R, Vita F, et al. Munc18-2 and syntaxin 3 control distinct essential steps in mast cell degranulation. J Immunol. 2014;192:41.

Cetica V, Santoro A, Gilmour KC, et al. STXBP2 mutations in children with familial haemophagocytic lymphohistiocytosis type 5. J Med Genet. 2010;47:595.

Cetica V, Sieni E, Pende D, et al. Genetic predisposition to hemophagocytic lymphohistiocytosis: report on 500 patients from the Italian registry. J Allergy Clin Immunol. 2016;137:188–96.e4.

Côte M, Ménager MM, Burgess A, et al. Munc18-2 deficiency causes familial hemophagocytic lymphohistiocytosis type 5 and impairs cytotoxic granule exocytosis in patient NK cells. J Clin Invest. 2009;119:3765–73.

Degar B. Familial hemophagocytic lymphohistiocytosis. Hematol Oncol Clin North Am. 2015;29:903–13.

Dieckmann NMG, Hackmann Y, Aricò M, Griffiths GM. Munc18-2 is required for syntaxin 11 localization on the plasma membrane in cytotoxic T-lymphocytes. Traffic. 2015;16:1330–41.

Esmaeilzadeh H, Bemanian MH, Nabavi M, et al. Novel patient with late-onset familial hemophagocytic lymphohistiocytosis with STXBP2 mutations presenting with autoimmune hepatitis, neurological manifestations and infections associated with hypogammaglobulinemia. J Clin Immunol. 2015;35:22–5.

Filipovich AH, Chandrakasan S. Pathogenesis of hemophagocytic lymphohistiocytosis. Hematol Oncol Clin North Am. 2015;29:895–902.

Gutierrez BA, Chavez MA, Rodarte AI, et al. Munc18-2, but not Munc18-1 or Munc18-3, controls compound and single-vesicle–regulated exocytosis in mast cells. J Biol Chem. 2018;293:7148–59.

Hackmann Y, Graham SC, Ehl S, et al. Syntaxin binding mechanism and disease-causing mutations in Munc18-2. Proc Natl Acad Sci. 2013;110:E4482.

Henter J-I, Aricò M, Egeler RM, et al. HLH-94: a treatment protocol for hemophagocytic lymphohistiocytosis. Med Pediatr Oncol. 1997;28:342–7.

Henter J-I, Horne A, Aricó M, et al. HLH-2004: diagnostic and therapeutic guidelines for hemophagocytic lymphohistiocytosis. Pediatr Blood Cancer. 2007;48:124–31.

Ishii E. Hemophagocytic lymphohistiocytosis in children: pathogenesis and treatment. Front Pediatr. 2016;4:47.

Jordan MB, Allen CE, Weitzman S, Filipovich AH, McClain KL. How I treat hemophagocytic lymphohistiocytosis. Blood. 2011;118:4041–52.

Machaczka M, Klimkowska M, Chiang SCC, et al. Development of classical Hodgkin's lymphoma in an adult with biallelic STXBP2 mutations. Haematologica. 2013;98:760.

Martin-Verdeaux S, Pombo I, Iannascoli B, et al. Evidence of a role for Munc18-2 and microtubules in mast cell granule exocytosis. J Cell Sci. 2003;116:325.

Meeths M, Entesarian M, Al-Herz W, et al. Spectrum of clinical presentations in familial hemophagocytic lymphohistiocytosis type 5 patients with mutations in STXBP2. Blood. 2010;116:2635–43.

Mosa MH, Nicolle O, Maschalidi S, et al. Dynamic formation of microvillus inclusions during enterocyte differentiation in Munc18-2–deficient intestinal organoids. Cell Mol Gastroenterol Hepatol. 2018;6:477–93.e1.

Nikiforow S. The role of hematopoietic stem cell transplantation in treatment of hemophagocytic lymphohistiocytosis. Hematol Oncol Clin North Am. 2015;29:943–59.

Pagel J, Beutel K, Lehmberg K, et al. Distinct mutations in STXBP2 are associated with variable clinical presentations in patients with familial hemophagocytic lymphohistiocytosis type 5 (FHL5). Blood. 2012;119:6016–24.

Seo JJ. Hematopoietic cell transplantation for hemophagocytic lymphohistiocytosis: recent advances and controversies. Blood Res. 2015;50:131–9.

Sieni E, Cetica V, Mastrodicasa E, et al. Familial hemophagocytic lymphohistiocytosis: a model for understanding the human machinery of cellular cytotoxicity. Cell Mol Life Sci. 2012;69:29–40.

Spessott WA, Sanmillan ML, McCormick ME, et al. Hemophagocytic lymphohistiocytosis caused by dominant-negative mutations in STXBP2 that inhibit

SNARE-mediated membrane fusion. Blood. 2015;125:1566–77.

Spessott WA, Sanmillan ML, McCormick ME, Kulkarni VV, Giraudo CG. SM protein Munc18-2 facilitates transition of Syntaxin 11-mediated lipid mixing to complete fusion for T-lymphocyte cytotoxicity. Proc Natl Acad Sci. 2017;114:E2176.

Stepensky P, Bartram J, Barth TF, et al. Persistent defective membrane trafficking in epithelial cells of patients with familial hemophagocytic lymphohistiocytosis type 5 due to STXBP2/MUNC18-2 mutations. Pediatr Blood Cancer. 2013;60:1215–22.

Tang Y-M, Xu X-J. Advances in hemophagocytic lymphohistiocytosis: pathogenesis, early diagnosis/differential diagnosis, and treatment. TheScientificWorldJOURNAL. 2011;11

Usmani GN, Woda BA, Newburger PE. Advances in understanding the pathogenesis of HLH. Br J Haematol. 2013;161:609–22.

Vogel GF, van Rijn JM, Krainer IM, et al. Disrupted apical exocytosis of cargo vesicles causes enteropathy in FHL5 patients with Munc18-2 mutations. JCI Insight. 2018;2

Zhao XW, Gazendam RP, Drewniak A, et al. Defects in neutrophil granule mobilization and bactericidal activity in familial hemophagocytic lymphohistiocytosis type 5 (FHL-5) syndrome caused by STXBP2/Munc18-2 mutations. Blood. 2013;122:109–11.

zur Stadt U, Rohr J, Seifert W, et al. Familial hemophagocytic lymphohistiocytosis type 5 (FHL-5) is caused by mutations in Munc18-2 and impaired binding to syntaxin 11. Am J Hum Genet. 2009;85:482–92.

Systemic Autoinflammation

▶ LUBAC Deficiencies

Systemic Lymphangiectasia

▶ LUBAC Deficiencies

S

T

T2K

▶ TBK1 Deficiency

TACI and CVID

Zoya Eskandarian[1,6] and
Bodo Grimbacher[1,2,3,4,5]
[1]Institute for Immunodeficiency, Center for
Chronic Immunodeficiency, Medical Center,
Faculty of Medicine, Albert-Ludwigs-University
of Freiburg, Freiburg, Germany
[2]DZIF – German Center for Infection Research,
Satellite Center Freiburg, Freiburg, Germany
[3]CIBSS – Centre for Integrative Biological
Signalling Studies, Albert-Ludwigs University,
Freiburg, Germany
[4]RESIST – Cluster of Excellence 2155 to
Hanover Medical School, Satellite Center
Freiburg, Freiburg, Germany
[5]Institute of Immunity and Transplantation, Royal
Free Hospital, University College London,
London, UK
[6]Faculty of Biology, Albert-Ludwigs-University
of Freiburg, Freiburg, Germany

Introduction

Common variable immunodeficiency (CVID) is one
of the most prevalent primary immunodeficiency
syndromes, affecting approximately 1 in 25,000
(Primary immunodeficiency diseases 1999). The
main immunological defect in CVID is a failure of
B cells to produce immunoglobulin. This antibody
deficiency predisposes patients to recurrent infections, most frequently of the respiratory tract
(Yong et al. 2011). Further clinical manifestations
may include autoimmunity, enteropathy, granulomatous disease, lymphoproliferation, or malignancy (Hammarstrom et al. 2000). Although
generally sporadic, approximately 10% of CVID
patients demonstrate familial clustering. Furthermore, it is well established that IgA deficiency
(IgAD) can also occur in family members of
patients with CVID (Vorechovsky et al. 2000).
These observations suggested a genetic background of disease. In the past decade, a growing
number of genes and mutations associated with
CVID/IgAD have been identified. Disease-
associated variants in *TNFRSF13B*, the gene
encoding transmembrane activator, and calcium
modulator cyclophilin ligand interactor (TACI)
are found in one allele of up to 10% of patients
with CVID (Bacchelli et al. 2011) but also in about
2% of healthy individuals. These variants have
therefore been classified as disease associated
rather than disease causing.

Transmembrane Activator and Calcium Modulator Cyclophilin Ligand Interactor (TACI)

TACI is a Tumor necrosis factor (TNF) receptor family member acts as a receptor for B cell-activating factor of the TNF family (BAFF) and a proliferation-inducing ligand (APRIL), both of which are expressed on multiple cell types (Schneider 2005; Ng et al. 2004). TACI is found on the surface of marginal zone B cells, CD27 memory B cell subsets, and plasma cells, as well as activated T cells (Novak et al. 2004a, b; Darce et al. 2007; Khare and Hsu 2001). TACI is important in immunoglobulin class switching (CSR), immunoglobulin production during T-independent immune responses, and regulation of B cell homeostasis (Seshasayee et al. 2003; Castigli et al. 2005a; von Bulow et al. 2001; Yan et al. 2001). TACI-deficient mice have low levels of serum immunoglobulins and an impaired antibody response to the type II T cell-independent antigens (Lee et al. 2009; Litinskiy et al. 2002). Briefly, in the T cell-independent pathway, BAFF and APRIL are released by cells of the innate immune system in response to microbial signals binding toll-like receptors (TLRs) and activating nuclear factor kappa-light-chain-enhancer of activated B cells (NFκB) by recruiting TNF receptor associated factor (TRAF) proteins through TACI and two receptors related to TACI: B cell maturation antigen (BCMA) and BAFF receptor (BAFF-R) (Balazs et al. 2002; He et al. 2007; Schneider 2005; He et al. 2010; Castigli et al. 2007). BAFF and APRIL elicit CSR by inducing the recruitment of Myeloid differentiation primary response 88 (MyD88) to TACI highly conserved cytoplasmic (THC) domain, different from the TIR domain of TLRs. Interaction of TACI with MyD88 initiates germline CH (constant heavy chain domain) gene transcription, AID expression, and CSR by activating NF-κB through a TLR-like signaling cascade which includes the MyD88- Interleukin-1 receptor-associated kinase 1 (IRAK) 1-IRAK4-TRAF6-TAK1-IKK signaling pathway. TACI also binds to CAML;

however, TACI may use CAML to enhance B cell proliferation, B cell survival and plasmacytoid differentiation independently of NF-κB and Activator protein 1 (AP-1), perhaps through a pathway involving NFAT (Castigli et al. 2007; Bossen et al. 2008). The human TACI gene (*TNFRSF13B*) locus is located on the short arm of chromosome 17, which is a common target for mutation and rearrangement. The TACI extracellular N-terminal domain is characterized by two cysteine-rich domains (CRDs) as the hallmark of the TNF receptor superfamily. CRDs contain six highly conserved cysteines that generate three intrachain disulfide bridges stabilizing the antiparallel β-strands (Bodmer et al. 2002; Banner et al. 1993). The first TACI CRD extends from amino acid 32 to amino acid 67. The second extends from amino acid 68 to amino acid 106 and binds APRIL and BAFF with high affinity (Hymowitz et al. 2005). Mutations in *TACI* have been identified in an estimated 8–10% of CVID patients (Castigli et al. 2005b; Salzer et al. 2005). These mutations are distributed throughout all regions of the TACI molecule: the A204bp frame shift and C104R are located in the extracellular domain, A181E in the transmembrane region, and S194X and R202H in the intracellular domain (Salzer et al. 2005). Among CVID patients, two *TACI* mutations are common: C104R which can abolish binding of BAFF and APRIL and A181E which might interfere with the capacity of the receptor to aggregate on ligand cross-linking (Castigli et al. 2005b). Alternatively, the mutated protein might be more accessible for proteolytic cleavage or to undergo a conformational change that might affect its capacity to signal (Castigli et al. 2005b). Apart from homozygosity in the abovementioned mutations, correlation between heterozygous mutation coding variants of C104R and A181E and CVID and IgAD has also been reported (Castigli et al. 2005b; Salzer et al. 2005). Heterozygous C104R or A181E mutations in *TNFRSF13B* impair removal of autoreactive B cells, weaken B cell activation, and convey CVID patients to an increased risk for autoimmunity (Romberg et al. 2015). C104R

TACI mutation causes a significant impairment of TACI function *in vivo* and *in vitro* because of haploinsufficiency (Lee et al. 2010). *TACI* mutations impaired the removal of autoreactive B cells at the central B cell tolerance checkpoint by imposing BCR and TLR defects in a dose-dependent manner in all subjects, regardless of CVID status (Romberg et al. 2013). It has been previously observed that the prevalence of autoimmunity is significantly lower in patients with biallelic mutations in *TNFRSF13B* than in patients with the specific monoallelic mutation, e.g., C104R (Salzer et al. 2009). This higher rate of autoimmunity in *TNFRSF13B* heterozygotes may arise because the wild-type *TACI* allele in heterozygotes may be able to promote the survival of autoreactive B cell clones better than any of the two mutated *TACI* alleles available in individuals with biallelic mutations. Subjects with two mutated *TACI* alleles had increased frequencies of autoreactive clones in all naive B cell compartments compared with CVID patients with a single *TACI* mutation (Salzer et al. 2009). However, in the absence of functional TACI, this increase in autoreactive B cells is accompanied by profound impairments of B cell activation after BCR, TLR7, and TLR9 triggering that are significantly worse than in subjects with a single *TACI* mutation (Sadanaga et al. 2007). Moreover, TLRs play an essential role in the development of autoimmunity. Hence, severe impairment of the function of TLR in individuals with TACI-deficiency is more likely to be protective against autoimmunity, despite profoundly impaired autoreactive B cell counter selection, leaving these individuals with an immunodeficient phenotype (Romberg et al. 2013).

Interestingly, the C104R and the A181E mutations have also been observed in healthy individuals at a frequency of about 1% each. Incomplete penetrance and familial segregation were demonstrated for heterozygous *TACI* sequence variants and imply that heterozygous mutations increase the risk but are neither necessary nor sufficient to cause CVID (Romberg et al. 2013). These facts strongly suggest the existence of modifying factors, which can either be of genetic nature but might also include epigenetic or environmental mechanisms such as DNA methylation and histone acetylation contributing to the CVID phenotype.

Clinical Presentation

Patients with defects in TACI might present with selective IgA deficiency or with common variable immunodeficiency (CVID). Penetrance is low; therefore, not all affected family members have significant symptoms or immunological abnormalities.

Management

Patients with significant hypogammaglobulinemia benefit from immunoglobulin supplementation to reduce the frequency and severity of infections. Antibiotic prophylaxis regimes might be considered. Preservation of lung function is a priority. Patients with CVID often developed bronchiectasis and impaired respiratory function.

Cross-References

▶ Clinical Presentation of Immunodeficiency, Primary Immunodeficiency
▶ Management of Immunodeficiency, Antibiotic Therapy
▶ Management of Immunodeficiency, IgG Replacement (IV)
▶ Management of Immunodeficiency, IgG Replacement (SC)

References

Bacchelli C, Buckland KF, Buckridge S, Salzer U, Schneider P, Thrasher AJ, Gaspar HB. The C76R transmembrane activator and calcium modulator cyclophilin ligand interactor mutation disrupts antibody production and B-cell homeostasis in heterozygous and homozygous mice. Am Acad Allergy Asthma Immunol. 2011; https://doi.org/10.1016/j.jaci.2011.02.037.

Balazs M, Martin F, Zhou T, Kearney J. Blood dendritic cells interact with splenic marginal zone B cells to initiate T-independent immune responses. Immunity. 2002;17:341–52.

Banner D, D'Arcy A, Janes W, Gentz R, Schoenfeld H, Broger CL, et al. Crystal structure of the soluble human 55 kd TNF receptor-human TNF beta complex: implications for TNF receptor activation. Cell Death Differ. 1993;73:431–45.

Bodmer J, Schneider P, Tschopp J. The molecular architecture of the TNF superfamily. Trends Biochem Sci. 2002;27:19–26.

Bossen C, et al. TACI, unlike BAFF-R, is solely activated by oligomeric BAFF and APRIL to support survival of activated B cells and plasmablasts. Blood. 2008;111:1004–12.

Castigli E, Wilson SA, Scott S, Dedeoglu F, Xu S, Lam KP, et al. TACI and BAFF-R mediate isotype switching in B cells. J Exp Med. 2005a;201:35–9.

Castigli E, Wilson SA, Garibyan L, Rachid R, Bonilla F, Schneider L, Geha RS. TACI is mutant in common variable immunodeficiency and IgA deficiency. Nat Genet. 2005b;37(8):829.

Castigli E, et al. Transmembrane activator and calcium modulator and cyclophilin ligand interactor enhances CD40-driven plasma cell differentiation. J Allergy Clin Immunol. 2007;120:885–91.

Darce JR, Arendt BK, Wu X, Jelinek DF. Regulated expression of BAFF-binding receptors during human B-cell differentiation. J Immunol. 2007;179:7276–86.

Hammarstrom ML, Vorechovsky I, Webster D. Selective IgA deficiency (SIgAD) and common variable immunode®ciency (CVID). J of Clin Exp Immunol. 2000;120:225–31.

He B, et al. Intestinal bacteria trigger T cell-independent immunoglobulin A2 class switching by inducing epithelial-cell secretion of the cytokine APRIL. Immunity. 2007;26:812–26.

He B, Santamaria R, Xu W, Cols M, Chen K, Puga I, Shan M, et al. The transmembrane activator TACI triggers immunoglobulin class switching by activating B cells through the adaptor MyD88. Nat Immunol. 2010; https://doi.org/10.1038/ni.1914.

Hymowitz S, Patel D, Wallweber H, Runyon S, Yan M, Yin J, et al. Structures of APRIL-receptor complexes: like BCMA, TACI employs only a single cysteine-rich domain for high affinity ligand binding. J Biol Chem. 2005;280:7218–27.

Khare SD, Hsu H. The role of TALL-1 and APRIL in immune regulation. Trends Immunol. 2001;22:61–3.

Lee JJ, Rauter I, Garibyan L, Ozcan E, Sannikova T, Dillon SR, et al. The murine equivalent of the A181E TACI mutation associated with common variable immunodeficiency severely impairs B-cell function. Blood. 2009;114:2254–62.

Lee JJ, Jabara HH, Garibyan L, Rauter I, Sannikova T, Dillon SR, Bram R, Geha RS. The C104R mutant impairs the function of transmembrane activator and calcium modulator and cyclophilin ligand interactor (TACI) through haploinsufficiency. J Allergy Clin Immunol. 2010;126(6):1234–41.e2.

Litinskiy MB, et al. DCs induce CD40-independent immunoglobulin class switching through BLyS and APRIL. Nat Immunol. 2002;3:822–9.

Ng LG, Sutherland APR, Newton R, et al. B cell activating factor belonging to the TNF family (BAFF)-R is the principal BAFF receptor facilitating BAFF costimulation of circulating T and B cells. J Immunol. 2004;173:807–17.

Novak AJ, Darce JR, Arendt BK, et al. Expression of BCMA, TACI, and BAFF-R in multiple myeloma: a mechanism for growth and survival. Blood. 2004a;103:689–94.

Novak AJ, Grote DM, Stenson M, et al. Expression of BLyS and its receptors in B-cell non-Hodgkin lymphoma: correlation with disease activity and patient outcome. Blood. 2004b;104:2247–53.

Primary immunodeficiency diseases. Report of an IUIS scientific committee. International Union of Immunological Societies. Clin Exp Immunol. 1999;118(suppl 1):1–28.

Romberg N, Chamberlain N, Saadoun D, Gentile M, Kinnunen T, Ng YS, Virdee M, et al. CVID-associated TACI mutations affect autoreactive B cell selection and activation. J Clin Invest. 2013;123(10):4283–93.

Romberg N, Virdee M, Chamberlain N, Oe T, Schickel J, Perkins T, Cantaert T, Rachid R, Rosengren S, Palazzo R, Geha R, Cunningham-Rundles C, Meffre E. TNF receptor superfamily member 13b (TNFRSF13B) hemizygosity reveals transmembrane activator and CAML interactor haploinsufficiency at later stages of B-cell development. J Allergy Clin Immunol. 2015; https://doi.org/10.1016/j.jaci.

Sadanaga A, et al. Protection against autoimmune nephritis in MyD88-deficient MRL/lpr mice. Arthritis Rheum. 2007;56(5):1618–1628. https://doi.org/10.1002/art.22571.

Salzer U, Chapel HM, Webster ADB, Pan-Hammarström Q, Schmitt-Graeff A, Schlesier M, Peter HH, Rockstroh JK, Schneider P, Schäffer AA, Hammarström L, Grimbacher B. Mutations in TNFRSF13B encoding TACI are associated with common variable immunodeficiency in humans. Nat Genet. 2005;37(8):820.

Salzer U, Bacchelli C, Buckridge S, Pan-Hammarström Q, Jennings S, Lougaris V, et al. Relevance of biallelic versus monoallelic TNFRSF13B mutations in distinguishing disease-causing from risk-increasing TNFRSF13B variants in antibody deficiency syndromes. Blood. 2009;113(9):1967–76.

Schneider P. The role of APRIL and BAFF in lymphocyte activation. Curr Opin Immunol. 2005;17:282–9.

Seshasayee D, Valdez P, Yan M, Dixit VM, Tumas D, Grewal IS. Loss of TACI causes fatal lymphoproliferation and autoimmunity, establishing TACI as an inhibitory BLyS receptor. Immunity, 2003;18:279–288.

von Bulow GU, van Deursen JM, Bram RJ. Regulation of the T-independent humoral response by TACI. Immunity. 2001;14:573–82.

Vorechovsky I, Cullen M, Carrington M, Hammarstrom L, Webster ADB. Fine mapping of IGAD1 in IgA deficiency and common variable immunodeficiency: identification and characterization of haplotypes shared by affected members of 101 multiple-case families. J Immunol. 2000;164:4408–16.

Yan M, Wang H, Chan B, Roose-Girma M, Erickson S, Baker T, et al. Activation and accumulation of B cells in TACI-deficient mice. Nat Immunol. 2001;2:638–43.

Yong FP, Thaventhiran JE, Grimbacher B. A rose is a rose but CVID is not CVID: common variable immunodeficiency (CVID), what do we know in 2011. Adv Immunol. 2011;111:46–107.

TBK1 Deficiency

Henry Y. Lu[1] and Stuart E. Turvey[2,3]

[1]Department of Pediatrics and Experimental Medicine Program, British Columbia Children's Hospital, The University of British Columbia, Vancouver, BC, Canada

[2]Division of Allergy and Clinical Immunology, Department of Pediatrics and Experimental Medicine Program, British Columbia Children's Hospital, The University of British Columbia, Vancouver, BC, Canada

[3]Willem-Alexander Children's Hospital, Leiden University Medical Center, Leiden, the Netherlands

Synonyms

NAK; T2K

Definition

TANK-binding kinase 1 (TBK1) is a serine-threonine kinase, which regulates various immune functions including the secretion of pro-inflammatory cytokines, cell growth, and proliferation, among others. Mutations affecting TBK1 lead to various disorders, where gain-of-function mutations can cause normal tension glaucoma and loss-of-function mutations can result in amyotrophic lateral sclerosis, frontotemporal dementia, or herpes simplex encephalitis.

Introduction

Please refer to the introductory section listed for ▶ UNC93B1 deficiency.

Molecular Genetics and Pathogenesis

Tumor necrosis factor (TNF) receptor-associated factor NF-κB activator (TANK)-binding kinase 1 (TBK1) is a serine-threonine kinase, which belongs to the "noncanonical IκB kinases" (IKKs) and has a crucial role in regulating type I IFN (Fitzgerald et al. 2003; Ahmad et al. 2016). It plays many functions, including induction of pro-inflammatory cytokine production in response to infection (Fitzgerald et al. 2003), autophagy (Stolz et al. 2014), pathogen elimination (Thurston et al. 2009; Wild et al. 2011; Pilli et al. 2012), and cell growth and proliferation (Clement et al. 2008). Interestingly, mutations in *TBK1* have been associated with a variety of neuroinflammatory diseases, depending on whether it is a gain-of-function or loss-of-function mutation. Gain-of-function mutations in *TBK1* have been linked to normal tension glaucoma (NTD), whereas loss-of-function mutations are associated with amyotrophic lateral sclerosis (ALS), frontotemporal dementia (FTD), and herpes simplex encephalitis (HSE) [reviewed in (Ahmad et al. 2016)].

Two cases of TBK1-mediated HSE susceptibility have been reported (Table 1) (Herman et al. 2012). Both patients possessed autosomal dominant (AD) mutations, leading to partial TBK1 deficiency. One patient was a young Polish girl carrying a heterozygous AD dominant negative mutation at nucleotide position 476 (c.476G>G/C). This

TBK1 Deficiency, Table 1 Known TBK1 mutations that cause HSE susceptibility

Mutation(s)	Inheritance	Gene expression	Protein expression	Functional impact	Molecular mechanism	No. HSE episodes	Age of episodes	References
p. G159A	AD	Unchanged	Unchanged	Partial	Dominant negative	1	7 years	Herman et al. (2012)
p. D50A	AD	↓	↓	Partial	Haploinsufficiency	1	11 months	Herman et al. (2012)

mutation led to a nonconservative replacement of glycine for alanine at amino acid position 159 (G159A) at the activation loop of the kinase, which caused a loss of kinase activity. Both parents of this girl were unaffected and had WT *TBK1*. The other patient was a young French girl carrying a heterozygous AD mutation at nucleotide position 149 (c.149A>A/C), leading to a nonconservative substitution of aspartic acid for alanine at amino acid position 50 (D50A) and haploinsufficiency (Herman et al. 2012). This girl's mother carried the same mutation but was healthy and her father was WT, indicating potential incomplete clinical penetrance. Both patients exhibited impaired responses to poly(I: C) stimulation based on measurement of signaling intermediates and IFN secretion (Herman et al. 2012).

Diagnosis

Please refer to the diagnosis section listed for ▶ UNC93B1 deficiency.

Prognostic Factors

Please refer to the prognosis section listed for ▶ UNC93B1 deficiency.

Treatment

Please refer to the treatment section listed for ▶ UNC93B1 deficiency.

Cross-References

- ▶ IRF3 deficiency
- ▶ TLR3 deficiency
- ▶ TRAF3 deficiency
- ▶ TRIF deficiency
- ▶ UNC93B1 deficiency

References

Ahmad L, Zhang SY, Casanova JL, Sancho-Shimizu V. Human TBK1: a gatekeeper of neuroinflammation. Trends Mol Med. 2016;22(6):511–27.

Clement JF, Meloche S, Servant MJ. The IKK-related kinases: from innate immunity to oncogenesis. Cell Res. 2008;18(9):889–99.

Fitzgerald KA, McWhirter SM, Faia KL, Rowe DC, Latz E, Golenbock DT, et al. IKKepsilon and TBK1 are essential components of the IRF3 signaling pathway. Nat Immunol. 2003;4(5):491–6.

Herman M, Ciancanelli M, Ou YH, Lorenzo L, Klaudel-Dreszler M, Pauwels E, et al. Heterozygous TBK1 mutations impair TLR3 immunity and underlie herpes simplex encephalitis of childhood. J Exp Med. 2012;209(9):1567–82.

Pilli M, Arko-Mensah J, Ponpuak M, Roberts E, Master S, Mandell MA, et al. TBK-1 promotes autophagy-mediated antimicrobial defense by controlling autophagosome maturation. Immunity. 2012;37(2):223–34.

Stolz A, Ernst A, Dikic I. Cargo recognition and trafficking in selective autophagy. Nat Cell Biol. 2014;16(6):495–501.

Thurston TL, Ryzhakov G, Bloor S, von Muhlinen N, Randow F. The TBK1 adaptor and autophagy receptor NDP52 restricts the proliferation of ubiquitin-coated bacteria. Nat Immunol. 2009;10(11):1215–21.

Wild P, Farhan H, McEwan DG, Wagner S, Rogov VV, Brady NR, et al. Phosphorylation of the autophagy receptor optineurin restricts Salmonella growth. Science. 2011;333(6039):228–33.

TC II

▶ TCN2 Deficiency

TC2

▶ TCN2 Deficiency

T-Cell Antigen Leu2

▶ CD8 Alpha (CD8A) Deficiency

T-Cell Receptor Alpha Deficiency (OMIM # 615387)

Jay J. Jin
Division of Pediatric Pulmonology, Allergy, and Sleep Medicine, Indiana University School of Medicine, Riley Hospital for Children at Indiana University Health, Indianapolis, IN, USA

Definition

T-cell receptor alpha deficiency is a rare immunodeficiency condition characterized by immune dysregulation, failure to thrive, lymphadenopathy, and hepatosplenomegaly.

Introduction/Background

The T-cell receptor (TCR) alpha subunit (TCRα), encoded by the T-cell receptor alpha gene locus (*TRA*, chromosome 14q11.2), is one of four multi-domain polypeptides that form the functional TCRs of the immune system. This gene locus is comprised of numerous gene segments and individual genes that undergo genomic rearrangement, transcription, and translation to form a functional TCRα subunit (Alcover et al. 2018). In 2011, two children were reported with a mutation in the TCR alpha constant gene (*TRAC*), which is within the *TRA* locus that resulted in an immunodeficiency phenotype (Morgan et al. 2011).

Functional TCRs are formed by pairing of either alpha with beta or gamma with delta subunits during a coordinated series of maturation events that take place in the thymus. T cells that complete this maturation process will thus express either alpha-beta TCRs (αβTCR) or gamma-delta TCRs (γδTCR). In humans, αβTCR expressing T cells (αβT cells) account for a predominance of the total CD3+ T cell population compared to γδTCR expressing T cells (γδT cells) and are generally implicated in the major functional roles of T cells (e.g., providing B-cell help and other T-cell-mediated immune responses). The αβT cells provide a tremendous diversity of antigen recognition capability due to the mechanisms of genomic recombination that take place within the alpha and beta subunit genes en route to the formation of a functional αβTCR (Shiromizu and Jancic 2018). Animal models with impaired TCRα expression highlight the importance of this subunit in the expression of a normal αβTCR at the cell surface. Mice that are genetically engineered to lack TCRα expression have a deficiency of αβT cell development, but not γδT cell development. Notably, the humoral immune response in these mice remains intact (Wen et al., 1994). Additionally, these mice often develop chronic colitis resembling human ulcerative colitis, thus implicating the absence αβT cells in the development of intestinal mucosal inflammation (Mombaerts et al. 1993). Perturbations in the maturation of T cells, genomic recombination of TCRs, or TCR signaling pathways are implicated in both severe-combined and combined immunodeficiencies and a growing number of immune dysregulation conditions (Bonilla et al. 2015).

In 2011, Morgan et al. presented two children with markedly reduced αβTCR expression due to a mutation in the T-cell receptor alpha constant region gene (*TRAC*). Detailed molecular characterization of the point mutation, which was distal to the final stop codon, indicated a drop out of exon 3 (of 4) from the final mRNA product of *TRAC*. Though the mutation resided within the *TRA* locus, both the TCRα subunit and the TCRβ subunit proteins were not detected by immunoblot from lymphocytes. Neither subunit could be seen on T-cell membranes using immunohistochemical techniques, which demonstrated that the *TRAC* was critical for proper expression and localization of both alpha and beta subunits.

Clinical Presentation (History/PE)

Two unrelated children from consanguineous families presented initially with recurrent respiratory tract infections, otitis media, candidiasis, diarrhea, and failure to thrive at 6 months and 15 months of age. During subsequent follow-up, the older child was also found to be susceptible to prolonged infections and viremia with herpes family viruses. Both children manifested a number of clinical features suggestive of immune dysregulation, including vitiligo, alopecia areata, organomegaly (liver and spleen), eczema, pityriasis rubra pilaris, and autoimmune hemolytic anemia. The younger of the two children developed bowel loop thickening and a mass at the porta hepatis without conclusive evidence for infection or malignancy. Lymphadenopathy was present in both children (Morgan et al. 2011).

Laboratory Findings/Diagnostic Testing

Morgan et al. noted that both children had strikingly similar immunologic phenotyping. Total CD3+ T cells were slightly decreased with a predominance of $\gamma\delta$T cells and near absence of $\alpha\beta$T cells. Markers for recent thymic emigrants (CD45+CD27+) were found within the CD3+$\gamma\delta$+ cells but not the CD3+$\gamma\delta$- cells. A small population of CD3low T cells expressed $\alpha\beta$TCRs, but the exact role of these cells was not clear. Despite the absence of $\alpha\beta$T cells, total immunoglobulin (Ig) G, IgA, IgM, and IgE levels were within age-appropriate reference ranges. The switched-memory B-cell population also developed appropriately and both children had protective responses to childhood vaccines (Morgan et al. 2011). These findings mirrored the observations in animal models of TCRα deficiency (Wen et al., 1994). Other lab findings were suggestive of underlying immune dysregulation with hypereosinophilia, low titer anti-nuclear antibodies, anti-tissue transglutaminase antibodies, and anti-thymocyte antibodies. Lymph node biopsies revealed follicle formation and germinal center architecture without evidence of neoplastic lymphoproliferation (Morgan et al. 2011).

Treatment/Prognosis

Long-term data on prognosis and evidence-based best practices for management are not currently available due to a paucity of reported cases.

The children identified by Morgan et al. did not succumb to severe infection, though both had frequent upper respiratory, lower respiratory, and gastrointestinal tract infections as well as a propensity for viral and fungal infections. Opportunistic and mycobacterial infections were not identified. Both children were noted to be relatively healthy for a number of years with anti-infective prophylaxis and intravenous immunoglobulin therapy. Other autoimmune manifestations were also managed accordingly. The presence of lymphadenopathy raised the question of malignancy risk, but no conclusions could be drawn from these two cases. Eventually both children did undergo matched sibling bone marrow transplant at age 6 and age 7 with reduced-intensity conditioning. Long-term follow-up information after bone marrow transplant was not provided (Morgan et al. 2011).

Cross-References

▶ CD3d, e and z Deficiencies
▶ ITK deficiency
▶ Lymphocyte-Specific Protein Tyrosine Kinase: LCK
▶ Mammalian Sterile 20-Like 1 (MST1) Deficiency
▶ MHC Class I, A Deficiency of
▶ MHC Class II, Deficiency of
▶ ZAP70 Deficiency (OMIM # 176947)

References

Alcover A, Alarcon B, Di Bartolo V. Cell biology of T cell receptor expression and regulation. Annu Rev Immunol. 2018;36:103–25.

Bonilla FA, Kahn DA, Ballas ZK, Chinen J, Frank MM, Hsu JT, et al. Practice parameter for the diagnosis and management of primary immunodeficiency. J Allergy Clin Immunol. 2015;136:1186–205.

Mombaerts P, Mizoguchi E, Grusby MJ, Glimcher LH, Bhan AK, Tonegawa S. Spontaneous development of inflammatory bowel disease in T cell receptor mutant mice. Cell. 1993;75:274–82.

Morgan NV, Goddard S, Cardno TS, McDonald D, Rahman F, Barge D, et al. Mutation in the TCRa subunit constant gene (TRAC) leads to a human immunodeficiency disorder characterized by lack of TCRab T cells. J Clin Invest. 2011;121(2):695–702.

Shiromizu CM, Jancic CC. γδ T lymphocytes: an effector cell in autoimmunity and infection. Front Immunol. 2018;9:2389.

Wen L, Roberts SJ, Viney JL, Wong FS, Mallick C, Findly RC, et al. Immunoglobulin synthesis and generalized autoimmunity in mice congenitally deficient in alpha beta(+) T cells. Nature. 1994;369(6482):65–658.

TCN2 Deficiency

Silvia Giliani
Department of Molecular and Translational Medicine, University of Brescia, Brescia, Italy

Synonyms

TC II; TC2

Definition

Transcobalamin II Deficiency (OMIM #275350) is a rare autosomal recessive disorder due to defects in the TCN2 gene encoding for trans-cobalamin (OMIM; 613441).

Introduction

Transcobalamin is a plasma globulin acting as transport protein for cobalamin (Cbl, vitamin B12), and its absence leads to impairment in Cbl absorption. Protein-free Cbl is usually first bound to haptocorrin and delivered from food to tissues through successive transport proteins and cell-surface receptors and transferred through intestinal cells to the bloodstream. Only TCN2 bound Cbl (holotranscobalamin) could enter the cell membrane through CD320 surface receptor (Alam et al. 2016) by receptor-mediated endocytosis. Once in the cell, Cbl is the key element in activating methionine synthetase, leading to the synthesis of methionine from homocysteine and then of S-adenosyl-methionine used to methylate DNA, RNA, and proteins. In parallel, the same methionine synthetase has a role in tetra-hydrofolate production, which is involved in nucleic acids and aminoacids synthesis or degra-dation. Moreover Cbl is a cofactor in the Krebs cycle, thus its absence affects one of the main cell energy source (Green et al. 2017).

Thus, it is clear that the lack of TCN2, the carrier of Cbl into the cell leads to deficiencies in many crucial cell functions based on nucleotides and fatty acids metabolism, such as growth and proliferation especially in newly generated blood cells. The main hematological manifestation is megaloblastic anemia resulting from impaired DNA synthesis and aberrant cell growth. Moreover, homocystein accumulation induces protein degradation and cell apoptosis, which could explain blood cells deficiencies, but the causes of neurological cell-specific impairment is at present not clear, even if the influence of Cbl deficiency on myelin homeosta-sis and neurons demyelination is known.

Clinical Presentation

TCN2 deficiency patients' symptoms usually become evident within the first months of life: failure to thrive, stomatitis, vomit, and diarrhea are the more common. Other symptoms are irritability, lethargy, neurological delays, and multi-lineage cytopenia giving rise to immunode-ficiency and bacterial and viral infections. The most common hematologic manifestations are megaloblastic anemia and neutropenia, but many cases begin as thrombocytopenia (Trakadis et al. 2014; Chao et al. 2017). Some cases onset as leukemia and few atypical cases have been reported, such as a presentation as Hemophagocytic Lymphohistiocytosis (HLH) in a 2-months-old patient.

The aspecific onset and the variability in the blood cell lineage affected by cytopenia frequently leads to a diagnostic delay.

Neurological and ophthalmological complications (speech impairment, motor disabilities, and retinopathy) usually are not evident at onset and are probably a result of inappropriate and delayed intervention (Trakadis et al. 2014).

Less than 50 cases are reported in literature, but the prevalence of TCN2 deficiency is actually uncertain.

Diagnosis

A diagnosis of TCN2 deficiency is suspected in patients with symptoms such as gastrointestinal problems, multilineage deficiency in blood cells, failure to thrive resembling immunodeficiency, and hematological disorder or B12 deficiency. Laboratory tests display methylmalonic aciduria (MMA) and homocystinuria, while serum Cbl may be normal: in fact the majority of circulating Clb is bound to haptocorrin, thus is not affected by TCN2 deficiency. The normal levels of Cbl drove to exclusion of nutritional deficiency. TCN2 can then be measured and has always been proven to be absent.

Newborn Screening (NBS) can give positive result in cases with C3 and C3/C2 acylcarnitine elevation (Trakadis et al. 2014), while in countries not including this test, could be seen only retrospectively (Chao et al. 2017).

As a rule, children with unexplained cytopenia in multiple lineages and gastrointestinal involvement must be considered for a TCN2 deficiency diagnosis and urine methylmalonic acid analyses should be performed (Chao et al. 2017), while a final diagnosis is achieved only through TCN2 gene sequencing.

Genetics

TCN2 gene is a housekeeping gene located on chromosome 22 and was initially characterized in 1991. Before 2003, only five mutations were described, while in recent years more variants have been characterized. Less than 50 cases are known in literature, and only 20 different mutations (Trakadis et al. 2014 for a review; Chao et al. 2017; Unal et al. 2015; Yildirim et al. 2017). The great majority is composed of nonsense or frameshift mutations coming from small or big indels, while only few cases are missense variants. Mutations usually lead to complete lack of TCN2 protein or interfere with the Cbl/TCN2 or TCN2/CD320 interaction. Most of the cases are homozygous, and a higher prevalence in the Turkish population seems to be related to a founder effect of the big deletion c.1106+1516_1222+1231del5304 (Yildirim et al. 2017; Unal et al. 2015).

Despite the few cases, some longitudinal evaluation on siblings or on patients bearing the same mutations has been performed, but no obvious genotype-phenotype correlation was established (Trakadis et al. 2014).

Some single nucleotide polymorphisms (SNPS) have been described which diminish the B12 levels in otherwise healthy individuals.

Treatment

The treatment of choice is idroxy-cobalamin (OHCbl) supplementation and must be administered for life in any of the oral, intramuscular, parenteral ways. This treatment is usually combined with folate supplementation and oral administration of betaine. Availability of different treatments in different countries makes it difficult to come to conclusion regarding which is the best administration way, even if IM-Cbl through all life seems to be the only durable treatment.

The dosage used is usually 1 mg of IM-Cbl and is normally sufficient for pancytopenia, methionine and total homocysteine plasma levels, and MMA urinary excretion normalization. It has been suggested that both the age of initiation (the earlier the better) and the way of administration (IM administration) could have an importance (Trakadis et al. 2014).

Overall, if the therapy is initiated early and is continuous, this could limit most severe symptoms, particularly permanent neurological and ophthalmological impairments, even if some late-onset symptoms, particularly neurological, could arise (Trakadis et al. 2014; Yildirim et al. 2017).

Early diagnosis is of utmost importance since it has been demonstrated that familiar cases usually have a better outcome due to early therapeutic intervention.

Cross-References

▶ Defects in B12 and Folate Metabolism (TCN2, SLC46A1 (PCFT Deficiency), MTHFD1)

References

Alam A, Woo JS, Schmitz J, Prinz B, Root K, Chen F, Bloch JS, Zenobi R, Locher KP. Structural basis of transcobalamin recognition by human CD320 receptor. Nat Commun. 2016;7:12100.

Chao MM, Illsinger S, Yoshimi A, Das AM, Kratz CP, Congenital Transcobalamin II. Deficiency: a rare entity with a broad differential. Klin Padiatr. 2017;229(6):335–57.

Green R, Allen LH, Bjørke-Monsen AL, Brito A, Guéant JL, Miller JW, Molloy AM, Nexo E, Stabler S, Toh BH, Ueland PM, Yajnik C. Vitamin B (12) deficiency. Nat Rev Dis Primers. 2017;3:17040.

Trakadis YJ, Alfares A, Bodamer OA, Buyukavci M, Christodoulou J, Connor P, Glamuzina E, Gonzalez-Fernandez F, Bibi H, Echenne B, Manoli I, Mitchell J, Nordwall M, Prasad C, Scaglia F, Schiff M, Schrewe B, Touati G, Tchan MC, Varet B, Venditti CP, Zafeiriou D, Rupar CA, Rosenblatt DS, Watkins D, Braverman N. Update on transcobalamin deficiency: clinical presentation, treatment and outcome. J Inherit Metab Dis. 2014;37(3):461–73.

Unal S, Rupar T, Yetgin S, Yaralı N, Dursun A, Gürsel T, Cetin M, Transcobalamin II. Deficiency in four cases with novel mutations. Turk J Haematol. 2015;32(4):317–22. Epub 2015 Apr 27

Yildirim ZK, Nexo E, Rupar T, Büyükavci M. Seven patients with transcobalamin deficiency diagnosed between 2010 and 2014: a single-center experience. J Pediatr Hematol Oncol. 2017;39(1):38–41.

TCN2: Transcobalamin II

▶ Defects in B12 and Folate Metabolism (TCN2, SLC46A1 (PCFT Deficiency), MTHFD1)

TERC Deficiency

Nicholas L. Rider
Section of Immunology, Allergy and Retrovirology, Department of Pediatrics, Baylor College of Medicine, Texas Children's Hospital, Houston, TX, USA

Introduction

TERC encodes the telomerase RNA component which functions as a template for telomere elongation (Feng et al. 1995). The gene is 451 nucleotides in length and is located at 3p26.2 (Feng et al. 1995). Human telomerase is a ribonucleoprotein complex which functions to maintain telomere length during normal cell division through controlled elongation thereby preventing shortening and ensuing cell cycle arrest and cell death (Du et al. 2009). Telomerase has two components: the reverse transcriptase (TERT) and the template RNA component, or TERC. Mono-allelic pathogenic mutations in *TERC* lead to dyskeratosis congenita, pulmonary fibrosis, and/or bone marrow failure in addition to susceptibilities to cutaneous malignant melanoma and leukemia (Armanios et al. 2005; Calado et al. 2009).

Clinical Relevance

Patients with *TERC* pathogenic mutations might develop dyskeratosis congenita (DC) (Mitchell et al. 1999). DC is characterized by progressive bone marrow failure, including aplastic anemia, and mucocutaneous symptoms such as abnormalities in skin pigmentation, dystrophic nails, and oral leukoplakia (Dokal 2000). It is important to note that a minority of DC patients present with mucocutaneous features; thus, the disease must be suspected in their absence by signs of marrow failure (Du et al. 2009). In addition to DC, *TERC* pathogenic mutations have been associated to idiopathic pulmonary fibrosis, in adult patients (Armanios 2012; Diaz de Leon et al. 2010).

Diagnosis

A diagnosis of DC should be suspected in anyone with aplastic anemia (AA), hypoplastic myelodysplastic syndrome or chronic cytopenias, dystrophic skin changes, and early graying of hair (Dokal 2000; Townsley et al. 2014). If autosomal dominant inheritance is noticed in family history, TERC deficiency should be suspected. Laboratory tests include measuring the mean telomere length (MTL) using age-matched ranges (Aubert et al. 2012). Decrease of MTL in peripheral blood supports the DC diagnosis (Alter et al. 2012). Short telomeres might be transiently found due to chronic inflammation. Detection of pathogenic mutations by gene sequencing analysis of telomerase genes (*DKC1*, *TERT*, *TERC*, and *TINF2*) provides with definitive diagnosis (Houben et al. 2008).

Treatment and Prognosis

TERC deficiency is one of a group of conditions called "telomeropathies," with an average age at death is presently noted to be 49 years (Shimamura and Alter 2010). The severity of presentation for those patients with a TERC defect is variable. Hematopoietic stem cell transplantation (HSCT) is potentially curative for disorders affecting bone marrow cells. Other adjunctive therapies include periodic red cell and platelet transfusion, and androgen therapy can aid in

maintaining telomere length (Dietz et al. 2011; Townsley et al. 2016). Lung transplant has been performed in patients with severe pulmonary disease.

Cross-References

▶ DKC1, Dyskeratosis Congenita/Hoyeraal-Hreidarsson Syndrome

References

Alter BP, Rosenberg PS, Giri N, Baerlocher GM, Lansdorp PM, Savage SA. Telomere length is associated with disease severity and declines with age in dyskeratosis congenita. Haematologica. 2012;97(3):353–9.

Armanios M. Telomerase and idiopathic pulmonary fibrosis. Mutat Res. 2012;730(1–2):52–8.

Armanios M, Chen JL, Chang YP, et al. Haploinsufficiency of telomerase reverse transcriptase leads to anticipation in autosomal dominant dyskeratosis congenita. Proc Natl Acad Sci U S A. 2005;102(44):15960–4.

Aubert G, Hills M, Lansdorp PM. Telomere length measurement-caveats and a critical assessment of the available technologies and tools. Mutat Res. 2012;730(1–2):59–67.

Calado RT, Regal JA, Hills M, et al. Constitutional hypomorphic telomerase mutations in patients with acute myeloid leukemia. Proc Natl Acad Sci U S A. 2009;106(4):1187–92.

Diaz de Leon A, Cronkhite JT, Katzenstein AL, et al. Telomere lengths, pulmonary fibrosis and telomerase (TERT) mutations. PLoS One. 2010;5(5):e10680.

Dietz AC, Orchard PJ, Baker KS, et al. Disease-specific hematopoietic cell transplantation: nonmyeloablative conditioning regimen for dyskeratosis congenita. Bone Marrow Transplant. 2011;46(1):98–104.

Dokal I. Dyskeratosis congenita in all its forms. Br J Haematol. 2000;110(4):768–79.

Du HY, Pumbo E, Ivanovich J, et al. TERC and TERT gene mutations in patients with bone marrow failure and the significance of telomere length measurements. Blood. 2009;113(2):309–16.

Feng J, Funk WD, Wang SS, et al. The RNA component of human telomerase. Science. 1995;269(5228):1236–41.

Houben JM, Moonen HJ, van Schooten FJ, Hageman GJ. Telomere length assessment: biomarker of chronic oxidative stress? Free Radic Biol Med. 2008;44(3):235–46.

T

Mitchell JR, Wood E, Collins K. A telomerase component is defective in the human disease dyskeratosis congenita. Nature. 1999;402(6761):551–5.

Shimamura A, Alter BP. Pathophysiology and management of inherited bone marrow failure syndromes. Blood Rev. 2010;24(3):101–22.

Townsley DM, Dumitriu B, Young NS. Bone marrow failure and the telomeropathies. Blood. 2014;124(18):2775–83.

Townsley DM, Dumitriu B, Liu D, et al. Danazol treatment for telomere diseases. N Engl J Med. 2016;374(20):1922–31.

Terminal Complement Complex

▶ C5b-C9 Deficiency

TERT

Nicholas L. Rider
Section of Immunology, Allergy and Retrovirology, Department of Pediatrics, Baylor College of Medicine, Texas Children's Hospital, Houston, TX, USA

Introduction

TERT encodes the catalytic subunit of the human telomerase (Cohen et al. 2007; Fu and Collins 2007). The gene is comprised by 16 exons and spans 35 kb, located on 5p15.33 (Meyerson et al. 1997; Cong et al. 1999). Human telomerase is a protein complex composed of two molecules of TERT, a reverse transcriptase enzyme, and two molecules of TERC, an RNA template. The role of telomerase is to regulate the telomere length and elongation in the cell division cycle. The length of chromosomal telomeres allows the initiation of cell cycle; and a consequence of short telomeres is cell death (Du et al. 2009). Pathogenic mutations in *TERT* lead to dyskeratosis congenita, pulmonary fibrosis, and/or bone marrow failure in addition to susceptibilities to

cutaneous malignant melanoma and leukemia (Armanios et al. 2005; Horn et al. 2013; Yamaguchi et al. 2005; Calado et al. 2009).

Clinical Relevance

Defects of human telomerase biology lead principally to dyskeratosis congenita (DC) (Mitchell et al. 1999). Patients with DC often present with progressive bone marrow failure and a triad of mucocutaneous findings which includes abnormal skin pigmentation, dystrophic nails, and leukoplakia of the oral mucosa (Dokal 2000). It is important to note that a minority of DC patients present with mucocutaneous features; thus, the disease must be suspected in their absence by signs of marrow failure (Du et al. 2009). In addition to DC, idiopathic pulmonary fibrosis, which appears histologically as interstitial pneumonitis and appears in adulthood, is a prominent clinical feature in patients with telomeropathies (Armanios 2012; Diaz de Leon et al. 2010). Lastly, *TERT* mutations have also been found to underlie the particularly severe form of DC, Hoyeraal-Hreidarsson (HH) syndrome which is noted phenotypically by intrauterine growth restriction, cerebellar hypoplasia, microcephaly, severe immunodeficiency, and early-life marrow failure (Khincha and Savage 2016).

Diagnosis

TERT deficiency presents with aplastic anemia (AA) or myelodysplastic syndrome (Townsley et al. 2014). Chronic cytopenias, including thrombocytopenia, anemia, or leukopenia, are initial manifestations, especially when detected in adulthood. Other manifestations include skin and nail dystrophy characteristics of DC (Dokal 2000). Family history of hematological or severe lung disease might reveal an autosomal-dominant mode of inheritance. Laboratory testing should include testing the mean telomere length (MTL) in peripheral blood leukocytes (Aubert et al. 2012). Reduction of MTL, as compared to age-matched controls, is consistent with telomerase-associated gene defect (Alter et al. 2012). Secondary causes of reduced MTL should be taken into consideration, such as the use of cytoreductive medications. Gene sequencing analysis of telomerase-associated genes (*DKC1*, *TERT*, *TERC*, and *TINF2*) might provide with definitive diagnosis (Houben et al. 2008).

Treatment and Prognosis

The definitive treatment of bone marrow disorders associated to TERT deficiency is hematopoietic stem cell transplantation (HSCT). A significant complication is the increased risk of developing pulmonary fibrosis due to chemotherapy. The use of danazol has been shown to decrease the rate of telomere shortening. Other measures include red blood cell transfusions for severe anemia and platelet transfusions for severe thrombocytopenia (Dietz et al. 2011; Townsley et al. 2016).

Current average life expectancy for DC is 49 years (Shimamura and Alter 2010). DC due to TERT or TERC deficiency appears to have milder disease manifestations than DC due to DKC1 deficiency.

Cross-References

▶ DKC1, Dyskeratosis Congenita/Hoyeraal-Hreidarsson Syndrome

References

Alter BP, Rosenberg PS, Giri N, Baerlocher GM, Lansdorp PM, Savage SA. Telomere length is associated with disease severity and declines with age in dyskeratosis congenita. Haematologica. 2012;97(3):353–9.

Armanios M. Telomerase and idiopathic pulmonary fibrosis. Mutat Res. 2012;730(1–2):52–8.

Armanios M, Chen JL, Chang YP, et al. Haploinsufficiency of telomerase reverse transcriptase leads to anticipation in autosomal dominant dyskeratosis congenita. Proc Natl Acad Sci U S A. 2005;102(44):15960–4.

Aubert G, Hills M, Lansdorp PM. Telomere length measurement-caveats and a critical assessment of the available technologies and tools. Mutat Res. 2012;730(1–2):59–67.

Calado RT, Regal JA, Hills M, et al. Constitutional hypomorphic telomerase mutations in patients with acute myeloid leukemia. Proc Natl Acad Sci U S A. 2009;106(4):1187–92.

Cohen SB, Graham ME, Lovrecz GO, Bache N, Robinson PJ, Reddel RR. Protein composition of catalytically active human telomerase from immortal cells. Science. 2007;315(5820):1850–3.

Cong YS, Wen J, Bacchetti S. The human telomerase catalytic subunit hTERT: organization of the gene and characterization of the promoter. Hum Mol Genet. 1999;8(1):137–42.

Diaz de Leon A, Cronkhite JT, Katzenstein AL, et al. Telomere lengths, pulmonary fibrosis and telomerase (TERT) mutations. PLoS One. 2010;5(5):e10680.

Dietz AC, Orchard PJ, Baker KS, et al. Disease-specific hematopoietic cell transplantation: nonmyeloablative conditioning regimen for dyskeratosis congenita. Bone Marrow Transplant. 2011;46(1):98–104.

Dokal I. Dyskeratosis congenita in all its forms. Br J Haematol. 2000;110(4):768–79.

Du HY, Pumbo E, Ivanovich J, et al. TERC and TERT gene mutations in patients with bone marrow failure and the significance of telomere length measurements. Blood. 2009;113(2):309–16.

Fu D, Collins K. Purification of human telomerase complexes identifies factors involved in telomerase biogenesis and telomere length regulation. Mol Cell. 2007;28(5):773–85.

Horn S, Figl A, Rachakonda PS, et al. TERT promoter mutations in familial and sporadic melanoma. Science. 2013;339(6122):959–61.

Houben JM, Moonen HJ, van Schooten FJ, Hageman GJ. Telomere length assessment: biomarker of chronic oxidative stress? Free Radic Biol Med. 2008;44(3):235–46.

Khincha PP, Savage SA. Neonatal manifestations of inherited bone marrow failure syndromes. Semin Fetal Neonatal Med. 2016;21(1):57–65.

Meyerson M, Counter CM, Eaton EN, et al. hEST2, the putative human telomerase catalytic subunit gene, is up-regulated in tumor cells and during immortalization. Cell. 1997;90(4):785–95.

Mitchell JR, Wood E, Collins K. A telomerase component is defective in the human disease dyskeratosis congenita. Nature. 1999;402(6761):551–5.

Shimamura A, Alter BP. Pathophysiology and management of inherited bone marrow failure syndromes. Blood Rev. 2010;24(3):101–22.

Townsley DM, Dumitriu B, Young NS. Bone marrow failure and the telomeropathies. Blood. 2014;124(18):2775–83.

Townsley DM, Dumitriu B, Liu D, et al. Danazol treatment for telomere diseases. N Engl J Med. 2016;374(20):1922–31.

Yamaguchi H, Calado RT, Ly H, et al. Mutations in TERT, the gene for telomerase reverse transcriptase, in aplastic anemia. N Engl J Med. 2005;352(14):1413–24.

T

THI

▶ Transient Hypogammaglobulinemia of Infancy

This Group of Primary Antibody Deficiencies Are also Known as Hyper IgM Syndromes (HIGMs)

▶ Immunoglobulin Class Switch Recombination Defects

3-Methylglutaconic Aciduria

Gesmar Rodrigues Silva Segundo
Pediatrics Allergy and Immunology,
Universidade Federal de Uberlandia, Uberlandia,
Brazil

Introduction

3-methylglutaconic aciduria (3-MGA-uria) is a nonspecific biochemical finding related with a group of inborn errors of metabolism, particularly mitochondrial disorders. 3-MGA is a branched-chain organic acid and intermediate of leucine degradation and the mevalonate shunt pathway. The clinical features of the 3-MGA-uria syndromes are varied and are classified into five types, each with substantial heterogeneity. In all types, with the exception of 3-MGA-uria type I, the activities of 3-methylglutaconyl-CoA hydratase and other enzymes of leucine degradation are normal, and the 3-MGA-uria is considered secondary to defects in phospholipid remodeling or integrity of mitochondrial membranes, leading to electron transport chain dysfunction. 3-MGA-uria type I is an inborn error of leucine metabolism, caused by variants in *AUH*. *AUH* encodes 3-methylglutaconyl-CoA hydratase, which catalyzes the fifth step of leucine catabolism, whereby 3-methylglutaconyl-CoA is

converted to 3-hydroxy-3-methylglutaryl-coenzyme A (Saunders et al. 2015; Wortmann et al. 2015).

3-MGA-uria type II, or Barth syndrome, is an X-linked recessive disorder caused by variants in *TAZ*, which encodes tafazzin, a cardiolipin trans-acylase in the inner mitochondrial membrane. 3-MGA-uria type III, or Costeff syndrome, is caused by variants in *OPA3*. Type V is caused by variants in *DNAJC19*, which encodes a mitochondrial cochaperone. DNAJC19 forms a complex with prohibitins (PHB) and lipid scaffolds in the inner membrane of the mitochondria that is necessary for mitochondrial morphogenesis, neuronal survival, and phospholipid remodeling. 3-MGA-uria type IV, the "unclassified type," includes all other forms of 3-MGA-uria with normal 3-methylglutaconyl-CoA hydratase enzyme activity. A diagnosis of 3-MGA-uria type IV is complicated by the large number of implicated genes, including those involved in mitochondrial DNA depletion syndromes, mitochondrial DNA deletion syndromes, MELAS, Smith-Lemli-Opitz syndrome, and glycogen storage disease type 1b. Recently, two more types were added, type VI, MEGDEL syndrome, caused by mutations in *SERAC1* and related with deafness and dystonia, and more recently, type VII associated with 3-MGA-uria, cataracts, neurological involvement, and neutropenia (MEGCANN) caused by homozygous or compound heterozygous mutation in the *CLPB* gene (Capo-Chichi et al. 2016; Kambus et al. 2015; Wortmann et al. 2015).

In this chapter we will discuss the disease caused by mutations in the gene CLPB, which codes for a member of the family of ATPases associated with various cellular activities (AAA(+) proteins) whose function remains unknown, due to the presence of severe congenital neutropenia in most cases associated with primary immunodeficiency diseases and recurrent infections.

Clinical Presentation

The first description of CLPB-mutated patients described 14 affected individuals with variable phenotype from mild presentation including cataracts and neutropenia but no neurological involvement or infections to severe phenotype associated with neonatal or prenatal onset of neurological disease (progressive brain atrophy, absence of development, movement disorder, seizures), severe neutropenia with progression into leukemia, and death in the first months of life. In this cohort, patients presented intellectual disability/developmental delay (12/14 individuals investigated), congenital neutropenia (10/14), brain atrophy (7/9), microcephaly (7/12), movement disorder (7/13), cataracts (5/10), and 3-MGA-uria (12/12 individuals) (Wortmann et al. 2015). Most affected individuals suffered regularly from serious, often life-threatening, infections. Subsequently, 12 more patients were published adding different levels of neurological impairment and also nephrocalcinosis, cardiomyopathy, and facial dysmorphisms (Capo-Chichi et al. 2015; Kanabus et al. 2015; Kykim et al. 2015; Saunders et al. 2015).

Laboratorial Findings

Clinical diagnosis of MEGCANN should be suspected in the presence of congenital cataracts and neurological involvement. All individuals had consistent and significant excretion of 3-MGA in their urine, amounting to 2–15 times over the limit of the reference range. Most of them demonstrated neutropenia ranging from moderate to severe, and others presented the neutropenia following infectious diseases. The bone marrow examination showed different alterations including a maturation arrest at the stage of the promyelocyte and an absence of mature neutrophils in the bone marrow of individuals. The presence of clinical manifestation and laboratorial alterations suggests that the disease and the genetic evaluation can confirm the diagnosis (Capo-Chichi et al. 2015).

Treatment and Prognosis

Apart from supportive therapy and neurologic medications, there are no specific therapeutic options for these affected patients. Neutropenia generally responds to G-CSF treatment; most of the patients in the case series also received continuous antibiotics and antimycotics. There is no enough data concerning the development of

hematologic malignancies in the follow-up; in these initial cases, two siblings not treated with G-CSF progressed one to an acute myeloid leukemia and another to a myelodysplastic syndrome/preleukemia; both died shortly after these diagnoses.

According the publications, the oldest affected patient alive is 18 years old, presenting a mild diagnosis, and most of them died early in life due to the severity of disease.

References

Capo-Chichi JM, Boissel S, Brustein E, Pickles S, Fallet-Bianco C, Nassif C, et al. Disruption of CLPB is associated with congenital microcephaly, severe encephalopathy and 3-methylglutaconic aciduria. J Med Genet. 2015;52:303–11.

Kanabus M, Shahni R, Saldanha JW, Murphy E, Plagnol V, Hoff WV, et al. Bi-allelic CLPB mutations cause cataract, renal cysts, nephrocalcinosis and 3-methylglutaconic aciduria, a novel disorder of mitochondrial protein disaggregation. J Inherit Metab Dis. 2015;38:211–9.

Kiykim A, Garncarz W, Karakoc-Aydiner E, Ozen A, Kiykim E, Yesil G, et al. Novel CLPB mutation in a patient with 3-methylglutaconic aciduria causing severe neurological involvement and congenital neutropenia. Clin Immunol. 2016;165:1–3.

Saunders C, Smith L, Wibrand F, Ravn K, Bross P, Thiffault I, et al. CLPB variants associated with autosomal-recessive mitochondrial disorder with cataract, neutropenia, epilepsy, and methylglutaconic aciduria. Am J Hum Genet. 2015;96:258–65.

Wortmann SB, Ziętkiewicz S, Kousi M, Szklarczyk R, Haack TB, Gersting SW, et al. CLPB mutations cause 3-methylglutaconic aciduria, progressive brain atrophy, intellectual disability, congenital neutropenia, cataracts, movement disorder. Am J Hum Genet. 2015;96:245–57.

Thymoma with Hypogammaglobulinemia

▶ Good Syndrome

TICAM1

▶ TRIF Deficiency

TIR Signaling Pathway Deficiency, HOIL1 Deficiency

Shan Yu Fung[1] and Stuart E. Turvey[2,3]
[1]BC Children's Hospital Research Institute, University of British Columbia, Vancouver, BC, Canada
[2]Division of Allergy and Clinical Immunology, Department of Pediatrics and Experimental Medicine Program, British Columbia Children's Hospital, The University of British Columbia, Vancouver, BC, Canada
[3]Willem-Alexander Children's Hospital, Leiden University Medical Center, Leiden, the Netherlands

Synonyms

HOIL1 deficiency; LUBAC deficiency

Introduction

HOIL1 (Heme-Oxidized IRP2 Ubiquitin Ligase 1) deficiency is a novel, rare autosomal recessive disorder caused by biallelic disabling mutations in the gene *HOIL1* (also known as *RBCK1*) with clinical characteristics of immunodeficiency, autoinflammation, and amylopectinosis. Currently, there are only three cases reported worldwide (Boisson et al. 2012). Patients with HOIL1 deficiency present recurrent pyogenic bacterial infections, episodes of noninfectious fever, autoinflammatory responses in the gastrointestinal tract and skin, hepatosplenomegaly, and glycogen storage dysfunction with amylopectin-like deposits in muscle tissues including cardiomyocytes. The detailed clinical manifestations are listed in Table 1.

HOIL1 together with HOIP (HOIL1 interacting protein, also known as RNF31) and SHARPIN (SHANK-associated RH domain-interacting protein) form a trimolecular complex named LUBAC (linear ubiquitin chain assembly complex). LUBAC catalyzes ubiquitin polymerization through N-terminal methionine (M1)-linkage to form linear polyubiquitin chains on specific proteins to regulate protein signal transduction (Iwai and Tokunaga 2009; Ikeda et al. 2011; Tokunaga et al. 2011). HOIP has the catalytic domain for linear ubiquitination while HOIL1 and SHARPIN are mainly for complex stabilization and ubiquitin binding to enhance LUBAC activity. It has been found that LUBAC plays an important role in TNFR (tissue necrosis factor receptor)-mediated NF-κB (nuclear factor kappa-light-chain-enhancer of activated B cells) signaling pathway (Iwai and Tokunaga 2009). NF-κB is one of the central transcription factors regulating both innate and adaptive immune responses (Li and Verma 2002). LUBAC adds linear ubiquitin chains to NEMO (also called IKKγ or NF-kappa-B essential modulator), a regulatory subunit of the IKK (IκB kinase) complex that phosphorylates the IκBα inhibitory subunit of NF-κB for subsequent degradation, leading to the activation of NF-κB. The linear ubiquitin chain serves as a linkage that brings the interacting proteins of the pathway together facilitating signal transduction. Based on this biology, it was anticipated that defects in LUBAC function would have a detrimental influence on NF-κB activation, impacting on both innate and adaptive immunity (Shimizu et al. 2015).

Two novel *HOIL1* mutations are reported, resulting in complete loss of HOIL1 protein expression. This in turn disrupts LUBAC formation and its function of linear ubiquitination. Ultimately, the NF-κB signaling is dysregulated in response to stimulation through TNFR pathways. Interestingly, HOIL1 deficiency can lead to both hypo- and hyper-immune responses depending on the cell types, suggesting HOIL1 may have multiple roles in different cells, accounting for the coexisting of immunodeficiency and autoinflammation.

Genetics and Diagnosis

To date, there are only three patients from two families reported to carry biallelic mutations in *HOIL1* (or *RBCK1*) that result in HOIL1 deficiency (Boisson et al. 2012). Two members of one family had compound heterozygous mutations, a single copy deletion of 31.799 kb in chromosome 20p.13 encompassing last three exons of

TIR Signaling Pathway Deficiency, HOIL1 Deficiency, Table 1 Clinical manifestations of HOIL1-deficient patients

	Family 1		Family 2
Clinical manifestations	Patient 1 (compound heterozygous)	Patient 2 (compound heterozygous)	Patient 3 (homozygous)
Immunodeficiency			
Recurrent bacterial infection	*Escherichia coli*	*Escherichia coli*	*Staphylococcus*
	Streptococcus pneumoniae	*Staphylococcus aureus*	*Enterococcus*
	Haemophilus influenzae	*Staphylococcus epidermidis*	*Malassezia furfur*
		S. pneumoniae	*Candida albicans*
		Pseudomonas aeruginosa	
Severe viral infection	No	No	CMV
Memory B-cell deficiency	Yes	Yes	NA
Hyper IgA	Yes	Yes	NA
Autoinflammation			
Fever	Yes	Yes	Yes
Skin rash	Yes	No	Yes
GI inflammation	Yes	Yes	Yes
Lymphadenopathy	Yes	Yes	No
Hepatosplenomegaly	Yes	Yes	Yes
Failure to thrive	Yes	Yes	Yes
Cardiomyopathy	Yes	Yes	Yes
Amylopectinosis	Yes	Yes	Yes
Muscle weakness	Yes	Yes	No
Respiratory distress	No	No	Yes
Treatments	Antibiotics, steroids, anti-TNF	Antibiotics, steroids, anti-TNF	Antibiotics, steroids, HSCT

CMV cytomegalovirus, *HSCT* hematopoietic stem cell transplantation, *NA* not available, *TNF* tissue necrosis factor

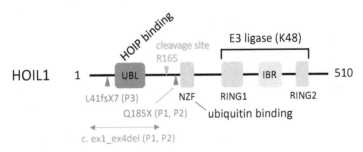

TIR Signaling Pathway Deficiency, HOIL1 Deficiency, Fig. 1 Schematic diagram of the HOIL1 domain structure with reported mutations in the domain. Patients 1 and 2 (P1 and P2) had compound heterozygous mutations with a single copy deletion (c. ex1_ex4del in *HOIL1*) and a nonsense mutation of p. Q185X; patient 3 (P3) had a homozygous frame shit of p. L41fsX7. *UBL* ubiquitin-like domain for HOIP binding, *NZF* Npl4 zinc finger domain for ubiquitin binding, RING1-IBR-RING2 domain is a E3 ligase catalytic region for K48-linked ubiquitination. HOIL1 can be cleaved by the human paracaspase MALT1 at R165

TRIB3 and the first four exons of *HOIL1* (del: *TRIB3*:g.-1272_*HOIL1*:g.9780del) and a nonsense mutant allele (c.533 C>T, p.Q185X) in the exon 5 of *HOIL1*. The third patient from a consanguineous family had the homozygous mutation with a deletion of two nucleotides (c.121_122delCT, p.L41fsX7) in exon 2 of *HOIL1*. These mutations are depicted in Fig. 1.

These mutations all resulted in the complete absence of HOIL1 protein.

Current diagnostic approach to HOIL1 deficiency is not well defined due to the limited number of affected individuals identified to date. In general, HOIL1 deficiency can lead to a complex clinical phenotype of immunodeficiency, auto-inflammation, and amylopectinosis (Boisson et al. 2012). Interestingly, it has been found that a patient with homozygous missense mutation in *HOIP* also presented a very similar clinical phenotype (Boisson et al. 2015). This clinical presentation should prompt sequencing of the three gene encoding elements of LUBAC – *HOIL1*, *HOIP*, and *SHARPIN*. Considering both HOIP and HOIL1 (together with SHARPIN) make up the LUBAC complex, which is essential for protein posttranslational modification of linear ubiquitination, it is likely that a more unified understanding of the clinical consequences of LUBAC deficiency will emerge with the description of additional affected patients (Aksentijevich and Zhou 2017).

Disease Mechanism

Since HOIL1 physically binds to HOIP and SHARPIN to form the trimolecular LUBAC complex, absence of HOIL1 has a detrimental impact on LUBAC function. First, the formation of the complex is critical to stabilize the individual components. It has been found that HOIL1 deficiency spontaneously reduces the levels of both HOIP and SHARPIN, leading to significant reduction in the catalytic activity of LUBAC (Boisson et al. 2012). In an analogous fashion, HOIP deficiency decreases HOIL1 and SHARPIN protein levels (Boisson et al. 2015). This phenomenon has also been seen in the context of HOIL1 cleavage by the human paracaspase MALT1 (mucosa-associated lymphoid tissue lymphoma translocation protein 1), where cleavage of HOIL1 disrupts LUBAC and significantly decreases HOIP level, down regulating the LUBAC activity of linear

ubiquitination (Klein et al. 2015). The impairment of LUBAC activity will ultimately dampen NF-κB activation, which is central to mount a variety of immune responses against infections.

Interestingly, HOIL1 deficiency caused a dysregulation of immune responses that is cell type specific. While the absence of HOIL1 results in the impairment of NF-κB activation and cytokine production in fibroblasts, HOIL1 deficiency can cause hyper immune responses (e.g., high cytokine production) to the same stimuli in myeloid cells, particularly monocytes (Boisson et al. 2012). This suggests that perhaps LUBAC has additional regulatory functions in monocytes, which have not yet been defined. It may be that these hyperinflammatory responses may account for the autoinflammation observed in all HOIL1 deficient patients.

HOIL1-deficient patients also displayed an unexpected clinical feature of amylopectinosis in muscle tissues, indicating some defects in the glycogen storage. This feature has never been found in other disorders associated with NF-κB dysregulation (Casanova et al. 2011; Picard et al. 2011). Although the mechanism remains to be defined, HOIL1 deficiency has become a new cause of amylopectinosis, in addition to the well-characterized glycogen branching enzyme (GBE) deficiency and phosphofructokinase (PFK) deficiency (Oldfors and DiMauro 2013).

Treatment

Today there are no targeted therapies for HOIL1 deficiency. Sadly, the three reported patients all died by age 8 years. The treatment options utilized included antibiotics for recurrent infections, systemic corticosteroids, and anti-TNFα therapy for inflammation (Boisson et al. 2012). One of the patients underwent the allogeneic hematopoietic stem cell transplantation (HSCT) at age 13 months with a graft from a matched unrelated donor, and no episodes of sepsis recorded posttransplant. Unfortunately, HSCT treatment did not resolve the amylopectinosis, and the patient eventually died of chronic myocarditis-associated sudden respiratory distress 3 years after HSCT (Boisson et al. 2012).

References

Aksentijevich I, Zhou Q. NF-kappaB pathway in auto-inflammatory diseases: dysregulation of protein modifications by ubiquitin defines a new category of autoinflammatory diseases. Front Immunol. 2017;8:399.

Boisson B, Laplantine E, Prando C, Giliani S, Israelsson E, Xu Z, et al. Immunodeficiency, autoinflammation and amylopectinosis in humans with inherited HOIL-1 and LUBAC deficiency. Nat Immunol. 2012;13(12):1178–86.

Boisson B, Laplantine E, Dobbs K, Cobat A, Tarantino N, Hazen M, et al. Human HOIP and LUBAC deficiency underlies autoinflammation, immunodeficiency, amylopectinosis, and lymphangiectasia. J Exp Med. 2015;212(6):939–51.

Casanova JL, Abel L, Quintana-Murci L. Human TLRs and IL-1Rs in host defense: natural insights from evolutionary, epidemiological, and clinical genetics. Annu Rev Immunol. 2011;29:447–91.

Ikeda F, Deribe YL, Skanland SS, Stieglitz B, Grabbe C, Franz-Wachtel M, et al. SHARPIN forms a linear ubiquitin ligase complex regulating NF-kappaB activity and apoptosis. Nature. 2011;471(7340):637–41.

Iwai K, Tokunaga F. Linear polyubiquitination: a new regulator of NF-kappaB activation. EMBO Rep. 2009;10(7):706–13.

Klein T, Fung SY, Renner F, Blank MA, Dufour A, Kang S, et al. The paracaspase MALT1 cleaves HOIL1 reducing linear ubiquitination by LUBAC to dampen lymphocyte NF-kappaB signalling. Nat Commun. 2015;6:8777.

Li Q, Verma IM. NF-kappaB regulation in the immune system. Nat Rev Immunol. 2002;2(10):725–34.

Oldfors A, DiMauro S. New insights in the field of muscle glycogenoses. Curr Opin Neurol. 2013;26(5):544–53.

Picard C, Casanova JL, Puel A. Infectious diseases in patients with IRAK-4, MyD88, NEMO, or IkappaBalpha deficiency. Clin Microbiol Rev. 2011;24(3):490–7.

Shimizu Y, Taraborrelli L, Walczak H. Linear ubiquitination in immunity. Immunol Rev. 2015;266(1):190–207.

Tokunaga F, Nakagawa T, Nakahara M, Saeki Y, Taniguchi M, Sakata S, et al. SHARPIN is a component of the NF-kappaB-activating linear ubiquitin chain assembly complex. Nature. 2011;471(7340):633–6.

TIR Signaling Pathway Deficiency, IRAK-4 Deficiency

Catherine M. Biggs[1] and Stuart E. Turvey[2,3]
[1]Department of Pediatrics, BC Children's Hospital, University of British Columbia, Vancouver, BC, Canada
[2]Division of Allergy and Clinical Immunology, Department of Pediatrics and Experimental Medicine Program, British Columbia Children's Hospital, The University of British Columbia, Vancouver, BC, Canada
[3]Willem-Alexander Children's Hospital, Leiden University Medical Center, Leiden, the Netherlands

Synonyms

Recurrent isolated invasive pneumococcal disease 1 (IPD1)

Definition

Interleukin-1 receptor associated kinase (IRAK-4) deficiency is an autosomal recessive disorder that impairs Toll/IL-1 receptor signaling pathways and leads to recurrent and/or severe pyogenic bacterial infections.

Introduction

Signaling through Toll-like receptors (TLR) and the interleukin-1 receptor (IL-1R) are critical for innate immunity and are collectively referred to as the Toll/IL-1R (TIR) signaling pathway (Puel et al. 2004). Both TLRs and the IL-1R share cytoplasmic sequence homology, and lead to activation of the IκB kinase (IKK) complex and the transcription factor NF-kappa B (NF-κB). NF-κB plays an essential role in regulating important cellular processes such as inflammation, stress responses, and survival (Awane et al. 1999). Interleukin-1 receptor associated kinase-4 (IRAK-4) is a protein kinase that acts upstream of the IKK complex to activate TIR signaling (Puel et al. 2004; Janssens and Beyaert 2003). Deficiency in IRAK-4 impairs signaling through all known TLRs except for TLR3 (Kim et al. 2007). First described in 2003, patients affected by IRAK-4 deficiency suffer from a narrow spectrum of invasive infections caused by pyogenic bacteria (Picard et al. 2003; Medvedev et al. 2003). Gram-positive organisms are the most frequently encountered and particularly *Streptococcus pneumoniae*; however, Gram-negative bacterial infections have also been reported (Ku et al. 2007).

Genetics

The *IRAK4* gene maps to chromosome 12q12 in humans and spans 13 exons in length. It encodes a protein consisting of 460 amino acids that is 52 kDa in size (von Bernuth et al. 2012). The protein contains an N-terminal death domain and a central kinase domain. It functions as a serine/threonine protein kinase (Li et al. 2002). Upon receptor binding by TLR agonists or IL-1/IL-18, the adaptor protein MyD88 is recruited and links TIR signaling with the IRAK complex. The IRAK complex consists of two protein kinases, IRAK-1 and IRAK-4, and two proteins without detectable kinase activity, IRAK-2 and IRAK-M (Akira and Takeda 2004). MyD88 binds to IRAK-4 via their shared death domains (Li et al. 2002; Suzuki et al. 2002). IRAK-4 and MyD88 then mediate activation of the NF-kB and mitogen-activated protein kinase pathways (Picard et al. 2007). These TIR signaling pathways, mediated through IRAK-4, lead to the synthesis of numerous inflammatory cytokines, including IL-1β, IL-6, IL-8, tumor necrosis factor (TNF)-α, interferon-α/β, and interferon λ (Picard et al. 2010).

IRAK-4 deficiency is inherited in an autosomal recessive manner, caused by homozygous or compound heterozygous mutations in the *IRAK4* gene. Both inherited and sporadic cases of IRAK-4

deficiency have been described (Picard et al. 2010). Affected patients have been reported to originate from 16 countries within five continents, including North America, Asia, Australia, Africa, and Europe (Picard et al. 2010; Ailal et al. 2012). Both missense mutations, as well as mutations leading to large deletions/early truncations of the protein, have been reported (Picard et al. 2010).

Disease

Patients with IRAK-4 deficiency suffer from both noninvasive and invasive pyogenic bacterial infections. The first bacterial infection occurs in most patients before 2 years of age, and can present as early as the neonatal period (Picard et al. 2010). Recurrent invasive infections with the same bacterial serotype have been reported (Szabo et al. 2007). Eighteen out of 48 patients suffered fatal invasive bacterial infections in the largest study of IRAK-4 deficiency, and those who died were all under 8 years of age (Picard et al. 2010). A clinical observation is that the susceptibility towards infections appears to decrease with age in IRAK-4-deficient patients, with invasive disease rare beyond 14 years of age (Picard et al. 2010; Frans et al. 2015). This has been attributed to maturation of other complimentary arms of the immune system that reconcile for this defect. In addition to pyogenic infections, delayed separation of the umbilical cord is another clinical feature seen in some patients with IRAK-4 deficiency (Takada et al. 2006).

The three most frequently isolated bacteria are *S. pneumoniae, Staphylococcus aureus*, and *Pseudomonas aeruginosa* (Ku et al. 2007; Picard et al. 2010). *S. pneumoniae* (commonly referred to as pneumococcus) accounts for the majority of invasive infections, and *S. aureus* for noninvasive disease (Picard et al. 2010; Grazioli et al. 2016). Other reported bacteria include *Shigella sonei*, other *Streptococcus* species, *Haemophilus influenzae* type B, *Clostridium septicum*, and *Neisseria meningitidis* (Medvedev et al. 2003; Chapel et al. 2005). Meningitis is the most common form of infection, and other forms of invasive disease that have been reported include sepsis and shock, arthritis, osteomyelitis, and deep-organ/tissue abscesses (Picard et al. 2010; Szabo et al. 2007; Chapel et al. 2005; Dilley et al. 2013; Ladhani et al. 2013). Noninvasive disease typically manifests as bacterial skin infections, which may require long courses of intravenous antibiotic therapy (Picard et al. 2010). Despite their acute sensitivity to pyogenic bacterial infections, IRAK-4-deficient patients do not experience an increased susceptibility to infections with other microorganisms, including viruses, fungi, parasites, and other types of bacteria (Picard et al. 2010).

Another striking quality of IRAK-4 deficiency is the blunted inflammatory response during an invasive infection. Patients may present with normal CRP levels, absence of fever, and normal/low leukocyte and neutrophil counts despite having an overwhelming infection. It should also be noted, however, that IRAK-4-deficient patients can also present with elevated CRP, white blood cell, and neutrophil levels as well as fever and pus formation at the site of infection, and therefore these features should not rule out the diagnosis (Picard et al. 2010).

Immunological evaluation in IRAK-4 deficiency typically reveals normal dendritic cell and monocyte, as well T, B, and NK cell numbers. T cell proliferation to mitogens is normal, and patients may have either normal or elevated immunoglobulin levels. Elevated IgE levels in conjunction with recurrent infections may lead to confusion of IRAK-4 deficiency for Hyper IgE syndrome (HIES); however, the degree of IgE elevation is typically modest in comparison to HIES caused by STAT3 deficiency (Picard et al. 2010; Frans et al. 2015). Antibody response to protein antigen vaccines is normal, whereas the response to glycan antigens, such as non-conjugated pneumococcal vaccines or allohemagluttinins, may be normal or impaired (Picard et al. 2010). This has been attributed to a decrease in IgM+IgD+CD27+ B Cells in IRAK-4-deficient patients, leading to impaired IgM responses to T-independent bacterial antigens (Maglione et al. 2014; Weller et al. 2012).

Diagnosis

IRAK-4 deficiency should be considered in patients presenting with recurrent or severe pyogenic bacterial infections, in particular those whose first infection occurs in early childhood, as well as those with a family history of invasive bacterial disease. Standard immunological evaluation is generally unrevealing, until further directed studies aimed at identifying a Toll-like receptor defect are performed. Evaluation typically demonstrates normal white blood cell and lymphocyte subset enumeration, and T cell proliferation. Immunoglobulin levels may be normal or elevated, and evaluation of the response to vaccines generally shows intact protein antigen vaccine titers, however, may reveal impaired polysaccharide antigen responses. Assessment of Toll-like receptor signaling can also aid in the diagnosis, and can be performed by measuring TNF-α or IL-6 production upon stimulation by Toll-like receptor agonists in whole blood or peripheral blood mononuclear cells (Picard et al. 2003; Deering and Orange 2006). This can be performed by enzyme-linked immunosorbent assay (ELISA) or by flow cytometry (Picard et al. 2003; Takada et al. 2006; Deering and Orange 2006). A more rapid assessment of IRAK-4 function can be performed by detecting the cleavage of membrane-bound L-selectin on granulocytes stimulated with TLR agonists on flow cytometry (von Bernuth et al. 2006). IRAK-4-deficient patients are identified by direct molecular sequencing of the *IRAK4* gene located on chromosome 12q12 (Picard et al. 2003). Sequencing of the *IRAK4* gene reveals biallelic mutations.

Treatment

The treatment of IRAK-4 deficiency involves prophylactic measures to prevent infection combined with prompt and aggressive evaluation and management at the first sign of infection. Prophylaxis in the form of antibiotics, immunizations, and in some cases gammaglobulin administration has been associated with a significant decrease in invasive bacterial infections (Picard et al. 2010). Patients should receive daily antimicrobial prophylaxis with an antibiotic that carries good Gram-positive, as well as some Gram-negative coverage, such as amoxicillin or sulfamethoxazole–trimethoprim. Despite receiving appropriate antibiotic prophylaxis and immunizations, those with IRAK-4 deficiency can still suffer from fatal invasive bacterial infections (McKelvie et al. 2014). Therefore, additional protection through the administration of gammaglobulin, either subcutaneously or intravenously, is recommended (Picard et al. 2011). If patients are unable to receive gammaglobulin prophylaxis, they should be immunized against encapsulated organisms such as *S. pneumoniae, N. meningitidis,* and *H. influenzae* type B. Consideration can be given to stopping the antimicrobial prophylaxis after 14 years of age, as the majority of infections occur before this age. When IRAK-4-deficient patients present with signs or symptoms concerning for a potential bacterial infection, bacterial cultures should be obtained and empiric antibiotics should be started as soon as possible.

References

Ailal F, Jouhadi Z, Jeddane L, Puel A, Picard C, Najib J, et al. About the first case of IRAK-4 deficiency in Morocco. J Clin Immunol. 2012;32:101.

Akira S, Takeda K. Toll-like receptor signalling. Nat Rev Immunol. 2004;4(7):499–511.

Awane M, Andres PG, Li DJ, Reinecker HC. NF-kappa B-inducing kinase is a common mediator of IL-17-, TNF-alpha-, and IL-1 beta-induced chemokine promoter activation in intestinal epithelial cells. J Immunol. 1999;162(9):5337–44.

Chapel H, Puel A, von Bernuth H, Picard C, Casanova JL. Shigella sonnei meningitis due to interleukin-1 receptor-associated kinase-4 deficiency: first association with a primary immune deficiency. Clin Infect Dis. 2005;40(9):1227–31.

Deering RP, Orange JS. Development of a clinical assay to evaluate toll-like receptor function. Clin Vaccine Immunol. 2006;13(1):68–76.

Dilley MA, Jones SM, Scurlock AM, Perry TT, Pesek RD. Pneumococcal meningitis in a patient with Irak-4 deficiency: a case of failed prophylactic therapy. J Allergy Clin Immunol. 2013;131(2):AB153.

Frans G, Moens L, Schrijvers R, Wuyts G, Bouckaert B, Schaballie H, et al. PID in disguise: molecular diagnosis of IRAK-4 deficiency in an adult previously misdiagnosed with autosomal dominant hyper IgE syndrome. J Clin Immunol. 2015;35(8):739–44.

Grazioli S, Hamilton SJ, McKinnon ML, Del Bel KL, Hoang L, Cook VE, et al. IRAK-4 deficiency as a cause for familial fatal invasive infection by *Streptococcus pneumoniae.* Clin Immunol. 2016;163:14–6.

Janssens S, Beyaert R. Functional diversity and regulation of different interleukin-1 receptor-associated kinase (IRAK) family members. Mol Cell. 2003;11(2):293–302.

Kim TW, Staschke K, Bulek K, Yao J, Peters K, Oh KH, et al. A critical role for IRAK4 kinase activity in Toll-like receptor-mediated innate immunity. J Exp Med. 2007;204(5):1025–36.

Ku CL, von Bernuth H, Picard C, Zhang SY, Chang HH, Yang K, et al. Selective predisposition to bacterial infections in IRAK-4-deficient children: IRAK-4-dependent TLRs are otherwise redundant in protective immunity. J Exp Med. 2007;204(10):2407–22.

Ladhani SN, Slack MPE, Andrews NJ, Waight PA, Borrow R, Miller E. Invasive pneumococcal disease after routine pneumococcal conjugate vaccination in children, England and Wales. Emerg Infect Dis. 2013;19(1):61–8.

Li S, Strelow A, Fontana EJ, Wesche H. IRAK-4: a novel member of the IRAK family with the properties of an IRAK-kinase. Proc Natl Acad Sci U S A. 2002;99(8):5567–72.

Maglione PJ, Simchoni N, Black S, Radigan L, Overbey JR, Bagiella E, et al. IRAK-4 and MyD88 deficiencies impair IgM responses against T-independent bacterial antigens. Blood. 2014;124(24):3561–71.

McKelvie B, Top K, McCusker C, Letenyi D, Issekutz TB, Issekutz AC. Fatal pneumococcal meningitis in a 7-year-old girl with interleukin-1 receptor activated kinase deficiency (IRAK-4) despite prophylactic antibiotic and IgG responses to *Streptococcus pneumoniae* vaccines. J Clin Immunol. 2014;34(3):267–71.

Medvedev AE, Lentschat A, Kuhns DB, Blanco JC, Salkowski C, Zhang S, et al. Distinct mutations in IRAK-4 confer hyporesponsiveness to lipopolysaccharide and interleukin-1 in a patient with recurrent bacterial infections. J Exp Med. 2003;198(4):521–31.

Picard C, Puel A, Bonnet M, Ku CL, Bustamante J, Yang K, et al. Pyogenic bacterial infections in humans with IRAK-4 deficiency. Science. 2003;299(5615):2076–9.

Picard C, von Bernuth H, Ku CL, Yang K, Puel A, Casanova JL. Inherited human IRAK-4 deficiency: an update. Immunol Res. 2007;38(1–3):347–52.

Picard C, von Bernuth H, Ghandil P, Chrabieh M, Levy O, Arkwright PD, et al. Clinical features and outcome of patients with IRAK-4 and MyD88 deficiency. Medicine. 2010;89(6):403–25.

Picard C, Casanova JL, Puel A. Infectious Diseases in Patients with IRAK-4, MyD88, NEMO, or IkBa deficiency. Clin Microbiol Rev. 2011 Jul;24(3):490–7.

Puel A, Picard C, Ku CL, Smahi A, Casanova JL. Inherited disorders of NF-kappaB-mediated immunity in man. Curr Opin Immunol. 2004;16(1):34–41.

Suzuki N, Suzuki S, Duncan GS, Millar DG, Wada T, Mirtsos C, et al. Severe impairment of interleukin-1 and Toll-like receptor signalling in mice lacking IRAK-4. Nature. 2002;416(6882):750–4.

Szabo J, Dobay O, Erdos M, Borbely A, Rozgonyi F, Marodi L. Recurrent infection with genetically identical pneumococcal isolates in a patient with interleukin-1 receptor-associated kinase-4 deficiency. J Med Microbiol. 2007;56(6):863–5.

Takada H, Yoshikawa H, Imaizumi M, Kitamura T, Takeyama J, Kumaki S, et al. Delayed separation of the umbilical cord in two siblings with interleukin-1 receptor-associated kinase 4 deficiency: rapid screening by flow cytometer. J Pediatr. 2006;148(4):546–8.

von Bernuth H, Ku CL, Rodriguez-Gallego C, Zhang SY, Garty BZ, Marodi L, et al. A fast procedure for the detection of defects in toll-like receptor signaling. Pediatrics. 2006;118(6):2498–503.

von Bernuth H, Picard C, Puel A, Casanova JL. Experimental and natural infections in MyD88- and IRAK-4-deficient mice and humans. Eur J Immunol. 2012;42(12):3126–35.

Weller S, Bonnet M, Delagreverie H, Israel L, Chrabieh M, Marodi L, et al. IgM(+)IgD(+)CD27(+)B cells are markedly reduced in IRAK-4-, MyD88-, and TIRAP- but not UNC-93B-deficient patients. Blood. 2012;120(25):4992–5001.

TIR Signaling Pathway Deficiency, MyD88 Deficiency

Catherine M. Biggs[1] and Stuart E. Turvey[2,3]
[1]Department of Pediatrics, BC Children's Hospital, University of British Columbia, Vancouver, BC, Canada
[2]Division of Allergy and Clinical Immunology, Department of Pediatrics and Experimental Medicine Program, British Columbia Children's Hospital, The University of British Columbia, Vancouver, BC, Canada
[3]Willem-Alexander Children's Hospital, Leiden University Medical Center, Leiden, the Netherlands

Definition

MyD88 deficiency is an autosomal recessive disorder characterized by recurrent and/or severe pyogenic bacterial infections and is caused by impaired Toll/IL-1 receptor signaling.

Introduction

The Toll-like receptor (TLR) and interleukin-1 receptor (IL-1R) signaling pathways play an essential role in the innate immune response (Puel et al. 2004). Collectively referred to as the Toll/IL-1R (TIR) signaling pathway, both TLRs and the IL-1R carry cytoplasmic sequence homology and cause downstream activation of the IκB kinase (IKK) complex and the transcription factor NF-kappa B (NF-κB). NF-κB regulates pathways that are critical to inflammatory, survival, and stress responses in the cell (Awane et al. 1999). MyD88 is an adaptor protein that connects signaling through the TIR family to downstream activation of both NF-κB and mitogen-activated protein kinase (MAPK) pathways (Janssens and Beyaert 2002; Medzhitov et al. 1998). Deficiency in MyD88 was first described in 2008, after patients presented with a similar clinical phenotype as those who are deficient in interleukin-1 receptor-associated kinase-4 (IRAK-4), however, did not have identified mutations in the *IRAK4* gene (von Bernuth et al. 2008). IRAK-4 is a protein kinase that acts upstream of the IKK complex to activate TIR signaling (Puel et al. 2004; Janssens and Beyaert 2003). Analogous to IRAK-4 deficiency, patients with defects in MyD88 suffer from a particular susceptibility towards invasive infections caused by pyogenic bacteria (Picard et al. 2003; Medvedev et al. 2003). Gram-positive organisms are the most frequently encountered; however, Gram-negative bacterial infections have also been reported (Ku et al. 2007).

Genetics

The *MyD88* gene maps to chromosome 3p21.3-3p22 in humans and spans five exons in length. It encodes a protein consisting of 296 amino acids that is 33 kDa in size (Bonnert et al. 1997). The protein contains a C-terminal region that carries sequence homology to the type I IL-IR cytoplasmic domain, while the N-terminal region carries a death domain that is shared with the IRAK family of proteins (Medzhitov et al. 1998; Bonnert et al. 1997).

Upon receptor binding by TLR agonists or IL-1/IL-18, the adaptor protein MyD88 is recruited and links TIR signaling with the IRAK complex. MyD88 binds to IRAK-4 via their shared death domains (Li et al. 2002; Suzuki et al. 2002). IRAK-4 and MyD88 then mediate activation of the NF-kB and MAPK pathways (Picard et al. 2007). Signaling through TIRs ultimately leads to the synthesis of numerous inflammatory cytokines, including IL-1β, IL-6, IL-8, tumor necrosis factor (TNF)-α, interferon-α/β, and interferon λ (Picard et al. 2010).

MyD88 deficiency is inherited in an autosomal recessive manner, caused by homozygous or compound heterozygous mutations in the *MyD88* gene. Both missense mutations leading to normal protein expression with functional impairment, as well as deletions causing decreased expression of a nonfunctional protein, have been described (von Bernuth et al. 2008). MyD88 deficiency has been reported in patients from both Europe and Asia (Picard et al. 2010; Giardino et al. 2016).

Disease

MyD88 deficiency is characterized by a propensity towards both noninvasive and invasive pyogenic bacterial infections. The presentation of MyD88 deficiency is a "phenocopy" of that seen in IRAK-4 deficiency, meaning that the two conditions can be nearly indistinguishable based on clinical features alone. The majority of MyD88-deficient patients suffer from their first bacterial infection before 2 years of age, often within the first 6 months of life (Picard et al. 2010). Approximately one-third of patients surveyed in the largest study of MyD88 deficiency experienced their first bacterial infection in the neonatal period (Picard et al. 2010). Invasive bacterial infections can be recurrent and fatal, with deaths typically occurring in early childhood before 8 years of age. It has also been appreciated in both MyD88 and IRAK4-deficient

patients that the risk of invasive bacterial disease appears to decrease with age (Picard et al. 2010). This has been attributed to maturation of other compensatory arms of the immune system that reconcile for this defect.

The three bacteria most commonly isolated from patients with MyD88 deficiency are *Streptococcus pneumoniae*, *Staphylococcus aureus*, and *Pseudomonas aeruginosa* (Picard et al. 2010). *Streptococcus pneumoniae* (or pneumococcus) accounts for the majority of invasive infections and *S. aureus* for noninvasive disease (Picard et al. 2010). While Gram-positive infections predominate, Gram-negative infections can also occur (Picard et al. 2010; Giardino et al. 2016). Other reported bacteria include β-hemolytic Streptococci as well as Gram-negative bacteria such as *Salmonella enteritidis*, *Haemophilus influenzae*, *Klebsiella pneumoniae*, *Moraxella catarrhalis*, *Escherichia coli*, and *Yersinia enterocolitica* (Picard et al. 2010; Giardino et al. 2016). Similar to IRAK-4 deficiency, meningitis is the most common form of infection, and other forms of invasive disease that have been reported include sepsis, arthritis, chronic intestinal yersiniosis, osteomyelitis, and deep inner organ/tissue abscesses (Picard et al. 2010; Giardino et al. 2016). Noninvasive disease typically manifested as lymphadenitis, as well as infections involving the skin or upper respiratory tract, locations that are noted to be common for necrotizing infections (Picard et al. 2010). Interestingly, patients with MyD88 deficiency have not displayed an increased propensity towards infections with other microorganisms, including parasites, fungi, viruses, and other types of bacteria.

Another notable feature of MyD88 deficiency is the diminished inflammatory response during an invasive infection. Patients may present without fever and may have normal CRP levels and normal/low leukocyte and neutrophil counts despite having an overwhelming infection. Conversely, it is also important to mention that patients with MyD88 deficiency can also demonstrate elevated CRP, white blood cell and neutrophil levels as well as fever and purulent debris at the site of infection; therefore, these features should not rule out the diagnosis (Picard et al. 2010).

Immunological evaluation in MyD88 deficiency typically demonstrates normal dendritic cell and monocyte as well as T, B, and NK cell numbers. T cell proliferation to mitogens is normal, and patients may have either normal or elevated immunoglobulin levels. Elevated IgE levels may be observed in MyD88 deficiency; however, the degree of IgE elevation is typically modest in comparison to hyper IgE syndrome caused by STAT3 deficiency (Picard et al. 2010; Frans et al. 2015). Antibody response to protein antigen vaccines is normal, whereas the response to glycan antigens, such as nonconjugated pneumococcal vaccines or allohemagluttinins, may be normal or impaired (Picard et al. 2010). This has been attributed to a decrease in IgM+IgD+CD27+ B Cells in IRAK-4-deficient patients, leading to impaired IgM responses to T-independent bacterial antigens (Maglione et al. 2014; Weller et al. 2012).

Diagnosis

Severe or recurrent pyogenic infections occurring in early childhood should prompt consideration of MyD88 deficiency. A standard immune workup is generally unrevealing; therefore, a high index of suspicion is required. When MyD88 deficiency is being considered in the differential diagnosis, further directed studies aimed at identifying a Toll-like receptor defect are performed. Evaluation usually demonstrates normal white blood cell and lymphocyte subset enumeration, T cell proliferation, normal or elevated immunoglobulin levels, and intact protein antigen vaccine titers, however may reveal impaired polysaccharide antigen responses. Definitive diagnosis is made by targeted molecular sequencing of the MyD88 gene, located on

chromosome 3p22 (von Bernuth et al. 2008). Toll-like receptor signaling analysis can also be helpful in making the diagnosis and can be performed by measuring specific cytokine production upon stimulation by Toll-like receptor agonists in whole blood or peripheral blood mononuclear cells (von Bernuth et al. 2008; Deering and Orange 2006). This can be performed by enzyme-linked immunosorbent assay (ELISA) or by flow cytometry (von Bernuth et al. 2008; Deering and Orange 2006; Takada et al. 2006). A rapid assessment of MyD88 function can also be performed by detecting the cleavage of membrane-bound L-selectin on granulocytes stimulated with TLR agonists on flow cytometry (von Bernuth et al. 2006). Sequencing of the *MyD88* gene reveals biallelic mutations.

Treatment

Treatment of MyD88 deficiency involves infection prophylaxis measures as well as prompt and aggressive evaluation and management of any suspected infections. Protection against infection warrants the routine use of prophylactic antibiotics, immunizations, and gammaglobulin administration. This regimen has been associated with a significant decrease in invasive bacterial infections (Picard et al. 2010). It is recommended that patients receive daily antimicrobial prophylaxis with an antibiotic that conveys good Gram-positive, as well as some Gram-negative coverage, such as amoxicillin or sulfamethoxazole–trimethoprim. It has been demonstrated in IRAK-4 deficiency that patients can still suffer from fatal invasive bacterial infections despite receiving appropriate antibiotic prophylaxis and immunizations (McKelvie et al. 2014). Given the similarities between IRAK-4 and MyD88 deficiency, it is therefore recommended that MyD88-deficient patients receive additional protection through the administration of gammaglobulin, either subcutaneously or intravenously. If patients are unable to receive gammaglobulin prophylaxis, they should be immunized against encapsulated organisms such as *S. pneumoniae, Neisseria meningitidis*, and *H. influenzae* type B. Consideration can be given to stopping the antimicrobial prophylaxis once patients reach young adulthood, as the majority of infections occur earlier in childhood. When MyD88-deficient patient present with signs or symptoms concerning for a potential bacterial infection, bacterial cultures should be obtained and empiric antibiotics should be started as soon as possible.

References

Awane M, Andres PG, Li DJ, Reinecker HC. NF-kappa B-inducing kinase is a common mediator of IL-17-, TNF-alpha-, and IL-1 beta-induced chemokine promoter activation in intestinal epithelial cells. J Immunol. 1999;162(9):5337–44.

Bonnert TP, Garka KE, Parnet P, Sonoda G, Testa JR, Sims JE. The cloning and characterization of human MyD88: a member of an IL-1 receptor related family. FEBS Lett. 1997;402(1):81–4.

Deering RP, Orange JS. Development of a clinical assay to evaluate toll-like receptor function. Clin Vaccine Immunol. 2006;13(1):68–76.

Frans G, Moens L, Schrijvers R, Wuyts G, Bouckaert B, Schaballie H, et al. PID in disguise: molecular diagnosis of IRAK-4 deficiency in an adult previously misdiagnosed with autosomal dominant hyper IgE syndrome. J Clin Immunol. 2015;35(8):739–44.

Giardino G, Gallo V, Somma D, Farrow EG, Thiffault I, D'Assante R, et al. Targeted next-generation sequencing revealed MYD88 deficiency in a child with chronic yersiniosis and granulomatous lymphadenitis. J Allergy Clin Immunol. 2016;137(5):1591.

Janssens S, Beyaert R. A universal role for MyD88 in TLR/IL-1R-mediated signaling. Trends Biochem Sci. 2002;27(9):474–82.

Janssens S, Beyaert R. Functional diversity and regulation of different interleukin-1 receptor-associated kinase (IRAK) family members. Mol Cell. 2003;11(2):293–302.

Ku CL, von Bernuth H, Picard C, Zhang SY, Chang HH, Yang K, et al. Selective predisposition to bacterial infections in IRAK-4-deficient children: IRAK-4-dependent TLRs are otherwise redundant in protective immunity. J Exp Med. 2007;204(10):2407–22.

Li SY, Strelow A, Fontana EJ, Wesche H. IRAK-4: a novel member of the IRAK family with the properties of an IRAK-kinase. Proc Natl Acad Sci U S A. 2002;99(8):5567–72.

Maglione PJ, Simchoni N, Black S, Radigan L, Overbey JR, Bagiella E, et al. IRAK-4 and MyD88 deficiencies impair IgM responses against T-independent bacterial antigens. Blood. 2014;124(24):3561–71.

McKelvie B, Top K, McCusker C, Letenyi D, Issekutz TB, Issekutz AC. Fatal pneumococcal meningitis in a 7-year-old girl with interleukin-1 receptor activated kinase deficiency (IRAK-4) despite prophylactic antibiotic and IgG responses to *Streptococcus pneumoniae* vaccines. J Clin Immunol. 2014;34(3):267–71.

Medvedev AE, Lentschat A, Kuhns DB, Blanco JC, Salkowski C, Zhang S, et al. Distinct mutations in IRAK-4 confer hyporesponsiveness to lipopolysaccharide and interleukin-1 in a patient with recurrent bacterial infections. J Exp Med. 2003;198(4):521–31.

Medzhitov R, Preston-Hurlburt P, Kopp E, Stadlen A, Chen CQ, Ghosh S, et al. MyD88 is an adaptor protein in the hToll/IL-1 receptor family signaling pathways. Mol Cell. 1998;2(2):253–8.

Picard C, Puel A, Bonnet M, Ku CL, Bustamante J, Yang K, et al. Pyogenic bacterial infections in humans with IRAK-4 deficiency. Science. 2003;299(5615):2076–9.

Picard C, von Bernuth H, Ku CL, Yang K, Puel A, Casanova JL. Inherited human IRAK-4 deficiency: an update. Immunol Res. 2007;38(1–3):347–52.

Picard C, von Bernuth H, Ghandil P, Chrabieh M, Levy O, Arkwright PD, et al. Clinical features and outcome of patients with IRAK-4 and MyD88 deficiency. Medicine. 2010;89(6):403–25.

Puel A, Picard C, Ku CL, Smahi A, Casanova JL. Inherited disorders of NF-kappaB-mediated immunity in man. Curr Opin Immunol. 2004;16(1):34–41.

Suzuki N, Suzuki S, Duncan GS, Millar DG, Wada T, Mirtsos C, et al. Severe impairment of interleukin-1 and Toll-like receptor signalling in mice lacking IRAK-4. Nature. 2002;416(6882):750–4.

Takada H, Yoshikawa H, Imaizumi M, Kitamura T, Takeyama J, Kumaki S, et al. Delayed separation of the umbilical cord in two siblings with interleukin-1 receptor-associated kinase 4 deficiency: rapid screening by flow cytometer. J Pediatr. 2006;148(4):546–8.

von Bernuth H, Ku CL, Rodriguez-Gallego C, Zhang SY, Garty BZ, Marodi L, et al. A fast procedure for the detection of defects in toll-like receptor signaling. Pediatrics. 2006;118(6):2498–503.

von Bernuth H, Picard C, Jin ZB, Pankla R, Xiao H, Ku CL, et al. Pyogenic bacterial infections in humans with MyD88 deficiency. Science. 2008;321(5889):691–6.

Weller S, Bonnet M, Delagreverie H, Israel L, Chrabieh M, Marodi L, et al. IgM(+)IgD(+)CD27(+)B cells are markedly reduced in IRAK-4-, MyD88-, and TIRAP- but not UNC-93B-deficient patients. Blood. 2012;120(25):4992–5001.

TLR3 Deficiency

Henry Y. Lu[1] and Stuart E. Turvey[2,3]
[1]Department of Pediatrics and Experimental
Medicine Program, British Columbia Children's
Hospital, The University of British Columbia,
Vancouver, BC, Canada
[2]Division of Allergy and Clinical Immunology,
Department of Pediatrics and Experimental
Medicine Program, British Columbia Children's
Hospital, The University of British Columbia,
Vancouver, BC, Canada
[3]Willem-Alexander Children's Hospital, Leiden
University Medical Center, Leiden, the
Netherlands

Synonyms

CD283; IIAE2

Definition

Toll-like receptor 3 (TLR3) is a pathogen recognition receptor, which recognizes dsRNA found in viruses to initiate the immune response. Deficiencies in TLR3 function caused by loss-of-function or hypomorphic mutations are linked to increased risk of developing herpes simplex encephalitis.

Introduction

Please refer to the introductory section listed for ▶ UNC93B1 deficiency.

Molecular Genetics and Pathogenesis

Five forms of Toll-like receptor 3 (TLR3) deficiency have been identified as the monogenic cause of isolated herpes simplex encephalitis (HSE) (Table 1). The first report to link TLR3 mutations to HSE identified two unrelated French children who each possessed the same heterozygous autosomal dominant (AD) cytosine to thymine substitution in the *TLR3* gene at nucleotide position 1660 (c.1660C>T) (Zhang et al. 2007). This led to a proline to serine substitution at residue 554 (P554S) in the ectodomain of TLR3. This dominant negative mutation resulted in a partial impairment of TLR3 signaling and responses in patient fibroblasts, but not peripheral blood mononuclear cells (PBMCs), as measured by induction of interferon (IFN)-β and IFN-γ (Zhang et al. 2007). Five relatives of these two children were also heterozygous for the mutation and HSV-1 seropositive, but had never suffered from HSE, suggesting incomplete clinical penetrance. Possible factors that may affect clinical penetrance include age at herpes simplex virus (HSV)-1 infection, size of viral inoculum, and modifier genes (Zhang et al. 2007).

A second report described the first autosomal recessive (AR) form of complete TLR3 deficiency in a young 19-year-old French male who developed HSE at 8 years of age (Guo et al. 2011). This patient carried two compound heterozygous mutations; one allele was the previously described P554S substitution, while the other allele carried a guanine to thymine substitution at nucleotide position 2236 (c.2236G>T), leading to premature termination of translation in the linker region of TLR3 (E746*) (Guo et al. 2011). Patient fibroblasts showed a complete lack of response to TLR3 stimulation. A third report aimed at identifying the proportion of children with HSE caused by deficiencies in TLR3, discovered three additional unique missense TLR3 alleles (Lim et al. 2014). These included a heterozygous G743D+R811I mutation in a patient born to Israeli consanguineous parents, heterozygous L360P mutation in a patient born to non-consanguineous Finnish parents, and homozygous R867Q mutation in a patient born to non-consanguineous Finnish parents.

Further studies employing these patient TLR3-deficient fibroblasts demonstrated the essential

TLR3 Deficiency, Table 1 Known TLR3 mutations associated with HSE

Mutation(s)	Inheritance	Gene expression	Protein expression	Functional impact	Molecular mechanism	No. HSE episodes	Age of episodes	References
p. P554S	AD	Unchanged	Truncated	Partial	Dominant negative	2	5 years, 6.5 years	Zhang et al. (2007)
p. P554S	AD	Unchanged	Truncated	Partial	Dominant negative	1	5 months	Zhang et al. (2007)
p. L360P	AD	Unchanged	Uncleaved	Partial	Dominant negative	3	2.5 years, 22 years, 28 years	Lim et al. (2014)
p. [G743D; R811I]	AD	Unchanged	↓	Partial	Haploinsufficiency	2	8 months, 35 years	Lim et al. (2014)
p. R867Q	AR	Unchanged	Unchanged	Partial	Homozygous for 1 hypomorphic allele	1	24 years onward	Lim et al. (2014)
p. [P554S]; [E746*]	AR	Unchanged	Abnormal glycosylation, truncated	Complete	Compound heterozygous	1	8 years	Lim et al. (2014)

role of TLR3 in protective immunity against herpes simplex virus type I (HSV-1) in the central nervous system (CNS) and redundancy in responses to other dsRNA viruses in the periphery (Guo et al. 2011). In addition, by deriving induced pluripotent stem cells (iPSCs) from TLR3-deficient patient dermal fibroblasts and polarizing them toward neural stem cells (NSCs), neurons, astrocytes, and oligodendrocytes, it was demonstrated that TLR3-deficient neurons are significantly more susceptible to HSV-1 infection (Lafaille et al. 2012). These studies played a large role in definitively establishing a causal relationship between TLR3 deficiencies and increased susceptibility to developing HSE.

Diagnosis

Please refer to the diagnosis section listed for ▶ UNC93B1 deficiency.

Prognostic Factors

Please refer to the prognosis section listed for ▶ UNC93B1 deficiency.

Treatment

Please refer to the treatment section listed for ▶ UNC93B1 deficiency.

Cross-References

▶ IRF3 Deficiency
▶ TBK1 Deficiency
▶ TRAF3 Deficiency
▶ TRIF Deficiency
▶ UNC93B1 Deficiency

References

Guo Y, Audry M, Ciancanelli M, Alsina L, Azevedo J, Herman M, et al. Herpes simplex virus encephalitis in a patient with complete TLR3 deficiency: TLR3 is otherwise redundant in protective immunity. J Exp Med. 2011;208(10):2083–98.

Lafaille FG, Pessach IM, Zhang SY, Ciancanelli MJ, Herman M, Abhyankar A, et al. Impaired intrinsic immunity to HSV-1 in human iPSC-derived TLR3-deficient CNS cells. Nature. 2012;491(7426):769–73.

Lim HK, Seppanen M, Hautala T, Ciancanelli MJ, Itan Y, Lafaille FG, et al. TLR3 deficiency in herpes simplex encephalitis: high allelic heterogeneity and recurrence risk. Neurology. 2014;83(21):1888–97.

Zhang SY, Jouanguy E, Ugolini S, Smahi A, Elain G, Romero P, et al. TLR3 deficiency in patients with herpes simplex encephalitis. Science. 2007;317(5844):1522–7.

TNF Receptor Associated Periodic Syndrome (TRAPS)

Michael F. McDermott
Leeds Institute of Rheumatic and Musculoskeletal Medicine (LIRMM), St James's University Hospital, Leeds, UK

Acronyms

CAPS	Cryopyrin-associated periodic syndrome
CRP	C-reactive protein.
ER	Endoplasmic reticulum
DMARDs	Disease-modifying anti-rheumatic drugs
FHF	Familial Hibernian fever
FMF	Familial Mediterranean fever.
IL-1β	Interleukin-1 beta
IL-6	Interleukin-6
IRE1	Inositol-requiring enzyme 1
LPS	Lipopolysaccharide
miR	microRNA
MKD	Mevalonate kinase deficiency
mROS	Mitochondrial ROS
NF-κB	Nuclear factor-kappaB
NSAIDs	Nonsteroidal anti-inflammatory drugs.
NLRP3	NACHT, LRR and PYD domains-containing protein 3.
ROS	Reactive oxygen species
SAA	Serum amyloid A
TLR	Toll-like receptor

TNF   Tumor necrosis factor
TNFR1   TNF receptor 1
UPR   Uunfolded protein response
XBP1   X-box binding protein 1

Definition

Tumor necrosis factor (TNF) receptor–associated periodic syndrome (TRAPS) is a rare autosomal dominant hereditary disease caused by loss-of-function mutations in *TNFRSF1A* gene, encoding TNF receptor 1 (TNFR1) (MIM# # 142680).

Introduction

The disease was originally termed familial Hibernian fever (FHF), following the first published clinical description of the condition by Williamson and colleagues in a Scottish-Irish family in 1982 (Williamson et al. 1982). FHF was found to be inherited in an autosomal dominant manner and the inflammatory attacks were accompanied by fevers, abdominal pain, skin rashes and joint pains, which bore some resemblance to typical attacks of familial Mediterranean fever (FMF). However, the duration of TRAPS attacks were much longer, and accompanied by myalgias, with centripetal migration and a prompt response to corticosteroids but relatively poor response to colchicine suggested differences from FMF. With the genetic identification of the disease-causing mutations of TRAPS, in 1999 (McDermott et al. 1999), it became apparent that TRAPS was not limited to a specific ethnic groups, but was present in most ethnicities (Lachmann 2011). The estimated incidence of TRAPS is 1/100,000 among populations of Northern-European ancestry. Furthermore, the disease was named TRAPS, as the new name reflected the molecular basis of the disorder.

Genetics

The *TNFRSF1A* gene, encoding TNF receptor 1 (TNFR1) was identified as the susceptibility gene for TRAPS, in 1999 (McDermott et al.

1999); most of the pathogenic mutations are heterozygous single-nucleotide missense variants localized in extracellular, cysteine rich domains of the 55 kDa (p55) receptor molecule. Two low penetrance TNFR1 variants, R92Q and P46, are associated with milder disease, with later onset, and amyloidosis has not been reported. The diagnosis of TRAPS depends on molecular genetic analysis.

Pathogenesis

The pathogenesis of TRAPS is complex; co-expression of the mutated and wild type receptor appears to be required in most cases. Unlike the pathophysiology of other hereditary fevers, for example cryopyrin-associated periodic syndrome (CAPS), where there is one predominant mechanism, in the case of TRAPS several alternative, but mutually non-exclusive, mechanisms have been proposed over the years. Intracellular retention of the mutated receptor is associated with several pathological responses including increased ER-stress, excessive mitochondrial reactive oxygen species (Bulua et al. 2011; Dickie et al. 2012) (mROS) and enhanced nuclear factor κB (NF-κB) activation. Other proposed pathogenic mechanisms include abnormal TNFR1 cleavage (McDermott et al. 1999); increased activation of nuclear factor kappa B (NF-κB)/mitogen-activated protein kinase; ligand-independent activation of mutant TNFR1. An important consequence of intracellular retention of TNFR1 is endoplasmic reticulum (ER) stress and an unfolded protein response (UPR) in affected cells. The physiological response of intracellular accumulation of misfolded protein is increased production of chaperone proteins, to help with trafficking of the mutated protein from the ER, thereby reducing the level of ER stress. Upregulation of UPR response genes has been reported in TRAPS patients (Bulua et al. 2011), with activation of ER-associated endonuclease, inositol-requiring enzyme 1 (IRE-1), which is one of the three ER stress sensors, resulting in hyper-responsiveness to lipopolysaccharide (LPS) and release of pro-inflammatory cytokines, IL-1β, TNF and IL-6.

More recent studies have suggested other mechanisms to explain LPS hyperresponsiveness, whereby activated IRE1 exerts its endonuclease function to target a number of mRNA and miR species, thereby constraining protein production and resolving ER stress (Maurel et al. 2014). Two miRNA species, in particular miR155 and miR146a, are specific targets of IRE1, and these two miRNA species have previously been identified as regulators of cellular response to LPS (Schulte et al. 2013).

Enhanced inflammatory cytokine production is mediated by sustained phosphorylation of JNK and p38, and maintained by ROS from dysfunctional mitochondria (Dickie et al. 2012). Furthermore, ROS may inactivate MAPK phosphatases and perpetuate MAPK activation (Kamata et al. 2005) in cells from patients with TRAPS. Increased JNK and p38 are associated with enhanced activation of nuclear factor κB (NF-κB), and augmented transcription of the pro-inflammatory cytokines.

In summary, several pathogenic mechanisms operate synergistically in TRAPS pathogenesis, including non-canonical UPR, dysregulated ROS and impaired autophagy. It is likely that some mechanisms are mutation and cell–type specific, thereby explaining some of the clinical heterogeneity of TRAPS and the underlying pathological processes.

Clinical Manifestations

Systemic Manifestations

Most patients report intermittent attacks of fever, with abdominal and/or chest pains due to serositis of the peritoneum/pleura, myalgia with or without overlying migratory rash, and arthralgia and/or arthritis. Most patients with TRAPS are symptomatic from childhood, with a minority of patients having continuous symptoms; furthermore, many of these patients exhibit biochemical evidence of an inflammatory response even in the absence of symptoms. Up to 15% of these patients developed potentially life-threatening systemic amyloidosis prior to the inauguration (initiation) of effective therapies.

Clinical Presentation and Features

The disease course in TRAPS varies from episodic flares in a majority of patients, continuous symptoms in a significant minority and clinically asymptomatic individuals with biochemical evidence of systemic inflammatory response (raised C-reactive protein and/or serum amyloid A). Most patients first develop symptoms during childhood but late presentations in adulthood has been reported.

Cutaneous Manifestations

A variety of cutaneous manifestations, such as erysipelas-like erythema, edematous plaques, discrete reticulate or serpiginous lesions in 70% of patients, and urticaria have been reported in TRAPS (Toro et al. 2000). Both dermal perivascular lymphocytic and monocytic infiltrates are seen on skin biopsies. At onset, erythematous macules or papules are present, but these tend to migrate in a centrifugal direction to form larger plaques at the limb extremities, or on the torso. MRI studies have demonstrated underlying muscle edema, and subsequent histological findings have shown this to be mainly due to monocytic fasciitis (Hull et al. 2002).

Musculoskeletal Manifestations

In addition to serositis abdominal pain may also originate from muscle involvement in the abdominal wall (Cantarini et al. 2010). Arthralgias are much more common than frank arthritis, and, are usually non-erosive, asymmetrical oligo- or monoarthritis with a predilection for larger joints. Periorbital edema, when present, is pathognomonic of TRAPS, and may be associated with uveitis or conjunctivitis.

Other Manifestations

Other clinical manifestations include aseptic meningitis, scrotal swelling and pain, and behavioral changes.

Clinical Data from Registries

A report from the Eurofever/Eurotraps registry describes the largest single cohort of adult (n = 105) and pediatric patients (n = 53) with TRAPS (Lachmann et al. 2014). The median age of symptom onset was 4.3 years, with some patients symptomatic from age 2 months; adult onset of TRAPS was seen in 22% with some up to the age of 63 years. The most commonly reported symptoms included fevers (88%), limb pain (85%), abdominal pain (74%) and rashes (63%). When the R92Q and P46L patients were analyzed separately a distinct disease phenotype, with a lower incidence of familial disease emerged, more headaches with fewer rashes and eye manifestations.

Laboratory Findings

Although routine laboratory tests are usually not diagnostic in patients with TRAPS, these usually reveal elevated acute phase response proteins during acute attacks, with associated neutrophilia and thrombocytosis, elevated C-reactive protein (CRP), erythrocyte sedimentation rate (ESR) and serum amyloid A (SAA), haptoglobin and fibrinogen levels. Although these variables may fluctuate considerably with attacks, in some patients they remain elevated, even between attacks. In untreated cases, there is often evidence of anemia of chronic disease with polyclonal hyper-gammaglobulinemia. As part of follow up, patients have regular testing CRP and SAA levels, if available, and routine blood counts. It is vital to check for development of amyloidosis by regular testing for proteinuria and amyloid scans, if available.

Diagnosis

There are no agreed clinical diagnostic criteria for TRAPS, unlike some other hereditary fevers such as FMF and CAPS. A diagnosis of TRAPS is mainly dependent on molecular analysis of *TNFRSF1A* gene. In an attempt to develop evidence-based clinical classification criteria for TRAPS and other hereditary fevers syndromes, clinical information from well-defined groups of patients with FMF, mevalonate kinase deficiency

(MKD), CAPS and TRAPS were analysed (Federici et al. 2015); patients were considered to be the 'gold standard' based on the presence of a confirmatory genetic test. In the case of TRAPS, only patients who had confirmed heterozygous *TNFRSF1A* mutations were included; patients with R92Q genotype, or uncertain variants were excluded. The clinical features most associated with TRAPS are shown in Table 1, as well as the score assigned to these features. A score ≥ 43 was highly suggestive of TRAPS. The overall sensitivity of these classification criteria was 56%, with a specificity of 84%. Although helpful, the low sensitivity of these classification criteria means that clinicians still rely heavily on genetic investigations to confirm the diagnosis of TRAPS. Advances in DNA sequencing technology has resulted in increased numbers of patients being diagnosed with TRAPS. In this regard one significant advantage of massive parallel sequencing over standard Sanger sequencing-based analysis is that cases of somatic mosaicism can be identified by this technology.

Treatment

The first choice of therapy for more severely affected patients is currently anti-interleukin (IL)-1 biological agents. Corticosteroids are very effective in treating patients with TRAPS but their use is limited due to long term toxicity. However, corticosteroids can be often used with or without non-steroidal anti-inflammatory drugs (NSAIDs) to terminate acute attacks. A short course of prednisolone (0.5–1 mg 1 mg/kg/d) given for 5–10 days is often sufficient in acute attacks. Patients with low penetrance mutations may respond to colchicine and generally have a more favorable response to TNF blockade. The general principles of TRAPS management have been proposed by a group of experts in the field of autoinflammatory diseases, with recommendations for management of CAPS, TRAPS and MKD (ter Haar et al. 2015). Treatment strategy is divided into two main groups: firstly therapeutic measures to deal with acute attacks

TNF Receptor Associated Periodic Syndrome (TRAPS), Table 1 Clinical features previously reported in TRAPS and features highly predictive of the disease

General and organ specific manifestations	Clinical features previously reported in TRAPS	Clinical features highly predictive of TRAPS[a]
Family history	Sporadic or AD	Family history (score 7)
Duration of fevers/ episode	1–3 weeks, continuous	> 6 days (score 19)
Cutaneous	Centrifugal migratory erythema, edematous plaques, annular and serpiginous patches, urticaria-like lesions	Typical migratory rash (score 18)
Musculoskeletal	Muscle cramps, migratory myalgias, fasciitis, arthralgias, oligo-monoarthritis, sacroileitis	Myalgia (score 6)
Gastrointestinal	Peritonitis-like picture, abdominal pain, vomiting	Absence of vomiting (ter Haar et al. 2015), absence of aphthous stomatitis (Ozen et al. 2017)
Ocular	Periorbital edema, conjunctivitis, ocular pain, uveitis	Periorbital edema (score 21),
Respiratory	Chest pain, pleurisy	Nil
Central nervous	Headache, aseptic meningitis, optic neuritis, behavioral abnormalities	Nil
Urogenital	Urethral strictures, scrotal pain	Nil
Cardiovascular	Pericarditis, myocarditis, ventricular tachycardia, restrictive cardiomyopathy, risk of myocardial infarction and arterial thrombosis	Nil
Lymphatic	Swollen and painful lymph nodes	Nil
Renal	Amyloidosis-related nephrotic syndrome	Nil
Autonomic nervous	Orthostatic hypotension, bowel disturbance	Nil

[a]A score equal and greater than 43 was highly suggestive of TRAPS

and then therapies used on a regular basis to control either subacute inflammation, symptomatic flares and, in the long run, prevent complications developing, such as amyloidosis.

Tumor Necrosis Factor (TNF) Inhibitors

Selective therapies targeting the TNF signaling pathway were the first biologic to be used in TRAPS. Etanercept proved to have limited efficacy despite biological plausibility. There are conflicting accounts regarding the effectiveness of etanercept in arresting or reversing the onset of renal amyloidosis, with some reports describing both the slowing and reversal of amyloidosis, but also the subsequent onset of proteinuria, with amyloid present on renal biopsy, while taking etanercept. A retrospective study that looked at treatment outcomes of 134 patients with hereditary fevers syndromes (FMF, MKD and TRAPS), included

47 patients with TRAPS. Out of 41 patients who received biologics, 54% received etanercept as a first agent whilst the rest received either anakinra (41%) or canakinumab (5%) (Ozen et al. 2017). Patients who were treated with anakinra were statistically more likely to achieve complete clinical and biochemical remission compared to patients who received etanercept.

Interleukin (IL)-1 and IL-6 Inhibitors

Over the years IL-1 blocking agents have become a favored treatment modality in TRAPS and a number of case reports describe sustained response to anakinra (Sacré et al. 2008). There has been a number of studies looking at the anti-IL-1β monoclonal antibody, canakinumab in patients with TRAPS. An open label phase II study, which included 19 patients, showed a rapid response to canakinumab, with the median time to remission being only 4 days (Gattorno et al. 2008).

These results were replicated in a much larger, phase III randomized controlled trial, which looked at the efficacy of canakinumab in patients with colchicine-resistant FMF, MKD and TRAPS. The first results of this trial were reported in 2016 (Benedetti et al. 2016) and the final publication in 2018 (De Benedetti et al. 2018). The primary objective of the trial was to show that canakinumab 150 mg by subcutaneous injection every 4 weeks, is superior to placebo in achieving a clinical response, defined as resolution of the index flare at Day 15 and no new disease flares over 16 weeks. In the case of TRAPS this was achieved by 45.5% of patients treated with canakinumab compared to 8.3% who received placebo (OR = 9.17, p = 0.005). Similar results were also seen for secondary objectives, which looked at the proportion of patients who achieved a physician global assessment (PGA) of disease activity <2 (minimal/none), a CRP $\leq$10 mg/L and an SAA level $\leq$ 10 mg/L at week 16. Compared to patients on placebo, canakinumab treated patients achieved statistically superior results in all 3 measures: PGA (OR = 23.79, p = 0.0028), CRP (OR = 6.64, p = 0.0149) and SAA (OR = 16.69, p = 0.0235).

In the 2018 paper it was further reported that significantly more patients on canakinumab had a complete response than the placebo group at week 16: 61% vs. 6% of patients with colchicine-resistant FMF (P < 0.001), 35% versus 6% of those with mevalonate kinase deficiency (P = 0.003), and 45% versus 8% of those with TRAPS (P = 0.006). After week 16, an extended dosing regimen (every 8 weeks) maintained disease control in 46% of patients with colchicine-resistant FMF, 23% of those with mevalonate kinase deficiency, and 53% of those with TRAPS. The most frequent adverse events were infections (173.3, 313.5, and 148.0 per 100 patient-years among patients with colchicine-resistant FMF, mevalonate kinase deficiency, and those with TRAPS, respectively), with no serious infections in the TRAPS cohort (0.0 per 100 patient-years). Considering the biological effects of *TNFRSF1A* mutations, it is quite plausible that biological therapies targeting IL-6 might

also be effective. Studies of tocilizumab in TRAPS have been limited, but reports suggest that it may also be effective for some patients.

Potential Novel Treatment Pathways

New small molecule inhibitors of NACHT, LRR and PYD domains-containing protein 3 (NLRP3), or the drugs that selectively target inositol-requiring enzyme/X-box binding protein 1 (IRE1/XBP1) axis might be options for future treatment of TRAPS. New small-molecule inhibitors of NLRP3 are currently in development and some have entered early clinical trials (Coll et al. 2015). Another potential novel therapeutic approach is to target the molecules implicated in ER stress and associated hyperinflammatory response and there are both animal models demonstrating the potential therapeutic benefits using this approach. Lastly, inhibition of XBP1, which provides a convergence point for both ER- stress and TLR-mediated inflammation, might prove to be a suitable target in the future (Savic et al. 2014).

Prognosis

Prior to the introduction of biologic response modifiers (biologics) for TRAPS, most of these patients were over-reliant on corticosteroids for symptomatic control. Furthermore, the initial favorable response to corticosteroids tends to decrease over time. In addition, 25% of patients carrying high- penetrance *TNFRSF1A* variants were considered to be at risk of developing amyloidosis but the more recent report from the Eurofever/Eurotraps registry found a 10% of incidence of amyloidosis (Cantarini et al. 2010).

References

Benedetti FD, Anton J, Gattorno M, Lachmann H, Kone-Paut I, Ozen S. A phase III pivotal umbrella trial of canakinumab in patients with autoinflammatory periodic fever syndromes (colchicine resistant FMF, HIDS/MKD and TRAPS). Ann Rheum Dis. 2016;75(Suppl 2):615–6.

Bulua AC, Simon A, Maddipati R, Pelletier M, Park H, Kim KY, Sack MN, Kastner DL, Siegel RM. Mitochondrial reactive oxygen species promote production of proinflammatory cytokines and are elevated in TNFR1-associated periodic syndrome (TRAPS). J Exp Med. 2011;208(3):519–33.

Cantarini L, Lucherini OM, Baldari CT, Laghi Pasini F, Galeazzi M. Familial clustering of recurrent pericarditis may disclose tumour necrosis factor receptor-associated periodic syndrome. Clin Exp Rheumatol. 2010;28(3):405–7.

Coll RC, Robertson AA, Chae JJ, Higgins SC, Muñoz-Planillo R, Inserra MC, Vetter I, Dungan LS, Monks BG, Stutz A, Croker DE, Butler MS, Haneklaus M, Sutton CE, Núñez G, Latz E, Kastner DL, Mills KH, Masters SL, Schroder K, Cooper MA, O'Neill LA. A small-molecule inhibitor of the NLRP3 inflammasome for the treatment of inflammatory diseases. Nat Med. 2015;21(3):248–55.

De Benedetti F, Gattorno M, Anton J, Ben-Chetrit E, Frenkel J, Hoffman HM, Koné-Paut I, Lachmann HJ, Ozen S, Simon A, Zeft A, Calvo Penades I, Moutschen M, Quartier P, Kasapcopur O, Shcherbina A, Hofer M, Hashkes PJ, Van der Hilst J, Hara R, Bujan-Rivas S, Constantin T, Gul A, Livneh A, Brogan P, Cattalini M, Obici L, Lheritier K, Speziale A, Junge G. Canakinumab for the treatment of autoinflammatory recurrent fever syndromes. N Engl J Med. 2018;378(20):1908–19.

Dickie LJ, Aziz AM, Savic S, Lucherini OM, Cantarini L, Geiler J, Wong CH, Coughlan R, Lane T, Lachmann HJ, Hawkins PN, Robinson PA, Emery P, McGonagle D, McDermott MF. Involvement of X-box binding protein 1 and reactive oxygen species pathways in the pathogenesis of tumour necrosis factor receptor-associated periodic syndrome. Ann Rheum Dis. 2012;71(12):2035–43.

Federici S, Sormani MP, Ozen S, Lachmann HJ, Amaryan G, Woo P, Koné-Paut I, Dewarrat N, Cantarini L, Insalaco A, Uziel Y, Rigante D, Quartier P, Demirkaya E, Herlin T, Meini A, Fabio G, Kallinich T, Martino S, Butbul AY, Olivieri A, Kuemmerle-Deschner J, Neven B, Simon A, Ozdogan H, Touitou I, Frenkel J, Hofer M, Martini A, Ruperto N, Gattorno M. Paediatric rheumatology international trials organisation (PRINTO) and Eurofever project. Evidence-based provisional clinical classification criteria for autoinflammatory periodic fevers. Ann Rheum Dis. 2015;74(5):799–805.

Gattorno M, Pelagatti MA, Meini A, Obici L, Barcellona R, Federici S, Buoncompagni A, Plebani A, Merlini G, Martini A. Persistent efficacy of anakinra in patients with tumor necrosis factor receptor-associated periodic syndrome. Arthritis Rheum. 2008;58(5):1516–20.

Hull KM, Wong K, Wood GM, Chu WS, Kastner DL. Monocytic fasciitis: a newly recognized clinical feature of tumor necrosis factor receptor dysfunction. Arthritis Rheum. 2002;46(8):2189–94.

Kamata H, Honda S, Maeda S, Chang L, Hirata H, Karin M. Reactive oxygen species promote TNFalpha-induced death and sustained JNK activation by inhibiting MAP kinase phosphatases. Cell. 2005;120(5):649–61.

Lachmann HJ. Clinical immunology review series: an approach to the patient with a periodic fever syndrome. Clin Exp Immunol. 2011;165(3):301–9.

Lachmann HJ, Papa R, Gerhold K, Obici L, Touitou I, Cantarini L, Frenkel J, Anton J, Kone-Paut I, Cattalini M, Bader-Meunier B, Insalaco A, Hentgen V, Merino R, Modesto C, Toplak N, Berendes R, Ozen S, Cimaz R, Jansson A, Brogan PA, Hawkins PN, Ruperto N, Martini A, Woo P, Gattorno M. Paediatric rheumatology international trials organisation (PRINTO), the EUROTRAPS and the Eurofever project. The phenotype of TNF receptor-associated autoinflammatory syndrome (TRAPS) at presentation: a series of 158 cases from the Eurofever/EUROTRAPS international registry. Ann Rheum Dis. 2014;73(12):2160–7.

Maurel M, Chevet E, Tavernier J, Gerlo S. Getting RIDD of RNA: IRE1 in cell fate regulation. Trends Biochem Sci. 2014;39(5):245–54.

McDermott MF, Aksentijevich I, Galon J, McDermott EM, Ogunkolade BW, Centola M, Mansfield E, Gadina M, Karenko L, Pettersson T, McCarthy J, Frucht DM, Aringer M, Torosyan Y, Teppo AM, Wilson M, Karaarslan HM, Wan Y, Todd I, Wood G, Schlimgen R, Kumarajeewa TR, Cooper SM, Vella JP, Amos CI, Mulley J, Quane KA, Molloy MG, Ranki A, Powell RJ, Hitman GA, O'Shea JJ, Kastner DL. Germline mutations in the extracellular domains of the 55 kDa TNF receptor, TNFR1, define a family of dominantly inherited autoinflammatory syndromes. Cell. 1999;97(1):133–44.

Ozen S, Kuemmerle-Deschner JB, Cimaz R, Livneh A, Quartier P, Kone-Paut I, Zeft A, Spalding S, Gul A, Hentgen V, Savic S, Foeldvari I, Frenkel J, Cantarini L, Patel D, Weiss J, Marinsek N, Degun R, Lomax KG, Lachmann HJ. International retrospective chart review of treatment patterns in severe familial Mediterranean fever, tumor necrosis factor receptor-associated periodic syndrome, and mevalonate kinase deficiency/hyperimmunoglobulinemia D syndrome. Arthritis Care Res (Hoboken). 2017;69(4):578–86.

Sacré K, Brihaye B, Lidove O, Papo T, Pocidalo MA, Cuisset L, Dodé C. Dramatic improvement following interleukin 1beta blockade in tumor necrosis factor receptor-1-associated syndrome (TRAPS) resistant to anti-TNF-alpha therapy. J Rheumatol. 2008;35(2):357–8.

Savic S, Ouboussad L, Dickie LJ, Geiler J, Wong C, Doody GM, Churchman SM, Ponchel F, Emery P, Cook GP, Buch MH, Tooze RM, McDermott MF. TLR dependent XBP-1 activation induces an autocrine loop in rheumatoid arthritis synoviocytes. J Autoimmun. 2014;50:59–66.

Schulte LN, Westermann AJ, Vogel J. Differential activation and functional specialization of miR-146 and miR-155 in innate immune sensing. Nucleic Acids Res. 2013;41:542–53.

ter Haar NM, Oswald M, Jeyaratnam J, Anton J, Barron KS, Brogan PA, Cantarini L, Galeotti C, Grateau G, Hentgen V, Hofer M, Kallinich T, Kone-Paut I, Lachmann

HJ, Ozdogan H, Ozen S, Russo R, Simon A, Uziel Y, Wouters C, Feldman BM, Vastert SJ, Wulffraat NM, Benseler SM, Frenkel J, Gattorno M, Kuemmerle-Deschner JB. Recommendations for the management of autoinflammatory diseases. Ann Rheum Dis. 2015;74(9):1636–44.

Toro JR, Aksentijevich I, Hull K, Dean J, Kastner DL. Tumor necrosis factor receptor-associated periodic syndrome: a novel syndrome with cutaneous manifestations. Arch Dermatol. 2000;136(12):1487–94.

Williamson LM, Hull D, Mehta R, Reeves WG, Robinson BH, Toghill PJ. Familial Hibernian fever. Q J Med. 1982;51(204):469–80.

TNFRSF4

▶ TNFRSF4 (OX40) Deficiency

TNFRSF4 (OX40) Deficiency

Robert P. Nelson
Divisions of Hematology and Oncology, Stem
Cell Transplant Program, Indiana University (IU)
School of Medicine and the IU Bren and Simon
Cancer Center, Indianapolis, IN, USA
Pediatric Immunodeficiency Clinic, Riley
Hospital for Children at Indiana University
Health, Indianapolis, IN, USA
Medicine and Pediatrics, Indiana University
School of Medicine, Immunohematology and
Transplantation, Indianapolis, IN, USA

Synonyms

CD134; TNFRSF4

Definition

Deficiency of tumor necrosis factor receptor superfamily, member 4 (TNFRSF4), previously called OX40, is associated to the development of childhood Kaposi sarcoma.

Introduction

The human OX-40 receptor (OX40R) cell surface antigen is a CD4+ T cell costimulatory receptor. The gene for its ligand *OX40L (TNFSF4)* was cloned by Godfrey et al., who found that it encodes protein gp34, a type II transmembrane antigen expressed by human T cell lymphotropic virus 1-infected cells. OX-40R ligation enhanced CD4+ T cell proliferation induced by phorbol myristate acetate (PMA), phytohemagglutinin (PHA), and anti-CD3 (Godfrey et al. 1994). Weinberg et al. adoptively transferred myelin basic protein (MBP)-specific encephalitogenic T helper cells into a murine host and found the central nervous system (CNS), but not the spleen or blood, to be enriched with the specific T cells. The donor cell number peaked on the 1st day of disease in the spinal cord and cerebrospinal fluid (CSF) and expressed OX40R. In contrast, the IL-2 receptor (CD25) and TH1 cytokine mRNA were enriched in all transferred T cells in all tissue sites (Weinberg et al. 1994). These findings suggested that the quantity, the activation state, and the level of lymphokine production at the site of inflammation determine the autoimmune potential of Ag-specific effector and that the OX40R-OX40L circuit plays a role in driving the autoreactivity. Support for the observations was provided by experiments that OX-40 immunotoxin ameliorates EAE without affecting peripheral T cells (Weinberg et al. 1996).

Function

Both the dose and affinity of antigen presented to lymphocytes are important for the regulation of IL-2, IL-4, and IFN-gamma production, which provide input that designates differentiation to TH1 and TH2 immune responses. Ligation of surface accessory receptors alters the dose of antigen required for differentiation and activation, and levels of expression of multiple accessory molecular pairs integrate with the number and affinity of peptide-MHC complexes (Weinberg et al. 1994). CD28 is a costimulatory molecule expressed constitutively on resting T cells, and

OX-40R is expressed on activated T cells. Costimulatory signals provided by OX40 alone appear to promote TH2 and to suppress TH1 differentiation, whereas simultaneous CD28 and OX-40 activation stimulate TH1 differentiation. Engagement of the OX40R with OX-40L or antibody agonists sends strong costimulatory signals to effector T cells. In humans, OX40R expression participates in regulation of autoimmune, alloimmune, and tumor immunity. Diabetes mellitus, multiple sclerosis, rheumatoid arthritis, inflammatory bowel disease, and autoimmune uveitis are all mediated by autoantigen-specific CD4+ T cells that rely in part on OX-40 costimulatory signals (Xiao et al. 2012). OX-40R is detectable on peripheral blood lymphocytes of haploidentical human transplant recipients who develop acute graft-versus-host disease (GvHD). Also, tumor antigen-specific OX40R+ lymphocytes are present within primary tumors and lymph nodes of patients with a number of human malignancies (Tittle et al. 1997; Petty et al. 2002).

The mechanism of autoimmune reactivity mediated by OX-40R is related to its expression on FOXp3 (+) regulatory T cells (Tregs). Absence of OX40R costimulation impairs CD4+ T cell-driven autoimmunity in FOXp3-deficient mice, and naive mice expressing OX40R are capable of expanding FOXp3 (+) Tregs, but the expanded Tregs are functionally impaired and phenotypically exhausted. Exogenous IL-2 agonists combined with OX40R can rescue exhausted Tregs, and the rescued cells are highly suppressive. Thus, OX40 promotes immune tolerance by interacting with Tregs. Recent evidence suggests that liver kinase B1 (LKB1) regulates the metabolic and functional fitness of Treg cells in the control of immune tolerance and homeostasis and the expression of immune regulatory molecules, including OX40 (Yang et al. 2017).

In humans, OX40L/OX40R signals are implicated in Treg dysfunction observed in human SLE (Jacquemin et al. 2018). Antigen-presenting cells from patients with active SLE mediate Treg dysfunction in an OX40L-dependent manner, and OX40L-expressing cells localize with Foxp3+ cells in active skin lesions (Jacquemin et al. 2018).

Clinical Manifestations

The OX40 deficiency belongs to the small group of combined immunodeficiency diseases, in that the clinical phenotype appears to be remarkably narrow and specific. OX40 defects segregate with a childhood form of Kaposi sarcoma (KS), an endothelial tumor that occurs rarely in persons infected with human herpes virus 8 (HHV-8) and very rarely in children (Stiller et al. 2014). HHV-8-infected endothelial cells express high levels of OX40L, suggesting that OX40 interaction is essential for anti-HHV-8 immunity. Classic KS of childhood that occurs has been associated in children with monogenic defects in OX40 (*TNFRSF4*), *WAS*, *IFNGR1*, and *STIM1*.

Three unrelated Turkish children with classic KS born to first-cousin parents included a female who developed disseminated cutaneous and mucosal KS at 2 years of age and expired within 3 months despite treatment with vincristine. Two other children described in the report developed milder forms of KS (Sahin et al. 2010). One was a 19-year-old Turkish woman diagnosed with classic KS at the age of 14, following successful treatment for visceral Leishmaniasis at the age of 9. Byun et al. reported an autosomal recessive OX40 deficiency in an otherwise healthy adult with a history of childhood-onset classic KS. The group found OX40L abundantly expressed in KS lesions, but the mutated OX40 protein in the patient was poorly expressed on the cell surface and failed to bind OX40L, resulting in complete functional OX40 deficiency (Byun et al. 2013).

Diagnoses and Laboratory Testing

Because KS occurs in human immunodeficiency virus (HIV) infection, testing for HIV infection is the first step prior to the initiation of and exhaustive molecular evaluation, in a patient with childhood KS. Flow cytometry to measure OX40 in T cells and/or gene sequencing analysis of the TNFRSF14 (OX40) gene might report defects to establish definitive diagnosis. HHV-8 viremia is expected to be positive.

Byun et al. described the genetic and immunological phenotypes of a patient with OX40 deficiency and demonstrated lower proportions of "nonnaive" T cell subsets compared to age-matched healthy controls. Memory CD4$^+$ T cell responses to recall antigens were impaired, as assessed by cytokine production and proliferative responses to a broad panel of recall antigens. Despite being vaccinated twice with BCG, PBMCs from this patient produced IFN-γ and IL-10 in similar quantities as healthy controls not vaccinated with BCG. The OX40-deficient patient showed protective antibody titers to tetanus toxoid, CMV, VZV, HSV-1, and EBV, although IFN-γ production in response to stimulation with the same antigens was low. There was a low frequency of circulating memory B cells. The proportion of CD10$^-$CD27$^+$ memory B cells within the total B cell population was lower and that of CD10$^-$CD27$^-$ naive B cells higher; however, the proportions of isotype-switched memory B cells were normal. These data, together with the lack of excessive infections with high-grade encapsulated organisms, suggest that antibody-mediated immunity is intact in OX40-deficient patients. There was low CD4+ T cell effector memory deficit with impaired CD4+ T cell responses to recall antigens. The proportion of effector memory CD8+ T cells was also diminished. These findings and detailed analyses suggest that human OX40 is necessary for robust CD4+ T cell memory and that it confers a rather specific protective immunity against HHV-8 infection in endothelial cells (Byun et al. 2013).

Treatment/Prognosis

The treatment of childhood KS depends on whether there is localized or disseminated disease. Systemic chemotherapy treatment (including doxorubicin, daunorubicin, paclitaxel, vincristine, etoposide, and bleomycin) is recommended in cases of pediatric KS with systemic disease, and intralesional chemotherapy (vinblastine, retinoic acid, radiotherapy) or surgical resection is used in cases of localized disease.

Referral to a tertiary center with expertise for the management of rare cancers and of immunodeficiency diseases is recommended.

Particular attention is given to address inflammatory conditions that require iatrogenic immunosuppression and anti-inflammatory therapy that exacerbate or synergistically add to the immunodeficiency's "potency" overall. Optimal, early high-complexity care requires consideration before morbid complications ensue. Antiviral prophylaxis to reduce burden of HHV-8 infection might be considered. In advanced-stage KS, chemotherapy with pegylated liposomal doxorubicin or paclitaxel is the most common treatment (Cesarman et al. 2019). The disorder is one that may be amenable to hematopoietic cell transplantation (HCT), given the indolent nature of HHV-8 infections, the presence of which would not be an absolute contraindication to HCT.

Cross-References

▶ STIM1 Deficiency
▶ Wiskott-Aldrich Syndrome Deficiency

References

Byun M, Ma CS, Akcay A, et al. Inherited human OX40 deficiency underlying classic Kaposi sarcoma of childhood. J Exp Med. 2013;210:1743–59.

Cesarman E, Damania B, Krown SE, Martin J, Bower M, Whitby D. Kaposi sarcoma. Nat Rev Dis Primers. 2019;5:9.

Godfrey WR, Fagnoni FF, Harara MA, Buck D, Engleman EG. Identification of a human OX-40 ligand, a costimulator of CD4+ T cells with homology to tumor necrosis factor. J Exp Med. 1994;180:757–62.

Jacquemin C, Augusto JF, Scherlinger M, et al. OX40L/OX40 axis impairs follicular and natural Treg function in human SLE. JCI Insight. 2018;3(24). pii: 122167. https://doi.org/10.1172/jci.insight.122167.

Petty JK, He K, Corless CL, Vetto JT, Weinberg AD. Survival in human colorectal cancer correlates with expression of the T-cell costimulatory molecule OX-40 (CD134). Am J Surg. 2002;183:512–8.

Sahin G, Palanduz A, Aydogan G, et al. Classic Kaposi sarcoma in 3 unrelated Turkish children born to consanguineous kindreds. Pediatrics. 2010;125:e704–8.

Stiller CA, Trama A, Brewster DH, et al. Descriptive epidemiology of Kaposi sarcoma in Europe. Report from the RARECARE project. Cancer Epidemiol. 2014;38:670–8.

Tittle TV, Weinberg AD, Steinkeler CN, Maziarz RT. Expression of the T-cell activation antigen, OX-40, identifies alloreactive T cells in acute graft-versus-host disease. Blood. 1997;89:4652–8.

Weinberg AD, Wallin JJ, Jones RE, et al. Target organ-specific up-regulation of the MRC OX-40 marker and selective production of Th1 lymphokine mRNA by encephalitogenic T helper cells isolated from the spinal cord of rats with experimental autoimmune encephalomyelitis. J Immunol. 1994;152:4712–21.

Weinberg AD, Bourdette DN, Sullivan TJ, et al. Selective depletion of myelin-reactive T cells with the anti-OX-40 antibody ameliorates autoimmune encephalomyelitis. Nat Med. 1996;2:183–9.

Xiao X, Gong W, Demirci G, et al. New insights on OX40 in the control of T cell immunity and immune tolerance in vivo. J Immunol. 2012;188:892–901.

Yang K, Blanco DB, Neale G, et al. Homeostatic control of metabolic and functional fitness of Treg cells by LKB1 signalling. Nature. 2017;548:602–6.

TNFS12: TWEAK Deficiency

Javier Chinen
Division of Allergy and Immunology, Department of Pediatrics, Baylor College of Medicine, Texas Children's Hospital, The Woodlands, TX, USA

Introduction

TNFS12 encodes a protein also known as TNF-related weak inducer of apoptosis or TWEAK. It contains seven exons and is located in chromosome 17p13.1 (Pradet-Balade et al. 2002; Chicheportiche et al. 1997). A deleterious mutation in this gene has been associated with an antibody deficiency.

TNFS12 is a member of the tumor necrosis factor superfamily (TNFS), involved in cytotoxicity and induction of apoptosis (Wang et al. 2013). TNFS12, through its receptor TWEAKR, is also a regulator of angiogenesis and promotes the proliferation of endothelial cells (Wiley et al. 2001). TNFSF12 is expressed in myeloid cells and T cells, and its expression is increased during inflammation.

Clinical Presentation

To date, three individuals of one family have been reported (Wang et al. 2013). They presented with recurrent respiratory infections since infancy, including pneumonias and sinusitis, and ear infections. Frequency of infections decreased during adulthood. Other medical problems included neutropenia, thrombocytopenia, and multiple warts. Laboratory testing results included undetectable or decreased serum levels of immunoglobulins IgM, IgG, and IgA and non-protective antibody titers of specific antibodies to childhood vaccines. B cells showed a predominance of the IgM+IgD+ naïve B cell phenotype. All three patients presented with a heterozygous mutation in exon 6 of the *TNFSF12* gene, resulting in an R145C change in the TNF homology domain. It was postulated that this mutation is in a protein domain that is essential for trimerization and ligand binding.

Molecular Mechanisms: In Vitro Studies

In experiments comparing wild-type TNFSF12 and the mutant R145C TNFS12, several observations demonstrated the deleterious effects of this mutation (Wang et al. 2013). R145C TNFSF12 failed to induce apoptosis in HT29 cells in the presence of gamma interferon. The mutant protein was expressed, secreted, and resulted in abnormally high molecular weight aggregates. The mutant protein was able to bind its receptor Fn14, but was unable to induce NFKB activation and cell death. R145C TNFSF12 also bound stronger to BAFF than wild-type TNFS12, and the heterodimer of BAFF with the mutant protein decreased the production of IgG and IgA.

Overall, the data suggested that this variant TNFSF12 may dominantly inhibit B cell survival and proliferation as well as Ig class switching by forming ineffective oligomers with BAFF.

Diagnosis

In patients with recurrent respiratory infections, immunology laboratory testing might indicate decreased serum levels of immunoglobulins IgG, IgM, and IgA. In addition, most B cells present with the naïve IgM+IgD+ phenotype. Because of the few numbers of patients reported, the immunological characteristics might not be well defined. The presence of several affected individuals within a family, an autosomal dominant pattern of inheritance, might suggest TNSF12 deficiency. Definite diagnosis is made with the detection of a pathogenic missense mutation in *TNSF12/TWEAK* gene. Because only the variant C145R of the protein has been characterized, new gene mutations should be investigated and their pathogenicity demonstrated.

Treatment and Prognosis

Patients with TNFS12 deficiency should receive immunoglobulin supplementation to reduce their risk of infections. Antibiotic prophylaxis should be considered.

Prognosis of these patients is not well defined, considering the limited number of individuals reported to date.

References

Chicheportiche Y, Bourdon PR, Xu H, Hsu Y, Scott H, Hession C, et al. TWEAK, a new secreted ligand in the tumor necrosis factor family that weakly induces apoptosis. J Biol Chem. 1997;272:32401–10.

Pradet-Balade B, Medema JP, Lopez-Fraga M, Lozano JC, Kolfschoten GM, Picard A, et al. An endogenous hybrid mRNA encodes TWE-PRIL, a functional cell surface TWEAK–APRIL fusion protein. EMBO J. 2002;21:5711–20.

Wang HY, Ma CA, Zhao Y, Fan X, Zhou Q, Edmonds P, et al. Antibody deficiency associated with an inherited autosomal dominant mutation in TWEAK. Proc Natl Acad Sci. 2013;110:5127–32.

Wiley SR, Cassiano L, Lofton T, Davis-Smith T, Winkles JA, Lindner V, et al. A novel TNF receptor family member binds TWEAK and is implicated in angiogenesis. Immunity. 2001;15:837–46.

TRAF3 Deficiency

Henry Y. Lu[1] and Stuart E. Turvey[2,3]
[1]Department of Pediatrics and Experimental Medicine Program, British Columbia Children's Hospital, The University of British Columbia, Vancouver, BC, Canada
[2]Division of Allergy and Clinical Immunology, Department of Pediatrics and Experimental Medicine Program, British Columbia Children's Hospital, The University of British Columbia, Vancouver, BC, Canada
[3]Willem-Alexander Children's Hospital, Leiden University Medical Center, Leiden, the Netherlands

Synonyms

CAP1; CD40bp; CRAF1; IIAE5; LAP1

Definition

Tumor necrosis factor (TNF) receptor-associated factor 3 (TRAF3) is an adaptor protein that facilitates signalling downstream of TNF receptors and Toll-like receptors. Mutations that impair TRAF3 have been associated with an enhanced susceptibility to developing herpes simplex encephalitis.

Introduction

Please refer to the introductory section listed for ▶ UNC93B1 deficiency.

Molecular Genetics and Pathogenesis

Tumor necrosis factor (TNF) receptor-associated factor 3 (TRAF3) belongs to a family of

TRAF3 Deficiency, Table 1 TRAF3 mutations that increase susceptibility to developing HSE

Mutation(s)	Inheritance	Gene expression	Protein expression	Functional impact	Molecular mechanism	No. of HSE episodes	Age of episodes	References
p. R118W	AD	Unchanged	↓	Partial	Dominant negative	1	4 years	Perez de Diego et al. (2010)

multifunctional intracellular proteins that act as important adaptor proteins for the recruitment and activation of protein kinases downstream of TNF receptors and receptors that lead to the induction of IFNs, including Toll-like receptor 3 (TLR3) (Hacker et al. 2011). In TLR3, TRAF3 interacts with TRIF and links proximal signaling with downstream regulatory kinases required for IRF activation, including TBK1 and IKKε (Oganesyan et al. 2006). This makes it a critical regulator of type I IFN production and the innate antiviral response.

There has only been one case of human TRAF3 deficiency described, and this was in an 18-year-old French girl who had suffered from herpes simplex encephalitis (HSE) at age 4 years (Table 1) (Perez de Diego et al. 2010). This was a *de novo* autosomal dominant (AD) heterozygous cytosine to thymine nucleotide substitution at position 352 (c.352C>T), which resulted in a non-conserved missense arginine to tryptophan substitution at amino acid position 118 (R118W). All family members of this patient did not possess this mutation and did not have a history of HSE. The R118W mutation led to decreased TRAF3 protein expression and impaired response to TLR3 agonists as measured by NF-κB activation and lack of IFN production.

Diagnosis

Please refer to the diagnosis section listed for
▶ UNC93B1 deficiency.

Prognostic Factors

Please refer to the prognosis section listed for
▶ UNC93B1 deficiency.

Treatment

Please refer to the treatment section listed for
▶ UNC93B1 deficiency.

Cross-References

▶ IRF3 Deficiency
▶ TBK1 Deficiency
▶ TLR3 Deficiency
▶ TRAF3 Deficiency
▶ UNC93B1 Deficiency

References

Hacker H, Tseng PH, Karin M. Expanding TRAF function: TRAF3 as a tri-faced immune regulator. Nat Rev Immunol. 2011;11(7):457–68.

Oganesyan G, Saha SK, Guo B, He JQ, Shahangian A, Zarnegar B, et al. Critical role of TRAF3 in the Toll-like receptor-dependent and -independent antiviral response. Nature. 2006;439(7073):208–11.

Perez de Diego R, Sancho-Shimizu V, Lorenzo L, Puel A, Plancoulaine S, Picard C, et al. Human TRAF3 adaptor molecule deficiency leads to impaired Toll-like receptor 3 response and susceptibility to herpes simplex encephalitis. Immunity. 2010;33(3): 400–11.

TRAF3-Interacting Protein 2 Deficiency

▶ Chronic Mucocutaneous Candidiasis, ACT1 Deficiency

Transient Hypogammaglobulinemia of Infancy

Javier Chinen
Division of Allergy and Immunology,
Department of Pediatrics, Baylor College of
Medicine, Texas Children's Hospital, The
Woodlands, TX, USA

Synonyms

THI

Definition

Transient hypogammaglobulinemia of infancy (THI) is defined by low serum IgG levels in infants, after excluding other known immunodeficiencies such as X-linked agammaglobulinemia (XLA) and secondary causes, such as protein-loss enteropathy. In THI, serum IgG levels usually reach normal range during childhood.

The International Union of Immunological Societies (IUIS) defines THI when a child presents with serum IgG and IgA levels lower than two standard deviations below the mean for age, with conserved ability to develop antibodies to vaccines (Bousfiha et al. 2018). The European Society for Immunodeficiencies (ESID) has a working definition of THI used for registry purposes (Seidel et al. 2019), for patients who present IgG below age-related normal value in the first 3 years of life, exclusion of defined causes of hypogammaglobulinemia, and spontaneous resolution at about the fourth birthday.

Because most children with THI would not achieve normal serum IgG levels before 1 year of age, the term transient hypogammaglobulinemia of childhood has been proposed as an alternative name for this condition (Swamy and Garcia-Putnam 2014).

Introduction

At birth, serum IgG levels mostly reflect maternal IgG that has crossed the placenta during the third trimester and only to a small part production of IgG levels by the infant (McGeady 1987). As maternal IgG is metabolized and decreases in peripheral blood, the infant IgG production increases. The lowest serum IgG level in an infant is expected to occur between 3 and 6 months of age. Taking in consideration that antibody production is normal, increased susceptibility to infections due to low immunoglobulin levels is not expected. When serum IgG levels remain low after 6 months of age, a diagnosis of hypogammaglobulinemia is made. Testing for primary and secondary immunodeficiencies should be considered. The diagnosis of THI is made *in retrospect*, when serum IgG levels spontaneously achieve normal range during follow-up.

Incidence

The frequency of THI is unknown. Most children with THI do not suffer from frequent infections. The ESID registry reports that up to 24% of children with hypogammaglobulinemia are diagnosed with THI (Schatorje et al. 2014). Males appear to be more affected than females.

Pathophysiology

The pathophysiology of THI is not well defined. Because of its temporary nature and the conserved ability to respond to antigens, it is postulated that there is an initial reduced number of antibody-producing cells as compared to normal infants. Proposed mechanisms to explain THI include decreased reserve of memory B cells (Eroglu et al. 2018), immature T cell signaling (Siemińska et al. 2018), suppression of IgG production by maternal antibodies with inhibitory properties (Keles et al. 2010), and nonpathogenic variations in genes related to immunodeficiency (Whelan et al. 2006).

Clinical Presentation

Infants and children under 5 years of age with THI are most commonly evaluated when they present with frequent infections, and the assessment of the immune response reveals low serum IgG with protective antibody titers to childhood vaccines. As mentioned above, it is necessary that other primary and secondary causes of immunodeficiency are ruled out. The most common infections at clinical presentation are upper and lower respiratory tract infections. Other associated infections are urinary tract infections, gastroenteritis, and invasive bacterial infections. It remains unclear whether these frequent infections can be attributed to hypogammaglobulinemia, considering that the antibody response is conserved. Physical exam findings are characteristic of the diagnosed infections.

In a minority of cases, THI patients are identified in infants without infections who are tested for serum immunoglobulin levels because of non-infection-related reasons, such as a family history of immunodeficiency or because serum protein studies suggest low globulin levels.

Differential Diagnosis

When low serum IgG levels are found in a child, primary and secondary causes of hypogammaglobulinemia should be ruled out. These causes include proteinuria, protein-loss enteropathy, IgG subclass deficiency, CVID, X-linked, and autosomal recessive agammaglobulinemia. The absence of antibody responses to childhood vaccines, decreased B cell counts, and low IgM levels are findings not consistent with a suspected THI diagnosis (Moschese et al. 2008).

Laboratory Testing

The laboratory testing of patients with suspected THI should be directed to confirm the hypogammaglobulinemia and ruled out known causes of low IgG levels:

- Quantitative immunoglobulins IgG, IgA, and IgM
- Quantitative IgG subclasses
- Antibody responses to childhood vaccines
- B cell enumeration
- Urine protein quantification
- Serum albumin and globulins

Management

If children with hypogammaglobulinemia suspected to be THI present with recurrent infections, they require frequent antibiotic courses. THI patients, similarly to other children, might also present with allergic inflammation and anatomical abnormalities that increase their risk of infections. The use of antibiotics at prophylactic regimens has been proposed to reduce the number of infections. Similarly, the use of immunoglobulin supplementation might reduce the frequency of infections (Dorsey and Orange 2006). These measures should be considered for limited periods of time, with reassessment of serum IgG levels and frequency of infections before continuation.

The resolution of THI is expected before 5 years of age, with an average of 27 months (Ozen et al. 2010). Serum immunoglobulin levels should be measured once a year or more frequently. Several studies have reported individuals reaching normal IgG levels by late childhood or adolescence (Ameratunga et al. 2019; Kidon et al. 2004). It is uncertain whether these reports describe a form of THI with extended recovery, a different syndrome, or represent variation of methods design, such as patient inclusion criteria and retrospective nature.

Cross-References

- ▶ CVID
- ▶ IgA Deficiency With or Without IgG Subclass Deficiencies
- ▶ X-linked Agammaglobulinemia (BTK Deficiency)

References

Ameratunga R, Ahn Y, Steele R, Woon ST. Transient hypogammaglobulinaemia of infancy: many patients recover in adolescence and adulthood. Clin Exp Immunol. 2019;198(2):224–32.

Bousfiha A, Jeddane L, Picard C, Ailal F, Bobby Gaspar H, Al-Herz W, et al. The 2017 IUIS phenotypic classification for primary immunodeficiencies. J Clin Immunol. 2018;38:129–43.

Dorsey MJ, Orange JS. Impaired specific antibody response and increased B-cell population in transient hypogammaglobulinemia of infancy. Ann Allergy Asthma Immunol. 2006;97:590–5.

Eroglu FK, Aerts Kaya F, Cagdas D, Özgür TT, Yılmaz T, Tezcan İ, Sanal Ö. B lymphocyte subsets and outcomes in patients with an initial diagnosis of transient hypogammaglobulinemia of infancy. Scand J Immunol. 2018;88(4):e12709.

Keles S, Artac H, Kara R, Gokturk B, Ozen A, Reisli I. Transient hypogammaglobulinemia and unclassified hypogammaglobulinemia: 'similarities and differences'. Pediatr Allergy Immunol. 2010;21(5):843–51.

Kidon MI, Handzel ZT, Schwartz R, Altboum I, Stein M, Zan-Bar I. Symptomatic hypogammaglobulinemia in infancy and childhood – clinical outcome and in vitro immune responses. BMC Fam Pract. 2004;5:23.

McGeady SJ. Transient hypogammaglobulinemia of infancy: need to reconsider name and definition. J Pediatr. 1987;110(1):47–50.

Moschese V, Graziani S, Avanzini MA, Carsetti R, Marconi M, La Rocca M, et al. A prospective study on children with initial diagnosis of transient hypogammaglobulinemia of infancy: results from the Italian Primary Immunodeficiency Network. Int J Immunopathol Pharmacol. 2008;21:343–52.

Ozen A, Baris S, Karakoc-Aydiner E, Ozdemir C, Bahceciler NN, Barlan IB. Outcome of hypogammaglobulinemia in children: immunoglobulin levels as predictors. Clin Immunol. 2010;137:374–83.

Schatorje EJ, Gathmann B, van Hout RW, de Vries E, PedPAD Consortium. The PedPAD study: boys predominate in the hypogammaglobulinaemia registry of the ESID online database. Clin Exp Immunol. 2014;176:387–93.

Seidel MG, Kindle G, Gathmann B, Quinti I, Buckland M, van Montfrans J, et al. The European Society for Immunodeficiencies (ESID) registry working definitions for the clinical diagnosis of inborn errors of immunity. J Allergy Clin Immunol Pract. 2019;7(6):1763–70.

Siemińska I, Rutkowska-Zapała M, Bukowska-Strakova K, Gruca A, Szaflarska A, Kobylarz K, Siedlar M, Baran J. The level of myeloid-derived suppressor cells positively correlates with regulatory T cells in the blood of children with transient hypogammaglobulinaemia of infancy. Cent Eur J Immunol. 2018;43(4):413–20.

Swamy GK, Garcia-Putnam R. Maternal immunization to benefit the mother, fetus, and infant. Obstet Gynecol Clin N Am. 2014;41:521–34.

Whelan MA, Hwan WH, Beausoleil J, Hauck WW, McGeady SJ. Infants presenting with recurrent infections and low immunoglobulins: characteristics and analysis of normalization. J Clin Immunol. 2006;26(1):7–11.

Translocation Three Four (TTF)

▶ Ras Homolog Family Member H (RHOH) Deficiency

Trichorrhexis Invaginata

▶ Comel-Netherton Syndrome (*SPINK5*)

TRIF Deficiency

Henry Y. Lu[1] and Stuart E. Turvey[2,3]
[1]Department of Pediatrics and Experimental Medicine Program, British Columbia Children's Hospital, The University of British Columbia, Vancouver, BC, Canada
[2]Division of Allergy and Clinical Immunology, Department of Pediatrics and Experimental Medicine Program, British Columbia Children's Hospital, The University of British Columbia, Vancouver, BC, Canada
[3]Willem-Alexander Children's Hospital, Leiden University Medical Center, Leiden, the Netherlands

Synonyms

TICAM1

Definition

Toll/IL-1R (TIR) domain-containing adaptor inducing IFN-b (TRIF) is a key adaptor protein, which facilitates signalling and activation of Toll-like receptors (TLRs) 3 and 4. Deficiencies in this protein have been linked to an increased predisposition to developing herpes simplex encephalitis.

Introduction

Please refer to the introductory section listed for ▶ UNC93B1 deficiency.

Molecular Genetics and Pathogenesis

Toll/IL-1R (TIR) domain-containing adaptor inducing IFN-β (TRIF) or TIR domain-containing adaptor molecule 1 (TICAM-1) is the sole adaptor protein for Toll-like receptor 3 (TLR3) (Oshiumi et al. 2003) and acts in mediating signaling for the MyD88-independent pathway of TLR4 (Yamamoto et al. 2003) as well as detecting cytosolic dsRNA via the DExD/H-box helicase complex DDX1-DDX21-DHX36 (Zhang et al. 2011). Physiologically, upon TLR3 activation, TRIF acts as a scaffold for the recruitment of other signalling proteins such as TRAF3, TBK1, RIP1, and IRF3 to facilitate downstream signalling processes (Jiang et al. 2004; Funami et al. 2008). This ultimately leads to the dsRNA-mediated activation of IFN-β through NF-κB, AP1, or IRF3 (Oshiumi et al. 2003).

Two forms of human TRIF deficiency have been linked to HSE (Table 1). Homozygous autosomal recessive (AR) TRIF nonsense mutations were identified in a boy born to consanguineous Saudi Arabian parents (Sancho-Shimizu et al. 2011). This mutation was a cytosine to thymine substitution at position 421 (c.421C>T), which led to premature termination of translation. The termination codon replaced an arginine residue at amino acid position 141 (R141*) and led to a complete absence of TRIF protein (Sancho-Shimizu et al. 2011).

The same report also identified a case of AD HSE susceptibility in a young girl of mixed European descent (French, Swiss, Portuguese) who had a heterozygous cytosine to thymine substitution at position 557 (c.557C>T), resulting in a serine to leucine substitution at amino acid position 186 (S186L) (Sancho-Shimizu et al. 2011). Incomplete clinical penetrance was evident in the heterozygous patient as the mother and maternal grandfather had the same mutations, were seropositive for HSV-1 infection, but had never developed HSE. Patient dermal fibroblasts from both patients showed an impaired ability to induce IFN-β, IFN-γ, and IL-6 upon poly(I:C) stimulation. The MyD88-independent arm of TLR4 signaling was abolished in the AR patient and partially disrupted in the AD patient. Both patients possessed a reduced capacity to activate the DExD/H-box helicases pathway. Overall, the TRIF deficiency was complete in the AR patient but partial in the AD patient (Sancho-Shimizu et al. 2011). Importantly, these patients also revealed the redundant roles of TRIF in both the TLR4 and DExD/H-box helicase pathways as

TRIF Deficiency, Table 1 Known TRIF mutations associated with predisposition to developing HSE

Mutation(s)	Inheritance	Gene expression	Protein expression	Functional impact	Molecular mechanism	No. of HSE episodes	Age of episodes	References
p. S186L	AD	Unchanged	Unchanged	Partial	Dominant negative	1	21 months	Sancho-Shimizu et al. (2011)
p. R141*	AR	Unchanged	Null	Complete	Homozygous for 1 null allele	1	2 years	Sancho-Shimizu et al. (2011)

both patients did not suffer from any other infections (Sancho-Shimizu et al. 2011).

Diagnosis

Please refer to the diagnosis section listed for ▶ UNC93B1 deficiency.

Prognostic Factors

Please refer to the prognosis section listed for ▶ UNC93B1 deficiency.

Treatment

Please refer to the treatment section listed for ▶ UNC93B1 deficiency.

Cross-References

▶ IRF3 Deficiency
▶ TBK1 Deficiency
▶ TLR3 Deficiency
▶ TRAF3 Deficiency
▶ UNC93B1 Deficiency

References

Funami K, Sasai M, Oshiumi H, Seya T, Matsumoto M. Homo-oligomerization is essential for Toll/interleukin-1 receptor domain-containing adaptor molecule-1-mediated NF-kappaB and interferon regulatory factor-3 activation. J Biol Chem. 2008;283(26):18283–91.

Jiang Z, Mak TW, Sen G, Li X. Toll-like receptor 3-mediated activation of NF-kappaB and IRF3 diverges at Toll-IL-1 receptor domain-containing adapter inducing IFN-beta. Proc Natl Acad Sci U S A. 2004;101(10):3533–8.

Oshiumi H, Matsumoto M, Funami K, Akazawa T, Seya T. TICAM-1, an adaptor molecule that participates in Toll-like receptor 3-mediated interferon-beta induction. Nat Immunol. 2003;4(2):161–7.

Sancho-Shimizu V, Perez de Diego R, Lorenzo L, Halwani R, Alangari A, Israelsson E, et al. Herpes simplex encephalitis in children with autosomal recessive and dominant TRIF deficiency. J Clin Invest. 2011;121(12):4889–902.

Yamamoto M, Sato S, Hemmi H, Hoshino K, Kaisho T, Sanjo H, et al. Role of adaptor TRIF in the MyD88-independent toll-like receptor signaling pathway. Science. 2003;301(5633):640–3.

Zhang Z, Kim T, Bao M, Facchinetti V, Jung SY, Ghaffari AA, et al. DDX1, DDX21, and DHX36 helicases form a complex with the adaptor molecule TRIF to sense dsRNA in dendritic cells. Immunity. 2011;34(6):866–78.

Trypanosomiasis: African Trypanosomiasis

▶ APOL-1 Variants, Susceptibility and Resistance to Trypanosomiasis

TTC7

▶ Immunodeficiency with Multiple Intestinal Atresias (TTC7A)

U

UNC13D Deficiency

Ivan K. Chinn
Section of Immunology, Allergy, and
Retrovirology, Texas Children's Hospital,
Houston, TX, USA
William T. Shearer Center for Human
Immunobiology, Texas Children's Hospital,
Houston, TX, USA
Department of Pediatrics, Baylor College of
Medicine, Houston, TX, USA

Introduction

UNC13D is located at 17q25 and encodes Munc13-4, a 120 kDa protein that is highly expressed in hematopoietic cells (Feldmann et al. 2003). The protein contains two Munc homology domains (MHDs) and two C2 domains (Holt et al. 2006; Ramadass and Catz 2016). Munc13-4 has the capacity to bind to Rab GTPases and soluble N-ethylmaleimide-sensitive factor-attachment protein receptors (SNAREs) (Ramadass and Catz 2016).

Molecular Function

Cytotoxic T cells and NK cells kill target cells by mobilizing secretory granules containing perforin and other agents, such as granzyme, to the cellular membrane and releasing the contents into the intercellular space at the immunologic synapse. This process is highly coordinated and regulated. Toward the beginning of the course of events, Munc13-4 promotes fusion of endosomes to form lytic granules (Tang and Xu 2011). Near the final steps of this pathway, Munc13-4 is directed toward secretory granules through its MHD domains (Holt et al. 2006). The protein then binds to Rab27a that is embedded within the membrane of the granule, priming the fusion of the granule with the cell membrane (Holt et al. 2006; Neeft et al. 2004). The Munc13-4–Rab27a complex tethers the granule to the membrane (Elstak et al. 2011). Defective binding of Munc13-4 to Rab27a is sufficient to impair cytotoxicity (Cetica et al. 2015; Netter et al. 2016). Fusion itself requires interactions between Munc13-4, Munc18-2, and syntaxin 11 (Ishii 2016). Munc13-4 is not required for granule docking (Feldmann et al. 2003). Binding of Ca^{2+} to both C2 domains is also necessary for cytolytic function (Bin et al. 2018). Loss of either C2 domain (or both) results in impaired Ca^{2+}-sensitive vesicle membrane fusion (Bin et al. 2018). Munc13-4 therefore further serves as a sensor for calcium-dependent degranulation (Bin et al. 2018).

Munc13-4 has key functions in other hematopoietic cells, as well. Consistent with its role in granule biology, the molecule regulates neutrophil reactive oxygen species production by nicotinamide adenine dinucleotide phosphate oxidase,

© Springer Science+Business Media LLC, part of Springer Nature 2020
I. R. Mackay et al. (eds.), *Encyclopedia of Medical Immunology*,
https://doi.org/10.1007/978-1-4614-8678-7

which is contained in specific intracellular vesicles (Monfregola et al. 2012). Munc13-4 deficiency results in impaired neutrophil intracellular and extracellular reactive oxygen species production (Monfregola et al. 2012). This process in neutrophils appears to be mediated through binding of Munc13-4 to Rab11 rather than Rab27a (Johnson et al. 2016). Munc13-4 also plays important roles in the function of other neutrophilic granules, such as azurophilic granules that contain myeloperoxidase, and endosomal maturation (Ramadass and Catz 2016). Munc13-4 additionally regulates exocytosis in mast cells and platelets (Ramadass and Catz 2016).

Presentation

Patients with biallelic loss of *UNC13D* most frequently present with familial hemophagocytic lymphohistiocytosis (HLH) type 3 within the first year of life with a median age of 4 months (Feldmann et al. 2003; Ishii 2016; Rudd et al. 2008; Sieni et al. 2011, 2012). Presentation may be delayed if the patient carries at least one hypomorphic variant that allows for residual protein expression or function (Rudd et al. 2008; Sieni et al. 2012). *UNC13D* deficiency is estimated to account for about 20–40% of familial HLH cases and varies by ethnic group (Gholam et al. 2011; Ishii 2016; Rudd et al. 2008; Sieni et al. 2012). HLH is characterized by fulfillment of at least five of the following eight criteria: fever; splenomegaly; cytopenia; hypertriglyceridemia and/or hypofibrinogenemia; hemophagocytosis in the bone marrow, spleen, or lymph nodes; deficient NK cell function; hyperferritinemia; and elevated levels of serum soluble CD25 (Henter et al. 2007). The most common findings in Munc13-4 deficiency consist of defective NK cell function (98%), splenomegaly (96%), thrombocytopenia (94%), and fever (89%) (Sieni et al. 2011). Central nervous system involvement was notable and reported in 60% of cases (49/81) in one large European cohort (Sieni et al. 2011).

Non-HLH presentations have been reported as rare cases. *UNC13D* deficiency can manifest as severe EBV-associated mononucleosis without HLH (Gray et al. 2017). Patients with Munc13-4 deficiency also carry increased susceptibility to other infections, perhaps due to impaired neutrophil function. Peripubertal growth arrest was reported in one individual that is corrected after hematopoietic stem cell transplantation (HSCT). The patient also had central nervous system inflammation, hypergammaglobulinemia, and low B-cell counts but did not develop HLH (Gray et al. 2017). In one family, *UNC13D* deficiency presented as recurrent hydrops fetalis (Bechara et al. 2011).

Diagnosis

Laboratory testing remains essential. *UNC13D* deficiency can be detected by decreased Munc13-4 expression in platelets using a flow cytometry assay (Murata et al. 2011; Shibata et al. 2018). Unlike perforin-deficient NK cells, which exhibit absent cytotoxicity, NK cells from patients with *UNC13D* deficiency demonstrate low to intermediate cytotoxicity (Marcenaro et al. 2006). In contrast to perforin deficiency, upregulation of CD107a on the surface of Munc13-4 deficient NK cells is abrogated (Marcenaro et al. 2006). CD107a testing is therefore strongly recommended for functional assessment of potential *UNC13D* deficiency (Rubin et al. 2017). This assay is not specific for loss of Munc13-4, however.

Genetic testing must be performed, but providers should be aware that *UNC13D* is known to carry pathogenic structural and deep intronic variants that may not be identified without specific instructions to the clinical genetics laboratory. These variants include the following: c.118-308C>T (Cichocki et al. 2014; Meeths et al. 2011; Seo et al. 2013; Qian et al. 2014), c.118-307G>A (Entesarian et al. 2013; Qian et al. 2014), a 253 kb Alu-mediated inversion (Meeths et al. 2011; Qian et al. 2014), and others (Santoro et al. 2008). The most frequent pathogenic variants in *UNC13D* have been reported to affect splicing (Santoro et al. 2008).

Treatment

Protocols have not been developed specifically for treatment of HLH due to *UNC13D* deficiency but instead apply to HLH in general. The initial HLH-94 protocol employed a combination of intravenous etoposide, oral or intravenous dexamethasone, and (if neurologic disease is present) intrathecal methotrexate (Henter et al. 1997). Subsequently, the HLH-2004 protocol was developed, which combines HLH-94 with the use of oral cyclosporine (Henter et al. 2007). Providers should be cognizant that cyclosporine use can be associated with the appearance of posterior reversible encephalopathy syndrome (Jordan et al. 2011). Adjunctive use of serotherapy has been reported to enhance outcomes (Filipovich and Chandrakasan 2015; Ishii 2016; Tang and Xu 2011). Supportive care with antibiotics and antifungal medications to minimize infections is necessary during treatment for HLH (Ishii 2016; Jordan et al. 2011). Patients may require additional support if bleeding or cardiac dysfunction is present (Jordan et al. 2011).

HSCT represents the only definitive therapy for this disease at this time (Rudd et al. 2008). Optimal strategies continue to be developed, as overall 5-year survival after HSCT in the HLH-94 study was only 54% (Henter et al. 1997; Nikiforow 2015). For all forms of HLH taken as a whole, survival is superior with use of reduced intensity conditioning after successful induction of HLH remission (Jordan et al. 2011; Nikiforow 2015; Seo 2015). Primary graft loss is common, and donor chimerism must be monitored closely (Jordan et al. 2011). Successful transplantation using umbilical cord blood stem cells has also been reported (Nikiforow 2015). For *UNC13D* deficiency, gene therapy may provide an excellent alternative definitive treatment option in the future (Dettmer et al. 2019).

Cross-References

▶ *PRF1* Deficiency
▶ *STX11* Deficiency
▶ *STXBP2* Deficiency

References

Bechara E, Dijoud F, de Saint Basile G, Bertrand Y, Pondarré C. Hemophagocytic lymphohistiocytosis with Munc13-4 mutation: a cause of recurrent fatal hydrops fetalis. Pediatrics. 2011;128:e251.

Bin N-R, Ma K, Tien C-W, et al. C2 domains of Munc13-4 are crucial for Ca^{2+}-dependent degranulation and cytotoxicity in NK cells. J Immunol. 2018;201:700.

Cetica V, Hackmann Y, Grieve S, et al. Patients with Griscelli syndrome and normal pigmentation identify RAB27A mutations that selectively disrupt MUNC13-4 binding. J Allergy Clin Immunol. 2015;135:1310–8.e1.

Cichocki F, Schlums H, Li H, et al. Transcriptional regulation of Munc13-4 expression in cytotoxic lymphocytes is disrupted by an intronic mutation associated with a primary immunodeficiency. J Exp Med. 2014;211:1079.

Dettmer V, Bloom K, Gross M, et al. Retroviral UNC13D gene transfer restores cytotoxic activity of T cells derived from familial hemophagocytic lymphohistiocytosis type 3 patients in vitro. Hum Gene Ther. 2019;30:975–84.

Elstak ED, Neeft M, Nehme NT, et al. The munc13-4–rab27 complex is specifically required for tethering secretory lysosomes at the plasma membrane. Blood. 2011;118:1570–8.

Entesarian M, Chiang SCC, Schlums H, et al. Novel deep intronic and missense UNC13D mutations in familial haemophagocytic lymphohistiocytosis type 3. Br J Haematol. 2013;162:415–8.

Feldmann J, Callebaut I, Raposo G, et al. Munc13-4 is essential for cytolytic granules fusion and is mutated in a form of familial hemophagocytic lymphohistiocytosis (FHL3). Cell. 2003;115:461–73.

Filipovich AH, Chandrakasan S. Pathogenesis of hemophagocytic lymphohistiocytosis. Hematol Oncol Clin North Am. 2015;29:895–902.

Gholam C, Grigoriadou S, Gilmour KC, Gaspar HB. Familial haemophagocytic lymphohistiocytosis: advances in the genetic basis, diagnosis and management. Clin Exp Immunol. 2011;163:271–83.

Gray PE, Shadur B, Russell S, et al. Late-onset non-HLH presentations of growth arrest, inflammatory arachnoiditis, and severe infectious mononucleosis, in siblings with hypomorphic defects in UNC13D. Front Immunol. 2017;8:944.

Henter J-I, Aricò M, Egeler RM, et al. HLH-94: a treatment protocol for hemophagocytic lymphohistiocytosis. Med Pediatr Oncol. 1997;28:342–7.

Henter J-I, Horne A, Aricó M, et al. HLH-2004: diagnostic and therapeutic guidelines for hemophagocytic lymphohistiocytosis. Pediatr Blood Cancer. 2007;48:124–31.

Holt OJ, Gallo F, Griffiths GM. Regulating secretory lysosomes. J Biochem. 2006;140:7–12.

Ishii E. Hemophagocytic lymphohistiocytosis in children: pathogenesis and treatment. Front Pediatr. 2016;4:47.

Johnson JL, He J, Ramadass M, et al. Munc13-4 is a Rab11-binding protein that regulates Rab11-positive

U

vesicle trafficking and docking at the plasma membrane. J Biol Chem. 2016;291:3423–38.

Jordan MB, Allen CE, Weitzman S, Filipovich AH, McClain KL. How I treat hemophagocytic lymphohistiocytosis. Blood. 2011;118:4041–52.

Marcenaro S, Gallo F, Martini S, et al. Analysis of natural killer-cell function in familial hemophagocytic lymphohistiocytosis (FHL): defective CD107a surface expression heralds Munc13-4 defect and discriminates between genetic subtypes of the disease. Blood. 2006;108:2316–23.

Meeths M, Chiang SCC, Wood SM, et al. Familial hemophagocytic lymphohistiocytosis type 3 (FHL3) caused by deep intronic mutation and inversion in UNC13D. Blood. 2011;118:5783–93.

Monfregola J, Johnson JL, Meijler MM, Napolitano G, Catz SD. MUNC13-4 protein regulates the oxidative response and is essential for phagosomal maturation and bacterial killing in neutrophils. J Biol Chem. 2012;287:44603–18.

Murata Y, Yasumi T, Shirakawa R, et al. Rapid diagnosis of FHL3 by flow cytometric detection of intraplatelet Munc13-4 protein. Blood. 2011;118:1225–30.

Neeft M, Wieffer M, de Jong AS, et al. Munc13-4 is an effector of Rab27a and controls secretion of lysosomes in hematopoietic cells. Mol Biol Cell. 2004;16:731–41.

Netter P, Chan SK, Banerjee PP, et al. A novel Rab27a mutation binds melanophilin, but not Munc13-4, causing immunodeficiency without albinism. J Allergy Clin Immunol. 2016;138:599–601.e3.

Nikiforow S. The role of hematopoietic stem cell transplantation in treatment of hemophagocytic lymphohistiocytosis. Hematol Oncol Clin North Am. 2015;29:943–59.

Qian Y, Johnson JA, Connor JA, et al. The 253-kb inversion and deep intronic mutations in UNC13D are present in North American patients with familial hemophagocytic lymphohistiocytosis 3. Pediatr Blood Cancer. 2014;61:1034–40.

Ramadass M, Catz SD. Molecular mechanisms regulating secretory organelles and endosomes in neutrophils and their implications for inflammation. Immunol Rev. 2016;273:249–65.

Rubin TS, Zhang K, Gifford C, et al. Perforin and CD107a testing is superior to NK cell function testing for screening patients for genetic HLH. Blood. 2017;129:2993–9.

Rudd E, Bryceson YT, Zheng C, et al. Spectrum, and clinical and functional implications of UNC13D mutations in familial haemophagocytic lymphohistiocytosis. J Med Genet. 2008;45:134.

Santoro A, Cannella S, Trizzino A, et al. Mutations affecting mRNA splicing are the most common molecular defect in patients with familial hemophagocytic lymphohistiocytosis type 3. Haematologica. 2008;93:1086.

Seo JJ. Hematopoietic cell transplantation for hemophagocytic lymphohistiocytosis: recent advances and controversies. Blood Res. 2015;50:131–9.

Seo JY, Song J-S, Lee K-O, et al. Founder effects in two predominant intronic mutations of UNC13D, c.118-

308C>T and c.754-1G>C underlie the unusual predominance of type 3 familial hemophagocytic lymphohistiocytosis (FHL3) in Korea. Ann Hematol. 2013;92:357–64.

Shibata H, Yasumi T, Shimodera S, et al. Human CTL-based functional analysis shows the reliability of a munc13-4 protein expression assay for FHL3 diagnosis. Blood. 2018;131:2016–25.

Sieni E, Cetica V, Santoro A, et al. Genotype–phenotype study of familial haemophagocytic lymphohistiocytosis type 3. J Med Genet. 2011;48:343.

Sieni E, Cetica V, Mastrodicasa E, et al. Familial hemophagocytic lymphohistiocytosis: a model for understanding the human machinery of cellular cytotoxicity. Cell Mol Life Sci. 2012;69:29–40.

Tang Y-M, Xu X-J. Advances in hemophagocytic lymphohistiocytosis: pathogenesis, early diagnosis/differential diagnosis, and treatment. Sci World J. 2011;11:697–708.

UNC93B

▶ UNC93B1 Deficiency

UNC93B1 Deficiency

Henry Y. Lu[1] and Stuart E. Turvey[2,3]
[1]Department of Pediatrics and Experimental Medicine Program, British Columbia Children's Hospital, The University of British Columbia, Vancouver, BC, Canada
[2]Division of Allergy and Clinical Immunology, Department of Pediatrics and Experimental Medicine Program, British Columbia Children's Hospital, The University of British Columbia, Vancouver, BC, Canada
[3]Willem-Alexander Children's Hospital, Leiden University Medical Center, Leiden, the Netherlands

Synonyms

IIAE1; UNC93B

OMIM: 610551

Definition

UNC93B1 is an endoplasmic reticulum (ER) protein that facilitates the delivery of nucleotide-sensing Toll-like receptors (TLRs), including TLR3, TLR7-9 from the ER to the endosome. UNC93B1 deficiency is characterized by mutations in UNC93B1 that increase a patient's susceptibility to developing herpes simplex encephalitis.

Introduction

Herpes simplex encephalitis (HSE) is the most common cause of fatal sporadic encephalitis among young children of the Western world (Levitz 1998; Wong et al. 2013). It arises as a rare life-threatening complication during primary herpes simplex virus type I (HSV-1) infection, where the virus progresses from nasal and oral epithelial cells to the central nervous system (CNS) via cranial nerves (Whitley 2006). Accounting to between 5% and 20% of all annual cases of encephalitis worldwide, this disease is often difficult to diagnose due to its highly variable clinical presentation, relative rarity, and lack of pathognomonic clinical findings (Whitley 1990; Sabah et al. 2012). It has an estimated incidence of between 1 in 250,000 and 1 in 500,000 cases per year (Whitley 2006). Patients who go undiagnosed or receive delayed treatment tend to suffer from severe permanent neurological sequelae such as recurrent seizures and neurological dysfunction (Guo et al. 2011). With mortality rates of 70% for untreated and 30% for treated patients (Levitz 1998), paired with high morbidity rates, improving the understanding of the etiology and pathogenesis of HSE is crucial to inform current and future clinical approaches.

HSE affects all age groups and does not occur with a seasonal pattern (Levitz 1998). It is an acute or subacute illness, which results in general and focal neurological deficits. Patients may present with a prodrome of malaise, headache (81%), fever (90%), nausea, and vomiting (46%) (Sabah et al. 2012). Patients with this medical history who then present with symptoms of acute and subacute

encephalopathy, including lethargy, delirium, and confusion, should raise suspicion for HSE. Typically, the most common symptoms of HSE include fever (90%), headache (81%), progressive behavioral changes (71%), focal epilepsy features such as olfactory hallucinations (67%), vomiting (46%), focal neurological features such as unilateral weakness (33%), and cognitive issues such as memory loss and confusion (24%) (Sabah et al. 2012; Whitley et al. 1982).

Recent exciting advances in our understanding of Toll-like receptors (TLRs) through the identification of patients with loss-of-function mutations have clearly defined the critical role of TLRs in innate immunity. More specifically, TLRs are a class of specialized receptors of the innate immune system that are crucial for sensing pathogen invasion and initiating inflammatory and defensive immune responses. This family of ten receptors in humans accomplishes this by recognizing specific molecular patterns across broad groups of pathogens. Individual TLRs recognize distinct yet limited repertoires of conserved microbial patterns. For example, TLR3 recognizes double-stranded RNA (dsRNA) in vivo and their synthetic analog polyinosinic:polycytidylic acid [poly(I:C)], an intermediate structure made during viral replication for many RNA and DNA viruses. Importantly, it was recently demonstrated that the TLR3-type I/II interferon (IFN) pathway in neurons and glial cells plays a nonredundant and imperative role in regulating immunity against HSV-1 in the CNS (Lafaille et al. 2012). Patients with inborn deficiencies in various components of this pathway have an enhanced predisposition to developing HSE, including ▶ TLR3 deficiency, ▶ TRIF deficiency, ▶ TRAF3 deficiency, ▶ TBK1 deficiency, ▶ UNC93B1 deficiency, and ▶ IRF3 deficiency (Fig. 1). Interestingly, these patients generally do not show evidence of other unusual infectious diseases nor inability to respond to them.

Molecular Genetics and Pathogenesis

UNC93B1 is an endoplasmic reticulum (ER) protein, which is essential for TLR3,

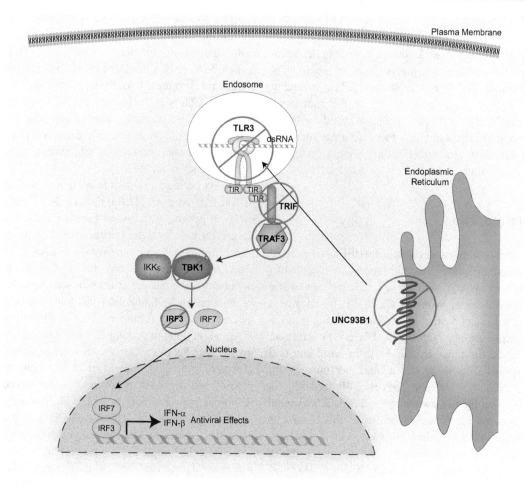

UNC93B1 Deficiency, Fig. 1 Schematic representation of the TLR3 signaling pathway and associated monogenic immune disorders linked to herpes simplex encephalitis HSE susceptibility. *dsRNA* double-stranded ribonucleic acid, *TIR* Toll/interleukin-1 receptor homology domain, *TLR3* Toll-like receptor 3, *TRIF* TIR domain-containing adaptor inducing IFN-β, *TRAF3* tumor necrosis factor (TNF) receptor-associated factor 3, *TBK1* TNF receptor-associated factor NF-κB activator (TANK)-binding kinase 1, *IFN* interferon, *IRF* IFN regulatory factor, *IKKε* inhibitor of nuclear factor kappa-B kinase subunit epsilon

TLR7, and TLR9 signaling via its physical interaction with TLRs in the ER (Brinkmann et al. 2007; Kim et al. 2008). It is unique in that it is the first protein to be identified that specifically acts in trafficking nucleotide-sensing TLRs (Kim et al. 2008). Defects in this gene have been associated with an enhanced predisposition to HSV-1 infections.

UNC93B1 deficiencies were the first primary immunodeficiencies to be identified as monogenic etiologies for HSE susceptibility (Casrouge et al.

2006). At the time, there were a series of reports that collectively demonstrated a potential genetic or familial basis of HSE based on the identification of two related patients with HSE in each of four unrelated families, who had intervals of years between HSE episodes affecting relatives in one or two generations (Lerner et al. 1983; Koskiniemi et al. 1995; Gazquez et al. 1996; Jackson et al. 2002). An epidemiological survey of pediatric HSE in France revealed a high frequency (13%) of affected individuals coming from consanguineous families (Casrouge et al. 2006). This raised suspicion for potential genetic HSE susceptibility.

Cells from two unrelated French children of consanguineous parents with HSE were found to be unresponsive to HSV-1, as measured by impaired IFN secretion by peripheral blood mononuclear cells (PBMCs), but normal responses to other viruses (Casrouge et al. 2006). This phenotype was highly similar to that of UNC93B1-deficient mice (Tabeta et al. 2006). Sequencing of this gene revealed one patient with a homozygous four-nucleotide deletion (CTTT) from positions 1034 to 1037 in exon 8 of *UNC93B1* (1034del4), while another patient possessed a homozygous guanine to adenine nucleotide substitution at position 781 (G>A) in exon 6 (Table 1) (Casrouge et al. 2006). Later, through the generation of induced pluripotent stem cells (iPSCs) from these patients and their subsequent differentiation into highly purified populations of neural stem cells (NSCs), neurons, astrocytes, and oligodendrocytes, it was discovered that *UNC93B1* was indispensable for neurons and oligodendrocytes to respond normally to HSV-1 (Lafaille et al. 2012).

Diagnosis

In suspected cases of HSE, workup should be initiated as soon as possible in order to minimize sequelae resulting from delayed treatment. There are no pathognomonic clinical findings associated with HSE. Patients who present with the more common HSE symptoms including fever, hemicranial headaches, abnormal language and behavioral patterns, memory defects, and seizures should raise suspicion for HSE (Tunkel et al. 2008). Focal neurological deficits, cerebrospinal fluid (CSF) pleocytosis, and computed tomography (CT) abnormalities are possible findings, but they may not be evident initially. Standard tests include (1) CSF polymerase chain reaction (PCR) for HSV, (2) magnetic resonance imaging (MRI) to look for edema in the temporal and/or inferior frontal lobes with high signal intensity in fluid

attenuation inversion recovery (FLAIR) and T2-weighted images (bilateral temporal lobe involvement is relatively pathognomonic), and (3) viral culture and antigen detection from brain biopsy specimens (if other tests are inconclusive) (Tunkel et al. 2008). Other tests include focal electroencephalographic (EEG) and serological evaluations of HSV-specific antibodies (for retrospective diagnosis) (Whitley 2006).

Prognostic Factors

A variety of factors should be taken into consideration when evaluating the potential outcome of a patient. This includes age (which can affect mortality, neurological sequelae, and recovery), clinical severity of illness, state of consciousness (alert, drowsy, stuporous, comatose), and the most important being the duration of illness prior to treatment (Tunkel et al. 2008; Marton et al. 1996). In addition, other potential prognostic factors such as low sodium levels, disorientation, and abnormal early CT scans have been reported (Riancho et al. 2013).

Treatment

Upon diagnosis or high suspicion of HSE, treatment should be initiated promptly. The treatment of choice for HSE patients is acyclovir (Tunkel et al. 2008; Whitley and Gnann 2002; Whitley and Kimberlin 2005). Even with the initiation of this antiviral, morbidity and mortality are still high. Initiation of therapy within 4 days of clinical onset of symptoms has been associated with a drop in mortality from 28% at 18 months to 8% (Tunkel et al. 2008). Despite this, relapses of HSE have also been reported after acyclovir therapy (Valencia et al. 2004). Corticosteroids in conjunction with acyclovir may be of benefit, but more validation is required (Kamei et al. 2005). As suggested by mouse models, recombinant IFN-α treatment may also be useful (Wintergerst et al. 1999). Enhanced understanding of the role of the TLR3/IRF3 axis through the study of rare human primary immunodeficiencies may eventually lead to novel treatment strategies.

UNC93B1 Deficiency, Table 1 UNC93B1 mutations linked to HSE susceptibility

Mutation(s)	Inheritance	Gene expression	Protein expression	Functional impact	Molecular mechanism	No. of HSE episodes	Age of episodes	References
c. 1034del4	AR	→	→	Complete	Homozygous for 1 null allele	3	11 months, 14 months, 3.5 year	Casrouge et al. (2006)
c. 781 G>A	AR	→	→	Complete	Homozygous for 1 null allele	2	5 year, 17 year	Casrouge et al. (2006)

Cross-References

▶ IRF3 Deficiency
▶ TBK1 Deficiency
▶ TLR3 Deficiency
▶ TRAF3 Deficiency
▶ TRIF Deficiency

References

Brinkmann MM, Spooner E, Hoebe K, Beutler B, Ploegh HL, Kim YM. The interaction between the ER membrane protein UNC93B and TLR3, 7, and 9 is crucial for TLR signaling. J Cell Biol. 2007;177(2):265–75.

Casrouge A, Zhang SY, Eidenschenk C, Jouanguy E, Puel A, Yang K, et al. Herpes simplex virus encephalitis in human UNC-93B deficiency. Science. 2006;314(5797):308–12.

Gazquez I, Jover A, Puig T, Vincente de Vera C, Rubio M. Familial herpes encephalitis. Lancet. 1996;347(9005):910.

Guo Y, Audry M, Ciancanelli M, Alsina L, Azevedo J, Herman M, et al. Herpes simplex virus encephalitis in a patient with complete TLR3 deficiency: TLR3 is otherwise redundant in protective immunity. J Exp Med. 2011;208(10):2083–98.

Jackson AC, Melanson M, Rossiter JP. Familial herpes simplex encephalitis. Ann Neurol. 2002;51(3):406–7.

Kamei S, Sekizawa T, Shiota H, Mizutani T, Itoyama Y, Takasu T, et al. Evaluation of combination therapy using acyclovir and corticosteroid in adult patients with herpes simplex virus encephalitis. J Neurol Neurosurg Psychiatry. 2005;76(11):1544–9.

Kim YM, Brinkmann MM, Paquet ME, Ploegh HL. UNC93B1 delivers nucleotide-sensing toll-like receptors to endolysosomes. Nature. 2008;452(7184):234–U80.

Koskiniemi M, Saarinen A, Klapper PE, Sarna S, Cleator G, Vaheri A. Familial herpes encephalitis. Lancet. 1995;346(8989):1553.

Lafaille FG, Pessach IM, Zhang SY, Ciancanelli MJ, Herman M, Abhyankar A, et al. Impaired intrinsic immunity to HSV-1 in human iPSC-derived TLR3-deficient CNS cells. Nature. 2012;491(7426):769–73.

Lerner AM, Levine DP, Reyes MP. Two cases of herpes simplex virus encephalitis in the same family. N Engl J Med. 1983;308(24):1481.

Levitz RE. Herpes simplex encephalitis: a review. Heart Lung. 1998;27(3):209–12.

Marton R, Gotlieb-Steimatsky T, Klein C, Arlazoroff A. Acute herpes simplex encephalitis: clinical assessment and prognostic data. Acta Neurol Scand. 1996;93(2–3):149–55.

Riancho J, Delgado-Alvarado M, Sedano MJ, Polo JM, Berciano J. Herpes simplex encephalitis: clinical presentation, neurological sequelae and new prognostic factors. Ten years of experience. Neurol Sci. 2013;34(10):1879–81.

Sabah M, Mulcahy J, Zeman A. Herpes simplex encephalitis. BMJ. 2012;344:e3166.

Tabeta K, Hoebe K, Janssen EM, Du X, Georgel P, Crozat K, et al. The Unc93b1 mutation 3d disrupts exogenous antigen presentation and signaling via toll-like receptors 3, 7 and 9. Nat Immunol. 2006;7(2):156–64.

Tunkel AR, Glaser CA, Bloch KC, Sejvar JJ, Marra CM, Roos KL, et al. The management of encephalitis: clinical practice guidelines by the Infectious Diseases Society of America. Clin Infect Dis. 2008;47(3):303–27.

Valencia I, Miles DK, Melvin J, Khurana D, Kothare S, Hardison H, et al. Relapse of herpes encephalitis after acyclovir therapy: report of two new cases and review of the literature. Neuropediatrics. 2004;35(6):371–6.

Whitley RJ. Viral encephalitis. N Engl J Med. 1990;323(4):242–50.

Whitley RJ. Herpes simplex encephalitis: adolescents and adults. Antivir Res. 2006;71(2–3):141–8.

Whitley RJ, Gnann JW. Viral encephalitis: familiar infections and emerging pathogens. Lancet. 2002;359(9305):507–13.

Whitley RJ, Kimberlin DW. Herpes simplex encephalitis: children and adolescents. Semin Pediatr Infect Dis. 2005;16(1):17–23.

Whitley RJ, Soong SJ, Linneman C Jr, Liu C, Pazin G, Alford CA. Herpes simplex encephalitis. Clin Assess JAMA. 1982;247(3):317–20.

Wintergerst U, Gangemi JD, Whitley RJ, Chatterjee S, Kern ER. Effect of recombinant human interferon alpha B/D (rHu-IFN-alpha B/D) in combination with acyclovir in experimental HSV-1 encephalitis. Antivir Res. 1999;44(1):75–8.

Wong T, Yeung J, Hildebrand KJ, Junker AK, Turvey SE. Human primary immunodeficiencies causing defects in innate immunity. Curr Opin Allergy Clin Immunol. 2013;13(6):607–13.

Unclassified Primary Antibody Deficiency (unPAD)

Esther de Vries
Tranzo, TSB, Tilburg University, Tilburg, the Netherlands
Laboratory for Medical Microbiology and Immunology, Elisabeth-Tweesteden Hospital, Tilburg, the Netherlands

Synonyms

CVID-like; Dysgammaglobulinemia

Definition

In primary antibody deficiency, one or more immunoglobulin isotypes (IgG, IgM, IgA), subclasses (IgG$_1$, IgG$_2$, IgG$_3$, IgG$_4$), and/or specific antibodies (anti-protein, anti-polysaccharide) in blood are decreased or (near) absent without an identifiable external cause such as severe protein loss (e.g., nephrotic syndrome, protein-losing enteropathy) or adverse events related to medication (e.g., steroids, biologicals, chemotherapy). This can occur in the context of a broader immune deficiency or restricted to antibodies only ("predominantly antibody deficiency" in the IUIS classification; e.g., Bousfiha et al. 2018). When B-lymphocytes in blood are also absent, X-linked or autosomal agammaglobulinemia are likely diagnoses. When B-lymphocytes in blood are present, and IgG as well as IgA and/or IgM are severely decreased in combination with decreased specific antibody responses, common variable immunodeficiency disorders (CVID) is a likely diagnosis. However, by far the largest, very heterogeneous group of primary antibody deficient patients suffers from an isolated or combined IgA, IgM, total IgG, and IgG subclass or specific antibody deficiency.

Although some are distinguished as separate subgroups (IgA deficiency, IgG subclass deficiency, specific antibody deficiency), these patients might be grouped together as "unclassified primary antibody deficiency (unPAD)" patients because their clinical presentation shows considerable overlap, and their immunological profile may develop from one type to another with time (Janssen et al. 2018).

Prevalence

The prevalence of unPAD is not fully known and varies considerably among the different subtypes. Isolated IgA deficiency may be as frequent as 1:500, whereas broader forms approaching the phenotype of CVID more likely have a prevalence of 1:10,000. Intermediate forms probably have a prevalence somewhere in between these extremes. Because patients are often not recognized in time, it may be that this is an underestimation of the prevalence in the population.

Clinical Presentation

Patients with unPAD often present with recurrent respiratory and/or ear-nose-throat (ENT) infections. It is important to relate the frequency, severity, and duration of such infections to what is considered normal in the patient's age group, especially when the infections are limited to the upper respiratory and ENT tract. In young children, this may be caused by ample exposure to respiratory viruses in day care; however, as children get older, these infections should subside. On the other hand, recurrent lower respiratory tract infections should always be a trigger to look for an underlying cause, especially when X-ray and/or culture-proven bacterial pneumonias have occurred. The cause of recurrent pneumonia is not always immune deficiency; also allergies, anatomical abnormalities, and cystic fibrosis can be the culprits. Distinguishing lower airway infections from bronchial hyperreactivity and asthma can be difficult at times; even more confusing, these can occur in patients in combination with unPAD. Also, immune deficiency becomes more likely in case of recurrent infections or "lung patients" in the family; it is known that CVID and CVID-like disease (unPAD) may show familial occurrence, and antibody deficiency with its sequelae is sometimes misdiagnosed as COPD. Similarly, when there is damage in the form of hearing loss and/or bronchiectasis, antibody deficiency becomes more likely.

Young children pose a specific problem. Babies are born with a high serum IgG level, originating from their mother through transplacental transfer in the third trimester of pregnancy. After birth, this maternal IgG slowly declines, while the infant's IgG production slowly increases, leading to a serum IgG nadir in the second and third trimester of the first year of life. This is physiological. However, in some children the increase of their own IgG production takes longer; sometimes they remain hypogammaglobulinemic for several years, but eventually end up with a normal immune system (Ameratunga et al. 2019; Sütçü et al. 2015). This is called transient hypogammaglobulinemia of infancy (THI), which can be difficult to distinguish from primary antibody deficiency. When IgM and IgA are also low, infections are severe, or when B-lymphocyte subpopulations are abnormal, complete recovery is less likely. It is important to follow such children closely, to treat bacterial infections in time to prevent organ damage, and to repeat immunological screening from time to time.

Genetics

As soon as a specific causally related genetic defect is identified, patients are no longer considered to have *unclassified* antibody deficiency. Thereafter they are classified according to the most suitable PAD subgroup. Since new gene defects are identified at a rapid pace nowadays, it is important to remain vigilant for these new developments in all patients originally identified as unclassified.

Immunological Phenotype

The unPAD patient group is very diverse, and some patients may show abnormalities in B-lymphocyte subsets reminiscent of the abnormalities found in subgroups of CVID patients. However, in most unPAD patients, lymphocyte subsets are relatively normal.

Diagnosis

Identification of antibody-deficient patients is relatively easy once the suspicion has arisen: IgG, IgA, IgM, and IgG subclasses as well as specific antibody responses can be determined in a small sample of blood. Not all hospitals in all countries offer every test, but in many cases these tests can be outsourced to hospitals with the appropriate laboratory facilities.

Therapy

Timely diagnosis is important, since antibody deficiency can and should be treated to prevent organ damage (hearing loss, bronchiectasis), decreased life quality (infections, chronic fatigue), and premature mortality. Depending on the severity, treatment should be focused on timely, adequate antibiotic treatment of acute infections, prolonged antibiotic prophylaxis, or immunoglobulin substitution.

Cross-References

▶ CVID
▶ IgA Deficiency With or Without IgG Subclass Deficiencies
▶ X-linked Agammaglobulinemia (BTK Deficiency)

References

Ameratunga R, Ahn Y, Steele R, Woon ST. Transient hypogammaglobulinaemia of infancy: many patients recover in adolescence and adulthood. Clin Exp Immunol. 2019;198(2):224–32.

Bousfiha A, Jeddane L, Picard C, Ailal F, Bobby Gaspar H, Al-Herz W, Chatila T, Crow YJ, Cunningham-Rundles C, Etzioni A, Franco JL, Holland SM, Klein C, Morio T, Ochs HD, Oksenhendler E, Puck J, Tang MLK, Tangye SG, Torgerson TR, Casanova JL, Sullivan KE. The 2017 IUIS phenotypic classification for primary immunodeficiencies. J Clin Immunol. 2018;38(1):129–43.

Janssen LMA, Basset P, Macken T, van Esch J, Prujit H, Knoops A, de Vries E, et al. Mild hypogammaglobulinemia can be a serious condition. Front Immunol. 2018;9:2384.

Sütçü M, Aktürk H, Salman N, Özçeker D, Gülümser-Şişko S, Acar M, Somer A. Transient hypogammaglobulinemia of infancy: predictive factors for late recovery. Turk J Pediatr. 2015;57(6):592–8.

U

V

Velocardiofacial Syndrome

▶ DiGeorge Anomaly (del22q11)

Warts, Hypogammaglobulinemia, Infections, Myelokathexis (WHIM) Syndrome

Kyla Jade Hildebrand
Division of Allergy & Immunology, Department
of Pediatrics, Faculty of Medicine, University of
British Columbia, Vancouver, BC, Canada
British Columbia Children's Hospital Research
Institute, Vancouver, BC, Canada

Synonyms

CXCL12 – Cysteine-X-cysteine chemokine
ligand 12; CXCR4 – Cysteine-X-cysteine chemokine receptor 4; HPV – Human Papillomavirus;
SDF-1 – Stromal cell-derived factor 1; WHIM –
Warts, hypogammaglobulinemia, infections,
myelokathexis

Introduction

Warts, hypogammaglobulinemia, infections,
myelokathexis (WHIM) syndrome is an autosomal
dominant combined immunodeficiency characterized by neutropenia, hypogammaglobulinemia,

and extensive infection with human papilloma
virus (HPV). The underlying genetic mutation is a
heterozygous defect in the chemokine receptor
4 (*CXCR4*) gene which has been mapped to
chromosome 2q22.

Background

In 1964, Zuelzer observed a new pattern of
granulocytopenia characterized by persistent
neutropenia and increased granulocyte reserve in
a 10-year-old female (Zuelzer et al. 1964). Zuelzer
coined the term myelokathexis (Kathexis ;=
retention) as he noted there was a failure of
mature neutrophils to leave the bone marrow,
resulting in hypercellularity. Of the neutrophils
noted to be in circulation, the morphology was
also noted to be unusual with a hypersegmented
nucleus and long filaments connecting the lobes
of the nucleus.

The term WHIM syndrome was suggested in
1990 after a particular phenotype was observed in
a family consisting of two sisters and their father
with a common presentation of chronic HPV
infections and recurrent sinopulmonary infections
associated with neutropenia and hypogammaglobulinemia (Wetzler et al. 1990). In
2003, Hernandez et al. identified the genetic mutation underlying WHIM syndrome consisting of a

© Springer Science+Business Media LLC, part of Springer Nature 2020
I. R. Mackay et al. (eds.), *Encyclopedia of Medical Immunology*,
https://doi.org/10.1007/978-1-4614-8678-7

truncated mutation of 12 cM on chromosome 2q21 affecting the cytoplasmic tail domain of the gene encoding CXCR4 (Hernandez et al. 2003). This group was the first to describe a genetic mutation in a chemokine receptor affecting its function leading to disease involving cell-mediated immunity to HPV infections.

Chemokine Receptor 4 (CXCR4)

CXCR4 is a gene that encodes for a G-protein-coupled chemokine receptor, CXCR4, that is, highly expressed in various stem cells and progenitor cells at an embryonic stage affecting hematopoietic, cardiovascular, nervous system, and reproductive development.

CXCR4 binds to its ligand C-X-C motif chemokine ligand 12 (CXCL12) to regulate bone marrow homeostasis and leukocyte trafficking in the peripheral blood. Additionally, CXCR4 has previously been characterized as a co-receptor for the human immunodeficiency virus. CXCL12, also known as stromal cell-derived factor 1 (SDF-1), is a ligand for CXCR4 and both the ligand and receptor are required for development of lymphocytes and myeloid cells. Heterozygous mutations of the CXCR4 receptor truncates the carboxy-terminus of the receptor, resulting in hyperresponsiveness of the CXCR4 receptor to its ligand, CXCL12, leading to a gain in function. Mature neutrophils accumulate in the bone marrow, as well as lymphocytes and monocytes, leading to a hypercellular marrow (Hernandez et al. 2003; Badolato and Donadieu 2017). Several *CXCR4* gene mutations have been sequenced including nonsense, deletion, insertion, and frame-shift mutations. A nonsense mutation resulting in an amino acid change pR334X accounts for the majority of *CXCR4* mutations reported in patients with WHIM syndrome to date (Badolato and Donadieu 2017).

Somatic mutations of *CXCR4* have been described affecting the intracellular tail of the CXCR4 receptor, leading to a presentation of Waldenstrom's macroglobulinemia.

Clinical Presentation and Pathophysiology

Sinopulmonary Infections

CXCR4 and CXCL12/SDF-1 are essential for the development of B lymphocytes and myeloid cells. Impaired numbers and/or function of B lymphocytes can lead to antibody deficiency manifesting as recurrent sinopulmonary infections. Recurrent otitis media and bacterial pneumonia can begin as early as infancy. Recurrent pneumonia can lead to bronchiectasis over time.

Human Papilloma Virus and Herpesviridae Infections

One of the hallmarks of WHIM syndrome is the susceptibility to HPV infections which is thought to be a result of a defect in the homeostasis and trafficking of dendritic cells, rather than an inability of lymphocytes to proliferate. HPV infections can range from verrucae vulgaris (warts) to cervical papillomatosis with severe cervical dysplasia and invasive cancer. Warts typically have an early onset in the first two decades of life and are located on the hands and feet, and occasionally the face and trunk. The number and severity of warts can be variable.

WHIM patients also experience herpes virus infections such as herpes simplex virus 1 and 2. Recurrent infections with Herpes simplex virus, Varicella-Zoster virus, Cytomegalovirus, and Epstein-Barr virus have been reported.

Infections as a Sequelae of Neutropenia

Neutropenia can predispose patients to skin infections such as cellulitis or abscesses, periodontal infections, suppurative adenitis. Septic arthritis, sepsis, and meningitis are rare but can also occur.

Congenital Heart Disease

Congenital heart disease has been reported as a manifestation of WHIM syndrome and, in particular, Tetralogy of Fallot. CXCR4 is a gene that encodes for a G-protein-coupled chemokine receptor that is highly expressed in various stem cells and progenitor cells at an embryonic stage affecting the cardiovascular system (Badolato and Donadieu 2017).

Lab Findings/Diagnostic Tests

WHIM syndrome is characterized by profound leukopenia and most notably, neutropenia. Lymphopenia and monocytopenia are also present. The neutrophils that are present function well: phagocytosis, chemotaxis, and bactericidal activity are often preserved. Although neutropenia is present, at times of infection, the neutrophil count may increase and normalize, but declines to low levels once the infection has resolved.

Lymphopenia is reflected by a reduction in the absolute numbers of B and T lymphocytes. B lymphocyte numbers are typically low with reduced class-switched subsets (CD27+). It is worth noting that although hypogammaglobulinemia is typically characteristic of this condition, immunoglobulin levels may be low or normal, and specific antibody titers to previous vaccines may be protective or absent. Hypogammaglobulinemia may affect all immunoglobulin isotypes. Specific antibody responses are often present following immunization with a vaccine, but sustained response over time may be diminished. Lymphocyte proliferation responses are usually impaired to both mitogen and antigen.

If bone marrow studies are performed, the marrow is typically hypercellular with a predominance of mature myeloid cells. Morphological abnormalities in the neutrophils include dense pyknotic lobes connected by long, thin filaments. Lymphoid, erythroid, and megakaryocytes are unaffected.

Gene sequencing for *CXCR4* mutations is diagnostic. Heterogeneity in clinical presentation can lead to delayed diagnosis. For example, warts are often not present until the second or third decade of life, and hematopoietic stem cell transplantation is a treatment option with the best outcomes reported if performed early in life (Badolato and Donadieu 2017).

Treatment

Treatment of patients with WHIM syndrome consists of managing acute infections and surveillance for long-term complications.

Most infections are not severe or invasive, and infections usually respond to oral antimicrobials. Sinopulmonary infections are treated with antimicrobials. The risk of bronchiectasis is very high, and for this reason, patients with WHIM syndrome are initiated on immunoglobulin replacement therapy, even if hypogammaglobulinemia is not present at the time of diagnosis. Patients with hypogammaglobulinemia and who lack specific antibody responses to previously administered vaccines are initiated on regular immunoglobulin replacement therapy with a dose of 400–600 mg/kg per 4-week interval (intravenous) or divided and delivered via the subcutaneous route. Immunoglobulin replacement therapy helps to prevent further sinopulmonary bacterial infections; however, it does not prevent or mitigate HPV infections. Antimicrobial prophylaxis may be helpful for patients experiencing recurrent bacterial skin infections.

Warts are typically resistant to treatment with usual therapies such as cryotherapy. Young patients with no preexisting HPV infections or lesions immunized with a quadravalent HPV vaccine were shown to confer protective immunity. Early immunization with HPV vaccines may be prophylactic in WHIM patients, with repeated boosters every 5 years to maintain immunity over time in the setting of reduced B cell function.

It is noteworthy that most patients with WHIM syndrome do not develop the typical infections associated with neutropenia. This finding may be partly explained by the bone marrow's ability to increase output of neutrophils at a time of infection or stress and minimize the risk of sepsis. Currently there is no strong evidence for the routine use of granulocyte colony stimulating factor (G-CSF) in the treatment of neutropenia associated with this condition. Most individuals with WHIM syndrome have normalization of the neutrophil count during an infection. G-CSF has no effect on lymphopenia, monocytopenia, or the severity of warts. Individuals with WHIM syndrome who do not normalize the absolute neutrophil count during an infection should be considered candidates for prophylactic G-CSF due to the increase risk of sepsis.

Patients must be monitored for malignancy from young age, as the risk of malignancy appears to increase in the third decade, particularly cancers related to HPV (anogenital and cervical cancers) and EBV-induced lymphoma. Lung disease is also closely monitored, with routine pulmonary function testing, and imaging including radiographs and computed tomography (CT) in the surveillance for bronchiectasis.

Plerixafor, a CXCR4 small molecule selective antagonist, is a new treatment currently in Phase III clinical trials in patients with WHIM syndrome. This drug has previously been approved by the Food and Drug Administration as a co-therapy with G-CSF in the management of patients with non-Hodgkin lymphoma and multiple myeloma for the hematopoietic stem cell mobilization prior to transplantation. Plerixafor blocks the ability of CXCL12 to permanently sustain the activation of CXCR4. Phase I and II clinical trials have demonstrated that this treatment can correct the panleukopenia in WHIM patients in a dose-dependent response. (https://clinicaltrials.gov/ct2/show/NCT02231879 – Accessed January 6, 2018).

Summary

WHIM syndrome is a rare primary immunodeficiency with a unique susceptibility to HPV infections. WHIM syndrome should be considered in the differential diagnosis of individuals with recurrent sinopulmonary or skin infections, warts or other HPV infections, or congenital heart disease where neutropenia and lymphopenia are also present. Supportive management with immunoglobulin replacement, and, in some patients, prophylaxis with antimicrobials or G-CSF, is the mainstays of treatment. Long-term surveillance includes close monitoring for bronchiectasis and malignancy. Hematopoietic stem cell transplantation may be beneficial if offered early in life. An additional treatment option with a CXCR4 selective antagonist remains under study.

Cross-References

▶ Thymoma with Hypogammaglobulinemia

References

Badolato R, Donadieu J. How I treat warts, hypogammaglobulinemia, infections, and myelokathexis syndrome. Blood. 2017;130(23):2491–8.

Hernandez P, Gorlin R, Lukens J, Taniuchi S, Bohinjec J, Francois F, et al. Mutations in the chemokine receptor gene CXCR4 are associated with WHIM syndrome, a combined immunodeficiency disease. Nat Genet. 2003;34(1):70–4.

Plerixafor versus G-CSF in the Treatment of People With WHIM Syndrome – Full Text View – ClinicalTrials. gov [Internet]. Clinicaltrials.gov. 2018 [cited 8 January 2018]. Available from: https://clinicaltrials.gov/ct2/show/NCT02231879

Wetzler M, Talpaz M, Kleinerman E, King A, Huh Y, Gutterman J, et al. A new familial immunodeficiency disorder characterized by severe neutropenia, a defective marrow release mechanism, and hypogammaglobulinemia. Am J Med. 1990;89(5):663–72.

Zuelzer W, Evans R, Goodman J. Myelokathexis – a new form of chronic granulocytopenia. N Engl J Med. 1964;270(14):699–704.

WAS Wiskott-Aldrich Syndrome

▶ Wiskott-Aldrich Syndrome Deficiency
▶ Wiskott-Aldrich Syndrome Protein-Interacting Protein (WIP) Deficiency

WHIM – Warts, Hypogammaglobulinemia, Infections, Myelokathexis

▶ Warts, Hypogammaglobulinemia, Infections, Myelokathexis (WHIM) Syndrome

WHIM Syndrome

Taco W. Kuijpers
Department of Pediatric Immunology, Rheumatology and Infectious Diseases, Emma Children's Hospital, Amsterdam University Medical Center (Amsterdam UMC), Amsterdam, The Netherlands

Background

Warts, hypogammaglobulinemia, infections, and myelokathexis (WHIM) syndrome was first described in 1990 by Wetzler et al. (1990; Kawai and Malech 2009). WHIM is a rare combined primary immunodeficiency disorder (PID) which in 2003 was identified to be caused by gain-of-function mutations in the gene for the chemokine receptor CXCR4 at chromosome 4q21 (Hernandez et al. 2003). CXCR4 is a member of the chemokine receptor superfamily of G-protein-coupled receptors (GPCRs) with a seven-transmembrane spanning domain structure (Allen et al. 2007). The N-terminal part of the molecule and the extracellular loops form a cup in which the ligand stromal-cell derived factor-1 (SDF1, CXCL12) can bind and generate an intramolecular change in the molecule that then transmits a signal via its C-terminal cytoplasmic tail.

The role of CXCL12 and CXCR4 is largely inferred from loss-of-function studies using constitutive or conditional mice deficient for *Cxcr4* and *Cxcr4*$^{-/-}$ chimeras (Ma et al. 1998; Tachibana et al. 1998). Mice deficient for *Cxcr4* die in utero or perinatally and display profound defects in the hematopoietic and nervous systems. Cxcr4-deficient mice have severely reduced B-lymphopoiesis, reduced myelopoiesis in fetal liver, and a virtual absence of myelopoiesis in bone marrow (Ma et al. 1998; Tachibana et al. 1998).

CXCR4 is expressed in developing vascular endothelial cells, and mice lacking *Cxcr4* or Sdf-1 have defective formation of the large vessels supplying the gastrointestinal tract. In addition, being defective in hematopoiesis as well as vascular development and cardiogenesis was first recognized in mice lacking Sdf-1 (Nagasawa et al. 1996). The Sdf1/Cxcr4 pair is thought to regulate the lymphoid trafficking of T cells and orchestrate B-cell homing, maturation, and differentiation in secondary lymphoid organs as well as direct plasma cells (PCs) toward specific niches in secondary lymphoid organs such as lymph nodes and the spleen, as well as the bone marrow (BM) (Okada et al. 2002; Hargreaves et al. 2001; Hauser et al. 2002).

Alternative Ligands: Atypical Receptors

CXCR4-mediated signaling is more complex as initially thought, as also macrophage migration inhibitory factor (MIF) and extracellular ubiquitin have been shown to bind CXCR4 and induce intracellular signaling (Bernhagen et al. 2007; Saini et al. 2011). Furthermore, the chemokine receptor ACKR3 (also known as CXCR7) has added to the complexity of CXCR4 signaling due to its ability to bind not only CXCL11 (I-TAC) but also CXCL12 (SDF-1) and to interact with MIF, regulating ligand availability for CXCR4 and evoking CXCL12- and MIF-triggered signaling independently from CXCR4 (Balabanian et al. 2005; Tarnowski et al. 2010). Interestingly, the endogenous, antimicrobial protein human β3-defensin (HBD-3) induced in and released by gut epithelial cells was identified as a natural antagonist of CXCR4, blocking CXCL12-induced CXCR4 signaling.

W

The β-defensins are a group of antimicrobial peptides present in mucosal epithelium of the lung and gut, which are also upregulated in the presence of HIV-1 and block HIV replication by direct binding of virions and blocking of the HIV co-receptor CXCR4 (Feng et al. 2006).

GPCRs, which signal via G proteins, induce various cellular functions including cell migration or leukocyte arrest and the atypical chemokine receptors (ACKRs), which are structurally homologous to the GPCRs but are unable to couple to G proteins (due to the absence of a cytosolic amino acid sequence, i.e., the DRYLAIV motif) and fail to induce classical chemokine signaling. Because ACKRs efficiently internalize their ligands, they can function as chemokine decoy receptors and may also concentrate chemokines in hard-to-reach domains to help guiding cell migration across cell layers.

In addition to homodimerization, CXCR4 can also form dimers with ACKR3 and other receptors (Sánchez-Martín et al. 2013). Upon ligand binding, CXCR4 is internalized by endocytosis and degraded in lysosomes (mediated by a degradation sequence in its C-terminus, i.e., the SSLKILSKGK motif). The homo- and hetero-dimerization of these receptors determine in part the membrane expression level, the signaling capacity of CXCR4, and its internalization and recycling capacity.

Pathophysiology

In humans, the chemokine receptor CXCR4 is expressed on most leukocyte subsets and functions to promote hematopoietic stem cell (HSC) and neutrophil homing to and retention in bone marrow. In contrast to the lack of Cxcr4 expression in the many murine models, in human patients the WHIM mutations alter the CXCR4 carboxyl terminus such that it enhances and prolongs receptor signaling (Kawai and Malech 2009; Dotta et al. 2019).

As a result, egress of normally produced and functional neutrophils from the bone marrow to the blood is impaired causing neutropenia in the circulation but an expansion of the pool of (over)differentiated neutrophils that do not have the typical multilobulated nuclear morphology of three to four lobes but increased to five or even six lobes (Kawai and Malech 2009; Dotta et al. 2019).

A similar mechanism of extensive retention in the bone marrow and additional resident (lymphoid) organs may also affect other leukocyte subsets and their homing behavior, hence explaining that WHIM patients usually may show panleukopenia, including T and B cells. Although differentiating B cells express CXCR4, the receptor disappears during activation in the peripheral compartment but gets re-expressed when a B cell gets poised toward the stage of an antibody-secreting plasma cell (PC). Thus, CXCR4 plays a central role in B-cell immune response, notably by promoting PC migration and maintenance in the bone marrow. The gain-of-function mutations in CXCR4 affect receptor desensitization. Interestingly, despite the lymphopenia, WHIM patients mount an immune response but fail to maintain the humoral memory over time. Although the Cxcr4 mutation intrinsically and locally promoted germinal center response and PC differentiation, antigen-specific PCs were barely detected in the BM. It was suggested that the early accumulation of immature plasmablasts may potentially occupy the niches for long-lived PCs, which indicate the inability of these PBs to generate a stable PC pool and/or give room to antibody-releasing long-lived PCs to populate the BM niche (Biajoux et al. 2016). Whatever the exact mechanism may be, fine-tuning of CXCR4 expression and desensitization is critically required for efficient PC differentiation and maintenance. Absence of such a regulatory process may account for the overall defective humoral immunity observed in WHIM patients.

Clinical Presentation, Differential Diagnosis, and Treatment

WHIM syndrome is a rare combined immunohematologic disorder characterized by chronic panleukopenia, including circulating neutrophils and B and T lymphocytes (Kawai and Malech 2009; Dotta et al. 2019). Despite this, patients show limited susceptibility to pathogens, with the notable exception of human papillomavirus and respiratory encapsulated bacteria (Kawai and Malech 2009). WHIM patients often present with frequent acute bacterial infections, especially infections of the pulmonary tract that may cause chronic morbidity, respiratory insufficiency, and in some cases premature death.

In addition, WHIM patients have marked difficulty clearing infections with human papillomavirus (HPV), a process in which CXCR4 may drive malignant transformation, and might be prevented by prior HPV immunization (Chow et al. 2010; Handisurya et al. 2010). These infections may result in recalcitrant and persistent cutaneous and anogenital warts that in several reported cases have evolved into cancer. Apart from HPV-induced carcinoma skin cancer, several deaths have also occurred due to malignancies associated with Epstein-Barr virus (EBV) infection (Beaussant Cohen et al. 2012). Other viral infections have not been described to form a major threat in patients diagnosed with WHIM syndrome.

Pathophysiological functions of CXCR4 in severe congenital neutropenia (SCN) have been particularly illustrated in the context of the WHIM syndrome, but also SCNs associated to *G6PC3* and *GATA2* genetic deficiencies were found to display CXCR4 dysfunctions similar to the WHIM syndrome without any germline *CXCR4* mutations (McDermott et al. 2010; Maciejewski-Duval et al. 2016). The molecular events and genetic anomalies accounting for CXCR4 dysfunctions remain largely unknown and can result from functional interplay between G6PC3 or GATA2 and the CXCL12/CXCR4 axis that can account for the neutropenia and immune dysfunctions. Additionally, dysfunctions of the CXCL12/CXCR4 axis might contribute to HPV-tumorigenesis (i.e., in WHIM syndrome and the heterozygous GATA2 defects) (Chow et al. 2010; Maciejewski-Duval et al. 2016), as well as the leukemic processes including the acute myeloid leukemia presented by some patients with SCN.

Therapies currently used to treat patients with WHIM syndrome are rather non-specific (antibiotics and IgG supplementation) and often expensive, such granulocyte colony-stimulating factor (G-CSF), a drug approved by the Food and Drug Administration (FDA) and European Medicines Agency (EMA) to treat severe congenital neutropenia.

In practice this G-CSF therapy is often following the initiation of prophylactic antibiotics and intravenous immunoglobulins (IVIG) to judge whether the infectious episodes in the WHIM patient have been sufficiently reduced and effectively covered prior to starting G-CSF as a further adjunct treatment. None of these measures have been formally evaluated for efficacy in WHIM syndrome. Thus, there continues to be a major unmet medical need for effective therapy in WHIM syndrome despite the availability and application of best therapy for neutropenia and hypogammaglobulinemia in these patients.

New Approaches

A specific small-molecule antagonist of CXCR4 – licensed as AMD3100 or plerixafor for HSC mobilization for stem cell transplantation in cancer – was considered a logical candidate for molecularly targeted treatment of WHIM syndrome. The goal of treatment would be to reduce CXCR4 signaling to normal, not to zero. Two recent short-term Phase I dose-escalation studies in a total of nine patients demonstrated that the drug could safely mobilize not only neutrophils but also all other leukocyte subsets that may be decreased in the blood of WHIM patients (Dale et al. 2011; McDermott et al. 2011) A Phase I study, conducted at the NIH, in three patients given plerixafor 0.02–0.04 mg/kg/d for 6 months demonstrated that these hematopoietic effects were durable (McDermott et al. 2014). Moreover, the frequency of infection was reduced, no new warts occurred during treatment, and several existing warts improved or resolved. Although these results are encouraging, these data leave open the question whether plerixafor is truly efficacious in WHIM syndrome, and a randomized, double-blinded, crossover trial described here to establish the long-term safety and clinical efficacy compared to G-CSF may never be possible because of the small number of patients to be treated. A recent follow-up report of the three WHIM patients for up to 52 months described the efficacy and long-term safety of plerixafor to improve pancytopenia, reduce the wart burden, and improve quality of life (McDermott et al. 2019).

There may be advantages of a CXCR4 antagonist above G-CSF. First, published evidence suggests that long-term, high-dose G-CSF therapy may be associated with the development of leukemia and myelodysplasia in SCN patients (Rosenberg et al. 2010). Whether or not this could also occur in WHIM patients is currently unknown. Patients have been described who due to G-CSF receptor mutations or the development of anti-G-CSF antibodies fail to respond to G-CSF with an increased absolute neutrophil count (ANC) (Connelly et al. 2012). Second, experience in WHIM patients is that these patients regularly complain about severe bone pain with the normal dosing of G-CSF of 5 ug/kg/day, which may be due to their increased retention of mature neutrophils in the marrow (myelokathexis), which is not expected and in fact minimized by the use of CXCR4 antagonists. Finally, G-CSF is not an effective treatment against warts commonly observed in WHIM syndrome, which might be more effectively covered with a therapy such as plerixafor which is directed at the receptor of virus entry into the activated keratinocyte (Meuris et al. 2016).

In WHIM syndrome question remains unanswered which part of the immune system may be more relevant to disease recovery (myeloid or lymphoid cells). A recent report on an intriguing case describes a patient with WHIM who was spontaneously cured by a process called "chromothripsis," a deletion and rearrangement process in chromosomes. The defective *CXCR4* (R334X) gene (as well as 163 other genes) was randomly deleted from one copy of chromosome 2 in a HSC that subsequently repopulated the myeloid but not the lymphoid lineage, leading to complete remission of the patient's clinical neutropenia and the clinical symptoms (McDermott et al. 2015). Whether CXCR4 ablation or blockade may help at a certain stage to repopulate the bone marrow in the setting of HSCT should be further explored.

References

Allen SJ, Crown SE, Handel TM. Chemokine: receptor structure, interactions, and antagonism. Annu Rev Immunol. 2007;25:787–820.

Balabanian K, Lagane B, Infantino S, Chow KY, Harriague J, Moepps B, Balabanian K, Lagane B, Infantino S. The chemokine SDF-1/CXCL12 binds to and signals through the orphan receptor RDC1 in T lymphocytes. J Biol Chem. 2005;280:35760–6.

Beaussant Cohen S, Fenneteau O, Plouvier E, Rohrlich PS, Daltroff G, Plantier I, Dupuy A, Kerob D, Beaupain B, Bordigoni P, Fouyssac F, Delezoide AL, Devouassoux G, Nicolas JF, Bensaid P, Bertrand Y, Balabanian K, Chantelot CB, Bachelerie F, Donadieu J. Description and outcome of a cohort of 8 patients with WHIM syndrome from the French Severe Chronic Neutropenia Registry. Orphanet J Rare Dis. 2012;7:71.

Bernhagen J, Krohn R, Lue H, Gregory JL, Zernecke A, Koenen RR, Dewor M, Georgiev I, Schober A, Leng L, Kooistra T, Fingerle-Rowson G, Ghezzi P, Kleemann R, McColl SR, Bucala R, Hickey MJ, Weber C, et al. MIF is a noncognate ligand of CXC chemokine receptors in inflammatory and atherogenic cell recruitment. Nat Med. 2007;13:587–96.

Biajoux V, Natt J, Freitas C, Alouche N, Sacquin A, Hemon P, Gaudin F, Fazilleau N, Espéli M, Balabanian K. Efficient plasma cell differentiation and trafficking require Cxcr4 desensitization. Cell Rep. 2016;17(1):193–205.

Chow KY, Brotin É, Ben Khalifa Y, Carthagena L, Teissier S, Danckaert A, Galzi JL, Arenzana-Seisdedos F, Thierry F, Bachelerie F. A pivotal role for CXCL12 signaling in HPV-mediated transformation of keratinocytes: clues to understanding HPV-pathogenesis in WHIM syndrome. Cell Host Microbe. 2010;8:523–33.

Connelly JA, Choi SW, Levine JE. Hematopoietic stem cell transplantation for severe congenital neutropenia. Curr Opin Hematol. 2012;19:44–51.

Dale DC, Bolyard AA, Kelley ML, Westrup EC, Makaryan V, Aprikyan A, Wood B, Hsu FJ. The CXCR4 antagonist plerixafor is a potential therapy for myelokathexis, WHIM syndrome. Blood. 2011;118:4963–6.

Dotta L, Notarangelo LD, Moratto D, Kumar R, Porta F, Soresina A, et al. Long-term outcome of WHIM syndrome in 18 patients: high risk of lung disease and HPV-related malignancies. J Allergy Clin Immunol Pract. 2019;7(5):1568–77.

Feng Z, Dubyak GR, Lederman MM, Weinberg A. Human beta defensin 3 – a novel antagonist of the HIV-1 coreceptor CXCR4. J Immunol. 2006;177:782–6.

Handisurya A, Schellenbacher C, Reininger B, Koszik F, Vyhnanek P, Heitger A, Kirnbauer R, Förster-Waldl E. A quadrivalent HPV vaccine induces humoral and cellular immune responses in WHIM immunodeficiency syndrome. Vaccine. 2010;28:4837–41.

Hargreaves DC, Hyman PL, Lu TT, Ngo VN, Bidgol A, Suzuki G, Zou YR, Littman DR, Cyster JG. A coordinated change in chemokine responsiveness guides plasma cell movements. J Exp Med. 2001;194:45–56.

Hauser AE, Debes GF, Arce S, Cassese G, Hamann A, Radbruch A, Manz RA. Chemotactic responsiveness toward ligands for CXCR3 and CXCR4 is regulated on plasma blasts during the time course of a memory immune response. J Immunol. 2002;169:1277–82.

Hernandez PA, Gorlin RJ, Lukens JN, Taniuchi S, Bohinjec J, Francois F, Klotman ME, Diaz GA. Mutations in the chemokine receptor gene CXCR4 are associated with WHIM syndrome, a combined immunodeficiency disease. Nat Genet. 2003;34:70–4.

Kawai T, Malech HL. WHIM syndrome: congenital immune deficiency disease. Curr Opin Hematol. 2009;16:20–6.

Ma Q, Jones D, Borghesani PR, Segal RA, Nagasawa T, Kishimoto T, Bronson RT, Springer TA. Impaired B-lymphopoiesis, myelopoiesis, and derailed cerebellar neuron migration in CXCR4- and SDF-1-deficient mice. Proc Natl Acad Sci U S A. 1998;95:9448–53.

Maciejewski-Duval A, Meuris F, Bignon A, Aknin ML, Balabanian K, Faivre L, Pasquet M, Barlogis V, Fieschi C, Bellanné-Chantelot C, Donadieu J, Schlecht-Louf G, Marin-Esteban V, Bachelerie F. Altered chemotactic response to CXCL12 in patients carrying GATA2 mutations. J Leukoc Biol. 2016;99:1065–76.

McDermott DH, De Ravin SS, Jun HS, Liu Q, Priel DA, Noel P, Takemoto CM, Ojode T, Paul SM, Dunsmore KP, Hilligoss D, Marquesen M, Ulrick J, Kuhns DB, Chou JY, Malech HL, Murphy PM. Severe congenital neutropenia resulting from G6PC3 deficiency with increased neutrophil CXCR4 expression and myelokathexis. Blood. 2010;116:2793–802.

McDermott DH, Liu Q, Ulrick J, Kwatemaa N, Anaya-O'Brien S, Penzak SR, Filho JO, Priel DA, Kelly C, Garofalo M, Littel P, Marquesen MM, Hilligoss D, Decastro R, Fleisher TA, Kuhns DB, Malech HL, Murphy PM. The CXCR4 antagonist plerixafor corrects panleukopenia in patients with WHIM syndrome. Blood. 2011;118:4957–62.

McDermott DH, Liu Q, Velez D, Lopez L, Anaya-O'Brien S, Ulrick J, Kwatemaa N, Starling J, Fleisher TA, Priel DA, Merideth MA, Giuntoli RL, Evbuomwan MO, Little P, Marquesen MM, Hilligoss D, DeCastro R, Grimes GJ, Hwang ST, Pittaluga S, Calvo KR, Stratton P, Cowen EW, Kuhns DB, Malech HL, Murphy PM, et al. A phase 1 clinical trial of long-term, low-dose treatment of WHIM syndrome with the CXCR4 antagonist plerixafor. Blood. 2014;123:2308–16.

McDermott DH, Gao J-L, Liu Q, Siwicki M, Martens C, Jacobs P, Velez D, Yim E, Bryke CR, Hsu N, Dai Z, Marquesen MM, Stregevsky E, Kwatemaa N, Theobald N, Long Priel DA, Pittaluga S, Raffeld MA, Calvo KR, Maric I, Desmond R, Holmes KL, Kuhns DB, Balabanian K, Bachelerie F, Porcella SF, Malech HL, Murphy PM. Chromothriptic cure of WHIM syndrome. Cell. 2015;160:686–99.

McDermott DH, Pastrana DV, Calvo KR, Pittaluga S, Velez D, Cho E, et al. Plerixafor for the treatment of WHIM syndrome. N Engl J Med. 2019;380(2):163–70.

Meuris F, Gaudin F, Aknin ML, Hémon P, Berrebi D, Bachelerie F. Symptomatic improvement in human papillomavirus-induced epithelial neoplasia by specific targeting of the CXCR4 chemokine receptor. J Invest Dermatol. 2016;136(2):473–80.

Nagasawa T, Hirota S, Tachibana K, Takakura N, Nishikawa S, Kitamura Y, Yoshida N, Kikutani H, Kishimoto T. Defects of B-cell lymphopoiesis and bone-marrow myelopoiesis in mice lacking the CXC chemokine PBSF/SDF-1. Nature. 1996;382:635–8.

Okada T, Ngo VN, Ekland EH, Förster R, Lipp M, Littman DR, Cyster JG. Chemokine requirements for B cell entry to lymph nodes and Peyer's patches. J Exp Med. 2002;196:65–75.

Rosenberg PS, Zeidler C, Bolyard AA, Alter BP, Bonilla MA, Boxer LA, Dror Y, Kinsey S, Link DC, Newburger PE, Shimamura A, Welte K, Dale DC. Stable long-term risk of leukaemia in patients with severe congenital neutropenia maintained on G-CSF therapy. Br J Haematol. 2010;150:196–9.

Saini V, Staren DM, Ziarek JJ, Nashaat ZN, Campbell EM, Volkman BF, Marchese A, Majetschak M. The CXC chemokine receptor 4 ligands ubiquitin and stromal cell-derived factor-1 function through distinct receptor interactions. J Biol Chem. 2011;286:33466–333477.

Sánchez-Martín L, Sánchez-Mateos P, Cabañas C. CXCR7 impact on CXCL12 biology and disease. Trends Mol Med. 2013;19:12–22.

Tachibana K, Hirota S, Iizasa H, Yoshida H, Kawabata K, Kataoka Y, Kitamura Y, Matsushima K, Yoshida N, Nishikawa S, Kishimoto T, Nagasawa T. The chemokine receptor CXCR4 is essential for vascularization of the gastrointestinal tract. Nature. 1998;393:591–4.

Tarnowski M, Grymula K, Liu R, Tarnowska J, Drukala J, Ratajczak J, Mitchell RA, Ratajczak MZ, Kucia M. Macrophage migration inhibitory factor is secreted by rhabdomyosarcoma cells, modulates tumor metastasis by binding to CXCR4 and CXCR7 receptors and inhibits recruitment of cancer-associated fibroblasts. Mol Cancer Res. 2010;8:1328–43.

Wetzler M, Talpaz M, Kleinerman ES, King A, Huh YO, Gutterman JU, Kurzrock R. A new familial immunodeficiency disorder characterized by severe neutropenia, a defective marrow release mechanism, and hypogammaglobulinemia. Am J Med. 1990;89:663–72.

W

Winged Helix Deficiency

Winged Helix Deficiency (FOXN1)

Sonia Joychan[1] and Panida Sriaroon[2]
[1]Division of Allergy and Immunology, University of South Florida/Johns Hopkins All Children's Hospital, Tampa, FL, USA
[2]Department of Pediatrics, Division of Allergy and Immunology, University of South Florida/ Johns Hopkins All Children's Hospital, Tampa, FL, USA

Synonyms

Alymphoid cystic thymic dysgenesis; FOXN1 deficiency; Nude SCID; Severe T cell immunodeficiency, congenital alopecia, nail dystrophy syndrome; Winged helix deficiency

Introduction/Background

FOXN1 encodes a transcription factor that is essential for the development of thymus and eccrine glands (Bonilla and Notarangelo 2015). This gene is a member of the forkhead gene family, which consists of a group of "winged helix" transcription factors that are involved in many aspects of cell development, metabolism, and aging (Palamaro et al. 2014). In fetal life, FOXN1 is expressed in mesenchymal and epithelial cells in the liver, lung, intestine, kidney, and urinary tract (Gallo et al. 2017). Postnatally, the gene is selectively expressed in thymic and skin epithelial cells (Palamaro et al. 2014).

The thymus is a primary lymphoid organ responsible for production of a diverse repertoire of immunocompetent T cells. FOXN1 is expressed in all thymic epithelial cells, which secrete chemokines such as CCL25, CCL21, and CXCL12 that are responsible for the recruitment of hematopoietic progenitors into thymus. FOXN1 also positively regulates expression of certain genes involved in antigen processing and presentation (Rota and Dhalla 2017). Although the exact molecular mechanisms of FOXN1 expression and function are not entirely understood, it is thought that activation of FOXN1 occurs through phosphorylation which leads to nuclear translocation, DNA binding through its forkhead domain, and transcription of genes involved in epithelial cell development. FOXN1 deficiency, characterized by defective thymic epithelial cells and a lack of normal T cell development and selection, results in a rare form of severe combined immunodeficiency (SCID) with athymia and consecutive absence or decrease in T cell count (T-B + NK+ SCID). Since FOXN1 is also required for the development of epithelial cells in the skin, hair, and nails, the animal model of loss-of-function Foxn1 with spontaneous phenotype of congenital alopecia is called the nude mouse (Rota and Dhalla 2017). In humans, the condition is also known as (Bonilla and Notarangelo 2015) nude SCID, (Palamaro et al. 2014) winged helix deficiency, (Gallo et al. 2017) alymphoid cystic thymic dysgenesis, and (Rota and Dhalla 2017) severe T cell immunodeficiency, congenital alopecia, and nail dystrophy syndrome.

Although the nude mouse phenotype of athymia, alopecia universalis, and nail dystrophy was first described by Flanagan in 1966 (Gallo et al. 2017), the molecular cause of this phenotype was not identified until the 1990s (Rota and Dhalla 2017). It was initially described as an autosomal recessive mutation in the winged helix nude (*Whn*) gene, which has since been renamed as forkhead box n1 (*FOXN1*) gene. Most of our knowledge on *FOXN1* is derived from murine models. Homozygous nude mice, "*nu/ nu* mice*,*" are hairless, have delayed growth, severe infertility, and die very early in life due to infectious complications (Gallo et al. 2017; Romano et al. 2012). There is no difference in the number of hair follicles present in the wild-type control and nude mouse (Gallo et al. 2017). However, the hair follicles in the nude mouse lack free sulfhydryl groups in the mid-follicle region resulting in coiling and an inability to penetrate the epidermis (Gallo et al. 2017; Romano et al. 2012). There is also an abnormal balance between proliferation and differentiation of keratinocytes in the hair follicles. In addition, nude mice are infertile with small ovaries, low egg, and immotile sperm, which may be due to hormonal changes including altered serum levels of estradiol, progesterone, and thyroxine. The nail dystrophy is attributed to loss of keratin 1 protein and abnormal expression of filaggrin in terminally differentiating keratinocytes of the nail matrix (Gallo et al. 2017). When thymic morphogenesis is disrupted early in development, significant changes take place including agenesis of the subcapsular, cortical, and medullary regions. Homozygous nude mice have profound T cell deficiency, and in the absence of normal T cell help, antibody production is compromised, rendering these mice susceptible to severe infections (Romano et al. 2012).

FOXN1 is located on chromosome 17q11.2 (Gallo et al. 2017) and is closely linked to the neurofibromatosis-1 gene (Palamaro et al. 2014). Only nine cases with three mutations have been reported in humans: R255X (founder variant from patients in Acerno, Southern Italy), S188 fs (Lebanese origin), and R320W (Gallo et al. 2017) (Rota and Dhalla 2017), which are located in different domains of the molecule and believed to result in loss of function of the protein.

Clinical Presentation

The human equivalent of the nude mouse phenotype was first described in 1996 in two Italian sisters who had congenital alopecia and nail dystrophy associated with a profound T cell immunodeficiency (Gallo et al. 2017). They were born to consanguineous parents, suggesting an autosomal recessive inheritance pattern. Only nine cases of nude SCID have been reported in the literature (Rota and Dhalla 2017), and all presented early in life with severe and recurrent, life-threatening infections. In addition to thymic aplasia and severe T cell deficiency, FOXN1 mutations are associated with congenital alopecia of the scalp, eyebrows, and eyelashes (Gallo et al. 2017; Rota and Dhalla 2017). The most common nail malformations are leukonychia and koilonychia. Leukonychia is characterized by a proximal

arciform pattern resembling a half-moon (Romano et al. 2012). Conversely, koilonychia is characterized by a longitudinal concavity of the nail plate with raised edges that create a "spoon-shape" appearance. Less frequently, canaliform dystrophy and Beau lines are seen. Central nervous system defects were found in two fetuses of the same family who carried the R255X mutation. One suffered from severe neural tube defects, including anencephaly and spina bifida; the other had milder abnormalities, including an enlarged interhemispheric fissure and absence of the cavum septi pellucidi and corpus callosum (Gallo et al. 2017). However, the role of FOXN1 in central nervous system development is still unclear as neurological abnormalities were not reported in murine models and were only seen in two of the fetuses who came from a single kindred, suggesting the possibility of another genetic etiology.

Six of the nine cases of nude SCID reported originated from Acerno, a town in southwestern Italy (Gallo et al. 2017). Fifty-five of the 843 inhabitants from this small community were heterozygous carriers of the R255X mutation, corresponding to 6.52% of the studied population. A genealogical study found that all of these carriers were linked in a seven-generational pedigree and derived from a single ancestral couple, dating back to the early nineteenth century. The majority of heterozygous carriers, 39 of 55, had evidence of nail dystrophy, primarily leukonychia, koilonychia, and Beau lines. One carrier had lymphopenia and absence of T cell receptor excision circles (TRECs).

Laboratory Findings/Diagnostic Testing

Nude SCID should be suspected in patients with the classic triad of severe T cell immunodeficiency associated with congenital alopecia universalis and nail dystrophy. Severe reductions in TRECs may be detected during newborn screening and are indicative of a T cell deficiency. There are no reports of FOXN1 deficiency being identified by newborn screening (Rota and Dhalla 2017). All nude SCID patients reported thus far have T cell lymphopenia with CD4+ T cells more severely reduced than CD8+ T cells (Gallo et al. 2017), impaired T cell responses to mitogen stimulation, and an oligoclonal T cell receptor repertoire. Other findings include expansion of the double negative (CD4-CD8-) αβ and γδ T cell populations and inefficient thymic T cell output as demonstrated by reduced TRECs, CD31+ recent thymic emigrants, and CD45RA+ naïve T cells, resulting in skewing toward a CD45RO+ memory phenotype (Rota and Dhalla 2017). NK and B cell numbers are typically normal. However, specific antibody production is compromised in the absence of T cell help (Gallo et al. 2017). Chest X-ray should be performed to evaluate for thymic hypoplasia or aplasia. Patients with FOXN1 deficiency are at risk of viral, fungal, and bacterial infections, including infections with opportunistic pathogens, and they should be actively screened and carefully monitored.

FOXN1 deficiency is an autosomal recessive disorder. Definitive diagnosis depends on genetic testing for mutations in *FOXN1*. Single gene Sanger sequencing or Next Generation Sequencing techniques, including targeted sequencing panels, may be used to identify a mutation (Rota and Dhalla 2017).

Treatment/Prognosis

FOXN1 deficiency requires prompt and appropriate definitive treatment. Patients in the past have received either hematopoietic stem cell transplantation (HSCT) or thymic transplantation, the latter is preferred and showed more favorable outcomes. Like other SCID conditions, it is critical to establish the diagnosis within a few weeks or months of life prior to development of life-threatening complications. Transplantation in earlier disease stages leads to significantly better outcomes (Gallo et al. 2017). While thymic transplantation (or HCST) may correct the underlying immune deficiency, it does not correct the associated alopecia or nail dystrophy.

Of the nine FOXN1-deficient patients reported in the literature, five have undergone transplantation,

three received human leukocyte antigen (HLA)-matched sibling/genoidentical HSCT at 5 months of age, and two underwent thymic transplantation at ages 9 and 14 months (Gallo et al. 2017). One of the HSCT recipients was alive, well, and infection-free when assessed 6 years after HSCT. This patient had an increase in numbers of CD3+, CD4+, and CD8+ T cells, but CD4+ CD45RA+ naïve lymphocytes were not regenerated, and lymphocyte proliferative responses to mitogens gradually declined after an initial recovery. The other two HSCT recipients died from post-transplant complications. HSCT-containing mature donor T cells can be offered to patients when an HLA-matched sibling or genoidentical donor is available (Rota and Dhalla 2017).

In the absence of proper thymic environment, thymic transplantation should be favored to expedite functional immune reconstitution (Rota and Dhalla 2017). Reconstitution of successful T cell lymphopoiesis was achieved in both FOXN1-deficient patients treated with thymic transplantation (Gallo et al. 2017). They had normal T cell numbers and thymic function as measured by either TREC-positive naïve CD4+ T cells or CD31+ recent thymic emigrants. The newly generated T cells demonstrated normal proliferative responses in vitro. Both patients had a diverse TCR repertoire and were able to produce specific antibody directed against T cell-dependent antigens. They were able to clear ongoing infections post-transplant and remained infection-free 3–5 years after the transplant. However, one patient later developed autoimmune hypothyroidism and vitiligo.

Experience from complete DiGeorge syndrome and this small cohort of FOXN1 deficiency suggest that HSCT may not result in long-lasting high-quality immune reconstitution. Thymic transplantation may, in fact, result in superior outcomes in patients with an underlying thymic defect as in FOXN1 deficiency. It is also suggested that these patients may need to be grouped as "congenital athymia" in the growing category of SCID cohort, implying the need to thymic transplant as the preferred therapeutic approach.

Summary

FOXN1 deficiency should be considered in the differential diagnosis of patients presenting with severe T cell immunodeficiency, especially in the context of congenital alopecia and nail dystrophy. Patients with suspected FOXN1 deficiency should be evaluated promptly for thymic transplantation or HSCT.

References

Bonilla F, Notarangelo L. Nathan and Oski's hematology and oncology of infancy and childhood. 8th ed. Philadelphia: Elsevier; 2015.

Gallo V, Cirillo E, Giardino G, Pignata C. FOXN1 deficiency: from the discovery to novel therapeutic approaches. J Clin Immunol. 2017;37(8):751–8.

Palamaro L, Romano R, Fusco A, Giardino G, Gallo V, Pignata C. FOXN1 in organ development and human diseases. Int Rev Immunol. 2014;33(2):83–93.

Romano R, Palamaro L, Fusco A, Iannace L, Maio S, Vigliano I, et al. From murine to human nude/SCID: the thymus, T-cell development and the missing link. Clin Dev Immunol. 2012;2012:467101.

Rota IA, Dhalla F. FOXN1 deficient nude severe combined immunodeficiency. Orphanet J Rare Dis. 2017;12(1):6.

WIP Wiskott-Aldrich Syndrome Protein-Interacting Protein

▶ Wiskott-Aldrich Syndrome Deficiency
▶ Wiskott-Aldrich Syndrome Protein-Interacting Protein (WIP) Deficiency

WIPF1 WAS/WASL Interacting Protein Family Member 1

▶ Wiskott-Aldrich Syndrome Protein-Interacting Protein (WIP) Deficiency

Wiskott-Aldrich Syndrome Deficiency

Michel J. Massaad
Department of Experimental Pathology, Immunology, and Microbiology, and Department of Pediatrics and Adolescent Medicine, American University of Beirut, Beirut, Lebanon
Department of Pediatrics, Division of Immunology, Boston Children's Hospital, Harvard Medical School, Boston, MA, USA

Synonyms

Arp actin-related protein; CDC42 cell division control protein 42; SH3 Src homology domain 3; SIN self-inactivating; WAS Wiskott-Aldrich syndrome; WIP Wiskott-Aldrich syndrome protein-interacting protein

Definition

Wiskott-Aldrich syndrome (WAS) is a rare X-linked primary immunodeficiency disorder that alters the normal dynamics of the actin cytoskeleton and thus affects the structure and function of hematopoietic cells resulting in thrombocytopenia, bloody diarrhea, eczema, recurrent infections, and an increased risk of autoimmunity and malignancies. The classical treatment for WAS patients includes prophylactic antibiotics and immunoglobulin replacement therapy; however, the ultimate cure is only achieved with allogeneic hematopoietic stem cell transplantation or autologous gene therapy to correct the patients' immune system.

Introduction/Background

Wiskott-Aldrich syndrome (WAS) is an X-linked primary immunodeficiency disorder (PID) that affects 1–10 per million male infants, resulting in a combination of thrombocytopenia often associated with small platelet size, bloody diarrhea, eczema, recurrent infections, fever, and an increased incidence of autoimmunity and malignancies. WAS is due to mutations in the *WAS* gene that encodes the WAS protein (WASp), with a strong genotype/phenotype correlation among the nature of the mutation, the level of the protein, and the severity of the disease. WASp is expressed exclusively in hematopoietic cells. It functions as an actin nucleation-promoting factor that relays surface signals to initiate filamentous actin (F-actin) polymerization through the actin-related protein (Arp)2/3 complex, thereby controlling the actin cytoskeleton dynamics and immune cell function (Massaad et al. 2013).

WASp is a multi-domain protein: it possesses an Ena-Vasp homology domain (EVH1) domain at the N-terminus, followed by a basic region (BR), CDC42/Rac GTPase binding domain (GBD), proline rich region (PPP), verprolin homology (V) domain, cofilin homology or central (C) domain, and a C-terminal acidic (A) domain (Fig. 1). The EVH1 domain is the binding site of the WASp-interacting protein (WIP), which exists in a constitutive complex with WASp, and is crucial for its stability, cellular localization, and activation. The biology of WASp is tightly controlled by WIP, as will be discussed in details in the chapter on WIP deficiency. The BR and GBD form intra-molecular interactions with the VCA domain that keep WASp in an auto-inhibited state in resting cells. The PPP is the binding site of many Src homology (SH)3 domain-containing proteins that play a role in both activation and inhibition of WASp. The VCA domain is the functional unit that interacts with and activates the Arp2/3 complex to initiate F-actin polymerization (Massaad et al. 2013).

Mechanism of WASp Activation

WASp exists in the cytoplasm of hematopoietic cells in a heteropolymeric complex that includes WIP and the guanine nucleotide exchange factor (GEF) dedicator of cytokinesis 8 (DOCK8) (Janssen et al. 2016). In resting cells, WASp is maintained in an inactive state due to the intra-molecular interactions between the BR/GBD and the VCA domain. Cellular activation leads to the conversion of cell division control protein 42 (CDC42) from an inactive GDP-bound form to an active GTP-bound form catalyzed by DOCK8 (Harada et al. 2012) that is bridged to WASp through a direct interaction with WIP (Janssen et al. 2016). The newly generated CDC42-GTP, along with phophatidylinositol (4,5)-biphosphate (PIP2), bind to the GBD and BR, respectively, with higher affinity than the VCA domain, resulting in a conformational change that liberates the VCA domain. Phosphorylation of tyrosine 291 in the GBD destabilizes the auto-inhibited conformation of WASp as well, and releases the VCA domain (Badour et al. 2004). The V domain is then free to bind a monomer of globular actin (G-actin), while the A domain interacts with the Arp2/3 complex and, together, they form the minimal nuclear unit that facilitates F-actin filament elongation (Fig. 1). WASp is recruited to sites of active actin polymerization through the interaction of the proline-rich domain of WASp with the SH3 domain of several adaptor and signaling proteins (Massaad et al. 2013), as shown in Fig. 1.

F-actin polymerization is diminished or dysregulated in hematopoietic cells from patients with *WAS* mutations that affect the levels of WASp or its actin-nucleation activity. Decreased or dysregulated actin polymerization leads to disruption of the structure of the actin cytoskeleton, immune synapse formation, cellular development, migration, and activation, as well as cytokine secretion by immune cells (Massaad et al. 2013; Rivers and Thrasher 2017), as detailed in Table 1.

Clinical Presentation/History (PE)

X-Linked Thrombocytopenia and WAS

The clinical presentation of WAS generally occurs within the first few months of life, but the diagnosis can be delayed especially in milder cases. Mutations in the *WAS* gene are associated with a broad range of clinical severity depending on the nature of the mutation and its effect on protein expression and function. In general, missense mutations in *WAS* that diminish but do not completely abolish WASp expression result in a

Wiskott-Aldrich Syndrome Deficiency, Fig. 1 WASp structure and function. WASp is a multi-domain protein that exists in the cytosol in complex with WIP and DOCK8 in an inactive state, maintained by the intra-molecular interactions between the BR/GBD and the VCA domain. Cellular activation leads to the conversion of CDC42-GDP to CDC42-GTP catalyzed by DOCK8. CDC42-GTP and PIP2 bind to the GBD and BR, respectively, resulting in a conformational change that liberates the VCA domain. Phosphorylation of tyrosine 291 in the GBD also releases the VCA domain. The VCA domain then interacts with G-actin and the Arp2/3 complex to initiate F-actin elongation. The binding of SH3 domain-containing proteins to the proline-rich region of WASp contributes to its activation or suppression. WIP Wiskott-Aldrich syndrome protein-interacting protein; DOCK8 dedicator of cytokinesis 8; EVH1 Ena-Vasp homology domain; BR basic region; GBD CDC42/Rac GTPase binding domain; PPP proline rich region; SH3 Src homology domain 3; V verprolin homology domain; C cofilin homology domain; A acidic domain; PIP2 phophatidylinositol(4,5)-biphosphate; CDC42 cell division control protein 42; GDP guanosine diphosphate; GTP guanosine triphosphate

relatively milder variant of the disease historically named X-linked thrombocytopenia (XLT) because it was described prior to cloning of the *WAS* gene and the recognition that mutations in *WAS* also result in XLT. XLT is characterized mainly by thrombocytopenia with small platelets, mild transient eczema, and minor infections. Although patients with XLT have an excellent long-term survival, they are still at a significant risk of episodes with serious bleeding, life-threatening infections, autoimmunity, and cancer, which should be considered when therapeutic decisions are taken (Albert et al. 2011). Splice site and nonsense mutations in *WAS* that abolish WASp expression or result in a truncated protein lacking the active VCA domain lead to the development of classical WAS, characterized by microthrombocytopenia, recurrent severe infections, eczema, and increased incidence of autoimmunity and malignancies (Candotti 2017; Massaad et al. 2013).

Thrombocytopenia

Thrombocytopenia is a distinctive feature of XLT and WAS, and could be the only clinical manifestation observed in XLT patients, or the earliest to manifest before other facets of the disease are recognized. It is due to a combination of ineffective thrombopoiesis and increased peripheral platelet clearance from the circulation, occasionally resulting in severe spontaneous or posttraumatic bleeding episodes most frequently in the gastrointestinal tract, intracranially, or orally. Platelets from XLT and WAS patients are generally small in size, have decreased F-actin content, are irregular in shape and structure, have a low metabolic activity, and aggregate poorly. Their abnormal shape and structure, as well as the reported presence of auto-autoantibodies that coat their surface, result in their phagocytosis by bone marrow and spleen macrophages. Splenectomy, which has been used in the treatment of patients with XLT and WAS, has been shown to improve the numbers and quality of circulating platelets in these patients.

Immunodeficiency

Both innate and adaptive immunity are defective in WAS patients (Table 1). Patients demonstrate

Wiskott-Aldrich Syndrome Deficiency, Table 1
Hematopoietic cell defects in Wiskott-Aldrich syndrome

Cellular component	Defect
T cells	T cell lymphopenia due to defective T cell development and output, and increased apoptosis Defective F-actin polymerization and immune synapse formation Decreased T cell migration Defective CD4 T cell activation, proliferation, and cytokine secretion Defective CD8 T cell tumor cell killing Defective regulatory T (Treg) cell function
B cells	Hyperproliferative and autoimmune Decreased marginal zone B cells Defective F-actin polymerization Decreased B cell migration Decreased regulatory B (Breg) cell development and function
Platelets	Decreased platelet production and increased clearance Small and irregular in shape Decreased activation and aggregation
Natural killer (NK) cells	Impaired localization of F-actin and disorganized immune synapse formation Impaired microtubule organization center and lytic granules polarization Decreased cytotoxic activity Decreased migration
Invariant natural killer (iNKT) cells	Decreased to absent in the periphery Decreased proliferation and cytokine secretion
Dendritic cells	Abnormal F-actin distribution and immune synapse formation Abnormal ruffle, filopodia, and lamellopodia formation Decreased migration Defective cytokine secretion
Monocytes/ macrophages	Decreased filopodia formation Defective podosome formation and cell polarization Defective migration Reduced apoptotic cell engulfment
Neutrophils	Defective F-actin polymerization and migration Defective degranulation and activation of respiratory burst

variable and selective T and B cell lymphopenia due to abnormal development and increased apoptosis. The most affected T cell compartments include naïve $CD4^+$ cells, cytotoxic $CD8^+$ cells, and T follicular helper cells (Tfh). Peripheral B cell count might be decreased in some young patients but are normal in adult patients, with a concomitant decrease in memory B cells and occasional expansion of the $CD21^{low}$ auto-reactive naïve-like population. Functionally, T cells from WAS patients exhibit cytoskeletal rearrangement defects that limit their ability to generate structured immune synapses (IS), which are important to maintain productive contacts with antigen-presenting cells (APC) and B cells to mount an efficient adaptive immune response, and with target cells to mediate their lysis. In addition, the T cells' capacity to migrate, proliferate, and upregulate activation markers and produce cytokines upon activation is severely diminished. B cells from WAS patients are hyperproliferative, exhibit cytoskeletal and migratory defects, fail to mount effective humoral immune responses especially against carbohydrate antigens and vaccines, and exhibit skewed rearrangements of immunoglobulin heavy chain variable region genes and lower frequency of somatic hypermutation. While part of the B cell defect is intrinsic, it is compounded by the poor ability of Tfh cells from WAS patients to drive antibody production by B cells.

NK cells from WAS and XLT patients are normal in numbers; however, they migrate poorly and are defective in their ability to polymerize F-actin and form stable IS conjugates with target cells, as well as polarize their microtubule organization center and lytic granules to the IS to mediate target cell lysis. Dendritic cells from WAS patients have decreased translocational mobility, and their ability to make stable IS and induce activation of T and NK cells is greatly reduced. In addition, monocytes/macrophages from WAS patients have reduced chemotactic and phagocytic abilities, and neutrophils fail to polymerize actin, adhere to surfaces, and exhibit reduced activation of respiratory burst.

The combinatory defects in innate and adaptive immune cells result in severe and recurrent bacterial (otitis, sinusitis, pneumonia, impetigo, cellulitis, abscesses, enterocolitis, urinary tract infections) viral (HSV, VZV, EBV, CMV, HPV) and fungal (candidiasis, aspergillosis) infections in WAS patients.

Atopy

One of the most common features of WAS is highly pruritic eczematous rash that fits the diagnostic criteria of atopic dermatitis. It affects up to 80% of the patients at some point in their lives and is often accompanied by eosinophilia and high serum IgE level. The eczema could be generalized and includes the face, scalp, arms, and legs or could be more limited to the diaper area and skin creases. Scratching the dry skin often leads to bleeding and provides an entry point for pathogens to cross the broken skin barrier and contribute to the infections that develop in the patients. Food allergy, asthma, and allergic rhinitis are also common is WAS patients. The atopy is associated with a Th1/Th2 imbalance and could be due to the inability of the patients' regulatory T cells (Treg) to keep Th2 cells in check.

Autoimmunity and Malignancies

WAS patients are at a high risk of developing autoimmunity, the most frequent manifestations including autoimmune cytopenia (hemolytic anemia, thrombocytopenia, neutropenia), inflammatory bowel disease, arthritis, vasculitis, and IgA nephropathy. While less frequent, autoimmune complications affecting the skin, muscle, eye, and liver have also been reported. Autoimmunity is mostly attributed to a defect in the function, but not numbers, of Treg cells, a population of T cells important for maintaining peripheral tolerance. In addition, WAS patients have an increase in the fraction of auto-reactive mature naive B cells, and a decrease in interleukin-10 (IL-10) secreting regulatory B cells (B10), both of which could also contribute to the establishment or maintenance of autoimmunity. In fact, multi-reactive auto-antibodies are commonly found in the serum of WAS patients, suggesting that the mechanisms of counter selection and control of self-reactive B lymphocytes may be defective.

Cancer development is a significant concern for WAS and XLT patients. The prevalence of malignancies is high (13–22%) mainly in WAS patients with a severe clinical presentation, especially those who had suffered from an autoimmune disease. While still present, this risk is reduced (5%) in XLT patients with a milder course of the disease. EBV-induced non-Hodgkin lymphoma is the most commonly diagnosed malignancy, but lymphoblastic leukemias, myelodysplasia, and myeloproliferative disorders have also been described. In addition, WAS patients tend to develop benign lymph node enlargements histologically characterized by follicular reactive hyperplasia, which represents further concern of potential malignant transformation. The development of malignancies has been attributed to defective IS formation and polarization of lytic granules by cytotoxic T cells and NK cells toward virally infected cells and cancer cells, which results in poor elimination of transformed cells and contributes to the aberrant immune surveillance in WAS patients.

Classification of XLT Versus WAS

A scoring system based on the severity of the clinical phenotype has been devised to help distinguish and classify patients as XLT or WAS (Zhu et al. 1997). Male patients who exhibit microthrombocytopenia solely are classified as XLT patients with a score of one, whereas those with additional mild transient eczema and minor infections are assigned a score of two. Patients who present with microthrombocytopenia, persistent but manageable eczema, and/or recurrent infections are classified as WAS patients with a score of three, while those with difficult-to-treat eczema and multiple severe infections are assigned a score of four. Both XLT and WAS patients who develop autoimmunity and/or malignancies at a later stage in life progress to a maximum score of five.

X-Linked Neutropenia

A third disorder termed X-linked neutropenia (XLN) is associated with missense mutations found exclusively in the GBD of WASp. Contrary to mutations that affect the level and/or function of

WASp resulting in XLT or WAS, XLN is due to mutations that decrease the affinity of the GBD to the VCA domain, and thus interfere with the auto-inhibited state of the protein resulting in a consti-tutively active form of WASp. Patients with XLN suffer from recurrent major bacterial infections, severe neutropenia, monocytopenia, and decreased NK and B cell numbers with no major platelet defect. In addition, they suffer from myelodysplasia due to abnormal F-actin formation during mitosis that results in the accumulation of multinucleated cells in the bone marrow, which undergo apoptosis (Thrasher and Burns 2010).

Laboratory Findings/Diagnostic Testing

Patients with XLT exhibit several clinical features and laboratory findings similar to those observed in patients with WAS, albeit with moderate sever-ities. The hallmark of XLT and WAS is thrombo-cytopenia with small mean platelet volume (MPV) and abnormal platelet surface structure. Serum immunoglobulin (Ig) levels are variable in the case of IgM, normal to high in the case of IgA, and high in the case of IgG, IgD, and IgE. Patients with WAS produce normal antibody responses to protein antigens but a selective anti-body defect to polysaccharide antigens. The ele-vated levels of IgE are usually associated with allergic diseases, which corroborate with the eczema observed in the patients, and could be due to an imbalance in Th1/Th2 cytokine produc-tion (Albert et al. 2011; Trifari et al. 2006).

Although WAS is often suspected in the case of young male patients with microthrombocytopenia, eczema, bloody diarrhea, and recurrent infections, a definite diagnosis is only achieved biochemically and/or genetically. The level of WASp expression in the patients' cells can be experimentally deter-mined in the laboratory using techniques such as flow cytometry and immunoblot analysis with an antibody highly specific to WASp, and compared to its level in healthy individuals. The advantage of flow cytometry is that it is readily available in most

clinical laboratories, requires a relatively small number of cells from the patients, and the levels of intracellular WASp can be simultaneously deter-mined in multiple cellular populations using sur-face markers for T cells, B cells, NK cells, neutrophils, and monocytes (Kanegane et al. 2017). However, the disadvantage of flow cytometry is that it cannot distinguish between normal and truncated WASp since it generates a signal proportional to the level of the protein pre-sent, rather than its structure. Immunoblotting can alternatively be used to determine the level and structure of WASp, as it identifies a band on a membrane that corresponds to the correct molecu-lar weight of WASp. The disadvantage of immu-noblotting is that it requires a relatively high number of cells from the patients and is generally performed in research laboratories and is thus not readily available to most centers.

Sequencing the *WAS* gene using Sanger or next-generation sequencing provides a genetic diagnosis for WAS deficiency. If the patient harbors a non-sense mutation that terminates protein expression, a splice-site mutation that results in the expression of an aberrant protein, or a previously reported missense mutation that affects the stability of the protein, then the genetic result would strongly sup-port WAS deficiency. If the patient harbors a novel missense mutation, then the effect of the mutation on protein expression would need to be investi-gated to achieve a formal diagnosis. The disadvan-tage of genetic sequencing is that it is not readily available to most laboratories and can only be performed commercially or on research basis.

Treatment/Prognosis

The prognosis of WAS and XLT with low WASp expression remains poor despite advances in diag-nosis and clinical care, due to the recurrence and severity of infections and bleeding episodes, as well as the elevated risk of autoimmunity and malignancies, especially later in life. Conven-tional management includes platelet transfusions to correct the thrombocytopenia and decrease the risks of bleeding episodes. However, platelet transfusions are short-lived, might lead to alloimmunization that could preclude engraftment after HSCT, and to the accumulation of abnormal platelets in the spleen, which results in its enlargement. Splenectomy has been shown to increase the level of platelets in the patients; however, T and B cell function is reduced and the risks of infections are increased following splenectomy, especially in patients who undergo HSCT, making it a less desirable intervention if HSCT is considered (Litzman et al. 1996). As an alternative to platelet transfusions, a thrombopoietin (TPO) receptor agonist (eltrombopag) can be used to promote the generation of mature platelets from megakaryocyte precursors, and was shown to increase the level of platelets and decrease the frequency of bleeding episodes while the patient was awaiting HSCT (Gabelli et al. 2017). The immunodeficiency observed in WAS and XLT patients is variable in presentation and severity; therefore, the risk and occurrence of serious infections are decreased by the regimented use of prophylactic antibiotics and intravenous immunoglobulin (IVIG) replacement therapy (Albert et al. 2011).

HSCT from a human leukocyte antigen-(HLA) identical related sibling or a matched unrelated donor (MUD) is the treatment of choice for WAS, and is most successful if performed in children under 5 years of age, and free of infections at the time of the transplant. The standard conditioning regiment to ensure high-level donor chimerism includes myeloablation with busulfan and immunosuppression with cyclophosphamide, and the highest degree of donor chimerism is observed for T cells, followed by B cells, then myeloid cells. HSCT with multi-lineage donor engraftment can correct all aspects of the disease. Contrary to that, low myeloid donor chimerism might poorly correct the thrombocytopenia, while reduced chimerism that leads to the coexistence of recipient and donor B cells with mostly donor T cells might result in the development of autoimmunity. Acute or chronic graft-versus-host disease (GVHD) is observed especially in the first year after HSCT but can persist longer, and is treated with immunosuppression. Patients with XLT have good long-term survival with conventional treatments. However, in cases with low mutant WASp expression, and in light of the possible development of severe infections, bleeding, autoimmunity, and lymphoproliferative disorders, HSCT can be considered especially for XLT patients for whom a matched sibling donor is available (Pai and Notarangelo 2010).

Gene therapy has been progressively ameliorated in the last decades for the treatments of patients with a number of PIDs. Consequently, it has been applied as an alternative to HSCT for WAS patients who do not have a matched donor, since the transplant from a mismatched donor is associated with a high rate of morbidity and mortality. The general approach consists of isolating autologous HSC from the patient, transducing them ex vivo with a modified viral vector that expresses functional *WAS* as a transgene, then re-infusing the corrected HSC back into the same patient. The initial gene therapy studies for WAS used γ-retroviral vectors with a strong promoter/enhancer long terminal repeat (LTR), and resulted in gene expression in lymphoid and myeloid cells with correction of cell function and platelet production, as well as net amelioration of the clinical symptoms. However, it was associated with the development of acute leukemia in the majority of the patients because of the preferential integration of γ-retroviral vectors in the vicinity of transcription start sites, promoters, and enhancer regions of active genes, resulting in the expansion of clones where the integrations occurred close to proto-oncogenes (LMO2, MDS1/EVI1, and MN1).

The genotoxic risk of γ-retroviral vectors was averted by the development of self-inactivating (SIN) lentiviral vectors that express *WAS* under the control of its own promoter. The novel lentiviral vectors have a high efficiency of transduction, randomly integrate in the genome and thus decrease the risk of insertional mutagenesis,

W

and express physiologic levels of WASp. A total of 21 patients treated with the lentiviral vectors showed expression of functional WASp in lymphoid cells, myeloid cells, and platelets. This resulted in the correction of the actin cytoskeleton defects, normalization of the patients' platelet numbers and T cell, B cell, and NK cell function, and clear clinical benefits as far as bleeding episodes, infections, autoimmunity, and eczema. Importantly, there have been no reports of any genotoxicity 3 years after the initiation of the studies, supporting the use of this new generation of lentiviral vectors in the gene therapy of WAS (Aiuti et al. 2013; Ghosh and Gaspar 2017).

Concluding Remarks

WAS is one of the most studied primary immunodeficiency disorders and represents a model for translational research from bench to bedside. While HSCT and gene therapy are considered the best options for a curative outcome, they are restricted to a limited number of centers and may require several months to be performed. Therefore, prophylactic antibiotics, IVIG therapy, platelet transfusions, and splenectomy in urgency are administered if transplantation is not possible or while the patient is awaiting transplant.

References

Aiuti A, Biasco L, Scaramuzza S, Ferrua F, Cicalese MP, Baricordi C, Dionisio F, Calabria A, Giannelli S, Castiello MC, Bosticardo M, Evangelio C, Assanelli A, Casiraghi M, Di Nunzio S, Callegaro L, Benati C, Rizzardi P, Pellin D, Di Serio C, Schmidt M, Von Kalle C, Gardner J, Mehta N, Neduva V, Dow DJ, Galy A, Miniero R, Finocchi A, Metin A, Banerjee PP, Orange JS, Galimberti S, Valsecchi MG, Biffi A, Montini E, Villa A, Ciceri F, Roncarolo MG, Naldini L. Lentiviral hematopoietic stem cell gene therapy in patients with Wiskott-Aldrich syndrome. Science. 2013;341:1233151.

Albert MH, Notarangelo LD, Ochs HD. Clinical spectrum, pathophysiology and treatment of the Wiskott-Aldrich syndrome. Curr Opin Hematol. 2011;18:42–8.

Badour K, Zhang J, Shi F, Leng Y, Collins M, Siminovitch KA. Fyn and PTP-PEST-mediated regulation of Wiskott-Aldrich syndrome protein (WASp) tyrosine phosphorylation is required for coupling T cell antigen receptor engagement to WASp effector function and T cell activation. J Exp Med. 2004;199:99–112.

Candotti F. Clinical manifestations and pathophysiological mechanisms of the Wiskott-Aldrich syndrome. J Clin Immunol. 2017;38:13.

Gabelli M, Marzollo A, Notarangelo LD, Basso G, Putti MC. Eltrombopag use in a patient with Wiskott-Aldrich syndrome. Pediatr Blood Cancer. 2017;64:1–3.

Ghosh S, Gaspar HB. Gene therapy approaches to immunodeficiency. Hematol Oncol Clin North Am. 2017;31:823–34.

Harada Y, Tanaka Y, Terasawa M, Pieczyk M, Habiro K, Katakai T, Hanawa-Suetsugu K, Kukimoto-Niino M, Nishizaki T, Shirouzu M, Duan X, Uruno T, Nishikimi A, Sanematsu F, Yokoyama S, Stein JV, Kinashi T, Fukui Y. DOCK8 is a Cdc42 activator critical for interstitial dendritic cell migration during immune responses. Blood. 2012;119:4451–61.

Janssen E, Tohme M, Hedayat M, Leick M, Kumari S, Ramesh N, Massaad MJ, Ullas S, Azcutia V, Goodnow CC, Randall KL, Qiao Q, Wu H, Al-Herz W, Cox D, Hartwig J, Irvine DJ, Luscinskas FW, Geha RS. A DOCK8-WIP-WASp complex links T cell receptors to the actin cytoskeleton. J Clin Invest. 2016;126:3837–51.

Kanegane H, Hoshino A, Okano T, Yasumi T, Wada T, Takada H, Okada S, Yamashita M, Yeh TW, Nishikomori R, Takagi M, Imai K, Ochs HD, Morio T. Flow cytometry-based diagnosis of primary immunodeficiency diseases. Allergol Int. 2017;67:43.

Litzman J, Jones A, Hann I, Chapel H, Strobel S, Morgan G. Intravenous immunoglobulin, splenectomy, and antibiotic prophylaxis in Wiskott-Aldrich syndrome. Arch Dis Child. 1996;75:436–9.

Massaad MJ, Ramesh N, Geha RS. Wiskott-Aldrich syndrome: a comprehensive review. Ann N Y Acad Sci. 2013;1285:26–43.

Pai SY, Notarangelo LD. Hematopoietic cell transplantation for Wiskott-Aldrich syndrome: advances in biology and future directions for treatment. Immunol Allergy Clin North Am. 2010;30:179–94.

Rivers E, Thrasher AJ. Wiskott-Aldrich syndrome protein: emerging mechanisms in immunity. Eur J Immunol. 2017;47:1857.

Thrasher AJ, Burns SO. WASP: a key immunological multitasker. Nat Rev Immunol. 2010;10:182–92.

Trifari S, Sitia G, Aiuti A, Scaramuzza S, Marangoni F, Guidotti LG, Martino S, Saracco P, Notarangelo LD, Roncarolo MG, Dupre L. Defective Th1 cytokine gene transcription in CD4$^+$ and CD8$^+$ T cells from Wiskott-Aldrich syndrome patients. J Immunol. 2006;177:7451–61.

Zhu Q, Watanabe C, Liu T, Hollenbaugh D, Blaese RM, Kanner SB, Aruffo A, Ochs HD. Wiskott-Aldrich syndrome/X-linked thrombocytopenia: WASP gene mutations, protein expression, and phenotype. Blood. 1997;90:2680–9.

Wiskott-Aldrich Syndrome Protein-Interacting Protein (WIP) Deficiency

Michel J. Massaad
Department of Experimental Pathology, Immunology, and Microbiology, and Department of Pediatrics and Adolescent Medicine, American University of Beirut, Beirut, Lebanon
Department of Pediatrics, Division of Immunology, Boston Children's Hospital, Harvard Medical School, Boston, MA, USA

Synonyms

CDC42 cell division control protein 42; RTI respiratory tract infections; WAS Wiskott-Aldrich syndrome; WIP Wiskott-Aldrich syndrome protein-interacting protein; WIPF1 WAS/WASL interacting protein family member 1

Definition

Wiskott-Aldrich syndrome protein-interacting protein deficiency is a rare autosomal recessive primary immunodeficiency disease characterized by failure to thrive, thrombocytopenia, eczematous rash, respiratory tract infections, enteritis, bloody diarrhea, and psychomotor delay. Treatment includes prophylactic antibiotic, antifungal, and antiviral therapy, immunoglobulin replacement, and platelet and red blood cell transfusions; however, cure is only achieved with hematopoietic stem cell transplantation.

Introduction/Background

The Wiskott-Aldrich syndrome protein-Interacting Protein (WIP) is encoded by the *WAS/WASL interacting protein family member 1* (*WIPF1*) gene located on chromosome 2. WIP deficiency results in a rare autosomal recessive primary immunodeficiency disease (PID) with a severe clinical course that manifests in the first few months of life, characterized by failure to thrive, thrombocytopenia, eczematous rash with infected papulovesicular and ulcerative lesions, viral bronchiolitis and pneumonia, viral enteritis, intermittent bloody diarrhea, and psychomotor delay (Lanzi et al. 2012; Pfajfer et al. 2017).

WIP was identified in a yeast two-hybrid screen using the Wiskott-Aldrich syndrome protein (WASp) as bait (Ramesh et al. 1997). It is a ubiquitously expressed 503 amino acid (a.a.) multidomain protein. At the N-terminus, it possesses a verprolin homology/actin-binding domain, followed by a proline-rich region, an NcK/CrkL binding region, and a C-terminal WASp-binding region (Anton et al. 2007). The N-terminal region of WIP interacts with the actin-binding protein profilin (Ramesh et al. 1997) and is believed to be the site where the guanine nucleotide exchange factor (GEF) dedicator of cytokinesis 8 (DOCK8) binds and initiates WASp activation (Janssen et al. 2016). Within the N-terminal region, the actin-binding domain (ABD; ^{43}KLKK^{54}) mediates the interaction of WIP with actin (Anton et al. 2003; Massaad et al. 2014). The interaction of WIP and filamentous actin (F-actin) is essential for the stability of the actin cytoskeleton and for the ability of T cells to migrate to secondary lymphoid organs and sites of infections where they mount an immune response (Massaad et al. 2014). The proline-rich region of WIP interacts with the actin-binding protein cortactin and enhances its actin-nucleation potential (Kinley et al. 2003). WIP a.a. 321–415 interact with the adaptor proteins NcK (Anton et al. 1998) and CrkL (Sasahara et al. 2002), which target a multimeric complex that includes WIP and WASp to the immunological synapse. The C-terminal WASp-binding region (a.a. 461–485) mediates the interaction of WIP with WASp (Volkman et al. 2002) and is primordial for WASp stabilization (Massaad et al. 2011).

WIP exists with WASp in a constitutive complex in which WIP serves as a chaperone for WASp. Mice in which *Wpif1* has been deleted (de la Fuente et al. 2007), patients with a nonsense mutation in *WIPF1* that abrogates WIP expression (Lanzi et al. 2012; Pfajfer et al. 2017), and patients with missense mutations in the WIP-binding Ena-Vasp homology (EVH1) domain of WASp have severely diminished levels or completely absent WASp. This highlights the importance of WIP for WASp stability, and hence its actin-nucleation function, which is important for the actin cytoskeleton dynamics and immune cell function.

WIP also interacts with another WASp family member, neuronal(N)-WASp (Martinez-Quiles et al. 2001); however, the interaction of WIP with N-WASp is dispensable for N-WASp stability (de la Fuente et al. 2007), which might be assumed by the interaction of N-WASp with the WIP- and CR16-homologous protein (WICH) (Kato et al. 2002).

Mechanistic Implication of WIP in WASp Activation and Actin Cytoskeleton Integrity

WIP exists in the cytoplasm of hematopoietic cells in a heteropolymeric complex that includes WASp and DOCK8, in which WIP bridges the two proteins together (Janssen et al. 2016). WASp is maintained in an inactive state in resting cells. Following cellular activation, the GEF DOCK8 converts the cell division control protein 42 (CDC42) from an inactive guanosine diphosphate(GDP)-bound form to an active guanosine triphosphate (GTP)-bound form (Harada et al. 2012). The newly generated CDC42-GTP binds to WASp and activates it to initiate F-actin filament elongation, as described in details in the chapter on Wiskott-Aldrich Syndrome (WAS) deficiency. Therefore, WIP plays a central role in the homeostasis and activation of WASp; on one hand, WIP binds to WASp and protects it from degradation, thus making it available for activation; on the other hand, WIP bridges the GEF DOCK8 and WASp, keeping the two proteins in close spatial proximity that favors the DOCK8-mediated activation of WASp.

The interaction of WIP with WASp serves not only to stabilize and activate WASp but also to recruit it to sites of cellular activation where actin polymerization is crucial. Through its interaction with NcK and CrkL, WIP targets WASp to the T cell receptor (TCR)/CD3 surface cluster in a mechanism that involves ZAP70 and SLP-76 (Sasahara et al. 2002). At the TCR, WASp mediates actin polymerization, important for the formation of productive immune synapses (IS) able to maintain stable contacts between T cells and antigen-presenting cells (APCs) to achieve efficient T cell activation. In addition, WIP facilitates the localization of WASp at podosomes in myeloid cells, thus favoring their directional migration (Chou et al. 2006).

The most extensively studied function of WIP is related to its role in WASp stability and activation. However, WIP plays a WASp-independent role in cytoskeletal integrity and dynamics. WIP interacts with F-actin at a site in the N-terminal region (^{43}KLKK^{54}) distant from the C-terminal WASp-interacting domain (Anton et al. 2003; Massaad et al. 2014). The interaction of WIP with F-actin is crucial for the stability of the F-actin network. Deletion of the ^{43}KLKK^{54} motif in WIP affects the integrity of the actin cytoskeleton, resulting in decreased migration of T cells in a transwell system in vitro, and to secondary lymphoid organs and sites of inflammation in vivo (Massaad et al. 2014). In addition, WIP associates with granzyme B in natural killer (NK) cells independently of WASp and is important for the polarization of perforin- and granzyme-containing lytic granules towards target cells to mediate their lysis (Krzewski et al. 2008).

Cellular Defects in WIP Deficiency

Our knowledge of the biochemical and mechanistic involvement of WIP in immune cell function is mostly derived from mice in which WIP has been deleted or modified, since only two patients with WIP deficiency have been reported so far (Lanzi et al. 2012; Pfajfer et al. 2017). Fortunately, the murine model of WIP deficiency faithfully mirrors the phenotype of the human disorder, and therefore, the biochemical and cellular defects observed in murine studies were instrumental to diagnose and study the patients.

WIP-Deficient T Cells

The total number of T cells in thymi from WIP-deleted (WIP$^{-/-}$) mice is decreased; however, their percentages in the thymi and in secondary lymphoid organs is not affected, indicating that WIP does not play a significant role in the development of T cells (Anton et al. 2002). Despite normal development, WIP$^{-/-}$ mouse T cells fail to proliferate, secrete interleukin (IL)-2, increase their F-actin content, polarize and extend actin-containing protrusions following TCR ligations, and form conjugate with superantigen-presenting B cells and anti-CD3 bilayers (Anton et al. 2002). In addition, WIP$^{-/-}$ T cells fail to migrate in a transwell system in vitro, and to lymphoid organs in vivo, in a mechanism that involves WASp (Gallego et al. 2005), and the actin-binding domain (^{43}KLKK^{54}) of WIP (Massaad et al. 2014). Deeper analysis of WIP$^{-/-}$ T cells revealed a gross failure in their ability to upregulate CD25 and respond to IL-2, due to a defect in the phosphorylation and signaling downstream of the signal transducer and activator of transcription (STAT) 5 (Le Bras et al. 2009). These data indicate that WIP is important for the proper dynamics of the actin cytoskeleton and migration of T cells, as well as the activation of T cells downstream of the TCR and chemokine receptors.

The two reported patients with WIP deficiency had variable T cell lymphopenia (Lanzi et al. 2012; Pfajfer et al. 2017). T cells isolated from one patient failed to proliferate when stimulated with an antibody that cross-links CD3, and this defect was not corrected by the addition of exogenous IL-2, which also failed to induce STAT5 phosphorylation (Lanzi et al. 2012), similar to what was observed in mouse WIP$^{-/-}$ T cells. In addition, T cells prepared from the patients were unable to migrate to a chemokine gradient in vitro (Lanzi et al. 2012, Pfajfer et al. 2017). Unstimulated T cells from one of the patients appeared abnormally large, and harbored aberrant shapes and reduced roundness. Upon chemokine stimulation, these cells emitted multiple actin-rich structures but failed to elongate and to assemble distinct leading and trailing edges, indicating a defect in the directional migration of the cells

(Pfajfer et al. 2017). Cytotoxic CD8$^+$ T cells isolated from one of the patients displayed aberrantly elongated shapes and actin-rich protrusions, and their capacity to secrete lytic granules and eliminate target cells was greatly reduced, most likely resulting from a failure to assemble productive IS (Pfajfer et al. 2017). These data demonstrate that WIP is necessary for the assembly of a reticulated actin meshwork ultrastructure and dynamics, primordial for T cell directional migration and activation.

WIP-Deficient B Cells

The development and peripheral distribution of B cells in WIP$^{-/-}$ mice is normal (Anton et al. 2002). However, B cells from WIP$^{-/-}$ mice display aberrant cytoskeletal architecture (Anton et al. 2002), and migrate poorly to lymph nodes in vivo, and to a chemokine gradient in vitro (Keppler et al. 2015). WIP$^{-/-}$ B cells hyperproliferate following stimulation and have increased levels of activation markers than their wild-type counterparts, suggesting that WIP plays a role in modulating the activation of B cells. In addition, WIP$^{-/-}$ B cells secrete high levels of IgE and IgM, normal levels of IgA, and normal to elevated levels of IgG despite decreased plasma cell differentiation (Anton et al. 2002; Keppler et al. 2015). WIP$^{-/-}$ B cells mount a normal immune response against T-independent antigens but fail to form germinal centers (GC) and mount an immune response against viral infections and T-dependent antigens, indicating that WIP is important for the ability of B cells to respond efficiently to viral infections and T-dependent immunization (Anton et al. 2002, Keppler et al. 2015).

The B cell receptor (BCR) and CD19 are immobilized in the B cell membrane by molecular interactions with the cortical actin cytoskeleton (Mattila et al. 2013). B cell activation results in cytoskeletal reorganization that releases BCR nanoclusters, which can diffuse laterally in the B cell membrane and interact with CD19, held in place by the CD81 tetraspanin network (Mattila et al. 2013). Immobilization of CD19 in the membrane is important for PI3K/AKT signaling

W

(Otero et al. 2001). Absence of WIP results in distortions in the cortical actin cytoskeleton that allow BCR diffusion but, at the same time, decreases the expression of CD81, resulting in abnormal lateral diffusion of CD19, and failure to support CD19 phosphorylation and CD19-mediated PI3K/AKT signaling downstream of the BCR, BAFFR, TLR4, CD40, CXCR4, and CXCR5 receptors (Keppler et al. 2015). In summary, the integrity of the actin cytoskeleton mediated by WIP is crucial to diminish the lateral diffusion of CD19 in the B cell membrane, thus favoring CD19 phosphorylation and activation of the PI3K/AKT complex, important for B cell homeostasis, survival, differentiation, and class-switch recombination.

Primary B cells from WIP-deficient patients were not analyzed; however, an Epstein-Barr virus (EBV)-transformed B cell line from one patient, and a normal EBV-B cell line in which WIP was knocked-down, emitted large filopodia and pseudopodia in various directions and failed to orient and polarize actin directionally in order to migrate towards a chemokine gradient (Pfajfer et al. 2017). This highlights the requirement for WIP in sustaining persistent actin-dependent B lymphocyte polarity, essential for chemokine-evoked directional motility.

WIP-Deficient NK Cells

WIP exists in activated murine NK cells in a complex that includes WASp, actin, and myosin IIA, the dissociation of which results in inhibition of cytotoxic activity (Krzewski et al. 2006). WIP also associates with granzyme B and is important for the polarization of perforin- and granzyme-containing lytic granules towards target cells to mediate their lysis, as cells in which WIP has been knocked down fail to lyse target cells despite normal conjugate formation (Krzewski et al. 2008).

NK cells isolated from one patient with WIP deficiency and expanded ex vivo demonstrated decreased expression of the activating receptors NKp30, NKp46, and NKG2D and a drastic reduction in cytolytic activity against target cells (Lanzi

et al. 2012). As NK cell cytolytic responses require actin cytoskeleton rearrangements for proper cell adhesion, IS formation, sustained signaling, and delivery of lytic granules to the target cell, the role WIP plays in this process is crucial for the function of cytolytic cells.

WIP-Deficient Platelets

$WIP^{-/-}$ mice are moderately thrombocytopenic, their platelets are coated with IgA antibodies, and they are cleared faster from the circulation when compared to their wild-type counterparts (Falet et al. 2009). In addition, signaling downstream of the collagen receptor glycoprotein VI (GPVI) is severely diminished in $WIP^{-/-}$ platelets, resulting in decreased P-selectin expression, integrin $\alpha IIb\beta 3$ activation, and actin assembly. Furthermore, GPVI shedding mediated by a specific anti-GPVI antibody and PLC-$\gamma 2$ phosphorylation and signaling downstream of GPVI were diminished in IgA-covered $WIP^{-/-}$ platelets, indicating that IgA antiplatelet antibodies target GPVI or a nearby receptor and negatively modulate GPVI signaling (Falet et al. 2009).

Both patients with WIP deficiency were severely thrombocytopenic requiring thrombopoietin receptor agonist treatment (Pfajfer et al. 2017) and platelet infusions (Lanzi et al. 2012; Pfajfer et al. 2017); however, the pathophysiology of the structure and function of the platelets were not investigated in the patients.

WIP-Deficient Myeloid Cells

Dendritic cells. WIP is important for the assembly of actin filaments, $\beta 2$-integrins, and vinculin into podosomes in mouse dendritic cells (DC) (Chou et al. 2006). Podosomes are highly dynamic structures that mediate transient adhesion followed by migration of DCs (Calle et al. 2006; Linder and Kopp 2005). They have a unique organization with actin filaments bundled in a conical core containing proteins, such as gelsolin, cortactin, the actin-nucleating factor Arp2/3 complex, and WASp (Calle et al. 2006), surrounded by a ring of integrins and integrin-associated proteins (Calle et al. 2006, Linder and Kopp 2005). In DCs,

WIP protects WASp from degradation and facilitates its localization to podosomes, thus favoring their maturation. Rather than podosomes, $WIP^{-/-}$ DCs assemble large focal contacts that adhere strongly to the substratum and have a lower turnover index, negatively affecting DC's directional migration and polarity (Chou et al. 2006).

Macrophages. WIP interacts with WASp in human macrophages. This association is important for podosome and phagocytic cup formation, as dissociating the complex or knocking down WIP impaired podosome formation, transendothelial migration, and the formation of a phagocytic cup important for the engulfment of pathogen (Tsuboi 2007; Tsuboi and Meerloo 2007). These data suggest that WIP plays a critical role in localizing WASp to podosome and phagocytic cups.

Mast cells. Mouse $WIP^{-/-}$ mast cells exhibit defects in the dynamic regulation of the actin cytoskeleton, decreased intracellular calcium flux, and impaired capacity to degranulate and secrete IL-6 after ligation of the immunoglobulin (Ig)E receptor (FcεRI) (Kettner et al. 2004). WIP interacts with the signaling molecule Syk following mast cell stimulation and protects it from degradation (Kettner et al. 2004). Therefore, in the absence of WIP, activation of Syk downstream of the FcεRI is severely diminished, resulting in cytoskeletal and functional defects in mast cells.

Fibroblasts. WIP regulates N-WASp-mediated actin polymerization, as well as filopodia and ruffle formation by human fibroblasts (Anton et al. 2003; Martinez-Quiles et al. 2001). In addition, mouse $WIP^{-/-}$ fibroblasts demonstrate increased levels of cytosolic G-actin, which sequester the serum response factor (SRF) transcription factor complex in the cytosol, leading to diminished expression or proteins important for the formation of focal adhesion (FA) and stress fiber assembly (Ramesh et al. 2014). These data demonstrate that WIP controls the dynamics of the actin cytoskeleton directly by modulating N-WASp-mediated actin polymerization and indirectly by controlling the expression of genes important for the assembly of stress fibers and adhesion of fibroblast.

Clinical Presentation/History (PE)

Taking into consideration that WIP and WASp form an inseparable unit in a common pathway, and that WIP tightly regulates WASp function, it was expected that WIP deficiency might display a disorder that closely resembles that of WAS deficiency. Long before two patients with WIP deficiency were identified and studied, it was documented that $WIP^{-/-}$ mice exhibited immunological abnormalities and pathological changes that mimic those observed in patients with WAS (Curcio et al. 2007). $WIP^{-/-}$ mice exhibit a marked granulocytosis coupled with a progressive severe central and peripheral T and B cell lymphopenia. The spleens isolated from aging $WIP^{-/-}$ mice are enlarged, with marked increase of red pulp and erythrocytes, and decrease of white pulp and lymphocytes. Of note is that a major defect in the T and B cell development was not reported in the original paper describing the immunological phenotype of $WIP^{-/-}$ mice (Anton et al. 2002), which might not have been obvious due to the young age of the mice used in that study. Ulcerative colitis was evident even in young mice, and this condition progressed with age to severe colitis aggravated by fibrosis and mucosal pseudopolyposis. Interstitial inflammation of the walls of the alveoli and signs of hypersensitive pneumonitis typically centered on bronchioles were also seen in $WIP^{-/-}$ mice. In addition, $WIP^{-/-}$ mice developed autoimmune kidney disease characterized by mild to severe mesangial proliferative glomerulonephritis and deposits of IgA, IgG, and complement C3. Furthermore, sera isolated from $WIP^{-/-}$ mice contained antibodies specific for nuclear and cytoplasmic antigens (Curcio et al. 2007). One or more of these symptoms are observed in patients with WAS, strongly supporting the hypothesis that there would be an overlap between the phenotypes of WIP and WAS deficiency.

WIP deficiency is a very rare disorder. Only two patients are reported, one being a girl with a clinical phenotype of WAS; however, since WAS is an X-linked disorder, she was unlikely to be a

W

WAS patient, and thus WIP deficiency was demonstrated (Lanzi et al. 2012), confirming the autosomal recessive mode of inheritance of this disorder. Each patient harbored a homozygous nonsense mutation in WIP (S434X and R125X) that abolished WIP protein expression and resulted in complete absence of WASp expression as well.

Both patients manifested the disease in the first month of life and suffered from failure to thrive and severe thrombocytopenia that required platelet transfusions. The female patient developed an eczematous rash, papulovesicular lesions on the scalp, and ulcerative lesions on the hard palate and tongue, indicative of an inflammatory process. *Staphylococcus epidermidis* and *Klebsiella pneumoniae* grew from the skin vesicular lesions. She developed respiratory distress, and a tracheal aspirate tested positive for respiratory syncytial virus. She also developed rotavirus enteritis and acute hepatitis. No clinical manifestations of autoimmunity or bleeding tendency were noted (Lanzi et al. 2012). She had a female sibling with a similar clinical picture who died of sepsis at 4 months of age before a genetic diagnosis was obtained (Lanzi et al. 2012). The male patient had bronchiolitis and viral pneumonia, as well as pneumonitis, highlighting the infectious and inflammatory nature of the lung manifestations. Cytomegalovirus was detected in his body fluids and the patient suffered from intermittent episodes of bloody diarrhea suggestive of inflammatory bowel disease. In addition, he experienced psychomotor delay of unknown etiology (Pfajfer et al. 2017).

The spectrum of clinical manifestations shared between the two WIP-deficient patients includes failure to thrive, thrombocytopenia, eczematous rash with infected papulovesicular and ulcerative lesions, severe respiratory tract infections (RTI), intermittent bloody diarrhea, and psychomotor delay. Although only two patients with WIP deficiency have been reported so far, it is clear that their clinical phenotype is reminiscent of the severe cases of WAS deficiency, highlighting the similarities between the two disorders.

Laboratory Findings/Diagnostic Testing

Patients with WIP deficiency exhibit several laboratory findings similar to those observed in patients with WASp deficiency (Massaad et al. 2013). Thrombocytopenia with bleeding episodes was a prominent feature in both patients described; however, unlike patients with WAS, the mean platelet volume (MPV) reported on one patient was normal (Lanzi et al. 2012; Pfajfer et al. 2017). Both patients suffered from cytopenia, which might be progressive in nature. The absolute numbers of T cells were severely diminished in both patients, and their residual T cells exhibited a memory phenotype and failed to proliferate upon cross-linking their TCR/CD3 complex, which was not corrected by addition of IL-2. The male patient suffered from thymus involution and low T-cell receptor excision circles and thymic emigrants, indicating that thymus development appeared abnormal, and providing a possible link with the T cell development defect. Both patients had low absolute numbers of B cells, but their IgG and IgM levels were normal to elevated, IgA levels were normal to low, and IgE levels were elevated in one of the patients tested. T and B cells failed to polarize their actin cytoskeleton and migrate to a chemokine gradient, while cytotoxic T cells failed to form IS and direct lytic granules towards target cells. Similar to NK cells from WAS patients, the absolute numbers of NK cells were elevated in both WIP-deficient patients, however, the NK cell from one patient tested expressed low levels of activation markers on their surface, and their cytolytic activity was defective.

WIP deficiency should be high on the differential for female patients presenting with a clinical picture of WAS, but also for male patients, especially if they descend from consanguineous families with a history suggestive of PID affecting male and female relatives. However, a definite diagnosis is only achieved biochemically and/or genetically. The level of WIP expression in the patients' cells can be determined by immunoblotting or flow cytometry (Lanzi et al. 2012, Pfajfer et al. 2017). Unfortunately, these tests are not commercially available and are done on research basis only. Sequencing the *WIPF1* gene using Sanger or next generation sequencing provides a genetic diagnosis for WIP deficiency. If the patient harbors a nonsense mutation that terminates protein expression or a splice-site mutation that results in the expression of an aberrant protein, then the genetic result would strongly support WIP deficiency. If the patient harbors a missense mutation, then the effect of the mutation on protein expression would need to be investigated to achieve a formal diagnosis. The disadvantage of genetic sequencing is that it is not readily available to most laboratories and can only be performed commercially or on research basis. Furthermore, since WIP is a rare disorder, the genetic diagnosis should always be supported through investigating the effect of the mutation on the protein level.

Treatment/Prognosis

WIP deficiency is a very severe disorder, and, similar to WASp deficiency, the prognosis would be poor if the patients are not diagnosed and treated early in life. The only two patients described in the literature had severe clinical manifestations that unveiled very early in life. Much of the treatment for WIP-deficient patients is based on the approaches used in the treatment of WAS. Conventional treatment includes wide-spectrum antibiotic therapy, fungal and viral prophylaxis, immunoglobulin replacement therapy, and platelet and red blood cell transfusions. Conventional therapy represents a temporary relieve for the patients' symptoms and a preventive measure against future infections. In addition, while platelet transfusions decrease the risks of bleeding episodes, platelet are short-lived, might lead to alloimmunization, and to the accumulation of abnormal platelets in the spleen, which results in its enlargement. If performed, splenectomy might increase the level of platelets in the patients; however, it might decrease the function of T and B cells and increase the risks of infections.

The specific antibody responses of WIP-deficient patients have not been measured; however, because of their similarities with WASp-deficient patients, and the faithful correlation between the murine model of WIP deficiency and the human disorder, it is likely that WIP-deficient patients would suffer from poor specific antibody responses that can be circumvented with immunoglobulin replacement therapy, which was given to the female patient.

Similar to WASp deficiency and most other PIDs, hematopoietic stem cell transplantation (HSCT) and, most likely in the future, gene therapy are the only curative approaches for patients with WIP deficiency. In general, HSCT from a human leukocyte antigen-(HLA) identical related sibling or a matched unrelated donor (MUD) are preferred in the treatment of WAS and are most successful if performed in children under 5 years of age and free of infections at the time of the transplant (Pai and Notarangelo 2010). The same would be expected for patients with WIP deficiency; however, since there are only two patients treated so far, more patients are needed to devise the best HSCT strategy to achieve the most desirable outcome. The female patient was transplanted from an unrelated cord blood donor at 4.5 months of age and was alive and well 16 months after the transplant, with >98% of T cells, >98% of B cells, 94% of NK cells, 50% of monocytes, and 41% of granulocytes of donor origin (Lanzi et al. 2012). The oral ulcerations resolved after HSCT, suggesting that they were secondary to deficient immune function. The clinical situation of the male patient was too severe for a fully conditioned allogeneic HSCT; instead, sequential infusions of peripheral lymphocytes and stem cells from the HLA-identical mother were performed at the 10th to 13th month of life, accompanied by sirolimus treatment during the first month. This resulted in sustained donor T cell and NK cell engraftment (CD3$^+$ cells: 61.5%; CD56$^+$ cells: 41.3% donor chimerism) but reduced donor B cell and myeloid cell engraftment (CD19$^+$ cells: 1.9%; CD33$^+$ cells: 0.4% donor chimerism), leading to complete clinical

W

stabilization regarding the infections 1 year following the treatment. However, he required platelet support by thrombopoietin receptor agonist treatment and sporadic platelet infusions because of severe thrombocytopenia that developed at the end of the infusion treatment (Pfajfer et al. 2017), likely the result of poor myeloid cell engraftment. In addition, the coexistence of recipient and donor B cells, with mostly donor T cells might result in the development of autoimmunity. Therefore, HSCT following myeloablative therapy may be more effective in the treatment of patients with WIP deficiency.

Concluding Remarks

WIP was identified as a binding partner for WASp, and its deficiency resulted in a similar phenotype in human patients and in murine models of the disease. The identification of WIP-deficient patients was greatly facilitated by the large body of knowledge on WAS patients and WIP$^{-/-}$ mice and represents a perfect example on how our knowledge of one disorder can help identify deficiencies in other members of the same pathway, which lead to a similar disorder. As in WASp deficiency and other PIDs, HSCT remains the best curative option and is best performed early in life to achieve the most desirable curative outcome.

Cross-References

▶ WAS Wiskott-Aldrich Syndrome

References

Anton IM, Lu W, Mayer BJ, Ramesh N, Geha RS. The Wiskott-Aldrich syndrome protein-interacting protein (WIP) binds to the adaptor protein Nck. J Biol Chem. 1998;273:20992–5.

Anton IM, de la Fuente MA, Sims TN, Freeman S, Ramesh N, Hartwig JH, Dustin ML, Geha RS. WIP deficiency reveals a differential role for WIP and the actin cytoskeleton in T and B cell activation. Immunity. 2002;16:193–204.

Anton IM, Saville SP, Byrne MJ, Curcio C, Ramesh N, Hartwig JH, Geha RS. WIP participates in actin reorganization and ruffle formation induced by PDGF. J Cell Sci. 2003;116:2443–51.

Anton IM, Jones GE, Wandosell F, Geha R, Ramesh N. WASP-interacting protein (WIP): working in polymerisation and much more. Trends Cell Biol. 2007;17:555–62.

Calle Y, Burns S, Thrasher AJ, Jones GE. The leukocyte podosome. Eur J Cell Biol. 2006;85:151–7.

Chou HC, Anton IM, Holt MR, Curcio C, Lanzardo S, Worth A, Burns S, Thrasher AJ, Jones GE, Calle Y. WIP regulates the stability and localization of WASP to podosomes in migrating dendritic cells. Curr Biol. 2006;16:2337–44.

Curcio C, Pannellini T, Lanzardo S, Forni G, Musiani P, Anton IM. WIP null mice display a progressive immunological disorder that resembles Wiskott-Aldrich syndrome. J Pathol. 2007;211:67–75.

de la Fuente MA, Sasahara Y, Calamito M, Anton IM, Elkhal A, Gallego MD, Suresh K, Siminovitch K, Ochs HD, Anderson KC, Rosen FS, Geha RS, Ramesh N. WIP is a chaperone for Wiskott-Aldrich syndrome protein (WASP). Proc Natl Acad Sci USA. 2007;104:926–31.

Falet H, Marchetti MP, Hoffmeister KM, Massaad MJ, Geha RS, Hartwig JH. Platelet-associated IgAs and impaired GPVI responses in platelets lacking WIP. Blood. 2009;114:4729–37.

Gallego MD, de la Fuente MA, Anton IM, Snapper S, Fuhlbrigge R, Geha RS. WIP and WASP play complementary roles in T cell homing and chemotaxis to SDF-1alpha. Int Immunol. 2005;18:221–32.

Harada Y, Tanaka Y, Terasawa M, Pieczyk M, Habiro K, Katakai T, Hanawa-Suetsugu K, Kukimoto-Niino M, Nishizaki T, Shirouzu M, Duan X, Uruno T, Nishikimi A, Sanematsu F, Yokoyama S, Stein JV, Kinashi T, Fukui Y. DOCK8 is a Cdc42 activator critical for interstitial dendritic cell migration during immune responses. Blood. 2012;119:4451–61.

Janssen E, Tohme M, Hedayat M, Leick M, Kumari S, Ramesh N, Massaad MJ, Ullas S, Azcutia V, Goodnow CC, Randall KL, Qiao Q, Wu H, Al-Herz W, Cox D, Hartwig J, Irvine DJ, Luscinskas FW, Geha RS. A DOCK8-WIP-WASp complex links T cell receptors to the actin cytoskeleton. J Clin Investig. 2016;126:3837–51.

Kato M, Miki H, Kurita S, Endo T, Nakagawa H, Miyamoto S, Takenawa T. WICH, a novel verprolin homology domain-containing protein that functions cooperatively with N-WASP in actin-microspike formation. Biochem Biophys Res Commun. 2002;291:41–7.

Keppler SJ, Gasparrini F, Burbage M, Aggarwal S, Frederico B, Geha RS, Way M, Bruckbauer A, Batista FD. Wiskott-Aldrich syndrome interacting protein deficiency uncovers the role of the co-receptor CD19 as a generic hub for PI3 kinase signaling in B cells. Immunity. 2015;43:660–73.

Kettner A, Kumar L, Anton IM, Sasahara Y, de la Fuente M, Pivniouk VI, Falet H, Hartwig JH, Geha RS. WIP regulates signaling via the high affinity receptor for immunoglobulin E in mast cells. J Exp Med. 2004;199:357–68.

Kinley AW, Weed SA, Weaver AM, Karginov AV, Bissonette E, Cooper JA, Parsons JT. Cortactin interacts with WIP in regulating Arp2/3 activation and membrane protrusion. Curr Biol. 2003;13:384–93.

Krzewski K, Chen X, Orange JS, Strominger JL. Formation of a WIP-, WASp-, actin-, and myosin IIA-containing multiprotein complex in activated NK cells and its alteration by KIR inhibitory signaling. J Cell Biol. 2006;173:121–32.

Krzewski K, Chen X, Strominger JL. WIP is essential for lytic granule polarization and NK cell cytotoxicity. In: Proceedings of the National Academy of Sciences of the United States of America, vol. 105; 2008. p. 2568–73.

Lanzi G, Moratto D, Vairo D, Masneri S, Delmonte O, Paganini T, Parolini S, Tabellini G, Mazza C, Savoldi G, Montin D, Martino S, Tovo P, Pessach IM, Massaad MJ, Ramesh N, Porta F, Plebani A, Notarangelo LD, Geha RS, Giliani S. A novel primary human immunodeficiency due to deficiency in the WASP-interacting protein WIP. J Exp Med. 2012;209:29–34.

Le Bras S, Massaad M, Koduru S, Kumar L, Oyoshi MK, Hartwig J, Geha RS. WIP is critical for T cell responsiveness to IL-2. Proc Natl Acad Sci USA. 2009;106:7519–24.

Linder S, Kopp P. Podosomes at a glance. J Cell Sci. 2005;118:2079–82.

Martinez-Quiles N, Rohatgi R, Anton IM, Medina M, Saville SP, Miki H, Yamaguchi H, Takenawa T, Hartwig JH, Geha RS, Ramesh N. WIP regulates N-WASP-mediated actin polymerization and filopodium formation. Nat Cell Biol. 2001;3:484–91.

Massaad MJ, Ramesh N, Le Bras S, Giliani S, Notarangelo LD, Al-Herz W, Geha RS. A peptide derived from the Wiskott-Aldrich syndrome (WAS) protein-interacting protein (WIP) restores WAS protein level and actin cytoskeleton reorganization in lymphocytes from patients with WAS mutations that disrupt WIP binding. J Allergy Clin Immunol. 2011;127(998–1005):e1–2.

Massaad MJ, Ramesh N, Geha RS. Wiskott-Aldrich syndrome: a comprehensive review. Ann N Y Acad Sci. 2013;1285:26–43.

Massaad MJ, Oyoshi MK, Kane J, Koduru S, Alcaide P, Nakamura F, Ramesh N, Luscinskas FW, Hartwig J, Geha RS. Binding of WIP to actin is essential for T cell actin cytoskeleton integrity and tissue homing. Mol Cell Biol. 2014;34:4343–54.

Mattila PK, Feest C, Depoil D, Treanor B, Montaner B, Otipoby KL, Carter R, Justement LB, Bruckbauer A, Batista FD. The actin and tetraspanin networks organize receptor nanoclusters to regulate B cell receptor-mediated signaling. Immunity. 2013;38:461–74.

Otero DC, Omori SA, Rickert RC. Cd19-dependent activation of Akt kinase in B-lymphocytes. J Biol Chem. 2001;276:1474–8.

Pai SY, Notarangelo LD. Hematopoietic cell transplantation for Wiskott-Aldrich syndrome: advances in biology and future directions for treatment. Immunol Allergy Clin N Am. 2010;30:179–94.

Pfajfer L, Seidel MG, Houmadi R, Rey-Barroso J, Hirschmugl T, Salzer E, Anton IM, Urban C, Schwinger W, Boztug K, Dupre L. WIP deficiency severely affects human lymphocyte architecture during migration and synapse assembly. Blood. 2017;130:1949–53.

Ramesh N, Anton IM, Hartwig JH, Geha RS. WIP, a protein associated with wiskott-aldrich syndrome protein, induces actin polymerization and redistribution in lymphoid cells. Proc Natl Acad Sci USA. 1997;94:14671–6.

Ramesh N, Massaad MJ, Kumar L, Koduru S, Sasahara Y, Anton I, Bhasin M, Libermann T, Geha R. Binding of the WASP/N-WASP-interacting protein WIP to actin regulates focal adhesion assembly and adhesion. Mol Cell Biol. 2014;34:2600–10.

Sasahara Y, Rachid R, Byrne MJ, de la Fuente MA, Abraham RT, Ramesh N, Geha RS. Mechanism of recruitment of WASP to the immunological synapse and of its activation following TCR ligation. Mol Cell. 2002;10:1269–81.

Tsuboi S. Requirement for a complex of Wiskott-Aldrich syndrome protein (WASP) with WASP interacting protein in podosome formation in macrophages. J Immunol. 2007;178:2987–95.

Tsuboi S, Meerloo J. Wiskott-Aldrich syndrome protein is a key regulator of the phagocytic cup formation in macrophages. J Biol Chem. 2007;282:34194–203.

Volkman BF, Prehoda KE, Scott JA, Peterson FC, Lim WA. Structure of the N-WASP EVH1 domain-WIP complex: insight into the molecular basis of Wiskott-Aldrich syndrome. Cell. 2002;111:565–76.

W

X

XIAP Deficiency

Ivan K. Chinn
Section of Immunology, Allergy, and
Retrovirology, Texas Children's Hospital,
Houston, TX, USA
William T. Shearer Center for Human
Immunobiology, Texas Children's Hospital,
Houston, TX, USA
Department of Pediatrics, Baylor College of
Medicine, Houston, TX, USA

Introduction

XIAP is located at Xq25 and encodes a 497 amino acid protein that is also sometimes known as BIRC4 (Yang et al. 2012). XIAP deficiency is therefore inherited as an X-linked recessive trait. The molecule is ubiquitously expressed and present in all hematopoietic cells (Yang et al. 2012; Latour and Aguilar 2015).

Molecular Function

The initial understanding of XIAP function focused upon its role in control of apoptosis. The molecule contains three baculovirus inhibitor of apoptosis repeat (BIR) domains (Yang et al. 2012). XIAP inhibits caspase-3, caspase-7, and caspase-9 in response to apoptotic stimuli, such as CD95 cross-linking (Deveraux et al. 1997;

Rigaud et al. 2006; Obexer and Ausserlechner 2014). BIR2 is necessary for direct inhibition of caspase-3 and caspase-7, while BIR3 is responsible for caspase-9 inhibition (Yang et al. 2012). SMAC/Diablo competitively binds to BIR2 and BIR3, releasing bound caspase molecules to increase the free levels of the proapoptotic molecules and promote cell death (Obexer and Ausserlechner 2014; Lalaoui and Vaux 2018).

Subsequent research has elucidated critical roles for XIAP in inflammatory responses and immune function. XIAP carries a C-terminal RING domain, which promotes proteasomal degradation of caspase-3 and SMAC/Diablo (Obexer and Ausserlechner 2014). This domain, however, also provides the molecule with important E3 ubiquitin ligase function (Yang et al. 2012). For example, upon NOD1/2 activation, RIPK2 and XIAP are recruited. XIAP binds to RIPK2 via its BIR2 domain and ubiquitylates RIPK2. This activity is critical for recruiting LUBAC to induce ubiquitylation of NEMO, which is necessary for canonical NF-κB activation (Estornes and Bertrand 2015). Binding of TAB1 to the BIR1 domain of XIAP activates TAK1 and subsequently both the MAP kinase (including JNK, p38, and ERK) and NF-κB (via IκB kinase kinase) pathways (Obexer and Ausserlechner 2014; Estornes and Bertrand 2015; Latour and Aguilar 2015; Lalaoui and Vaux 2018). Ubiquitylated RIPK2 serves as a scaffold to potentiate formation of this TAB-TAK1 complex. Aside from its role in NOD signaling, XIAP has

© Springer Science+Business Media LLC, part of Springer Nature 2020
I. R. Mackay et al. (eds.), *Encyclopedia of Medical Immunology*,
https://doi.org/10.1007/978-1-4614-8678-7

been shown to mediate BCL10-dependent Dectin-1 induction of the NF-κB and MAP kinase pathways, cytokine production, and phagocytosis (Latour and Aguilar 2015). In mouse models, XIAP inhibits RIPK1- and RIPK3-controlled TNF-α production and inflammation (Latour and Aguilar 2015). XIAP has further been proposed to downregulate NLRP3 inflammasome activity, but cIAP1 and cIAP2 may possess similar redundant roles (Estornes and Bertrand 2015; Lalaoui and Vaux 2018). XIAP is downregulated by apoptosis-related protein in the TGF-β signaling pathway (ARTS) (Vasudevan and Don Ryoo 2015).

hypomorphic genetic change has been associated with isolated dysgammaglobulinemia (Nishida et al. 2015). Another hypomorphic pathogenic variant resulted in granulomatous lymphocytic interstitial lung disease and granulomatous hepatitis in the absence of detectable EBV infection (Steele et al. 2016). Affected cases do not appear to carry increased risk for the appearance of lymphoma (Aguilar and Latour 2015). Of note, although XIAP deficiency is inherited in an X-linked recessive manner, erythema nodosum, gastrointestinal disease, and HLH have been observed in female carriers (Dziadzio et al. 2015; Latour and Aguilar 2015).

Presentation

XIAP deficiency typically presents as lymphoproliferative disease, hemophagocytic lymphohistiocytosis (HLH), or very early- or early-onset Crohn's-like inflammatory bowel disease (Rigaud et al. 2006; Speckmann et al. 2013; Nielsen and LaCasse 2017). Two of the three manifestations can occur simultaneously (Speckmann et al. 2013). Most affected cases consist of male children who present early in life (Latour and Aguilar 2015). Splenomegaly represents the most common clinical manifestation (nearly 60% of cases) (Latour and Aguilar 2015). Lymphoproliferative disease and HLH are often, but not always, associated with EBV infection (Rigaud et al. 2006; Speckmann et al. 2013). HLH can also be triggered by CMV or HHV-6 (Latour and Aguilar 2015). Some patients may present with recurrent fevers and splenomegaly or "severe infectious mononucleosis" without fulfilling the criteria for HLH (Speckmann et al. 2013). Overall survival approximates 80% (Latour and Aguilar 2015).

Other disease manifestations have been reported. Hypogammaglobulinemia occurs in some patients (Rigaud et al. 2006; Rezaei et al. 2011; Speckmann et al. 2013). Erythema nodosum, arthritis, recurrent skin abscesses, hepatitis, nephritis, and anterior uveitis have also been observed (Speckmann et al. 2013; Dziadzio et al. 2015; Latour and Aguilar 2015). At least one

Diagnosis

Early diagnosis can provide the opportunity for timely treatment to reduce mortality and morbidity (Nielsen and LaCasse 2017). Absence of XIAP protein by either flow cytometry or western blotting remains pathognomonic, but not all pathogenic variants lead to abnormal protein expression (Rigaud et al. 2006; Speckmann et al. 2013). Patients with XIAP deficiency have variable numbers of NKT and mucosal-associated invariant T (MAIT) cells, and normal numbers of these cells cannot be used to exclude the diagnosis (Rigaud et al. 2006; Rezaei et al. 2011; Latour and Aguilar 2015). Cytotoxic T- and NK-cell function is not generally impaired (Rigaud et al. 2006). HLH that results from XIAP deficiency is characterized by elevated serum levels of IL-6, neopterin, IFN-γ, and TNF-α, which can also be seen in patients with other forms of HLH (Wada et al. 2014). A markedly elevated serum level of IL-18, however, distinguishes XIAP deficiency-driven HLH from other causes of HLH (Wada et al. 2014). XIAP deficiency can sometimes be determined by increased CD95-induced apoptosis in T-cell blasts or EBV-transformed B cells or increased activation-induced cell death in T cells (Rigaud et al. 2006; Latour and Aguilar 2015). This finding can be variable, however (Ammann et al. 2014). Rather, because XIAP is essential for NOD2 signaling, quantitative or qualitative XIAP deficiency can be confirmed by diminished monocyte production of TNF-α in response to lipidated muramyl peptide (L18-MDP) (Ammann et al. 2014; Latour and Aguilar 2015). Genetic testing is fully indicated for diagnostic purposes, but functional testing can sometimes be necessary for confirmation of variant pathogenicity (Nielsen and LaCasse 2017).

Treatment

Hematopoietic stem cell transplantation (HSCT) provides the only definitive treatment for XIAP deficiency. Use of myeloablative or intermediate intensity conditioning is associated with remarkably poor survival and is not recommended (Marsh et al. 2013). Use of reduced intensity conditioning (RIC) was found to result in 55% survival after HSCT, and remission of HLH at the time of HSCT further correlated with improved survival (Marsh et al. 2013). Greatest survival (about 90%) has been observed with use of RIC in patients in remission of HLH at the time of transplantation (Marsh et al. 2013; Chellapandian et al. 2016; Ono et al. 2017). One interesting case reported an excellent outcome after HSCT in a patient with uncontrolled HLH using minimal intensity conditioning and adjunctive use of anti-CD45 antibodies together with a high dose of donor stem and T cells (Worth et al. 2013).

Cross-References

▶ Blau Syndrome
▶ LUBAC Deficiencies
▶ Neonatal-Onset Multisystem Inflammatory Disease (NOMID)
▶ NF-kB Essential Modulator (NEMO)

References

Aguilar C, Latour S. X-linked inhibitor of apoptosis protein deficiency: more than an X-linked lymphoproliferative syndrome. J Clin Immunol. 2015;35:331–8.

Ammann S, Elling R, Gyrd-Hansen M, et al. A new functional assay for the diagnosis of X-linked inhibitor of apoptosis (XIAP) deficiency. Clin Exp Immunol. 2014;176:394–400.

Chellapandian D, Krueger J, Schechter T, et al. Successful allogeneic hematopoietic stem cell transplantation in XIAP deficiency using reduced-intensity conditioning. Pediatr Blood Cancer. 2016;63:355–7.

Deveraux QL, Takahashi R, Salvesen GS, Reed JC. X-linked IAP is a direct inhibitor of cell-death proteases. Nature. 1997;388:300–4.

Dziadzio M, Ammann S, Canning C, et al. Symptomatic males and female carriers in a large Caucasian kindred with XIAP deficiency. J Clin Immunol. 2015;35:439–44.

Estornes Y, Bertrand MJM. IAPs, regulators of innate immunity and inflammation. Semin Cell Dev Biol. 2015;39:106–14.

Lalaoui N, Vaux D. Recent advances in understanding inhibitor of apoptosis proteins [version 1; peer review: 2 approved]. F1000Res. 2018;7:1889.

Latour S, Aguilar C. XIAP deficiency syndrome in humans. Semin Cell Dev Biol. 2015;39:115–23.

Marsh RA, Rao K, Satwani P, et al. Allogeneic hematopoietic cell transplantation for XIAP deficiency: an international survey reveals poor outcomes. Blood. 2013;121:877–83.

Nielsen OH, LaCasse EC. How genetic testing can lead to targeted management of XIAP deficiency-related inflammatory bowel disease. Genet Med. 2017;19:133–43.

Nishida N, Yang X, Takasaki I, et al. Dysgammaglobulinemia associated with Glu349del, a hypomorphic XIAP mutation. J Investig Allergol Clin Immunol. 2015;25:205–13.

Obexer P, Ausserlechner MJ. X-linked inhibitor of apoptosis protein – a critical death resistance regulator and therapeutic target for personalized cancer therapy. Front Oncol. 2014;4:197.

Ono S, Okano T, Hoshino A, et al. Hematopoietic stem cell transplantation for XIAP deficiency in Japan. J Clin Immunol. 2017;37:85–91.

Rezaei N, Mahmoudi E, Aghamohammadi A, Das R, Nichols KE. X-linked lymphoproliferative syndrome: a genetic condition typified by the triad of infection, immunodeficiency and lymphoma. Br J Haematol. 2011;152:13–30.

Rigaud S, Fondanèche M-C, Lambert N, et al. XIAP deficiency in humans causes an X-linked lymphoproliferative syndrome. Nature. 2006;444:110–4.

Speckmann C, Lehmberg K, Albert MH, et al. X-linked inhibitor of apoptosis (XIAP) deficiency: the spectrum of presenting manifestations beyond hemophagocytic lymphohistiocytosis. Clin Immunol. 2013;149:133–41.

Steele CL, Doré M, Ammann S, et al. X-linked inhibitor of apoptosis complicated by granulomatous lymphocytic interstitial lung disease (GLILD) and granulomatous hepatitis. J Clin Immunol. 2016;36:733–8.

Vasudevan D, Don Ryoo H. Regulation of cell death by IAPs and their antagonists. Curr Top Dev Biol. 2015;114:185–208.

Wada T, Kanegane H, Ohta K, et al. Sustained elevation of serum interleukin-18 and its association with hemophagocytic lymphohistiocytosis in XIAP deficiency. Cytokine. 2014;65:74–8.

Worth AJJ, Nikolajeva O, Chiesa R, Rao K, Veys P, Amrolia PJ. Successful stem cell transplant with antibody-based conditioning for XIAP deficiency with refractory hemophagocytic lymphohistiocytosis. Blood. 2013;121:4966–8.

Yang X, Miyawaki T, Kanegane H. SAP and XIAP deficiency in hemophagocytic lymphohistiocytosis. Pediatr Int. 2012;54:447–54.

X-linked Agammaglobulinemia (BTK Deficiency)

Vassilios Lougaris and Alessandro Plebani
Pediatrics Clinic and Institute for Molecular Medicine A. Nocivelli, Department of Clinical and Experimental Sciences, University of Brescia and ASST-Spedali Civili of Brescia, Brescia, Italy

Definition

X-linked agammaglobulinemia (XLA; OMIM#300755) is a rare primary immunodeficiency with an incidence ranging from 1:100,000 to 1:200,000, depending on ethnicity, and is characterized by reduced serum levels of all immunoglobulin classes in the absence of peripheral B cells (peripheral B cells <2%). XLA is caused by mutations in the gene encoding for Bruton's tyrosine kinase (BTK).

Pathogenesis

While XLA was first described in 1952 by Colonel OC Bruton (1952), the underlying genetic cause was not identified until 1993 (Tsukada et al. 1993; Vetrie et al. 1993). Bruton's tyrosine kinase, which is deficient in XLA, is a member of the Tec family of kinases (Vihinen et al. 1997).

Normally, B cells are generated in the bone marrow starting from pluripotent lymphocyte progenitors. They acquire specific phenotypic features and upregulate the expression of specific genes in order to proceed from the pro-B cell to the pre-B cell maturational stage in the bone marrow (Matthias and Rolink 2005). This step is characterized by the expression of the pre-B cell receptor (pre-BCR) on the cell surface (Clark et al. 2005).

BTK is a kinase that acts downstream of the BCR in B cells. Thus, mutations in *BTK* do not allow for this maturational step to take place, and B cell maturation is blocked early in the bone marrow at the pro-B to pre-B stage. Consequently, peripheral B cells are absent, immunoglobulin levels are very low for all classes, and there is no humoral response to recall antigens. BTK deficiency specifically affects the B cell lineage, resulting in reduced size of lymph nodes and tonsils, tissues normally highly populated by B cells. Both number and function of T cells are not affected. *BTK* maps on the X chromosome, and therefore affected patients are males; mutations can be both familiar and de novo ones; in the first case, mothers of affected individuals with only one allele affected are healthy carriers.

Clinical Presentation

Maternal immunoglobulins are transferred to the fetus through the placenta and protect affected patients for the first 6–9 months of life. Upon the progressive catabolism of maternal immunoglobulins, patients develop increase susceptibility to infections and usually present recurrent bacterial infections, mainly of the upper and lower respiratory tract. Invasive infections, such as meningitis, may also occur. In some cases, affected patients may remain asymptomatic for the first year of life. Rarely, XLA might be diagnosed in adolescence or early adulthood. These cases are characterized by partial B cell development and production of immunoglobulins associated with missense mutations resulting in BTK expression with partial protein function.

Common infections observed in XLA patients include recurrent otitis media, sinusitis, bronchitis, pneumonia, and gastrointestinal infections (Conley and Howard 2002). Etiology and frequency of these infections vary depending on the cohort of patients investigated; nonetheless, infections of the upper and lower respiratory tract remain the most frequent ones (Lederman and Winkelstein 1985; Plebani et al. 2002).

Among the bacterial infectious agents, encapsulated pyogenic bacteria such as *Streptococcus pneumoniae*, *Haemophilus influenzae*, and *Staphylococcus aureus* are the most frequently isolated ones. In the case of septicemia, the most frequently isolated pathogens belong to the *Pseudomonas* species, followed by *H. influenzae*, *S. pneumoniae*, and *S. aureus*. Septic arthritis and bacterial meningitis mainly caused by *H. influenzae* and *S. pneumoniae* might be observed.

Unfortunately, it is well established that even upon XLA diagnosis and initiation of immunoglobulin replacement treatment, affected patients present recurrent respiratory infections of the lower tract, leading to the development of bronchiectasis (Lederman and Winkelstein 1985; Plebani et al. 2002).

Frequent infections of the gastrointestinal tract also occur, even upon regular Ig replacement treatment commencement (Lederman and Winkelstein 1985; Plebani et al. 2002). The most frequently isolated pathogen is *Giardia lamblia*, often not responsive to treatment, leading in some cases to chronic diarrhea and malabsorption. Similar clinical findings are caused by *Campylobacter jejuni* infections that can however be accompanied by skin manifestations and fever. Finally, *Salmonella* species have also been described as cause of gastrointestinal symptoms in XLA patients (Lederman and Winkelstein 1985; Plebani et al. 2002).

The clinical history of XLA may be complicated not only by bacterial but also by viral infections, mainly by enterovirus, namely, poliovirus, echovirus, and coxsackie virus. Vaccine-associated poliomyelitis after live attenuated oral vaccine (Sabin) has been reported and is associated with a high mortality rate. Neurotropic enteroviral infections may present with atypical clinical features, such as ataxia, paresthesias, loss of cognitive skills, and neurosensorial hearing loss. Enteroviral meningoencephalitis in XLA patients tends to manifest slowly throughout the years, although fulminating infection with fever, headache, and seizures has also been reported (Halliday et al. 2003; Misbah et al. 1992; Wilfert et al. 1977). One of the main diagnostic problems is the isolation of the enterovirus, since PCR techniques do not always detect the virus in the CSF samples. CSF findings on the other hand may be suggestive of viral infection, although in many cases CSF may be almost normal. Treatment consists in high-dose IVIG, and in some isolated cases, intrathecal IgG administration has been performed, with variable results. Pleconaril treatment has also been implemented in enteroviral infections of the CNS in XLA, in association with high-dose IVIG. Chronic enteroviral infection eventually results in cerebral edema, diffuse inflammation, and progressive cerebral atrophy (Halliday et al. 2003; Plebani et al. 2002).

Arthritis has been reported in almost 20% of XLA patients (Lederman and Winkelstein 1985; Plebani et al. 2002). Clinical presentation may be indistinguishable from rheumatoid arthritis. In some cases, an infectious agent may be isolated from joint fluid, although in the majority of the cases, no isolates are found. Since these joint symptoms tend to respond to IVIG therapy, the hypothesis of a possible infectious cause is strong.

A peculiar hematologic finding in XLA is neutropenia that may be present in variable percentages (Buckley and Rowlands 1973; Cham et al. 2002; Farrar et al. 1996). Neutropenia is typically found at diagnosis of XLA, and neutrophil counts tend to normalize upon Ig replacement treatment.

Diagnosis

Laboratory investigation in patients with XLA shows low to undetectable immunoglobulin serum levels and severely reduced peripheral B cells (<2%). Clinical suspicion, together with suggestive immunological work-up, indicates testing of BTK expression testing by means of flow cytometry. Definitive diagnosis requires molecular analysis of the *BTK* gene. Once a pathogenic mutation is defined, carrier diagnosis, prenatal diagnosis, and other family testing might be discussed.

Management

Immunoglobulin replacement therapy is essential in XLA as in all humoral immunodeficiencies. While in the past, intramuscular administration was used, currently two options are available: intravenous or subcutaneous. Normally, a dose of 400 mg/kg/dose every 3–4 weeks is sufficient to maintain trough serum IgG levels >500 mg/dl that should be able to reduce the number of infectious episodes, especially that of invasive infections.

Although the overall infections rate is reduced in XLA upon Ig replacement therapy initiation, many patients may present recurrent respiratory infections during follow-up, ultimately leading to lung complications, with the development of bronchiectasis and chronic lung disease (Plebani et al. 2002). Antibiotics are frequently used, both in the case of acute infections and in terms of prophylactic regimen. Malignancy, especially gastrointestinal cancers, seems to present an increased incidence in XLA. Finally, lymphoid malignancies have been reported but percentages vary in the different cohorts of patients.

References

Bruton OC. Agammaglobulinemia. Pediatrics. 1952; 9:722–8.

Buckley RH, Rowlands DT Jr. Agammaglobulinemia, neutropenia, fever, and abdominal pain. J Allergy Clin Immunol. 1973;51:308–18.

Cham B, Bonilla MA, Winkelstein J. Neutropenia associated with primary immunodeficiency syndromes. Semin Hematol. 2002;39:107–11.

Clark MR, Cooper AB, Wang LD, Aifantis I. The pre-B cell receptor in B cell development: recent advances, persistent questions and conserved mechanisms. Curr Top Microbiol Immunol. 2005;290:87–103.

Conley ME, Howard V. Clinical findings leading to the diagnosis of X-linked agammaglobulinemia. J Pediatr. 2002;141:566–71.

Farrar JE, Rohrer J, Conley ME. Neutropenia in X-linked agammaglobulinemia. Clin Immunol Immunopathol. 1996;81:271–6.

Halliday E, Winkelstein J, Webster ADB. Enteroviral infections in primary immunodeficiency (PID): a survey of morbidity and mortality. J Infect. 2003;46:1–8.

Lederman HM, Winkelstein JA. X-linked agammaglobulinemia: an analysis of 96 patients. Medicine (Baltimore). 1985;64:145–56.

Matthias P, Rolink AG. Transcriptional networks in developing and mature B cells. Nat Rev Immunol. 2005;5:497–508.

Misbah SA, Spickett GP, Ryba PCJ, Hockaday JM, Kroll JS, Sherwood C, Kurtz JB, Moxon ER, Chapel HM. Chronic enteroviral meningoencephalitis in agammaglobulinemia – case-report and literature-review. J Clin Immunol. 1992;12:266–70.

Plebani A, Soresina A, Rondelli R, Amato GM, Azzari C, Cardinale F, Cazzola G, Consolini R, De Mattia D, Dell'Erba G, Duse M, Fiorini M, Martino S, Martire B, Masi M, Monafo V, Moschese V, Notarangelo LD, Orlandi P, Panei P, Pession A, Pietrogrande MC, Pignata C, Quinti I, Ragno V, Rossi P, Sciotto A, Stabile A, Italian Pediatric Group for XLA-AIEOP. Clinical, immunological, and molecular analysis in a large cohort of patients with X-linked agammaglobulinemia: an Italian multicenter study. Clin Immunol. 2002;104:221–30.

Tsukada S, Saffran DC, Rawlings DJ, Parolini O, Allen RC, Klisak I, Sparkes RS, Kubagawa H, Mohandas T, Quan S, et al. Deficient expression of a B cell cytoplasmic tyrosine kinase in human X-linked agammaglobulinemia. Cell. 1993;72:279–90.

Vetrie D, Vorechovský I, Sideras P, Holland J, Davies A, Flinter F, Hammarström L, Kinnon C, Levinsky R, Bobrow M, et al. The gene involved in X-linked agammaglobulinaemia is a member of the src family of protein-tyrosine kinases. Nature. 1993;361: 226–33.

Vihinen M, Mattsson PT, Smith CI. BTK, the tyrosine kinase affected in X-linked agammaglobulinemia. Front Biosci. 1997;2:d27–42.

Wilfert CM, Buckley RH, Mohanakumar T, Griffith JF, Katz SL, Whisnant JK, Eggleston PA, Moore M, Treadwell E, Oxman MN, Rosen FS. Persistent and fatal central-nervous-system echovirus infections in patients with agammaglobulinemia. N Engl J Med. 1977;296:1485–9.

X-Linked Hyper-IgM Syndrome: CD40Ligand Deficiency (OMIM # 308230)

M. Teresa de la Morena
Department of Pediatrics and Division of
Immunology, Seattle Children's Hospital and
University of Washington, Seattle, WA, USA

Introduction/Background

Deficiency in CD40Ligand (CD40L) causes a combined immunodeficiency affecting both cellular and humoral immunity. Mutations in the *CD40LG* gene causes the X-linked form of hyper-IgM (XHIGM) syndrome, called hyper-IgM type 1. This is a rare primary immunodeficiency with an estimated frequency of 1:1,000,000 (Winkelstein et al. 2003). The *CD40LG* gene is located on chromosome Xq26. In 1993, five different research groups identified CD40 ligand (CD40L) as causative of XHIGM (Allen et al. 1993; Aruffo et al. 1993; DiSanto et al. 1993; Fuleihan et al. 1993; Korthauer et al. 1993).

The protein encoded by *CD40LG*, CD40L (CD154), is tightly regulated and expressed when T cells are activated during an immune response. CD40L, on activated T cells, is capable of binding CD40, constitutively expressed on the surface of B cells. CD40L/CD40 binding permits an effective antibody response through two mechanisms: class-switch recombination (CSR) and somatic hypermutation. During CSR, the constant region of the mu (μ) heavy chain is replaced by a different immunoglobulin constant region: alpha, gamma, or epsilon. This induces B cells to "switch" from producing IgM to producing IgA, IgG, or IgE. This change in immunoglobulin isotype modifies the biologic property of the antibody molecule, defined by the constant region, while maintaining the variable region properties that allows for antigen binding. The second mechanism, somatic hypermutation, introduces mutations within the variable region of the antibody molecule, improving the quality of the antibody response by producing high affinity antibody molecules for a particular antigen. Finally, class switched memory B cells are subsequently generated which are quickly recruited upon re-encounter with the antigen (Notarangelo et al. 2006). In addition to isotype switching, CD40L enables priming of T lymphocytes and CD40L binding of CD40 on macrophages and dendritic cells activates them (Jain et al. 1999).

Clinical Presentation

Patients with XHIGM are susceptible to bacterial, viral, and opportunistic infections, can develop autoimmune manifestations, and have high risk of malignancies (Levy et al. 1997; Winkelstein et al. 2003; Lee et al. 2013; Cabral-Marques et al. 2014; Leven et al. 2016; De la Morena et al. 2017).

Over 80% of XHIGM patients come to medical attention during infancy with recurrent respiratory diseases (otitis media, sinusitis, and pneumonia). Approximately 40% of patients may present with *Pneumocystis jirovecii* pneumonia before the first year of life. Viruses that contribute to lower respiratory tract infections include cytomegalovirus (CMV), adenovirus, parainfluenza, and respiratory syncytial virus (RSV).

Gastrointestinal (GI) manifestations are noted in almost 40% of patients, with chronic diarrhea being a common complaint and contributing to failure to thrive in young children. Infectious and noninfectious enteritis/colitis is common. Unique pathogens reported contributing to GI morbidity and mortality include CMV, adenovirus, Norovirus, *Salmonella* sp., *Isospora* sp., *Blastocytis hominis*, and Giardia among others. Importantly, *Cryptosporidium* may cause liver disease. Liver and bile duct pathology including sclerosing cholangitis, cirrhosis, and/or liver failure are significant contributors to the limited life expectancy for XHIGM patients and can be seen in the absence of *Cryptosporidium* infection. In countries where BCG is standard of care, BCG infections were reported in up to 30% of patients with XHIM as their first manifestation.

Oral ulcers are frequently associated with chronic or intermittent neutropenia, by far the most commonly encountered hematologic complication, with hemolytic anemia and parvovirus-induced red cell aplasia also reported.

Central nervous system manifestations occur in approximately 10% of patients and may contribute to developmental delay. Progressive neurodegenerative encephalopathies caused by JC (John Cunningham) viruses or of unknown etiology have been reported.

Patients with CD40L deficiency can develop malignancies. Neuroendocrine tumors involving the gastrointestinal tract and pancreas are the most frequently encountered malignancies and are associated with high mortality. These tumors include hepatocarcinoma, cholangiocarcinoma, rectal carcinoma, leukemia, and lymphoma.

Finally, case reports of osteopenia and fractures in XHIGM suggest a potential role for CD40L in osteoclastogenesis (Lopez-Granados et al. 2007).

Patients with XHIGM have no syndromic features that might be diagnosed in the physical exam. Most physical findings are consequences of the clinical manifestations described above. Importantly, those with liver disease may have hepatomegaly associated hepatitis, while those with cirrhosis and portal hypertension may have associated features including splenomegaly. It is noteworthy that lymphadenopathy is not a common physical finding.

Diagnosis and Laboratory Testing

The laboratory findings common to most XHIM patients include low or borderline levels of IgG, absent IgA with elevated or normal levels of IgM. It is important to note that IgM levels can vary depending on the age of the child.

Antibody responses to routine childhood vaccinations are usually absent, while iso-hemagglutinins are usually normal or elevated. Standard flow cytometric analyses of peripheral blood lymphocytes, including T, B, and NK

populations are normal. In contrast, B cell sub-populations flow analysis demonstrates a lack of class switched memory B cells (CD27+ IgM−), which may resemble patients with common variable immunodeficiency (CVID). Thus, mutations in CD40L should be ruled out in male patients with clinical phenotypes of XHIGM who carry the diagnosis of CVID. Proliferation studies to mitogens will be normal but in vitro studies have demonstrated poor INF-γ and TNF-α production.

Histological analysis of lymph nodes demonstrates a lack germinal center formation (De la Morena 2016).

Diagnosis is made when pathogenic mutations are found in CD40L gene sequencing, available through several commercial laboratories. Functional flow cytometry studies aim to identify CD40L expression on activated T lymphocytes. Most patients with XHIGM will not express CD40L. These flow analysis studies confirm T cell activation by staining for other activation markers such as CD69 and CD25. Importantly, use of anti-human CD40L monoclonal antibody alone can miss up to 30% of CD40L mutations, because patient with mutations located in the intracytoplasmic tail of CD40L may have CD40L surface expression and therefore appear normal.

Treatment

Patients with XHIGM require management by their primary care practitioner in conjunction with a clinical immunologist. Gammaglobulin replacement therapy, either intravenous (IVIG) or subcutaneous, is recommended for all patients. In addition, prompt treatment with appropriate antimicrobial therapy for bacterial infections should be instituted. Similarly, use of ganciclovir for cytomegalovirus infection needs to be initiated as soon as possible, given its associated high mortality. Furthermore, treatment of other viral infections for which effective therapies are available should be pursued as soon as the diagnosis is established and in severe cases, even empirically suspected.

Prevention of opportunistic infections includes use of appropriate antimicrobial prophylaxis against *Pneumocystis jirovecii* pneumonia with trimethoprim-sulfamethoxazole. For patients with reported adverse reactions to this medication, alternative therapies include pentamidine, dapsone, or atovaquone.

Patients with CD40 deficiency are treated similar to those XHIGM. Gammaglobulin replacement therapy, either intravenous (IVIG) or subcutaneous, is recommended for all patients. Treat bacterial and viral infections promptly with appropriate antimicrobial therapy; a prolonged course may be necessary. Antimicrobial prophylaxis is recommended to prevent *Pneumocystis jirovecii* pneumonia and trimethoprim-sulfamethoxazole may be used with caution, given the tendency for neutropenia. Prevention against *Cryptosporidium* spp. infection is based on hygiene measures. The parasite is waterborne; toddlers and young children are especially vulnerable. It is important to recognize that alcohol-based sanitizers are not effective, and it is recommended hand washing with soap and water. Swimming in waterparks, rivers, lakes, or drinking from water fountains should be avoided. Nitazoxanide and paromomycin have been used for treatment but do not eradicate the pathogen from immunocompromised hosts. However, evidence-based anti-cryptosporidial prophylactic regimens are not established for patients with XHIGM and its use is variable among specialists.

XHIGM patients with chronic or intermittent neutropenia may develop oral ulcers. While there are no evidence-based indications for use of human recombinant-granulocyte colony-stimulating-factor (rhG-CSF) in patients with XHIGM, recurrent infections and oral ulcers and periodontal infections do benefit from use of rhG-CSF. The length of therapy with rhG-CSF is not established. The potential risk for malignant transformation with rhG-CSF is an unproven concern that may limit its indefinite use; otherwise asymptomatic moderately neutropenic patients may prefer expectant treatment of oral infections.

The long-term prognosis for XHIGM remains poor, with an estimated median survival from time of diagnosis of 25 years (Levy et al. 1997; De la Morena et al. 2017). The morbidity and mortality related to this condition has prompted the application of allogeneic hematopoietic stem cell transplantation (HCT) as the only current curative therapeutic option (Gennery et al. 2004). In a recent retrospective international study of 176 patients with XHIGM, 67 patients had undergone HCT. Posttransplant survival was reported as >80% at 10 years, with most deaths occurring within 1 year of transplant. However, long-term survival was similar between those undergoing HCT versus those treated with conventional therapies alone. In contrast, a study from Japan comparing long-term outcomes of 29 patients with XHIGM undergoing transplantation to 27 patients treated with medical regimens and suggested greater overall survival in HCT recipients (Mitsui-Sekinaka et al. 2015). Early age at transplantation, similar to transplantation outcomes for other primary immunodeficiency disorders, was associated with improved long-term survival. Liver and pulmonary disease at time of transplantation has been associated with poor survival. Transplant variables such as hematopoietic stem cells source (bone marrow, cord, or mobilized peripheral stem cells), stem cell donor relationship (related vs unrelated), conditioning regimen (ablative vs. non-myeloablative), and engraftment did not influence survival. Graft vs. host disease has been reported in up to 40% of patients (De la Morena et al. 2017). Liver transplantation with and without HCT has been performed in patients with XHIGM associated end-stage liver disease with variable success. Malignancy associated with XHIGM is associated with high mortality (De la Morena et al. 2017).

Research studies have suggested the use of recombinant CD40L (rCD40L) as a potential therapeutic intervention. Three patients with XHIGM have been treated thus far demonstrating adequate IFN-γ and TNF-α production by mitogen-activated T-cells (Jain 1995). rCD40L is not currently available clinically and the long-term utility of this approach remains to be

X

determined. Finally, similarly to other monogenic primary immune deficiency diseases, gene therapy experimental approaches may provide an alternative option for patients in the future (Hubbard et al. 2016).

References

Allen RC, Armitage RJ, Conley ME, Rosenblatt H, Jenkins NA, Copeland NG, et al. CD40 ligand gene defects responsible for X-linked hyper-IgM syndrome. Science. 1993;259:990–3.

Aruffo A, Farrington M, Hollenbaugh D, Li X, Milatovich A, Nonoyama S, et al. The CD40 ligand, gp39, is defective in activated T cells from patients with Xlinked hyper-IgM syndrome. Cell. 1993;72:291–300.

Cabral-Marques O, Klaver S, Schimke LF, Ascendino EH, Khan TA, Pereira PV, et al. First report of the Hyper-IgM syndrome Registry of the Latin American Society for immunodeficiencies: novel mutations, unique infections, and outcomes. J Clin Immunol. 2014;34:146–56.

De la Morena MT. Clinical phenotypes of hyper IgM-syndromes. J Allergy Clin Immunol Pract. 2016;4:1023–36.

De la Morena MT, Leonard D, Torgerson TR, Cabral-Marques O, Slatter M, Aghamohammadi A, et al. Long-term outcomes of 178 patients with X-linked hyper-IgM syndrome treated with or without hematopoietic cell transplantation. J Allergy Clin Immunol. 2017;139:1282–92.

DiSanto JP, Bonnefoy JY, Gauchat JF, Fischer A, de Saint Basile G. CD40 ligand mutations in x-linked immunodeficiency with hyper-IgM. Nature. 1993;361:541–3.

Fuleihan R, Ramesh N, Loh R, Jabara H, Rosen RS, Chatila T, et al. Defective expression of the CD40 ligand in X chromosome-linked immunoglobulin deficiency with normal or elevated IgM. Proc Natl Acad Sci USA. 1993;90:2170–3.

Gennery AR, Khawaja K, Veys P, Bredius RG, Notarangelo LD, Mazzolari E, et al. Treatment of CD40 ligand deficiency by hematopoietic stem cell transplantation: a survey of the European experience, 1993-2002. Blood. 2004;103:1152–7.

Hubbard N, Hagin D, Sommer K, Song Y, Khan I, Clough C, et al. Targeted gene editing restores regulated CD40L function in X-linked hyper-IgM syndrome. Blood. 2016;127(21):2513–22.

Jain A, Atkinson TP, Lipsky PE, Slater JE, Nelson DL, Strober W. Defects of T-cell effector function and postthymic maturation in X-linked hyper-IgM syndrome. J Clin Invest. 1999;103:1151–8.

Korthauer U, Graf D, Mages HW, Briere F, Padayachee M, Malcolm S, et al. Defective expression of T-cell CD40 ligand causes X-linked immunodeficiency with hyper-IgM. Nature. 1993;361:539–41.

Lee WI, Huang JL, Yeh KW, Yang MJ, Lai MC, Chen LC, et al. Clinical features and genetic analysis of Taiwanese patients with the hyper IgM syndrome phenotype. Pediatr Infect Dis J. 2013;32:1010–6.

Leven E, Maffucci P, Ochs H, Scholl P, Buckley R, Fuleihan R, et al. Hyper IgM syndrome: a report from the USIDENT Registry. J Clin Immunol. 2016;36:490–501.

Levy J, Espanol-Boren T, Thomas C, Fischer A, Tovo P, Bordigoni P, et al. Clinical spectrum of X-linked hyper-IgM syndrome. J Pediatr. 1997;131:47–54.

Lopez-Granados E, Temmerman ST, Wu L, Reynolds JC, Follmann D, Liu S, et al. Osteopenia in X-linked hyperIgM syndrome revelas a regulatory role for CD40 ligand in osteoclastogenesis. PNAS. 2007;104(12):5056–61.

Mitsui-Sekinaka K, Imai K, Sato H, Tomizawa D, Kajiwara M, Nagasawa M, et al. Clinical features and hematopoietic stem cell transplantations for CD40 ligand deficiency in Japan. J Allergy Clin Immunol. 2015;136:1018–24.

Notarangelo LD, Lanzi G, Peron S, Durandy A. Defects of class-switch recombination. J Allergy Clin Immunol. 2006;117:855–64.

Winkelstein JA, Marino MC, Ochs H, et al. The X-linked hyper-IgM syndrome: clinical and 1161 immunologic features of 79 patients. Medicine (Baltimore). 2003;82(6):373–84.

X-Linked Immunodeficiency with Magnesium Defect, Epstein-Barr Virus Infection, and Neoplasia (XMEN Disease)

▶ MAGT1 Deficiency

X-Linked Neutropenia/ Myelodysplasia

Eli Mansour and Denise Leite-Caldeira
Division of Clinical Immunology and Allergy, Department of Clinical Medicine, State University of Campinas (UNICAMP), Campinas, Brazil

Synonyms

Neutropenia with myelodysplasia; X-linked severe congenital neutropenia

Definition

X-linked neutropenia (OMIM #300299) is an X-linked form of severe non-syndromic congenital neutropenia, caused by mutation in the *WASP* gene (OMIM *300392) mapped to the short arm of the X chromosome, Xp11.23.

Introduction

X-linked neutropenia (XLN) is a rare severe congenital neutropenia (SCN) due to an activating mutation of *WASP* gene. As a result, the gene product Wiskott-Aldrich syndrome protein (*WASP*) is overactive. Mutations of the *WASP* gene are responsible for three distinct phenotypes: X-linked thrombocytopenia (XLT), classic Wiskott-Aldrich syndrome (WAS), and XLN. XLN is characterized by profound neutropenia, associated with monocytopenia and T lymphopenia, and an increased risk of myelodysplasia (MDS) and acute myeloid leukemia (AML). XLN is a rare cause of severe congenital neutropenias affecting about 2% of cases (Ochs 2009; Skokowa et al. 2017; Spoor et al. 2019).

Pathogenesis and Genetics

WASP is an important signaling molecule, expressed exclusively in the cytoplasm of hematopoietic cells, transducing upstream signals and inducing reorganization of the actin cytoskeleton vital for cell movement, vesicular trafficking, and immune cell functioning (Ochs 2009; Spoor et al. 2019).

Mutations in the *WASP* gene, leading to complete absence of WASP, cause the WAS phenotype, whereas mutations leading to decreased WASP cause the milder phenotype XLT (Ochs 2009; Spoor et al. 2019).

WASP gene mutations causing XLN are biologically different. In XLN, a gain-of-function mutation in GTPase-binding domain of WASP results in a constitutively active WASP (CA-WASP). CA-WASP causes disruption in cell division and chromosomal instability, by the generation of high levels of cytoplasmic polymerized F-actin. Excess cytoplasmic F-actin may lead to increased viscosity and perturbed mitosis. As a consequence of chromosomal instabilities, XLN shows profound congenital neutropenia, monocytopenia, T cell lymphopenia, and an increased risk of MDS and AML (Ochs 2009; Moulding et al. 2012; Spoor et al. 2019).

Clinical Presentation

XLN patients suffer from reduced myelopoiesis and severe congenital neutropenia and may have fever and recurrent bacterial infections. The skin and the respiratory and digestive tracts are most commonly affected (Moulding et al. 2012; Errante et al. 2013). However, despite severe neutropenia, XLN patients have lower risk of infections compared to other SCN causes, and the risk of infection in XLN does not correlate with peripheral blood neutrophil numbers. It has been shown that in some of these patients with defective myelopoiesis but a normal neutrophil number in saliva suggests a compensatory effect (Keszei et al. 2018). Most importantly, Keszei et al. showed that peripheral neutrophils are hyperactive and exhibited increased migration to tissues, which explain the milder phenotype. In addition, gingivitis and periodontitis are rare compared to other SCN (Keszei et al. 2018). Monocytopenia and T lymphopenia may occur, as well as impaired B cell proliferation (Moulding et al. 2012; Errante et al. 2013).

Apart from the immune system defects, XLN patients show a higher risk of bone marrow cell dysplasia (giant megakaryocytes, micromegakaryocytes, hypogranularity, reduced granulopoiesis, and excessive number of blasts) and myeloid leukemia (Skokowa et al. 2017; Spoor et al. 2019.

Diagnosis

Medical and family history and a careful exam are important, and if possible previous exams can be helpful to determine if neutropenia is acute or chronic, permanent or intermittent (Dale 2016).

X

Laboratory findings in patients with X-linked congenital neutropenia show an absolute neutrophil count (ANC) <500/mm³. Monocytopenia and T lymphopenia, as well as impaired B cell proliferation, may be found. In patients with severe congenital neutropenia, bone marrow evaluation can be useful and can help to rule out MDS, AML, and aplastic anemia (Errante et al. 2013; Dale 2016; Skokowa et al. 2017).

Genetic analysis is increasingly important in confirming the diagnosis in most primary immunodeficiency diseases. Clinical features presented by the patient can help to determine which gene should be tested. In this XLN, *WAS* sequencing must be done when an X-linked inheritance is suspected. Barth syndrome is another X-linked disorder with neutropenia, shortness of breath, and symptoms of heart failure. Sequencing of *TAZ* may confirm the diagnosis (Dale 2016; Skokowa et al. 2017; Kobayashi et al. 2018).

Treatment

General preventive measures such as skin and oral hygiene, supportive care, and aggressive broad-spectrum antibiotics to treat infections may be indicated. Antibiotic prophylaxis with sulfamethoxazole-trimethoprim (SMX-TMP), if needed, decreases the frequency of infection but is now considered secondary to G-CSF (Kuruvilla and de la Morena 2013; Spoor et al. 2019).

The treatment of choice is recombinant granulocyte colony-stimulating factor (G-CSF), a myeloid growth factor, to stimulate the development and function of neutrophils. G-CSF is given subcutaneously, daily, on alternate days, or three times per week. It was reported that XLN patients have a good response to low/median doses (1–3 μg/kg per day). The most common adverse events are related to the initiation of G-CSF: bone pain, headache, and myalgias. Splenomegaly, thrombocytopenia, and osteopenia/osteoporosis may occur. While controversial, AML and MDS were reported as secondary effects of G-CSF use (Dale 2016; Keszei et al. 2018; Spoor et al. 2019).

Hematopoietic stem cell transplantation (HSCT) can be indicated in exceptional cases. HSCT is recommended for severe cases, such as SCN unresponsive to G-CSF, WAS, and XLT, or for the treatment of AML or MDS (Oshima et al. 2015; Skokowa et al. 2017; Spoor et al. 2019).

Neutropenia patients should receive all inactivated vaccines and annual inactivated influenza vaccine. Live viral vaccines are recommended. Live bacterial vaccines, like BCG, should be avoided (Sobh and Bonilla 2016).

References

Dale DC. How I diagnose and treat neutropenia. Curr Opin Hematol. 2016;23:1–4.

Errante PR, Josias Brito Frazão JB, Condino Neto A. Congenital neutropenia. Braz J Allergy Immunol. 2013;1:23–38.

Keszei M, Record J, Kritikou JS, et al. Constitutive activation of WASp in X-linked neutropenia renders neutrophils hyperactive. J Clin Invest. 2018;128:4115–31.

Kobayashi M, Yokoyama K, Shimizu E, et al. Phenotype-based gene analysis allowed successful diagnosis of X-linked neutropenia associated with a novel WASp mutation. Ann Hematol. 2018;97:367–9.

Kuruvilla M, de la Morena MT. Antibiotic prophylaxis in primary immune deficiency disorders. J Allergy Clin Immunol Pract. 2013;1:573–82.

Moulding DA, Moeendarbary E, Valon L, et al. Excess F-actin mechanically impedes mitosis leading to cytokinesis failure in X-linked neutropenia by exceeding Aurora B kinase error correction capacity. Blood. 2012;120:3803–11.

Ochs HD. Mutations of the Wiskott–Aldrich syndrome protein affect protein expression and dictate the clinical phenotypes. Immunol Res. 2009;44:84–8.

Oshima K, Imai K, Albert MH, Bittner TC, et al. Hematopoietic stem cell transplantation for X-linked thrombocytopenia with mutations in the WAS gene. J Clin Immunol. 2015;35:15–21.

Skokowa J, Dale DC, Touw IP, et al. Severe congenital neutropenias. Nat Rev Dis Primers. 2017;3:17032.

Sobh A, Bonilla FA. Vaccination in primary immunodeficiency disorders. J Allergy Clin Immunol Pract. 2016;4:1066–75.

Spoor J, Farajifard H, Rezaei N. Congenital neutropenia and primary immunodeficiency diseases. Crit Rev Oncol Hematol. 2019;133:149–62.

X-Linked Severe Congenital Neutropenia

▶ X-Linked Neutropenia/Myelodysplasia

Z

ZAP70 Deficiency (OMIM # 176947)

Lisa J. Kobrynski
Children's Healthcare of Atlanta, Department of
Pediatrics, Emory University School of Medicine,
Atlanta, GA, USA

Introduction/Background

Deficiency in the Zeta-chain-associated protein kinase (ZAP70) causes a combined immunodeficiency affecting both cellular and humoral immunity. ZAP70 is a 70kD syk-related tyrosine kinase, encoded on chromosome 2q11.2. ZAP-70 is expressed in T and NK cells and exists in an autoinhibitory state. TCR stimulation occurs after the presentation of antigen bound to MHC on the surface of the antigen presenting cell (APC) to the TCR-CD3 receptor on the surface of a T cell. This causes phosphorylation of the immunoreceptor activating motifs (ITAM) associated with the CD3γ, δ, and ϵ intracellular chains. Then the ITAM on the CD3 ζ chain dimer is phosphorylated as well. Tyrosine phosphorylation by Lck (protein kinase) leads to recruitment of ZAP-70. Binding of both SH2 domains of ZAP-70 causes alignment of the CD3-ζ chains. Then, phosphorylation of ZAP70 by Lck stabilizes the molecule in an active conformational state by causing a structural change in ZAP70 with dissociation of the SH2 linker domain from the kinase domain (Yan et al. 2013) (Fig. 1). The activated ZAP70 permits downstream phosphorylation of several intracellular signaling molecules such as the linker of activation in T cells (LAT) and SLP -76, another linker protein. LAT associates with lipid rafts in the cytoplasm and is important for directing transmission of signals from membrane complexes to intracellular downstream targets. SLP-76 binds and activates phospholipase C-γ (PLCγ), guanine-nucleotide exchange factors (GEF), and Tec kinases (e.g., Itk). These molecules drive the activation of gene transcription in the nucleus through two main pathways. PLCγ cleaves phosphatidylinositol bisphosphate (PIP$_2$) forming diacylglycerol (DAG) and inositol triphosphate (IP$_3$). Subsequently, protein kinase C and calcineurin activate NF$\kappa\beta$ and NFAT respectively, which upregulate genes leading to cell proliferation and differentiation. Most of the disease-causing mutations appear to be clustered in the kinase domain of the ZAP70 gene (Chan2016).

ZAP-70 Function

In the absence of ZAP70, CD3+CD4+ cell development is normal, but there is a lack of CD3+CD8+ cell development in the thymus. The absence of ZAP70 was shown to abolish the progression of CD4+CD8+ DP T cells to CD8+ SP T cells (Katamura et al. 1999). In addition, ZAP70 appears to be important in negative selection of autoreactive T cells in the thymus (Negishi et al. 1995). In patients with ZAP70 deficiency,

© Springer Science+Business Media LLC, part of Springer Nature 2020
I. R. Mackay et al. (eds.), *Encyclopedia of Medical Immunology*,
https://doi.org/10.1007/978-1-4614-8678-7

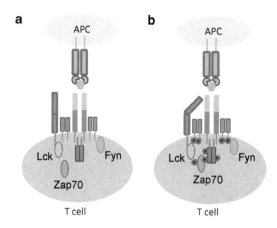

ZAP70 Deficiency (OMIM # 176947), Fig. 1 (**a**) TCR binding of antigen presented with MHC by APC causes phosphorylation of ITAMs on CD3γ, δ and ε intracellular chains. (**b**) ZAP70 is activated by phosphorylation through Lck. ZAP70 binds the phosphorylated ITAMs of the CD3ζ chain

peripheral T cells do not proliferate after stimulation with mitogens or anti-CD3 antibodies. However, they do proliferate after stimulation with a protein kinase C activator and a Ca2+ ionophore, which bypass the TCR complex.

Clinical Presentation

A combined immune deficiency in humans due to inactive ZAP70 was described in 1994 (Chan et al. 1994). A compound heterozygous mutation resulted in decreased production of an inactive ZAP70 protein. This mutation caused a frameshift leading to a premature stop codon in the ZAP70 kinase domain. Although ZAP70 mRNA could be detected the resulting ZAP70 protein was inactive (Elder et al. 1994).

This patient had an unusual combined immune deficiency characterized by a profound decrease in peripheral CD8+ T cells and absent proliferation of CD4+ T cells after stimulation with mitogens or CD3. The NK function and serum immunoglobulins were normal, but there was no antigen-specific antibody production. Further

analysis of ZAP70 protein expression in the parents and siblings was consistent with autosomal recessive inheritance. (Elder et al. 1994).

In a Mennonite community patients with a homozygous splice site mutation had production of an unstable ZAP70 protein due to the insertion of three additional amino acids in the protein. Homozygous individuals also displayed a combined immunodeficiency due to a selective T cell defect while heterozygous carriers were unaffected (Arpaie et al. 1994).

Other phenotypes have been noted. Chan et al. reported a novel clinical phenotype due to a compound heterozygous missense mutation. One mutation caused a decrease of ZAP70 binding to the CD3 ζ chain, while the mutation on the other allele acted as an activating mutation for ZAP-70. The clinical phenotype was the early onset of autoimmune disease (within the first year of life). Two affected siblings had early onset of multisystem autoimmune diseases (nephrotic syndrome, bullous pemphigoid, colitis, and autoimmune hemophilia). Hematopoietic cell transplant (HCT) resulted in correction of the immune defect and the autoimmunity (Chan et al. 2016).

Late onset of immune deficiency without autoimmunity due to a homozygous hypomorphic mutation in ZAP70 also been described (Picard et al. 2009). In this patient, a 78 base pair insertion, at the 3′ end of exon 7 (inside intron 7) combined with a homozygous single base pair mutation caused a premature stop codon. This patient had a lower expression of ZAP70 protein compared to controls presumably due to rapid degradation of the shortened protein. The abnormal product lacks an active kinase domain and exhibits decreased TCR signaling. Clinical symptoms were milder than those seen patients with a complete absence of ZAP70 activity. The reported patient had a decrease in both CD4+ and CD8+ T cells, with normal serum IgG subclasses, increased IgE, and low-specific IgG to diphtheria, polio, and *Streptococcus pneumoniae*. The milder phenotype may result from the presence of a small percentage of T cells expressing WT ZAP70 capable of providing a small amount of TCR-induced signaling (Picard et al. 2009).

Diagnosis and Laboratory Testing

Patients with a combined immunodeficiency due to homozygous or compound heterozygous mutations in ZAP70 generally have low/absent CD8+ cells and normal numbers of CD4+ cells measured in peripheral blood by flow cytometry. Serum immunoglobulins can be normal, but specific antibody responses are absent likely due to dysfunction of CD4+ T cells. Indeed, CD4+ cell proliferation in response to mitogens and antigens is decreased. Newborn screening using detection of TREC in newborn dried blood spots is unlikely to identify infants with ZAP70 deficiency (Grazoli et al. 2014). Detection of mutations in both alleles, either those known to be associated with ZAP70 deficiency or those predicted to cause a deleterious mutation, is diagnostic for ZAP70 deficiency. Thus, ZAP70 would be expected to be inherited in an autosomal recessive fashion.

Treatment/Prognosis

Correction of the combined immune defect in ZAP70 deficiency due to either homozygous or compound heterozygous mutations in ZAP-70 can be achieved through HCT. Due to the presence of nonfunctional CD4+ T cells, pretransplant conditioning is generally required for successful correction of the immune deficiency. Gene transfection using both retroviral and lentiviral vectors in mouse and human cells has been shown to correct the defect (Steinberg et al. 2000; Adjali et al. 2005). At this time, there are no published clinical trials for gene therapy.

Cross-References

▶ CD8 Alpha (CD8A) Deficiency

References

Adjali O, Marodon G, Steinberg M, et al. In vivo correction of ZAP-70 immunodeficiency by intrathymic gene transfer. J Clin Invest. 2005;115(8):2287–95.

Arpaie E, Shahar M, Dadi H, et al. Defective T cell receptor signaling and CD8+ thymic selection in humans lacking Zap=70 kinase. Cell. 1994;76:947–58.

Chan AC, Kadlecek TA, Elder ME, et al. ZAP-70 deficiency in an autosomal recessive form of severe combined immunodeficiency. Science. 1994;264:1599–601.

Chan AY, Punwani D, Kadlecek TA, et al. A novel human autoimmune syndrome caused by combined hypomorphic and activating mutations in ZAP-70. J Exp Med. 2016;213(2):155–65.

Elder ME, Lin D, Clever J, et al. Human severe combined immunodeficiency due to a defect in ZAP-70, a T cell tyrosine kinase. Science. 1994;264(5165):1596–9.

Grazoli S, Bennett M, Hildebrand KJ, et al. Limitation of TREC-based newborn screening for ZAP70 severe combined immune deficiency. Clin Immunol. 2014;153:209–10.

Katamura K, Tai G, Tachibana T, et al. Existence of activated and memory CD4+ T cells in peripheral blood and their skin infiltration in CD8 deficiency. Clin Exp Immunol. 1999;115:124–30.

Negishi I, Motoyama N, Nakayama K, et al. Essential role for ZAP-70 in both positive and negative selection of thymocytes. Nature. 1995;376:435–8.

Picard C, Dogniaux S, Chemin K, et al. Hypomorphic mutation of ZAP70 in human results in a late onset immunodeficiency and no autoimmunity. Eur J Immunol. 2009;39:1966–76.

Steinberg M, Swainson L, Schwarz K, et al. Retrovirus-mediated transduction of primary ZAP-70-deficient human T cells results in the selective growth advantage of gene-corrected cells: implications for gene therapy. Gene Ther. 2000;7(16):1392–400.

Yan Q, Barros PR, Visperas S, et al. Structural basis for activation of ZAP-70 by phosphorylation of the SH2-kinase linker. Mol Cell Biol. 2013;33:2188–201.

Z

CPSIA information can be obtained
at www.ICGtesting.com
Printed in the USA
LVHW060917100122
708179LV00003B/4